MULTILINGUAL DICTIONARY OF MEDICAL EMERGENCIES

English-French-Spanish-Italian-Croatian

SECOND ENGLISH EDITION

Edita Ciglenečki

INTRODUCTION-L'INTRODUCTION-INTRODUCCIÓN-INTRODUZIONE-UVOD

English

The audience for this dictionary includes medical professionals working in multilingual environments; global health professionals in tourist areas; professionals in public health, humanitarian medicine, emergency disaster management, rescue teams and frequent travellers disposed to any kind of danger or health risk and therefore in the need of medical assistance while in some foreign speaking country. In emergency situations even small misunderstandings can lead to the loss of valuable time and consequently lives, therefore this dictionary is created in very practical time-saving and easy-to-understand way for both medical professionals and their patients. Instead of one classical A to Z alphabetical order, it consists of several topics where terms regarding each topic are organized alphabetically. The topics start from very basic subjects of numbers and orientation and proceed with terminology concerning accidents and disasters, parts of the human body, injuries, symptoms and diseases, pharmacy, medical facilities, medical procedures, diagnostics, pregnancy and obstetrics.

Consisting of over 3000 medical terms in five languages, this book is a valuable tool for medical students on exchange programs and can serve as a basic medical dictionary for translators.

Français

Pratique et facile à consulter, ce dictionnaire médical propose plus de 3000 termes médicaux en français, anglais, espagnol, italien et croate, couvrant l'essentiel de la pratique médicale: orientation dans le temps et dans l'espace; les types des accidents, catastrophes et détresse; parties du corps humain; les symptômes, blessures et maladies; pharmacie; établissements médicaux, procédures et soins; examens médicaux, grossesse et obstétrique.

Español

Este diccionario médico español-inglés- francés-italiano-croata, proporciona de forma breve, clara y suficiente unos 3000 términos médicos que cubren orientación en el tiempo y espacio; accidentes y catástrofes; partes del cuerpo humano; síntomas, heridas y enfermedades; farmacia; facilidades médicas, procedimientos y asistencia médica; exámenes médicos; embarazo y obstetricia.

Italiano

Questo dizionario contiene più di 3000 termini medici in italiano, inglese, francese, spagnolo e croato ed è stato concepito come un manuale compatto di facile comprensione di terminologia medica dall'orientamento nel tempo e spazio; gli accidenti, catastrofi e angoscia; parti del corpo umano; i sintomi, ferite e malattie; farmacia; istituzioni, procedure e cure di medicina ed esami medici, alla gravidanza e ostetricia.

Hrvatski

Ovaj rječnik sastoji se od preko 3000 medicinskih pojmova na hrvatskom, engleskom, francuskom, španjolskom i talijanskom jeziku, prikazanih na jednostavan i razumljiv način koji obuhvaća orijentaciju u prostoru i vremenu; nesreće, katastrofe i pogibeljne situacije; dijelove ljudskog tijela; ozljede, simptome i bolesti; ljekarništvo; medicinske ustanove, njegu i postupke; dijagnostiku te trudnoću i porodništvo.

CONTENTS-CONTENU-CONTENIDO-CONTENUTO-SADRŽAJ

MULTILINGUAL DICTIONARY OF MEDICAL EMERGENCIES

English-French-Spanish-Italian-Croatian

English	French	Spanish	Italian	Croatian
NUMBERS:	**NUMÉROS:**	**NÚMEROS:**	**NUMERI:**	**BROJEVI:**
Zero	Zéro	Cero	Zero	Nula
One	Un	Uno	Uno	Jedan
Two	Deux	Dos	Due	Dva
Three	Trois	Tres	Tre	Tri
Four	Quatre	Cuatro	Quattro	Četiri
Five	Cinq	Cinco	Cinque	Pet
Six	Six	Seis	Sei	Šest
Seven	Sept	Siete	Sette	Sedam
Eight	Huit	Ocho	Otto	Osam
Nine	Neuf	Nueve	Nove	Devet
Ten	Dix	Diez	Dieci	Deset
Eleven	Onze	Once	Undici	Jedanaest
Twelve	Douze	Doce	Dodici	Dvanaest
Thirteen	Treize	Trece	Tredici	Trinaest
Fourteen	Quatorze	Catorce	Quattordici	Četrnaest
Fifteen	Quinze	Quince	Quindici	Petnaest
Sixteen	Seize	Dieciséis	Sedici	Šesnaest
Seventeen	Dix-sept	Diecisiete	Diciassette	Sedamnaest
Eighteen	Dix-huit	Dieciocho	Diciotto	Osamnaest
Nineteen	Dix-neuf	Diecinueve	Diciannove	Devetnaest
Twenty	Vingt	Veinte	Venti	Dvadeset
Twenty-one	Vingt et un	Veintiuno	Ventuno	Dvadest i jedan
Twenty-two	Vingt-deux	Veintidós	Ventidue	Dvadeset i dva
Thirty	Trente	Treinta	Trenta	Trideset
Forty	Quarante	Cuarenta	Quaranta	Četrdeset
Fifty	Cinquante	Cincuenta	Cinquanta	Pedeset
Sixty	Soixante	Sesenta	Sessanta	Šezdeset
Seventy	Soixante-dix	Setenta	Settanta	Sedamdeset
Eighty	Quatre-vingts	Ochenta	Ottanta	Osamdeset
Ninety	Quatre-vingt-dix	Noventa	Novanta	Devedeset
Hundred	Cent	Cien	Cento	Sto
One hundred and one	Cent un	Ciento uno	Centouno	Sto jedan
One hundred and twenty-three	Cent vingt-trois	Ciento veintitrés	Centoventitre	Sto dvadeset i tri
Twohundred	Deux cents	Doscientos	Duecento	Dvjesto
Three hundred	Trois cents	Trescientos	Trecento	Tristo
Four hundred	Quatre cents	Cuatrocientos	Quattrocento	Četristo
Five hundred	Cinq cents	Quinientos	Cinquecento	Petsto
Six hundred	Six cents	Seiscientos	Seicento	Šesto
Seven hundred	Sept cents	Setecientos	Settecento	Sedamsto
Eight hundred	Huit cents	Ochocientos	Ottocento	Osamsto
Nine hundred	Neuf cents	Novecientos	Novecento	Devetsto
Thousand	Mille	Mil	Mille	Tisuća
Two thousand	Deux mille	Dos mil	Duemila	Dvije tisuće
Million	Million	Millón	Un milione	Milijun
Milliard (billion)	Milliard	Mil millones (miliarda)	Un miliardo	Milijarda
ORIENTATION IN TIME:	**ORIENTATION DANS LE TEMPS:**	**ORIENTACIÓN EN EL TIEMPO:**	**ORIENTAMENTO NEL TEMPO:**	**ORIJENTACIJA U VREMENU:**
Yesterday	Hier	Ayer	Ieri	Jučer
Today	Aujourd'hui	Hoy	Oggi	Danas
Tomorrow	Demain	Día de mañana	Domani	Sutra
Year	Année	Año	Anno	Godina
Month	Mois	Mes	Mese	Mjesec
Week	Semaine	Semana	Settimana	Tjedan
Day	Jour	Día	Giorno	Dan
Hour	Heure	Hora	Ora	Sat
Minute	Minute	Minuto	Minuto	Minuta
Second	Seconde	Segundo	Secondo	Sekunda
Morning	Matin	Mañana	Mattina	Jutro (prijepodne)
Afternoon	Après-midi	Tarde	Pomeriggio	Poslijepodne
Evening	Soir	Anochecer	Sera	Večer
Night	Nuit	Noche	Notte	Noć
ORIENTATION IN SPACE:	**ORIENTATION DANS L'ESPACE:**	**ORIENTACIÓN EN EL ESPACIO:**	**ORIENTAMENTO NELLO SPAZIO:**	**ORIJENTACIJA U PROSTORU:**
Up (above)	En haut (au-dessus)	Arriba	Su	Gore (iznad)
Down (below)	En bas (au-dessous)	Abajo	In basso	Dolje (ispod)
Left	Gauche	Izquierda	Sinistra	Lijevo
Right	Droite	Derecha	Destra	Desno
In front	Devant	Enfrente	Davanti	Ispred
Behind	Derrière	Detrás	Dietro	Iza
Inside	Dedans	Dentro	Dentro	Unutra
Outside	Dehors	Fuera	Fuori	Vani

English	French	Spanish	Italian	Croatian
ACCIDENTS, CATASTROPHES AND DISTRESS:	**LES ACCIDENTS, CATASTROPHES ET DÉTRESSE:**	**ACCIDENTES, CATÁSTROFES Y ANGUSTIA:**	**GLI ACCIDENTI, CATASTROFI E ANGOSCIA:**	**NESREĆE, KATASTROFE I POGIBELJNE SITUACIJE:**
ABC weapons	Arme nucléaire, biologique et chimique (NBC)	Armas atómicas, biológicas y químicas (ABQ)	Armi nucleari, biologiche e chimiche (NBC)	Atomsko biološko i kemijsko oružje
Air attack	Attaque aérienne	Ataque aéreo	Incursione area	Zračni napad
Airplane crash	Accident aérien	Accidente de aviación	Incidente aereo	Pad aviona
Alarm	Alarme	Alarma	Allarme	Uzbuna
Alarm signal	Signal d'alarme	Señal de alarma	Segnale di allarme	Znak za uzbunu
Atomic bomb (A-bomb)	Bombe atomique (bombe A)	Bomba atómica (bomba A)	Bomba atomica (bomba A)	Atomska bomba
Atomic weapons	Arme atomique	Arma atómica	Arma atomica	Atomsko oružje
Attack	Attaque	Ataque	Attaco	Napad
Avalanche	Avalanche	Avalancha	Valanga	Lavina
Bacteria	Bacteria	Bacteria	Batterio	Bakterija
Biological weapon	Arme biologique	Arma biológica	Arma biologica	Biološko oružje
Bomb	Bombe	Bomba	Bomba	Bomba
Bullet	Balle	Bala	Pallottola	Metak
Call for help	Appel à l'aide	Llamada de socorro	Chiamata di aiuto	Poziv u pomoć
Car accident	Accident automobile (accident de la route)	Accidente automovilístico (siniestro de tráfico)	Incidente stradale	Automobilska nesreća
Cave	Grotte	Cueva	Grotta	Špilja
Chemical pollution	Pollution chimique	Polución química	Inquinamento chimico	Kemijsko zagađenje
Chemical weapon	Arme chimique	Arma química	Arma chimica	Kemijsko oružje
Civil defense	Sécurité civile	Protección civil	Difesa civile	Civilna zaštita
Cobalt bomb	Bombe salée	Bomba de cobalto	Bomba al cobalto (bomba gamma, bomba G)	Kobaltna bomba
Cold weapon	Arme de contact	Arma blanca	Arma bianca	Hladno oružje
Collision	Collision	Colisión	Collisione	Sudar
Conventional weapon	Arme conventionnelle	Arma convencional	Arma convenzionale	Konvencionalno oružje
Dirty bomb	Bombe radiologique (bombe sale)	Bomba sucia	Bomba sporca	Prljava bomba
Domestic accident	Accident domestique	Accidente doméstico	Infortunio domestico	Nesreća u kući
Drowned person	Noyé	Ahogado	Annegato	Utopljenik
Drowning	Noyade	Ahogamiento	Annegamento	Utapanje
Earthquake	Séisme (tremblement de terre)	Terremoto	Terremoto	Potres
Electric shock	Électrisation (électrocution)	Choque eléctrico	Folgorazione (elettrocuzione)	Strujni udar
Enriched uranium	Uranium enrichi	Uranio einriquecido	Uranio arricchito	Obogaćeni uranij
Epidemic	Épidémie	Epidemia	Epidemia	Epidemija
Explosion	Explosion	Explosión	Esplosione	Eksplozija
Explosive	Explosif	Explosivo	Esplosivo	Eksploziv
Fall	Chute	Caída	Cadutta (cascata)	Pad
Fight	Combat	Pelea	Combattimento	Tučnjava
Fire	Feu	Fuego	Fuoco	Vatra
Fire (conflagration)	Incendie	Incendio (fuego)	Incendio (fuoco)	Požar
Firearm	Arme à feu	Arma de fuego	Arma da fuoco	Vatreno oružje
Flood	Inondation	Inundación	Inondazione	Poplava
Heat stroke	Coup de chaleur	Golpe de calor	Colpo di calore	Toplotni udar
Helicopter (chopper)	Hélicoptère	Helicóptero	Elicottero	Helikopter
"Help!"	"Aide!"	"¡Socorro!"	"Aiuto!"	"U pomoć!"
Hidrogen bomb (H-bomb)	Bombe à hydrogène (bombe H)	Bomba de hidrógeno (bomba H)	Bomba all'idrogeno (bomba H)	Hidrogenska bomba
Homicide (murder)	Homicide (assassinat)	Homicídio (asesinato)	Omicidio (uccisione)	Ubojstvo
Hostage	Otage	Rehén	Ostaggio	Taoc (talac)
Human trafficking	Trafic d'êtres humains	Trata de personas	Traffico di esseri umani	Trgovina ljudima
Hurricane	Ouragan	Huracán	Uragano	Uragan
Ice	Glace	Hielo	Ghiaccio	Led
Iceberg	Iceberg	Témpano de hielo	Ghiacciaio	Ledenjak
Icebreaker	Brise-glace	Rompehielos	Rompighiaccio	Ledolomac
Invasion	Invasion	Invasión	Invasione	Invazija
Kidnapping	Enlèvement (rapt)	Secuestro	Rapimento	Otmica
Lake	Lac	Lago	Lago	Jezero
Land	Terre	Tierra	Terra	Kopno
Land mine	Mine terrestre	Mina terrestre	Mina terrestre	Kopnena mina
Laser weapon	Arme de laser	Arma láser	Armi laser	Lasersko oružje
Lava	Lave	Lava	Lava	Lava
Lifebelt (lifebuoy)	Bouée couronne	Boya salvavidas	Boa di salvataggio	Pojas za spašavanje
Lifeboat	Canot de secours	Bote salvavidas	Scialuppa	Čamac za spašavanje
Lifejacket (life vest)	Gilet de sauvetage	Chaleco salvavidas	Giubbotto di salvataggio	Prsluk za spašavanje
Marine salvage	Sauvetage en mer	Salvamento marítimo	Salvataggio navale	Spašavanje broda
Mine	Mine	Mina	Mina	Mina
Mine clearance (demining)	Déminage	Desminado (eliminación de minas)	Eliminazione di mine (sminamento)	Razminiranje

English	French	Spanish	Italian	Croatian
Mine field	Champ de mines	Campo minero	Campo minato	Minsko polje
Mountain	Montagne	Montaña	Montagna	Planina
Naval mine	Mine marine (mine sous-marine)	Mina marina	Mina navale	Morska mina
Neurotoxin	Neurotoxine	Neurotoxina	Neurotossina	Živčani otrov (neurotoksin)
Neutron bomb	Bombe à neutrons	Bomba de neutrones (bomba N)	Bomba al neutrone (bomba N)	Neutronska bomba
Nuclear accident	Accident nucléaire	Accidente nuclear	Accidente nucleare	Nuklearna nesreća
Nuclear waste (radioactive waste)	Déchet radioactif (déchet nucléaire)	Desechos nucleares	Scoria nucleare (scoria radioattiva)	Nuklearni otpad (radioaktivni otpad)
Nuclear weapon	Arme nucléaire	Arma nuclear	Arma nucleare	Nuklearno oružje
Nuclear weapons testing	Essai nucléaire	Prueba nuclear (ensayo nuclear)	Test nucleare	Nuklearni pokus
Occupational accident	Accident du travail	Accidente laboral	Infortunio sul lavoro	Nesreća na radu
Pandemic	Pandémie	Pandemia	Pandemia	Pandemija
Parachute	Parachute	Paracaídas	Paracadute	Padobran
Physical assault	Attaque physique	Asalto físico	Attacco fisico	Tjelesni napad
Pirate	Pirate	Pirata	Pirata	Gusar
Pirate attack	Attaque de pirates	Ataque de piratas	Attacco dei pirati	Gusarski napad
Plutonium	Plutonium	Plutonio	Plutonio	Plutonij
Poison gas	Gaz toxique	Gas tóxico	Gas tossico	Bojni otrov (otrovni plin)
Radiation	Rayonnement	Radiación	Radiazione	Zračenje
Rape (violation)	Viol	Violación	Violenza sessuale	Silovanje
Refugee	Réfugié	Refugiado	Rifugiato	Izbjeglica
Refugee camp	Camp de réfugiés	Campamento para refugiados	Campo per rifugiati	Izbjeglički logor
Rescuer	Sauveur	Salvador (rescatador)	Salvatore	Spasilac
River	Rivière	Río	Fiume	Rijeka
Robbery	Vol	Robo	Rapina	Pljačka
Rock	Roche	Roca	Roccia	Stijena
Rope	Corde	Cuerda	Cordone	Uže
Ruins	Ruine	Ruinas	Macerie (rovine)	Ruševine
Salvage	Sauvetage	Salvamento	Salvataggio	Spašavanje
Sand storm	Tempête de sable	Tormenta de arena	Tempesta di sabbia	Pješčana oluja
Sea	Mer	Mar	Mare	More
Sea ice	Banquise	Banquisa (hielo marino)	Banchisa (ghiaccio marino; banchiglia)	Santa leda
Search	Recherche	Búsqueda	Ricerca	Potraga
Search and rescue dog	Chien de sauvetage	Perro de búsqueda y rescate	Cane da ricerca e salvataggio	Pas za traganje i spašavanje
Search and rescue team	Équpie de recherche et sauvetage	Equipo de búsqueda y rescate	Squadra di ricerca e salvataggio	Ekipa za traganje i spašavanje
Shark attack	Attaque de requin	Ataque de tiburón	Attacco di squalo	Napad morskog psa
Shelter	Abri	Abrigo	Rifugio	Sklonište
Ship	Navire	Barco	Nave	Brod
Ship wreck	Épave de navire	Buque naufragado	Relitto	Olupina broda
Shrapnel	Shrapnel	Metralla	Shrapnel	Šrapnel
Sinking of a ship	Naufrage du navire	Hundimiento de un barco	Affondamento della nave	Potonuće broda
Slavery	Esclavage	Esclavitud	Schiavitù (prigionia)	Ropstvo
Snow	Neige	Nieve (zapada)	Neve	Snijeg
Snow storm	Tempête de neige	Nevasca (ventisca de nieve)	Bufera di neve (nevicata)	Snježna mećava
SOS call	Appel SOS	Llamada de SOS	SOS richiesta	SOS poziv
Storm	Tempête	Tormenta (tempestad)	Tempesta	Nevrijeme (oluja)
Stranding of a ship	Échouage du navire	Encallamiento de barco	Incaglio di nave	Nasukavanje broda
Strategic nuclear weapon	Arme nucléaire stratégique	Arma nuclear estratégica	Arma nucleare strategica	Strateško nuklearno oružje
Stroke (hit, blow)	Coup	Golpe	Colpo (botta)	Udarac
Suicide	Suicide	Suicidio	Suicidio	Samoubojstvo
Tactical nuclear weapon	Arme nucléaire tactique (mini-nuke)	Arma nuclear táctica	Arma nucleare tattica	Taktičko nuklearno oružje
Terrorist	Terroriste	Terrorista	Terrorista	Terorist
Terrorist attack	Attaque terroriste	Ataque terrorista	Attentato terroristico	Teroristički napad
Terrorist cell	Cellule terroriste (cellule dormante)	Célula terrorista	Cellula terroristica	Teroristička ćelija
Thunderclap	Foudre	Trueno	Percossa dal fulmine	Udar groma
Tidal wave	Onde de marée	Ola de marea	Onda di marea	Plimni val
Traffic accident	Accident sur la voie publique	Accidente de tráfico	Incidente di traffico	Prometna nesreća
Tsunami	Tsunami (raz-de-marée)	Tsunami (maremoto)	Tsunami	Tsunami
Typhoon	Typhon	Tifón	Tifone	Tajfun
Uranium	Uranium	Uranio	Uranio	Uranij
Victim	Victime	Víctima	Vittima	Žrtva
Virus	Virus	Virus	Virus	Virus
Volcanic eruption	Éruption volcanique	Erupción volcánica	Eruzione vulcanica	Erupcija vulkana
War	Guerre	Guerra	Guerra	Rat
Water	Eau	Agua	Acqua	Voda

English	French	Spanish	Italian	Croatian
Waterspout	Trombe marine	Managa de agua (tromba marina)	Tromba marina	Morska pijavica
Weapon	Arme	Arma	Arma	Oružje
Weapon of mass destruction	Arme de destruction massive	Armas de destrucción masiva	Arma di distruzione di massa	Oružje za masovno uništavanje
PARTS OF THE HUMAN BODY :	PARTIES DU CORPS HUMAIN:	PARTES DEL CUERPO HUMANO:	PARTI DEL CORPO UMANO:	DIJELOVI LJUDSKOG TIJELA:
Abdominal aorta	Aorte abdominale	Aorta abdominal	Aorta addominale	Abdominalna aorta
Abdominal oblique muscle	Muscle oblique de l'abdomen	Músculo oblicuo del abdomen	Musculo obliquo dell'abdome	Kosi trbušni mišić
Abdominal wall	Face de la cavité abdominale	Pared abdominal	Parete addominale	Trbušna stijenka
Acetabulum	Acetabulum	Acetábulo	Cotile (acetabolo)	Čašica zdjelične kosti (acetabulum)
Acetylcholine	Acétylcholine	Acetilcolina	Acetilcolina	Acetilkolin
Acoustic nerve (vestibulocochlear nerve)	Nerf vestibulocochléaire (nerf auditif)	Nervio auditivo (nervio vestibulococlear, nervio estatoacústico)	Nervo vestibolococleare (nervo stato-acustico)	Slušni živac
Adam's apple	Pomme d'Adam	Nuez de Adán	Pomo d'Adamo	Adamova jabučica
Adductor muscle	Muscle adducteur	Músculo aductor	Muscolo adduttore	Mišić primicač
Adenohypophysis	Adénohypophyse	Adenohipófisis	Adenoipofisi	Adenohipofiza
Adrenal gland	Glande surrénale	Glándula suprarrenal	Surrene	Nadbubrežna žlijezda
Adrenalin (adrenaline)	Adrénaline	Adrenalina	Adrenalina	Adrenalin
Agglutinin	Agglutinine	Aglutinina	Agglutinine	Aglutinin
Agglutinogen	Agglutinogène	Aglutinógeno	Agglutinogeno	Aglutinogen
Albumin	Albumine	Albúmina	Albumina	Albumin
Aldosterone	Aldostérone	Aldosterona	Aldosterone	Aldosteron
Alveolus	Alvéole	Alvéolo	Alveolo	Alveola
Amino acid	Acide aminé	Aminoácido	Amminoacido	Aminokiselina
Ammonia	Ammoniac	Amoníaco	Ammoniaca	Amonijak
Ankle joint	Cheville (cou-de pied)	Tobillo	Caviglia	Skočni zglob (gležanj)
Antidiuretic hormone (vasopressin)	Hormone antidiurétique (vasopressine)	Hormona anidiurética (arginina vasopresina)	Ormone antidiuretico (vasopressina)	Antidiuretski hormon (vazopresin)
Anus	Anus	Ano	Ano	Čmar (anus)
Anvil (incus)	Enclume	Yunque	Incudine	Nakovanj
Aorta	Aorte	Aorta	Aorta	Aorta
Aortic valve	Valve aortique	Válvula sigmoidea aórtica	Valvola semilunare aortica	Polumjesečasti aortni zalistak
Aponeurosis	Aponévrose	Aponeurosis	Aponeurosi	Široka plosnata tetiva (aponeuroza)
Arachnoid mater	Arachnoïde	Aracnoides	Aracnoide	Paučinasta ovojnica (arachnoidea)
Arm	Bras	Brazo	Braccio	Ruka
Armpit (axilla, underarm)	Aisselle	Sobaco (axila)	Ascella	Pazuh (aksila)
Arteriole	Artériole	Arteriola	Arteriola	Arteriola
Artery	Artère	Arteria	Arteria	Arterija
Articular capsule (joint capsule)	Capsule articulaire	Cápsula articular	Capsula articolare	Zglobna čahura
Astrocyte	Astrocyte	Astrocito	Astrocita	Astrocit
Atrioventricular node	Noeud atrio-ventriculaire	Nódulo auriculoventricular	Nodo atrioventricolare	Atrioventrikularni čvor
Auditory canal (ear canal)	Conduit auditif externe (canal auriculaire)	Conducto auditivo externo	Meato acustico esterno	Slušni kanal
Back	Dos	Espalda	Schiena (dorso)	Leđa
Bartholin's gland	Glande de Bartholin	Glándula de Bartolino	Ghiandola di Bartolini	Bartolinova žlijezda
Basophil granulocyte	Granulocyte basophile	Basófilo	Granulocita basofilo	Bazofilni granulocit
Belly (abdomen)	Abdomen	Abdomen (panza)	Addome (ventre, pancia)	Trbuh (abdomen)
Biceps brachii muscle	Muscle biceps brachial	Músculo bíceps braquial	Muscolo bicipite brachiale	Dvoglavi mišić nadlaktice
Biceps femoris muscle	Muscle biceps fémoral	Músculo bíceps crural	Bicipite femorale	Dvoglavi bedreni mišić
Bile duct	Voie biliaire	Vía biliar	Coledoco	Žučovod
Bilirubin	Bilirubine	Bilirrubina	Bilirubina	Bilirubin
Blood	Sang	Sangre	Sangue	Krv
Blood group	Groupe sanguin	Grupo sanguíneo	Gruppo sanguigno	Krvna grupa
Blood group A	Groupe sanguin A	Grupo sanguíneoA	Gruppo sanguigno A	Krvna grupa A
Blood group AB	Groupe sanguin AB	Grupo sanguíneo AB	Gruppo sanguigno AB	Krvna grupa AB
Blood group B	Groupe sanguin B	Grupo sanguíneo B	Gruppo sanguigno B	Krvna grupa B
Blood group 0	Groupe sanguin 0	Grupo sanguíneo 0	Gruppo sanguigno 0	Krvna grupa 0
Blood vessel	Vaisseau sanguin	Vaso sanguíneo	Vaso sanguigno	Krvna žila
Body fluid	Fluide corporel	Fluido corporal	Fluido corporale	Tjelesna tekućina
Bone	Os	Hueso	Osso	Kost
Bone marrow	Moelle osseuse	Médula ósea	Midollo osseo	Koštana srž
Brachialis muscle	Muscle brachial	Braquial anterior	Muscolo brachiale	Nadlaktični mišić
Brain	Cerveau	Cerebro	Cervello	Mozak
Brain marrow	Moelle du cerveau	Médula cerebral	Midollo cerebrale	Moždana srž
Brain stem	Tronc cérébral	Tronco del encéfalo	Tronco encefalico	Moždano stablo
Brain ventricle	Ventricule cérébral	Ventrículo cerebral	Ventricolo cerebrale	Moždana klijetka
Breast	Sein	Mama	Mammella	Dojka
Breastbone (sternum)	Sternum	Esternón	Sterno	Prsna kost (sternum)

English	French	Spanish	Italian	Croatian
Bronchiole	Bronchiole	Bronquiolo	Bronchiolo	Bronhiola
Bronchus	Bronche	Bronquio	Bronco	Dušnica (bronh)
Bulbourethral gland (Cowper's gland)	Glande de Cowper (glande bulbo-uretrale)	Glándula bulbouretral (glándula de Cowper)	Ghiandola bulbouretrale (ghiandola di Cowper)	Bulbouretralna žlijezda (Cowperova žlijezda)
Bundle of His	Faisceau de His	Haz de His	Fascio di His	Hisov snopić
Calcaneus	Calcanéus (calcanéum)	Calcáneo	Calcagno	Petna kost (kalkaneus)
Calcitonin	Calcitonine	Calcitonina	Calcitonina	Kalcitonin
Calf	Mollet	Pantorrilla	Polpaccio	List
Canal of Schlemm	Canal de Schlemm	Canal de Schlemm	Canale di Schlemm	Schlemmov kanal
Canine tooth	Canine	Canino (diente colmillo)	Canino	Očnjak (kanin)
Capillary	Capillaire	Capilar	Capillare	Kapilara
Carbohydrate	Hidrate de carbone (glucide)	Carbohidrato	Carboidrato (glucide)	Ugljikohidrat
Cardiac atrium	Oreillette	Aurícula cardíaca (atrio)	Atrio	Srčana pretklijetka (atrij)
Cardiac muscle (myocardium)	Myocarde	Miocardio	Miocardio	Srčani mišić (miokard)
Cardiac ventricle	Ventricule cardiaque	Ventrículo cardíaco	Ventricolo cardiaco	Srčana klijetka
Carpus	Carpe	Carpo	Carpo	Zapešće
Cartilage	Cartilage	Cartílago	Cartilagine	Hrskavica
Cartilage ring	Cartilage cricoïde	Cartílago circoides	Anello cartilagineo	Hrskavični prsten
Catecholamine	Catécholamine	Catecolamina	Catecolamina	Katekolamin
Cell	Cellule	Célula	Cellula	Stanica
Cementum	Cément	Cemento dental	Cemento	Zubni cement
Cerebellum	Cervelet	Cerebelo	Cervelletto	Mali mozak
Cerebral cortex	Cortex cérébral (écorce cérébrale)	Corteza cerebral	Corteccia cerebrale	Moždana kora
Cerebrospinal fluid	Liquide cérébro-spinal	Líquido cefalorraquídeo (líquido cerebrospinal)	Liquido cefalora-chidiano (liquor, liquido cerebrospinale)	Moždana tekućina (likvor)
Cerebrum (telencephalon)	Télencéphale (cerveau)	Telencéfalo	Telencefalo (cervello)	Veliki mozak (telencefalon)
Cheek	Joue	Mejilla (carrillo)	Guancia	Obraz
Chest	Torse	Pecho	Torace	Grudište (prsa)
Chin	Menton	Barbilla (mentón)	Mento	Brada
Cholesterol	Cholestérol	Colesterol	Colesterolo	Kolesterol
Choroid	Choroïde	Coroides	Coroide	Žilnica
Ciliary muscle	Muscle ciliaire	Músculo ciliar	Muscolo ciliare	Cilijarni mišić
Clitoris	Clitoris	Clítoris	Clitoride	Dražica (klitoris)
Coccygeal vertebra	Vertèbre coccygienne	Vértebra coccígea	Vertebra coccigea	Trtični kralježak
Cochlea	Cochlée	Cóclea (caracol)	Coclea	Pužnica
Collagen	Collagène	Colágeno	Collagene	Kolagen
Collarbone (clavicle)	Clavicule	Clavícula	Clavicola	Ključna kost (klavikula)
Cornea	Cornée	Córnea	Cornea	Rožnica
Coronary artery	Artère coronaire	Arteria coronaria	Arteria coronaria	Koronarna arterija
Corpus luteum	Corps jaune	Cuerpo lúteo (cuerpo amarillo)	Corpo luteo	Žuto tijelo
Corticosteroid	Corticostéroïde	Corticosteroide	Corticosteroide	Kortikosteroid
Corticosterone	Corticostérone	Corticosterona	Corticosterone	Kortikosteron
Corticotropin (adrenocorticotropic hormone)	Hormone corticotrope (adrenocorticotropic hormone, ACTH)	Hormona adrenocorticotropa (corticotropina, corticotrofina)	Corticotropina (ormone adrenocorticotropo)	Kortikotropin
Cortisol	Cortisol (hydro-cortisone)	Cortisol (hidrocortisona)	Cortisolo	Kortizol
Cortisone	Cortisone	Cortisona	Cortisone	Kortizon
Cranial nerve	Nerf crânien	Nervio craneal	Nervo cranico	Moždani živac
Crown ofa tooth	Couronne de la dent	Corona del diente	Corona del dente	Kruna zuba
Deltoid muscle	Muscle deltoïde	Músculo deltoides	Muscolo deltoide	Rameni mišić (deltoideus)
Dendrite	Dendrite	Dendrita	Dendrite	Dendrit
Dental pulp	Pulpe dentaire	Pulpa dentaria	Polpa dentaria	Središte zuba (pulpa)
Dentin	Dentine (ivoire)	Dentina	Dentina	Zubni dentin
Deoxyribonucleic acid (DNA)	Acide désoxyribonucléique	Ácido desoxirribonucleico	Acido desossiribonucleico (DNA)	Dezoksiribonukleinska kiselina (DNK)
Diaphragm	Diaphragme	Diafragma	Muscolo diaframma	Ošit (dijafragma)
Diencephalon	Diencéphale	Diencéfalo	Diencefalo	Međumozak
Duodenum	Duodénum	Duodeno	Duodeno	Dvanaesnik (duodenum)
Dura mater	Dure-mère	Duramadre	Dura madre (pachimeninge)	Tvrda moždana ovojnica
Ear	Oreille	Óido	Orecchio	Uho
Eardrum (tympanic membrane)	Tympan	Tímpano	Timpano (membrana timpanica)	Bubnjić
Earwax (cerumen)	Cire de l'oreille (cérumen)	Cerumen (cerilla)	Cerume	Ušna mast (ušna smola, cerumen)
Ejaculatory duct	Canal éjaculateur	Conducto eyaculador	Dotto eiaculatore	Sjemenovod
Elastin	Élastine	Elastina	Elastina	Elastin
Elbow	Coude	Codo	Gomito	Lakat
Elbow joint	Articulation oléocranienne	Articulación del codo	Articolazione del gomito	Lakatni zglob
Electrolyte	Électrolyte	Electrolito	Elettrolita	Elektrolit
Eosinophil	Éosinophile	Eosinófilo	Eosinofilo	Eozinofil

English	French	Spanish	Italian	Croatian
Epididymis	Épididyme	Epidídimo	Epididimo	Pasjemenik
Erythrocyte (red blood cell)	Érythrocyte (hématie, globule rouge)	Eritrocito (glóbulo rojo)	Eritrocita (globulo rosso)	Eritrocit (crveno krvno tjelešce)
Estradiol	Estradiol	Estradiol	Estradiolo	Folikulin (estradiol)
Estrogen	Estrogène	Estrógeno	Estrogeno	Estrogen
Ethmoid bone	Os ethmoïde	Hueso etmoides	Osso etmoide	Sitasta kost (etmoidna kost)
Eye	Oeil	Ojo	Occhio	Oko
Eye orbit	Orbite de l'oeil	Órbita	Orbita oculare	Očna šupljina
Eyeball	Globe oculaire	Globo ocular	Bulbo oculare	Očna jabučica
Eyebrow	Sourcils	Ceja	Sopracciglio	Obrva
Eyelash	Cil	Pestaña	Ciglia	Trepavica
Eyelid	Paupière	Párpado	Palpebra	Kapak
Face	Visage	Cara (faz)	Viso	Lice
Fallopian tube (oviduct)	Trompe de Fallope	Trompa de Falopio (tuba uterina, oviducto)	Tuba di Falloppio	Jajovod
Fat	Matière grasse	Grasa	Lipidi	Mast
Fat tissue	Tissu adipeux (masse grasse)	Tejido graso (tejido adiposo)	Tessuto adiposo	Masno tkivo
Fibrin	Fibrine	Fibrina	Fibrina	Fibrin
Fibrinogen	Fibrinogène	Fibrinógeno	Fibrinogeno	Fibrinogen
Fibroblast	Fibroblaste	Fibroblasto (célula fija)	Fibroblasto	Fibroblast
Fibula (calf bone)	Fibula (péroné)	Peroné (fibula)	Perone (fibula)	Lisna kost (fibula)
Finger	Doigt	Dedo de la mano	Dito della mano	Ručni prst
Foot	Pied	Pie	Piede	Stopalo
Forearm	Avant-bras	Antebrazo	Avambraccio	Podlaktica
Forefinger	Index	Dedo índice	Dito indice	Kažiprst
Forehead	Front	Frente	Fronte	Čelo
Foreskin (prepuce)	Prépuce	Prepucio	Prepuzio	Prepucij
Frontal bone	Os frontal	Hueso frontal	Osso frontale	Čeona kost
Gall (bile)	Bile	Bilis	Bile	Žuč
Gall bladder	Vésicule biliaire (cholécyste)	Vesícula biliar	Cistifellea	Žućni mjehur
Gas	Gaz	Gas	Gas	Plin
Gastric acid	Acide gastrique	Ácido gástrico	Acido gastrico	Želučana kiselina
Gastric juice	Suc gastrique	Jugo gástrico	Succo gastrico	Želučani sok
Gastric mucous membrane	Muqueuse gastrique	Mucosa estomacal	Mucosa gastrica	Želučana sluznica
Gland	Glande	Glándula	Ghiandola	Žlijezda
Glans	Gland	Glande	Glande	Glavić
Globulin	Globuline	Globulina	Globulina	Globulin
Glomerulus	Glomérule	Glomérulo	Glomerulo	Glomerul
Glucagon	Glucagon	Glucagón	Glucagone	Glukagon
Glucocorticoid	Glucocorticoïde	Glucocorticoide	Glucocorticoide	Glukokortikoid
Glucose	Glucose	Glucosa	Glucosio	Glukoza
Gluteal muscle	Muscle glutéal	Músculo glúteo	Muscolo gluteo	Sjedni mišić
Glycogen	Glycogène	Glucógeno	Glicogeno	Glikogen
Gonadotrophin	Gonadotrophine	Gonadotropina	Gonadotropina	Gonadotropin
Granulocyte	Granulocyte (polynucléaire)	Granulocito	Granulocita	Granulocit
Groin	Aine	Ingle	Inguine	Prepona
Growth hormone (somatotrophin)	Hormone de croissance (somatotropine)	Hormona de crecimiento somatotropa	Somatotropina	Hormon rasta (somatotropin)
Gullet (oesophagus)	Oesophage	Esófago	Esofago	Jednjak
Gums (gingiva)	Gencive	Encía	Gengiva	Desni
Hair	Poil	Pelo	Pelo	Dlaka
Hair	Cheveu	Cabello	Capelli	Kosa
Hammer (malleus)	Marteau (malléus)	Martillo (malleus)	Martello	Čekić (malleus)
Hand	Main	Mano	Mano	Šaka
Hard palate	Palais osseux	Paladar óseo	Palato duro (volta palatina)	Tvrdo nepce
Head	Tête	Cabeza	Testa	Glava
Heart	Coeur	Corazón	Cuore	Srce
Heart valve (cardiac valve)	Valve cardiaque	Válvula cardiaca (válvula de corazón)	Valvola cardiaca	Srčani zalistak
Heel	Talon	Talón (calcañar)	Tallone	Peta
Hemoglobin	Hémoglobine	Hemoglobina	Emoglobina	Hemoglobin
Hip bone	Os coxal	Hueso coxal	Osso dell'anca	Kost kuka
Hip joint	Hanche	Articulación de la cadera	Articolazione dell'anca	Kuk (zglob kuka)
Hormone	Hormone	Hormona	Ormone	Hormon
Hymen	Hymen	Himen	Imene	Djevičnjak (himen)
Hyoid bone (lingual bone)	Os hyoïde (os lingual)	Hueso hioides	Osso ioide	Podjezična kost
Hypophysis (pituitary gland)	Hypophyse (glande pituitaire)	Hipófisis (glándula pituitaria)	Ipòfisi (ghiandola pituitaria)	Hipofiza
Hypothalamus	Hypothalamus	Hipotálamo	Ipotalamo	Hipotalamus
Ileum	Iléon (ileum)	Íleon	Ileo	Ileum
Ilium	Ilion (ilium)	Ilion	Osso iliaco	Crijevna kost
Immunoglobulin	Immunoglobuline	Inmunoglobulina	Immunoglobulina	Imunoglobulin
Incisor	Incisive	Incisivo	Incisivo	Sjekutić (inciziv)
Inferior vena cava	Veine cave inférieure	Vena cava inferior	Vena cava inferiore	Donja šuplja vena

English	French	Spanish	Italian	Croatian
Innominate bone (pelvis)	Bassin osseux	Pelvis	Bacino	Zdjelica
Insulin	Insuline	Insulina	Insulina	Inzulin
Intercostal muscle	Muscle intercostal	Músculo intercostal	Muscolo intercostale	Međurebreni mišić
Interstitial fluid	Liquide interstitiel	Líquido intersticial (líquido tisular)	Liquido extracellulare	Međustanična tekućina
Intervertebral disc	Disque intervertébral	Disco intervertebral	Disco intervertebrale	Međukralježnični disk
Intestinal juice	Suc intestinal	Jugo intestinal	Succo intestinale	Crijevni sok
Intestinal villus	Villosité intestinale	Vellosidad intestinal	Villo intestinale	Crijevna resica
Intestine	Intestin	Intestin	Intestino	Crijevo
Iris	Iris	Iris	Iride	Šarenica
Ischium	Ischium	Isquión	Ischio	Sjedna kost
Jaw	Mâchoire	Quijada	Scheletro della bocca	Čeljust
Jejunum	Jéjunum	Yeyuno	Digiuno	Jejunum
Joint	Articulation	Articulación	Articolazione	Zglob
Joint cartilage	Cartilage articulaire	Cartílago articular	Cartilagine articolare	Zglobna hrskavica
Keratin	Kératine	Queratina	Cheratina	Keratin
Kidney	Rein	Riñón	Rene	Bubreg
Knee	Genou	Rodilla	Ginocchio	Koljeno
Kneecap (patella)	Rotule (patella)	Rótula (patela)	Rotula (patella)	Iver (patela)
Lachrymal bone	Os lacrymal (unguis)	Unguis (hueso lacrimal)	Osso lacrimale	Suzna kost
Lachrymal gland	Glande lacrymale	Glándula lagrimal	Ghiandola lacrimale	Suzna žlijezda
Large intestine (colon)	Gros intestin (côlon)	Intestino grueso (colon)	Intestino crasso (colon)	Debelo crijevo
Larynx	Larynx	Laringe	Laringe	Grkljan
Leg	Membre inférieur	Miembro inferior	Arto inferiore	Noga
Lens	Cristallin	Cristalino	Cristallino	Leća
Leukocyte	Leucocyte	Leucocito	Leucocita	Leukocit
Ligament	Ligament	Ligamento	Legamento	Ligament
Lip	Lèvre	Labio	Labbro	Usna
Little finger (pinky)	Auriculaire (petit doigt)	Dedo meñique	Mignolo	Mali prst
Liver	Foie	Hígado	Fegato	Jetra
Loin	Lombes	Espalda baja	Lombo	Križa
Lower jaw (mandible)	Mandibule	Mandíbula	Mandibola	Donja čeljust (mandibula)
Lower leg	Jambe	Pierna	Gamba	Potkoljenica
Lumbar vertebra	Vertèbre lombale	Vértebra lumbar	Vertebra lombare	Slabinski kralježak (lumbalni kralježak)
Lung	Poumon	Pulmón	Polmone	Plućno krilo
Lungs	Poumons	Pulmones	Polmoni	Pluća
Luteinisin g hormone	Hormne lutéinisante	Hormona luteinizante (lutropina)	Ormone luteinizzante	Luteinizirajući hormon
Lymph	Lymphe	Linfa	Linfa	Limfa
Lymph gland (lymph node)	Ganglion lymphatique (noeud lymphatique)	Ganglio linfático	Linfonodo	Limfna žlijezda
Lymph vessel	Vaisseau lymphatique	Vaso linfático	Vaso linfatico	Limfna žila
Lymphocyte	Lymphocyte	Linfocito	Linfocita	Limfocit
Masseter muscle	Muscle masséter	Músculo masetero	Muscolo massetere	Žvakaći mišić
Medulla oblongata	Moelle allongée (medulla oblongata, bulbe rachidien, myélencéphale)	Bulbo raquídeo (médula oblongada, miencéfalo)	Bulbo (midollo allungato, encefalo)	Produžena moždina
Melanin	Mélanine	Melanina	Melanina	Melanin
Melanotropin	Hormone mélanotrope (mélanocortine, mélanotropine)	Melanotropina	Ormone melanotropo	Melanotropin
Melatonin	Mélatonine (hormone du sommeil)	Melatonina	Melatonina	Melatonin
Meninx	Méninge	Meninge	Meninge	Moždana ovojnica
Meniscus	Ménisque	Menisco	Menisco	Zglobni menisk
Metacarpal bone	Os métacarpe	Hueso del metacarpo	Osso metacarpale	Kost pesti (metakarpalna kost)
Metacarpus	Métacarpe	Metacarpo	Metacarpo	Pest (metakarpus)
Metatarsal bone	Os du métatarse	Hueso del metatarso	Osso metatarsale	Kost donožja (metatarzalna kost)
Metatarsus	Métatarse	Metatarso	Metatarso	Donožje (metatarzus)
Middle ear	Oreille moyenne	Oído medio	Orecchio medio	Srednje uho
Middle finger	Majeur	Dedo corazón	Dito medio	Srednji prst
Milk tooth	Dent temporaire	Diente de leche	Dente da latte	Mliječni zub
Mineralcorticoid	Minéralcorticoïde	Mineralocorticoide	Mineralcorticoide	Mineralkortikoid (Na-hormon)
Mitral valve (bicuspid valve)	Valve mitrale (valve bicuspide)	Válvula bicúspide (válvula mitral)	Valvola mitrale (valvola bicuspide)	Mitralni zalistak (bikuspidalni zalistak)
Molar	Molaire	Molar	Molare	Kutnjak (molar)
Monocyte	Monocyte	Monocito	Monocita	Monocit
Mouth	Bouche	Boca	Bocca	Usta
Mouth cavity (oral cavity)	Cavité buccale	Cavidad bucal (cavidad oral)	Cavità orale	Usna šupljina
Mucous membrane	Muqueuse	Mucosa	Membrana mucosa	Sluznica
Mucus	Mucus	Moco	Muco	Sluz
Muscle	Muscle	Músculo	Muscolo	Mišić

English	French	Spanish	Italian	Croatian
Muscular fascia	Fascia musculaire (périmysium)	Fascia profunda	Fascia muscolare	Mišićna fascija
Nail	Ongle	Uña	Unghia	Nokat
Nape (occiput)	Nuque	Nuca	Nuca	Zatiljak
Nasal bone	Os nasal	Hueso proprio de la nariz (hueso nasal)	Osso nasale	Nosna kost
Nasolacrimal duct (tear duct)	Canal lacrymonasal (canal lacrimal, canal des larmes)	Conducto nasolagrimal	Canale naso-lacrimale	Suzno-nosni kanal
Navel (belly button)	Ombilic (nombril)	Ombligo (pupo)	Ombelico	Pupak
Neck	Cou	Cuello	Collo	Vrat
Nerve	Nerf	Nervio	Nervo	Živac
Nipple	Mamelon (papille)	Pezón	Capezzolo	Bradavica
Noradrenaline	Noradrénaline	Noradrenalina	Noradrenalina	Noradrenalin
Nose	Nez	Nariz	Naso	Nos
Nostril	Narine	Narina	Narice	Nosnica
Occipital bone	Os occipital	Hueso occipital	Osso occipitale	Zatiljna kost
Optic nerve	Nerf optique	Nervio óptico	Nervo ottico	Vidni živac
Organ	Organe	Órgano	Organo	Organ
Ovary	Ovaire	Ovario	Ovaia	Jajnik
Ovum	Ovule	Óvulo	Uovo	Jajašce
Oxytocin	Ocytocine (oxytocine)	Oxitocina	Ossitocina	Oksitocin
Palate	Palaise	Paladar	Palato	Nepce
Palatine bone	Os palatin	Hueso palatino	Osso palatino	Nepčana kost
Palm	Paume	Palma	Palmo	Dlan
Pancreas	Pancréas	Páncreas	Pancreas	Gušterača
Pancreatic juice	Suc pancréatique	Jugo pancreático	Succo pancreatico	Sok gušterače
Parasympathetic nervous system	Système nerveux parasympatique (système vagal)	Sistema nervioso parasimpático	Sistema nervoso parasimpatico	Parasimpatikus
Parathyroid gland	Parathyroïde	Glándula paratiroides	Paratiroide	Doštitnjača
Parathyroid hormone	Parathormone (hormone parathyroïdienne)	Parathormona (hormona paratiroidea, paratirina)	Paratormone (ormone paratiroideo)	Paratireoidni hormon
Parietal bone	Os pariétal	Hueso parietal	Osso parietale	Tjemena kost
Parietal pleura	Plèvre pariétale	Pleura parietal	Pleura parietale	Porebrica (parijetalna pleura)
Pectoralis major muscle	Muscle grand pectoral	Músculo pectoral mayor	Muscolo grande pettorale	Veliki prsni mišić
Pectoralis minor muscle	Muscle petit pectoral	Músculo pectoral menor	Muscolo piccolo pettorale	Mali prsni mišić
Penis	Pénis	Pene (falo)	Pene	Penis
Pericardium	Péricarde	Pericardio	Pericardio	Osrčje (perikard)
Perineum	Périnée	Periné (perineo)	Perineo	Međica (perineum)
Peritoneum	Péritoine	Peritoneo	Peritoneo	Potrbušnica (peritoneum)
Phalanx bone	Phalange	Falange	Falange	Kost prsta (falanga)
Pharynx (gullet, gorge)	Pharynx	Faringe	Faringe	Ždrijelo
Phospholipid	Phospholipide	Fosfolípido	Fosfolipide	Fosfolipid
Pia mater	Pie-mère	Piamadre	Pia madre	Meka moždana ovojnica
Pineal body (pineal gland, epiphysis)	Glande pinéale (épiphyse)	Glándula pineal (epífisis)	Ghiandola pineale (epifisi)	Pinealna žlijezda (epifiza)
Pinna (auricle)	Pavillon auriculaire	Pabellón auricular (aurícula)	Padiglione auricolare	Ušna školjka
Plasma	Plasma sanguin	Plasma sanguíneo	Plasma	Plazma
Pleura	Plèvre	Pleura	Pleura (pleure)	Pleura
Pore	Pore	Poro	Poro	Pora
Portal vein	Veine porte	Vena porta	Vena porta	Portalna vena
Premolar	Prémolaire	Premolar	Premolare	Pretkutnjak (premolar)
Progesterone	Progestérone	Progesterona	Progesterone	Progesteron
Prostate	Prostate	Próstata	Prostata	Prostata
Protein	Protéine	Proteína	Proteina	Bjelančevina (protein)
Pubis (pubic bone)	Os pubien	Pubis	Pube (osso pubico)	Stidna kost
Pulmonary artery	Artère pulmonaire	Arteria pulmonar (tronco pulmonar, tronco de las pulmonares)	Arteria polmonare	Plućna arterija
Pupil	Pupille	Pupila	Pupilla	Zjenica
Quadriceps femoris muscle	Muscle quadriceps fémoral	Músculo cuádriceps crural	Muscolo quadricipite femorale	Četveroglavi bedreni mišić
Radius	Radius	Radio	Radio	Palčana kost
Rectus abdominis muscle	Muscle droit de l'abdomen	Músculo recto mayor del abdomen	Muscolo retto dell'addome	Ravni trbušni mišić
Retina	Rétine	Retina	Rètina	Mrežnica (retina)
Rh factor negative	Système Rhésus négatif	Factor Rh negativo	Fattore Rh negativo	Negativan Rh faktor
Rh factor positive	Système Rhésus positif	Factor Rh positivo	Fattore Rh positivo	Pozitivan Rh faktor
Rhomboid muscle	Muscle rhomboïde	Músculo romboides	Muscolo romboide	Romboidni mišić
Rib	Côte	Costilla	Costola (costa)	Rebro
Rib cage	Cage thoracique	Caja torácica	Gabbia toracica	Grudni koš
Ribonucleic acid	Acide ribonucléique (ARN)	Ácido ribonucleico (ARN)	Acido ribonucleico (ARN)	Ribonukleinska kiselina
Ring finger	Annulaire	Dedo anular	Anulare	Prstenjak
Root of a tooth	Racine dentaire	Raíz del diente	Radice del dente	Korijen zuba
Sacral vertebra	Vertèbre sacrale	Vértebra sacra	Vertebra sacrale	Krstačni kralježak (sakralni kralježak)

English	French	Spanish	Italian	Croatian
Saliva (spit, slobber)	Salive	Saliva	Saliva	Slina (pljuvačka)
Salivary gland	Glande salivaire	Glándula salival	Ghiandola salivare	Žlijezda slinovnica
Scalp	Cuir chevelu	Cuero cabelludo (capa capilar)	Cuoio capelluto	Vlasište
Sclera	Sclère	Eclerótica	Sclera	Bjeloočnica
Sebaceous gland	Glande sébacée	Glándula sebácea	Ghiandola sebacea	Žlijezda lojnica
Sebum	Sébum	Sebo cutáneo	Sebo	Loj
Semen	Sperme	Semen (esperma)	Sperma	Sperma
Semimembranosus muscle	Muscle semi-membraneux	Músculo semimembranoso	Muscolo semimembranoso	Poluopnasti mišić
Seminal vesicle	Vésicule séminale (glande vésiculeuse)	Vesícula seminal	Vescicola seminale	Sjemena vrećica
Semitendinosus muscle	Muscle semi-tendineux	Músculo semitendinoso	Muscolo semitendinoso	Polutetivni mišić
Sesamoid bone	Os sésamoïde	Hueso sesamoide	Osso sesamoide	Sezamska kost
Sex gland (gonad)	Gonade	Gónada	Gonade	Spolna žlijezda
Shinbone (tibia)	Tibia	Tibia	Tibia	Goljenica (tibija)
Shoulder	Épaule	Hombro	Spalla	Rame
Shoulder blade (scapula)	Omoplate (scapula)	Omóplato (escápula)	Scapola (omoplata)	Lopatica (skapula)
Shoulder joint	Complexe articulaire de l'épaule	Articulación del hombro	Articolazione della spalla	Rameni zglob
Sigmoid colon	Côlon sigmoïde	Colon sigmoide	Sigma (colon sigmoideo)	Sigmoidni dio debelog crijeva
Sinus	Sinus	Seno	Seno	Sinus
Skeleton	Squelette	Esqueleto	Scheletro	Kostur
Skin	Peau	Piel	Pelle (cute)	Koža
Skull	Crâne	Calavera (cráneo)	Cranio	Lubanja
Skull base	Base du crâne	Base del cráneo	Base del cranio	Baza lubanje
Small intestine	Intestin grêle	Intestino delgado	Intestino tenue (piccolo intestino)	Tanko crijevo
Smooth muscle	Muscle lisse	Músculo liso	Tessuto muscolare liscio	Glatki mišić
Soft palate	Voile du palais	Úvula	Palato molle	Meko nepce
Sole	Plante	Planta del pie	Pianta del piede	Taban
Sperm (spermatozoon)	Spermatozoïde	Espermatozoide	Spermatozoo	Spermij
Sphenoid bone	Os sphénoïde	Hueso esfenoides	Osso sfenoide	Klinasta kost (leptirasta kost)
Sphincter	Sphincter	Esfínter	Sfintere	Kružni mišić (sfinkter)
Spinal cord	Moelle épinière (moelle spinale)	Médula espinal	Midollo spinale	Kralježnična moždina
Spinal nerve	Nerf spinal	Nervio espinal	Nervo spinale	Spinalni živac
Spine (spinal column, backbone)	Colonne vertébrale (rachis)	Columna vertebral	Columna vertebral	Kralježnica
Spleen	Rate	Bazo	Milza	Slezena
Stirrup (stapes)	Étrier	Estribo	Staffa (columella)	Stremen
Stomach	Estomac	Estómago	Stomaco	Želudac
Stool (feces)	Fèces	Excrementos (heces)	Feci	Stolica (feces, izmet)
Striated muscle	Muscle strié	Músculo estriado	Muscolo striato	Poprečno-prugasti mišić
Superior vena cava	Veine cave supérieure	Vena cava superior	Vena cava superiore	Gornja šuplja vena
Sweat	Sueur	Sudor	Sudore	Znoj
Sweat gland	Glande sudoripare (sudorale)	Glándula sudorípara	Ghiandola sudoripara	Žlijezda znojnica
Sympathetic nervous system	Système nerveux orthosympathique (système nerveux sympathique)	Sistema nervioso simpático	Sistema nervoso simpatico	Simpatikus
Synapse	Synapse	Sinapsis	Sinapsi (bottone sinaptico)	Sinapsa
Synovial bursa	Bourse séreuse	Bursa (bolsa sinovial)	Borsa sierosa	Sluzna vreća (bursa)
Synovial fluid (synovia)	Liquide synovial	Líquido sinovial	Liquido sinoviale (sinovia)	Zglobna tekućina (sinovijalna tekućina)
Synovial membrane	Membrane synoviale	Membrana sinovial	Membrana sinoviale	Sinovijalna opna
Tailbone (coccyx)	Coccyx	Cóccix (coxis)	Coccige	Trtica
Tailor's muscle (sartorius muscle)	Muscle couturier (muscle sartorius)	Músculo sartorio	Muscolo sartorio	Krojački mišić
Tarsal bone	Os du tarse	Hueso del tarso	Osso tarsale	Kost zastoplja (kost tarzusa)
Tarsus	Tarse	Tarso	Tarso	Zastoplje
Taste bud	Papille gustative	Papila gustativa	Papilla gustativa	Okusni pupoljak
Tear	Larme	Lágrima	Lacrima	Suza
Temple	Tempe	Sien	Tempia	Sljepoočnica
Temporal bone	Os temporal	Hueso temporal	Osso temporale	Sljepoočna kost
Tendon (sinew)	Tendon	Tendón	Tendine	Tetiva
Testicle	Testicule	Testículo	Testicolo	Jaje (mudo, testis)
Testosterone	Testostérone	Testosterona	Testosterone	Testosteron
Thalamus	Thalamus	Tálamo	Talamo	Talamus
Thigh	Cuisse	Muslo (región femoral)	Coscia	Natkoljenica (bedro)
Thighbone (femur)	Os de la cuisse (fémur)	Fémur	Femore	Bedrena kost (femur)
Thoracic aorta	Aorte thoracique	Aorta torácica	Aorta toracica	Torakalna aorta
Thoracic vertebra	Vertèbre thoracique	Vértebra torácica	Vertebra toracica	Leđni kralježak (grudni ili torakalni kralježak)

English	French	Spanish	Italian	Croatian
Throat	Gorge	Garganta	Gola	Grlo
Thrombocyte	Thrombocyte	Plaqueta (trombocito)	Trombocita (piastrina)	Trombocit
Thumb	Pouce	Dedo pulgar (pólice)	Pollice	Palac
Thymus	Thymus	Timo	Timo	Grudna žlijezda (timus)
Thyroid	Thyroïde	Tiroides	Tiroide	Štitnjača
Thyroid-stimulating hormone (TSH, thyrotropin)	Thyréostimuline (thyréotropine)	Tirotropina (TSH, hormona estimulante de la tiroides)	Tirotropina (ormone tireostimolante)	Tireotropin (TSH)
Thyroxine	Thyroxine	Tiroxina (tetrayodotironina, T4)	Tiroxina	Tiroksin
Tissue	Tissu	Tejido	Tessuto	Tkivo
Toe	Orteil	Dedo del pie	Dito del piede	Nožni prst
Tongue	Langue	Lengua	Lingua	Jezik
Tonsil	Tonsille	Amígdala	Tonsille	Krajnik
Tooth	Dent	Diente	Dente	Zub
Tooth enamel	Émail dentaire	Esmalte dental	Smalto	Zubna caklina
Trapezius muscle	Muscle trapèze	Músculo trapecio	Muscolo trapezio	Trapezni mišić
Triceps brachii muscle	Muscle triceps brachial	Músculo tríceps braquial	Muscolo tricipite del braccio	Troglavi mišić nadlaktice
Triceps surae muscle	Muscle triceps sural	Músculo tríceps sural	Muscolo tricipite della sura	Troglavi mišić potkoljenice
Tricuspid valve	Valve tricuspide	Válvula tricúspide	Valvola tricuspide	Trolisni zalistak
Triglyceride	Triglycéride	Triglicérido	Trigliceride	Triglicerid
Triiodothyronine	Triiodothyronine	Triiodotironina	Triiodotironina	Trijodtironin
Trunk (torso)	Tronc	Tronco	Tronco	Trup (torzo)
Tympanic cavity	Cavité tympanique	Cavidad timpánica	Cassa del timpano	Bubnjište
Ulna	Ulna (cubitus)	Cúbito (ulna)	Ulna (cubito)	Lakatna kost (ulna)
Upper arm	Partie supérieure du bras	Parte superior del brazo	Barccio	Nadlaktica
Upper arm bone (humerus)	Humérus	Húmero	Omero	Nadlaktična kost (humerus)
Upper back	Parti supérieur du dos	Espalda superior	Schiena alto	Gornji dio leđa
Upper jaw (maxilla)	Os maxillaire	Hueso maxilar superior (maxila)	Osso mascellare	Gornja čeljust (maksila)
Urea	Urée (carbamide)	Urea	Urea	Mokraćevina (urea, ureja)
Ureter	Uretère	Uréter	Uretere	Mokraćovod (ureter)
Urethra	Urètre	Uretra	Uretra	Vanjska mokraćna cijev (uretra)
Urinary bladder	Vessie	Vejiga urinaria	Vescica urinaria	Mokraćni mjehur
Urine	Urine	Orina	Urina	Mokraća (urin)
Vagina	Vagin	Vagina (colpos)	Vagina	Rodnica (vagina)
Valve (valvula)	Valve	Válvula	Valvola	Zalistak
Vein	Veine	Vena	Vena	Vena
Ventricle	Ventricule	Ventrículo	Ventricolo	Klijetka
Venule	Veinule (vénule)	Vénula	Venula	Venula
Vermiform appendix (cecal appaendix)	Appendice iléo-caecal (appendice, appendice vermiforme)	Apéndice vermiforme (apéndice cecal, apéndice)	Appendice vermiforme	Slijepo crijevo (crvuljak)
Vertebra	Vertèbre	Vértebra	Vertebra	Kralježak
Vertex (crown of head)	Vertex	Vértice craneal	Vertice della testa	Tjeme
Vestibule	Vestibule	Vestíbulo	Vestibolo	Predvorje (vestibulum)
Visceral pleura	Plèvre viscérale	Pleura visceral	Pleura viscerale	Poplućnica (visceralna pleura)
Vocal chord	Corde vocale	Cuerda vocal	Corda vocale	Glasnica
Vomer	Vomer	Vómer	Vomere	Raonik (vomer)
Vulva	Vulve	Vulva	Vulva	Stidnica
Windpipe (trachea)	Trachée	Tráquea	Trachea	Dušnik
Womb (uterus)	Utérus	Matriz (útero, seno materno)	Utero	Maternica (uterus)
Wrist	Poignet	Muñeca	Polso	Ručni zglob
Wrist bone (carpal bone)	Os du carpe	Hueso del carpo	Osso carpale	Kost zapešća (karpalna kost)
Zygoma (cheekbone, malar bone)	Os zygomatique (zygoma)	Hueso cigomático (malar)	Osso zigomatico	Sponična kost

SYMPTOMS, INJURIES AND DISEASES:	LES SYMPTÔMES, BLESSURES ET MALADIES:	SÍNTOMAS, HERIDAS Y ENFERMEDADES:	I SINTOMI, FERITE E MALATTIE:	SIMPTOMI, OZLJEDE I BOLESTI:
Abdominal aortic aneurysm	Anévrisme de l'aorte abdominale	Aneurisma de aorta abdominal	Aneurisma dell'aorta addominale	Aneurizma abdominalne aorte
Abdominal colic	Colique abdominale	Cólico abdominal	Colica addominale	Trbušna kolika (abdominalna kolika)
Abdominal pain	Douleur abdominale	Dolor abdominal	Dolore addominale	Bol u trbuhu
Abdominal wall tension	Tension de la paroi stomacale	Tensión de la pared abdominal	Tensione di parete addominale	Napetost trbušne stijenke
Aberrant pancreas	Pancréas aberrant	Pancreas aberrante	Pancraes aberrante	Aberantni pankreas
Abnormal flexibility	Flexibilité anormale	Flexibilidad anormal	Movimento anormale	Abnormalna gibljivost
Abnormal twisting of the intestines (volvulus)	Volvulus	Retorcimiento anormal del intestino (vólvulo)	Volvolo	Zapletaj crijeva

English	French	Spanish	Italian	Croatian
Abnormally heavy menstrual period (menorrhagia)	Cycle menstruel anormalement excessice (ménorragie)	Pérdida de sangre ma-yor durante la menstruación (menorragia)	Anormale perdita di sangue durante il ciclo mestruale(menorragia)	Abnormalno velik gubitak krvi tijekom mjesečnice (menoragija)
Abnormally large intake of food (hyperphagia)	Prise excessive d'aliments (hyperphagie)	Ingestas descontroladas de alimentos (hiperfagia)	Aumento incontrollato di assunzione di cibo (iperfagia)	Prekomjerno jedenje (hiperfagija)
Aboulia (disorder of diminished motivation)	Aboulie	Abulia	Abulia	Abulija (poremećaj umanjene motivacije)
Abrasion	Écorchure	Abrasión (escoriación)	Abrasione (escoriazione)	Ojedina (abrazija)
Abscess	Abcès	Absceso	Ascesso	Apsces
Absence in development of an organ (aplasia of an organ)	Arrêt du développement d'un organe (aplasie d'un organe)	Desarrollo detenido de un órgano (aplasia de un órgano)	Mancato sviluppo di un organo (aplasia di un organo)	Nerazvijenost organa (aplazija organa)
Absence of menstrual period (amenorrhea)	Absence des règles (aménorrhée)	Ausencia de la men-struación (amenorrea)	Assenza di mestrua-zioni (amenorrea)	Izostanak mjesečnice (amenoreja)
Absence of pulse	Absence de pouls	Pérdida de pulso	Perdita di polso	Gubitak pulsa
Acariasis	Acariase	Acariasis	Acariasi	Akarijaza
Accelerated basal metabolism	Metabolisme de base accéléré	Metabolismo basal acelerado	Metabolismo basale accelerato	Ubrzan bazalni metabolizam
Accelerated pulse rate	Fréquence du pouls accélérée	Pulso acelerado	Polso accelerato	Ubrzani puls
Achilles tendon overuse injury	Tendinite achilléenne chronique	Tendinitis por sobreuso en el tendón de Aquiles	Tendinopatia Achille da overuse	Sindrom prenaprezanja Ahilove tetive
Achilles tendon rupture	Rupture du tendon d'Achille	Ruptura del tendón de Aquiles	Rottura del tendine di Achille	Puknuće Ahilove tetive
Achillodynia (Achilles tendinitis)	Tendinite du tendon d'Achille	Tendinitis de Aquiles	Tendinopatia achillea (achillodinia)	Ahilodinija (tendinitis Ahilove tetive)
Achlorhydria	Achlorhydrie	Aclorhidria	Acloridria	Aklorhidrija
Achondroplasia	Achondroplasie	Acondroplasia	Acondroplasia	Ahondroplazija
Acidosis	Acidose	Acidosis	Acidosi	Acidoza
Acne	Acné	Acné	Acne	Akne
Acne vulgaris	Acné papulo-pustuleuse	Acné común (acne vulgaris)	Acne volgare (acne)	Vulgarne akne
Acoustic neuroma	Neurome acoustique	Neuroma acústico	Neuroma dell'acustico	Neurom slušnog živca
Acrocyanosis	Acrocyanose	Acrocianosis	Acrocianosi	Akrocijanoza
Acromegaly	Acromégalie	Acromegalia	Acromegalia	Akromegalija
Acrophobia (fear of heights)	Acrophobie (peur des hauteurs)	Acrofobia (miedo a las alturas)	Acrofobia (paura dei luoghi elevati)	Akrofobija (strah od visine)
Actinic keratosis	Kératose actinique	Queratosis actínica	Cheratosi solare	Aktinička keratoza
Actinomycosis	Actinomycose	Actinomicosis	Actinomicosi	Aktinomikoza
Acute abdomen	Abdomen aigu	Abdomen agudo	Addome acuto	Akutni abdomen
Acute appendicitis	Appendicite aiguë	Apendicitis aguda	Appendicite acuta	Akutna upala crvuljka
Acute gastric dilatation	Dilatation aiguë de l'estomac	Dilatación aguda del estómago	Dilatazione gastrica acuta	Akutna dilatacija želuca
Acute kidney failure	Insuffisance rénale aiguë	Insuficiencia renal aguda	Insufficienza renale acuta	Akutno zatajenje bubrega
Acute lymphoblastic leukemia	Leucémie lymphoblastique aiguë	Leucemia linfoblástica aguda	Leucemia acuta linfoblastica	Akutna limfatična leukemija
Acute myeloid leukemia (AML)	Leucémie aiguë myéloblastique	Leucemia mieloide aguda	Leucemia mieloide acuta	Akutna mijeloična leukemija
Acute pain	Douleur aiguë	Dolor agudo	Dolore acuto	Akutna bol
Acute pulmonary heart	Coeur pulmonaire aigu	Cor pulmonale agudo	Cuore polmonare acuto	Akutno plućno srce
Addiction	Dépendance (addiction)	Adicción (dependencia)	Dipendenza	Ovisnost
Addison's disease	Maladie d'Addison	Enfermedad de Addison	Morbo di Addison	Addisonova bolest
Adenocarcinoma	Adénocarcinome	Adenocarcinoma	Adenocarcinoma	Adenokarcinom
Adenoma	Adénome	Adenoma	Adenoma	Adenom
Adenopathy	Adénopathie	Adenopatía	Adenopatia	Adenopatija
African trypanosomiasis (sleeping sickness)	Maladie du sommeil (trypanosomiase africaine)	Tripanosomiasis africana (enfermedad del sueño)	Tripanosomiasi africana (malattia del sonno)	Afrička tripanosomijaza (bolest spavanja)
Age-related hearing loss (presbycusis)	Perte de l'audition liée à l'age (presbyacousie)	Trastorno de la capacidad para oír de las personas envejecen (presbiacusia)	Perdita dell'udito dovuta all'avanzamento dell'età (presbiacusia)	Staračka nagluhost (prezbiakuzija)
Age-related long-sightedness (presbyopia)	Mauvaise vision de près liée à l'âge (presbytie)	Vista cansada por la edad (presbiopía)	Presbiopia (presbitismo)	Staračka dalekovidnost (prezbiopija)
Agenesis (absence of an organ)	Agénésie	Agenesia (ausencia de un órgano)	Agenesia (mancanza di un organo)	Agenezija (nedostatak jednog organa)
Agnail (hangnail)	Envie de l'ongle	Padrastro	Pipita	Zanoktica
Agranulocytosis	Agranulocytose	Agranulocitosis	Agranulocitosi	Agranulocitoza
AIDS (acquired immune deficiency syndrome)	SIDA (syndrome d'immunodéficience acquise)	SIDA (síndrome de inmunodeficiencia adquirida)	SIDA (sindrome da ImmunoDeficienza Acquisita, AIDS)	SIDA (sindrom stečene imunodeficijencije, AIDS)
Air embolism (gas embolism)	Embolie gazeuse	Embolia gaseosa	Embolia gassosa	Zračna embolija
Albinism	Albinisme	Albinismo	Albinismo	Albinizam
Albuminuria	Albuminurie	Albuminuria	Albuminuria	Albuminurija
Alcohol poisoning	Empoisonnement par l'alcool	Intoxicación por alcohol	Avvelenamento da alcool	Trovanje alkoholom
Alcoholic cardiomyopathy	Cardiomyopathie alcoolique	Miocardiopatía alcohólica	Miocardiopatia alcolica	Alkoholna kardiomiopatja

English	French	Spanish	Italian	Croatian
Alcoholic cirrhosis	Cirrhose alcoolique	Cirrosis alcohólica	Cirrosi alcolica	Alkoholna ciroza
Alcoholism	Alcoolisme	Alcoholismo	Alcolismo	Alkoholizam
Aldosteronism (hyperaldosteronism)	Hyperaldostéronisme	Aldosteronismo (hiperaldosteronismo)	Iperaldosteronismo	Aldosteronizam
Algodystrophy	Algodystrophie	Algodistrofia	Algodistrofia	Algodistrofija
Alkali poisoning	Empoisonnement par alcalis	Intoxicación por álcalis	Avvelenamento da alcali	Trovanje alkalima
Alkalosis	Alcalose	Alcalosis	Alcalosi	Alkaloza
Allergic contact dermatitis	Dermite de contact allergique	Dermatitis alérgica de contacto	Dermatite allergica	Alergijski kontaktni dermatitis
Allergic conjunctivitis	Conjonctivite allergique	Conjuntivitis alérgica	Congiuntivite allergica	Alergijski konjuktivitis
Allergic rhinitis	Rhinite allergique	Rinitis alérgica	Rinite allergica	Alergijski rinitis
Allergy	Allergie	Alergia	Allergia	Alergija
Alopecia	Alopécie	Alopecia	Alopecia	Ćelavost
Alopecia areata	Alopécie areata	Alopecia areata	Alopecia areata	Alopecia areata
Alopecia universalis	Alopécie universalis	Alopecia areata universal	Alopecia universale	Opća alopecija
Altitude sickness (acute mountain sickness)	Mal aigu des montagnes	Mal de montaña (mal de altura)	Mal di montagna	Visinska bolest
Alzheimer's diesase	Maladie d'Alzheimer	Enfermedad de Alzheimer	Morbo di Alzheimer	Alzheimerova bolest
Amebiasis (amebic dysentery)	Amibiase (dysenterie amibienne)	Disentería amebiana (amebiasis)	Amebiasi	Amebijaza
Amnesia	Amnésie	Amnesia	Amnesia	Amnezija
Amputation	Amputation	Amputación	Amputazione	Amputacija
Amyloidosis	Amylose (amyloïdose, maladie orpheline)	Amiloidosis	Amiloidosi	Amiloidoza
Amyotrophic lateral sclerosis	Sclérose latérale amyotrophique (maladie de Charcot)	Esclerosis lateral amiotrófica	Sclerosi laterale amiotrofica	Amiotrofična lateralna skleroza
Anal abscess	Abcès anale	Absceso anal	Ascesso anale	Analni apsces
Anal atresia	Atrésie anale	Atresia anal	Atresia anale	Atrezija anusa
Anal bleeding	Saignement anal (rectorragie)	Pérdida de sangre a través del ano (rectorragia)	Perdita di sangue dall'ano (rettoragia, proctorragia)	Krvarenje iz analnog otvora
Anal fissure	Fissure anale	Fisura anal	Fissura anale	Analna fisura
Anal fistula	Fistule anale	Fístula anal	Fistola anale	Analna fistula
Analgesia (loss of pain sensation)	Analgésie	Analgesia	Analgesia	Analgezija (neosjetljivost na bol)
Anaphylactic shock	Choc anaphylactique	Choque anafiláctico	Anafilassi	Anafilaktični šok
Anaplastic carcinoma	Carcinome anaplastique	Carcinoma anaplásico	Carcinoma anaplastico	Anaplastični karcinom
Ancylostomiasis	Ankylostomose	Anquilostomiasis	Anchilostomiasi	Ankilostomijaza
Androblastoma (Sertoli-Leydig cell tumor)	Androblastome (tumeur à cellule de Sertoli et Leydig)	Tumor de células de Sertoli-Leydig (arrenoblastoma)	Androblastoma	Androblastom (tumor Sertoli-Leydigovih stanica)
Anemia	Anémie	Anemia	Anemia	Slabokrvnost (anemija)
Anemia of chronic disease	Anémie des maladies chroniques	Anemia de enfermedades crónicas	Anemia da malattia cronica	Anemija kronične bolesti
Anencephaly	Anencéphalie	Anencefalia	Anencefalia	Anencefalija
Aneurysm (aneurism)	Anévrisme (anévrysme)	Aneurisma	Aneurisma	Aneurizma
Aneurysm rupture	Rupture d'anévrisme	Ruptura del aneurisma	Rottura di aneurisma	Prsnuće aneurizme
Angina	Angine	Angina	Angina	Angina
Angina pectoris	Angine de poitrine (angor)	Angina de pecho (angor, angor pectoris)	Angina pectoris	Angina pektoris
Angioedema (angioneurotic edema)	Oedème de Quincke (angio-oedème)	Angioedema (edema de Quincke)	Angioedema (edema di Quincke, edema angioneurotico)	Angioedem (Quinckeov edem, angioneurotski edem)
Angioma	Angiome	Angioma	Angioma	Angiom
Angiosarcoma	Angiosarcome	Angiosarcoma	Angiosarcoma	Angiosarkom
Anisakiasis	Anisakiase	Anisakiasis (anisakidosis)	Anisakidosi	Anisakijaza
Ankle arthrosis	Arthrose de cheville	Artrosis de tobillo	Artrosi di caviglia	Artroza skočnog zgloba
Ankle distortion	Distorsion de la cheville	Distorsión del tobillo	Distorsione alla caviglia	Uganuće skočnog zgloba
Ankle impingement syndrome	Conflit antérieur de la cheville	Pinzamiento anterolateral del tobillo	Sindrome da impingement della caviglia	Prednji sindrom sraza gornjeg nožnog zgloba
Ankylosing spondylitis (Bechterew's syndrome)	Spondylarthrite ankylosante (morbus Bechterew)	Espondilitis anquilosante (morbus Bechterew)	Spondilite anchilosante	Ankilozantni spondilitis (Bechterewov sindrom)
Ankylosis (joint stiffness)	Ankylose	Anquilosis	Anchilosi	Ankiloza (ukočenje zgloba)
Anorexia	Anorexie	Anorexia	Anoressia	Anoreksija
Ant sting	Piqûre de fourmi	Picadura de hormiga	Puntura di formiche	Ugriz mrava
Anterior cruciate ligament rupture (ACL rupture)	Rupture du ligament croisé antéro-externe (rupture du LCA)	Ruptura de ligamento cruzado anterior	Rottura del legamento crociato anteriore del ginocchio	Razdor prednje ukrižene sveze koljenskog zgloba
Anthracosis	Anthracose	Antracosis	Antracosi	Antrakoza
Anthrax	Charbon	Carbunco (ántrax)	Antrace	Antraks (bedrenica, crni prišt)
Anuria (passage of urine < 100 ml in 24 hours)	Anurie (volume urinaire < 100 ml par 24 heures)	Anuria (menos de 100ml de orina en 24h)	Anuria (produzione di urina < 100 ml nelle 24 ore)	Anurija (lučenje urina < 100 ml u 24 sata)
Anxiety	Anxiété	Ansiedad	Ansia (ansietà)	Nemir (anksioznost)
Aortic aneurysm	Anévrisme de l'aorte	Aneurisma de aorta	Aneurisma aortico	Aneurizma aorte
Aortic dissection	Dissection aortique	Disección aórtica	Dissecazione aortica	Disekcija aorte
Aortic valve stenosis	Sténose valvulaire aortique	Estenosis de la válvula aórtica	Stenosi aortica	Stenoza aortnog ušća

English	French	Spanish	Italian	Croatian
Aortoiliac occlusive disease (Leriche's syndrome)	Maladie occlusive aorto-iliaque	Síndrome de Leriche	Sindrome di Leriche	Lericheov sindrom
Aphtha (mouth ulcer)	Aphte (ulcère de la muqueuse buccale)	Afta (úlcera en la mucosa oral)	Afta (ulcera all'interno della cavità orale)	Afte (ulceracija sluznice usta)
Aplasia	Aplasie	Aplasia	Aplasia	Aplazija
Aplastic anemia	Anémie aplasique	Anemia aplásica	Anemia aplastica	Aplastična anemija
Apoplexy	Apoplexie (attaque d'apoplexie)	Apoplejía (golpe apoplético)	Apoplessia	Moždano krvarenje (apopleksija)
Appetite	Appétit	Apetito	Appetito	Apetit
Appetite changes	Changements d'appétit	Cambios en el apetito	Cambiamenti nell'appetito	Promjene apetita
Aquaphobia	Aquaphobie	Acuafobia	Idrofobia	Hidrofobija
Arrhythmia	Arythmie	Arrítmia	Aritmia	Aritmija
Arrhytmogenic right ventricular dysplasia	Dysplasie ventriculair droite arythmogène	Displasia arritmogénica ventricular derecha	Displasia ventricolare destra aritmogena	Aritmogena displazija desne klijetke
Arsenic poisoning	Empoisonnement à l'arsenic	Envenenamiento por arsénico	Avvelenamento da arsenico	Trovanje arsenom
Arterial bleeding	Hémorragie artérielle	Hemorragia arterial	Emorragia arteriosa	Arterijsko krvarenje
Arterial embolism	Embolie artérielle	Embolia arterial	Embolia dell'arteria	Arterijska embolija
Arteriosclerosis	Artérosclérose	Arteriosclerosis	Arteriosclerosi	Arterioskleroza
Arthrogryposis	Arthrogrypose	Artrogriposis	Artrogriposi	Artrogripoza
Arthropathy	Arthropathie	Artropatía	Artropatia	Artropatija
Arthrosis (osteoarthritis, degenerative arthritis)	Arthrose (arthropathie chronique dégénérative)	Artrosis	Artrosi	Artroza (osteoartritis, degenerativni artritis)
Asbestos poisoning	Empoisonnement par l'amiante	Envenenamiento por asbesto	Avvelenamento da amianto	Trovanje azbestom
Asbestosis	Asbestose (amiantose)	Asbestosis	Asbestosi	Azbestoza
Ascaridosis	Ascaridiose	Ascaridiasis	Ascaridiasi	Askaridijaza
Ascites	Ascite	Ascitis	Ascite	Ascites
Aspergilloma (mycetoma, fungus ball)	Aspergillome	Aspergiloma (micetoma)	Aspergilloma (micetoma)	Aspergilom
Aspergillosis	Aspergillose	Aspergilosis	Aspergillosi	Aspergiloza
Asphyxia	Asphyxie	Asfixia	Asfissia	Asfiksija
Asthma	Asthme	Asma	Asma	Astma
Astigmatism	Astigmatisme	Astigmatismo	Astigmatismo	Astigmatizam
Astrocytoma	Astrocytome	Astrocitoma	Astrocitoma	Astrocitom
Atherosclerosis	Athérosclérose	Ateroesclerosis	Aterosclerosi	Ateroskleroza
Athetosis	Athétose	Atetosis	Atetosi	Atetoza
Athlete's foot (tinea pedis)	Pied d'athlète (tinea pedis)	Tiña del pie (pie de atleta, tinea pedis)	Piede d'atleta (tinea pedis)	Atletsko stopalo (gljivična infekcija stopala, tinea pedis)
Athlete's heart (cardiac hypertrophy)	Hypertrophie cardiaque du sportif (coeur d'athlète)	Corazón de atleta (hipertrofia del corazón del deportista)	Cuore dell'atleta (ipertrofia cardiaca da sport)	Sportsko srce
Atony (atonia)	Atonie	Atonía	Atonia muscolare	Atonija
Atopic dermatitis	Dermatite atopique	Dermatitis atópica	Neurodermite (dermatite atopica)	Atopijski dermatitis
Atrial fibrillation	Fibrillation auriculaire	Fibrilación auricular	Fibrillazione atriale	Atrijska fibrilacija
Atrial septal defect	Communication inter-auriculaire	Comunicación interauricular	Difetto del setto interatriale	Atrijski septalni defekt
Atrioventricular block (AV block)	Bloc auriculo-ventriculaire	Bloqueo auriculoventricular	Blocco atrioventricolare	Atrijskoventrikularni blok
Atrophy	Atrophie	Atrofia	Atrofia	Atrofija
Attention deficit disorder	Trouble déficit de l'attention	Trastorno por déficit de atención	Disturbo della concentrazione	Poremećaj koncentracije
Atypical pneumonia	Pneumonie atypique	Neumonía atípica	Polmonite atipica	Atipična upala pluća
Autism	Autisme	Autismo	Autismo	Autizam
Autoimmune disease	Maladie auto-immune	Enfermedad autoinmune	Malattia autoimmunitaria	Autoimunološka bolest
Aviophobia (fear of flying)	Aerophobie (peur de l'avion)	Aerofobia (miedo a volar)	Aviofobia (paura di volare)	Aerofobija (strah od letenja)
Avitaminosis	Avitaminose	Avitaminosis	Avitaminosi	Avitamonoza
Baby colic	Coliques de bébé	Cólico del recién nacido	Coliche del neonato	Novorođenačke kolike
Back pain (dorsalgia)	Mal de dos (dorsalgie)	Dolor de espalda (dorsalgia)	Mal di schiena (dorsopatia)	Bol u leđima (dorzopatija)
Bacteremia	Bactériémie	Bacteriemia (bacteremia)	Batteriemia	Bakterijemija
Bacterial conjunctivitis	Conjonctivite bactérienne	Conjuntivitis bacteriana	Congiuntivite batterica	Bakterijski konjuktivitis
Bacterial endocarditis	Endocardite bactérienne	Endocarditis bacteriana	Endocardite batterica	Bakterijski endokarditis
Bacterial infection	Infection bactérienne	Infección bacteriana	Infezione batterica	Bakterijska infekcija
Bacterial pneumonia	Pneumonie bactérienne	Neumonía bacteriana	Polmonite batterica	Bakterijska upala pluća
Bacterial vaginosis	Vaginose bactérienne	Vaginosis bacteriana	Infezione della vagina batterica (vaginosi)	Bakterijska infekcija rodnice (bakterijska vaginoza)
Bacteriuria	Bactériurie	Bacteriuria	Batteriuria	Bakteriurija
Bad breath (halitosis)	Mauvaise heleine (halitose)	Mal aliento (halitosis)	Odore sgradevole dell'alito (alitosi, bromopnea)	Zadah iz usta (halitoza)
Balance disorder	Trouble de l'équilibre	Trastorno del equilibrio	Disturbo dell'equilibrio	Poremećaj ravnoteže
Ball-shaped aneurysm of the brain artery	Anévrisme intracrânien en forme de sac	Aneurisma cerebral arterial sacular	Aneurisma cerebrale sferica	Kuglasta aneurizma arterije mozga

English	French	Spanish	Italian	Croatian
Barotrauma	Barotraumatisme	Barotraumatismo (barotrauma)	Barotrauma	Barotrauma
Bartonellosis	Bartonellose	Bartonelosis	Bartonellosi	Bartoneloza
Basal cell carcinoma	Carcinome basocellulaire	Carcinoma de células basales (basilioma)	Basalioma (carcinoma basocellulare)	Karcinom bazalnih stanica (bazaliom)
Base of skull fracture (basal skull fracture)	Fracture de la base du crâne	Fractura de la base del cráneo	Frattura della base del cranio	Prijelom baze lubanje
Basedow Graves disease	Maladie de Basedow	Enfermedad de Graves Basedow	Morbo di Basedow-Graves	Basedowljeva bolest
Basophilia	Basophilie	Basofilia	Basofilia	Bazofilija
Bedsore (decubitus ulcer)	Escarre (plaie de lit, ulcère de décubitus)	Úlcera de decúbito	Piaga da decubito (decubito)	Dekubitus
Behavioral disorder	Trouble du comportement	Trastorno del comportamiento	Disturbo dell'umore	Poremećaj ponašanja
Behçet's disease	Maladie de Behçet	Síndrome de Behçet	Sindrome di Behçet	Behçetova bolest
Bell's palsy	Paralysie de Bell	Parálisis de Bell	Paralisi di Bell	Bellova paraliza
Bell's phenomenon	Phénomène de Bell	Fenómeno de Bell	Fenomeno di Bell	Bellov fenomen
Benign positional vertigo	Vertige paroxystique positionnel bénin	Vértigo posicional paroxístico benigno	Cupololitiasi (canalolitiasi)	Benigna pozicijska vrtoglavica
Benign prostatic hyperthroph	Hypertrophie bénigne de la prostate	Hiperplasia benigna de próstata	Ipertrofia prostatica benigna	Benigna hipertrofija prostate
Benign tumor	Tumeur bénigne	Tumor benigno	Tumore benigno	Dobroćudni tumor (benigni tumor)
Bile duct atresia	Atrésie biliaire	Atresia biliar	Atresia biliare	Atrezija žučnih vodova
Biliary cirrhosis	Cirrhose biliaire	Cirrosis biliar	Cirrosi biliare	Bilijarna ciroza
Biliary colic	Colique biliaire	Cólico biliar	Colica biliare	Žučna kolika
Biot's respiration	Respiration de Biot	Respiración de Biot	Respiro di Biot	Biotovo disanje
Bipolar disorder (manic-depressive psychosis)	Trouble bipolaire (psychose maniaco-dépressive)	Trastorno bipolar (psicosis maníaco-depresiva)	Psicosi maniaco-depressiva	Bipolarni poremećaj (manično-depresivna psihoza)
Bird flu (influenza virus A subtype H5N1)	Grippe aviaire (influenzavirus A sous-type H5N1)	Gripe aviar H5N1	Influenza aviaria H5N1	Ptičja gripa podtip H5N1
Birthmark (nevus)	Grain de beauté (naevus)	Nevus (nevo)	Voglia (neo, nevo)	Madež (nevus)
Bite	Morsure	Mordedura	Morsicatura	Ugriz
Bite by rabies infected animal	Morsure d'un animal infecté par le virus de la rage	Mordedura de un animal enfermo de rabia	Morsicatura di animale rabbioso	Ugriz bijesne životinje
Bite wound	Blessure par morsure	Herida por mordedura	Ferita da morso	Ugrizna rana
Black stool (melena)	Selles noir (melanea, méléna)	Heces negras (melena)	Feci picee (melena)	Crna stolica (melena)
Black widow bite	Morsure de veuve noire	Mordedura de viuda negra	Morso della vedova nera	Ugriz crne udovice
Bladder stone (urolithiasis)	Calcul urinaire (urolithiase)	Cálculo en el tracto urinario (urolitiasis)	Calcolo urinario (urolitiasi)	Kamenac mokraćnog mjehura
Blast-syndrome	Syndrome de blast	Síndrome por explosion	Lesioni da scoppio (blast-syndrome)	Blast-sindrom
Blastoma	Blastome	Blastoma	Blastoma	Blastom
Blastomycosis	Blastomycose	Blastomicosis	Blastomicosi	Blastomikoza
Bleeding (haemorrhage)	Saignement (hémorragie)	Desangramiento (hemorragia)	Emorragia	Krvarenje (hemoragija)
Bleeding into joint space (hemarthrosis)	Épanchement de sang à l'intérieur d'une articulation (hémarthrose)	Sangrado interno de las articulaciones (hemartrosis)	Emartro	Krvarenje u zglob (hemartroza)
Bleeding into the fallopian tube (hematosalpinx)	Collection de sang dans la trompe de Fallope (hématosalpinx)	Colección de sangre en la trompa de Falopio (hematosalpinx)	Flusso di sangue nella tuba di Falloppio	Krvarenje u jajovod (hematosalpinks)
Blepharitis	Blépharite	Blefaritis	Blefarite	Blefaritis
Blindness	Cécité	Ceguera	Cecità	Sljepoća
Blister	Phlyctène (ampoule, cloque)	Ampolla	Vescichetta (bolla)	Plik
Blister (corn)	Cor (cal)	Ampolla (callo)	Callo (vescica, bolla)	Žulj (plik, kurje oko)
Bloating and gases (flatulence)	Ballonnements et vesse (flatulence)	Hinchazón y gases (flatulencia, ventosidad)	Gonfiezza e venti (flatulenza)	Nadutost i vjetrovi
Blood clot (thrombus)	Caillot sanguin (thrombus)	Coágulo sanguíneo (trombo)	Trombo	Krvni ugrušak (tromb)
Blood in cerebrospinal fluid	Sang dans le liquide cérébro-spinal	Sangre en el líquido cefalorraquídeo	Sangue al liquido cerebrospinale	Krv u likvoru
Blood in sputum (hemoptysis)	Sang dans l'expectoration (hémoptysie)	Sangre en el esputo (hemoptisis)	Sangue nello sputo (emottisi)	Krvavi iskašljaj (hemoptiza)
Blood in stool (hematochezia)	Sang dans les selles (hématochézie)	Sangre en las heces (hematochezia)	Sangue nelle feci (ematochezia)	Krv u stolici (hematohezija)
Blood in urine (hematuria)	Sang dans les urines (hématurie)	Sangre en la orina (hematuria)	Ematuria	Krv u urinu (hematurija)
Blood pressure fall	Pression artérielle effondrée	Caída de la presión arterial	Abbassamento della pressione del sangue	Pad krvnog tlaka
Blood vessel diseases	Maladies des vaisseaux sanguins	Enfermedades de los vasos sanguíneos	Malattie dei vasi sanguigni	Bolesti krvnih žila

English	French	Spanish	Italian	Croatian
Blount's disease	Maladie de Blount	Enfermedad de Blount (tibia vara)	Síndrome di Blount	Blountova bolest
Bone bending (bone torsion)	Torsion osseuse	Torsión del hueso	Torsione dell'osso	Savijanje kosti
Bone tuberculosis	Tuberculose des os	Tuberculosis ósea	Tubercolosi delle ossa	Tuberkuloza kosti
Borderline personality disorder	Personnalité borderline	Trastorno límite de la personalidad	Disturbo borderline di personalità	Granični poremećaj osobnosti
Bornholm disease (epidemic myalgia)	Maladie de Bornholm (myalgie épidémique)	Enfermedad de Bornholm (mialgía epidémica)	Malattia di Bornholm (mialgia epidemica)	Bornholmska bolest (epidemijska mialgija)
Borreliosis	Borréliose	Borreliosis	Borreliosi	Borelioza
Botryoid sarcoma	Sarcome botryoïde	Sarcoma botrioide	Sarcoma botrioide	Botrioidni sarkom
Botulism	Botulisme	Botulismo	Botulismo	Botulizam
Bouchard's nodes	Nodules de Bouchard	Nudosidades de Bouchard	Noduli di Bouchard	Bouchardovi čvorići
Bow legs (genu varum)	Genu varum	Genu varum	Ginocchio varo (genu varum)	Genu varum
Bowen's disease (squamous cell carcinoma in situ)	Maladie de Bowen	Enfermedad de Bowen	Morbo di Bowen	Bowenova bolest
Brachial syndrome	Brachialgie	Síndrome braquial	Brachialgia	Brahijalni sindrom bolne nadlaktice
Brain abscess	Abcès cérébral	Absceso cerebral	Ascesso cerebrale	Apsces mozga
Brain compression	Compression cérébrale	Compresión cerebral	Compressione cerebrale	Kompresija mozga
Brain concussion	Commotion cérébrale	Conmoción cerebral	Commozione cerebrale	Potres mozga
Brain development anomaly	Anomalie du développement cérébral	Malformación del desarrollo cerebral	Anomalia di sviluppo del sistema nervoso	Anomalija u razvoju mozga
Brain laceration	Lacération cérébrale	Laceración cerebral	Lacerazione cerebrale	Laceracija mozga
Breast cancer	Cancer du sein	Cáncer de mama	Cancro della mammella	Rak dojke
Breast carcinoma	Carcinome du sein	Carcinoma de mama	Carcinoma mammario	Karcinom dojke
Breast pain (mastalgia)	Douleur au sein (mastodynie)	Dolor en la mama (mastalgia)	Dolore al seno (mastalgia)	Bol u dojci (mastalgija)
Breathing difficulty	Difficulté de respiration	Dificultad de respiración	Respirazione difficoltosa	Otežano disanje
Breathing sound due to blockage in the airway (stridor)	Bruit anormal émis lors de la respiration (stridor)	Estridor	Rumore durante la respirazione (stridore)	Glasno otežano disanje (stridor)
Brenner tumour	Tumeur de Brenner	Tumor de Brenner	Tumore di Brenner	Brennerov tumor
Brill's disease	Maladie de Brill-Zinserr (typhus résurgent)	Enfermedad de Brill	Malattia di Brill-Zinsser	Brillova bolest (Brill-Zinsserova bolest)
Brodie abscess	Abcès de Brodie	Absceso de Brodie	Ascesso di Brodie	Brodijev apsces
Broken ankle (ankle fracture)	Fracture de la cheville	Fractura de tobillo	Frattura della caviglia	Prijelom gležnja
Broken big toe (fractured hallux)	Fracture du gros orteil	Fractura de los huesos del dedo gordo del pie	Frattura dell'alluce	Prijelom falange nožnog palca
Broken bone (bone fracture)	Fracture des os	Fractura de hueso	Frattura	Prijelom kosti (fraktura kosti)
Broken collar bone (clavicle fracture)	Fracture de la clavicule	Fractura de clavícula	Frattura della clavicola	Prijelom ključne kosti
Broken elbow (olecranon fracture)	Fracture de l'olécrâne	Fractura de olécranon	Frattura dell'olecrano	Prijelom lakatnog vrha (prijelom olekranona)
Broken fibula (fibula fracture)	Fracture de la fibula	Fractura del peroné	Frattura della fibula	Prijelom lisne kosti
Broken finger (finger fracture)	Fracture du doigt	Fractura de falange del dedo	Frattura della falange del dito	Prijelom članka prsta
Broken foot (metatarsal fracture)	Fracture métatarsienne	Fractura de metatarso	Frattura del metatarso	Prijelom kosti stopala
Broken forearm (fractured ulna and radius)	Fracture du radius et du cubitus	Fractura de radio y cúbito	Frattura di radio e ulna	Prijelom obje podlaktične kosti
Broken heel bone (calcaneus fracture)	Fracture du calcanéus	Fractura del calcáneo	Frattura del calcagno	Prijelom petne kosti
Broken knee cap (patellar fracture)	Fracture de rotule	Fractura de la rótula	Frattura della rotula	Prijelom ivera (prijelom patele)
Broken lower leg bones (fractured tibia and fibula)	Fracture du tibia et de la fibula	Fractura de tibia y peroné	Frattura di tibia e perone	Prijelom obje kosti potkoljenice
Broken navicular bone (navicular fracture)	Fracture du scaphoïde	Fractura de escafoides (fractura navicular)	Frattura dell'osso navicolare	Prijelom navikularne kosti
Broken pelvis (pelvis fracture)	Fracture du bassin	Fractura de pelvis	Frattura del bacino	Prijelom zdjelice
Broken rib (rib fracture)	Fracture de côte	Fractura de costilla	Frattura della costola	Prijelom rebra
Broken shinbone (tibia fracture)	Fracture du tibia	Fractura de tibia	Frattura della tibia	Prijelom goljenične kosti
Broken shoulder blade (scapula fracture)	Fracture de la scapula	Fractura de escápula	Frattura della scapola	Prijelom lopatice
Broken thighbone (femur fracture)	Fracture du fémur	Fractura de fémur	Frattura del femore	Prijelom bedrene kosti
Broken ulna (ulna fracture)	Fracture de l'ulna	Fractura de cúbito	Frattura dell'ulna	Prijelom lakatne kosti

English	French	Spanish	Italian	Croatian
Broken upper arm (humerus fracture)	Fracture de l'humérus	Fractura del húmero	Frattura dell'omero	Prijelom nadlaktice
Broken vertebral body (vertebral corpus fracture)	Fracture du plateau vertébral	Fractura de cuerpo vertebral	Frattura del corpo vertebrale	Prijelom trupa kralješka
Bronchial carcinoid	Carcinoïde bronchiale	Carcinoide bronquial	Carcinoide bronchiale	Karcinoid bronha
Bronchial carcinoma	Carcinome bronchique	Carcinoma bronquial	Carcinoma bronchiale	Karcinom bronha
Bronchiectasis	Bronchectasie (dilatation des bronches)	Bronquiectasia	Bronchiectasia	Bronhiektazije
Bronchopleural fistula	Fistule bronchopleurale	Fístula bronco-pleural	Fistola broncopleurica	Bronhopleuralna fistula
Bronchopneumonia	Bronchopneumonie	Neumonía bronquial	Broncopolmonite	Bronhopneumonija
Bronchospasm	Bronchospasme	Broncoespasmo	Broncospasmo	Bronhospazam
Brown urine	Urine marron	Orina de color marrón	Urina marrone	Smeđi urin
Brucellosis	Brucellose (fièvre de Malte, fièvre méditerranéenne)	Brucelosis	Brucellosi	Bruceloza (malteška ili sredozemna groznica, Bangova bolest)
Bruise (ecchymosis)	Ecchymose	Moretón (equimosis)	Ammaccatura (ecchimosi)	Modrica (ekhimoza)
Buerger's disease (thromboangiitis obliterans)	Maladie de Buerger (thromboangéite oblitérante)	Enfermedad de Buerger (tromboangeítis obliterante)	Morbo di Buerger	Buergerova bolest
Bulging eyes (exophthalmos)	Exophtalmie (proptose)	Exoftalmos	Esoftalmo	Izbuljene oči (egzoftalmus)
Bulimia	Boulimie	Bulimia	Bulimia	Bulimija
Bundle branch block	Bloc de branche	Bloqueo de rama	Blocco di branca	Blok grane Hisovog snopića
Bunion	Hallux valgus	Bunión (hallux valgus)	Alluce valgo	Čukalj
Burn	Brûlure	Quemadura	Ustione	Opeklina
Burning sensation	Sensation cuisante	Sensación de ardor	Sensazione bruciante	Pečenje (žarenje)
Burping (belching)	Rot (renvoi, éructation)	Eructo	Eruttazione	Podrigivanje
Byssinosis (Monday fever)	Byssinose	Bisinosis (fiebre del lunes)	Bissinosi	Bisinoza
Cachexia	Cachexie	Caquexia	Cachessia	Kaheksija
Cadmium poisoning	Empoisonnement au cadmium	Envenenamiento por cadmio	Avvelenamento da cadmio	Trovanje kadmijem
Calcification	Calcification	Calcificación	Calcificazione	Ovapnjenje (kalcifikacija)
Callosity (thickening)	Callosité	Callosidad (callo)	Callosità (callo)	Zadebljanje kože
Candidiasis (thrush)	Candidiase	Candidiasis	Candidosi (candidiasi)	Kandidijaza
Capillary hemangioma (infantile hemangioma, strawberry hemangioma)	Hémangiome capillaire	Hemangioma capilar (marca de fresa)	Emangioma capillare	Kapilarni hemangiom
Carbon monoxide poisoning	Empoisonnement au monoxyde de carbone	Intoxicación por monóxido de carbono	Avvelenamento da monossido di carbonio	Trovanje ugljičnim monoksidom
Carbuncle	Anthrax	Ántrax (carbunco)	Carbonchio (pustola)	Karbunkul
Carcinoid	Carcinoïde	Carcinoide	Carcinoide	Karcinoid
Carcinoid syndrome	Syndrome carcinoïde	Síndrome carcinoide	Sindrome da carcinoide	Karcinoidni sindrom
Carcinoma	Carcinome	Carcinoma	Carcinoma	Karcinom
Carcinosis	Carcinose	Carcinosis	Carcinosi (carcinomatosi, cancerosi)	Karcinoza
Cardiac arrest (cardiopulmonary arrest)	Arrêt cardiaque (arrêt ventilatoire, arrêt cardio-respiratoire)	Paro cardiaco (parada cardiorrespiratoria)	Arresto cardiaco	Zastoj srca (srčani arest)
Cardiac arrhythmia	Arythmie cardiaque	Arrítmia cardíaca	Aritmia cardiaca	Srčana aritmija
Cardiac asthma (paroxysmal nocturnal dyspnea)	Dyspnée chez un cardiaque	Disnea paroxística nocturna	Dispnea parossistica notturna	Srčana astma (paroksizmalna dispneja)
Cardiac decompensation	Décompensation cardiaque	Descompensación cardíaca	Decompensazione cardiaca	Srčana dekompenzacija
Cardiogenic shock	Choc cardiogénique	Choque cardiogénico	Shock cardiogeno	Kardiogeni šok
Cardiomyopathy	Cardiomyopathie	Miocardiopatía	Cardiomiopatia	Kardiomiopatija
Cardiotoxicity	Cardiotoxicité	Cardiotoxicidad	Cardiomiopatia tossica	Toksična kardiomiopatija
Carpal tunnel syndrome	Syndrome du canal carpien	Síndrome del túnel carpiano	Sindrome del tunnel carpale	Sindrom karpalnog tunela
Cat bite	Morsure de chat	Mordedura de gato	Morsicatura di gatto	Ugriz mačke
Cat cry syndrome (5p minus syndrome, Lejeune's syndrome)	Maladie du cri du chat (syndrome de Lejeune)	Síndrome del maullido del gato (síndrome de Lejeune)	Sindrome del grido di gatto	Sindrom mačjeg krika
Catalepsy	Catalepsie	Catalepsia	Catalessia	Katalepsija
Cataplexy	Cataplexie	Cataplexia (cataplejía)	Cataplessia	Katapleksija
Cataract	Cataracte	Catarata	Cataratta	Mrena (katarakta)
Catarrh	Catarrhe	Catarro	Catarro	Katar
Cavernous hemangioma	Cavernome (angiome caverneux)	Hemangioma cavernoso	Emangioma cavernoso	Kavernozni hemangiom
Cellulitis	Cellulite	Celulitis	Cellulite	Celulitis
Cephalocele	Céphalocèle	Cefalocele	Cefalocèle	Cefalokela
Cercaria	Cercaire	Cercaria	Cercaria	Cerkarija
Cerebral aneurysm	Anévrisme intra-crânien	Aneurisma cerebral	Aneurisma cerebrale	Cerebralna aneurizma
Cerebral contusion	Contusion cérébrale	Contusión cerebral	Contusione cerebrale	Nagnječenje mozga
Cerebral edema	Oedème cérébral	Edema cerebral	Edema cerebrale	Edem mozga
Cerebral palsy	Infirmité motorice cérébrale	Parálisis cerebral	Paralisi cerebrale infantile	Cerebralna paraliza
Cerebrovascular anomaly	Anomalie cérébrovasculaire	Malformación arteriovenosa cerebral	Anomalia cerebrovascolare	Anomalija moždanih krvnih žila

English	French	Spanish	Italian	Croatian
Cervical cancer	Cancer du col utérin	Cáncer del cuello uterino (cáncer cervical)	Cancro della cervice uterina	Rak grlića maternice
Cervical carcinoma	Carcinome du col utérin	Carcinoma del cuello uterino	Carcinoma della cervice uterina	Karcinom grlića maternice
Cervical dysplasia	Dysplasie du col de l'utérus	Displasia del cuello uterino	Displasia cervicale	Cervikalna displazija
Cervical erosion	Érosion du col de l'utérus	Erosión cervical	Erosione cervicale	Cervikalna erozija
Cervical polyp	Polype au col de l'utérus	Pólipo cervical	Polipo cervicale	Polip na grliću maternice
Cervical rib	Côte cervicale	Costilla cervical	Costa cervicale	Vratno rebro
Cervicobrachial syndrome	Syndrome cervico-brachial	Síndrome cérvico-braquial	Sindrome cervico-brachiale (sindrome spalla-mano)	Sindrom vrat-rame (cervikobrahijalni sindrom)
Cervicocephal syndrome	Syndrome cervical	Síndrome cervical	Sindrome cervicale	Cervikocefalni sindrom
Chagas disease (American trypanosomiasis)	Maladie de Chagas (trypanosomiase américaine)	Enfermedad de Chagas (tripanosomiasis americana)	Malattia di Chagas	Chagasova bolest (americka tripanosomijaza)
Chalicosis	Chalicose	Calicosis	Calicosi	Kalikoza
Chancre	Chancre	Chancro	Sifiloma	Čankir
Chancroid (soft chancre)	Chancre mou (chancrelle)	Chancroide (chancro blando)	Ulcera venerea (cancroide)	Meki čankir
Changes in consciousness	Changements de conscience	Cambios en la conciencia	Alterazione della conoscenza	Promjene stanja svijesti
Changes in moles	Changements dans les grains de beauté	Cambios en los lunares	Cambiamenti di nevi	Promjene na madežima
Changes in mucous membrane	Changement de la muqueuse	Cambios en la membrana mucosa	Cambiamenti della mucosa	Promjene na sluznici
Changes in olfactory sensation	Changements des sensations olfactives	Cambios en la sensibilidad olfatoria	Cambiamenti delle sensazoni olfattive	Promjene osjeta mirisa
Changes in shape of bones	Changements dans la forme des os	Cambios en la forma de los huesos	Cambiamenti nella forma delle ossa	Promjene oblika kosti
Changes in tactile sensation	Changements des sensations tactiles	Cambios en la sensibilidad táctil	Cambiamenti della sensazione tattile	Promjene osjeta dodira
Changes in taste sensation	Changements de sensation de goût	Cambios en la sensación de sabores	Cambiamenti nelle sensazioni del gusto	Promjene osjeta okusa
Charcot-Marie-Tooth disease	Maladie de Charcot-Marie-Tooth	Enfermedad de Charcot-Marie Tooth	Malattia di Charcot-Marie-Tooth	Bolest Charcot-Marie-Tooth
Chemical conjunctivitis	Conjonctivite chimique	Conjuntivitis química	Congiuntivite irritativa da agenti chimici	Kemijski konjuktivitis
Chemical injuries	Altération d'origine chimique	Lesiones químicas	Ferita chimica	Kemijske ozljede
Chemical warfare poisoning	Intoxcation par arme chimique	Intoxicación por armas químicas	Avvelenamento da armi chimiche	Trovanje kemijskim oružjem
Chest pain	Douleur thoracique	Dolor torácico	Dolore toracico	Bol u prsištu
Chicken-pox	Varicelle	Varicela	Varicella	Vodene kozice (varičela)
Chikungunya	Chikungunya	Chikungunya	Chikungunya	Chikungunya virusna bolest
Chilblain (perniosis)	Engelure	Sabañón	Perniosi	Smrzotina
Childhood infectious diseases	Maladies infectieuses des enfants	Enfermedades infantiles contagiosas	Malattie infettive dei bambini	Dječje zarazne bolesti
Chlamydia infection	Infection à Chlamydia	Infección por clamidia	Infezione da clamidia	Klamidijska infekcija
Choking (suffocation)	Suffocation	Atragantamiento	Soffocamento (soffocazione, asfissia)	Gušenje
Cholangiocellular carcinoma	Cholangiocarcinome	Carcinoma de las vías biliares (colangiocarcinoma)	Colangiocarcinoma (carcinoma colangiocellulare)	Kolangiocelularni karcinom
Cholera	Choléra	Cólera	Colera	Kolera
Chondroblastoma	Chondroblastome	Condroblastoma	Condroblastoma	Hondroblastom
Chondroma	Chondrome	Condroma	Condroma	Hondrom
Chondromalacia patellae (runner's knee, patello-femoral pain syndrome)	Chondromalacie rotulienne	Chondromalacia rotuliana (síndrome patelo-femoral)	Sindrome del dolore patello-femorale (ginocchio del corridore)	Hondromalacija patele (trkačko koljeno, sindrom patelofemoralne boli)
Chondromyxoid fibroma	Fibrome chondromyxoïde	Fibroma condromixoide	Fibroma condromixoide	Hondromiksoidni fibrom
Chondrosarcoma	Chondrosarcome	Condrosarcoma	Condrosarcoma	Hondrosarkom
Choreoathetosis	Choréoathétose	Coreoatetosis	Coreoatetosi	Koreoatetoza
Choriocarcinoma	Choriocarcinome	Coriocarcinoma	Coriocarcinoma	Koriokarcinom
Chromoblastomycosis (chromomycosis, Pedroso's disease)	Chromomycose	Cromomicosis (cromoblastomicosis)	Cromomicosi (cromoblastomicosi)	Kromomikoza
Chronic cerebrospinal venous insufficiency	Insuffisance veineuse cérébro-spinale chronique	Insuficiencia venosa cerebro-espinal crónica	Insufficienza venosa cronica cerebrospinale	Kronična cerebrospinalna venozna insuficijencija
Chronic fatigue syndrome	Syndrome de fatigue chronique	Síndrome de fatiga crónica	Sindrome da fatica cronica	Sindrom kroničnog umora
Chronic lymphocytic leukemia	Leucémie lymphoïde chronique	Leucemia linfocítica crónica	Leucemia linfatica cronica	Kronična limfocitna leukemija
Chronic myeloid leukemia	Leucémie myéloïde chronique	Leucemia mieloide crónica	Leucemia mieloide cronica	Kronična mijeloična leukemija
Chronic obstructive pulmonary disease	Bronchopneumopathie chronique obstructive	Enfermedad pulmonar obstructiva crónica	Bronchite cronica	Kronična opstruktivna plućna bolest
Chronic pain	Douleur chronique	Dolor crónico	Dolore cronico	Kronična bol

English	French	Spanish	Italian	Croatian
Chronic paroxysmal hemicrania (Sjaastad syndrome)	Hémicrânie paroxystique chronique	Hemicránea crónica paroxismal	Emicrania cronica parossistica	Kronična paroksizmalna hemikranija (Sjaastadov sindrom)
Chronic renal failure	Insuffisance rénale chronique	Insuficiencia renal crónica	Insufficienza renale cronica	Kronično zatajenje bubrega
Chylothorax	Chylothorax	Quilotórax	Chilotorace	Hilotoraks
Claustrophobia (fear of closed space)	Claustrophobie	Claustrofobia (miedo a los espacios cerrados)	Claustrofobia (paura di luoghi chiusi)	Klaustrofobija (strah od zatvorenog prostora)
Cleft lip and palate	Fente labiale et fente palatine	Labio leporino (fisura labial)	Labbro leporino	Rascjep usne i nepca
Clonorchiasis	Clonorchiase	Clonorquiasis (clonorquiosis)	Clonorchiasi	Klonorkijaza
Clostridium perfringens toxic infection	Toxi-infection à Clostridium perfringens	Tóxico-infección por Clostridium perfringens	Tossinfezione da Clostridium perfringens	Toksična infekcija Clostridium perfringensom
Club foot (talipes equinovarus)	Pied-bot (pied-bot équin)	Pie equinovaro (talipes equinovarus, pie bot, pie retorcido)	Piede equino (talipes equinovarus)	Čopavo stopalo (uvrnuto stopalo, pes equinovarus)
Cluster headache	Algie vasculaire de la face	Cefalea en racimos	Cefalea a grappolo	Cluster glavobolja
Coagulation factor deficiency	Déficit en facteur de la coagulation	Deficiencia de factor de coagulación	Carenza di fattore di coagulazione	Manjak faktora koagulacije
Coarctation of the aorta	Coarctation de l'aorte	Coartación de la aorta	Coartazione dell'aorta	Koarktacija aorte
Coccidioidomycosis (San Joaquin Valley fever)	Coccidioïmycose (fièvre de la vallée de San Joaquin, fièvre du désert)	Coccidioidomicosis	Coccidiomicosi	Kokcidioidomikoza (San Joaquin Valley vrućica)
Coccygodynia	Coccygodynie (douleur coccygienne)	Coccigodinia (dolor de coxis)	Coccigodinia	Kokcigodinija
Coeliac disease (celiac disease)	Maladie coeliaque	Celiaquía (enfermedad celíaca)	Celiachia (malattia caliacha)	Celijakija
Colic	Colique	Cólico	Colica	Kolika
Collapse	Collapsus	Colapso	Collasso	Kolaps
Colon diverticulum	Diverticule du côlon	Divertículo del colon	Diverticolo del colon	Divertikul na debelom crijevu
Colon polyp	Polype du côlon	Pólipo de colon	Polipo del colon	Polip na debelom crijevu
Colorado tick fever (mountain tick fever)	Fièvre à tiques du Colorado (fièvre à tiques des montagnes)	Fiebre del Colorado por garrapatas (fiebre de montaña americana por garrapatas)	Febbre da zecca del Colorado	Groznica planinskog krpelja
Coma	Coma	Coma	Coma	Koma
Comminuted fracture	Fracture comminutive	Fractura cominuta	Frattura comminuta	Kominutivni prijelom kosti
Common cold	Rhume	Resfriado común (resfrío)	Infreddatura (raffreddore)	Prehlada (hunjavica)
Compartment syndrome	Syndrome des loges	Síndrome compartimental	Sindrome compartimentale	Sindrom fascijalnog prostora
Confusion	Confusion	Confusión	Confusione (disordine)	Smetenost
Congenital aneurysm of arteries at the base of the brain	Anévrisme congénital de l'artère à la base du cerveau	Aneurisma congénito arterial de la base del cerebro	Aneurisma arteriosa congenita alla base dell'encefalo	Urođena aneurizma arterija baze mozga
Congenital dysplasia of the hip (congenital hip dislocation)	Luxation congénitale de la hanche	Displasia congénita de la cadera (luxación congénita de cadera)	Lussazione congenita dell'anca (displasia dell'anca)	Urođeno iščašenje kuka (kongenitalna displazija kuka)
Congenital heart defect	Malformation congénitale du coeur	Malformación cardiaca congénita	Difetto cardiaco congenito	Urođena srčana greška
Congenital heart disease (congenital cardiopathy)	Cardiopathie congénitale	Cardiopatía congénita	Cardiopatia congenita	Urođena srčana bolest (kongenitalna kardiopatija)
Congenital pyloric stenosis	Sténose congénitale du pylore	Estenosis congénita del píloro	Stenosi pilorica congenita	Urođena stenoza pilorusa
Conjunctival foreign body	Conjonctivite due à un corps étranger	Conjuntivitis por cuerpo extraño	Congiuntivite irritativa da corpi estranei	Konjuktivitis izazvan stranim tijelom
Constipation (obstipation)	Constipation	Estreñimiento	Stitichezza (costipazione)	Zatvor (opstipacija)
Contact dermatitis	Dermite de contact	Dermatitis de contacto	Dermatite da contatto	Kontaktni dermatitis
Contracture	Contracture	Contractura	Contrattura	Kontraktura
Contusion	Contusion	Contusión	Contusione	Nagnječenje (zgnječenje, kontuzija)
Convulsions	Convulsions	Convulsiones	Convulsioni	Konvulzije
Coronary disease	Maladie coronarienne	Enfermedad coronaria	Coronaropatia	Koronarna bolest (koronaropatija)
Cough	Toux	Tos	Tosse	Kašalj
Cradle cap (infantile seborrhoeic dermatitis)	Dermite séborrhéique infantile	Dermatitis seborreica infantil	Dermatite seborroica infantile	Tjemenica (dojenačka seboreja)
Cranial neuralgia	Névralgie des nerfs crâniens	Neuralgia craneal	Nevralgia del nervo cranico	Neuralgija moždanih živaca
Crepitation	Crépitation	Crepitación	Crepitazione	Krepitacija

English	French	Spanish	Italian	Croatian
Creutzfeldt-Jakob disease (so called "mad cow disease")	Maladie de Creutzfeldt-Jakob	Enfermedad de Creutzfeldt-Jakob	Malattia di Creutzfeldt-Jakob (cosiddetta "malattia della mucca pazza")	Creutzfeldt-Jakobova bolest (tzv. "kravlje ludilo")
Crimean-Congo hemorrhagic fever	Fièvre hémorragique de Congo-Crimée	Fiebre hemorrágica de Crimea-Congo	Febbre emorragica Crimean-Congo	Krimska hemoragijska groznica
Crohn's disease	Maladie de Crohn	Enfermedad de Crohn	Malattia di Crohn	Crohnova bolest
Crotch itch (tinea cruris)	Eczéma marginé de hebra	Tiña crural (tinea cruris)	Tinea cruris	Gljivična infekcija prepona (tinea cruris)
Croup (acute obstructive laryngitis)	Croup (laryngotrachéo-bronchite)	Crup (laringotraqueo-bronquitis)	Croup (laringite acuta ostruttiva)	Krup (akutni opstruktivni laringitis)
Crush-syndrome	Syndrome d'écrasement	Síndrome de aplastamiento (síndrome de crush)	Sindrome da schiacciamento	Crush-sindrom
Crust (scab)	Croûte	Costra	Crosta (escara)	Krasta
Cryptococcosis	Cryptococcose	Criptococcosis	Criptococcosi	Kriptokokoza
Cryptogenic cirrhosis	Cirrhose cryptogénique	Cirrosis criptogénica	Cirrosi criptogenica	Kriptogena ciroza
Cryptorchidism	Cryptorchidie	Criptorquidismo	Criptorchidismo	Retencija testisa (kriptorhizam)
Cushing's syndrome (hypercorticism)	Syndrome de Cushing (hypercorticisme)	Síndrome de Cushing (hipercortisolismo)	Sindrome di Cushing (ipercortisolismo)	Cushingov sindrom (hiperkortikolizam)
Cut wound	Plaie par objet tranchant	Herida por corte	Ferita da taglio	Rezna rana (posjekotina)
Cutaneous leishmaniasis (Oriental sore)	Leishmaniose cutanée (bouton d'Orient)	Leishmaniasis cutánea (uta)	Leishmaniosi cutanea	Orijentalni ulkus (kožna lišmenijaza)
Cyanide poisoning	Empoisonnement au cyanure	Envenenamiento por cianuro	Avvelenamento da cianuro	Trovanje cijanidom
Cyanosis	Cyanose	Cianosis	Cianosi	Cijanoza
Cyst	Kyste	Quiste	Cisti (ciste)	Cista
Cystadenocarcinoma	Cystadénocarcinome	Cistadenocarcinoma	Cistadenocarcinoma	Cistadenokarcinom
Cystadenofibroma	Cystadénofibrome	Cistadenofibroma	Cistadenofibroma	Cistadenofibrom
Cystadenoma	Cystadénome	Cistadenoma	Cistadenoma	Cistadenom
Cystic fibrosis	Mucoviscidose (fibrose kystique)	Fibrosis quística (mucoviscidosis)	Fibrosi cistica	Cistična fibroza
Cysticercosis	Cysticercose	Cisticercosis	Cisticercosi	Cisticerkoza
Cystoma	Kystome	Cistoma	Cistoma	Cistom
Daltonism	Daltonisme	Daltonismo	Daltonismo	Daltonizam
Dancer's foot (pes equinus)	Pied equin	Pie equino	Piede equino	Balerinsko stopalo (pes equinus)
Dancer's tendinitis (flexor hallucis tendinitis)	Tendinite des danseurs (fléchisseur de l'hallux tendinite)	Tendinitis del flexor hallucis longus	Tendinite del flessore lungo dell'alluce	Tendinitis plesača (tendinitis dugog pregibača palca)
Dandruff	Pellicule	Caspa	Forfora	Perut
Day blindness (hemeralopia)	Héméralopie	Falta de visión en luz brillante (hemeralopia)	Emeralopia	Kokošje sljepilo (hemeralopija)
Deafness	Surdité	Sordera	Sordità	Gluhoća
Death	Mort	Muerte	Morte	Smrt
Decompression sickness (diver's disease, caisson disease)	Maladie de décompression (maladie des plongeurs, maladie des caissons)	Síndrome de decompresión (enfermedad de los buzos, mal de presión)	Malattia di decompressione (sindrome di Caisson)	Dekompresijska bolest (kesonska bolest)
Decreased body temperature (hypothermia)	Température corporelle basse (hypothermie)	Temperatura corporal baja (hipotermía)	Bassa temperatura corporea (ipotermia)	Snižena temperatura tijela (hipotermija)
Decreased production of urine (oliguria)	Raréfaction du volume des urines (oligurie)	Disminución de producción de orina (oliguria)	Diminuita escrezione urinaria (oliguria)	Smanjeno izlučivanje urina (oligurija)
Dehydration	Déshydratation	Deshidratación	Disidratazione	Dehidracija
Delayed puberty	Puberté tardive	Retraso de la pubertad	Pubertà tardiva	Zakašnjeli pubertet
Delirium	Delirium	Delirio	Delirio	Delirij
Dementia	Démence	Demencia	Demenza	Demencija
Demineralization	Déminéralisation	Desmineralización	Demineralizzazione	Demineralizacija
Dengue fever	Dengue (grippe tropicale, dengue hémorragique)	Dengue	Dengue	Dengue groznica
Dental caries	Carie dentaire	Caries	Carie dentaria	Zubni karijes
Dental plaque (dental tartar)	Plaque dentaire	Placa dental	Placca (tartaro)	Zubni kamenac
Depression	Dépression	Depresión	Depressione	Depresija
DeQuervain syndrome	Syndrome de DeQuervain (ténosynovite de DeQuervain)	Síndrome de DeQuervain	Sindrome di De Quervain	Sindrom bubnjarskog palca (Morbus DeQuervain)
Dermatitis herpetiformis (Duhring's disease)	Dermatite herpétiforme	Dermatitis herpetiforme (enfermedad de Duhring)	Dermatite erpetiforme di Duhring	Duhringova bolest (dermatitis herpetiformis)
Dermatomycosis	Dermatomycose	Dermatomicosis	Dermatomicosi	Dermatomikoza
Dermatomyositis	Dermatomyosite	Dermatomiositis	Dermatomiosite	Dermatomiozitis
Dermoid cyst	Kyste dermoïde	Quiste dermoide	Cisti dermoide	Dermoidna cista
Development anomalies	Anomalies de développement	Anomalías del desarrollo	Anomalie di sviluppo	Razvojne anomalije
Diabetes	Diabète	Diabetes	Diabete	Dijabetes
Diabetes insipidus	Diabète insipide	Diabetes insípida	Diabete insipido	Dijabetes insipidus

English	French	Spanish	Italian	Croatian
Diabetes mellitus	Diabète sucré	Diabetes mellitus (diabetes sacarina)	Diabete mellito	Dijabetes melitus
Diabetes mellitus type 1	Diabète sucré de type 1 (diabète insulino-dépendant)	Diabetes mellitus tipo 1	Diabete mellito di tipo 1	Dijabetes melitus tip 1
Diabetes mellitus type 2	Diabète sucré de type 2 (diabète insulinorésistant)	Diabetes mellitus tipo 2	Diabete mellito di tipo 2	Dijabetes melitus tip 2
Diabetic coma	Coma diabétique	Coma diabético	Coma diabetico	Dijabetična koma
Diabetic ketoacidosis	Cétoacidose diabétique	Cetoacidosis diabética	Chetoacidosi diabetica	Dijabetična ketoacidoza
Diabetic nephropathy	Néphropathie diabétique	Nefropatía diabética	Nefropatia diabetica	Dijabetična nefropatija
Diabetic neuropathy	Neuropathie diabétique	Neuropatía diabética	Neuropatia diabetica	Dijabetična neuropatija
Diabetic retinopathy	Rétinopathie diabétique	Retinopatía diabética	Retinopatia diabetica	Dijabetična retinopatija
Diaphragmatic hernia	Hernie diaphragmatique	Hernia diafragmática	Ernia diaframmatica	Dijafragmalna kila
Diaphyseal humeral fracture	Fracture diaphysaire de l'humérus	Fractura diafisaria del húmero	Frattura diafisaria dell'omero	Prijelom nadlaktice u području dijafize
Diaphyseal tightbone fracture	Fracture de la diaphyse fémorale	Fractura de la diáfisis del fémur	Frattura della diafisi femorale	Prijelom dijafize bedrene kosti
Diarrhea	Diarrhée	Diarrea	Diarrea	Proljev (dijarea)
Difficult defecation (tenesmus)	Difficulté à déféquer (ténesme)	Dificultad para la defecación (tenesmo rectal)	Difficoltà a defecare (tenesmo)	Otežano pražnjenje crijeva (otežana defekacija)
Difficult urination (dysuria)	Difficulté à uriner (dysurie)	Dificultad al orinar (disuria)	Emissione di urine con difficoltà (disuria)	Otežano usporeno mokrenje (dizurija)
Difficult swallowing (dysphagia)	Difficulté de deglutition (dysphagie)	Dificultad para tragar (disfagia)	Difficoltà a deglutire (disfagia)	Otežano gutanje (disfagija)
Dilated cardiomyopathy	Cardiomyopathie dilatée	Miocardiopatía dilatada	Cardiomiopatia dilatativa	Dilatacijska kardiomiopatija
Diphtheria	Diphtérie	Difteria	Difterite	Difterija
Discarthrosis (degenerative disc disease)	Arthrose du disque intervertébral	Discartrosis	Discartrosi (discopatia degenerativa)	Diskartroza
Discharge	Sécrétion (suintement, écoulement)	Flujo (descarga, secreción)	Fuoriuscita (scolo)	Iscjedak
Diseases of the aorta	Maladies de l'aorte	Enfermedades de la aorta	Malattie dell'aorta	Bolesti aorte
Dislocated ankle joint	Luxation de la cheville	Luxación del tobillo	Lussazione della caviglia	Iščašenje skočnog zgloba
Dislocated fragments	Fragments deboîtées	Dislocación de los fragmentos	Dislocazione dei frammenti	Dislokacija ulomaka
Dislocated shoulder	Luxation de l'épaule	Luxación del hombro	Lussazione della spalla	Iščašenje ramena
Dislocation (luxation)	Déboîtement (luxation)	Luxación (lujación, dislocación)	Lussazione	Iščašenje (dislokacija, luksacija)
Dislocation of a hip	Luxation de la hanche	Luxación de la cadera	Lussazione dell'anca	Iščašenje kuka
Disorientation	Désorientation	Desorientación	Disorientamento	Dezorijentiranost
Disseminated intravascular coagulation	Coagulation intravasculaire disséminée	Coagulación intravascular diseminada	Coagulazione intravascolare disseminata	Diseminirana intravaskularna koagulacija
Distal radial fracture	Fracture de l'extrémité inferieure du radius (fracture de Pouteau-Colles)	Fractura distal del radio	Frattura di Pouteau-Colles (frattura delle metafisi radiali distali)	Prijelom palčane kosti loco typico
Diverticulitis	Diverticulite	Diverticulitis	Diverticolite	Divertikulitis
Diverticulosis	Diverticulose	Enfermedad diverticular	Diverticolosi	Divertikuloza
Diverticulum	Diverticule	Divertículo	Diverticolo	Divertikul
Dizziness (vertigo)	Vertige	Vértigo	Capogiro (vertigine)	Vrtoglavica
Dog bite	Morsure de chien	Mordedura de perro	Morsicatura di cane	Ugriz psa
Double vision (diplopia)	Vision double (diplopie)	Visión doble (diplopía)	Visione doppia (diplopia)	Dvoslike
Down syndrome	Syndrome de Down	Síndrome de Down	Sindrome di Down	Downov sindrom (mongoloidizam)
Dracunculiasis	Dracunculose	Dracunculiasis	Dracunculiasi	Drakunkulijaza
Drooling (ptyalism, sialorrhea, slobbering)	Hypersialorrhée (ptyalisme)	Sialorrea (ptialismo)	Sbavando (ptialismo, scialorrea)	Slinjenje
Drooping of the upper eyelid (blepharoptosis)	Abaissement de la paupière supérieure (blépharoptose)	Despredimiento del párpado superior (blefaroptosis)	Spostamento della palpebra (palpebra calante, blefaroptosi)	Spušteni kapak (blefaroptoza)
Drowning	Noyade	Ahogamiento	Affogamento	Utapanje
Drug addiction	Toxicomanie	Adicción a las drogas (drogodependencia)	Tossicodipendenza (tossicomania)	Ovisnost o drogama
Drug allergy	Allergie aux médicaments	Alergia al medicamento	Allergia a farmaci	Alergija na lijekove
Drug overdose	Surdose de drogue	Sobredosis por droga	Overdose di droga	Predoziranje drogom
Dry cough	Toux sèche	Tos seca (tos perruna)	Tosse secca	Suhi kašalj
Dry eyes (keratoconjuctivitis sicca)	Oeil sec (kérato-conjonctivite sèche)	Sequedad de los ojos (xeroftalmia)	Occhi secchi (xeroftalmia)	Suhe oči (kseroftalmija)
Dry gangrene	Gangrène sèche	Gangrena seca	Gangrena secca	Suha gangrena
Dry mouth (xerostomia)	Sècheresse de la bouche (xèrostomie)	Sequedad de la boca (xerostomía)	Scarsa secrezione salivare (xerostomia)	Suha sluznica usta
Duchenne muscular dystrophy	Myopathie de Duchenne	Distrofia muscular de Duchenne	Distrofia di Duchenne	Duchenneova mišićna distrofija
Ductus arteriosus (ductus Botalli shunt)	Canal artériel	Ductus arteriosus (conducto arterioso de Botal)	Dotto arterioso di Botallo	Ductus Botalli
Dull pain	Douleur sourde	Dolor sordo	Dolore ottuso	Tupa bol
Dullness in limbs	Membres sourds	Torpeza en las extremidades	Ottusità alle estremità	Tupost u udovima
Duodenal atresia	Atrésie duodénale	Atresia duodenal	Atresia duodenale	Atrezija dvanaesnika
Duodenal diverticulum	Diverticule duodenal	Divertículo duodenal	Diverticolo duodenale	Divertikul na dvanaesniku
Duodenal ulcer	Ulcère du doudénum	Úlcera duodenal	Ulcera duodenale	Čir na dvanaesniku

English	French	Spanish	Italian	Croatian
Dupuytren's contracture	Contracture de Dupuytren	Contractura de Dupuytren	Malattia di Dupuytren	Dupuytrenova kontraktura
Dust allergy	Allergie à la poussière	Alergia al polvo	Allergia a polvere	Alergija na prašinu
Dwarfism (nanism)	Nanisme	Enanismo	Nanismo	Patuljasti rast (nanizam)
Dyschondroplasia	Dyschondroplasie	Discondroplasia	Discondroplasia	Dishondroplazija
Dysentery (flux)	Dysenterie	Disentería	Dissenteria	Dizenterija
Dysgerminoma	Dysgerminome	Disgerminoma	Disgerminoma	Disgerminom
Dyshidrosis	Dyshidrose	Eczema dishidrótico	Disidrosi	Dishidroza
Dyslexia	Dyslexie	Dislexia	Dislessia	Disleksija
Dyspepsia (upset stomach)	Dyspepsie	Dispepsia (indigestión)	Dispepsia	Dispepsija (nervozni želudac)
Dystonia	Dystonie	Distonía	Distonia	Distonija
Dystrophy	Dystrophie	Distrofia	Distrofia	Distrofija
Ear bleeding	Saignement de l'oreille	Hemorragia de oído (otorragia)	Fuoriuscita di sangue dall'orecchio (otorragia)	Krvarenje iz uha
Ear pain (otalgia)	Mal à l'oreille (otalgie)	Dolor en oído (otalgia)	Dolore auricolare (otalgia)	Bol u uhu (otalgija)
Early symptom (prodrome)	Phase prodromique	Síndrome prodrómico	Sindrome prodromica	Predsimptom bolesti prije nego se bolest razvije
Eating disorder	Trouble de conduite alimentaire	Trastorno alimentario	Disturbo del comportamento alimentare	Poremećaj ishrane
Ebola hemorrhagic fever	Fièvre Ébola	Fiebre hemorrágica viral de Ébola	Ebola	Groznica Ebola
Echinococcosis (hydatid disease)	Échinococcose	Hidatidosis (equinocosis)	Echinococcosi (idatidosi)	Ehinokokoza
Echolalia	Écholalie	Ecolalia	Ecolalia	Eholalija
Echopraxia (involuntary repetition ofthe observed movements of another person)	Échopraxie (tendance spontanée à répéter les mouvements d'une autre personne)	Ecopraxia (repetición de los movimientos de otra persona)	Ecoprassia (imitazione spontanea di movimenti osservati)	Ehopraksija (nevoljno ponavljanje tuđih pokreta)
Ectopic pregnancy (extrauterine pregnancy)	Grossesse extra-utérine	Embarazo ectópico	Gravidanza ectopica	Izvanmaternična trudnoća (ektopična trudnoća)
Eczema	Eczéma	Eccema (eczema)	Eczema	Ekcem
Edema	Oedème	Edema (hidropesía)	Edema	Edem
Edwards syndrome (trisomy 18)	Syndrome d'Edwards (trisomie 18)	Síndrome de Edwards (trisomía del 18)	Sindrome di Edwards	Trisomija 18D (Edwardsov sindrom)
Eisenmenger's syndrome	Syndrome d'Eisenmenger	Síndrome de Eisenmenger	Sindrome di Eisenmenger	Eisenmengerov sindrom
Elbow arthrosis	Arthrose du coude	Artrosis de codo	Artrosi di gomito	Artroza lakta
Elbow dislocation (luxation of the elbow)	Luxation du coude	Luxación del codo	Lussazione del gomito	Iščašenje lakta
Electric shock burn	Brûlure électrique	Quemadura eléctrica	Ustione da corrente elettrica	Opeklina od strujnog udara
Electrical injuries (electric shock)	Électrisation	Lesiones por corriente eléctrica	Folgorazione (elettrocuzione)	Ozljede električnom strujom (strujni udar)
Electromagnetic hypersensitivity	Sensibilité éléctromagnétique	Hipersensibilidad electromagnética	Elettrosensibilità	Elektromagnetska hipersenzibilnost
Elephantiasis (lymphedema)	Éléphantiasis (filariose lymphatique)	Elefantiasis	Elefantiasi	Elefantijaza (limfedem)
Elevated body temperature	Élévation de la température du corps	Aumento en la temperatura corporal	Temperatura corporea elevata	Povišena tjelesna temperatura
Embolism	Embolie	Embolia	Embolismo (embolia)	Embolija
Embryonal carcinoma	Carcinome embryonnaire	Carcinoma embrional	Carcinoma embrionale	Embrionalni karcinom
Emphysema	Emphysème	Enfisema	Enfisema	Emfizem
Empyema	Empyème	Empiema	Empiema	Empijem
Encephalocele	Encéphalocèle	Encefalocele	Encefalocele	Encefalokela
Encephalopathy	Encéphalopathie	Encefalopatía	Encefalopatia	Encefalopatija
Enchondroma	Enchondrome	Encondroma	Encondroma	Enhondrom
Encopresis	Encoprésie	Encopresis	Enconpresi	Enkopreza
Endocardial fibroelastosis	Fibroélastose endocardique	Fibroelastosis endocardial	Fibroelastosi endocardica	Fibroelastoza endokarda
Endometrial carcinoma	Carcinome de l'endomètre	Carcinoma de endometrio	Carcinoma endometriale	Karcinom endometrija
Endometrial hyperplasia	Hyperplasie endométriale	Hiperplasia endometrial	Iperplasia endometriale	Hiperplazija endometrija
Endometrial polyp (uterine polyp)	Polype utérin	Pólipo endometrial	Polipo endometriale	Polip maternice
Endometriosis	Endométriose	Endometriosis	Endometriosi	Endometrioza
Endotoxic shock	Choc endotoxique	Choque endotoxico	Shock endotossico	Endotoksični šok
Enlarged liver (hepatomegaly)	Augmentation du foie (hépatomégalie)	Aumento del tamaño del hígado (hepatomegalia)	Aumento di volume del fegato (epatomegalia)	Povećanje jetre (hepatomegalija)
Enlarged lymph nodes (lymphadenopathy)	Augmentation d'un ganglion lymphatique (lymphadénopathie)	Aumento de volumen de los ganglios linfáticos (linfadenopatía)	Ingrossamento dei linfonodi (linfoadenopatia)	Povećanje limfnih čvorova (limfadenopatija)
Enlarged pupils	Pupilles dilatées	Pupilas dilatadas	Pupille dilatate	Proširene zjenice
Enlarged tongue (macroglossia)	Augmentation de la langue (macroglossie)	Lengua más grande de lo normal (macroglosia)	Eccessiva crescita della lingua (macroglossia)	Uvećani jezik (makroglosija)
Enthesopathy	Enthésiopathie	Entesopatía	Entesopatia	Entezopatija
Eosinophilia	Éosinophilie	Eosinofilia	Eosinofilia	Eozinofilija
Ependymoma	Épendymome	Ependimoma	Ependimoma	Ependimom
Epicondylar elbow fracture	Fracture du condyle huméral	Fractura de epicóndilo humeral	Frattura dell'epicondilo omerale	Prijelom kondila nadlaktične kosti

English	French	Spanish	Italian	Croatian
Epidemic typhus (louse-borne typhus)	Typhus épidémique (typhus à poux, typhus européen)	Tifus exantemático epidémico	Tifo esantematico (tifo epidemico)	Trbušni tifus (epidemjski tifus, pjegavac)
Epidural bleeding	Hémorragie épidurale	Hemorragia epidural	Emorragia epidurale	Epiduralno krvarenje
Epidural hematoma	Hématome épidural	Hematoma epidural	Ematoma epidurale	Epiduralni hematom
Epigastric pain	Douleur épigastrique	Dolor epigástrico	Gastralgia	Bol u epigastriju
Epilepsy	Épilepsie	Epilepsia	Epilessia	Epilepsija
Epiphyseolysis capitis femoris	Épiphysiolyse de l'extrémité supérieure du fémur	Epifisario de la cabeza femoral (epifisiolisis capitis femoris)	Epifisiolisi della testa femorale	Epifizeoliza glave bedrene kosti
Epispadias	Épispadias	Epispadia	Epispadia	Epispadija
Epithelial carcinoma	Carcinome épithélial	Carcinoma epitelial	Carcinoma epiteliale	Karcinom pokrovnog epitela
Erysipelas (Ignis sacer, St. Anthony's fire)	Érysipèle (érésipèle)	Erisipela	Erisipela	Crveni vjetar (vrbanac, erizipel)
Erysipeloid	Erysipéloïde	Erisipeloide	Erisipeloide	Erizipeloid
Erythromelalgia (acromelalgia)	Érythromelalgie	Eritromelalgia	Eritromelalgia	Eritromelalgija
Erythroplakia (erythroplasia)	Érythroplasie	Eritroplasia	Eritroplachia (eritroplasia)	Eritroplazija
Erythroplasia of Queyrat	Érythroplasie de Queyrat	Eritroplasia de Queyrat	Eritroplasia di Queyrat	Eritroplazija Queyrat
Esophageal atresia	Atrésie de l'oesophage	Atresia esofágica	Atresia esofagea	Atrezija jednjaka
Esophageal stenosis	Sténose oesophagienne	Estenosis esofágica	Stenosi esofagea	Stenoza jednjaka
Esophageal varices	Varices oesophagiennes	Varices esofágicas	Varici esofagee	Proširene vene jednjaka (flebektazije)
Essential hypertension	Hypertension artérielle essentielle	Hipertensión esencial	Ipertensione arteriosa essenziale	Esencijalna hipertenzija
Estrogen deficiency	Carence oestrogénique	Deficiencia de estrógenos	Carenza di estrogeno	Manjak estrogena
Ewing's sarcoma	Sarcome d'Ewing	Sarcoma de Ewing	Sarcoma di Ewing	Ewing sarkom (endoteliosarkom)
Exanthem	Exanthème	Exantema	Esantema	Egzantem
Exanthema subitum (roseola infantum, sixth disease)	Roséole (exanthème subit, sixième maladie)	Roséola (exantema súbito)	Sesta malattia (roseola infantum, esantema subitum)	Rozeola infantum (egzantema subitum, šesta bolest)
Exasperation	Exaspération (irritation)	Exasperación	Esasperazione (irritazione)	Razdražljivost
Excessive hunger (polyphagia)	Faim excessive (polyphagie)	Aumento anormal de la necesidad de comer (polifagia)	Aumento incontrollato dell'appetito (polifagia)	Neumjerena glad
Excessive secretion of saliva (hypersalivation)	Sécrétion de la salive excessive	Excesiva producción de saliva (hipersalivación)	Produzione di saliva eccessiva (ipersalivazione)	Pojačano lučenje sline (hipersalivacija)
Excessive sweating (hyperhidrosis)	Sudation excessive (hyperhidrose)	Excesiva producción de sudor (hiperhidrosis)	Aumento della sudorazione (iperidrosi)	Prekomjerno znojenje (hiperhidroza)
Exostosis	Exostose	Exostosis	Esostosi	Egzostoza
Expectoration of blood (hemoptysis)	Rejet de sang issu des voies aériennes (hémoptysie)	Expectoración de sangre (hemoptisis)	Espettorazione di sangue (emottisi)	Iskašljavanje krvi (hemoptiza, hemoptoja)
Explosive wound	Blessure par explosion	Lesión por explosión	Ferita esplosiva	Eksplozivna rana
Expulsion of undigested food from stomack to the mouth (regurgitation)	Retour à la bouche du contenu de l'estomac (régurgitation)	Regreso del contenido alimentario a través del esófago (regurgitación)	Risalita di alimenti dallo stomaco alla bocca (rigurgito)	Vraćanje hrane iz želuca u usta (regurgitacija)
Extensor tendinitis (inflammation of the extensor tendons of the toes)	Tendinite des extenseurs des orteils	Tendinitis de los extensores de los dedos	Tendinite dei estensori delle dita del piede	Tendinitis ekstenzora prstiju stopala
External abdominal wall hernia	Hernie de la paroi abdominale (hernie abdominale externe)	Hernia de la pared abdominal	Ernia esterna addominale	Kila vanjske trbušne stijenke
External bleeding	Saignement externe (hémorragie externe)	Sangrado externo (hemorragia externa)	Emorragia esterna	Vanjsko krvarenje
Extrajoint rheumatism	Rhumatisme extraarticulaire	Reumatismo extraarticular	Reumatismo extra-articolare	Izvanzglobni reumatizam
Facial spasm	Spasme facial	Espasmo facial	Spasmo facciale	Grč mišića lica
Familial Mediterranean fever	Fièvre méditerranéenne familiale	Fiebre mediterránea familiar	Febbre mediterranea familiare	Obiteljska mediteranska groznica
Farmer's lung	Maladie du poumon de fermier	Pulmón de granjero	Febbre da fieno	Farmerska pluća
Farsightedness (hyperopia)	Hypermétropie	Hipermetropía	Ipermetropia	Dalekovidnost
Fat embolism	Embolie de cholestérol	Embolismo graso	Embolia adiposa	Masna embolija
Fatigue (exhaustion, lethargy)	Fatigue (affaiblissement)	Cansancio (fatiga, letargo, astenia)	Stanchezza (fatica, astenia)	Iscrpljenost (umor, fatigo)
Fatty liver metamorphosis	Stéatose hépatique	Metamorfosis grasa del hígado	Metamorfosi grassa del fegato	Masna metarmofoza jetre
Favus	Favus	Tiña favosa (favus, tinea favosa)	Tinea favosa	Tinea favosa (favus)
Feather allergy	Allergie aux plumes	Alergia a las plumas	Allergia alle piume	Alergija na perje
Febrile convulsions	Convulsion hyperthermique	Convulsiones febriles	Convulsioni febbrili	Febrilne konvulzije
Femoral neck fracture	Fracture du col du fémur	Fractura de cuello del fémur	Frattura del collo del femore	Prijelom vrata bedrene kosti
Fetal alcohol syndrome	Syndrome d'alcoolisation foetale	Síndrome de alcoholismo fetal	Sindrome alcolica fetale	Fetusni alkoholni sindrom
Fever	Fièvre	Fiebre	Febbre	Groznica (vrućica)
Fibrinoid necrosis	Nécrose fibrinoïde	Necrosis fibrinoide	Necrosi fibrinoide	Fibrinoidna nekroza

English	French	Spanish	Italian	Croatian
Fibroadenoma	Fibroadénome	Fibroadenoma	Fibroadenoma	Fibroadenom
Fibrocystic breast disease	Mastopathie fibrocystique	Mastitis quística crónica (enfermedad fibroquística)	Mastopatia fibrocistica	Fibrocistična bolest dojke
Fibroma	Fibrome	Fibroma	Fibroma	Fibrom
Fibromyalgia	Fibromyalgie	Fibromialgia	Fibromialgia	Fibromialgija
Fibrosarcoma (fibroblastic sarcoma)	Fibrosarcome	Fibrosarcoma	Fibrosarcoma	Fibrosarkom
Fibrosis	Fibrose	Fibrosis	Fibrosi	Fibroza
Fibrous dysplasia	Dysplasie fibreuse	Displasia fibrosa	Displasia fibrosa	Fibrozna displazija
Fibrous histiocytoma	Histiocytome fibreux	Histiocitoma fibroso	Fibroistiocitoma benigno	Fibrozni histiocitom
Filariasis	Filariose	Filariasis	Filariasi	Filarijaza
Finger clubbing (digital clubbing)	Hippocratisme digital (doigts en baguettes de tambour)	Acropaquia (hipocratismo digital)	Dita ippocratiche (dita a bacchetta di tamburo)	Batićasti prsti
First menstrual cycle (menarche)	Première période de menstruations (ménarche)	Primera menstruación (menarquia)	Primo flusso mestruale (menarca)	Prva mjesečnica (menarha)
Fish poisoning	Empoisonnement du poisson	Intoxicación por pescado	Avvelenamento da pesci	Trovanje ribom
Fistula	Fistule	Fístula	Fistola	Fistula
Flaccid muscle (untoned muscle)	Muscle flasque (hypotonie musculaire)	Músculo flácido	Muscolo flaccido	Mlohavi mišić
Flat foot (pes planus)	Pied plat (pes planus)	Pie plano (pes planus, arcos vencidos)	Piede piatto (pes planus)	Spušteno stopalo (pes planus)
Floating kidney (nephroptosis, renal ptosis)	Syndrome du rein flottant (néphroptose)	Riñón flotante (ptosis renal, nefroptosis)	Spostamento del rene (ptosi renale, nefroptosi)	Spušteni bubreg (putujući bubreg, nefroptoza)
Floppy infant syndrome	Syndrome du bébé mou	Síndrome de bebé flácido	Sindrome del bambino flaccido	Sindrom mlohavog djeteta
Flu (influenza)	Grippe (influenza)	Gripe (gripa, influenza)	Influenza	Gripa (influenca)
Foamy sputum	Crachat spumeux	Esputo espumoso	Sputo schiumoso	Pjenušavi ispljuvak
Folliculitis	Folliculite	Foliculitis	Follicolite	Folikulitis
Food allergy	Allergie alimentaire	Alergia a alimentos	Allergia alimentare	Alergija na hranu
Food aversion	Aversion pour la nourriture	Aversión por la comida	Ripugnanza al cibo	Gađenje prema hrani
Food poisoning	Empoisonnement alimentaires	Intoxicación alimentaria	Avvelenamento da cibo	Trovanje hranom
Foot arthrosis	Arthrose du pied	Artrosis del pie	Artrosi al piede	Artroza stopala
Foot deformity	Difformité du pied	Deformidad del pie	Difetto del piede	Deformacija stopala
Forearm tendinitis	Tendinite de l'avant-bras	Tendinitis en el antebrazo	Tendinite dell'avambraccio	Veslačka podlaktica (tendinitis podlaktice)
Foreign body in ear	Corps étranger dans l'oreille	Cuerpo extraño en el oído	Corpo estraneo nell'orecchio	Strano tijelo u uhu
Foreign body in nose	Corps étranger dans le nez	Cuerpo extraño en la nariz	Corpo estraneo nel naso	Strano tijelo u nosu
Fournier gangrene	Gangrène de Fournier	Gangrena de Fournier	Gangrena di Fournier	Fournierova gangrena
Fracture with displacement	Fracture à déplacement	Fractura-dislocación	Frattura con dislocazione	Prijelom kosti s pomakom
Freiberg's disease	Maladie de Freiberg	Enfermedad de Freiberg	Malattia di Freiberg	Freibergova bolest
Frequent urination	Miction fréquente	Micción frecuente	Urinazione frequente (pollachiuria)	Učestalo mokrenje
Frequent urination at night (nocturia)	Excrétion urinaire à prédominance nocturne (nycturie)	Emisión excesiva de orina durante la noche (nicturia)	Urinazione notturna (nicturia)	Noćno mokrenje (nokturija)
Frigidity	Frigidité	Frigidez	Frigidità	Frigidnost
Frostbite	Gelure	Congelamiento	Congelamento	Ozeblina
Frozen shoulder (adhesive capsulitis of shoulder)	Épaule bloquée (périarthrite scapulo-humérale)	Capsulitis adhesiva del hombro	Capsulite adesiva	Sindrom bolnog ramena (adhezivni kapsulitis ramena, smrznuto rame)
Fungal infection	Infection fongique	Infección por hongos	Infezione fungina	Gljivična infekcija
Fungal osteomyelitis	Ostéomyélite fongique	Osteomielitis micótica	Osteomielite fungale	Gljivični osteomijelitis
Fur allergy	Allergie aux animaux à poils	Alergia al pelo de los animales	Allergia a pello di animali	Alergija na životinjsku dlaku
Furuncle (boil)	Furoncle	Forúnculo (furúnculo)	Foruncolo	Furunkul (čir na koži)
Gaining weight	Grossissement	Engorde (ganar peso)	Ingrossamento (divenire grosso)	Debljanje
Galactorrhea	Galactorrhée	Galactorrea	Galattorrea	Galaktoreja
Gallbladder hydrops	Hydrops de la vésicule biliaire	Hidrops vesicular	Idrope della colecisti	Hidrops žučnog mjehura
Gallstone (cholelithiasis)	Calcul biliaire (cholélithiase)	Cálculo biliar (litiasis biliar)	Calcolo biliare	Žučni kamenac (holelitijaza)
Gambling addiction (ludomania)	Jeu pathologique (jeu compulsif)	Adicción a jugar (ludopatía, ludomanía)	Giocco d'azzardo patologico	Ovisnost o kockanju (ludopatija)
Gangrene	Gangrène	Gangrena	Cancrena	Gangrena
Gas gangrene	Gangrène gazeuse	Gangrena gaseosa	Gangrene gassosa	Plinska gangrena
Gas poisoning	Empoisonnement au gaz	Envenenamiento por gas	Avvelenamento da gas	Trovanje plinom
Gastric carcinoma	Carcinome de l'estomac	Carcinoma gástrico	Carcinoma gastrico	Karcinom želuca
Gastric ulcer	Ulcère de l'estomac	Úlcera gástrica	Ulcera gastrica	Čir na želucu
Gastroenteritis	Gastroentérite	Gastroenteritis	Gastroenterite	Gastroenteritis
Generalized edema (anasarca)	Oedème généralisé (anasarque)	Anasarca	Edema diffuso (anasarca)	Generalizirani edem (anasarka)
Genital herpes	Herpès génital	Herpes genital	Herpes genitalis	Genitalni herpes

English	French	Spanish	Italian	Croatian
Genital wart	Verrue génitale	Verruga genital (condiloma acuminata)	Condiloma	Genitalna bradavica (venerična bradavica)
German measles (rubella)	Rubéole	Rubéola	Rosolia	Rubeola (crljenac)
Giant cell arteritis (temporal arteritis)	Artérite giganto-cellulaire (maladie de Horton, artérite temporale)	Arteritis de células gigantes (arteritis de la temporal)	Arterite temporale (arterite di Horton)	Arteritis divovskih stanica (temporalni arteritis)
Gigantism	Gigantisme	Gigantismo	Gigantismo	Divovski stas
Gigantocellular tumor (osteoclastoma)	Tumeur à cellules géantes	Tumor de células gigantes (osteoclastoma)	Osteoclastoma (tumore a cellule giganti)	Gigantocelularni tumor (osteoklastom)
Glanders	Morve	Muermo	Morva umana	Sakagija
Glaucoma	Glaucome	Glaucoma	Glaucoma	Glaukom
Glioblastoma	Glioblastome	Glioblastoma	Glioblastoma	Glioblastom
Glioma	Gliome	Glioma	Glioma	Gliom
Gliosis	Gliose	Gliosis	Gliosi	Glioza
Glomerulonephritis	Gloméluronéphrite	Glomerulonefritis	Glomerulonefrite	Glomerulonefritis
Glomus tumor (glomangioma)	Tumeur glomique (glomangiome)	Tumor glómico (glomangioma)	Glomangioma (paraganglioma)	Glomus-tumor
Glucose in urine (glycosuria)	Sucre dans les urines (glycosurie)	Azúcar en orina (glucosuria)	Glicosuria (mellituria)	Šećer u urinu (glikozurija)
Gluten intolerance	Intolérance au gluten	Intolerancia al gluten	Intolleranza al glutine	Nepodnošenje glutena
Goiter	Goitre	Bocio (coto)	Gozzo	Guša (struma)
Gonadoblastoma	Gonadoblastome	Gonadoblastoma	Gonadoblastoma	Gonadoblastom
Gonorrhea	Gonorrhée (blennorragie, chaude-pisse)	Gonorrea (blenorragia, blenorrea)	Gonorrea (blenorragia)	Gonoreja (kapavac, triper)
Goodpasture's syndrome	Syndrome de Goodpasture (maladie des anti-corps anti-membrane basale glomérulaire)	Síndrome de Goodpasture	Sindrome di Goodpasture	Goodpastureov sindrom
Gout (gouty arthritis)	Goutte	Gota (enfermedad gotosa)	Gotta	Ulozi (giht)
Granulocytosis	Polynucléose	Granulocitosis	Granulocitosi	Granulocitoza
Granulomatous inflammation	Inflammation granulomateuse	Inflamación granulomatosa	Infiammazione granulomatosa	Granulomatozna upala (granulom)
Granulosa cell tumor	Tumeur de la granulosa	Tumor de células de la granulosa (tumor de teca-granulosa)	Follicoloma	Granuloza tumor
Green stool	Selles vertes	Heces verdes	Feci di colore verde	Zelenkasta stolica
Greenstick fracture	Fracture en bois vert	Fractura en rama verde	Frattura a legno verde	Prijelom mlade kosti
Groin pain syndrome	Pubalgie du sportif	Síndrome de dolor inguinal	Pubalgia dello sportivo	Sindrom bolnih prepona
Guillain-Barré syndrome	Syndrome de Guillain-Barré	Síndrome de Guillain-Barré	Sindrome di Guillain-Barré	Guillain-Barréov sindrom
Gunshot wound	Blessure par balle	Herida de bala	Ferita da arma da fuoco	Prostrijelna rana
Gymnastics lower back pain	Lombalgie du gymnaste	Espalda del gimnasta	Lombalgia dell'atleta	Gimnastičarska bolna križa
Gynecomastia	Gynécomastie	Ginecomastia	Ginecomastia	Ginekomastija
Haglund's disease	Maladie de Haglund	Enfermedad de Haglund (deformidad de Haglund)	Malattia di Haglund (deformità di Haglund)	Haglundova bolest
Hallucination	Hallucination	Alucinación	Allucinazione	Halucinacija
Hand and finger joints dislocation	Luxation des doigts et du poignet	Luxaciones de la mano y los dedos	Lussazioni delle atricolazioni della mano e delle dita	Iščašenje zglobova šake i prstiju
Hand arthrosis	Arthrose de le main	Artrosis de mano	Artrosi della mano	Artroza šake
Hand fibrositis	Fasciite de la main (fasciite palmaire)	Fibrositis de la mano	Fibrosite di mano	Fibrozitis šake
Hand tremor	Tremblement des mains	Temblor en las manos	Tremore delle mani	Drhtanje ruku
Hand-arm vibration syndrome (vibration white finger)	Syndrome des vibrations du système main-bras	Vibraciones mano brazo (dedo blanco inducido por vibraciones)	Sindrome da vibrazioni mano-braccio	Vibracijski sindrom šaka-ruka
Hard of hearing	Surdité partielle	Corto de oído (parcialmente sordo)	Sordità parziale	Nagluhost
Hashimoto's disease	Thyroïdite de Hashimoto	Tiroiditis de Hashimoto	Tiroidite di Hashimoto	Hashimotov sindrom
Head and brain injuries	Blessures à la tête et blessures du cerveau	Lesiones de la cabeza y del cerebro	Lesioni della testa e del cervello	Ozljede glave i mozga
Headache	Mal de tête (céphalée)	Dolor de cabeza	Mal di testa	Glavobolja
Hearing disorder	Trouble de l'audition	Trastorno de la audición	Disturbo dell'udito	Poremećaj sluha
Hearing loss	Perte d'ouïe	Pérdida de la capacidad auditiva	Perdita di udito	Gubitak sluha
Heart attack (myocardial infarction)	Infarctus du myocarde	Infarto de miocardio	Infarto miocardico acuto	Infarkt miokarda
Heart disease (cardiopathy)	Maladie cardiaque (cardiopathie)	Enfermedad del corazón (cardiopatía)	Malattia del cuore (cardiopatia)	Srčana bolest (kardiopatija)
Heart murmur	Souffle cardiaque	Soplo del corazón	Soffio cardiaco	Šum na srcu
Heart valve diseases	Maladies des valves cardiaques	Enfermedades de las válvulas del corazón	Malattie delle valvole cardiache	Bolesti srčanih zalistaka
Heartburn	Brûlure de l'estomac (pyrosis)	Ardor de estómago (acidez, pirosis)	Bruciore di stomaco (pirosi)	Žgaravica
Heavy metal poisoning	Empoisonnement aux métaux lourds	Envenenamiento por metales pesados	Intossicazione da metalli pesanti	Trovanje teškim metalima
Heberden's nodes	Nodules d'Heberden	Nódulos de Heberden	Noduli di Heberden	Heberdenovi čvorići

English	French	Spanish	Italian	Croatian
Heel spur (calcaneal spur)	Éperon de talon (epine calcaneenne)	Espuela de talón (espuela calcánea)	Spina nel calcagno (spina calcaneare)	Petni trn
Hemangioendothelioma	Hémangio-endothéliome	Hemangioendotelioma	Emangioendotelioma	Hemangioendoteliom
Hemangioma	Hémangiome	Hemangioma	Emangioma	Hemangiom
Hematoma	Hématome	Hematoma	Ematoma	Hematom
Hemivertebrae	Hémivértèbre	Hemivértebra	Emivertebra	Hemivertebra
Hemochromatosis	Hémochromatose	Hemocromatosis	Emocromatosi	Hemokromatoza
Hemoglobin in urine (hemoglobinuria)	Hémoglobine dans l'urine (hémoglobinurie)	Hemoglobina en orina (hemoglobinuria)	Presenza di emoglobina nelle urine (emoglobinuria)	Hemoglobin u urinu (hemoglobinurija)
Hemolytic anemia	Anémie hémolytique	Anemia hemolítica	Anemia emolitica	Hemolitična anemija
Hemophilia	Hémophilie	Hemofilia	Emofilia	Hemofilija
Hemophiliac arthropathy	Arthropathie hémophile	Artropatía hemofílica	Artropatia emofilica	Hemofilična artropatija
Hemopneumothorax	Hémopneumothorax	Hemoneumotórax	Emopneumotorace	Hemopneumotoraks
Hemorrhagic brain infarction	Infarctus cérébral hémorragique	Infarto cerebral hemorrágico	Ictus emorragico	Hemoragijski infarkt mozga
Hemorrhagic fever with renal syndrome (Korean hemorrhagic fever)	Fièvre hémorragique avec syndrome rénal (fièvre hémorragique de Corée)	Fiebre hemorrágica con síndrome renal (fiebre hemorrágica coreana)	Febbre emorragica con sindrome renale (febbre emorragica coreana)	Hemoragijska groznica s renalnim sindromom (korejska hemoragijska groznica)
Hemorrhoids	Hémorroïdes	Hemorroides	Emorroidi	Hemoroidi
Hemosiderosis	Hémosidérose	Hemosiderosis	Emosiderosi	Hemosideroza
Hemothorax	Hémothorax	Hemotórax	Emotorace	Hemotoraks
Hepatic echinococcosis	Échinococcose hépatique	Hidatidosis hepática	Echinococcosi epatica	Ehinokokoza jetre
Hepatic tuberculosis	Tuberculose hépatique	Tuberculosis hepática	Tubercolosi epatica	Tuberkuloza jetre
Hepatitis A	Hépatite A	Hepatitis A	Epatite virale A	Hepatitis A
Hepatitis B	Hépatite B	Hepatitis B	Epatite virale B	Hepatitis B
Hepatitis C	Hépatite C	Hepatitis C	Epatite virale C	Hepatitis C
Hepatitis D	Hépatite D	Hepatitis D	Epatite virale D	Hepatitis D
Hepatitis E	Hépatite E	Hepatitis E	Epatite virale E	Hepatitis E
Hepatocellular adenoma	Adénome hépatocellulaire	Adenoma hepático (adenoma hepatocelular)	Adenoma epatocellulare	Hepatocelularni adenom
Hepatocellular carcinoma	Carcinome hépatocellulaire	Carcinoma hepatocelular	Carcinoma epatocellulare	Hepatocelularni karcinom
Hepatorenal syndrome	Syndrome hépato-rénal	Síndrome hepatorrenal	Sindrome epato-renale	Hepatorenalni sindrom
Hereditary ataxia	Ataxie héréditaire	Ataxia de Friidreich (ataxia hereditaria)	Atassia ereditaria	Heredoataksija
Hereditary multiple exostoses	Maladie des exostoses multiples	Exostosis múltiple hereditaria	Esostosi multipla ereditaria	Multiple egzostoze
Hermaphroditism	Hermaphrodisme	Hermafroditismo	Ermafroditismo	Dvospolnost
Hernia	Hernie	Hernia	Ernia	Kila (bruh, hernija)
Hernia sack	Sac herniaire	Saco de hernia (saco herniario)	Sacco dell'ernia	Kilna vreća
Herpangina (mouth blisters)	Herpangine	Herpangina	Erpangina (faringite vescicolare)	Herpangina
Herpes simplex	Herpès (infection herpétique)	Herpes simple	Herpes simplex	Herpes simpleks
Herpes zoster	Zona	Herpes zóster (herpes zona)	Herpes zoster	Herpes zoster
Hiatus hernia	Hernie hiatale	Hernia de hiato	Ernia iatale	Hijatusna kila
Hiccup	Hoquet	Hipo	Singhiozzo	Štucavica
High arches (pes cavus)	Pied creux	Pie cavo (pes cavus)	Piede cavo (pes cavus)	Izdubljeno stopalo (pes excavatus)
High blood cholesterol (hyper-cholesterolemia)	Cholésterol sanguin élevée (hypercholestérolémie)	Colesterol elevado de la sangre (hipercolesterolemia)	Eccesso di colesterolo nel sangue (ipercolesterolemia)	Povišeni kolesterol u krvi (hiperkolesterolemija)
High blood pressure (hypertension)	Pression artérielle élevée (hypertension artérielle)	Incremento de la presión sanguínea (hipertensión)	Ipertensione arteriosa sistemica	Visoki krvni tlak (hipertenzija)
High blood sugar (hyperglicemia)	Taux de sucre dans le sang élevé (hyperglycémie)	Cantidad excesiva de glucosa en la sangre (hiperglucemia, hiperglicemia)	Eccesso di glucosio nel sangue (iperglicemia)	Povišeni šećer u krvi (hiperglikemija)
Hip arthrosis	Arthrose de hanche (coxarthrose)	Artrosis de cadera (coxartrosis)	Artrosi di anca	Artroza kuka (koksartroza)
Hirschsprung's disease (congenital aganglionic megacolon)	Maladie de Hirschsprung (mégacolôn)	Enfermedad de Hirschsprung (megacolon agangliónico)	Malattia di Hirschsprung (malattia di Mya)	Hirschsprungova bolest (kongenitalni aganglionarni megakolon)
Hirsutism	Hirsutisme	Hirsutismo	Irsutismo	Hirzutizam
Histoplasmosis (Darling's disease)	Histoplasmose	Histoplasmosis	Istoplasmosi	Histoplazmoza
Hives (urticaria)	Urticaire	Urticaria	Orticaria	Koprivnjača (urtikarija)
Hoarseness	Enrouement	Ronquera	Raucedine	Promuklost
Hodgkin's disease	Maladie de Hodgkin	Enfermedad de Hodgkin	Linfoma di Hodgkin	Hodgkinova bolest
Hoffa's disease	Maladie de Hoffa	Enfermedad de Hoffa	Sindrome di Hoffa	Morbus Hoffa
Horseshoe kidney (renal fusion)	Rein en fer à cheval	Riñón de herradura (fusión en los riñones)	Rene a ferro di cavallo (fusione renale)	Potkovičasti bubreg
Hot flushes	Bouffée de chaleur	Sofocos	Vampata di calore	Valovi vrućine (valunzi)
Human bite	Morsure humaine	Mordedura humana	Morsicatura di uomo	Ugriz čovjeka (ljudski ugriz)
Human papilloma virus (HPV) infection	Infection par le virus du papillome humain (VPH)	Infeccion por el virus del papilom humano (VPH)	Infezione da Papilloma Virus Umano (HPV)	Infekcija humanim papiloma virusom (HPV)

English	French	Spanish	Italian	Croatian
Humeral neck fracture	Fracture du col de l'humérus	Fractura de cuello del húmero	Frattura del collo dell'omero	Prijelom vrata nadlaktične kosti
Hunchback	Bossu	Joroba	Gibbo (gobba, gibbosità)	Grba
Hunger	Faim	Hambre	Fame	Glad
Huntington's chorea (Huntington's disease)	Chorée de Huntington (maladie de Huntington)	Enfermedad de Huntington (corea de Huntington)	Malattia di Huntington	Huntingtonova koreja
Hyaline membrane disease (infant respiratory distress syndrome)	Maladie des membranes hyalines (détresse respiratoire néonatale)	Enfermedad de la membrana hialina (síndrome de distrés respiratorio)	Sindrome da distress respiratorio del neonato (malattia da membrane ialine polmonari)	Bolest hijaline membrane (respiratorni sindrom novorođenčeta)
Hydremia	Hydrémie	Hidremia	Idremia	Hidremija
Hydrocele	Hydrocèle	Hidrocele	Idrocele	Hidrokela
Hydrocephalus	Hydrocéphalie	Hidrocefalia	Idrocefalo	Hidrocefalus
Hydronephrosis	Hydronéphrose	Hidronefrosis	Idronefrosi	Hidronefroza
Hydrops	Hydrops	Hidrops	Idrope	Hidrops
Hydrothorax	Hydrothorax	Hidrotórax	Idrotorace	Hidrotoraks
Hygroma	Hygroma	Higroma	Igroma	Higrom
Hyperactivity	Hyperactivité	Hiperactividad	Iperattività	Hiperaktivnost
Hypercalcemia	Hypercalcémie	Hipercalcemia	Ipercalcemia	Hiperkalcijemija
Hyperinsulinism	Hyperinsulinisme	Hiperinsulinismo	Iperinsulinismo	Povišen inzulin u krvi (hiperinzulinizam)
Hyperkalemia	Hyperkaliémie	Hiperpotasemia (hipercalemia)	Iperkaliemia	Hiperkalijemija
Hyperparathyroidism	Hyperparathyroïdie	Hiperparatiroidismo	Iperparatiroidismo	Hiperparatireoidizam
Hyperpituitarism	Hyperpituitarisme	Hiperpituitarismo	Iperpituitarismo	Hiperpituitarizam
Hyperthermia	Hyperthermie	Hipertermia	Ipertermia	Hipertermija
Hyperthropic osteoarthropaty (Pierre Marie-Bamberger syndrome)	Ostéo-arthropathie hypertrophiante de Pierre Marie (syndrome de Marie-Bamberger)	Osteoartropatía hipertrófica (enfermedad de Bamberger-Marie)	Osteoartropatia ipertrofizzante (sindrome di Pierre Marie-Bamberger)	Osteoartropatija hipertrofika Pierre Marie
Hyperthyroidism	Hyperthyroïdie	Hipertiroidismo	Ipertiroidismo	Hipertireoza
Hypertrophic cardiomyopathy	Cardiomyopathie hypertrophique	Miocardiopatía hipertrófica	Cardiomiopatia ipertrofica	Hipertrofijska kardiomiopatija
Hypertrophic pyloric stenosis	Sténose hypertrophique du pylore	Estenosis pilórica hipertrófica	Stenosi ipertrofica del piloro	Hipertrofijska stenoza pilorusa
Hypertrophy	Hypertrophie	Hipertrofia	Ipertrofia	Hipertrofija
Hyperuricemia	Hyperuricémie	Hiperuricemia	Iperuricemia	Hiperurikemija
Hyperventilation	Hyperventilation	Hiperventilación	Iperventilazione	Hiperventilacija
Hypervitaminosis	Hypervitaminose	Hipervitaminosis	Ipervitaminosi	Hipervitaminoza
Hypervolemia (increased level of fluid in the blood)	Hypervolémie (augmentation du volume de sang dans les vaisseaux)	Hipervolemia (aumento del volumen de sangre en la circulación)	Ipervolemia (aumento del volume ematico circolante)	Hipervolemija (porast volumena krvi u optoku)
Hyphema	Hyphème	Hipema	Ifema	Hifema
Hypoalbuminemia	Hypoalbuminémie	Hipoalbuminemia	Ipoalbuminemia	Hipoalbuminemija
Hypocalcemia	Hypocalcémie	Hipocalcemia	Ipocalcemia	Hipokalcijemija
Hypochondria	Hypocondrie	Hipocondría	Ipocondria	Hipohondrija
Hypochromic anemia	Anémie hypochrome	Anemia hipocrómica	Anemia ipocromica	Hipokromna anemija
Hypoglycemia	Hypoglycémie	Hipoglicemia	Ipoglicemia	Hipoglikemija
Hypoinsulinism	Hypoinsulinisme	Hipoinsulinismo	Ipoinsulinemia	Hipoinzulinizam
Hypokalemia	Hypokaliémie	Hipocaliemia	Ipokaliemia	Hipokalijemija
Hypoparathyroidism	Hypoparathyroïdie	Hipoparatiroidismo	Ipoparatiroidismo	Hipoparatireodizam
Hypopituitarism	Hypopituitarisme	Hipopituitarismo	Ipopituitarismo	Hipopituitarizam
Hypospadias	Hypospadias	Hipospadias	Ipospadia	Hipospadija
Hypotension and syncope	Hypotension et syncope	Hipotensión y síncope	Ipotensione e sincope	Hipotenzija i sinkope
Hypothermia	Hypothermie	Hipotermia	Ipotermia	Pothlađenost (hipotermija)
Hypothyroidism	Hypothyroïdie	Hipotiroidismo	Ipotiroidismo	Hipotireoza
Hypotonia	Hypotonie	Hipotonía	Ipotonia	Hipotonija
Hypovolemic shock	Choc hypovolémique	Choque hipovolémico	Shock ipovolemico	Hipovolemički šok
Hypoxia	Hypoxie	Hipoxia	Ipossia	Hipoksija
Hysteria	Hystérie	Histeria	Isteria (isterismo)	Histerija
Idiopathic pulmonary fibrosis	Fibrose pulmonaire idiopathique	Fibrosis pulmonar idiopática	Fibrosi polmonare idiopatica	Plućna idiopatska fibroza
Ileus	Iléus	Íleo	Ileo	Ileus
Iliotibial band friction syndrome	Syndrome de la bandelette iliotibiale (syndrome de l'essuie glace)	Síndrome de fricción de la banda iliotibial	Sindrome della benderella ileotibiale	Sindrom trenja iliotibijalnog traktusa
Imbecility	Imbécillité	Imbecilidad	Imbecillità	Slaboumnost
Immunodeficiency	Immunodéficience	Inmunodeficiencia	Immunodeficienza	Sniženi imunitet
Impacted cerumen	Bouchon de cérumen	Tapón de cerumen	Tappo di cerume	Ceruminozni čep
Impetigo	Impétigo	Impétigo	Impetigine	Impetigo
Impotency	Impotence	Impotencia	Impotenza	Impotencija
Inability to urinate	Incapacité d'uriner	Incapacidad para orinar	Mancata secrezione di urina	Nemogućnost mokrenja
Incomplete fracture	Fracture incomplète	Fractura incompleta	Frattura incompleta (infrazione)	Nepotpuni prijelom kosti (napuknuće kosti)
Incontinence	Incontinence	Incontinencia	Incontinenza	Inkontinencija

English	French	Spanish	Italian	Croatian
Increased distance between two organs or parts of the body (hypertelorism)	Élargissement de la distance des organes (hypertélorisme)	Aumento de la separación de los organos (hipertelorismo)	Aumento della distanza fra due parti del corpo (ipertelorismo)	Povećan razmak izmedu dva organa ili dijela tijela (hipertelorizam)
Increased hair loss	Perte de cheveux excessive	Aumento de la cáida del cabello	Aumento di perdita di capelli	Pojačano opadanje kose
Increased hairiness (hypertrichosis)	Pilosité excessive (hypertrichose)	Exceso de cabello (hipertricosis)	Aumento della pelosità (ipertricosi)	Pojačana dlakavost
Increased sensitivity to stimuli of the senses (hyperesthesia)	Hypersensibilité aux stimuli extérieurs (hyperesthésie)	Sensación exagerada de los estímulos táctiles (hiperestesia)	Ippersensibilità ai normali stimoli esterni (iperestesia)	Preosjetljivost na podražaj (hiperestezija)
Increased thirst senasation (polydipsia)	Soif excessive (polydipsie)	Aumento anormal de la sed (polidipsia)	Aumento del senso della sete (polidipsia)	Pojačan osjećaj žeđi (polidipsija)
Indigestion	Indigestion	Indigestión	Indigestione	Probavne smetnje
Infarct	Infarctus	Infarto	Infarto	Infarkt
Infected mosquito bite	Piqûre de moustique infecté	Picadura de mosquito infectado	Puntura di zanzara infetta	Ugriz zaraženog komarca
Infected tick bite	Piqûre de tique infectée	Picadura de garrapata infectada	Morsicatura di zecca infetta	Ugriz zaraženog krpelja
Infection	Infection	Infección	Infezione (malattia infettiva)	Infekcija
Infection of the bone or bone marrow (osteomyelitis)	Infection osseuse ou de la moelle osseuse (ostéomyélite)	Infección del hueso o médula ósea (osteomielitis)	Infezione dell'apparato osteo-articolare (osteomielite)	Infekcija kosti ili koštane srži (osteomijelitis)
Infectious arthritis (septic arthritis)	Arthrite septique	Artritis infecciosa (artritis séptica)	Artrite settica	Infekcijski artritis (septički artritis)
Infectious erythema (fifth disease)	Érythème infectieux (cinquième maladie)	Eritema infeccioso (quinta enfermedad)	Eritema infettivo (quinta malattia)	Infektivni eritem (peta bolest)
Infectious mononucleosis (Pfeiffer's disease, kissing disease, glandular fever)	Mononucléose infectieuse (maladie du baiser, maladie des amoureux)	Mononucleosis infecciosa (fiebre glandular, enfermedad de Pfeiffer)	Mononucleosi infettiva (malattia del bacio)	Mononukleoza (bolest poljupca)
Infertility (sterility)	Infertilité (stérilité)	Infertilidad	Sterilità (infecondità)	Neplodnost (sterilitet)
Infestation with head lice (pediculosis)	Infestation par des poux (pédiculose)	Infestación por piojos (pediculosis)	Infestazione da pidocchi (pediculosi)	Infestacija ušima (ušljivost, pedikuloza)
Infestation with intestinal parasitic warms (helminthiasis)	Infestation par des vers parasites intestinaux (helminthiase)	Infestación de gusanos (helmintiasis)	Infestazione da vermi (elmintiasi)	Infestacija crijevnim parazitima (helmintijaza)
Infestation with pubic lice (phthiriasis)	Infestation par des poux du pubic (phtiriase)	Infestación por ladilla (ftiriasis)	Infestazione da pidocchi del pube (ftiriasi)	Infestacija stidnim ušima (ftirijaza)
Inflammation	Inflammation	Inflamación	Infiammazione (flogosi)	Upala
Inflammation of the appendix (appendicitis)	Inflammation de l'appendice iléo-caecal (appendicite)	Inflamación del apéndice (apendicitis)	Infiammazione dell'appendice vermiforme (appendicite)	Upala slijepog crijeva (apendicitis)
Inflammation of the arterial walls (arteritis)	Inflammation des parois des artères (artérite)	Inflamación de las arterias (arteritis)	Infiammazione delle arterie (arterite)	Upala stijenke arterije (arteritis)
Inflammation of the brain (encephalitis)	Inflammation du cerveau (encéphalite)	Inflamación del encéfalo (encefalitis)	Infiammazione del cervello (encefalite)	Upala mozga (encefalitis)
Inflammation of the breast (mastitis)	Inflammation de la mamelle (mastite)	Inflamación del seno (mastitis)	Infiammazione della mammella (mastite)	Upala dojke (mastitis)
Inflammation of the bronchi (bronchitis)	Inflammation des bronches des poumons (bronchite)	Inflamación de los bronquios (bronquitis)	Infiammazione dei bronchi (bronchite)	Upala bronhija (bronhitis)
Inflammation of the bronchioles (bronchiolitis)	Inflammation des petites bronches (bronchiolite)	Inflamación de los bronquiolos (bronquiolitis)	Infiammazione dei bronchioli (bronchiolite)	Upala bronhiola (bronhiolitis)
Inflammation of the conjunctiva (conjunctivitis)	Inflammation de la conjonctive (conjonctivite)	Inflamación de la conjuntiva (conjuntivitis)	Infiammazione della congiuntiva (congiuntivite)	Upala sluznice oka (konjuktivitis)
Inflammation of the cornea (keratitis)	Inflammation de la cornée (kératite)	Inflamación de la córnea (queratitis)	Infiammazione della cornea (cheratite)	Upala rožnice (keratitis)
Inflammation of the cornea and conjunctiva (keratoconjunctivitis)	Inflammation de la conjonctive et de la cornée (kératoconjonctivite)	Inflamación de la córnea y de la conjuntiva (queratoconjuntivitis)	Infiammazione della cornea e della congiutiva (cheratocongiuntivite)	Upala rožnice i sluznice oka (keratokonjuktivitis)
Inflammation of the endocardium (endocarditis)	Inflammation de l'endocarde (endocardite)	Inflamación del endocardio (endocarditis)	Infiammazione dell'endocardio (endocardite)	Upala srčane ovojnice (endokarditis)
Inflammation of the endometrium (endometritis)	Inflammation de l'endomètre (endométrite)	Inflamación del endometrio (endometritis)	Infiammazione dell'endometrio (endometrite)	Upala endometrija maternice (endometritis)
Inflammation of the entheses (enthesitis)	Inflammation de l'enthèse (enthésite)	Inflamación de la zona de inserción de un músculo (entesitis)	Infiammazione dell'inserzione di muscolo (entesite)	Upala hvatišta mišića (entezitis)
Inflammation of the epididymis (epididymitis)	Inflammation de l'épididyme (épididymite)	Inflamación del epidídimo (epididimitis)	Infiammazione dell'epididimo (epididimite)	Upala pasjemenika (epididimitis)
Inflammation of the epiglottis (epiglottitis)	Inflammation de l'épiglotte (épiglottite)	Inflamación de la epiglotis (epiglotitis)	Infiammazione del'epiglottide (epiglottite)	Upala epiglotisa (epiglotitis)
Inflammation of the fascia (fasciitis)	Inflammation du fascia (fasciite)	Inflamación de la fascia (fascitis)	Infiammazione della fascia (fascite)	Upala fascije (fasciitis)
Inflammation of the gall bladder (cholecystitis)	Inflammation de la vésicule biliaire (cholécystite)	Inflamación de la vesícula biliar (colecistitis)	Infiammazione della colecisti (colecistite)	Upala žučnog mjehura (holecistitis)
Inflammation of the glans penis (balanitis)	Inflammation du gland du pénis (balanite)	Inflamación del glande del pene (balanitis)	Infiammazione della testa del glande (balanite)	Upala glavića penisa (balanitis)

English	French	Spanish	Italian	Croatian
Inflammation of the gums (gingivitis)	Inflammation de la gencive (gingivite)	Inflamación de las encías (gingivitis)	Infiammazione dei tessuti gengivali (gengivite)	Upala desni (gingivitis)
Inflammation of the heart muscle (myocarditis)	Inflammation du myocarde (myocardite)	Inflamación del miocardio (miocarditis)	Infiammazione del miocardio (miocardite)	Upala srčanog mišića (miokarditis)
Inflammation of the inner ear (labyrinthitis)	Inflammation de l'oreille interne (labyrinthite, otite interne)	Inflamación del laberinto del oído interno (laberintitis)	Infiammazione di labirinto nell'orecchio interno (labirintite)	Upala labirinta u unutarnjem uhu (labirintitis)
Inflammation of the joint (arthritis)	Inflammation des articulations (arthrite)	Inflamación de una articulación (artritis)	Infiammazione articolare (artrite)	Upala zgloba (artritis)
Inflammation of the kidney (nephritis)	Inflammation du rein (néphrite)	Inflamación del riñón (nefritis)	Infiammazione dei reni (nefrite)	Upala bubrega (nefritis)
Inflammation of the larynx (laryngitis)	Inflammation du larynx (laryngite)	Inflamación de la laringe (laringitis)	Infiammazione della laringe (laringite)	Upala glasnica (laringitis)
Inflammation of the liver (hepatitis)	Inflammation du foie (hépatite)	Inflamación del hígado (hepatitis)	Infiammazione del fegato (epatite)	Upala jetre (hepatitis)
Inflammation of the lung (pneumonia)	Inflammation des poumons (pneumonie)	Inflamación de los pulmones (neumonía, pulmonía, neumonitis)	Infiammazione dei polmoni (polmonite)	Upala pluća (pneumonija)
Inflammation of the lymph node (lymphadenitis)	Inflammation des ganglions (adénite, lymphadénite)	Inflamación de los ganglios linfáticos (linfadenitis)	Infiammazione delle ghiandole linfatiche (linfoadenite)	Upala limfnog čvora (limfadenitis)
Inflammation of the meninges (meningitis)	Inflammation des méninges (méningite)	Inflamación de las meninges (meningitis)	Infiammazione delle meningi (meningite)	Upala moždanih ovojnica (meningitis)
Inflammation of the middle layer of the eye (uveitis)	Inflammation de l'uvée (uvéite)	Inflamación de la lámina intermedia del ojo (uveítis)	Infiammazione della tunica media dell'occhio (uveite)	Upala srednje ovojnice oka (uveitis)
Inflammation of the mouth mucous lining (stomatitis)	Inflammation de la muqueuse buccale (stomatite)	Inflamación de la mucosa bucal (estomatitis)	Infiammazione delle mucose della bocca (stomatite)	Upala sluznice usta (stomatitis)
Inflammation of the muscles (myositis)	Inflammation du tissu musculaire (myosite)	Inflamación del músculo esquelético (miositis)	Infiammazione del tessuto muscolare (miosite)	Upala mišića (miozitis)
Inflammation of the nerve (neuritis)	Inflammation du nerf (névrite)	Inflamación del nervio (neuritis)	Infiammazione del nervo (neurite, nevrite)	Upala živca (neuritis)
Inflammation of the pancreas (pancreatitis)	Inflammation du pancréas (pancréatite)	Inflamación del páncreas (pancreatitis)	Infiammazione del pancreas (pancreatite)	Upala gušterače (pankreatitis)
Inflammation of the parametrium (parametritis)	Inflammation du paramètre (paramétrite)	Inflamación del parametrio (parametritis)	Infiammazione del parametrio (parametrite)	Upala parametrija (parametritis)
Inflammation of the paranasal sinuses (sinusitis)	Inflammation du sinus (sinusite)	Inflamación de los senos paranasales (sinusitis)	Infiammazione dei seni paranasali (sinusite)	Upala sinusa (sinusitis)
Inflammation of the pericardium (pericarditis)	Inflammation du péricarde (péricardite)	Inflamación del pericardio (pericarditis)	Infiammazione del pericardio (pericardite)	Upala osrčja (perikarditis)
Inflammation of the peritoneum (peritonitis)	Inflammation du péritoine (péritonite)	Inflamación del peritoneo (peritonitis)	Infiammazione dela sierosa peritoneale (peritonite)	Upala potrbušnice (peritonitis)
Inflammation of the pleura (pleuritis)	Inflammation de la plèvre (pleurésie)	Inflamación de la pleura (pleuritis, pleuresía)	Infiammazione della pleura (pleurite)	Upala plućne ovojnice (pleuritis)
Inflammation of the prostate gland (prostatitis)	Inflammation de la prostate (prostatite)	Inflamación de la próstata (prostatitis)	Infiammazione della ghiandola prostatica (prostatite)	Upala prostate (prostatitis)
Inflammation of the retina (retinitis)	Inflammation de la rétine (rétinite)	Inflamación de la retina (retinitis)	Infiammazione della retina (retinite)	Upala mrežnice (retinitis)
Inflammation of the salivary gland (sialadenitis)	Inflammation des glandes salivaires (sialoadénite)	Inflamación de las glándulas salivales (sialadenitis)	Infiammazione delle ghiandole salivari (sialadenite)	Upala žlijezda slinovnica (sialadenitis)
Inflammation of the skin (dermatitis)	Inflammaton de la peau (dermatite)	Inflamación de la piel (dermatitis)	Infiammazione della pelle (dermatite)	Upala kože (dermatitis)
Inflammation of the stomach lining (gastritis)	Inflammation de la paroi de l'estomac (gastrite)	Inflamación de la mucosa gástrica (gastritis)	Infiammazione della mucosa gastrica (gastrite)	Upala želučane sluznice (gastritis)
Inflammation of the synovial fluid sac (bursitis)	Inflammation de la bourse séreuse articulaire (hygroma, bursite)	Inflamación de la bursa (bursitis)	Infiammazione della borsa sierosa di un'articolazione (borsite)	Upala sluzne vreće (burzitis)
Inflammation of the synovial membrane (synovitis)	Inflammation de la gaine synoviale (synovite)	Inflamación de la membrana sinovial (sinovitis)	Infiammazione della membrana sinoviale (sinovite)	Upala tetivne ovojnice (sinovitis)
Inflammation of the synovium and tendon (tenosynovitis)	Inflammation d'un tendon et de sa gaine synoviale (ténosynovite)	Inflamación de un tendón y de su vaina (tenosinovitis)	Infiammazione di tendine e di guaina tendinea (tenosinovite)	Upala tetive s ovojnicom (tenosinovitis)
Inflammation of the tendon (tendinitis, tendonitis)	Inflammation d'un tendon (tendinite)	Inflamación de un tendón (tendinitis)	Infiammazione del tendine (tendinite)	Upala tetive (tendinitis)
Inflammation of the testes (orchitis)	Inflammation des testicules (orchite)	Inflamación del testículo (orquitis)	Infiammazione dei testicoli (orchite)	Upala testisa (orhitis)
Inflammation of the thymus (thymitis)	Inflammation du thymus	Inflamación del timo (timitis)	Infiammazione del timo	Upala prsne žlijezde (timitis)
Inflammation of the thyroid gland (thyroiditis)	Inflammation de la glande thyroïde (thyroïdite)	Inflamación de la glándula tiroides (tiroiditis)	Infiammazione della tiroide (tiroidite)	Upala štitnjače (tireoiditis)

English	French	Spanish	Italian	Croatian
Inflammation of the tonsils (tonsillitis)	Inflammation des tonsilles (tonsillite)	Inflamación de las amígdalas palatinas (amigdalitis)	Infiammazione delle tonsille (tonsillite)	Upala krajnika (tonzilitis)
Inflammation of the urethra (urethritis)	Inflammation de l'urètre (urétrite)	Inflamación de la uretra (uretritis)	Infiammazione dell'uretra (uretrite)	Upala sluznice mokraćne cijevi (uretritis)
Inflammation of the urinary bladder (cystitis)	Inflammation de la vessie (cystite)	Inflamación de la vejiga urinaria (cistitis)	Infiammazione della vescica urinaria (cistite)	Upala mokraćnog mjehura (cistitis)
Inflammation of the vagina (vaginitis)	Inflammation du vagin (vaginite)	Inflamación de la vagina (vaginitis)	Infiammazione della vagina (vaginite)	Upala rodnice (vaginitis)
Inflammation of the vein (phlebitis)	Inflammation des veines (phlébite)	Inflamación de las venas (flebitis)	Infiammazione delle vene (flebite)	Upala vena (flebitis)
Inflammation of the vulva (vulvitis)	Inflammation de la vulve (vulvite)	Inflamación de la vulva (vulvitis)	Infiammazione della vulva (vulvite)	Upala stidnice (vulvitis)
Inflammation of the windpipe (tracheitis)	Inflammation de la trachée (trachéite)	Inflamación de la tráquea (traqueitis)	Infiammazione della trachea (tracheite)	Upala dušnika (traheitis)
Ingrown nail (onychocryptosis, unguis incarnatus)	Ongle incarné (onychocryptose)	Uña encarnada (onicocriptosis)	Unghia incarnita (onicocriptosi)	Urasli nokat (ungvis inkarnatus)
Inguinal hernia	Hernie inguinale	Hernia inguinal	Ernia inguinale	Preponska kila
Insecticide poisoning	Empoisonnement au insecticide	Envenenamiento por insecticidas	Avvelenamento da insetticidi	Trovanje insekticidima
Insomnia	Insomnie	Insomnio	Insonnia	Nesanica
Intermittent claudication	Claudication intermittente	Claudicación intermitente	Claudicatio intermittens	Intermitentna klaudikacija
Internal bleeding	Saignement interne (hémorragie interne)	Sangrado interno (hemorragia interna)	Emorragia interna	Unutarnje krvarenje
Interstitial lung disease	Maladie pulmonaire interstitielle	Enfermedad pulmonar intersticial	Pneumopatia interstiziale	Intersticijska bolest pluća
Interstitial nephritis	Néphrite interstitielle	Nefritis intersticial	Nefrite interstiziale	Intersticijska upala bubrega
Intestinal atresia	Atrésie intestinale	Atresia intestinal	Atresia intestinale	Crijevna atrezija
Intestinal tuberculosis	Tuberculose intestinale	Tuberculosis intestinal	Tubercolosi intestinale	Tuberkuloza crijeva
Intracerebral hematoma	Hématome intracérébral	Hematoma intracerebral	Ematoma cerebrale	Intracerebralni hematom
Intracerebral hemorrhage	Hémorragie intracérébrale	Hemorragia intracerebral	Emorragia cerebrale	Intracerebralno krvarenje
Intracranial hypertension	Hypertension intra-crânienne	Hipertensión intracraneal	Elevata pressione intracranica	Intrakranijalna hipertenzija
Inverted nipple	Téton ombiliqué	Pezón invertido	Capezzolo invertito	Uvučena bradavica
Involuntary swearing (coprolalia)	Tic de langage à dire des mots vulgaires (coprolalie)	Expresión vocal involuntaria de obscenidades (coprolalia)	Coprolalia	Nekontrolirano psovanje (koprolalija)
Ionising irradiation	Irradiation ionisante	Exposición a las radiaciones ionizantes	Esposizione alle radiazioni ionizzanti	Ionizirajuća ozračenost
Iridodialysis (coredialysis)	Iridodialyse	Iridodiálisis	Iridodialisi	Iridodijaliza
Iritis	Iritis	Iritis	Irite	Iritis
Iron deficiency anemia (sideropenic anemia)	Anémie ferriprive	Anemia ferropénica	Anemia da carenza di ferro	Anemija radi deficita željeza (sideropenična anemija)
Iron poisoning	Empoisonnement au fer	Intoxicación por hierro	Avvelenamento da ferro	Trovanje željezom
Irritable bowel syndrome (spastic colon)	Côlon irritable (côlon spastique)	Síndrome de intestino irritable (colon irritable, colon espástico)	Sindrome del colon irritabile (colon spastico)	Sindrom iritabilnog crijeva (spastični kolon)
Irritant contact dermatitis	Dermite de contact irritative	Dermatitis irritante de contacto	Dermatite irritativo da contatto	Iritantni kontaktni dermatitis
Irritated knee (jumper's knee, patellar tendinopathy)	Genou du sauteur (tendinite rotulienne)	Rodilla de saltador (tendinopatía rotuliana)	Peritendite rotulea (ginocchio del saltatore)	Podraženo koljeno (skakačko koljeno)
Ischemia	Ischémie	Isquemia	Ischemia	Ishemija
Ischemic heart disease	Ischémie myocardique	Isquemia miocárdica (angina de pecho)	Ischemia miocardica	Ishemijska bolest srca
Ischemic limbs	Ischémie des membres	Isquemia de miembros	Ischemia degli arti	Ishemični udovi
Ischemic ulceration	Ulcère ischémique	Úlcera isquémica	Ulcera ischemica	Ishemična ulceracija
Isosporiasis	Isosporose	Isosporiasis	Isosporiasi	Izosporijaza
Itching	Prurit	Prurito (picazón, comezón, rasquiña)	Prurito (pizzicore)	Svrbež
Jaundice (icterus)	Ictère (jaunisse)	Ictericia	Ittero (itterizia)	Žutica (ikterus)
Jellyfish sting burn	Brûlure de méduse	Quemadura de medusa	Ustione da medusa	Opeklina od meduze
Joint contracture	Contracture articulaire	Contractura articular	Contrattura articolare	Kontraktura zgloba
Joint distortion	Distorsion articulaire	Distorsión articular	Distorsione	Uganuće zgloba (distorzija zgloba)
Joint pain (arthralgia)	Douleur articulaire (arthralgie)	Dolor en articulación (artralgia)	Articolazione doloroso (artralgia)	Bol u zglobu (artralgija)
Joint stiffness	Raideur articulaire	Rigidez de las articulaciones	Rigidità dell'articolazione	Zakočenost zgloba
Juvenile osteochondrosis	Ostéochondrose juvénile	Osteocondrosis juvenil	Osteocondrite dissecante	Juvenilna osteohondroza
Juvenile rheumatoid arthritis	Arthrite chronique juvénile	Artritis juvenil	Artrite idiopatica giovanile	Mladenački reumatoidni artritis (juvenilni reumatoidni artritis)
Kala-azar (black fever)	Kala azar (fièvre noire)	Kala azar (fiebre negra)	Kala-azar (febbre d'Assam, splenomegalia infantile)	Kala-azar
Kaposi's sarcoma	Sarcome de Kaposi	Sarcoma de Kaposi	Sarcoma di Kaposi	Kaposijev sarkom (endoteliosarkom)

English	French	Spanish	Italian	Croatian
Kawasaki disease	Maladie de Kawasaki	Enfermedad de Kawasaki	Sindrome di Kawasaki	Kawasakijeva bolest (mukokutani limfoglandularni sindrom)
Keloid	Chéloïde	Queloide	Cheloide	Keloid
Keratosis	Kératose (kératodermie)	Keratosis	Cheratosi	Keratoza
Kernicterus	Kernictère	Kernicterus (encefalopatía neonatal bilirrubínica)	Kernittero (encefalopatia bilirubinica)	Žutica moždanih jezgri
Kidney failure (renal insufficiency)	Insuffisance rénale	Fallo renal (insuficiencia renal)	Insufficienza renale	Zatajenje bubrega (insuficijencija bubrega)
Kidney stone (nephrolithiasis)	Calcul rénal (néphrolithiase, lithiase urinaire)	Piedra en el riñon (cálculo renal, litiasis renal)	Calcolosi renale (nefrolitiasi)	Bubrežni kamenac (nefrolitijaza)
Kidney transplatation	Transplantation rénale	Transplante de riñón	Trapianto renale	Transplantacija bubrega
Kienböck's disease	Maladie de Kienböck	Enfermedad de Kienböck	Morbo di Kienböck	Kienböckova bolest
Kleptomania	Cleptomanie	Cleptomanía	Cleptomania	Kleptomanija
Knee arthrosis	Arthrose du genou (gonarthrose)	Artrosis de rodilla (gonartrosis)	Artrosi di ginocchio	Artroza koljena (gonartroza)
Knee dislocation (luxation of the knee)	Luxation du genou	Luxación de la rodilla	Lussazione del ginocchio	Iščašenje koljena
Knock knees (genu valgum)	Genou cagneux (genu valgum, genou en X)	Genu valgo	Ginocchio valgo	Genu valgum
Knot (lump)	Nodule	Nudo	Nodo (nodulo)	Kvržica
Köhler disease	Maladie de Köhler	Enfermedad de Köhler	Malattia di Köhler	Köhlerova bolest
Koplik's spots	Signe de Koplik	Manchas de Koplik	Macchie di Koplik	Koplikove pjege
Kuru	Kuru	Kuru (muerte de la risa)	Kuru	Kuru (smrtni smijeh)
Kussmaul breathing	Respiration de type Kussmaul	Respiración de Kussmaul	Respiro di Kussmaul	Kussmaulovo disanje
Kyphoscoliosis	Cypho-scoliose	Cifoescoliosis	Cifoscoliosi	Kifoskolioza
Kyphosis	Cyphose	Cifosis	Cifosi	Kifoza
Laceration (tear)	Lacération	Laceración	Lacerazione (strappo)	Razderotina
Lack of coordination of muscle movements (ataxia)	Trouble de coordination des mouvements musculaires (ataxie)	Descoordinación en el movimientos musculares (ataxia)	Disturbo della coordinazione muscolare (atassia)	Poremećaj koordinacije mišićnih pokreta (ataksija)
Lactose intolerance	Intolérance au lactose	Intolerancia a la lactosa	Intolleranza al lattosio	Nepodnošenje laktoze (netolerancija laktoze)
Lambliasis (giardiasis)	Lambliase (giardiase)	Giardiasis (lambliasis)	Giardiasi (lambliasi)	Lamblijaza (giardijaza)
Laryngospasm	Laryngospasme	Laringoespasmo	Laringospasmo	Laringospazam
Lassa fever	Fièvre de Lassa	Fiebre de Lassa	Febbre di Lassa	Groznica Lassa
Lazy eye (amblyopia)	Mal-voyance (amblyopie)	Ojo vago (ambliopía)	Ambliopia	Slabovidnost
Lead poisoning	Empoisonnement au plomb	Envenenamiento por plomo	Avvelenamento da piombo (saturnismo)	Trovanje olovom
Leakage of cerebrospinal fluid through the ear	Écoulement de liquide cérébrospinal par l'oreille (otoliquorrhée)	Salida de líquido cerebroespinal por el oído (otoliquorrea)	Perdita di liquido cerebrospinale dall'orechio (otoliquorrea)	Curenje likvora na uho (cerebrospinalna otoreja)
Leakage of cerebrospinal fluid through the nose	Écoulement de liquide cérébrospinal par le nez (rhinoliquorrhée)	Salida de líquido cerebroespinal por la nariz (rinoliquorrea)	Perdita di liquido cerebrospinale dal naso (rinoliquorrea)	Curenje likvora na nos (cerebrospinalna rinoreja)
Learning disability	Trouble de l'apprentissage	Dificultad del aprendizaje	Disturbo di apprendimento	Poremećaj učenja
Leg varicose veins	Varices des membres inférieurs	Venas varicosas de las piernas	Varici degli arti inferiori	Proširene vene na nogama
Legg-Calvé-Perthes disease	Maladie de Legg-Calvé-Perthes (ostéochondrite primitive de hanche)	Síndrome de Legg-Calvé-Perthes	Malattia di Legg-Perthes-Calvé	Legg-Calvé-Perthesova bolest
Leiomyoma	Léiomyome	Leiomioma	Leiomioma	Lejomiom
Leiomyosarcoma	Leiomyosarcome	Leiomiosarcoma	Leiomiosarcoma	Lejomiosarkom
Leishmaniasis	Leishmaniose	Leishmaniasis	Leishmaniosi	Lišmenijaza
Leprosy	Lèpre	Lepra	Lebbra	Lepra (guba)
Leptospirosis	Leptospirose	Leptospirosis	Leptospirosi	Leptospiroza
Leukemia	Leucémie	Leucemia	Leucemia	Leukemija
Leukocytosis	Leucocytose	Leucocitosis	Leucocitosi	Leukocitoza
Leukodystrophy	Leucodystrophie	Leucodistrofia	Leucodistrofia	Leukodistrofija
Leukoplakia	Leucoplasie	Leucoplaquia	Leucoplachia	Leukoplakija
Leukorrhea	Leucorrhée	Leucorrea	Leucorea	Bijelo pranje
Lichen planus	Lichen plan	Liquen plano	Lichen planus	Lišaj (lichen planus)
Ligament rupture (torn ligament)	Rupture ligamentaire	Ruptura de ligamento	Rottura del legamento	Puknuće ligamenta
Ligament sprain	Déchirure ligamentaire	Desgarro de ligamento	Stiramento del legamento	Istegnuće ligamenta
Limited joint mobility	Mobilité atriculaire limitée	Rango de movimiento articular limitado	Ridotta mobilità articolare	Ograničena pokretljivost zgloba
Limping	Boitlement	Cojera	Zoppicamento	Šepanje
Lipodystrophy	Lipodystrophie	Lipodistrofia	Lipodistrofia	Lipodistrofija
Lipoma	Lipome	Lipoma	Lipoma	Lipom
Liposarcoma	Liposarcome	Liposarcoma	Liposarcoma	Liposarkom
Listeriosis	Listériose	Listeriosis	Listeriosi	Listerioza
Lithium poisoning	Empoisonnement au lithium	Intoxicación por litio	Avvelenamento da litio	Trovanje litijem

English	French	Spanish	Italian	Croatian
Little league elbow syndrome (LLE syndrome)	Syndrome du tunnel cubital	Síndrome del túnel cubital	Sindrome del tunnel cubitale	Sindrom kopljaškog lakta
Liver abscess	Abcès hépatique	Absceso hepático	Ascesso epatico	Apsces jetre
Liver cirrhosis	Cirrhose hépatique	Cirrosis hepática	Cirrosi	Ciroza jetre
Liver insufficiency	Insuffisance hépatique	Fallo hepático (insuficiencia hepática)	Insufficienza epatica	Zatajenje jetre
Long-lasting painful erection (priapism)	Érection persistente douloureuse (priapisme)	Erección sostenida y dolorosa (priapismo)	Erezione persistente dolorosa (priapismo)	Dugotrajna bolna erekcija (prijapizam)
Lordosis	Lordose	Lordosis	Lordosi	Lordoza
Loss of appetite	Perte d'appétit	Pérdida del apetito	Mancanza dell'appetito	Gubitak apetita
Loss of half of a field of vision (hemianopsia)	Perte de la vue dans une moitié du champ visuel (hémianopsie)	Pérdida de la mitad del campo visual (hemianopsia)	Perdita di metà di campo visivo (emianopsia)	Gubitak polovice vidnog polja (hemianopsija)
Loss of language ability (aphasia)	Perte d'habileté d'expression du langage (mutisme, aphasie)	Pérdida de capacidad de producir lenguaje (afasia)	Perdita di abilità di produzione del linguaggio verbale (afasia)	Gubitak sposobnosti govora (afazija)
Loss of olfaction (anosmia)	Perte de la sensibilité aux odeurs (anosmie)	Pérdida del sentido del olfato (anosmia)	Incapacità di percipire gli odori (disosmia)	Gubitak osjeta mirisa
Loss of strenght (asthenia)	Affaiblissement de l'organisme (asthénie)	Pérdida de fuerza muscular (astenia)	Riduzione della forza muscolare (astenia)	Gubitak mišićne snage (astenija)
Loss of the sense of taste (ageusia)	Perte du sens du goût (agueusie)	Pérdida del sentido del gusto (ageusia)	Incapacità di percipire i sapori (ageusia)	Gubitak osjeta okusa
Loss of the sense of touch	Perte du sens du toucher	Pérdida del sentido del tacto	Perdita di senso di tocco	Gubitak osjeta dodoira
Low back pain (lumbago, lumbosacral syndrome)	Lombalgie	Dolor de espalda baja (lumbalgia)	Lombaggine	Križobolja (lumbosakralni sindrom)
Low blood pressure (hypotension)	Baisse de la pression artérielle (hypotension artérielle)	Presión sanguínea baja (hipotensión)	Bassa pressione arteriosa (ipotensione)	Nizak krvni tlak (hipotenzija)
Low semen volume (oligospermia)	Présence de spermatozoïdes en quantité faible (oligospermie)	Bajo volumen de semen (oligospermia)	Produzione di pochi spermatozoi (oligospermia)	Manjak sperme (oligospermija)
Luetic osteomyelitis	Ostéomyélite syphilitique	Osteomielitis luética	Osteomielite luetica	Luetični osteomijelitis
Lung abscess	Abcès pulmonaire	Absceso pulmonar	Ascesso polmonare	Apsces pluća
Lupus erythematosus	Lupus érythémateux	Lupus eritematoso sistémico	Lupus eritematoso sistemico	Sistemski lupus eritematozus
Luxating patella (trick knee, floating patella)	Luxation de la rotule	Luxación de la rótula	Lussazione della rotula	Iščašenje čašice
Lyme disease (lyme borreliosis)	Maladie de Lyme	Enfermedad de Lyme (borreliosis de Lyme)	Malattia di Lyme (borreliosi di Lyme)	Lajmska bolest (Lajmska borelioza)
Lymphangioma	Lymphangiome	Linfangioma	Linfangioma	Limfangiom
Lymphangiosarcoma	Lymphangiosarcome	Linfangiosarcoma	Linfangiosarcoma	Limfangiosarkom
Lymphatic leukemia	Leucémie lymphoïde	Leucemia linfática	Leucemia linfatica	Limfatična leukemija
Lymphedema	Lymphoedème	Linfedema	Linfedema	Limfedem (zastoj limfe)
Lymphocytic choriomeningitis	Chorioméningite lymphocytaire	Coriomeningitis linfocítica	Coriomeningite linfocitaria	Limfocitni koriomeningitis
Lymphoma	Lymphome	Linfoma	Linfoma	Limfom
Macular degeneration	Dégénérescence maculaire	Degeneración macular	Degenerazione maculare	Degeneracija makule
Madelung's deformity	Déformation de Madelung	Deformidad de Madelung	Deformità di Madelung	Madelungov deformitet
Malabsorption	Malabsorption	Malabsorción	Malassorbimento	Malapsorpcija
Malaria	Malaria	Malaria (paludismo)	Malaria	Malarija
Malignant hypertension	Hypertension artérielle maligne	Hipertensión maligna	Ipertensione maligna	Maligna hipertenzija
Malignant mixed tumor	Tumeur mixte malin	Tumor mixto maligno	Tumore misto maligno	Mješoviti maligni tumor
Malignant tumor (cancer)	Tumeur maligne (cancer)	Tumor maligno (cáncer)	Tumore maligno	Zloćudni tumor (maligni tumor, rak)
Mandibular dislocation	Luxation temporo-mandibulaire	Dislocación de la mandibula	Lussazione della mandibola	Iščašenje vilice
Mania	Manie	Manía	Mania	Manija
Marburg hemorrhagic fever	Fièvre hémorragique de Marbourg	Fiebre hemorrágica de Marburgo	Febbre emorragica di Marburg	Marburška hemoragijska groznica
Marfan syndrome	Syndrome de Marfan	Síndrome de Marfan	Sindrome di Marfan	Marfanov sindrom
Mastopathy	Mastopathie	Mastopatía	Mastopatia	Mastopatija
McCune-Albright syndrome	Syndrome de McCune-Albright	Síndrome de McCune-Albright	Sindrome di McCune-Albright-Sternberg	Albrightov sindrom
Measles	Rougeole (1re maladie)	Sarampión	Morbillo	Ospice (morbili)
Mechanic icterus (bile duct obstruction)	Ictère par obstruction des voies biliaires	Ictericia obstructiva	Ittero ostruttivo	Mehanički ikterus
Mechanical injuries	Lésions mécaniques	Lesiones mecánicas	Lesioni meccaniche	Mehaničke ozljede
Medication overdose	Surdose du médicament	Sobredosis de medicamentos	Overdose di farmaci	Predoziranje lijekom
Medullary carcinoma	Carcinome médullaire	Carcinoma medular	Carcinoma midollare	Medularni karcinom
Medulloblastoma	Médulloblastome	Meduloblastoma	Medulloblastoma	Meduloblastom
Megacolon	Mégacolôn	Megacolon	Megacolon	Megakolon
Megaloblastic anemia	Anémie mégaloblastique	Anemia megaloblástica	Anemia megaloblastica	Megaloblastična anemija (anemija radi deficita vitamina)
Melanoma	Mélanome	Melanoma	Melanoma	Melanom

English	French	Spanish	Italian	Croatian
Melasma (chloasma faciei)	Chleuasme (chloasma)	Melasma (cloasma)	Melasma	Kloazma (melazma)
Melioidosis (Whitmore disease)	Mélioïdose	Melioidosis	Melioidosi	Melioidoza
Memory loss	Perte de mémoire	Pérdida de la memoria	Perdita di memoria	Gubitak pamćenja
Meniere's disease	Maladie de Menière	Enfermedad de Menière	Sindrome di Menière	Menierova bolest
Meningioma	Méningiome	Meningioma	Meningioma	Meningeom
Meningocele	Méningocèle	MeningoceleOsteoporosis	Meningocele	Meningokela
Meningoencephalocele	Méningoencphalocèle	Meningoencefalocele	Meningoencefalocele	Meningoencefalokela
Meningomyelocele	Myéloméningocèle	Mielomeningocele	Mielomeningocele	Meningomijelokela
Meniscal disease	Meniscopathie	Meniscopatia	Meniscopatia	Meniskopatija
Meniscus rupture (meniscus tear)	Rupture du ménisque	Ruptura de menisco	Rottura del menisco	Razdor meniskusa
Menopause	Ménopause	Menopausia	Menopausa	Menopauza (klimakterij)
Menstrual disorder	Troubles du cycle menstruel	Trastorno menstrual	Disturbi mestruali	Menstrualne smetnje
Mental retardation	Retard mental (handicap mental)	Retraso mental	Ritardo mentale	Mentalna retardacija
Mercury poisoning	Empoisonnement au mercure	Envenenamiento por mercurio	Avvelenamento da mercurio	Trovanje živom
Mesothelioma	Mésothéliome	Mesotélioma	Mesotelioma	Mezoteliom
Metabolic acidosis	Acidose métabolique	Acidosis metabólica	Acidosi metabolica	Metabolička acidoza
Metal fume fever	Fièvre des métaux	Fiebre de los vapores metálicos	Febbre da inalazione di fumi metallici	Metalna groznica
Metastasis	Métastase	Metástasis	Metastasi	Metastaza
Metatarsalgia (Morton's neuroma)	Métatarsalgie	Metatarsalgia	Metatarsalgia	Metatarzalgija (Mortonova metatarzalgija)
Meteoropathy	Météoropathie	Meteoropatía	Meteoropatia	Meteoropatija
Methanol poisoning	Empoisonnement au méthanol	Intoxicación por metanol	Avvelenamento da metanolo	Trovanje metanolom
Migraine	Migraine	Migraña (jaqueca)	Emicrania	Migrena
Milia (milk spots)	Milium (grutum, acné miliaire)	Milium (milia)	Acne miliare	Milije (dječje akne)
Miliaria rubra (sweat rash)	Miliarie rouge	Miliaria rubra (sarpullido por el calor)	Miliaria rubra	Milijarija rubra
Mitral stenosis	Sténose mitrale	Estenosis mitral	Stenosi mitralica	Stenoza mitralnog ušća
Mixed tumor	Tumeur mixte	Tumor mixto	Tumore misto	Mješoviti tumor
Molluscum contagiosum	Molluscum contagiosum	Molusco contagioso	Mollusco contagioso	Molusk
Monocytic leukemia	Leucémie monocytique	Leucemia monocítica	Leucemia monocitica	Monocitična leukemija
Mood swing	Saute d'humeur	Oscilaciones del humor	Cambiamento d'umore	Promjene raspoloženja
Morquio's syndrome (mucopolysaccharidosis IV)	Maladie de Morquio (mucopolysaccharidose type IV)	Enfermedad de Morquio (mucopolisacaridosis tipo IV)	Malattia di Morquio (mucopolisaccaridosi IV)	Sindrom Morquio (mukopolisaharidoza tip IV)
Motor neurone disease	Maladie du motoneurone	Enfermedad de la motoneurona	Malattia del motoneurone	Bolest motornog neurona
Movement ability	Capacité de mouvement	Capacidad de movimiento	Abilità di muoversi	Sposobnost kretanja
Movement disorder	Trouble du mouvement	Trastorno de movimiento	Disordine del movimento	Poremećaj kretanja
Movement inability	Incapacité de se mouvoir	Incapacidad de movimiento	Mancanza di movimento	Nemogućnost kretanja
MRSA	SARM	SARM	MSSA (MRSA)	MRSA
Mucocele	Mucocèle	Mucocele	Mucocele	Mukocela
Mucopolysaccharidosis	Mucopolysaccharidose	Mucopolisacaridosis	Mucopolisaccaridosi	Mukopolisaharidoza
Mucus in stool	Mucus dans les selles	Moco en las heces	Muco nelle feci	Sluzava stolica
Multiple sclerosis	Sclérose en plaques	Esclerosis múltiple	Sclerosi multipla	Multipla skleroza
Multiple system atrophy	Atrophie multisystématisée	Atrofia multisistémica	Atrofia multi-sistemica	Multipla sistemska atrofija
Mumps (epidemic parotitis)	Oreillons (parotidite virale)	Paperas (parotiditis)	Parotite (orecchioni)	Zaušnjaci (mumps, parotitis)
Murine typhus (endemic typhus)	Typhus murin	Tifus endémico murino	Tifo murino (tifo endemico)	Štakorski pjegavac
Muscle pain (myalgia)	Douleur musculaire (myalgie)	Dolor muscular (mialgia)	Dolore muscolare (mialgia)	Bol u mišiću (mijalgija)
Muscle rupture	Rupture musculaire	Ruptura muscular	Rottura muscolare	Rastrgnuće mišića (ruptura mišića)
Muscle strain (muscle pull)	Déchirure musculaire (claquage)	Desgarro muscular	Strappo muscolare	Istegnuće mišića (distenzija mišića)
Muscle twitch (fasciculation)	Fasciculation musculaire	Crispar del músculo (fasciculación)	Scossa muscolare (fasciciolazione)	Trzanje mišića
Muscular contracture	Contracture musculaire	Contractura muscular	Contrattura muscolare	Kontraktura mišića
Muscular cramp (spasm)	Crampe musculaire (spasme)	Espasmo muscular (calambre)	Spasmo muscolare	Mišićni grč (spazam)
Muscular dystrophy	Dystrophie musculaire	Distrofia muscular	Distrofia muscolare	Mišićna distrofija
Muscular fibrositis	Fibrosite musculaire	Fibrositis (reumatismo muscular)	Fibrosite muscolare	Fibrozitis mišića
Muscular hypotonia	Hypotonie musculaire	Hipotonía muscular	Ipotonia muscolare	Mišićna hipotonija
Mushroom poisoning	Empoisonnement par des champignons	Envenenamiento por setas	Avvelenamento da funghi	Trovanje gljivama
Myasthenia gravis	Myasthénie grave	Miastenia gravis	Miastenia gravis	Miastenija gravis
Mycetoma	Mycétome	Micetoma	Micetoma	Micetoma
Mycosis	Mycose	Micosis	Micosi	Mikoza

English	French	Spanish	Italian	Croatian
Myelodysplastic syndrome	Syndrome myélodysplasique	Síndrome mielodisplásico (preleucemia)	Sindrome mielodisplasica	Mijelodisplastični sindrom
Myeloid leukemia	Leucémie myéloïde	Leucemia mieloide	Leucemia mieloide	Mijeloična leukemija
Myoblastoma	Rhabdomyome granocellulaire	Mioblastoma	Mioblastoma	Mioblastom
Myoclonic twitches (myoclonus)	Myoclonie	Mioclono	Mioclono	Miokloničko trzanje (mioklonus)
Myogelosis	Myogélose	Miogelosis	Miogelosi	Miogeloza
Myoma	Myome	Mioma	Mioma	Miom
Myosarcoma	Myosarcome	Miosarcoma	Miosarcoma	Miosarkom
Myositis ossificans	Myosite ossifiante	Miositis osificante	Miosite ossificante	Osificirajući miozitis
Myositis ossificans progressiva	Myosite ossifiante progressive	Miositis osificante progresiva	Miosite ossificante progressiva	Progresivno okoštavanje mišića
Myxedema	Myxoedème	Mixedema	Mixedema	Miksedem
Myxoma	Myxome	Mixoma	Mixoma	Miksom
Myxosarcoma	Myxosarcome	Mixosarcoma	Mixosarcoma	Miksosarkom
Nail biting (onychophagia)	Se ronger les ongles (onychophagie)	Comerse las uñas (onicofagia)	Abitudine di mangiare le unghie (onicofagia)	Griženje noktiju (onikofagija)
Narcolepsy	Narcolepsie (maladie de Gélineau)	Narcolepsia (síndrome de Gelineau, epilepsia del sueño)	Narcolessia	Narkolepsija
Nasal congestion (stuffy nose)	Congestion nasale	Congestión nasal	Congestione nasale	Začepljeni nos
Nasal polyp	Polype nasal	Pólipo nasal	Polipo nasale	Polip u nosu (nosni polip)
Nasal secretion (mucus)	Mucus nasal	Moco (mucus) nasal	Muco nasale	Sekrecija iz nosa
Nasal septum deviation	Déviation du septum nasal	Desviación del tabique nasal	Deviazione del setto nasale	Devijacija nosnog septuma
Natural death	Mort naturelle	Muerte natural	Morte naturale	Prirodna smrt
Nausea	Nausée	Náusea	Nausea	Mučnina
Neck myalgia	Myalgie cervicale	Mialgia cervical	Mialgia cervicale	Mijalgični sindrom vrata
Neck varicose veins	Varice dans le cou	Varices del cuello	Vene varicose del collo	Proširene vratne vene
Necrosis	Nécrose	Necrosis	Necrosi	Nekroza
Necrotizing fasciitis	Fasciite nécrosante	Fascitis necrotizante	Fascite necrotizzante	Nekrotizirajući fasciitis
Neonatal jaundice	Ictère néonatal	Ictericia del recién nacido	Ittero neonatale	Novorođenačka žutica
Nephrosis	Néphrose	Nefrosis	Nefrosi	Nefroza
Nephrotic syndrome	Syndrome néphrotique	Síndrome nefrótico	Sindrome nefrosica	Nefrotski sindrom
Nerve compression (pinched nerve)	Compression du nerf	Compresión del nérvio	Compressone del nervo	Kompresija živca (ukliješten živac)
Nerve lesion	Lésion du nerf	Lesión de nervio	Lesione del nervo	Oštećenje živca (lezija živca)
Neuralgia	Névralgie	Neuralgia	Nevralgia	Neuralgija
Neurasthenia	Neurasthénie	Neurastenia	Nevrastenia	Neurastenija
Neurinoma	Neurinome	Neurinoma	Neurinoma (Schwannoma)	Neurinom
Neuroblastoma	Neuroblastome	Neuroblastoma	Neuroblastoma	Neuroblastom
Neuroborreliosis	Neuroborréliose	Neuroborreliosis	Neuroborreliosi	Neuroborelioza
Neurofibromatosis type 1 (Von Recklinghausen's disease)	Neurofibromatose de type 1 (maladie de Von Recklinghausen)	Neurofibromatosis de tipo 1 (enfermedad de Von Recklinghausen)	Neurofibromatosi di tipo1 (malattia di von Recklinghausen)	Von Recklinghausenova bolest
Neurogenic shock	Choc neurogénique	Choque neurogénico	Shock neurogeno	Neurogeni šok
Neuroma	Neurome	Neuroma	Neuroma	Neurom
Neuropathy	Neuropathie	Neuropatía	Neuropatia	Neuropatija
Neurosis	Névrose (neurose)	Neurosis	Nevrosi	Neuroza
Night blindness (nyctalopia)	Cécité nocturne (héméralopie)	Ceguera nocturna (nictalopia)	Cecità notturna (nictalopia)	Noćno sljepilo
Night sweats	Sueurs nocturnes	Sudor nocturno	Sudore notturno	Noćno znojenje
Nocturnal leg cramps	Crampes nocturnes des jambes	Calambres nocturnos en las piernas	Crampo notturno alle gambe	Noćni grčevi u nogama
Nodular goiter	Goitre multinodulaire	Bocio nodular	Gozzo multinodulare	Čvorasta guša (nodularna struma)
Non-Hodgkin's lymphoma	Lymphome non-Hodgkinien	Linfoma no-Hodgkin	Linfoma non Hodgkin	Non-Hodgkinov limfom
Non-ionising irradiation	Irradiation non-ionisante	Irradiación no-ionizante	Irradiazione non ionizzante	Neionizirajuća ozračenost
Nonpassage of urine	Arrêt de la sécrétion d'urine	Supresión de la secreción de orina	Soppressione della secrezione di urina	Prestanak lučenja urina
Nose bleeding (epistaxis)	Saignement de nez (épistaxis)	Pérdida de sangre por la nariz (epistaxis)	Epistassi (rinorragia)	Krvarenje iz nosa (epistaksa)
Nuchal rigidity (stiff neck)	Raideur de nuque (raideur méningée)	Rigidez de nuca (cuello rígido)	Rigidità nucale	Kočenje šije (ukočeni vrat)
Numbness in limbs	Engourdissements dans les membres (paresthésie)	Adormecimiento de las extremidades	Parestesie delle estremità	Utrnulost udova
Nummular dermatitis	Dermatite nummulaire	Dermatitis numular	Dermatite nummulare	Numularni dermatitis
Nystagmus	Nystagmus	Nistagmo	Nistagmo	Nistagmus
Obesity	Obésité	Obesidad	Obesità	Debljina (gojaznost)
Oblique fracture	Fracture oblique	Fractura obliqua	Frattura obliqua	Kosi prijelom kosti
Obstructive lesion of the small intestine	Lésion obstructive de l'intestin grêle	Lesión obstructiva del intestino delgado	Lesione ostruttiva dell'intestino tenue	Opstruktivna lezija tankog crijeva
Obstructive shock	Choc obstructive	Choque obstructivo	Shock ostruttivo	Opstruktivni šok
Occipital neuralgia (Arnold's neuralgia)	Nèvralgie occipitale	Síndrome occipital (neuralgia occipital)	Nevralgia occipitale (nevralgia di Arnold)	Okcipitalna neuralgija

English	French	Spanish	Italian	Croatian
Occupational disease	Maladie professionnelle	Enfermedad profesional	Malattia professionale	Profesionalno oboljenje
Oligodendroglioma	Oligodendrocytome	Oligodendroglioma	Oligodendroglioma	Oligodendrogliom
Oligomenorrhea	Oligoménorrhée	Oligomenorrea	Oligomenorrea	Oligomenoreja
Onchocerciasis (river blindness)	Onchocercose (cécité des rivières)	Oncocercosis	Oncocercosi (cecità fluviale)	Onkocerkijaza (riječno sljepilo)
Open fracture (compound fracture)	Fracture ouverte	Fractura abierta	Frattura aperta (frattura esposta)	Otvoreni prijelom kosti
Optic nerve edema	Oedème du nerf optique	Edema del nervio óptico	Papilledema (edema del nervo ottico)	Otok očnog živca (zastojna papila)
Orbital cellulitis	Cellulite orbitale	Celulitis orbital	Cellulite orbitale	Celulitis orbite
Oroya fever (Carrion's disease)	Fièvre d'Oroya (maladie de Carrion)	Fiebre de la Oroya (enfermedad de Carrión, verruga peruana)	Febbre di Oroya	Oroya groznica (Carrionova bolest)
Osgood-Schlatter disease (rugby knee)	Maladie d'Osgood-Schlatter	Enfermedad de Osgood-Schlatter	Sindrome di Osgood-Schlatter	Osgood-Schlatterova bolest
Osteitis fibrosa cystica	Ostéite fibrokystique	Ostéitis fibrosa quística	Osteitis fibrosa cistica	Fibrozna cistična upala kosti
Osteochondroma	Ostéochondrome	Osteocondroma	Osteocondroma	Osteohondrom
Osteogenesis imperfecta (brittle bone disease)	Ostéogenèse imparfaite	Osteogénesis imperfecta (huesos de cristal)	Osteogenesi imperfetta	Osteogeneza imperfekta (staklaste kosti)
Osteoma	Ostéome	Osteoma	Osteoma	Osteom
Osteomalacia	Ostéomalacie	Osteomalacia	Osteomalacia	Osteomalacija
Osteopetrosis (marble bone disease)	Ostéopétrose (os de marbre)	Osteopetrosis (enfermedad de los huesos de marmol)	Osteopetrosi (malattia delle ossa di marmo)	Osteopetroza (zadebljane kosti, bolest mramornih kostiju)
Osteoporosis	Ostéoporose	Osteoporosis	Osteoporosi	Osteoporoza
Osteosarcoma	Ostéosarcome	Osteosarcoma	Osteosarcoma	Osteosa
Osteosclerosis	Ostéosclérose	Osteosclerosis	Osteosclerosi	Osteoskleroza
Ovarian cyst	Kyste ovarien	Quiste ovárico	Cisti ovarica	Cista na jajniku
Ovulation pain (mittelschmerz)	Douleurs ovulatoires (mittelschmerz)	Ovulación dolorosa	Dolore ovulatorio (mittelschmerz)	Bolna ovulacija (mittelschmerz)
Paget's disease	Maladie de Paget	Enfermedad de Paget	Morbo di Paget	Pagetova bolest
Pain	Douleur	Dolor	Dolore	Bol
Pain syndrome	Syndrome de douleur	Síndrome doloroso	Sindrome dolorosa	Bolni sindrom
Painful menstruation (dysmenorrhea)	Règle douloureuse (dysménorrhée)	Menstruación dolorosa (dismenorrea)	Mestruazione dolorosa (dismenorrea)	Bolna menstruacija (dismenoreja)
Painful sexual intercourse (dyspareunia)	Douleur lors du rapport sexuel (dyspareunie)	Relación sexual dolorosa (coitalgia, dispareunia)	Dolore durante rapporto sessuale (dispareunia)	Bol pri snošaju
Painful swallowing (odynophagia)	Déglutition douloureuse (odynophagie)	Dolor al tragar (odinofagia)	Deglutizione dolorosa (odinofagia)	Bolno gutanje (odinofagija)
Painful urination (strangury)	Urination douloureuse (strangurie)	Micción dolorosa (angurria)	Minzione dolorosa (stranguria)	Bol pri mokrenju (strangurija)
Paleness (pallor)	Pâleur	Palidez	Pallore	Bljedilo
Palpitation	Palpitation	Palpitación	Cardiopalmo (palpitazione)	Lupanje srca (palpitacije)
Pancreatic cyst	Kyste du pancréas	Quiste de páncreas	Cisti pancreatica	Cista na gušterači
Pancreatic lipomatosis	Lipomatose du pancréas	Lipomatosis pancreática (reemplazo graso del páncreas)	Lipomatosi pancreatica	Lipomatoza gušterače (masna infiltracija gušterače)
Panic attack	Crise de panique	Ataque de pánico	Attaco di panico	Napadaj panike
Panner's disease	Maladie de Panner	Enfermedad de Panner	Malattia di Panner	Pannerova bolest
Papillary carcinoma	Carcinome papillaire	Carcinoma papilar	Carcinoma papillare	Papilarni karcinom
Papilloma	Papillome	Papiloma	Papilloma	Papilom
Pappataci fever (phlebotomus fever, sandfly fever)	Fièvre pappataci (fièvre à phlébotomes)	Fiebre pappataci	Febbre da pappataci (febbre da Flebotomi)	Papatači-groznica
Paracetamol poisoning	Intoxication par le paracétamol	Intoxicación por paracetamol	Avvelenamento da paracetamolo	Trovanje paracetamolom
Paracoccidioidomycosis (Brazilian blastomycosis)	Paracoccidioidose brésilienne	Paracoccidioidomicosis	Paracoccidioidimicosi (blastomicosi sudamericana)	Parakokcidioidomikoza (brazilska blastomikoza)
Paragonimiasis	Paragonimiase humaine	Paragonimosis (paragonimiasis)	Paragonimiasi	Paragonimijaza
Paralysis	Paralysie	Parálisis	Paralisi	Paraliza (oduzetost, kljenut)
Paralysis of all limbs and torso (quadriplegia, tetraplegia)	Paralysie des quatre membres (tétraplégie)	Parálisis en brazos y piernas (tetraplejía, cuadriplejia)	Paralisi dei arti superiori e inferiori(quadriplegia)	Oduzetost gornjih i donjih ekstremiteta i torza(kvadriplegija, tetraplegija)
Paralysis of lower extremities (paraplegia)	Paralysie des membres inférieurs (paraplégie)	Parálisis de la parte inferior del cuerpo (paraplejía)	Paralisi di parte inferiore del corpo (paraplegia)	Oduzetost donjih ekstremiteta (paraplegija)
Paralysis of one half of a body (hemiplegia)	Paralysie de la moitié du corps (hémiplégie)	Parálisis de una mitad lateral de cuerpo (hemiplejía)	Paralisi di una metà del corpo (emiplegia)	Oduzetost jedne polovine tijela (hemiplegija)
Paralysis of symmetrical parts of the body (diplegia)	Paralysie des régions symétriques du corps (diplégie)	Parálisis de partes simétricas del cuerpo (diplejía)	Paralisi di una parte di corpo simmetrica (diplegia)	Oduzetost simetričnih dijelova tijela (diplegija)
Paranoia	Paranoïa	Paranoia	Paranoia	Paranoja
Parasitic disease (parasitosis)	Maladie parasitique (parasitose)	Enfermedad parasitaria (parasitosis)	Malattia parassitaria (parassitosi)	Parazitarna bolest (parazitoza)
Paratyphoid fever	Fièvre paratyphoïde	Fiebre paratifoidea	Febbre paratifoide	Trbušni paratifus

English	French	Spanish	Italian	Croatian
Paresis	Parésie	Paresis	Paresi	Pareza
Parkinson's disease	Maladie de Parkinson	Enfermedad de Parkinson	Morbo di Parkinson	Parkinsonova bolest
Paronychia	Paronychie	Paroniquia	Paronichia	Paronihija
Partial dislocation (subluxation)	Luxation incomplète (subluxation)	Desplazamiento de una articulación (subluxación)	Lussazione incompleta (sublussazione)	Djelomična dislokacija (subluksacija)
Passage of large volumes of urine (polyuria)	Sécrétion d'urine en quantité abondante (polyurie)	Gasto urinario excesivo (poliuria)	Aumentata emissione di urina (poliuria)	Učestalo mokrenje velikih količina mokraće (poliurija)
Passing gas (flatulence, farting)	Pet (flatulence, vesse)	Tener gases (flatulencia)	Miscela di gas (flatulenza)	Puštanje vjetra (flatulencija, plinovi)
Patau syndrome (trisomy 13)	Syndrome de Patau (trisomie 13)	Síndrome de Patau (trisomía en el par 13)	Sindrome di Patau	Trisomija 13D (Patauov sindrom)
Patent ductus arteriosus (persistent ductus arteriosus)	Persistance du canal artériel	Ductus arterioso persistente (conducto arterioso persistente)	Dotto arterioso persistente (ductus arteriosus persistente)	Otvoreni ductus arteriosus (Ductus arteriosus persistens)
Pectus excavatum	Thorax en entonnoir (pectus excavatum)	Pecho hundido (pectus excavatum)	Torace a imbuto (petto escavato)	Udubljena prsa (ljevkasta prsa)
Pellegrini-Stieda disease	Maladie de Pellegrini-Stieda	Enfermedad de Pellegrini-Stieda	Malattia di Pellegrini-Stieda	Bolest Pellegrini-Stieda
Pelvic inflammatory disease	Maladie pelvienne inflammatoire	Enfermedad pélvica inflamatoria	Malattia infiammatoria pelvica	Upalna bolest zdjelice
Pemphigus	Pemphigus	Pénfigo	Pemfigo	Pemfigus
Perforated eardrum (tympanorrhexis)	Perforation du tympan	Perforación del tímpano	Perforazione del timpano	Puknuće bubnjića (perforacija bubnjića, timpanoreksija)
Perforated ulcer	Perforation d'ulcère	Úlcera perforada	Ulcera perforata	Puknuće čira (perforacija ulkusa)
Perianal abscess	Abcès périanal	Absceso perianal	Ascesso perianale	Perianalni apsces
Pericardial carcinosis	Carcinose péricardique	Carcinosis pericárdica	Carcinosi pericardiale	Karcinoza perikarda
Pericardial effusion (hydropericard)	Épanchement péricardique	Derrame pericárdico	Idropericardio	Hidroperikard
Pericardial tamponade (cardiac tamponade)	Tamponnade cardiaque	Tamponamiento cardíaco (tamponamiento pericárdiaco)	Tamponamento cardiaco	Tamponada perikarda
Perinephric abscess	Abcès périnéphrique	Absceso perinéfrico	Ascesso perinefrico	Paranefritički apsces
Periodic breathing (Cheyne-Stokes respiration)	Respiration Cheynes-Stokes	Respiración periódica (respiración de Cheynes-Stokes)	Respiro di Cheyne-Stokes	Periodično disanje (Cheyne-Stokesovo disanje)
Periodontitis	Parodontite	Periodontitis (piorrea)	Parodontite	Parodontoza
Peripheral nerve lesion	Lésion du nerf périphérique	Lesión de nervio periférico	Lesione del nervo periferico	Oštećenje perifernog živca
Peritoneal carcinosis	Carcinose péritonéale	Carcinosis peritoneal	Carcinosi peritoneale	Karcinoza peritoneuma
Pernicious anemia	Anémie pernicieuse	Anemia perniciosa	Anemia perniciosa	Perniciozna anemija
Personality changes	Changements de personnalité	Cambios de personalidad	Cambiamenti di personalità	Promjene osobnosti
Personality disorder	Trouble de la personnalité	Trastorno de personalidad	Disturbo di personalità	Poremećaj osobnosti
Pes calcaneus	Pied calcanéus	Pie calcáneo	Piede calcaneo	Petno stopalo
Pes valgus	Pied valgus	Pie valgo	Piede piatto valgo (pes valgus)	Izvrnuto stopalo (pes valgus)
Petechia	Pétéchie	Petequia	Petecchia	Petehije
Peyronie's disease (induratio penis plastica)	Maladie de La Peyronie	Enfermedad de La Peyronie (induración plástica del pene)	Induratio penis plastica (malattia di Peyronie)	Plastična induracija penisa
Phantom pain	Douleur du membre fantôme	Dolor del miembro fantasma	Dolore fantomatico	Fantomska bol
Phenylketonuria	Phénylcétonurie	Fenilcetonuria	Fenilchetonuria	Fenilketonurija
Pheochromocytoma	Phéochromocytome	Feocromocitoma	Feocromocitoma	Feokromocitom (tumor srži nadbubrežne žlijezde)
Phimosis	Phimosis	Fimosis	Fimosi	Fimoza
Phlebothrombosis	Phlébothrombose	Flebotrombosis	Flebotrombosi	Flebotromboza
Phlegmon	Phlegmon	Flegmón	Flemmone	Flegmona
Phobia	Phobie	Fobia	Fobia	Fobija
Photophobia (fear of light)	Photophobie (crainte de la lumière)	Fotofobia (intolerancia a la luz)	Fotofobia	Fotofobija (strah od svjetla)
Pig flu (swine influenza, influenzavirus A subtype H1N1)	Gripe porcine	Gripe porcina (influenza porcina, gripe del cerdo)	Influenza suina	Svinjska gripa
Pigeon chest (pectus carinatum)	Pectus carinatum	Pectus carinatum	Petto carenato	Kokošja prsa
Pilonidal cyst	Kyste pilonidal	Quiste pilonidal	Cisti pilonidale	Pilonidalna cista
Pinta	Pinta	Pinta	Pinta	Pinta
Plague (pest)	Peste	Peste	Peste (pestilenza)	Kuga
Plantar fasciitis	Fasciite plantaire	Fascitis plantar	Fasciosi plantare	Plantarni fasciitis
Plasmacytoma (multiple myeloma)	Plasmocytome (myélome multiple)	Plasmacitoma (mieloma múltiple)	Mieloma multiplo	Plazmocitom (multipli mijelom)
Pleural carcinosis	Carcinose pleurale	Carcinosis pleural	Carcinosi pleurica	Karcinoza pleure
Pneumoconiosis	Pneumoconiose	Neumoconiosis	Pneumoconiosi	Pneumokonioza

English	French	Spanish	Italian	Croatian
Pneumocystis pneumonia (pneumocystosis)	Pneumocystose	Neumonía por Pneumocystis	Polmonite da Pneumocisti	Pneumocistična upala pluća
Pneumothorax	Pneumothorax	Neumotórax	Pneumotorace	Pneumotoraks
Poisoning (toxication)	Empoisonnement (toxicité)	Envenenamiento (intoxicación)	Avvelenamento (intossicazione)	Trovanje
Poliomyelitis (polio, infantile paralysis)	Poliomyélite (polio, paralysie spinale infantile)	Poliomielitis (parálisis infantil)	Poliomielite (polio, paralisi infantile)	Dječja paraliza (polio, poliomijelitis)
Pollen allergy	Allergie au pollen	Alergia al polen	Allergia da poline	Alergija na pelud
Polycystic kidney disease	Rein polykystique	Enfermedad poliquística renal	Rene policistico	Policistični bubreg
Polycythemia	Polycythémie	Policitemia	Policitemia	Policitemija
Polydactyly	Polydactylie	Polidactilia	Polidattilia	Polidaktilija
Polymyalgia rheumatica	Polymyalgia rheumatica	Polimialgia reumática	Polimialgia reumatica	Reumatska polimialgija
Polymyositis	Polymyosite	Polimiositis	Polimiosite	Polimiozitis
Polyp	Polype	Pólipo	Polipo	Polip
Popliteus syndrome	Syndrome poplité douloureux	Tendinitis poplítea	Tendinite del popliteo	Sindrom m. popliteusa
Porphyria	Porphyrie	Porfiria	Porfiria	Porfirija
Portal hypertension	Hypertension portale	Hipertensión portal	Ipertensione portale	Portalna hipertenzija
Post-necrotic cirrhosis	Cirrhose postnecrotique	Cirrosis postnecrótica	Cirrosi post-necrotica	Postnekrotična ciroza
Post-thrombotic syndrome	Syndrome post-thrombotique	Síndrome postrombótico	Sindrome post trombotica	Posttrombotički sindrom
Post-traumatic headache	Céphalée post-traumatique	Cefalea postraumática	Cefalea post-traumatica	Posttraumatska glavobolja
Posterior ankle impingement syndrome	Conflit postérieur de la cheville	Síndrome de pinzamiento posterior del tobillo	Sindrome da impingement posteriore di caviglia	Sindrom sraza stražnjeg nožnog zgloba
Posttraumatic stress disorder	Trouble de stress post-traumatique	Trastorno por estrés postraumático	Disturbo post traumatico da stress	Posttraumatski stresni poremećaj (PTSP)
Postural back pain	Lombalgie posturale	Dolor de espalda postural	Mal di schiena su base posturale	Posturalna križobolja
Postural edema	Oedème postural	Edema postural	Edema posturale	Posturalni edem (statički edem)
Precocious puberty (premature puberty)	Puberté précoce	Pubertad precoz	Pubertà precoce (pubertà prematura)	Preuranjeni pubertet
Preiser disease	Maladie de Preiser	Enfermedad de Preiser	Sindrome di Preiser	Morbus Preiser
Premature ejaculation	Éjaculation précoce	Eyaculación precoz	Eiaculazione precoce	Prijevremena ejakulacija
Premature sexual development of the opposite sex	Développement sexuel prématuré du sexe opposé	Desarrollo sexual prematuro del sexo opuesto	Prematuro sviluppo sessuale del sesso opposto	Prerano spolno fizičko sazrijevanje suprotnog spola
Premature sexual development of the same sex	Développement sexuel prématuré du même sexe	Desarrollo sexual prematuro del mismo sexo	Prematuro sviluppo sessuale dello stesso sesso	Prerano splono fizičko sazrijevanje istog spola
Premenstrual syndrome (PMS)	Syndrome prémenstruel (SPM)	Síndrome premenstrual	Sindrome premestruale	Predmenstruacijski sindrom (PMS)
Primary amoebic meningoencephalitis	Méningo-encéphalite amibienne primaire	Meningoencefalitis amebiana primaria	Meningoencefalite amebica primaria	Primarni amebni meningoencefalitis
Prinzmetal's angina	Angine de Prinzmetal	Angina de Prinzmetal	Angina di Prinzmetal	Prinzmetalova angina
Proctitis	Proctite	Proctitis	Proctite	Proktitis
Productive cough	Toux productive	Tos productiva	Tosse produttiva	Produktivni kašalj
Progressive muscular dystrophy	Dystrophie musculaire progressive	Distrofia muscular progresiva	Distrofia muscolare progressiva	Progresivna mišićna distrofija
Prostate cancer	Cancer de la prostate	Cáncer de próstata	Cancro della prostata	Rak prostate
Prostate carcinoma	Carcinome de la prostate	Carcinoma de próstata	Carcinoma della prostata	Karcinom prostate
Proteinuria (presence of proteins in urine)	Protéinurie (excès de protéines dans l'urine)	Proteinuria	Proteinuria	Bjelančevine u urinu (proteinurija)
Pseudoepitheliomatous hyperplasia	Hyperplasie pseudo-épithéliomateuse	Hiperplasia pseudoepiteliomatosa	Iperplasia pseudoepiteliomatosa	Pseudoepiteliematozna hiperplazija
Psittacosis (parrot fever)	Psittacose	Psitacosis (fiebre del loro)	Psittacosi (psittacornitosi)	Psitakoza
Psoriasis	Psoriasis	Psoriasis	Psoriasi	Psorijaza
Psoriatic arthritis	Arthrite psoriatique	Artritis psoriásica	Artrite psoriasica	Psorijatični artritis
Psychic changes	Changements psychiques	Cambios psíquicos	Alterazioni dello stato psishico	Psihičke promjene
Psychoneurosis	Psychonévrose	Psiconeurosis	Psiconevrosi (nevrosi)	Psihoneuroza
Psychopathy	Psychopathie	Psicopatía	Psicopatia	Psihopatija
Psychosis	Psychose	Psicosis	Psicosi	Psihoza
Pulmonary alveolar proteinosis	Protéinose alvéolaire pulmonaire	Proteinosis alveolar pulmonar	Proteinosi alveolare polmonare	Alveolarna proteinoza pluća
Pulmonary atelectasis	Atélectasie pulmonaire	Atelectasia pulmonar	Atelectasia polmonare	Atelektaza pluća
Pulmonary congestion	Congestion pulmonaire	Congestión pulmonar	Congestione polmonare	Plućna kongestija
Pulmonary echinococcosis	Échinococcose pulmonaire	Hidatidosis pulmonar	Echinococcosi polmonare	Ehinokokoza pluća
Pulmonary edema	Oedème pulmonaire	Edema pulmonar	Edema polmonare	Plućni edem
Pulmonary embolism	Embolie pulmonaire	Embolia pulmonar	Embolia polmonare	Plućna embolija
Pulmonary heart disease	Coeur pulmonaire	Enfermedad cardíaca pulmonar (cor pulmonale)	Cuore polmonare	Plućno srce
Pulmonary hypertension	Hypertension artérielle pulmonaire	Hipertensión arterial pulmonar	Ipertensione arteriosa polmonare	Plućna hipertenzija

English	French	Spanish	Italian	Croatian
Pulmonary hypoplasia	Hypoplasie pulmonaire	Hipoplasia pulmonar	Ipoplasia del tronco polmonare	Hipoplazija plućnog režnja
Pulmonary infarction	Infarctus pulmonaire	Infarto pulmonar	Infarto polmonare	Infarkt pluća
Pulmonary tuberculosis	Tuberculose pulmonaire	Tuberculosis pulmonar	Tubercolosi polmonare	Tuberkuloza pluća
Pulmonary valve stenosis	Sténose de la valve pulmonaire	Estenosis de la válvula pulmonar	Stenosi polmonare	Stenoza plućnog ušća (pulmonalna stenoza)
Pulsing pain	Douleur pulsatile	Dolor pulsante	Dolore pulsante	Pulsirajuća bol
Purpura	Purpura	Púrpura	Porpora	Purpura
Pus	Pus	Pus	Pus	Gnoj
Pus in sputum	Crachat purulent	Esputo que contiene pus	Presenza di pus nello sputo	Gnojni ispljuvak
Pus in urine (pyuria)	Présence de pus dans l'urine (pyurie)	Presencia de pus en la orina (piuria)	Presenza di pus nelle urine (piuria)	Gnoj u urinu (piurija)
Pustule	Pustule	Pústula	Pustola	Gnojni mjehurić
Pyelonephritis (kidney infection)	Pyélonéphrite (infection bactérienne des voies urinaires hautes)	Pielonefritis (infección urinaria alta)	Pielonefrite	Pijelonefritis (infekcija bubrega)
Pyloric stenosis	Sténose du pylore	Estenosis del píloro	Stenosi pilorica	Stenoza pilorusa (pilorostenoza)
Pylorospasm	Spasme du pylore	Pilorospasmo	Pilorospasmo	Pilorospazam
Pyonephrosis	Pyonéphrose (pus dans le rein)	Pionefrosis	Pionefrosi	Pionefroza
Pyromania	Pyromanie	Piromanía	Piromania	Piromanija
Q fever	Fièvre Q	Fiebre Q	Febbre Q	Q-groznica
Quinsy (peritonsillar abscess)	Abcès périamygdalien	Absceso peritonsilar	Ascesso peritonsillare	Gnojna upala krajnika
Rabies	Rage	Rabia	Rabbia	Bjesnoća (rabies)
Radial head fracture (radial capitulum fracture)	Fracture de la tête radiale	Fractura de la cabeza del radio	Frattura del capitello radiale	Prijelom glavice palčane kosti
Radiation poisoning	Empoisonnement par radiations	Envenenamiento por radiación	Avvelenamento da radiazione	Trovanje zračenjem
Radioactive irradiation	Irradiation par rayons radioactifs (contamination radioactive)	Irradiación radioactiva	Irradiazione radioattiva	Radioaktivna ozračenost
Radioulnar synostosis	Synostose radio-ulnaire	Sinostosis radiocubital	Sinostosi radio-ulnare	Radioulnarna sinostoza
Radius fracture	Fracture du radius	Fractura del radio	Frattura del radio	Prijelom palčane kosti
Rapid breathing (tachypnea)	Respiration accélérée (tachypnée)	Respiración rápida (taquipnea)	Aumento del ritmo respiratorio (tachipnea)	Ubrzano disanje (tahipnea)
Rash (eruption, eczema)	Rash (eczéma)	Sarpullido (erupción, eccema)	Sfogo (eruzione cutanea)	Osip
Rat bite	Morsure de rat	Mordedura de rata	Morsicatura di ratto	Ugriz štakora
Rat-bite fever	Fièvre de la morsure de rat	Fiebre por mordedura de rata	Febbre da morso di ratto	Groznica štakorskog ugriza
Raynaud's disease	Maladie de Raynaud	Enfermedad de Raynaud	Sindrome di Raynaud	Raynaudova bolest
Reactive arthritis (Reiter's syndrome)	Arthrite réactive (syndrome de Reiter)	Síndrome de Reiter (artritis reactiva)	Sindrome di Reiter	Reiterov sindrom
Rectal prolapse	Prolapsus rectal	Prolapso rectal	Prolasso del retto	Prolaps rektuma
Red colored stool	Selles rouges	Heces de color rojo	Feci di colore rosso	Crvena stolica
Red urine	Urine rouge	Orina de color rojo	Urina di colore rosso	Crveni urin
Redness of the skin (erythema)	Érythème (rougeur de la peau)	Enrojecimiento de la piel (eritema)	Eritema	Crvenilo kože (eritem)
Refracturing (repeated fracture)	Fracture répétée	Fractura repetida	Frattura ripetuta	Opetovani prijelom kosti
Relapsing fever	Fièvre récurrente	Fiebre reincidente	Febbre ricorrente	Povratna groznica
Renal agenesis	Agénésie rénale	Agenesia renal	Agenesia renale	Agenezija bubrega
Renal cell carcinoma (hypernephroma)	Carcinome à cellules rénales	Carcinoma de células renales	Carcinoma a cellule renali	Hipernefrom
Renal colic	Colique néphrétique	Cólico nefrítico (cólico renal)	Colica renale	Bubrežna kolika (renalna kolika)
Renal cyst	Kyste rénal	Quiste de riñón	Cisti renale	Cista na bubregu
Renal rickets	Rachitisme rénal	Raquitismo renal	Rachitismo renale	Bubrežni rahitis
Renal tuberculosis	Tuberculose rénale	Tuberculosis renal	Tubercolosi dei reni	Tuberkuloza bubrega
Renal tubular acidosis	Acidose tubulaire rénale	Acidosis tubular renal	Acidosi renale tubulare	Renalna tubularna acidoza
Renovacsular hypertension	Hypertension rénovasculaire	Hipertensión renovascular	Ipertensione renale	Renovaskularna hipertenzija
Repetitive strain injury (cumulative trauma disorder)	Lésion due à un surmenage répétitif	Síndrome de sobreuso	R.S.I (Repetitive Strain Injury)	Sindrom prenaprezanja
Respiratory alkalosis	Alcalose respiratoire	Alcalosis respiratoria	Alcalosi respiratoria	Respiratorna alkaloza
Respiratory distress syndrome	Syndrome de détresse respiratoire	Síndrome de distrés respiratorio	Sindrome da distress respiratorio	Respiratorni distres sindrom
Restrictive cardiomyopathy	Cardiomyopathie restrictive	Cardiomiopatía restrictiva	Cardiomiopatia restrittiva	Restriktivna kardiomiopatija
Reticuloendothelial sarcoma	Sarcome réticuloendothélial	Reticulosarcoma (sarcoma reticuloendotelial)	Reticoloendotelioma (reticolosarcoma)	Retikuloendotelijalni sarkom
Retinal ablation (retinal detachment)	Décollement de la rétine	Desprendimiento de retina	Distacco di retina	Odvajanje mrežnice (ablacija retine)
Retinal artery occlusion	Occlusion de l'artère de la rétine	Oclusión de la arteria de la retina	Occlusione arteria retinica	Blokada mrežnične arterije

English	French	Spanish	Italian	Croatian
Retinal degeneration	Dégénérescence de la rétine	Degeneración retinal	Degenerazione della retina	Degeneracija mrežnice
Retinitis pigmentosa (retinal pigment epithelium dystrophy)	Rétinite pigmentaire	Retinitis pigmentosa	Retinite pigmentosa	Pigmentna distrofija mrežnice
Retinopathy of prematurity (retrolental fibroplasia)	Rétinopathie du prématuré	Retinopatía de la prematuridad	Retinopatia del prematuro	Retrolentalna fibroplazija
Retroperitoneal fibrosis (Ormond's disease)	Fibrose rétropéritonéale (maladie d'Ormond)	Fibrosis retroperitoneal	Fibrosi retroperitoneale	Retroperitonealna fibroza (Ormondova bolest)
Retroverted uterus	Utérus rétroversé	Retroversión del útero	Retroflessione uterina	Retrovertirani uterus
Reye's syndrome	Syndrome de Reye	Síndrome de Reye	Sindrome di Reye	Reyeov sindrom
Rh incompatibility (hemolytic disease of the newborn)	Maladie hémolytique du nouveau-né	Enfermedad hemolítica del recién nacido (incompatibilidad Rh)	Eritroblastosi fetale (malattia emolitica del neonato)	Rh-inkompatibilnost (hemolitička bolest novorođenčeta)
Rhabdomyoma	Rhabdomyome	Rabdomioma	Rabdomioma	Rabdomiom
Rhabdomyosarcoma	Rhabdomyosarcome	Rabdomiosarcoma	Rabdomiosarcoma	Rabdomiosarkom
Rheumatic fever	Rhumatisme articulaire aigu (maladie de Bouillaud)	Fiebre reumática	Febbre reumatica	Reumatska groznica
Rheumatic heart disease	Cardite rhumatismale	Cardiopatía reumática	Cardiopatia reumatica	Reumatska bolest srca
Rheumatoid arthritis	Arthrite rhumatoïde	Artritis reumatoide	Artrite reumatoide	Reumatoidni artritis
Rhinitis	Rhinite	Rinitis	Rinite	Rinitis
Rickets (rachitis)	Rachitisme	Raquitismo	Rachitismo	Rahitis
Rickettsiosis	Rickettsiose	Rickettsiosis	Rickettsiosi	Rikecioza
Riedel's thyroiditis	Thyroïdite de Riedel	Tiroiditis de Riedel	Tiroidite di Riedel	Riedelov tireoiditis
Rift Valley fever	Fièvre de la vallée du Rift	Fiebre de Rift Valley	Febbre della Rift Valley	Rift Valley groznica
Ringing in ears (tinnitus)	Acouphène	Pitidos en el oído (acúfeno, tinnitus)	Ronzio auricolare (acufene, tinnito)	Zujanje u ušima (tinitus)
Rosacea	Rosacée (couperose)	Rosácea	Rosacea	Rozacea
Rotator cuff rupture (rotator cuff tear)	Rupture de la coiffe des rotateurs	Ruptura del manguito rotador	Rottura della cuffia dei rotatori	Razdor rotatorne manžete ramenog zgloba
Rotten tooth	Dent pourri	Diente podrido	Dente guasto	Pokvareni zub
Runny nose (rinorrhea)	Écoulement par le nez (rhinorhée)	Goteo nasal (rinorrea)	Naso che cola (rinorrea)	Curenje iz nosa (rinoreja)
Rupture	Rupture	Ruptura (rotura)	Rottura	Prsnuće (puknuće, razdor, ruptura)
Rupture of urinary bladder	Rupture de la vessie	Ruptura de la vejiga urinaria	Rottura della vescica urinaria	Rascjep mokraćnog mjehura
Ruptured spleen	Rupture de la rate	Ruptura del bazo	Rottura della milza	Ruptura slezene
Salicylate poisoning	Empoisonnement au salicylate	Intoxicación por salicilatos	Avvelenamento da salicilati	Trovanje salicilatima
Salmonellosis	Salmonellose	Salmonelosis	Salmonellosi	Salmoneloza
Sarcoidosis (sarcoid, Besnier-Boeck disease)	Sarcoïdose (maladie de Besnier-Boeck-Schaumann)	Sarcoidosis (enfermedad de Besnier-Boeck)	Sarcoidosi	Sarkoidoza
Sarcoma	Sarcome	Sarcoma	Sarcoma	Sarkom
Sarcomatoid mesothelioma	Mésothéliome sarcomatoïde	Mesotélioma sarcomatoide	Mesotelioma sarcomatoide	Mezoteliosarkom
Sarcopenia	Sarcopénie	Sarcopenia	Sarcopenia	Sarkopenija
Scabies (the itch)	Gale (mal de Sainte-Marie)	Arador de la sarna (escabiosis)	Scabbia (rogna)	Svrab (skabijes)
Scar	Cicatrice	Cicatriz	Cicatrice (sfregio)	Ožiljak
Scarlet fever	Scarlatine (fièvre écarlate)	Escarlatina (fiebre escarlata)	Scarlattina	Šarlah (skarlatina)
Schistosomiasis (snail fever)	Schistosomiase (bilharziose)	Esquistosomiasis (bilharziasis)	Schistosomiasi	Šistosomijaza
Schizophrenia	Schizophrénie	Esquizofrenia	Schizofrenia	Šizofrenija
Sciatica	Sciatique	Ciática	Sciatica	Išijas
Scleroderma	Sclérodermie	Esclerodermia	Sclerodermia	Sklerodermija
Sclerosing adenosis	Adénose sclérosante	Adenosis esclerosante	Adenosi sclerosante	Sklerozirajuća adenoza
Scoliosis	Scoliose	Escoliosis	Scoliosi	Skolioza
Scorpion sting	Piqûre de scorpion	Picadura de escorpión	Puntura di scorpione	Ugriz škorpiona
Scotoma	Scotome	Escotoma	Scotoma	Skotom
Scratch	Égratignure	Rasguño	Graffio (graffiatura)	Ogrebotina
Scrub typhus (Japanese river fever, Tsutsugamushi fever)	Fièvre fluviale du Japon (typhus à chiques)	Tsutsugamushi (fiebre fluvial japonesa, tifus de los matorrales)	Tsutsugamushi (tifo fluviale giapponese)	Japanska riječna groznica (Tsutsugamushi groznica)
Scurvy	Scorbut	Escorbuto	Scorbuto	Skorbut
Seasickness	Mal de mer	Mal de mar	Mal di mare	Morska bolest
Sebaceous cyst (wen)	Kyste sébacé	Quiste sebáceo	Cisti sebacea	Lojna cista
Seborrhea	Séborrhée	Seborrea	Seborrea	Seboreja
Seborrheic keratosis	Kératose séborrhéïque	Queratosis seborreica	Cheratosi seborroica	Seboreična keratoza
Secondary hypertension (inessential hypertension)	Hypertension secondaire	Hipertensión secundaria	Ipertensione arteriosa secondaria	Sekundarna hipertenzija
Self-harm	Automutilation	Autolesión (automutilación)	Autolesionismo	Samoozljeđivanje
Semicoma	Semi-coma	Semicoma	Semi-coma	Semikoma
Sensation of fear	Sensation de peur	Sensación de miedo	Senso della paura	Osjećaj straha
Sensitivity to pain (algesia)	Sensibilité à la douleur (algésie)	Sensibilidad al dolor (algesia)	Sensibilità al dolore (algesia)	Osjetljivost na bol (algezija)

English	French	Spanish	Italian	Croatian
Separated shoulder (acromioclavicular dislocation)	Luxation acromio-claviculaire	Luxación de la articulación acromioclavicular	Lussazione acromio-clavicolare	Iščašenje akromio-klavikularnog zgloba
Sepsis	Sepsis	Sepsis	Sepsi	Sepsa
Septic shock	Choc septique	Choque séptico	Shock settico	Septički šok
Septicemia	Septicémie	Septicemia	Setticemia	Septikemija
Sever's disease	Maladie de Sever	Enfermedad de Sever	Malattia di Sever	Severova bolest
Severe acute respiratory syndrome (SARS)	Syndrome respiratoire aigu sévère (SRAS)	Síndrome respiratorio agudo severo (SRAS, SARS)	SARS (Sindrome Acuta Respiratoria Severa)	Sindrom akutne respiratorne insuficijencije (SARS)
Sexual addiction	Sexualité compulsive	Adicción sexual	Dipendenza sessuale	Ovisnost o seksu
Sexual differentiation disorder	Trouble de la différenciation sexuelle	Trastorno de la diferenciación sexual	Disordine della differenziazione sessuale	Poremećaj spolne diferencijacije
Sexually transmitted disease	Maladie vénérienne	Enfermedad de transmisión sexual	Malattia sessualmente trasmissibile	Spolno prenosiva bolest
Shallow breathing	Respiration superficielle	Respiración superficial	Respirazione superficiale	Površinsko plitko disanje
Sharp pain	Douleur tranchante	Dolor afilado	Dolore tagliente	Oštra bol
Shedding of the skin (desquamation)	Desquamation	Desquamación	Perdita dello strato superiore della pelle (desquamazione)	Ljuštenje kože (deskvamacija)
Shellfish poisoning	Intoxication par des coquillages	Intoxicación por mariscos	Avvelenamento da molluschi	Trovanje školjkašima
Shigellosis (bacillary dysentery)	Shigellose	Shigelosis	Shigellosi	Šigeloza
Shin splints	Périostite tibiale	Dolor en las espinillas	Sindrome da stress tibiale mediale	Trkačka potkoljenica
Shivering	Frissonnement	Escalofrío (tiritón)	Brivido	Zimica (tresavica)
Shock	Choc	Choque (shock)	Collaso circolatorio (shock)	Šok
Shortness of breath (dyspnea)	Difficulté respiratoire (dyspnée)	Falta de aire (disnea)	Fame d'aria (dispnea, respirazione difficoltosa)	Zaduha (nedostatak daha, dispneja)
Shortsightedness (myopia)	Myopie	Miopía	Miopia	Kratkovidnost
Shoulder arthrosis	Arthrose de l'épaule	Artrosis del hombro	Artrosi gleno-omerale	Artroza ramena
Shoulder impingement syndrome (subacromial impingement syndrome)	Syndrome du conflit sous-acromial	Síndrome del conflicto subacromial	Sindrome da conflitto subacromiale (impingement sub-acromiale)	Sindrom sraza ramena (subakromijalni sindrom sraza)
Shuffling gait	Démarche traînante	Marcha arrastrando los pies	Barcollamento	Teturav nesiguran hod
Sickle-cell disease (sickle-cell anemia)	Drépanocytose (anémie à cellules falciformes)	Anemia falciforme (anemia drepanocítica)	Anemia drepanocitica	Anemija srpastih stanica
Siderosis	Sidérose	Siderosis	Siderosi	Sideroza
Sight disorder	Trouble de la vue	Trastorno de la visión	Disturbo della vista	Poremećaj vida
Silicosis	Silicose	Silicosis	Silicosi	Silikoza
Silo-filler's disease	Maladie des ouvriers des silos	Enfermedad de los ensiladores	Malattia dei riempitori dei silos	Silosna pluća
Simple bone fracture	Fracture simple	Fractura simple	Frattura semplice	Jednostavni prijelom kosti
Sinus headache	Douleur des sinus (sinusite)	Dolor de cabeza por sinusitis	Sinusite	Sinusna glavobolja
Sister Mary Joseph nodule	Nodule de Soeur Marie Joseph (métastase cutanée ombilicale)	Nódulo de la hermana María José	Nodulo di Suor Maria Giuseppa	Čvor sestre Mary Joseph (umbilikalna metastaza)
Sjögren's syndrome	Syndrome de Sjögren	Síndrome de Sjögren	Sindrome di Sjögren	Sjögrenov sindrom
Skin color changes	Changements de couleur de la peau	Cambios en el color de la piel	Cambiamento di colore della pelle	Promjene boje kože
Sleep apnea	Apnée du sommeil	Apnea del sueño	Sindrome delle apnee nel sonno	Noćna desaturacija
Sleeping disorder	Trouble du sommeil	Trastorno del sueño	Disturbo del sonno	Poremećaj spavanja
Sleepwalking (somnambulism)	Somnabulisme	Sonambulismo (noctambulismo)	Sonnambulismo	Mjesečarenje (somnambulizam)
Slow basal metabolism	Métabolisme basal diminué	Metabolismo basal lento	Basso metabolismo basale	Usporen bazalni metabolizam
Slow breathing rate (bradypnea)	Respiration ralentie (bradypnée)	Descenso de la frecuencia respiratoria (bradipnea)	Riduzione della frequenza respiratoria (bradipnea)	Usporeno disanje (bradipneja)
Slow psychophysiological responses	Réponses psychophysiologiques lentes	Respuestas psicofisiológicas lentas	Lentezza psicofisica	Psihofizička usporenost
Slow pulse rate (bradycardia)	Rythme cardiaque bas (bradycardie)	Descenso de la frecuencia cardiaca (bradicardia)	Riduzione della frequenza cardiaca (bradicardia)	Usporen puls (bradikardija)
Small intestine diverticulum	Diverticule de Meckel	Divertículo de Meckel	Diverticolo di Meckel	Divertikul tankog crijeva
Small pupils	Pupilles diminuées	Pupilas pequeñas	Pupille costrette	Sužene zjenice
Smallpox	Variole (petite vérole)	Viruela	Variola vera (vaiolo)	Velike boginje (crne boginje, variola vera)
Snake bite	Morsure de vipère	Mordedura de víbora	Morsicatura di serpenti	Ugriz zmije
Sneezing	Éternuement	Estornudo	Starnuto	Kihanje
Sniffing (sniffle)	Renifler	Sorberse la nariz (moqueo)	Tirare su col naso	Šmrcanje
Soft fibroma (fibroma molle, acrochordon)	Molluscum pendulum (acrochordon)	Fibroma blando (fibroma molle)	Mollusco pendule (fibroma molle)	Kožni privjesak (mekani fibrom)
Somnolence	Somnolence	Somnolencia	Sonnolenza	Pospanost (somnolencija)

English	French	Spanish	Italian	Croatian
Sopor	Sopor	Sopor	Stupor	Sopor
Sore throat (inflammation of the throat, pharyngitis)	Mal à la gorge (inflammattion du pharinx, pharingite)	Mal de garganta (inflamación de la faringe, faringitis)	Mal di gola (infiammazione della faringe, faringite)	Upala grla (grlobolja, faringitis)
Spanish flu	Grippe espagnole	Gripe española	Influenza spagnola	Španjolska gripa
Spasm (cramp)	Spasme (crampe)	Espasmo (calambre)	Spasmo (contrazione involontaria)	Grč (spazam)
Spastic arching position (opisthotonus)	Contracture sur les muscles extenseurs de sorte que le corps est incurvé en arrière (opisthotonos)	Contracción del cuerpo entero de tal manera que se mantiene encorvado hacia atrás (opistótonos)	Iperestenzione della regione posteriore del tronco (opistotono)	Izvijanje misića vrata i leđa u luk (opistotonus)
Speech difficulty (dysphasia)	Trouble de l'apprentissage du langage (dysphasie)	Trastorno del lenguaje (disfasia)	Disturbo del linguaggio verbale (afasia)	Otežan govor (disfazija)
Spermatocele	Spermatocèle	Espermatocele	Spermatocele (cisti spermatica)	Spermatokela (cista epididimisa
Spider angioma (spider nevus)	Angiome stellaire	Angioma en araña (angioma aracnoideo)	Angioma a ragno	Paukoliki angiom (spider nevus)
Spider bite	Piqûre d'araignée	Picadura de araña	Morsicatura di ragno	Ugriz pauka
Spina bifida	Spina bifida	Espina bífida	Spina bifida	Spina bifida
Spinal deformity	Difformité spinale	Deformidad vertebral	Degenerazione spinale	Deformacija kralježnice
Spinal disc herniation	Hernie discale	Hernia discal	Ernia del disco	Hernija intervertrebralnog diska
Spinal shock	Choc spinal	Choque espinal	Shock spinale	Spinalni šok
Spiral fracture	Fracture en spirale	Fractura espiral	Frattura a spirale	Spiralni prijelom kosti
Splenomegaly	Splénomégalie	Esplenomegalia	Splenomegalia	Splenomegalija
Split foot (lobster claw foot, ectrodactyly)	Pince de homard (aplasie digitale, ectrodactylie)	Ectrodactilia en pie	Lobster-claw deformità di piede	Lobster Claw stopalo
Spondylitis	Spondilite	Espondilitis	Spondilite	Spondilitis
Spondylolisthesis	Spondylolisthésis	Espondilolistesis	Spondilolistesi	Spondilolisteza
Spondylosis	Spondylose	Espondilosis	Spondilosi	Spondiloza
Spontaneous fractures	Fractures spontanées	Fracturas espontáneas	Fratture spontanee	Spontane frakture
Sporotrichosis	Sporotrichose	Esporotricosis	Sporotricosi	Sporotrihoza
Sports injury	Blessure de sportif	Lesión deportiva	Trauma sportivo	Sportska ozljeda
Sprengel's deformity	Anomalie de Sprengel	Deformidad de Sprengel	Deformità di Sprengel	Sprengelova bolest (scapula alta)
Squamous cell carcinoma (planocellular carcinoma)	Carcinome spinocellulaire	Carcinoma de células escamosas	Carcinoma a cellule squamose	Planocelularni karcinom
Stab wound	Coup de couteau	Estocada	Ferita da punta	Ubodna rana
Staphylococcal food poisoning	Intoxication alimentaire staphylococcique	Intoxicación alimentaria por estafilococo dorado	Intossicazione alimentare da stafilococco	Stafilokokno trovanje hranom
Starvation	Famine	Inanición	Inedia	Izgladnjelost
Stenosis of pulmonary artery	Sténose de l'artère pulmonaire	Estenosis de la arteria pulmonar	Stenosi dell'arteria polmonare	Stenoza plućne arterije
Stiffness	Raideur	Agarrotamiento	Rigidità	Ukočenost
Stomach cancer (gastric cancer)	Cancer de l'estomac	Cáncer de estómago (cáncer gástrico)	Cancro dello stomaco (cancro gastrico)	Rak želuca
Stomach growling (borborygmus)	Gargouillements (borborygme)	Sonidos de tripas (borborigmo)	Borborigmo	Kruljenje u želucu
Strabismus	Strabisme	Estrabismo	Strabismo	Razrokost (strabizam)
Strain (sprain, pull)	Déchirure	Desgarro	Stiramento	Istegnuće
Strangulation	Strangulation (étranglement)	Estrangulamiento	Strangolamento (strozzamento)	Davljenje
Streptococcal pharyngitis	Pharyngite streptococcique	Faringitis por estreptococo	Faringite streptococcica	Streptokokna angina
Stress fracture	Fracture de fatigue	Fractura por estrés	Frattura da stress	Prijelom zamora
Stress urinary incontinence	Incontinence urinaire d'effort	Incontinencia urinaria por estrés	Incontinenza urinaria da sforzo	Stres-inkontinencija urina
Stroke (cerebrovascular accident)	Attaque cérébrale (accident vasculaire cérébral)	Derrame cerebral (accidente cerebrovascular)	Colpo apoplettico	Moždani udar
Stupor	Stupeur	Estupor	Stupore	Stupor
Stye (chalazion)	Chalazion	Orzuelo	Calazio	Ječmenac
Subarachnoid hemorrhage	Hémorragie sous arachnoïdienne	Hemorragia subaracnoidea	Emorragia subaracnoidea	Subarahnoidalno krvarenje
Subcutaneous emphysema	Emphisème sous-cutané	Enfisema subcutáneo	Enfisema sottocutaneo	Potkožni emfizem
Subdural hematoma	Hématome subdural	Hematoma subdural	Ematoma subdurale	Subduralni hematom
Subdural hemorrhage	Subdural hemorrhage	Hemorragia subdural	Emorragia subdurale	Subduralno krvarenje
Sudden infant death syndrome (crib death, cot death)	Syndrome de mort subite du nourrisson	Síndrome de muerte súbita del lactante (muerte en cuna)	Sindrome della morte improvvisa del lattante	Sindrom iznenadne smrti dojenčeta
Sudeck's atrophy	Atrophie de Sudeck	Atrofia de Sudeck	Atrofia di Sudeck	Sudeckova distrofija
Sunstroke (heat stroke)	Coup de soleil (insolation)	Insolación	Insolazione (colpo di sole)	Sunčanica
Supracondylar femoral fracture	Fracture supracondylienne du fémur	Fractura supracondilar del fémur	Frattura sovracondiloidea del femore	Suprakondilarni prijelom bedrene kosti
Supracondylar humerus fracture	Fracture supracondylienne de l'humérus	Fractura supracondilar del húmero	Frattura sovracondiloidea di omero	Suprakondilarni prijelom nadlaktice
Supramaleolar fracture of tibia and fibula	Fracture tibia péroné sus-malléolaire	Fractura supramaleolar de tibia y peroné	Frattura del terzo distale di tibia e perone	Supramaleolarni prijelom potkoljenice

English	French	Spanish	Italian	Croatian
Surgical shock (postoperative shock)	Choc post-opératoire	Choque quirúrgico	Shock chirurgico	Kirurški šok
Suspension of external breathing (apnea)	Arrêt respiratoire (apnée)	Falta de respiración (apnea)	Assenza di respirazione (apnea)	Zastoj disanja (apnea)
Sweating	Sudation	Transpiración (sudación)	Sudorazione (traspirazione)	Znojenje
Swelling	Gonflement (enflure)	Hinchazón	Gonfiore	Oteklina
Swimmer's knee	Syndrome du brasseur aux genoux	Rodilla de nadador de pecho (bursitis de la pata de ganso)	Ginocchio del nuotatore a rana (stiramento cronico del legamento mediale)	Plivačko koljeno
Syncope	Syncope	Síncope	Sincope	Sinkopa
Syndactyly	Syndactylie	Sindactilia	Sindattilia	Sindaktilija
Synovial sarcoma	Sarcome synovial	Sarcoma sinovial	Sarcoma sinoviale	Sinovijalni sarkom
Synovioma	Synoviome	Sinovioma	Sinovioma	Sinoviom
Syphilis	Syphilis (vérole)	Sífilis	Sifilide (lue)	Sifilis (lues)
Syringomyelia	Syringomyélie	Siringomielia	Siringomielia	Siringomijelija
Tachycardia	Tachycardie	Taquicardia	Tachicardia	Tahikardija
Tarsal tunnel syndrome	Syndrome du canal tarsien	Síndrome del túnel tarsiano	Sindrome del tunnel tarsale	Sindrom tarzalnog kanala
Tendinosis (chronic tendon injury)	Tendinose	Tendinosis (lesión crónica del tendón)	Tendinosi	Tendinoza (kronična ozljeda tetive)
Tendinous fibrositis	Fibrosite du tendon	Fibrositis de tendón	Fibrosi tendinea	Fibrozitis tetive
Tendon rupture (torn tendon)	Rupture du tendon	Ruptura del tendón	Rottura del tendine	Puknuće tetive
Tendon strain	Déchirure au tendon	Desgarro de tendón	Stiramento del tendine	Istegnuće tetive (distenzija tetive)
Tennis elbow	Épicondylite latérale	Codo del tenista (epicondilitis lateral)	Gomito del tennista (epicondilite)	Teniski lakat
Tension headache	Céphalée de tension	Cefalea tensional	Cefalea di tipo tensivo	Tenzijska glavobolja
Teratocarcinoma	Tératocarcinome	Teratocarcinoma	Teratocarcinoma	Teratokarcinom
Teratoma	Tératome	Teratoma	Teratoma	Teratom
Testicular dysgenesis	Dysgénésie testiculaire	Disgénesis testicular	Disgenesia gonadica	Testikularna disgeneza
Testicular torsion	Torsion testiculaire	Torsión testicular	Torsione del testicolo	Torzija testisa
Tetanus	Tétanos	Tétanos (tétano)	Tetano	Tetanus (zli grč)
Tetany	Tétanie	Tetania	Tetania	Tetanija
Tetralogy of Fallot	Tétralogie de Fallot	Tetralogía de Fallot	Tetralogia di Fallot	Fallotova tetralogija
Thalassemia	Thalassémie	Talasemia	Talassemia	Talasemija
Thallium poisoning	Empoisonnement au thallium	Envenenamiento por talio	Avvelenamento da tallio	Trovanje talijem
Thermal injuries	Lésions thermiques	Lesiones térmicas	Lesioni termiche	Termičke ozljede
Thermal wound	Blessure thermique	Herida térmica	Ferita termica	Termička rana
Thermonuclear injuries	Lésions provoquées par une explosion thermonucléaire	Lesiones por una explosión termonuclear	Ferite provocate da esplosioni termonucleari	Termonuklearne ozljede
Thirst	Soif	Sed	Sete	Žeđ
Thoracic aortic aneurysm	Anévrisme aortique thoracique	Aneurisma de aorta torácica	Aneurisma dell'aorta toracica	Aneurizma torakalne aorte
Thoracic outlet syndrome	Syndrome de traversée thoraco-cervico-brachiale	Síndrome del estrecho torácico	Sindrome dello stretto toracico superiore	Torakalni sindrom
Thrombocytopenia	Thrombocytopénie	Trombocitopenia	Trombocitopenia	Trombocitopenija
Thromboembolism	Accident thromboembolique	Tromboembolismo	Tromboembolia	Tromboembolija
Thrombophlebitis	Thrombophlébite	Tromboflebitis	Tromboflebite	Tromboflebitis
Thrombosis	Thrombose	Trombosis	Trombosi	Tromboza
Thrombotic thrombocytopenic purpura	Purpura thrombotique thrombocytopénique	Púrpura trombocitopénica trombótica	Porpora trombotica trombocitopenica	Trombotska trombocitopenična purpura
Thrush (oral candidiasis)	Candidose orale	Candidiasis oral (muguet oral)	Mughetto (moniliasi orale)	Sor (oralna kandidijaza)
Thumb joint arthritis	Rhizarthrose	Rizartrosis	Rizartrosi (artrosi dell'articolazione alla base del police)	Rizartroza
Thyroglossal duct cyst	Kyste du canal thyréoglosse	Quiste tirogloso	Cisti del dotto tiroglosso	Cista na tireoglosnom vodu
Thyroid cyst	Kyste thyroïdien	Quiste de tiroides	Cisti tiroidea	Cista na štitnjači
Thyrotoxicosis	Thyréotoxicose	Tirotoxicosis	Tireotossicosi	Tireotoksikoza (tireotoksična oluja)
Tibia stress fracture	Fracture de fatigue du tibia	Fractura por estrés de la tibia	Frattura da stress della tibia	Prijelom zamora goljenične kosti
Tibialis posterior syndrome	Syndrome tibial postérieur	Síndrome del tibial posterior	Periostite tibiale (sindrome del muscolo tibiale posteriore)	Sindrom stražnjeg tibijalnog mišića
Tibialis posterior tendinitis	Tendinopathie du tibial postérieur	Tendinopatía tibial posterior	Tendinite del muscolo tibiale posteriore	Tendinitis stražnjeg tibijalnog mišića
Tic	Tic	Tic	Tic	Tik
Tick-borne meningoencephalitis	Méningoencéphalite à tique	Meningoencefalitis de garrapata	Encefalite trasmessa da zecche	Krpeljni meningoencefalitis
Tight hamstrings syndrome	Hamstring syndrome	Síndrome de isquiosurales cortos	Sindrome degli ischio-crurali (sindrome dell'hamstring)	Sindrom stražnje lože natkoljenice (sindrom hamstringsa)
'Tight shoes' sensation	Sensation des chaussures très serré	Sensación de "zapatos apretados"	Senso delle scarpe troppo strette	Osjećaj "tijesnih cipela"

English	French	Spanish	Italian	Croatian
Tinea capitis (scalp ringworm)	Teigne (tinea capitis)	Tiña de la cabeza (tinea capitis)	Tigna (tinea capitis)	Gljivična infekcija vlasišta (tinea capitis)
Tinea corporis	Tinea corporis	Tiña corporal (tinea corporis)	Tinea corporis	Tinea corporis
Tinea versicolor (pityriasis versicolor, haole rot)	Pityriasis versicolor	Tiña versicolor (pitiriasis versicolor)	Pitiriasi versicolor (tinea versicolor)	Pitirijaza (svjetlije mrlje na osunčanoj koži, Tinea versicolor)
Tingling	Fourmillement	Hormigueo	Intormentire	Trnjenje
Tonic-clonic seizure	Crise tonico-clonique	Crisis tónico-clónica	Crisi tonico-clonica	Toničko-klonički napadaj
Toothache	Mal de dents	Dolor de muelas	Mal di denti	Zubobolja
Tourette's syndrome	Syndrome de Tourette	Síndrome de Tourette	Sindrome di Tourette	Touretteov sindrom
Toxocariasis	Toxocarose	Toxocariasis	Toxocariasi	Toksokarijaza
Toxoplasmosis	Toxoplasmose	Toxoplasmosis	Toxoplasmosi	Toksoplazmoza
Trachoma	Trachome	Tracoma	Tracoma	Trahom
Transitional cell carcinoma	Carcinome à cellules de transition	Carcinoma de células transicionales	Carcinoma transizionale	Tranzicionalni karcinom
Transposition of aorta	Transposition de l'aorte	Transposición de la aorta	Trasposizione dell'aorta	Transpozicija aorte
Transposition of pulmonary artery	Transposition de l'artère pulmonaire	Transposición de la arteria pulmonar	Trasposizione dell'arteria polmonare	Transpozicija plućne arterije
Transposition of the great vessels	Transposition des gros vaisseaux	Transposición de los grandes vasos	Trasposizione dei grossi vasi	Transpozicija velikih žila
Transverse colon	Côlon transverse	Colon transverso	Colon trasverso	Poprečno debelo crijevo
Transverse fracture	Fracture transversale	Fractura transversal	Frattura trasversale	Poprečni prijelom kosti
Traumatic shock	Choc traumatique	Choque traumático	Shock traumatico	Traumatski šok
Traveller's thrombosis (economy class syndrome)	Thrombose du voyageur	Síndrome de la clase turista	Sindrome della classe economica	Sindrom ekonomske klase
Tremor	Tremblement	Temblor	Tremito (tremore)	Drhtanje (tremor)
Trichinosis (trichinellosis)	Trichinose	Triquinelosis (triquinosis)	Trichinosi	Trihinoza (trihineloza)
Trichomonas vaginalis	Trichomonas vaginalis	Trichomonas vaginalis	Trichomonas vaginalis	Trihomonazni vaginitis
Trichomoniasis	Trichomoniase	Trichomoniasis	Trichomoniasi	Trihomonijaza
Trifascicular block	Bloc trifasciculaire	Bloqueo trifascicular	Blocco trifascicolare	Trifascikularni blok
Trigeminal neuralgia	Névralgie du trijumeau (névralgie trigéminale)	Neuralgia del trigémino	Nevralgia del trigemino	Neuralgija trigeminusa
Trypanosomiasis	Trypanosomiase	Tripanosomiasis	Tripanosomiasi	Tripanosomijaza
Tuberculosis (TBC)	Tuberculose	Tuberculosis (tisis, TBC)	Tubercolosi (tisi)	Tuberkuloza (sušica, TBC)
Tuberculous arthritis	Arthrite tuberculeuse	Artritis tuberculosa	Artrite tubercolare	Tuberkulozni artritis
Tuberculous lymphadenitis	Lymphadénite tuberculeuse	Tuberculosis ganglionar (linfadenitis tubercular)	Linfadenite tubercolare	Tuberkuloza limfnih čvorova
Tuberculous spondylitis (Pott disease)	Mal de Pott (tuberculose vertébrale)	Espondilitis tuberculosa	Spondilite tubercolare (morbo di Pott)	Tuberkulozni spondilitis (Pottova bolest)
Tubular adenoma	Adénome tubulaire	Adenoma tubular	Adenoma tubulare	Tubularni adenom
Tularemia (rabbit fever)	Tularémie	Tularemia (fiebre de los conejos)	Tularemia (febbre dei conigli)	Tularemija (zečja groznica)
Tumor (tumour)	Tumeur	Tumor	Tumore	Tumor
Tungiasis (nigua, pique)	Sarcopsyllose	Tungiasis	Tungiasi (tunga penetrans)	Tungijaza
Turner syndrome	Syndrome de Turner	Síndrome de Turner	Sindrome di Turner	Turnerov sindrom
Twinging pain	Élancement	Dolor tipo punzada	Dolore pungente	Probadajuća bol
Typhoid fever (typhoid)	Fièvre typhoïde (typhus abdominal)	Fiebre tifoidea (fiebre entérica)	Febbre tifoide (tifo)	Tifusna groznica (tifus)
Ulcer	Ulcère	Úlcera (llaga)	Ulcera (ulcerazione)	Čir (ulkus)
Ulcerative colitis	Colite ulcéreuse	Colitis ulcerosa	Rettocolite ulcerosa	Ulcerozni kolitis
Umbilical hernia	Hernie ombilicale	Hernia umbilical	Ernia ombelicale	Pupčana kila (umbilikalna hernija)
Unclear urine (foggy urine)	Urine opaque	Orina turbia	Urine torbide	Mutni urin
Unconsciousness	Absence de la conscience	Inconsciencia	Incoscienza (stato di incoscienza)	Nesvjestica
Uncontrolled eye movement (opsoclonus)	Mouvements involontaires anarchiques des globes oculaires (opsoclonus)	Movimientos involuntarios y rápidos de los ojos (opsoclonus)	Movimenti incontrollati degli occhi (opsoclono)	Nekontrolirani pokreti očiju (opsoklonus)
Underfedness (malnutrition)	Malnutrition	Desnutrición	Sottopeso (grave magrezza)	Neuhranjenost
Undescended testicle	Absence de descente des testicules	Descenso incompleto de testículo	Mancata discesa del testicolo	Nespušteni testis
Unequal size of pupils (anisocoria)	Différence de taille entres les pupilles (anisocorie)	Asimetría del tamaño de las pupilas (anisocoria)	Diseguaglianza del diametro delle pupille (anisocoria)	Nejednaka veličina zjenica (anizokorija)
Upper and/or lower jaw fracture (broken upper/lower jaw)	Fracture du maxillaire et/ou de la mandibule	Fractura de maxilar y/o mandíbula	Frattura della mascella e/o della mandibola	Prijelom gornje i/ili donje čeljusti
Upper respiratory tract infection	Infection respiratoire haute	Infección respiratoria alta	Infezione del tratto respiratorio superiore	Infekcija gornjih dišnih puteva
Uremia (autointoxication due to kidney failure)	Urémie (le taux de l'urée dans le sang)	Uremia (acumulación en la sangre de los productos tóxicos por un fallo renal)	Uremia (accumulo nel sangue di sostanze azotate a causa dell'insufficienza renale)	Uremija (autointoksikacija radi nelučenja urina)
Ureteral stone (ureterolithiasis)	Calcul dans l'uretère	Cálculo en el uréter (ureterolitiasis)	Calcolo ureterale	Ureteralni kamenac (ureterolitijaza)

English	French	Spanish	Italian	Croatian
Urge to vomit	Envie de vomir	Ganas de vomitar	Impulso a vomitare	Podražaj na povraćanje
Urinary burning	Brûlures à la miction	Ardor al orinar	Bruciore urinario	Pećenje za vrijeme mokrenja
Urinary incontinence	Incontinence urinaire	Incontinencia urinaria	Incontinenza urinaria	Urinarna inkotinencija
Urinary retention (ischuria)	Rétention d'urine	Retención de orina	Ritenzione urinaria	Zastoj urina (urinarna retencija)
Urination disorder	Trouble de la miction	Trastorno de la micción	Disturbo della minzione	Poremećaj mokrenja
Urogenital neoplasm	Tumeur du système uro-génital	Tumor urogenital	Neoplasie del tratto urogenitale	Urogenitalni tumor
Urogenital tuberculosis	Tuberculose urogénitale	Tuberculosis urogenital	Tubercolosi urogenitale	Urogenitalna tuberkuloza
Uterine bleeding (metrorrhagia)	Saignement de l'utérus (métrorragie)	Pérdida de sangre uterina (metrorragia)	Perdita di sangue al di fuori della mestruazione (metrorragia)	Krvarenje iz maternice (metroragija)
Uterine prolapse (fallen womb)	Prolapsus de l'utérus	Prolapso del útero	Prolasso uterino	Prolaps maternice (spuštena maternica)
Vaginal discharge	Pertes vaginales	Flujo vaginal	Fuoriuscita vaginale	Vaginalni iscjedak
Vaginal spasm (vaginismus)	Spasme vaginal (vaginisme)	Espasmo vaginal (vaginismo)	Spasmo di vagina (vaginismo)	Grč rodnice (vaginizam)
Van Neck disease	Maladie de Van Neck-Odelberg	Enfermedad de Van Neck	Malattia di Van Neck	Morbus Van Neck
Varicocele	Varicocèle	Varicocele	Varicocele	Varikokela
Varicose veins	Varices	Varices	Varicosi (varici, malattia varicosa)	Proširene vene
Vasomotor rhinitis	Rhinite vasomotrice	Rinitis vasomotora	Rinite vasomotoria	Vazomotorni rinitis
Venous bleeding	Saignement veineux	Sangrado venoso (hemorragia venosa)	Emorragia venosa	Vensko krvarenje
Venous thrombosis	Thrombose veineuse	Trombosis venosa	Trombosi venosa	Venska tromboza
Venous ulcer (varicose ulcer)	Ulcère veineux	Úlcera varicosa	Ulcera varicosa	Varikozni ulcer (venski ulcer)
Ventricular fibrillation	Fibrillation ventriculaire	Fibrilación ventricular	Fibrillazione ventricolare	Ventrikularna fibrilacija
Ventricular hypertrophy	Hypertrophie ventriculaire	Hipertrofia ventricular	Ipertrofia ventricolare	Ventrikularna hipertrofija
Ventricular septal defect	Communication inter-ventriculaire	Comunicación interventricular	Difetto del setto ventricolare	Ventrikularni septalni defekt
Vibration disease	Maladie des vibrations	Enfermedad de las vibraciones	Malattia da vibrazioni	Vibracijska bolest
Violent death	Mort violente	Muerte violenta	Morte violenta	Nasilna smrt
Viral conjuctivitis	Conjonctivite virale	Conjuntivitis viral	Congiuntivite virale	Virusni konjuktivitis
Viral hemorrhagic fever	Fièvre hémorragique virale	Fiebre hemorrágica viral	Febbre emorragica	Virusna hemoragijska groznica
Viral hepatitis	Hépatite virale	Hepatitis viral	Epatite virale	Virusni hepatitis
Viral infection	Infection virale	Infección viral	Infezione virale	Virusna infekcija
Viral pneumonia	Pneumonie virale	Neumonía viral	Polmonite virale	Virusna upala pluća
Vitamin A deficiency	Carence en vitamine A	Carencia de vitamina A	Carenza di vitamina A	Manjak vitamina A
Vitamin B1 deficiency	Carence en vitamine B1	Carencia de vitamina B1	Carenza di vitamina B1	Manjak vitamina B1
Vitamin B2 deficiency	Carence en vitamine B2	Carencia de vitamina B2	Carenza di vitamina B2	Manjak vitamina B2
Vitamin B3 deficiency	Carence en vitamine B3	Carencia de vitamina B3	Carenza di vitamina B3	Manjak vitamina B3
Vitamin B12 deficiency	Carence en vitamine B12	Carencia de vitamina B12	Carenza di vitamina B12	Manjak vitamina B12
Vitamin C deficiency	Carence en vitamine C	Carencia de vitamina C	Carenza de vitamina C	Manjak vitamina C
Vitamin D deficiency	Carence en vitamine D	Carencia de vitamina D	Carenza de vitamina D	Manjak vitamina D
Vitamin deficiency	Carence en vitamine	Carencia de vitamina	Carenza di vitamine	Manjak vitamina
Vitamin K deficiency	Carence en vitamine K	Carencia de vitamina K	Carenza de vitamina K	Manjak vitamina K
Vitiligo	Vitiligo	Vitíligo	Vitiligine	Vitiligo
Vocal chords polyp	Polype des cordes vocales	Pólipo de las cuerdas vocales	Polipo della corda vocale	Polip na glasnicama
Voice changes	Changements de voix	Cambios en la voz	Cambiamento di voce	Promjene glasa
Volkmann's ischemic contracture	Syndrome de Volkmann	Contractura isquémica de Volkmann	Contrattura ischemica di Volkmann	Volkmannova ishemična kontraktura
Vomiting	Vomissement	Vómito (emesis)	Vomito (emetismo)	Povraćanje
Vomiting of blood (hematemesis)	Vomissement de sang (hématémèse)	Vómito de sangre (hematemesis)	Emesi emorragica (ematemesi)	Povraćanje krvi (hematemeza)
Vomiting without nausea (cerebral vomiting)	Vomissement en fusée sans effort	Vómito sin náusea (vómito cerebral)	Vomito senza nausea (vomito a getto, vomito cerebrale)	Povraćanje bez mučnine (povraćanje u luku, cerebralno povraćanje)
Warfare gases poisoning	Intoxication par gaz de combat	Intoxicación por armas gaseosas	Avvelenamento da gas tossico	Trovanje bojnim otrovima
Warm sweaty palms	Paumes des mains chaudes et humides	Palmas de las manos calientes y mojadas	Palmi delle mani caldi e sudati	Topli i vlažni dlanovi
Wart	Verrue	Verruga	Verruca	Bradavica (virusna bradavica)
Watery eyes	Yeux larmoyants	Ojos llorosos	Occhi lacrimosi	Suzenje očiju
Watery stool	Selles aqueuses	Heces acuosas	Consistenza acquosa delle feci	Vodenasta stolica
Weakness	Faiblesse	Debilidad	Debolezza	Slabost
Weight loss (weight reduction)	Amaigrissement	Pérdida de peso	Dimagramento	Mršavljenje
West Nile fever	Fièvre du Nil occidental	Fiebre del Nilo Occidental	Febbre del Nilo occidentale	Groznica zapadnog Nila
Wet gangrene	Gangrène humide	Gangrena húmeda	Gangrena umida	Vlažna gangrena

English	French	Spanish	Italian	Croatian
Whipple's disease	Maladie de Whipple	Enfermedad de Whipple	Morbo di Whipple	Whippleova bolest
Whitlow (felon)	Panaris	Panadizo	Patereccio	Panaricij
Whooping cough (pertussis)	Coqueluche	Tos ferina (coqueluche)	Pertosse	Hripavac (pasji kašalj, pertussis)
Wilm's tumor (nephroblastoma)	Tumeur de Wilms (néphroblastome)	Tumor de Wilms (nefroblastoma)	Tumore di Wilms (nefroblastoma)	Wilmsov tumor (nefroblastom)
Withdrawal	Sevrage	Síndrome de abstinencia	Crisi d'astinenza	Apstinencijska kriza
Wound (injury, lesion)	Plaie	Herida	Ferita	Rana
Wrinkle	Ride	Arruga	Ruga	Bora
Wrist arthrosis	Arthrose du poignet	Artrosis de muñeca	Artrosi di polso	Artroza ručnog zgloba
Wry neck (torticollis)	Torticolis	Torticolis	Torcicollo	Krivi vrat (tortikolis)
Xanthelasma	Xanthelasma	Xantelasma	Xantelasma	Ksantelazma
Xanthoma	Xanthome	Xantoma	Xantoma	Ksantom
Yawn	Bâillement	Bostezo	Sbadiglio	Zijevanje
Yaws (pian)	Pian	Pian (frambesia)	Framboesia	Frambezija
Yellow fever	Fièvre jaune	Fiebre amarilla	Febbre gialla	Žuta groznica
Yellow stool	Selles jaunes	Heces amarillas	Feci gialle	Žuta stolica
Yolk sac tumor (endodermal sinus tumor)	Tumeur du sac vitellin	Tumor de saco vitelino	Tumore del sacco vitellino	Tumor žumanjčane vreće (endodermalni sinus tumor)
Zika fever	Fièvre Zika	Fiebre del Zika	Febbre Zika	Zika groznica
Zoonosis	Zoonose	Zoonosis	Zoonosi	Zoonoza
PHARMACY:	PHARMACIE:	FARMACIA:	FARMACIA:	LJEKARNA:
Activated carbon	Charbon actif	Carbón activado	Carbone attivo	Aktivni ugljen
Adrenaline	Adrénaline	Adrenalina	Adrenalina	Adrenalin
Aerosol	Aérosol	Aerosol	Aerosol	Aerosol
After meal	Après-repas	Después de una comida	Dopo il pasto	Nakon jela
Alcohol	Alkohol	Alcol	Alcool	Alcohol
Almond oil	Huile d'amande	Aceite de almendras dulces	Olio di mandorla	Bademovo ulje
Aminophylline	Aminophylline	Aminofilina	Aminofillina	Aminofilin
Ampicillin	Ampicilline	Ampicilina	Ampicillina	Ampicilin
Ampoule	Ampoule	Ampolla (recipiente)	Ampolla (fiala)	Ampula
Analgesic (painkiller)	Analgésique	Analgésico	Analgesico	Analgetik
Anesthetic	Anesthésique	Anestésico	Anestetico	Anestetik
Antacid	Antiacide	Antiácido	Antiacido	Antacid
Anti-diabetic drug	Médicament antidiabétique	Antidiabético	Antidiabetico	Antidiabetik
Anti-inflammatory	Anti-inflammatoire	Antiinflamatory (antiflogístico)	Antinfiammatorio	Protuupalno
Anti-obesity medication	Médicament anti-obésité	Fármaco antiobesidad	Dimagrante (farmaco antiobesità)	Dijetetsko sredstvo
Antialcoholic drug	Médicament contre la dépendance à l'alcool	Fármaco antialcohólico	Farmaco anti-alcol	Antialkoholik
Antiallergic drug	Antiallergique	Antialérgico	Farmaco antiallergico	Antialergik
Antianemic	Médicament antianémique	Antianémico	Farmaco antianemico	Antianemik
Antiarrhythmic agent	Agent antiarythmique	Agente antiarrítmico	Farmaco antiaritmico	Antiaritmik
Antibiotic	Antibiotique	Antibiótico	Antibiotico	Antibiotik
Anticoagulant	Anticoagulant	Anticoagulante	Anticoagulante	Antikoagulans
Anticonvulsant	Antiépileptique (anticonvulsivant)	Anticonvulsivo (antiepiléptico)	Anticonvulsante	Antiepileptik (antikonvulziv)
Antidepressant	Antidépresseur	Antidepresivo	Antidepressivo	Antidepresiv
Antidiarrhoeal drug	Médicament antidiarrhéique	Antidiarréico	Antidiarroici	Antidiaroik
Antidote	Antidote	Antídoto	Antidoto	Antidot
Antiemetic and motion sickness drug	Antiémétique	Antiemético	Antiemetico	Lijek protiv mučnine i povraćanja
Antihelminthic	Antihelminthique	Antihelmíntico	Antielmintici	Antihelmintik
Antihemorrhagic (hemostatic)	Hémostatique	Hemostático	Emostatico	Hemostatik
Antihistamine	Antihistaminique	Antihistamínico	Antistaminico	Antihistaminik
Antihypertensive drug	Antihypertenseur	Antihipertensivo	Farmaco antiipertensivo	Antihipertenziv
Antimalarial drug	Antimalarique	Antimalárico	Antimalarico	Antimalarik
Antimycotic	Antimycosique	Antimicótico (antifúngico)	Antimicotico	Antimikotik
Antioxidant	Antioxydant	Antioxidante	Antiossidante (sostanza antiossidante)	Antioksidans
Antiperspirant	Déodorant	Desodorante	Antidiaforetico	Antiperspirant
Antiprotozoal agent	Médicament antiprotozoal	Antiprotozoario	Farmaco antiprotozoico	Antiprotozoik
Antipsychotic	Antipsychotique	Antipsicótico	Antipsicotico	Antipsihotik
Antipyretic	Antipyrétique	Antipirético	Antipiretico	Antipiretik
Antirheumatic drug	Médicament antirhumatismal	Antireumático	Antireumatico	Antireumatik
Antiseptic	Antiseptique	Antiséptico	Antisettico	Antiseptik
Antiserum	Antisérum	Antisuero	Antisiero	Antiserum
Antitoxin	Antitoxine	Antitoxina	Antitossina	Protuotrov
Antitubercular agent	Antituberculeux	Fármaco tuberculostático	Farmaco antitubercolare	Antituberkulotik
Antiviral drug	Médicament antiviral	Fármaco antiviral	Farmaco antivirale	Antivirusni lijek
Aspirin	Aspirine	Aspirina	Aspirina	Aspirin
At noon	À midi	A mediodía	A mezzogiorno	U podne
Atropine	Atropine	Atropina	Atropina	Atropin

English	French	Spanish	Italian	Croatian
Bandage	Bandage	Venda	Bendaggio	Zavoj
Barbiturate	Barbiturique	Barbitúrico	Barbiturico	Barbiturat
Blood pressure meter (sphygmomanometer)	Tensiomètre (sphygmomanomètre)	Tensiómetro (esfigmomanómetro)	Misuratore di pressione (sfigmomanometro)	Tlakomjer
Boric acid	Acide borique	Ácido bórico	Acido borico	Borova otopina
Bronchodilator	Bronchodilatateur	Broncodilatador	Broncodilatatore	Bronhodilatator
Caffeine	Caféine	Cafeína	Caffeina	Kofein
Calcium	Calcium	Calcio	Calcio	Kalcij
Capsule	Gélule	Cápsula	Capsula	Kapsula
Cardiotonic agent	Médicament cardiotonique	Cardiotónico	Cardiotonico	Kardiotonik
Castor oil	Huile de ricin	Aceite de ricino	Olio di ricino	Ricinusovo ulje
Cephalosporin	Céphalosporine	Cefalosporina	Cefalosporina	Cefalosporin
Chamomile	Camomille	Manzanilla	Camomilla	Kamilica
Chemotherapy	Chimiothérapie	Quimioterapia	Chemioterapia	Kemoterapija
Chloramphenicol	Chloramphénicol	Cloranfenicol	Cloramfenicolo	Kloramfenikol
Chlorine	Chlore	Cloro	Cloro	Klor
Cobalt	Cobalt	Cobalto	Cobalto	Kobalt
Codeine	Codéine	Codeína	Codeina	Kodein
Compress	Compresse	Compresa	Compressa	Oblog
Condom	Préservatif	Preservativo (condón, profiláctico)	Preservativo (profilattico, condom)	Prezervativ (kondom)
Contact lenses	Lentilles de contact	Lentes de contacto (lentillas, pupilentes)	Lenti a contatto	Kontaktne leće
Contact lenses cleaning solution	Solution nettoyante pour lentilles	Solución limpiadora de lentes de contacto	Soluzione per pulizia lenti a contatto	Tekućina za čišćenje kontaktnih leća
Contraceptive	Contraceptif	Anticonceptivo	Contraccettivo	Kontraceptiv
Contraceptive foam	Mousse contraceptive	Espuma anticonceptiva	Schiuma anticoncezionale	Kontracepcijska pjena
Contraceptive pill (oral contraceptive)	Contraception orale	Píldora anticonceptiva	Pillola anticoncezionale	Kontracepcijska pilula
Contraceptive sponge	Éponge contraceptive	Esponja anticonceptiva	Spugna contraccettiva	Kontracepcijska spužva
Copper	Cuivre	Cobre	Rame	Bakar
Corticosteroid	Corticostéroïde	Corticosteroide	Corticosteroide	Kortikosteroid
Cotton-wool	Ouate (coton hydrophile)	Algodón hidrófilo	Ovatta	Vata
Cytostatic	Cytostatique	Citostático	Citostatico	Citostatik
Dental floss	Fil dentaire	Seda dental (hilo dental)	Filo interdentale	Zubni konac
Denture cleaning solution	Solution nettoyante pour les prothèses	Solución limpiadora de dentadura	Soluzione per pulizia dentiera	Tekućina za čišćenje umjetnog zubala
Diaphragm (Dutch cap)	Diaphragme	Diafragma	Diaframma	Dijafragma
Digestive	Médicament digestif	Digestivo	Digestivo	Digestiv
Diuretic	Diurétique	Diurético	Diuretico	Diuretik
Dose	Dose	Dosis	Dose	Doza
Drops	Gouttes	Gotas	Gocce	Kapi (kapljice)
Drug allergy	Allergie à un médicament	Alergia al medicamento	Allergia a medicamento	Alergija na lijek
Drug side-effects	Effets indésirables d'un médicament	Reacción adversa a medicamento	Effetti indesiderati da farmaco	Nuspojave lijeka
Ear drops	Gouttes auriculaires	Gotas óticas	Gocce per il mal di orecchi	Kapi za uši
Emulsion	Émulsion	Emulsión	Emulsione	Emulzija
Enema (clyster)	Clystère	Enema (clisma)	Clistere	Klizma (klistir)
Erythromycin	Érythromycine	Eritromicina	Eritromicina	Eritromicin
Essential oil	Huile essentielle	Aceite esencial	Olio essenziale (olio eterico)	Eterično ulje
Expectorant	Expectorant	Expectorante	Espettorante	Sredstvo za iskašljavanje
Eye drops	Collyre (gouttes ophtalmiques)	Colirio	Collirio	Kapi za oči
Fentanyl	Fentanyl	Fentanilo	Fentanyl	Fentanil
Foam	Mousse	Espuma	Schiuma (spuma)	Pjena
For external application	Pour l'application externe	De uso externo	Per l'applicazione esterna	Za vanjsku primjenu
Gauze sponge	Gaze	Gasa	Garza	Gaza
Gel	Gel	Gel	Gel	Gel
Gentamicin	Gentamicine	Gentamicina	Gentamicina	Gentamicin
Glasses	Lunettes de vue	Gafas	Occhiali	Naočale
Glucose	Glucose	Glucosa	Glucosio	Glukoza
Gram (gramme)	Gramme	Gramo	Grammo	Gram
Hard contact lens	Lentille de contact rigide	Lente de contacto duro	Lente a contatto rigida	Tvrda kontaktna leća
Heparin	Héparine	Heparina	Eparina	Heparin
Herbal tea	Tisane	Tisana (infusión de hierbas)	Tisana (infuso di erbe)	Biljni čaj
Home pregnancy test	Test de grossesse	Prueba de embarazo	Test di gravidanza ad uso domiciliare	Kućni test za trudnoću
Hormone replacement therapy	Hormonothérapie de substitution	Terapia de sustitución hormonal	Terapia ormonale sostitutiva	Hormonalna nadomjesna terapija
Hot water bottle	Bouillotte	Bolsa de agua caliente (guatero)	Bouillotte (bouilloire)	Termofor
Hypnotic (soporific)	Hypnotique (somnifère)	Hipnótico	Ipnotico	Hipnotik
Immunoglobulin	Immunoglobuline	Inmunoglobulina	Immunoglobulina	Imunoglobulin
Immunosuppressive	Immunosuppresseur	Inmunosupresor	Immunosoppressivo	Imunosupresiv
In the evening	Le soir	Por la noche	La sera	Na večer

English	French	Spanish	Italian	Croatian
In the morning	Le matin	Por la mañana	Di mattina	U jutro
Incontinence pads (adult diapers)	Slip d'incontinence	Pañal para adultos	Assorbenti per l'incontinenza	Pelene za inkontinenciju
Inhalation	Inhalation	Inhalación	Inalazione (farmaco per inalazioni)	Inhalacija
Injection	Injection	Inyección	Iniezione	Injekcija
Insect repellent	Répulsif d'insectes	Repelente de insectos	Insettifugo	Sredstvo protiv insekata
Insulin	Insuline	Insulina	Insulina	Inzulin
Interferon	Interféron	Interferón	Interferone	Interferon
International System of Units	Système international d'unités	Sistema Internacional de Unidades	Sistema internazionale di unità di misura	Sustav međunarodnih mjernih jedinica
Iodine	Iode	Yodo (iodo)	Iodio (tintura di iodio)	Jod
Iron	Fer	Hierro (fierro)	Ferro	Željezo
Jojoba oil	Huile de jojoba	Aceite de jojoba	Olio di jojoba	Jojobino ulje
Laxative	Laxatif	Laxante	Lassativo	Laksativ
Lip balm	Tube de soin pour lèvres	Bálsamo de labios	Burrocacao	Grožđana mast
Liquid powder	Poudre fluide	Polvo liquido	Polvere liquido	Tekući puder
Litre	Litre	Litro	Litro	Litra
Lotion	Lotion	Loción	Lozione	Losion
Lubricant	Lubrifiant	Lubricante	Lubrificante	Lubrikant
Magnesium	Magnésium	Magnesio	Magnesio	Magnezij
Manganese	Manganèse	Manganeso	Manganese	Mangan
Medical cannabis	Cannabis médical	Cannabis medicinal	Cannabis terapeutica	Medicinski kanabis
Medication (remedy, drug)	Médicament	Medicamento (fármaco)	Medicamento (farmaco, rimedio)	Lijek
Methadone	Méthadone	Metadona	Metadone	Metadon
Microgram	Microgramme	Microgramo	Microgrammo	Mikrogram
Milligram (milligramme)	Milligramme	Miligramo	Milligrammo	Miligram
Millilitre	Millilitre	Mililitro	Millilitro	Mililitar
Mineral	Minéral	Mineral	Minerale	Mineral
Mineral oil	Huile minérale	Aceite mineral	Olio minerale	Mineralno ulje
Molybdenum	Molybdène	Molibdeno	Molibdeno	Molibden
'Morning -after' pill (postcoital contraception, emergency contraception)	Pilule du lendemain (contraception postcoïtale, contraception d'urgence)	Anticonceptivo de emergencia (contracepción poscoital)	Pillola del "giorno do-ppo" (contraccezione postcoitale, contraccezione di emergenza)	Pilula za "dan poslije" (postkoitalna kontracepcija, hitna kontracepcija)
Morphine	Morphine	Morfina	Morfina	Morfin
Mosquito repellent	Répulsif antimoustiques	Repelente de mosquitos	Repellente antizanzare	Sredstvo protiv komaraca
Mouthwash liquid	Eau dentifrice	Enjuague bucal (colutorio)	Collutorio	Tekućina za ispiranje usne šupljine
Mucolytic	Mucolytique	Mucolítico	Mucolitico	Mukolitik
Muscle relaxant	Myorelaxant	Relajante muscular (miorrelajante)	Miorilassante	Miorelaksator
Nasal drops	Gouttes nasales	Gotas nasales	Gocce nasali	Kapi za nos
Needle	Aiguille	Aguja	Ago	Igla
Nicotine gum	Gomme à la nicotine	Goma de mascar de nicotina	Gomma da masticare antifumo	Nikotinska guma za žvakanje
Nicotine patch	Timbre à la nicotine	Parche de nicotina	Cerotto antifumo	Nikotinski flaster
Non-steroidal antiinflammatory drug	Anti-inflammatoire non stéroïdien	Antiinflamatorio no esteroideo	Farmaco anti-infiammatore non steroide-FANS	Nesteroidni antireumatik
Nutrient	Nutriment (élément nutritif)	Nutrimento (nutriente)	Sostanza nutriente (sostanza nutritiva)	Nutritiv
Nystatin	Nystatine	Nistatina	Nistatina	Nistatin
Ointment (fat)	Pommade	Ungüento (pomada)	Pomata (unguento)	Pomada (mast)
Omega-3 fatty acid	Acides gras oméga-3	Ácido graso omega 3	Omega-3 acidi grassi	Omega-3 masne kiseline
On empty stomach (before the meal)	À jeun	En ayunas	A digiuno	Na tašte
Opioid	Opioïde	Opioide	Oppioide	Opijat (opioid)
Orally	Par voie orale	Por vía oral	Oralmente (per via orale, per bocca)	Na usta
Overdose	Surdose	Sobredosis	Sovradosaggio	Predoziranje
Oxycodone	Oxycodone	Oxicodona	Ossicodone	Oksikodon
Paracetamol	Paracétamol	Paracetamol	Paracetamolo	Paracetamol
Paraffin	Paraffine	Parafina	Paraffina	Parafin
Paste	Pâte	Pasta	Pasta	Pasta
Pastille (lozenge)	Pastille	Pastilla	Pasticca (pastiglia)	Tableta za sisanje (pastila)
Penicillin	Pénicilline	Penicilina	Penicilina	Penicilin
Pharmacist	Pharmacien	Farmacéutico	Farmacista	Ljekarnik
Phosphorus	Phosphore	Fósforo	Fosforo	Fosfor
Phytotherapy	Phytothérapie	Fitoterapia	Fitoterapia	Fitoterapija
Piece	Morceau	Pieza	Pezzo (porzione)	Komad
Plaster (adhesive strip)	Pansement	Tira adhesiva sanitaria	Cerotto	Flaster
Poison	Poison	Veneno	Veleno	Otrov
Potassium	Potassium	Potasio	Potassio	Kalij
Potion	Potion	Poción	Pozione	Ljekoviti napitak
Powder	Poudre	Polvo	Polverina (polvere)	Prašak (puder)

English	French	Spanish	Italian	Croatian
Prescription	Ordonnance médicale	Receta	Prescrizione (rimedio prescritto)	Recept
Psychostimulant	Psychostimulant	Psicoestimulante	Psicostimulanti	Psihostimulans
Purgative	Purgatif	Purgante (purgativo)	Purgante (purga)	Purgativ
Rectal	Rectal	Rectal	Rettale	Rektalno
Rinsing	Rinçage	Lavado	Sciacquatra (risciacquatura)	Ispiranje
Salicylate	Salicylate	Salicilato	Salicilato	Salicilat
Saline solution	Solution physiologique	Suero fisiológico	Soluzione fisiologica	Fiziološka otopina
Sanitary pads (sanitary napkins)	Serviette hygiénique (protège-slip)	Toalla sanitaria (compresa, pantiprotector)	Assorbenti igienici	Higijenski ulošci
Scales	Balance	Balanza	Bilancia	Vaga
Sedative	Sédatif	Sedativo	Sedativo (calmante)	Sedativ
Serum	Sérum	Suero	Siero	Serum
Skin cream	Crème	Crema	Crema	Krema
Soap	Savon	Jabón	Sapone	Sapun
Sodium	Sodium	Sodio	Sodio	Natrij
Soft contact lens	Lentille de contact souple	Lente de contacto blanda	Lente a contatto morbida	Meka kontaktna leća
Solution	Solution	Soluto	Soluzione	Otopina
Spasmolytic	Spasmolytique	Espasmolítico	Spasmolitico	Spazmolitik
Spermicide	Spermicide	Espermicida	Spermicida	Spermicid
Spoon	Cuillère	Cuchara	Cucchiaio	Žlica
Spray	Spray	Rociada	Spruzzo (vaporizzato)	Sprej
Sublingual administration	Sublingual	Vía sublingual	Sublinguale	Pod jezik
Sugar substitute	Édulcorant	Edulcorante artificial	Dolcificante artificiale	Umjetno sladilo
Sulphonamide	Sulfamidé	Sulfonamida	Sulfamidici (sulfonamidici)	Sulfonamid
Sulphur	Soufre	Azufre	Zolfo	Sumpor
Sunscreen (sunblock)	Crème solaire	Protector solar	Filtro solare (crema solare ad alta protezione)	Sredstvo za zaštitu od sunca
Suppository	Suppositoire	Supositorio	Supposta	Čepić
Syringe	Seringue	Jeringa	Siringa per iniezioni	Šprica
Syrup	Sirop	Jarabe	Sciroppo	Sirup
Tablet	Comprimé	Comprimido	Compressa (pasticca, tavoletta)	Dražeja (tableta)
Tampon	Tampon hygiénique	Tampón	Tampone	Tampon
Tetracycline	Tétracycline	Tetraciclina	Tetraciclina	Tetraciklin
Thermometer	Thermomètre	Termómetro	Termometro	Toplomjer
Tincture	Teinture	Tintura	Tintura	Tinktura
Tonic	Tonique	Tónico	Tonico (ricostituente)	Tonik
Tooth paste	Dentifrice	Pasta de dientes (dentífrico)	Dentifricio	Pasta za zube
Tramadol	Tramadol	Tramadol	Tramadolo	Tramal
Urinary antiseptic	Antiseptique urinaire	Antiséptico de las vías urinarias	Antisettico urinario	Uroantiseptik
Vaccine	Vaccin	Vacuna	Vaccino	Cjepivo
Vaginal suppository	Ovule (suppositoire vaginal)	Supositorio vaginal	Candelette	Vaginaleta
Vasodilatator	Vasodilatateur	Vasodilatador	Vasodilatatore	Vazodilatator
Viagra (sildenafil citrate)	Viagra (citrate de sildénafil)	Viagra	Viagra (citrato di sildenafil)	Viagra
Vial	Fiole	Frasquito	Bottiglietta (boccetta)	Bočica
Vitamin	Vitamine	Vitamina	Vitamina	Vitamin
Vitamin A (retinol)	Vitamine A (rétinol)	Vitamina A (retinol)	Vitamina A (retinolo)	Vitamin A (retinol)
Vitamin B1 (thiamin)	Vitamine B1 (thiamine)	Vitamina B1 (tiamina)	Vitamina B1 (tiamina)	Vitamin B1 (tiamin)
Vitamin B2 (riboflavin)	Vitamine B2 (riboflavine)	Vitamina B2 (riboflavina)	Vitamina B2 (riboflavina)	Vitamin B2 (riboflavin)
Vitamin B3 (niacin)	Vitamine B3 (nicotinamide, PP)	Vitamina B3 (niacina, vitamina PP)	Vitamina B3 (niacina, vitamina PP)	Vitamin B3 (niacin)
Vitamin B4 (adenine)	Vitamine B4 (adénine)	Vitamina B4 (adenina)	Vitamina B4 (adenina)	Vitamin B4 (adenin)
Vitamin B5 (pantothenic acid)	Vitamine B5 (acide pantothénique)	Vitamina B5 (ácido pantoténico)	Vitamina B5 (acido pantotenico, vitamina W)	Vitamin B5 (pantotenska kiselina)
Vitamin B6 (pyridoxine)	Vitamine B6 (pyridoxine)	Vitamina B6 (piridoxina)	Vitamina B6 (piridossina)	Vitamin B6 (piridoksin)
Vitamin B7 (inositol)	Vitamine B7 (inositol)	Vitamina B7 (inositol)	Vitamina B7 (inositolo)	Vitamin B7 (inozitol)
Vitamin B8 (biotin)	Vitamine B8 (biotine)	Vitamina B8 (biotina)	Vitamina B8 (biotina)	Vitamin B8 (biotin)
Vitamin B9 (folic acid)	Vitamine B9 (acide folique)	Vitamina B9 (ácido fólico)	Vitamina B9 (acido folico)	Vitamin B9 (folna kiselina)
Vitamin B10 (factor-R)	Vitamine B10 (vitamine R)	Vitamina B10 (vitamina R)	Vitamina B10 (vitamina R)	Vitamin B10 (faktor-R)
Vitamin B11 (factor-S)	Vitamine B11 (carnitine)	Vitamina B11 (vitamina S)	Vitamina B11 (vitamina S)	Vitamin B11 (faktor-S)
Vitamin B12 (cobalamin)	Vitamine B12 (cobalamine)	Vitamina B12 (ciancobalamina)	Vitamina B12 (cobalamina)	Vitamin B12 (kobalamin)
Vitamin C (L-ascorbic acid)	Vitamine C (acide ascorbique)	Vitamine C (enantiómero L de ácido ascórbico)	Vitamina C (acido L-ascorbico)	Vitamin C (L-askorbinska kiselina)
Vitamin D2 (ergocalciferol)	Vitamine D2 (ergocalciférol)	Vitamina D2 (ergocalciferol)	Vitamina D2 (ergocalciferolo)	Vitamin D2 (ergokalciferol)
Vitamin D3 (cholecalciferol)	Vitamine D3 (cholécalciférol)	Vitamina D3 (colecalciferol)	Vitamina D3 (colecalciferolo)	Vitamin D3 (kolekalciferol)
Vitamin D4	Vitamine D4	Vitamina D4	Vitamina D4 (diidroergocalciferolo)	Vitamin D4
Vitamin D5 (sitocalciferol)	Vitamine D5 (sitocalciférol)	Vitamina D5 (sitocalciferol)	Vitamina D5 (sitocalciferolo)	Vitamin D5 (sitokalciferol)
Vitamin E (tocopherol)	Vitamine E (tocophérol)	Vitamina E (alfatocoferol)	Vitamina E (tocoferolo)	Vitamin E (tokoferol)
Vitamin F (linoleic acid)	Vitamine F (acide linoléique)	Ácido linoleico	Vitamina F (acido linoleico)	Vitamin F (linoleična kiselina)

English	French	Spanish	Italian	Croatian
Vitamin J (choline)	Vitamine J (choline)	Vitamina J (colina)	Vitamina J (colina)	Vitamin J (kolin)
Vitamin K (phylloquinone)	Vitamine K (phylloquinone)	Vitamina K (filoquinona)	Vitamina K (fillochinone)	Vitamin K (filokinon)
Vitamin L1 (anthranilic acid)	Vitamine L1 (acide anthranilique)	Vitamina L1 (ácido antranílico)	Vitamina L1 (acido antranilico)	Vitamin L1 (antranilna kiselina)
Vitamin P (flavonoids)	Vitamine P (flavonoïde)	Vitamina P (flavonoide)	Vitamina P (flavonoidi)	Vitamin P (flavonoidi)
Water-soluble tablets	Comprimé effervescent	Solubilizantes (comprimidos dispersables en agua)	Compresse solubili	Šumeće tablete
Zinc	Zinc	Zinc (cinc)	Zinco	Cink
Zinc ointment	Pommade à l'oxyde de zinc	Pasta de óxido de zinc	Zinco pasta	Cinkova pasta

MEDICAL FACILITIES, PROCEDURES AND CARE:	ÉTABLISSEMENTS MÉDICAUX, PROCÉDURES ET SOINS:	FACILIDADES MÉDICAS, PROCEDIMIENTOS Y ASISTENCIA MÉDICA:	ISTITUZIONI, PROCEDURE E CURE DI MEDICINA:	MEDICINSKE USTANOVE, ZAHVATI I NJEGA:
Administration of drugs	Administration des médicaments	Administración de fármacos	Somministrazione dei farmaci	Davanje lijekova
Airway (cannula)	Canule	Cánula	Cannula	Kanila
Alarm	Alarme	Alarma	Allarme	Uzbuna (alarm)
Ambu bag valve mask	Respirateur manuel type Ambu	Bolsa Ambú de ventilación manual	Pallone autoespandibile	Ambu balon s maskom
Ambulance	Ambulance	Ambulancia	Autoambulanza	Kola hitne pomoći
Ambulance (clinic)	Infirmerie	Enfermería	Ambulanza	Ambulanta
Amputation	Amputation	Amputación	Amputazione	Amputacija
Anesthesia	Anesthésie	Anestesia	Anestesia	Anestezija (narkoza)
Arthrodesis	Arthrodèse	Artrodesis	Artrodesi	Artrodeza
Artificial respiration	Ventilation artificielle	Respiración artificial	Respirazione artificiale	Umjetno disanje
Autopsy	Autopsie	Autopsia	Autopsia	Obdukcija
Balance training	Entraînement de l'equilibre	Entrenamiento del equilibrio	Esercizi di equilibrio	Trening ravnoteže
Bath (wash)	Laver	Darse un baño	Lavare (fare il bagno)	Kupati
Bathroom	Salle de bains	Cuarto de baño	Bagno	Kupaonica
Bed	Lit	Cama	Letto	Krevet
Bed rest	Repos au lit	Guardar cama	Riposo a letto	Mirovanje u krevetu
Bite	Mordre	Morder	Addentare	Zagristi
Blanket	Couverture	Manta (cobija)	Schiavina	Deka
Blood donation	Don de sang	Donación de sangre	Donazione del sangue	Darovanje krvi (donacija krvi)
Body positioner	Coussin de positionnement	Almohada de posicionamiento	Posizionatore	Udlaga za pozicioniranje
Breakfast	Petit déjeuner	Desayuno	Colazione	Doručak
Breast implant	Implant mammaire	Implante de mama	Protese mammaria	Umetak za dojku
Breathing exercises	Exercice de respiration	Ejercicios de respiración	Esercizi di respirazione	Vježbe disanja
Bypass	Pontage	By-pass	Bypass	Premosnica
Calling of the time of death	Détermination de l'heure de la mort	Determinación del tiempo de muerte	Proclamazione del tempo della morte	Proglašenje vremena smrti
Cardiology	Cardiologie	Cardiología	Cardiologia	Kardiologija
Catheter	Cathéter	Catéter	Catetere	Kateter
Cause of death	Cause de la mort	Causa de muerte	Causa di morte	Uzrok smrti
Cauterization	Cautérisation	Cauterización	Cauterizzazione	Kauterizacija
Chamber -pot	Pot de chambre	Orinal	Vaso da notte (pitale)	Noćna posuda
Chemotherapy	Chimiothérapie	Quimioterapia	Chemioterapia	Kemoterapija
Circumcision	Circoncision	Circoncisión	Circoncisione	Obrezivanje
Cleansing	Purification	Purificación	Purificazione	Pročišćavanje
Close	Fermer	Cerrar	Chiudere	Zatvoriti
Contagious	Contagieux (contagieuse)	Contagioso	Contagioso (infettivo)	Zarazno
Corpse	Cadavre	Cadáver	Cadavere (salma)	Leš
Cover	Couverture	Cubrecama (colcha, manta)	Coperta	Pokrivač
CPR mask	Masque de réanimation	Máscara de reanimación	Maschera per rianimazione	Maska za oživljavanje
Crutch	Béquille	Muleta	Gruccia (stampella)	Štaka
Cryoextraction	Cryo-extraction	Crío-extracción	Crioestrazione	Krioekstrakcija
Cytology	Cytologie	Citología	Citologia	Citologija
Debris	Débris	Materia de desperdicio	Rottami	Otpad (otpadni proizvod)
Defecation	Défécation	Defecación	Defecazione	Pražnjenje stolice (defekacija)
Defibrillation	Défibrillation	Desfibrilación	Defibrillazione	Defibrilacija
Defibrillator	Défibrillateur	Desfibrilador	Defibrillatore	Defibrilator
Dental crown	Couronne	Corona	Corona	Zubna krunica
Dental extraction	Extraction dentaire	Exodoncia dental	Estrazione del dente	Vađenje zuba
Dental filling	Composite dentaire	Empaste (emplomadura)	Otturazione odontoiatrica	Zubna plomba
Dentist	Dentiste	Dentista	Dentista	Stomatolog (zubar)
Dentures	Dentier	Prótesis dental	Protesi dentale	Umjetno zubalo
Dermatology	Dermatologie	Dermatología	Dermatologia	Dermatologija
Diagnosis	Diagnostic	Diagnóstico	Diagnosi	Dijagnoza
Dialysis	Dialyse	Diálisis	Dialisi	Dijaliza
Die	Mourir	Morir	Morire	Umrijeti
Diet	Régime alimentaire	Régimen (dieta)	Dieta (regime dietetico)	Dijeta
Digestion	Digestion	Digestión	Digestione	Probava

English	French	Spanish	Italian	Croatian
Dining-room	Salle à manger	Comedor	Sala da pranzo (cenàcolo)	Blagavaonica
Dinner (supper)	Dîner (souper)	Cena	Cena	Večera
Doctor (physician)	Médecin	Médico	Dottore/dottoressa (medico)	Liječnik
Doctor's office	Bureau du médecin	Consultorio de médico	Ufficio del medico	Liječnička ambulanta
Donor	Donneur	Donante	Donatore/donatrice	Davalac (donator)
Door	Porte	Puerta	Porta	Vrata
Drain tube	Drain	Sonda de drenaje	Tubo di drenaggio	Dren
Drainage	Drainage	Drenaje	Drenaggio	Drenaža
Dressing	Pansement	Apósito	Fasciatura (bendaggio)	Previjanje
Drill	Perceuse	Taladro	Trapano (trivella)	Bušilica
Dynamometer	Dynamomètre	Dinamómetro	Dinamometro	Dinamometar
Electrode	Électrode	Electrodo	Elettrodo	Elektroda
Electrode conductive gel	Gel électroconductif	Gel conductor	Gel elettro-conduttivo	Kontaktni gel za elektrode
Electrosurgery	Électrochirurgie	Electrocirugía	Elettrochirurgia	Elektrokirurgija
Electrotherapy	Électrothérapie	Electroterapia	Elettroterapia	Elektroterapija
Elevator	Ascenseur	Elevador	Ascensore	Dizalo
Emergency medical services	Aide médicale urgente	Servicios médicos de emergencia	Servizio di urgenza ed emergenza medica	Hitna služba
Endotracheal tube	Sonde d'intubation endotrachéale	Sonda endotraqueal	Tubo endotracheale	Endotrahealna kanila
Escape chair	Chaise d'évacuation	Silla de evacuación	Sedia portantina	Sjedalica za evakuaciju
Exercise	Exercice	Ejercicio	Esercizio	Vježbanje
Facelift (rhytidectomy)	Lifting facial (rhytidectomie, lissage, remodelage)	Estiramiento de la cara (ritidectomía)	Lift facciale (ritidectomia)	Lifting lica (ritidektomija)
Feeding tube	Sonde d'alimentation	Sonda de alimentación	Sonda gastrica per nutrizione	Sonda za hranjenje
First aid	Premiers secours	Primeros auxilios	Primo soccorso	Prva pomoć
First aid kit	Trousse de secours	Botiquín de primeros auxilios	Cassetta di pronto soccorso	Kutija prve pomoći
Gastric lavage (stomach pumping)	Lavage gastrique	Lavado gástrico	Lavanda gastrica	Ispiranje želuca
General anesthesia	Anesthésie générale	Anestesia general	Anestesia generale	Opća anestezija
General practitioner	Médecin généraliste (médecin omnipraticien)	Médico de cabecera	Medico di medicina generale (medico di famiglia)	Liječnik opće prakse
Germs	Germes	Gérmenes	Germi	Klice
Gerontology	Gérontologie	Gerontología	Gerontologia	Gerontologija
Get changed	Se changer	Cambiarse	Cambiarsi	Presvući se
Goniometer	Goniomètre	Goniómetro	Goniometro	Goniometar
Gynecology	Gynécologie	Ginecología	Ginecologia	Ginekologija
Head immobilizer	Immobiliseur de tête	Inmovilizador de cabeza	Fermacapo	Imobilizator glave
Health insurance	Assurance maladie	Seguro de salud	Assicurazione sanitaria	Zdravstveno osiguranje
Hearing assist device	Appareil acoustique	Audífono	Apparecchio acustico	Slušni aparat
Heel and elbow protectors	Talonnières et coudières	Protectores talón/codo antiescaras	Talloniere e gomitiere antidecubito	Zaštitnici za pete i laktove
Heimlich maneuver (abdominal thrusts)	Méthode de Heimlich	Maniobra de Heimlich	Manovra di Heimlich	Heimlichov zahvat
Hospital	Hôpital	Hospital	Ospedale (policlinico)	Bolnica
Hospital trolley	Chariot	Camilla	Carrello	Kolica
Hydrotherapy	Hydrothérapie	Hidroterapia	Idroterapia	Hidroterapija
Immunology	Immunologie	Inmunología	Immunologia	Imunologija
Incontinence pad	Protège-matelas	Sábana de hule para la incontinencia	Proteggi materasso cerato	Gumirano platno
Infectious disease unit	Salle maladies infectieuses	Pabellón de enfermedades infecciosas	Reparto di malattie infettive	Zarazni odjel
Infusion	Perfusion	Infusión	Infusione	Infuzija
Infusion stand	Pied à perfusion	Intravenoso poste	Piantana portaflebo	Stalak za infuziju
Injection	Injection	Inyección	Iniezione	Injekcija
Intensive care	Soins intensifs	Cuidados intensivos	Terapia intensiva	Intenzivna njega
Intensive care unit	Unité de soins intensifs	Unidad de cuidados intensivos	Stanza da terapia intensiva	Jedinica intenzivne njege
Internal medicine	Médicine interne	Medicina interna	Medicina interna	Interna medicina
Intubation	Intubation	Intubación	Intubazione	Intubacija
Kegel exercise	Exercice de Kegel	Ejercicios de Kegel	Esercizi di Kegel	Kegelove vježbe
Laparoscopic surgery	Laparoscopie (coelioscopie)	Cirugía laparoscópica	Chirurgia laparoscopica	Laparoskopska operacija
Laryngeal mask airway	Masque laryngé	Máscara laríngea	Maschera laringea	Laringealna maska
Laryngoscope	Laryngoscope	Laringoscopio	Laringoscopio	Laringoskop
Laundry	Blanchisserie	Lavandería	Lavanderia	Večeraj
Light	Lumière	Luz	Luce	Svjetlo
Liposuction	Liposuccion	Liposucción	Liposuzione	Liposukcija
Litter bin	Poubelle	Papelera	Pattumiera	Kanta za smeće
Liver dialysis	Dialyse hépatique	Diálisis de hígado	Dialisi epatica	Dijaliza jetre
Lobotomy	Lobotomie	Lobotomía	Lobotomia	Lobotomija
Local anesthesia	Anesthésie locale	Anestesia local	Anestesia locale	Lokalna anestezija
Lunch	Déjeuner	Almuerzo	Pranzo	Ručak

English	French	Spanish	Italian	Croatian
Manometer cuff	Brassard du manomètre	Manguito de presión arterial	Manicotto di sfigmomanometro	Manšeta tlakomjera
Manual de fibrillator	Défibrillateur manuel	Desfibrilador manual	Defibrillatore manuale	Ručni defibrilator
Mattress	Matelas	Colchón	Materasso	Madrac
Medical center	Centre médical	Centro médico	Centro di medicina	Medicinski centar
Morgue (mortuary)	Morgue	Depósito de cadáveres (morgue)	Obitorio (mortorio)	Mrtvačnica
Nasal cannula	Canule nasale	Cánula nasal	Cannula nasale	Nosna kanila
Neck immobilizer	Support de cou	Collar cervical	Collare cervicale	Imobilizator vrata
Neurology	Neurologie	Neurología	Neurologia	Neurologija
Night table (bedside table)	Table de chevet (table de nuit)	Mesilla de noche	Comodino	Noćni ormarić
Nightgown	Chemise de nuit	Camisón	Camicia da notte	Spavačica
Nurse	Infirmier	Enfermera	Infermiera/infermiere	Medicinska sestra
Nursing (care)	Soins de santé	Asistencia (cuidado)	Assistenza infermieristica	Njega
Occupational therapist	Ergothérapeute	Terapeuta ocupacional	Terapista occupazionale	Radni terapeut
Oncology	Oncologie (cancérologie)	Oncología	Oncologia	Onkologija
Open	Ouvrir	Abrir	Aprire	Otvoriti
Operating room	Bloc opératoire	Quirófano	Sala operatoria	Operacijska sala
Operation (surgery)	Opération chirurgicale	Operación quirúrgica	Operazione (intervento chirurgico)	Operacija
Ophtalmology ward	Salle d'ophtalmologie	Sala de oftalmología	Reparto di oftalmologia	Očni odjel
Oropharyngeal airway	Canule de Guedel	Cánula orofaríngea (tubo de Mayo, cánula de Guédel)	Cannula oro-faringea	Orofaringealna kanila
Orthopedics	Orthopédie	Ortopedia	Ortopedia	Ortopedija
Otorhinolaryngology	Oto-rhino-laryngologie	Otorrinolaringología	Otorinolaringoiatria	Uho-grlo-nos
Overbed table	Table de lit	Mesa para cama	Carrello servitore	Stolić za serviranje hrane
Oxygen mask	Masque à oxygène	Máscara de oxígeno	Maschera dell'ossigeno	Maska za kisik
Oxygen storage tank	Réservoir d'oxygène	Tanque de oxígeno	Serbatoio di ossigeno	Boca s kisikom
Pacemaker	Stimulateur cardiaque (pacemaker, pile)	Marcapasos	Cardiostimolatore (stimolatore cardiaco)	Električni stimulator srca
Palpation	Palpation	Palpación	Palpazione	Pregled pipanjem (palpacija)
Pathology	Pathologie	Patología	Patologia	Patologija
Patient	Patient (malade)	Paciente	Paziente (ammalato)	Bolesnik
Patient's room	Chambre de malade	Cuarto del paciente	Camera di malato	Bolesnička soba
Pediatrics	Pédiatrie	Pediatría	Pediatria	Pedijatrija
Percussion	Percussion	Percusión	Percussione	Pregled kucanjem (perkusija)
Percutaneous coronary intervention (coronary angioplasty)	Angioplastie coronaire (dilatation transluminale)	Intervención coronaria percutánea	Angioplastica coronarica	Perkutana koronarna angioplastika
Pessary	Pessaire (pessus)	Pesario	Pessario	Pesar
Physical therapy	Physiothérapie	Fisioterapia	Fisioterapia	Fizikalna terapija
Physiotherapist	Physiothérapeute	Fisioterapeuta	Fisioterapista	Fizioterapeut
Pillow	Oreiller	Almohada	Cuscino	Jastuk
Plaster cast (immobilization plaster)	Plâtre pour immobilisation rigide	Escayola de inmovilización	Bendaggio gessato	Gipsana udlaga
Plastic surgery of the abdomen ("tummy tuck", abdominoplasty)	Opération de chirurgie esthétique de la paroi abdominale (abdominoplastie)	Cirugía estética del abdomen (abdominoplastia)	Procedura di chirurgia plastica dell'addome (addominoplastica)	Plastična operacija trbuha (abdominoplastika)
Plastic surgery of the breasts (mammoplasty)	Opération de chirurgie esthétique des seins (mammoplastie)	Cirugía estética de los senos (mamoplastia)	Procedura di chirurgia plastica del seno (mastoplastica)	Plastična operacija dojke (mastoplastika)
Plastic surgery of the eyelid (blepharoplasty)	Opération de chirurgie esthétique des paupières (blépharoplastie)	Cirugía estética de los párpados (blefaroplastia)	Procedura di chirurgia plastica della palpebra (blefaroplastica)	Plastična operacija očnog kapka (blefaroplastika)
Plastic surgery of the nose (rhinoplasty)	Opération de chirurgie esthétique du nez (rhinoplastie)	Cirugía estética de la nariz (rinoplastia)	Procedura di chirurgia plastica del naso (rinoplastica)	Plastična operacija nosa (rinoplastika)
Postural drainage	Drainage postural	Drenaje postural	Drenaggio posturale	Drenažni položaj
Primary health care	Soins de santé primaire	Atención primaria de salud	Assistenza sanitaria primaria	Primarna zdravstvena zaštita
Protect gloves	Gants à usage unique	Guantes desechables	Guanti protettivi	Zaštitne rukavice
Protection cap	Charlotte à usage unique	Gorra desechable	Cuffietta protettiva	Zaštitna kapa
Protection face mask	Masque de protection	Mascarilla desechable	Mascherina di protezione	Zaštitna maska za lice
Protection gown	Blouse de protection	Gabacha desechable	Camicia protettiva	Zaštitna navlaka za odjeću
Protection shoe cover	Sur-chaussures à usage unique	Cubrezapatos	Sovrascarpe protettive	Zaštitna navlaka za obuću
Psychiatry	Psychiatrie	Psiquiatría	Psichiatria	Psihijatrija
Psychologist	Psychologue	Psicólogo	Psicologo	Psiholog
Pulmonary ward	Salle de pneumologie	Sala de neumología	Reparto polmonare	Plućni odjel
Pyjamas (pajamas)	Pyjama	Pijama (piyama)	Pigiama	Piđama
Quarantine	Quarantaine	Cuarentena	Quarantena	Karantena
Radiation	Radiation	Radiación	Radiazione	Zračenje
Radiology	Radiographie	Radiología	Radiologia	Radiologija

English	French	Spanish	Italian	Croatian
Reanimation	Réanimation	Reanimación	Rianimazione	Oživljavanje (reanimacija)
Reception office	Réception	Mostrador de recepción	Accettazione	Prijemni ured
Recipient of an organ	Receveur de greffe	Receptor de un órgano	Ricevente di trapianto	Primatelj organa
Recover (heal)	Se remettre (se guérir)	Reponerse (recuperarse)	Sanare (guarire, recuperare)	Ozdraviti
Recovery	Guérison	Recuperación	Guarigione (ristabilimento)	Oporavak
Rehabilitation (rehab)	Réhabilitation	Rehabilitación	Riabilitazione	Rehabilitacija
Remission	Rémission	Fase de remisión	Remissione	Stadij mirovanja bolesti (remisija)
Renal dialysis	Dialyse rénale	Diálisis renal	Dialisi renale	Dijaliza bubrega
Respirator	Appareil respiratoire	Aparato respiratorio	Respiratore	Aparat za disanje (respirator)
Rhinology	Rhinologie	Rinología	Rinologia	Rinologija
Rinse	Rincer	Lavar	Sciacquare	Isprati
Scalpel	Scalpel	Escalpelo	Scalpello	Skalpel
Scissors	Ciseau	Tijeras	Forbici	Škare
Semi -intensive care	Soins semi-intensifs	Cuidados semi-intensivos	Terapia semi-intensiva	Poluintenzivna njega
Sheet	Drap	Sábana	Lenzuolo	Plahta
Shunt	Pontage (shunt)	Shunt	Shunt	Spoj (skretnica)
Slippers	Chausson	Pantuflas	Ciabatte	Šlape
Sonde	Sonde	Sonda	Sonda	Sonda
Spit	Cracher	Escupir	Sputare	Pljunuti
Sponge	Éponge	Esponja	Spugna	Spužva
Sterile (aseptic)	Stérile	Estéril	Sterile	Sterilno
Sterilization	Stérilisation	Esterilización	Sterilizzazione	Sterilizacija
Stethoscop	Stéthoscope	Estetoscopio	Stetofonendoscopio	Stetoskop
Storage	Stockage	Almacenaje	Deposito (magazzino)	Spremište
Stretcher	Civière	Camilla enrollable	Barella (lettiga)	Nosila
Suction catheter	Cathéter à succion	Catéter de succión	Tubo d'aspirazione	Usisni kateter
Suction unit (aspirator)	Appareil à succion	Aspirador	Aspiratore di secreti	Aspirator
Surgery	Chirurgie	Cirugía	Chirurgia	Kirurgija
Surgical opening of a direct airway on the neck (tracheostomy)	Ouverture chirurgicale dans la trachée (trachéotomie)	Incisión quirúrgica en la tráquea (traqueotomía)	Incisione chirurgica della trachea (tracheotomia)	Kirurško otvaranje dišnog puta (traheotomija)
Surgical opnening of the cranium (craniotomy)	Ouverture chirurgicale du crâne (craniotomie)	Abertura quirúrgica en el cráneo (craneotomía)	Apertura chirurgica del cranio (craniotomia)	Kirurški zahvat otvaranja lubanje (kraniotomija)
Surgical procedure of formation of stoma (colostomy)	Formation chirurgicale de la stomie (colostomie)	Exteriorización de una parte de intestino a través de la cavidad abdominal (colostomía)	Formazione chirurgica di stomia (colostomia)	Kirurški zahvat formiranja stome (kolostomija)
Surgical procedure on a joint (arthrotomy)	Ouverture chirurgicale d'une articulation (arthrotomie)	Incisión quirúrgica de una articulación (artrotomía)	Apertura chirurgica di un articolazione (artrotomia)	Kirurški zahvat na zglobu (artrotomija)
Surgical procedure on the middle ear (stapedectomy)	Ablation chirurgicale de l'étrier (stapédectomie)	Cirugía del oído medio (stapedectomía)	Intervento chirurgico dell'orecchio medio (stapedectomia)	Kirurški zahvat na srednjem uhu (stapedektomija)
Surgical procedure on the spine (laminectomy)	Résection chirurgicale des lames vertébrales (laminectomie)	Extirpación quirúrgica de parte de una vértebra (laminectomía)	Asportazione chirurgica della lamina di vertebre (laminectomia)	Kirurški zahvat na kralježnici (laminektomija)
Surgical procedure on the thalamus (thalamotomy)	Ablation chirurgicale d'une partie du thalamus (thalamotomie)	Cirugía del tálamo (talamotomía)	Intervento chirurgico delle connessioni talamiche (talamotomia)	Kirurški zahvat na talamusu (talamotomija)
Surgical removal of a breast (mastectomy)	Enlèvement chirurgical d'un sein (mastectomie)	Remoción quirúrgica de seno (mastectomía)	Asportazione chirurgica della mammella (mastectomia)	Kirurško odstranjenje dojke (mastektomija)
Surgical removal of a hemorrhoid (hemorrhoidectomy)	Ablation chirurgicale des hémorroïdes (hémorroïdectomie)	Extirpación quirúrgica de las hemorroides (hemorroidectomía)	Asportazione chirurgica delle emorroidi (emorroidectomia)	Kirurško odstranjenje hemeroida (hemoroidektomija)
Surgical removal of a lobe of some organ (lobectomy)	Ablation chirurgicale d'un lobe d'organe (lobectomie)	Extirpación quirúrgica de un lóbulo de un órgano (lobectomía)	Asportazione chirurgica di struttura lobale di un organo (lobectomia)	Kirurško odstranjenje režnja nekog organa (lobektomija)
Surgical removal of a testicle (orchidectomy)	Amputation chirurgicale d'un ou des deux testicules (orchidectomie, orchiectomie)	Extirpación quirúrgica del testículo (orquidectomía)	Asportazione chirurgica del testicolo (orchiectomia)	Kirurško odstranjenje testisa (orhidektomija)
Surgical removal of adenoids (adenoidectomy)	Ablation chirurgicale des végétations adénoïdes (adénoïdectomie)	Extirpación quirúrgica de las adenoides (adenoidectomía)	Asportazione chirurgica delle adenoidi (adenoidectomia)	Kirurško odstranjenje trećeg krajnika (adenoidektomija)
Surgical removal of one or both adrenal glands (adrenalectomy)	Ablation chirurgicale d'une ou des deux glandes surrénales (adrenalectomie)	Extirpación quirúrgica de una glándula suprarrenal (adrenalectomía)	Asportazione chirur-gica di uno o etrambi surreni(surrenectomia, adrenalectomia)	Kirurško odstranjenje nadbubrežne žlijezde (adrenalektomija)
Surgical removal of stones (lithotomy)	Extraction chirurgicale des pierres de la vessie (lithotomie)	Extracción quirúrgica de los cálculos (litotomía)	Asportazione chirurgica di calcolo (litotomia)	Kirurško odstranjenje kamenca (litotomija)
Surgical removal of the aneurysm (aneurysmectomy)	Résection chirurgicale d'une poche anévrismale (anevrismectomie)	Extirpación quirúrgica de un aneurisma (aneurismectomía)	Asportazione chirurgica della sacca aneurismatica (aneurismectomia)	Kirurško odstranjenje aneurizme (aneurizmektomija)

English	French	Spanish	Italian	Croatian
Surgical removal of the gallbladder (cholecystectomy)	Enlèvement chirurgical de la vésicule biliaire (cholécystectomie)	Extracción quirúrgica de la vesícula biliar (colecistectomía)	Asportazione chirur-gica della colecisti (colecistectomia)	Kirurško odstranjenje žučnog mjehura (kolecistektomija)
Surgical removal of the larynx (laryngectomy)	Ablation chirurgicale du larynx (laryngectomie)	Extirpación quirúrgica de la laringe (laringectomía)	Asportazione chirurgica della laringe (laringectomia)	Kirurško odstranjenje grkljana (laringektomija)
Surgical removal of the pancreas (pancreatectomy)	Ablation chirurgicale du pancréas (pancréatectomie)	Extirpación quirúrgica del páncreas (pancreatectomía)	Asportazione chirurgica del pancreas (pancreatectomia)	Kirurško odstranjenje gušterače (pankreatektomija)
Surgical removal of the prostate gland (prostatectomy)	Ablation chirurgicale de la prostate (prostatectomie)	Extirpación quirúrgica de la próstata (prostatectomía)	Asportazione chirurgica della prostata (prostatectomia)	Kirurško odstranjenje prostate (prostatektomija)
Surgical removal of the spleen (splenectomy)	Ablation chirurgicale de la rate (splénectomie)	Extirpación quirúrgica del bazo (esplenectomía)	Asportazione chirurgica della milza (splenectomia)	Kirurško odstranjenje slezene (splenektomija)
Surgical removal of the stomach (gastrectomy)	Ablation chirurgicale de l'estomac (gastrectomie)	Extirpación quirúrgica del estómago (gastrectomía)	Asportazione chirurgica dello stomaco (gastrectomia)	Kirurško odstranjenje želuca (gastrektomija)
Surgical removal of the thymus (thymectomy)	Ablation chirurgicale du thymus (thymectomie)	Extirpación quirúrgica del timo (timectomía)	Asportazione chirurgica del timo (timectomia)	Kirurško odstranjenje prsne žlijezde (timektomija)
Surgical removal of the thyroid gland (thyroidectomy)	Ablation chirurgicale de la thyroïde (thyroïdectomie, isthmectomie)	Extirpación quirúrgica de la glándula tiroides (tiroidectomía)	Asportazione chirurgica della tiroide (tiroidectomia)	Kirurško odstranjenje štitne žlijezde (tiroidektomija)
Surgical removal of the uterus (hysterectomy)	Enlèvement chirurgical de l'uterus (hystérectomie)	Extracción quirúrgica del útero (histerectomía)	Asportazione chirurgica dell'utero (isterectomia)	Kirurško odstranjenje maternice (histerektomija)
Surgical removal of the vermiform appendix (appendectomy)	Ablation chirurgicale de l'appendice iléocaecal (appendicectomie)	Extirpación quirúrgica del apéndice cecal (apendicectomía)	Asportazione chirurgica dell'appendice (appendicectomia)	Kirurško odstranjenje slijepog crijeva (apendektomija)
Surgical removal of tonsils (tonsillectomy)	Ablation chirurgicale des amygdales palatines (amygdalectomie, tonsillectomie)	Extracción quirúrgica de las amígdalas (tonsilectomía)	Asportazione chirurgica delle tonsille (tonsillectomia)	Kirurško odstranjenje krajnika (tonzilektomija)
Surgical removal of uterine myomas (myomectomy, fibroidectomy)	Ablation chirurgicale des fibromes utérins (myomectomie)	Extirpación quirúrgica de los fibromas uterinos (miomectomía)	Asportazione chirurgica di fibromi nell'utero (miomectomia)	Kirurško odstranjenje mioma u maternici (miomektomija)
Surgical sterilization of a man (vasectomy)	Ligature des canaux déférents des testicules (vasectomie)	Esterilización quirúrgica masculina (vasectomía)	Vasectomia	Kirurška sterilizacija muškarca (vazektomija)
Surgical sterilization of a woman (tubal ligation)	Stérilisation chirurgicale au femme (ligature des trompes)	Esterilizatióm quirúrgica femenina (ligadura de trompas)	Chiusura delle tube	Kirurška sterilizacija žene (podvezivanje jajovoda)
Table (desk)	Table	Mesa (escritorio)	Tavolo (scrivania)	Stol
Tea	Thé	Té	Tè	Čaj
Teeth polishing	Vernis à dents	Pulidor de los dientes	Pulitura dei denti	Poliranje zuba
Test tube	Tube à essai	Tubo de ensayo	Provetta	Epruveta
Therapy	Thérapie (traitement curatif)	Tratamiento (terapia)	Terapia	Liječenje (terapija)
Toilet (lavatory)	Toilette (cabinet)	Servicio	Vaso sanitario	Nužnik
Traction	Traction	Tracción	Trazione	Trakcija
Transfusion	Transfusion	Transfusión	Trasfusione	Transfuzija
Transplantation	Greffe (transplantation)	Trasplante	Trapianto	Presađivanje (transplantacija)
Transurethral resection of the prostate	Résection transurétrale de la prostate	Resección transuretral de la próstata	Resezione transuretrale della prostata	Transuretralna resekcija prostate
Trauma	Trauma	Trauma	Trauma	Trauma
Trendelenburg position	Position de Trendelenburg	Posición de Trendelenburg	Posizione di Trendelenburg	Trendelenburgov položaj
Tweezers	Brucelles	Pinzas	Pinzette	Pinceta
Urination (voiding)	Miction	Micción	Urinazione	Mokrenje (uriniranje)
Urological catheter	Cathéter urologique	Catéter urinario	Catetere vescicale	Urinarni kateter
Urology	Urologie	Urología	Urologia	Urologija
Using a toilet	Aller aux toilettes	Ir al servicio	Uso del gabinetto	Obaviti nuždu
Vaccination (inoculation)	Vaccination (inoculation)	Vacunación	Vaccinazione (inoculazione)	Cijepljenje
Vaccination schedule	Calendrier des vaccinations	Calendario de vacunación	Calendario vaccinale	Kalendar cijepljenja
Vacuum mattress	Matelas immobilisateur à dépression	Colchón al vácio	Materassino a depressione	Vakumirani madrac
Visit	Visite	Visita	Visita	Posjeta
Visitor	Visiteur	Visitante	Ospite (visitatore/visitatrice)	Posjetitelj
Vital signs monitor	Moniteur de signes vitaux	Monitor de signos vitales	Monitor per parametri vitali	Monitor za praćenje vitalnih znakova
Waiting -room	Salle d'attente	Sala de espera	Sala d'aspetto	Čekaonica
Walker (walking frame)	Déambulateur (cadre de marche, gadot)	Andador	Deambulatore (tutore per disabili)	Hodalica
Ward	Salle	Sala (pabellón)	Padiglione (reparto)	Odjel
Wardrobe (cupboard, cabinet)	Armoire	Armario	Armadio (credenza)	Ormar
Wash basin	Cuvette	Palangana (ajofaina)	Secchia	Lavor
Water	Eau	Agua	Acqua	Voda
Wheelchair	Fauteuil roulant (charriot, charrette)	Silla de ruedas	Sedia a rotelle (carrozzella)	Invalidska kolica

English	French	Spanish	Italian	Croatian
Window	Fenêtre	Ventana	Finestra	Prozor
Wound stitching	Suture de la plaie	Suturar la herida	Suturare la ferita	Šivanje rane

MEDICAL EXAMS:	**EXAMENS MÉDICAUX:**	**EXÁMENES MÉDICOS:**	**ESAMI MEDICI:**	**MEDICINSKE PRETRAGE:**
Abdominal ultrasound	Échographie abdominale	Ecografía abdominal (ultrasonido abdominal)	Ecografia addominale	Ultrazvuk abdomena
Agglutination tests	Test d'agglutination	Análisis de aglutinación	Test di agglutinazione	Test aglutinacije
Alkaline phosphatase	Phosphatase alcaline	Fosfatasa alcalina	Fosfatasi alcalina totale	Alkalna fosfataza
Alpha -fetoprotein test (AFP test)	Test d'alpha-foetoprotéine	Prueba de alfa-fetoproteína	Test alfa-fetoproteina	Alfafetoproteinski test (AFP)
Amniocentesis	Amniocentèse	Amniocentesis	Amniocentesi	Amniocenteza
Angiography	Angiographie	Angiografía	Angiografia	Angiografija
Anoscopy	Anuscopie	Anoscopía	Anoscopia	Anoskopija
Antibiogram	Antibiogramme	Antibiograma	Antibiogramma	Antibiogram
Aortography	Aortographie	Aortografía	Aortografia	Aortografija
Arteriography	Artériographie	Arteriografía	Arteriografia	Arteriografija
Arthroscopy	Arthroscopie	Artroscopia	Artroscopia	Artroskopija
Aspartate transaminase (SGOT)	Aspartate transaminase (SGOT)	Aspartato aminotransferasa (AST, transaminasa glutámico-oxalacética GOT)	Aspartato transaminasi (SGOT)	Transaminaze u serumu
Audiometry	Audiométrie	Audiometría	Audiometria	Audiometrija
Barium enema	Lavement baryté	Enema de bario con doble contraste	Indagini radiologiche del colon con clisma opaco a doppio contrasto	Rendgensko snimanje debelog crijeva i rektuma s kontrastom barija
Barium meal (upper gastrointestinal series)	Radiographie de l'abdomen en bouillie de sulfate de baryum	Radiografía de esófago, estómago y duodeno tomada con comida baritada	Radiografia gastroduodenale con pasto baritato	Rendgensko snimanje želuca i dvanaesnika barijevom kašom
Benzidine stool test	Analyse fécale de benzidine	Prueba de la bencidina	Prova della benzidina	Benzidinski test stolice
Biochemical blood tests	Analyse de biochimie du sang	Exámenes bioquímicos de sangre	Test biochimici di sangue	Biokemijske pretrage krvi
Biomarker	Biomarqueur	Marcador biológico	Biomarcatore	Biomarker
Biopsy	Biopsie	Biopsia	Biopsia	Biopsija
Blood culture	Hémoculture	Hemocultivo	Emocoltura	Mikrobiološki pregled krvi (hemokultura)
Blood gas test	Prélèvement des gaz du sang	Prueba de gases en la sangre	Analisi dei gas nel sangue (emogas analisi)	Analiza plinova u krvi
Blood pressure monitoring	Monitoring de la pression artérielle	Monitorización de la presión arterial	Misurazione della pressione arteriosa	Mjerenje krvnog pritiska
Blood sugar concetration (glucose level)	Taux de la glycémie	Concentración de glucosa en sangre	Concentrazione del glucosio nel plasma	Šećer u krvi
Blood urea nitrogen test (BUN)	Azote d'urée dans le sang	Nitrógeno ureico en sangre (BUN)	Azoto ureico nel sangue (BUN)	Ostatni dušik u krvi (urea nitrogen test)
Bone densitometry (dual energy X-ray absorpriometry)	Ostéodensitométrie	Densitometría ósea	Densità minerale ossea	Denzitometrija kostiju (apsorpciometrija kostiju)
Bone marrow biopsy	Biopsie ostéomédullaire	Biopsia de médula ósea	Biopsia del midollo osseo	Biopsija koštane srži
Bone scintigraphy	Scintigraphie osseuse	Gammagrafía ósea	Scintigrafia ossea	Scintigrafija kostiju
Bone X-ray (bone radiography)	Radiographie des os	Radiografía de hueso (radiografía ósea)	Radiografia ossea	Rendgensko snimanje kostiju
Brain ventricle biopsy	Biopsie d'un ventricule cérébral	Biopsia cerebral	Biopsia cerebrale (biopsia dei ventricoli cerebrali)	Biopsija moždanih klijetki (ventrikulopunkcija)
Breast examination	Examen du sein	Exploración física de mama	Esame della mammella	Pregled dojke
Breast ultrasound	Échographie mammaire	Ecografía de mama (ultrasonido de mama)	Ecografia mammaria	Ultrazvuk dojke
Bromsulphalein liver function test	Test de la bromesulfonephtaléine	Prueba de la función hepática con bromosulfaleína	Test dela bromosulfaleina di funzionalità epatica	Brom-sulfalein test funkcije jetre
Bronchography	Bronchographie	Broncografía	Broncografia	Bronhografija
Bronchoscopy	Bronchoscopie	Broncoscopia	Broncoscopia	Bronhoskopija
CA 125 (cancer antigen 125)	Antigène de cancer CA 125	Marcador tumoral CA 125	CA 125 (antigene di carcinoma 125)	CA 125 (karcinomski antigen 125)
CA 19-9 (carbohydrate antigen)	Antigène de cancer CA 19-9 (antigène d'hydrate de carbone)	CA 19-9 (antígeno carbohidrato 19-9)	CA 19-9 (antigene carboidratico)	CA 19-9 (karbohidratni antigen)
Carcinoembryonic antigen (CEA)	Antigène carcinoembryonnaire (ACE)	Antígeno carcinoembrionario	Antigene carcino-embrionario (CEA)	Karcinoembrionski antigen (CEA)
Cardiac catheterization (heart cath, angiocardiography)	Cathétérisme cardiaque	Cateterismo cardíaco	Cateterismo cardiaco (angiocardiografia)	Kateterizacija srca (angiokardiografija)
Cardiac ultrasound (echocardiography)	Échocardiographie	Ecocardiografía	Ecocardiografia	Ultrazvuk srca (ehokardiografija)
Cardiotocography	Cardiotocographie	Cardiotocografía	Cardiotocografia	Kardiotokografija

English	French	Spanish	Italian	Croatian
Catheter angiography	Angiographie interventionnelle utilisant un cathéter	Angiografía por catéter	Angiografia con cateterismo	Kateterska angiografija
Central venous pressure (CVP)	Pression veineuse centrale	Presión venosa central	Pressione venosa centrale	Centralni venozni pritisak (CVP)
Cephalometry	Céphalométrie	Cefalometría	Cefalometria	Cefalometrija
Cerebral angiography	Angiographie cérébrale	Angiografía cerebral	Angiografia cerebrale	Cerebralna angiografija
Cerebrospinal fluid analysis	Analyse du liquide céphalo-rachidien	Análisis del líquido cefalorraquídeo	Analisi del liquido cerebro-spinale	Pregled likvora
Cerebrospinal fluid culture	Culture du liquide cérébro-spinal	Cultivo de líquido cefalorraquídeo	Coltura del liquor	Mikrobiološki pregled likvora
Cervical conization	Conisation	Conización	Conizzazione	Konizacija
Chest X-ray	Radiographie de thorax	Radiografía de tórax	Radiografia del torace	Rendgensko snimanje srca i pluća
Cholangiography	Cholangiographie	Colangiografía	Colangiografia	Kolangiografija
Colonoscopy	Colonoscopie	Colonoscopía	Colonscopia	Kolonoskopija
Colposcopy	Colposcopie	Colposcopia	Colposcopia	Kolposkopija
Complete blood count	Hémogramme (numération formule sanguine)	Hemograma (conteo sanguíneo completo)	Emocromo (analisi del sangue, esame emocromocitometrico)	Kompletna krvna slika
Computed tomography (CT)	Tomodensitométrie (TDM)	Tomografía computada	Tomografia computerizzata (TC)	Kompjuterizirana tomografija (CT)
Contrast medium	Produit de contraste	Medio de contraste	Mezzo di contrasto	Kontrast
Coronary catheterization (coronarography)	Coronarographie	Coronariografía	Coronarografia	Koronarografija
Cystography	Cystographie	Cistografía	Cistografia	Cistografija
Cystoscopy	Cystoscopie	Cistoscopia	Cistoscopia	Cistoskopija
Defecography	Défécographie	Defecografía	Defecografia	Defekografija
Dental X-ray	Radiographie dentaire	Radiografía dental	Radiografia dentale	Rendgensko snimanje zuba
Dermatoscopy (dermoscopy)	Dermatoscopie (dermoscopie)	Dermatoscopia	Dermatoscopia (dermoscopia)	Dermatoskopija (dermoskopija)
Differential diagnosis	Diagnostic différentiel	Diagnóstico diferencial	Diagnosi differenziale	Diferencijalna dijagnoza
Digital subtraction angiography	Angiographie numérique	Angiografía de sustracción digital	Angiografia digitale a sottrazione	Digitalna supstrakcijska angiografija
Dilated fundus examination	Fond d'oeil	Exámen dilatado de fundus	Esame del fundus oculi	Pregled očnog fundusa
DNA analysis	Analyse de l'ADN	Análisis de DNA	Analisi del DNA	DNK analiza
Doppler echocardiography	Échocardiographie-doppler	Ecocardiografía doppler	Ecocardiografia doppler	Ultrazvuk srca s dopplerom
Drug induced pupillary dilatation	Dilatation des pupilles provoquée par les médicaments	Dilatación pupilar inducida por fármacos	Dilatazione delle pupille provocando con tropicamide	Širenje zjenica potaknuto lijekovima
Echoencephalography	Échoencéphalographie	Ecoencefalografia	Ecoencefalografia	Ehoencefalografija
Electrocardiography (ECG)	Électrocardiographie (ECG)	Electrocardiografía (ECG, EKG)	Elettrocardiografia	Elektrokardiografija (EKG)
Electroencephalography (EEG)	Électro-encéphalographie (EEG)	Electroencefalografía	Elettroencefalografia	Elektroencefalografija (EEG)
Electromyography (EMG)	Électromyographie	Electromiografía	Elettromiografia	Elektromiografija (EMG)
Electroneurography	Électroneurographie	Electroneurografía	Elettroneurografia	Elektroneurografija
Electroretinography	Électrorétinographie	Electrorretinografía	Elettroretinografia	Elektroretinografija
Endometrial biopsy	Biopsie endométriale	Biopsia endometrial	Biopsia endometriale	Biopsija endometrija
Endoscopic retrograde cholangiopancreatography (ERCP)	Cholangiopancréatographie rétrograde endoscopique	Colangiopancreatografía retrógrada endoscópica	Colangio-pancreatografia endoscopica retrograda	Endoskopska retrogradna kolangiopankreatografija (ERCP)
Endoscopy	Endoscopie	Endoscopia	Endoscopia	Endoskopija
Enteroscopy	Entéroscopie	Enteroscopia	Enteroscopia	Enteroskopija
Ergometry test	Ergométrie	Ergometría	Ergometria (ECG sotto sforzo)	Test opterećenja (ergometrija)
Erythrocyte sedimentation rate	Vitesse de sédimentation	Velocidad de sedimentación globular	Velocità di eritrosedimentazione	Sedimentacija eritrocita
Esophageal manometry	Manométrie oesophagienne	Manometría esofágica	Manometria esofagea	Manometrija jednjaka
Esophagogastroduodeno-scopy	Endoscopie oeso-gastro-duodénale	Esofagogastroduodenosco-pia	Esofagogastroduodenosco-pia	Ezofagogastrodoudenosko-pija
Fine needle aspiration biopsy	Forage-biopsie	Punción aspiración con aguja fina	Agoaspirato (biopsia mediante ago sottile)	Punkcijsko-aspiracijska biopsija
Fluoroscopy	Fluoroscopie	Fluoroscopia	Fluoroscopia	Fluoroskopija
Functional magnetic resonance imaging (functional MRI)	Imagerie par résonance magnétique fonctionnelle (IRMf)	Imagen por resonancia magnética funcional (IRMf)	Risonanza magnetica funzionale	Funkcionalna magnetska rezonancija (FMR)
Gastric juice chemical examination	Analyse chimique du suc gastrique	Análisis químico del jugo gástrico	Esame chimico di succo gastrico	Kemijski pregled želučanog soka
Gastroscopy	Gastroscopie	Gastroscopia	Gastroscopia	Gastroskopija
Glasgow coma scale	Échelle de Glasgow	Escala de coma de Glasgow	Punteggio del coma di Glasgow	Glasgowska skala kome
Glucose urine test	Test du sucre dans les urines	Examen de glucosa en orina	Glucosio nelle urine	Šećer u urinu
Gonioscopy	Gonioscopie	Gonioscopia	Gonioscopia	Gonioskopija
Gynecological examination	Examen gynécologique	Examen ginecológico	Esame ginecologico	Ginekološki pregled

English	French	Spanish	Italian	Croatian
HbsAg (Hepatitis B surface antigen)	Antigène HbsAg (antigène de surface du virus de l'hépatite B)	HbsAg (antígeno de superficie de la hepatitis B)	HbsAg (antigene di superficie dell'epatite B)	HbsAg (hepatitis B površinski antigen)
Hematocrit	Hématocrite	Hematocrito	Ematocrito	Hematokrit
Hepatobiliary scintigraphy with technetium -99m	Scintigraphie hépato-biliaire au Technétium 99m	Gammagrafía hepatobiliar con tecnecio 99m	Scintigrafia epatobiliare con tecnezio -99m	Scintigrafija jetre i žučnih vodova radioaktivnim izotopima
High intensity focused ultrasound	Ultrasons focalisés de haute intensité	Ultrasonido focalizado de alta intensidad (HIFU)	Ultrasuono ad alta intensità focalizzato	Fokusirani ultrazvuk visokog intenziteta
Hysterescopy	Hystéroscopie	Histeroscopia	Isteroscopia	Histeroskopija
Hysterosalpingography	Hystérosalpingographie	Histerosalpingografía	Isterosalpingografia	Rendgensko snimanje maternice i jajovoda
Indirect Coombs test	Réaction de Coombs indirecte	Prueba de Coombs indirecta	Test di Coombs indiretto	Indirektni Coombsov test
Intravenous biligraphy	Biligraphie intraveineuse	Biligrafía intravenosa	Biligrafia venosa	Intravenozna biligrafija
Intravenous pyelography	Urographie intra-veineuse	Urografía intravenosa	Urografia intravenosa (pielografia intravenosa)	Intravenozna pijelografija (i.v. Urografija)
Iodine -131 thyroid test	Fixation thyroïdienne de l'iode 131	Captación tiroidea de 131 yodo	Test di captazione tiroidea dello iodio 131	Test štitnjače na provodljivost radioaktivnog joda 131
Joint X-ray (arthrography)	Arthrographie	Artrografía	Artrografia	Rendgensko snimanje zgloba
Karyotype	Caryotype	Cariotipo	Cariotipo	Kariotip
Kidney biopsy	Biopsie rénale	Biopsia renal	Biopsia renale	Biopsija bubrega
Laboratory (lab)	Laboratoire	Laboratorio	Laboratorio	Laboratorij
Laboratory tests	Analyse médicale (examens de biologie médicale)	Pruebas de laboratorio	Esami di laboratorio	Laboratorijske pretrage
Laparoscopy	Laparoscopie	Laparoscopia	Laparoscopia	Laparoskopija
Laryngoscopy	Laryngoscopie	Laringoscopia	Laringoscopia	Laringoskopija
Liver biopsy	Biopsie du foie	Biopsia hepática	Biopsia epatica	Biopsija jetre
Liver function tests	Explorations fonctionnelles hépatiques	Pruebas de función hepática	Test di funzionalità epatica	Funkcionalne pretrage jetre
Liver ultrasound	Échographie du foie (échographie hépatique)	Ecografía hepática (ultrasonido hepático)	Ecografia epatica	Ultrazvuk jetre
Lumbar myelography	Myélographie lombaire	Mielografía lumbar	Mielografia lombare	Lumbalna mijelografija
Lumbar puncture	Ponction lombaire (rachicentèse)	Punción lumbar	Puntura lombare (rachicentesi)	Lumbalna punkcija
Lung scintigraphy	Scintigraphie pulmonaire	Gammagrafía pulmonar	Scintigrafia polmonare	Scintigrafija pluća
Lymph node biopsy	Biopsie du ganglion lymphatoque	Biopsia de ganglio linfático	Biopsia del linfonodo	Biopsija limfnog čvora
Lymphography (lymphangiography)	Lymphographie	Linfografía	Linfangiografia (linfografia)	Limfografija
Magnetic resonance imaging (MRI)	Imagerie par résonance magnétique (IRM)	Imagen por resonancia magnética (IRM)	Imaging a risonanza magnetica (risonanza magnetica tomografica)	Magnetska rezonancija (MR)
Magnetoencephalography (MEG)	Magnétoencéphalographie	Magnetoencefalografía	Magnetoencefalografia	Magnetoencefalografija (MEG)
Mammography	Mammographie	Mamografía	Mammografia (mastografia)	Mamografija
Mantoux test (PPD test)	Test Mantoux (test PPD)	Test de Mantoux (PPD)	Mantoux test	Tuberkulinski kožni test
Mediastinoscopy	Médiastinoscopie	Mediastinoscopia	Mediastinoscopia	Medijastinoskopija
Microbiological culture	Culture microbiologique	Cultivo	Coltura di microrganismi	Mikrobiološki pregled (kultura)
Myelography	Myélographie	Mielografía	Mielografia	Mijelografija
Ophtalmoscopy	Ophtalmoscopie	Oftalmoscopia	Oftalmoscopia	Oftalmoskopija
Oral cholecystography	Cholécystographie orale	Colecistografía oral	Colecistografia orale	Rendgensko snimanje žučnog mjehura s kontrastom (peroralna kolecistografija)
Oral glucose tolerance test (OGTT)	Test de tolérance orale au glucose (TTOG)	Test de tolerancia oral a la glucosa	Test orale di tolleranca al glucosio (OGTT, curva da carico orale di glucosio)	Oralni test tolerancije na glukozu (OGTT)
Otoscopy	Otoscopie	Otoscopía	Otoscopia	Otoskopija
Pancreas ultrasound	Échographie du pancréas	Ecografía de páncreas (ultrasonido de páncreas)	Ecografia pancreatica	Ultrazvuk gušterače
Papanicolau test (Pap test)	Test PAP	Prueba de Papanicolau	Test di Papanicolau (Pap test)	Papa-test (Papanicolaouova klasifikacija)
Partial thromboplastin time (PTT)	Temps de céphaline activée (TCA)	Tiempo de tromboplastina parcial activado	Tempo di tromboplastina parziale	Parcijalno tromboplastinsko vrijeme (PTT)
Patch test	Patch test	Prueba de emplasto (prueba del parche)	Patch test	Kožni alergološki test flasterom
Patellar reflex	Réflexe rotulien	Reflejo patelar	Riflesso patellare	Patelarni refleks
Pelvigraphy	Pelvigraphie	Pelvigrafía	Pelvigrafia	Rendgensko snimanje zdjelice i porođajnog kanala
Pelvimetry	Pelvimétrie	Pelvimetria	Pelvimetria	Pelvimetrija
Perimetry	Périmétrie	Campimetría (perimetría)	Perimetria	Perimetrija

English	French	Spanish	Italian	Croatian
Phenolsulfonphthalein test (PSP test)	Épruve à la phénosulfonphtaléine	Prueba de la fenolsulfonftaleína	Test alla fenolsulfonftaleina	Fenolsulfoftaleinski test (PSP-test)
Phlebography	Phlébographie	Flebografia	Flebografia	Venografija (flebografija)
Plethysmography	Pléthysmographie	Pletismografia	Pletismografia	Pletizmografija
Pleural biopsy	Biopsie pleurale	Biopsia pleural	Biopsia pleurica	Biopsija pleure
Pneumoencephalography	Encéphalographie gazeuse	Neumoencefalografia	Pneumoencefalografia	Pneumoencefalografija
Polysomnography (sleep study)	Polysomnographie (polygraphie du sommeil)	Polisomnografia	Polisonnografia	Polisomnografija (viseparametarski test u pracenju procesa sna)
Positron emission tomography	Tomographie par émission de positrons	Tomografia por emisión de positrones	Tomografia ad emissione di positroni	Pozitronska emisijska tomografija (PET)
Post-void residual urine volume	Volume urinaire résiduel	Volumen residual de orina	Volume urinario residuo	Ostatni urin (rezidualni urin)
Pregnancy test	Test de grossesse	Pruebas de embarazo	Test di gravidanza	Test na trudnoću
Prostate specific antigen	Antigène prostatique spécifique	Antígeno prostático específico	Semenogelasi (antigene prostatico specifico)	Prostatični specifični antigen (PSA)
Prothrombin time	Taux de prothrombine	Tiempo de protrombina	Tempo di protrombina	Protrombinski indeks
Pulmonary angiography	Angiographie pulmonaire	Angiografía pulmonar	Angiografia polmonare	Pulmonalna angiografija
Pulse monitoring	Prise de pouls	Comprobación del pulso	Misurazione del polso	Mjerenje pulsa
Pyelography	Urographie	Urografia	Urografia	Pijelografija (urografija)
Radioisotope scanning (nuclear medicine)	Médicine nucléaire	Medicina nuclear	Medicina nucleare	Radioizotopna dijagnostika
Rapid strep test	Test de diagnostic rapide du streptocoque	Prueba rápida para estreptococo	Test rapido dello streptococco	Brzi test na streptokok (strep-test)
Rectal examination	Toucher rectal	Tacto rectal	Esplorazione rettale	Rektalni pregled
Rectoscopy	Rectoscopie	Rectoscopia	Rettoscopia	Rektoskopija
Refractometry	Réfractométrie	Refractomería	Rifrattometria	Ispitivanje refrakcije
Renal scintigraphy	Scintigraphie rénale	Gammagrafia renal	Scintigrafia renale	Scintigrafija bubrega
Renal ultrasound	Échographie rénale	Ecografia renal (ultrasonido renal)	Ecografia renale	Ultrazvuk bubrega
Retrograde pyelography	Urétéro-pyélographie rétrograde	Pielografía retrógrada	Pielografia retrograda	Retrogradna pijelografija
Rose Waaler test	Réaction de Waaler Rose	Test de Waaler-Rose	Rose Waaler test	Rose Waaler test
Semen analysis	Spermogramme	Espermiograma	Spermiogramma	Spermogram
Serology blood tests	Analyse sérologique	Pruebas de serología	Esami sierologici	Serološke pretrage na antitijela
Serum albumin	Albumine dans le sang	Albúmina en la sangre	Seroalbumina	Albumin u serumu
Serum bilirubin	Diagnostic différentiel pour bilirubine sérique	Análisis de bilirrubina sérica	Test della bilirubina	Bilirubin u serumu
Serum protein electrophoresis	Électrophorèse des protéines	Electroforesis de proteínas séricas	Elettroforesi delle sieroproteine	Elektroforeza proteina u serumu
Sialography	Sialographie	Sialografia	Sialografia (scialografia)	Sijalografija
Sigmoidoscopy	Sigmoïdoscopie	Sigmoidoscopia	Sigmoidoscopia	Sigmoidoskopija
Skin allergy testing (prick test)	Test de la piqûre	Test cutaneos de alergia (prick)	Test cutaneo per le allergie "prick test"	Alergološko testiranje kože (prick test)
Skin biopsy	Biopsie de peau	Biopsia de piel	Biopsia cutanea	Biopsija kože
Skull X-ray (craniography)	Craniographie	Craneografia	Craniografia	Rendgensko snimanje lubanje
Speech audiometry	Audiométrie vocale	Audiometría del habla	Audiometria di discorso	Govorna audiometrija
Spinal angiography	Angiographie spinale	Angiografía espinal	Angiografia spinale	Spinalna angiografija
Spine X-ray (spine radiography)	Radiographie de la colonne vertébrale	Radiografía de la columna vertebral (radiografía vertebral)	Radiografia della colonna vertebrale	Rendgensko snimanje kralježnice
Spirometry (vital capacity test)	Spirométrie	Espirometría	Spirometria (pneumometria)	Spirometrija (mjerenje vitalnog kapaciteta)
Spleen scintigraphy with technetium -99m	Scintigraphie splénique au Technétium 99m	Gammagrafía de bazo con tecnecio 99m	Scintigrafia splenica con tecnezio -99m	Scintigrafija slezene radioaktivnim izotopima
Sputum culture	Culture de crachat	Cultivo de esputo	Coltura di sputo	Mikrobiološki pregled ispljuvka
Stereotactic biopsy	Biopsie stéréotaxique	Biopsia estereotáctica	Biopsia stereotassica	Stereotaktična biopsija
Suboccipital myelography	Myélographie sous-occipitale	Mielografia cervical suboccipital	Mielografia sotto-occipitale	Subokcipitalna mijelografija
Suboccipital puncture	Ponction sous-occipitale	Punción suboccipital	Puntura suboccipitale	Subokcipitalna punkcija
Thoracoscopy	Thoracoscopie	Toracoscopia	Toracoscopia	Torakoskopija
Throat swab culture	Culture de gorge avec le coton-tige	Exudado faríngeo	Coltura di gola	Mikrobiološki pregled brisa grla
Thyroid biopsy	Biopsie thyroïdienne	Biopsia de tiroides	Biopsia della tiroide	Biopsija štitnjače
Thyroid blood tests	Taux d'hormones thyroïdiennes dans le sang	Concetración de hormonas tiroideas en sangre	Test di ormoni tiroidei nel sangue	Test na hormone štitnjače u krvi
Thyroid scintigraphy	Scintigraphie thyroïdienne	Gammagrafia tiroidea	Scintigrafia tiroidea	Scintigrafija štitnjače
Thyroid ultrasound	Échographie thyroïdienne	Ecografia de la tiroides (ultrasonido de la tiroides)	Ecografia della tiroide	Ultrazvuk štitnjače
Tomography	Tomographie	Tomografia	Tomografia	Tomografija
Tonometry	Tonométrie oculaire	Tonometría	Tonometria	Tonometrija oka
Transthoracic percutaneous fine needle aspiration	Ponction transthoracique percutanée à l'aiguille fine	Punción transtorácica aspirativa con aguja ultrafina	Agoaspirato polmonare percutaneo transtoracico	Perkutana transtorakalna punkcija pluća

English	French	Spanish	Italian	Croatian
Tumor marker	Marqueur tumoral	Marcador tumoral	Marker tumorale	Tumorski marker
Tympanocentesis	Tympanocentese	Timpanocentesis	Timpanocentesi	Timpanocenteza
Tympanometry	Tympanométrie	Timpanometría	Timpanometria	Timpanometrija
Ultrasound (medical ultrasonography)	Échographie	Ultrasonografia (ecografía)	Ecografia	Ultrazvuk
Ultrasound of the gallbladder and bile ducts	Échographie la vésicule biliaire et les voies biliaires	Ecografía de vesícula y vías biliares	Ecografia colecisti e vie biliari	Ultrazvuk žuči i žučnih vodova
Urea breath test	Test respiratoire à l'urée	Prueba del aliento con urea	Test del respiro (urea breath test)	Urea izdisajni test
Urea clearance test	Épruve d'élimination de l'urée sanguine	Prueba de aclaramiento de urea sanguínea	Urea clearance (clearance dell'urea)	Urea klirens
Ureteroscopy	Urétéroscopie	Ureteroscopía	Ureteroscopia	Ureteroskopija
Urethrography	Urétrographie	Uretrografia	Uretrografia	Uretrografija
Urine chemical analysis	Analyse chimique de l'urine	Análisis químico de orina	Analisi chimiche delle urine	Kemijska analiza urina
Urine culture	Uroculture	Urocultivo	Urinocoltura	Mikrobiološki pregled mokraće (urinokultura)
Urine protein test	Protéines dans les urines	Proteínas en la orina	Proteine nelle urine	Bjelančevine u urinu
Urine specific gravity	Poids spécifique de l'urine	Gravedad específica de la orina	Esame delle urine peso specifico	Specifična težina urina
Urobilinogen in urine	Urobilinogène dans les urines	Urobilinógeno en orina	Urobilinogeno nelle urine	Urobilinogen u urinu
Vaginal swab culture	Culture vaginale	Cultivo vaginal	Coltura vaginale	Mikrobiološki pregled brisa rodnice
Ventriculography	Ventriculographie	Ventriculografia	Ventricolografia	Ventrikulografija
Weber test	Test de Weber	Prueba de Weber	Prova di Weber	Weberov test
X-ray (radiography)	Radiographie	Radiografia	Radiografia	Rendgen
PREGNANCY AND OBSTETRICS:	GROSSESSE ET OBSTÉTRIQUE:	EMBARAZO Y OBSTETRICIA:	GRAVIDANZA ED OSTETRICIA:	TRUDNOĆA I PORODNIŠTVO:
Abortifacients	Médicaments abortifs	Fármacos abortivos	Farmaci abortivi	Abortivni lijekovi
Abortion (pregnancy termination)	Avortement	Aborto inducido	Interruzione di gravidanza (aborto)	Prekid trudnoće (abortus)
Absence of menstrual period (amenorrhea)	Absence des règles (aménorrhée)	Ausencia de la menstruación (amenorrea)	Assenza di mestru-azioni (amenorrea)	Izostanak mjesečnice (amenoreja)
Amniocentesis	Amniocentèse	Amniocentesis	Amniocentesi	Amniocenteza
Amnioscopy	Amnioscopie	Amnioscopia	Amnioscopia	Amnioskopija
Amniotic fluid	Liquide amniotique	Líquido amniótico	Liquido amniotico	Plodna voda (amnijska tekućina)
Amniotic sac	Amnios (sac amniotique)	Saco amniótico	Amnios	Vodenjak
Artificial insemination	Insémination artificielle	Inseminación artificial	Fecondazione assistita (fecondazione artificiale)	Umjetna oplodnja
Biological parent	Parent biologique	Padre biológico	Genitore biologico	Biološki roditelj
Biophysical profile of the fetus	Profil biophysique foetal	Perfil biofísico fetal	Profilo biofisico fetale	Biofizikalni profil fetusa
Birth canal	Canal utérin	Canal del parto	Canale del parto	Porodni kanal
Blastocyst	Blastocyste	Blastocisto	Blastocisti	Blastocista
Bleeding (haemorrhage)	Saignement (hémorragie)	Desangramiento (hemorragia)	Emorragia	Krvarenje (hemoragija)
Body length of a newborn	Taille corporelle du nouveau-né	Talla de un neonato	Lunghezza di neonato	Dužina novorođenčeta
Braxton Hicks contractons	Fausse contraction (contraction de Braxton Hicks)	Contracción de Braxton Hicks	False contrazioni (contrazioni di Braxton Hicks)	Lažni trudovi
Breast	Sein	Mama	Mammella	Dojka
Breast pump	Tire-lait	Sacaleches	Pompa tiralatte	Pumpica za izdajanje
Breathing	Respiration	Respiración	Respirazione	Disanje
Breech	Siège	Nalga	Culatta (deretano)	Zadak
Breech position	Présentation podalique (présentation du siège)	Posición de nalgas	Posizione podalica del feto	Stav zatkom
Cardiotocography	Cardiotocographie	Cardiotocografia	Cardiotocografia	Kardiotokografija
Cervical dilation	Dilatation cervicale	Dilatación del cuello uterino	Dilatazione della cervice uterina	Otvaranje ušća maternice
Cesarean section (C-section)	Césarienne	Cesárea	Taglio cesareo	Carski rez
Chadwick's sign	Signe de Chadwick	Signo de Chadwick	Segno del Chadwick (tinta bluastra alla vagina)	Hiperemična sluznica rodnice (Chadwickov znak)
Childbirth	Accouchement (naissance)	Parto	Parto	Porod
Choriocarcinoma	Choriocarcinome	Coriocarcinoma	Coriocarcinoma	Koriokarcinom
Chorion	Chorion	Corion	Corion (corio)	Korion
Chorion-gonadotrophin	Gonadotrophine chorionique	Gonadotropina coriónica	Gonadotropina corionica	Korion-gonadotropin
Chorionic villi	Villosités choriales	Vellosidades coriónicas	Villi coriali	Korionske resice
Chorionic villus sampling	Choriocentèse	Muestra de vellosidades coriónicas	Villocentesi	Uzorak korionskih resica
Conception	Conception (fécondation)	Fecundación (fertilización)	Concezione	Začeće (oplodnja)
Contracted pelvis	Bassin contracté	Pelvis contraída	Pelvi ristretto	Sužena zdjelica
Cordocentesis	Cordocentèse	Cordocentesis	Cordocentesi	Kordocenteza
Curettage	Curetage	Legrado	Raschiamento (curetage)	Kiretaža

English	French	Spanish	Italian	Croatian
Cut	Couper	Cortar	Tagliare (intersecare)	Presjeći
Delivery room	Salle d'accouchement	Sala de partos	Sala parto	Rađaona
Diaper	Couche-culotte	Pañal	Pannolino	Pelena
Dizygotic twins (biovular twins)	Jumeaux dizygotes	Gemelos dicigóticos (mellizos)	Gemelli fraterni (gemelli dizigoti)	Dvojajčani blizanci
Duration of contraction	Durée de la contraction utérine	Duración de las contracciones uterinas	Durata di contrazioni	Trajanje truda
Duration of pregnancy	Durée de la grossesse	Duración del embarazo	Durata della gravidanza	Trajanje trudnoće
Eclampsia	Éclampsie	Eclampsia	Eclampsia	Eklampsija
Ectopic pregnancy (extrauterine pregnancy)	Grossesse extra-utérine	Embarazo ectópico	Gravidanza ectopica	Izvanmaternična trudnoća (ektopična trudnoća)
Edema	Oedème	Edema (hidropesía)	Edema	Edem
Egg donation	Donneuse d'ovule	Donación de ovocitos	Ovodonazione	Donacija jajašca
Ejaculation	Éjaculation	Eyaculación	Eiaculazione	Ejakulat
Embryo	Embryon	Embrión	Embrione	Embrij (zametak)
Endometrial hyperplasia	Hyperplasie endométriale	Hiperplasia endometrial	Iperplasia endometriale	Hiperplazija maternice
EPH gestosis (preeclampsia)	Pré-éclampsie	Preeclampsia	Preeclampsia (gestosi)	EPH-gestoze (preeklampsija)
Episiotomy	Épisiotomie	Episiotomía	Episiotomia	Kirurško proširenje porođajnog kanala (epiziotomija)
Excessive secretion of saliva (hypersalivation)	Sécrétion de la salive excessive	Excesiva producción de saliva (hipersalivación)	Produzione di saliva eccessiva (ipersalivazione)	Pojačano lučenje sline (hipersalivacija)
Expulsion of placenta	Expulsion du placenta	Expulsión de la placenta	Espulsione della placenta	Istiskivanje posteljice i ovoja
Expulsion of the baby	Expulsion du bébé	Expulsión del producto	Espulsione del feto	Istiskivanje ploda
Fallopian tube (oviduct)	Trompes de Fallope	Trompa de Falopio (tuba uterina, oviducto)	Ovidotto (ovidutto)	Jajovod
Father	Père	Padre	Padre	Otac
Fetal anomalies (fetal abnormalities)	Anomalies foetales	Anomalías fetales	Anomalie di sviluppo fetale (anomalie fetali)	Anomalije fetusa
Fetal hypotrophy	Hypotrophie foetale	Hipotrofia fetal	Ipotrofia fetale	Fetalna hipotrofija
Fetal pH-metry	pH-métrie foetale	pH-metría fetal	pH-metria fetale	Fetalna pH-metrija
Fetal weight (birth mass)	Poids de naissance	Peso al nacer	Peso di neonato	Težina ploda (porođajna težina)
Fetoscopy	Foetoscopie	Fetoscopia	Fetoscopia	Fetoskopija
Fetus	Foetus	Feto	Feto	Fetus
Forceps	Forceps	Fórceps	Forcipe	Forceps (kliješta)
Full term birth	Accouchement à terme	Parto a término	Parto a termine	Ročni porod
Gestational diabetes	Diabète gestationnel	Diabetes gestacional	Diabete gestazionale	Gestacijski dijabetes
Graafian follicle	Follicule de Graaf	Folículo de Graaf	Follicolo di Graaf	Graafov folikul
Gynecology	Gynécologie	Ginecología	Ginecologia	Ginekologija
Habitual abortion (recurrent miscarriage)	Avortement à répétition	Aborto habitual	Aborto abituale	Habitualni pobačaj
Head	Tête	Cabeza	Testa	Glavica
Hemolytic disease of the newborn	Maladie hémolytique du nouveau-né	Enfermedad hemolítica del recién nacido (eritroblastosis fetal)	Eritroblastosi fetale (malattia emolitica del neonato)	Hemolitička bolest novorođenčeta
High blood pressure (hypertension)	Pression artérielle élevée (hypertension artérielle)	Incremento de la presión sanguínea (hipertensión)	Ipertensione arteriosa sistemica	Visoki krvni tlak (hipertenzija)
Hymen	Hymen	Himen	Imene	Djevičnjak (himen)
Hypertrophy of uterus	Hypertrophie de l'utérus	Hipertrofia del útero	Ipertrofia dell'utero	Hipertrofija maternice
Implantation	Implantation	Implatación	Impianto	Implantacija (usađivanje)
In vitro fertilisation	Fécondation in vitro	Fecundación in vitro	Fertilizzazione in vitro	Oplodnja in vitro
Incubator	Couveuse (incubateur)	Incubadora	Incubatrice	Inkubator
Infection	Infection	Infección	Infezione	Infekcija
Infertility	Stérilité	Infertilidad	Sterilità	Neplodnost (sterilitet)
Inflammation of the fetal membranes (chorioamnionitis)	Chorioamnionite	Infección de las membranas placentarias (corioamnionitis)	Infiammazione del sacco amniotico (corioamniosite)	Upala plodovih ovoja (korioamnionitis)
Inflammation of the urinary bladder (cystitis)	Inflammation de la vessie (cystite)	Inflamación de la vejiga urinaria (cistitis)	Infiammazione della vescica urinaria (cistite)	Upala mokraćnog mjehura (cistitis)
Inner membrane of the uterus (endometrium)	Muqueuse utérine (endomètre)	Mucosa interior del útero (endometrio)	Mucosa interna dell'utero (endometrio)	Sluznica maternice (endometrij)
Intensity of contractions	Intensité des contractions utérines	Intensidad de contracciones uterinas	Intensità di contrazione	Snaga trudova
Intracytoplasmatic sperm injection	Injection intracytoplasmique de spermatozoïdes	Inyección intracitoplasmática de espermatozoides	Iniezione intracitoplasmatica dello spermatozoo	Intracitoplazmatska spermalna injekcija
Labor contraction frequency	Fréquence des contractions utérines	Frecuencia de las contracciones uterinas	Frequenza di contrazioni uterine	Frekvencija trudova
Labor contractions	Contractions utérines du travail	Contracciones del trabajo de parto (contracciones uterinas)	Contrazioni del travaglio	Trudovi
Lactation	Lactation	Lactancia	Lattazione	Dojenje (laktacija)
Lactiferous duct	Canal galactophore	Conducto mamario (conducto galactóforo)	Dotto galattoforo	Mliječni vod

English	French	Spanish	Italian	Croatian
Leg varicose veins	Varices des membres inférieurs	Venas varicosas de las piernas	Varici degli arti inferiori	Proširene vene na nogama
Lithopedion (stone baby)	Lithopédion (enfant pétrifié)	Litopedion	Lithopedion	Litopedion (okamenjeno dijete)
Lochia	Lochies	Loquios	Lochi	Lohija (iscjedak u babinjama)
Macrosomia (big baby syndrome)	Macrosomie foetale	Macrosomía fetal	Macrosomia fetale	Fetalna hipertrofija
Maternity blues (baby blues)	Baby blues	Baby blues (leve depresión post parto)	Sindrome del terzo giorno (baby blues)	Labilno psihičko raspoloženje (baby blues)
Maternity hospital	Maternité	Hospital de maternidad	Clinica ostetrica	Rodilište
Meconium	Méconium	Meconio	Meconio	Mekonij
Meconium aspiration syndrome	Syndrome d'aspiration méconiale	Síndrome de aspiración de meconio	Sindrome da aspirazione di meconio	Mekonijalni aspiracijski sindrom
Meconium ileus	Iléus méconial	Enfermedad de Hirsch-sprung (megacolon agangliónico)	Malattia di Hirsch-sprung (ostruzione del colon congenita)	Mekonijalni ileus
Meconium peritonitis	Péritonite méconiale	Peritonitis meconial	Peritonite da meconio	Mekonijalni peritonitis
Medically assisted procreation	Procréation médicalement assistée	Reproducción asistida	Procreazione assistita	Medicinski potpomognuta oplodnja
Medication that suppresses premature labor (tocolytic)	Médicament pour interrompre le déclenchement du travail (tocolytique)	Fármaco utilizado para suprimir el trabajo de parto prematuro (tocolítico)	Farmaco con lo scopo di arrestare le contrazioni uterine (tocolisi)	Lijek za sprečavanje trudova (tokolitik)
Menopause	Ménopause	Menopausia	Menopausa	Menopauza (klimakterij)
Menstrual cycle	Cycle menstruel	Ciclo menstrual	Ciclo mestruale	Menstruacijski ciklus
Menstruation	Règle (menstruation)	Menstruación (período)	Mestruazione	Menstruacija
Microcephaly	Microcéphalie	Microcefalia	Microcefalia	Mikrocefalija (sitnoglavost)
Midwife	Sage-femme	Matrona (matrón)	Ostetrica (levatrice)	Babica
Mifepristone	Mifépristone	Mifepristona	Mifepristone	Mifepriston
Monozygotic twins (identical twins)	Jumeaux monozygotes	Gemelos monocigóticos	Gemelli identici (gemelli monozigoti)	Jednojajčani blizanci
Morula	Morula	Mórula	Morula	Morula
Mother	Mère	Madre	Madre	Majka
Multigravida	Multipare	Multigrávida	Pluripara	Višerotkinja
Multiple pregnancy	Grossesse multiple	Embarazo múltiple	Gravidanza gemellare	Blizanačka trudnoća
Nausea	Nausée	Náusea	Nausea	Mučnina
Navel (belly button)	Ombilic (nombril)	Ombligo (pupo)	Ombelico	Pupak
Neck	Cou	Cuello	Collo	Vrat
Neonatology	Néonatologie	Neonatología	Neonatologia	Neonatologija
Newborn (infant)	Nouveau-né	Neonato (recién nacido)	Neonato	Novorođenče
Nipple	Mamelon (papille)	Pezón	Capezzolo	Bradavica
Nuchal scan (nuchal translucency)	Clarté nucale	Traslucencia nucal	Translucenza nucale	Nuhalna translucencija
Obstetrician	Obstétricien	Tocólogo (obstetra)	Ostetrico	Porodničar (opstetičar)
Obstetrics	Obstétrique	Obstetricia	Ostetricia	Porodništvo
Oogenesis	Ovogenèse	Ovogénesis	Ovogenesi	Ovogeneza (oogeneza)
Ovarian hyperemia	Hyperhémie ovarienne	Hiperemia del ovario	Iperemia dell'ovaio	Hiperemija jajnika
Ovary	Ovaire	Ovario	Ovaia (ovario)	Jajnik
Ovulation	Ovulation	Ovulación	Ovulazione	Ovulacija
Ovum	Ovule	Óvulo	Uovo	Jajašce
Parent	Géniteur	Padre (primario)	Genitore	Roditelj
Pathological birth	Accouchement pathologique	Parto patológico	Parto patologico	Patološki porod
Pelvimetry	Pelvimétrie	Pelvimetría	Pelvimetria	Pelvimetrija
Placenta	Placenta	Placenta	Placenta	Posteljica (placenta)
Placenta accreta	Placenta accreta	Placenta accreta	Placenta accreta	Prirasla posteljica (placenta accreta)
Placenta previa	Placenta praevia	Placenta previa	Placenta previa	Placenta previja
Placental abruption	Abruption placentaire (rupture placentaire)	Desprendimiento prematuro de placenta	Distacco di placenta (abruptio placentae)	Abrupcija posteljice
Placental estrogen	Oestrogène placentaire	Estrógeno de la placenta	Estrogeno placentare	Estrogen placente
Placental progesterone	Progestérone placentaire	Progesterona de placenta	Progesterone placentare	Progesteron placente
Plagiocephaly	Plagiocéphalie	Plagiocefalia	Plagiocefalia	Plagiocefalija
Postmature birth	Naissance après terme	Parto postérmino	Parto post-termine	Poslijeročni porod
Postnatal (postpartum period, puerperium)	Post-partum	Puerperio	Puerperio	Babinje (puerperij)
Postnatal depression (postpartum depression)	Dépression post-natale (dépression post-partum)	Depresión postparto (depresión postnatal)	Depressione post-partum	Postporođajna depresija
Postpartum psychosis	Psychose puerpérale	Psicosis postparto	Psicosi post-partum	Puerperalna psihoza
Pregnancy	Grossesse	Embarazo	Gravidanza (gestazione)	Trudnoća
Pregnancy risk factors	Facteurs de risque de la grossesse	Agentes teratogénicos	Rischio teratogenico	Teratogeni faktori rizika
Premature birth	Prématurité	Parto pretérmino	Parto pretermine	Prijevremeni porod
Premature rupture of membranes	Rupture prématurée des membranes	Ruptura prematura de membrana	Rottura precoce delle membrane	Prijevremeno prsnuće vodenjaka
Preterm newborn	Nouveau-né prématuré	Recién nacido pre-término	Neonato pretermine	Nedonošće
Primigravida	Primigeste	Primigesta	Primipara	Prvorotkinja

English	French	Spanish	Italian	Croatian
Progesterone	Progestérone	Progesterona	Progesterone	Progesteron
Prolactin	Prolactine	Prolactina	Prolattina	Prolaktin
Prolonged birth	Accouchement prolongé	Parto prolongado	Parto prolungato	Produljeni porod
Puerperal fever	Fièvre puerpérale	Fiebre puerperal	Febbre puerperale	Puerperalna groznica (babinja groznica)
Puerperal mastitis	Mammite puerpérale	Mastitis puerperal	Mastite puerperale	Puerperalni mastitis
Puerperal sepsis	Septicémie puerpérale	Sepsis puerperal	Sepsi puerperale	Puerperalna sepsa
Push	Pousser	Empujar	Spingere	Tiskati
Pyelonephritis	Pyélonéphrite	Pielonefritis	Pielonefrite	Pijelonefritis
Quadruplets	Quadruplés	Cuatrillizos	Quattro gemelli	Četvorci
Rupture of membranes	Rupture des membranes	Ruptura de membrana	Rottura delle membrane	Prsnuće vodenjaka
Semen (sperm)	Sperme	Semen (esperma)	Seme (sperma)	Sjemena tekućina (sperma)
Sperm bank	Banque du sperme	Banco de semen	Banca del seme	Banka sperme
Sperm viability	Viabilité du sperme	Viabilidad de espermatozoides	Sopravvivenza di spermatozoo	Životna sposobnost spermija
Spermatozoon (sperm cell)	Spermatozoïde	Espermatozoide	Spermatozoo	Spermij
Spontaneous abortion (miscarriage)	Fausse couche	Aborto espontáneo	Aborto spontaneo	Spontani pobačaj
Stage of birth	Stade du travail	Etapas del parto	Fase del parto	Porodno doba
Stillborn	Mort-né	Nacido muerto	Nato morto	Mrtvorođenče
Suckling	Succion	Succión	Suzione	Sisanje
Surgical removal of the uterus (hysterectomy)	Enlèvement chirurgical de l'uterus (hystérectomie)	Extracción quirúrgica del útero (histerectomía)	Asportazione chirurgica dell'utero (isterectomia)	Kirurško odstranjenje maternice (histerektomija)
Surrogate mother (womb mother)	Mère porteuse	Madre de alquiler	Surrogazione di maternità	Surogat majka (zamjenska majka)
TORCH infections	Infections TORCH	Infecciones TORCH	Complesso TORCH	TORCH infekcije
Transverse fetal position	Position transversale du foetus	Feto posición transversal	Posizione del feto trasversale	Kosi položaj ploda
Twins	Jumeaux	Gemelos	Gemelli	Blizanci
Ultrasound (medical ultrasonography)	Échographie	Ultrasonografía (ecografía)	Ecografia	Ultrazvuk
Umbilical cord	Cordon ombilical	Cordón umbilical	Funicolo ombelicale	Pupkovina (pupčana vrpca)
Umbilical cord prolapse	Prolapsus du cordon ombilical	Prolapso del cordón umbilical	Prolasso del funicolo ombelicale	Ispala pupkovina (prolaps pupkovine)
Urinary incontinence	Incontinence urinaire	Incontinencia urinaria	Incontinenza urinaria	Urinarna inkotinencija
Urinary retention (ischuria)	Rétention d'urine	Retención de orina	Ritenzione urinaria	Zastoj urina (urinarna retencija)
Uterine anomalies	Malformations utérines	Malformaciones uterinas	Anomalie uterine	Anomalije maternice
Vacuum extractor (ventouse)	Vacuum extractor	Aspirador al vacío	Aspiratore a vuoto	Vakuumski ekstraktor
Vagina	Vagin	Vagina	Vagina	Rodnica
Vomiting	Vomissement	Vómito (emesis)	Vomito (emetismo)	Povraćanje
Water birth	Accouchement dans l'eau	Parto en agua	Parto nell'acqua	Porod u vodi
Womb (uterus)	Utérus	Útero (matriz, seno materno)	Utero	Maternica (uterus)

DICTIONNAIRE MULTILINGUE DES URGENCES MÉDICALES

Français-Anglais-Espagnol-Italien-Croate

Français	Anglais	Espagnol	Italien	Croate
NUMÉROS:	**NUMBERS:**	**NÚMEROS:**	**NUMERI:**	**BROJEVI:**
Zéro	Zero	Cero	Zero	Nula
Un	One	Uno	Uno	Jedan
Deux	Two	Dos	Due	Dva
Trois	Three	Tres	Tre	Tri
Quatre	Four	Cuatro	Quattro	Četiri
Cinq	Five	Cinco	Cinque	Pet
Six	Six	Seis	Sei	Šest
Sept	Seven	Siete	Sette	Sedam
Huit	Eight	Ocho	Otto	Osam
Neuf	Nine	Nueve	Nove	Devet
Dix	Ten	Diez	Dieci	Deset
Onze	Eleven	Once	Undici	Jedanaest
Douze	Twelve	Doce	Dodici	Dvanaest
Treize	Thirteen	Trece	Tredici	Trinaest
Quatorze	Fourteen	Catorce	Quattordici	Četrnaest
Quinze	Fifteen	Quince	Quindici	Petnaest
Seize	Sixteen	Dieciséis	Sedici	Šesnaest
Dix-sept	Seventeen	Diecisiete	Diciassette	Sedamnaest
Dix-huit	Eighteen	Dieciocho	Diciotto	Osamnaest
Dix-neuf	Nineteen	Diecinueve	Diciannove	Devetnaest
Vingt	Twenty	Veinte	Venti	Dvadeset
Vingt et un	Twenty-one	Veintiuno	Ventuno	Dvadest i jedan
Vingt-deux	Twenty-two	Veintidós	Ventidue	Dvadeset i dva
Trente	Thirty	Treinta	Trenta	Trideset
Quarante	Forty	Cuarenta	Quaranta	Četrdeset
Cinquante	Fifty	Cincuenta	Cinquanta	Pedeset
Soixante	Sixty	Sesenta	Sessanta	Šezdeset
Soixante-dix	Seventy	Setenta	Settanta	Sedamdeset
Quatre-vingts	Eighty	Ochenta	Ottanta	Osamdeset
Quatre-vingt-dix	Ninety	Noventa	Novanta	Devedeset
Cent	Hundred	Cien	Cento	Sto
Cent un	One hundred and one	Ciento uno	Centouno	Sto jedan
Cent vingt-trois	One hundred and twenty-three	Ciento veintitrés	Centoventitre	Sto dvadeset i tri
Deux cents	Two hundred	Doscientos	Duecento	Dvjesto
Trois cents	Three hundred	Trescientos	Trecento	Tristo
Quatre cents	Four hundred	Cuatrocientos	Quattrocento	Četristo
Cinq cents	Five hundred	Quinientos	Cinquecento	Petsto
Six cents	Six hundred	Seiscientos	Seicento	Šesto
Sept cents	Seven hundred	Setecientos	Settecento	Sedamsto
Huit cents	Eight hundred	Ochocientos	Ottocento	Osamsto
Neuf cents	Nine hundred	Novecientos	Novecento	Devetsto
Mille	Thousand	Mil	Mille	Tisuća
Deux mille	Two thousand	Dos mil	Duemila	Dvije tisuće
Million	Million	Millón	Un milione	Milijun
Milliard	Milliard (billion)	Mil millones (miliarda)	Un miliardo	Milijarda
ORIENTATION DANS LE TEMPS:	**ORIENTATION IN TIME:**	**ORIENTACIÓN EN EL TIEMPO:**	**ORIENTAMENTO NEL TEMPO:**	**ORIJENTACIJA U VREMENU:**
Hier	Yesterday	Ayer	Ieri	Jučer
Aujourd'hui	Today	Hoy	Oggi	Danas
Demain	Tomorrow	Día de mañana	Domani	Sutra
Année	Year	Año	Anno	Godina
Mois	Month	Mes	Mese	Mjesec
Semaine	Week	Semana	Settimana	Tjedan
Jour	Day	Día	Giorno	Dan
Heure	Hour	Hora	Ora	Sat
Minute	Minute	Minuto	Minuto	Minuta
Seconde	Second	Segundo	Secondo	Sekunda
Matin	Morning	Mañana	Mattina	Jutro (prijepodne)
Après-midi	Afternoon	Tarde	Pomeriggio	Poslijepodne
Soir	Evening	Anochecer	Sera	Večer
Nuit	Night	Noche	Notte	Noć
ORIENTATION DANS L'ESPACE:	**ORIENTATION IN SPACE:**	**ORIENTACIÓN EN EL ESPACIO:**	**ORIENTAMENTO NELLO SPAZIO:**	**ORIJENTACIJA U PROSTORU:**
En haut (au-dessus)	Up (above)	Arriba	Su	Gore (iznad)
En bas (au-dessous)	Down (below)	Abajo	In basso	Dolje (ispod)
Gauche	Left	Izquierda	Sinistra	Lijevo
Droite	Right	Derecha	Destra	Desno
Devant	In front	Enfrente	Davanti	Ispred
Derrière	Behind	Detrás	Dietro	Iza
Dedans	Inside	Dentro	Dentro	Unutra
Dehors	Outside	Fuera	Fuori	Vani

Français	Anglais	Espagnol	Italien	Croate
LES ACCIDENTS, CATASTROPHES ET DÉTRESSE:	**ACCIDENTS, CATASTROPHES AND DISTRESS:**	**ACCIDENTES, CATÁSTROFES Y ANGUSTIA:**	**GLI ACCIDENTI, CATASTROFI E ANGOSCIA:**	**NESREĆE, KATASTROFE I POGIBELJNE SITUACIJE:**
"Aide!"	"Help!"	"¡Socorro!"	"Aiuto!"	"U pomoć!"
Abri	Shelter	Abrigo	Rifugio	Sklonište
Accident aérien	Airplane crash	Accidente de aviación	Incidente aereo	Pad aviona
Accident automobile (accident de la route)	Car accident	Accidente automovilístico (siniestro de tráfico)	Incidente stradale	Automobilska nesreća
Accident domestique	Domestic accident	Accidente doméstico	Infortunio domestico	Nesreća u kući
Accident du travail	Occupational accident	Accidente laboral	Infortunio sul lavoro	Nesreća na radu
Accident nucléaire	Nuclear accident	Accidente nuclear	Accidente nucleare	Nuklearna nesreća
Accident sur la voie publique	Traffic accident	Accidente de tráfico	Incidente di traffico	Prometna nesreća
Alarme	Alarm	Alarma	Allarme	Uzbuna
Appel à l'aide	Call for help	Llamada de socorro	Chiamata di aiuto	Poziv u pomoć
Appel SOS	SOS call	Llamada de SOS	SOS richiesta	SOS poziv
Arme	Weapon	Arma	Arma	Oružje
Arme à feu	Firearm	Arma de fuego	Arma da fuoco	Vatreno oružje
Arme atomique	Atomic weapons	Arma atómica	Arma atomica	Atomsko oružje
Arme biologique	Biological weapon	Arma biológica	Arma biologica	Biološko oružje
Arme chimique	Chemical weapon	Arma química	Arma chimica	Kemijsko oružje
Arme conventionnelle	Conventional weapon	Arma convencional	Arma convenzionale	Konvencionalno oružje
Arme de contact	Cold weapon	Arma blanca	Arma bianca	Hladno oružje
Arme de destruction massive	Weapon of mass destruction	Armas de destrucción masiva	Arma di distruzione di massa	Oružje za masovno uništavanje
Arme de laser	Laser weapon	Arma láser	Armi laser	Lasersko oružje
Arme nucléaire	Nuclear weapon	Arma nuclear	Arma nucleare	Nuklearno oružje
Arme nucléaire stratégique	Strategic nuclear weapon	Arma nuclear estratégica	Arma nucleare strategica	Strateško nuklearno oružje
Arme nucléaire tactique (mini-nuke)	Tactical nuclear weapon	Arma nuclear táctica	Arma nucleare tattica	Taktičko nuklearno oružje
Arme nucléaire, biologique et chimique (NBC)	ABC weapons	Armas atómicas, biológicas y químicas (ABQ)	Armi nucleari, biologiche e chimiche (NBC)	Atomsko biološko i kemijsko oružje
Attaque	Attack	Ataque	Attaco	Napad
Attaque aérienne	Air attack	Ataque aéreo	Incursione area	Zračni napad
Attaque de pirates	Pirate attack	Ataque de piratas	Attacco dei pirati	Gusarski napad
Attaque de requin	Shark attack	Ataque de tiburón	Attacco di squalo	Napad morskog psa
Attaque physique	Physical assault	Asalto físico	Attacco fisico	Tjelesni napad
Attaque terroriste	Terrorist attack	Ataque terrorista	Attentato terroristico	Teroristički napad
Avalanche	Avalanche	Avalancha	Valanga	Lavina
Bacteria	Bacteria	Bacteria	Batterio	Bakterija
Balle	Bullet	Bala	Pallottola	Metak
Banquise	Sea ice	Banquisa (hielo marino)	Banchisa (ghiaccio marino; banchiglia)	Santa leda
Bombe	Bomb	Bomba	Bomba	Bomba
Bombe à hydrogène (bombe H)	Hidrogen bomb (H-bomb)	Bomba de hidrógeno (bomba H)	Bomba all'idrogeno (bomba H)	Hidrogenska bomba
Bombe à neutrons	Neutron bomb	Bomba de neutrones (bomba N)	Bomba al neutrone (bomba N)	Neutronska bomba
Bombe atomique (bombe A)	Atomic bomb (A-bomb)	Bomba atómica (bomba A)	Bomba atomica (bomba A)	Atomska bomba
Bombe radiologique (bombe sale)	Dirty bomb	Bomba sucia	Bomba sporca	Prljava bomba
Bombe salée	Cobalt bomb	Bomba de cobalto	Bomba al cobalto (bomba gamma, bomba G)	Kobaltna bomba
Bouée couronne	Lifebelt (lifebuoy)	Boya salvavidas	Boa di salvataggio	Pojas za spašavanje
Brise-glace	Icebreaker	Rompehielos	Rompighiaccio	Ledolomac
Camp de réfugiés	Refugee camp	Campamento para refugiados	Campo per rifugiati	Izbjeglički logor
Canot de secours	Lifeboat	Bote salvavidas	Scialuppa	Čamac za spašavanje
Cellule terroriste (cellule dormante)	Terrorist cell	Célula terrorista	Cellula terroristica	Teroristička ćelija
Champ de mines	Mine field	Campo minero	Campo minato	Minsko polje
Chien de sauvetage	Search and rescue dog	Perro de búsqueda y rescate	Cane da ricerca e salvataggio	Pas za traganje i spašavanje
Chute	Fall	Caída	Cadutta (cascata)	Pad
Collision	Collision	Colisión	Collisione	Sudar
Combat	Fight	Pelea	Combattimento	Tučnjava
Corde	Rope	Cuerda	Cordone	Uže
Coup	Stroke (hit, blow)	Golpe	Colpo (botta)	Udarac
Coup de chaleur	Heat stroke	Golpe de calor	Colpo di calore	Toplotni udar
Déchet radioactif (déchet nucléaire)	Nuclear waste (radioactive waste)	Desechos nucleares	Scoria nucleare (scoria radioattiva)	Nuklearni otpad (radioaktivni otpad)
Déminage	Mine clearance (demining)	Desminado (eliminación de minas)	Eliminazione di mine (sminamento)	Razminiranje
Eau	Water	Agua	Acqua	Voda

Français	Anglais	Espagnol	Italien	Croate
Échouage du navire	Stranding of a ship	Encallamiento de barco	Incaglio di nave	Nasukavanje broda
Électrisation (électrocution)	Electric shock	Choque eléctrico	Folgorazione (elettrocuzione)	Strujni udar
Enlèvement (rapt)	Kidnapping	Secuestro	Rapimento	Otmica
Épave de navire	Ship wreck	Buque naufragado	Relitto	Olupina broda
Épidémie	Epidemic	Epidemia	Epidemia	Epidemija
Équipe de recherche et sauvetage	Search and rescue team	Equipo de búsqueda y rescate	Squadra di ricerca e salvataggio	Ekipa za traganje i spašavanje
Éruption volcanique	Volcanic eruption	Erupción volcánica	Eruzione vulcanica	Erupcija vulkana
Esclavage	Slavery	Esclavitud	Schiavitù (prigionia)	Ropstvo
Essai nucléaire	Nuclear weapons testing	Prueba nuclear (ensayo nuclear)	Test nucleare	Nuklearni pokus
Explosif	Explosive	Explosivo	Esplosivo	Eksploziv
Explosion	Explosion	Explosión	Esplosione	Eksplozija
Feu	Fire	Fuego	Fuoco	Vatra
Foudre	Thunderclap	Trueno	Percossa dal fulmine	Udar groma
Gaz toxique	Poison gas	Gas tóxico	Gas tossico	Bojni otrov (otrovni plin)
Gilet de sauvetage	Lifejacket (life vest)	Chaleco salvavidas	Giubbotto di salvataggio	Prsluk za spašavanje
Glace	Ice	Hielo	Ghiaccio	Led
Grotte	Cave	Cueva	Grotta	Špilja
Guerre	War	Guerra	Guerra	Rat
Hélicoptère	Helicopter (chopper)	Helicóptero	Elicottero	Helikopter
Homicide (assassinat)	Homicide (murder)	Homicidio (asesinato)	Omicidio (uccisione)	Ubojstvo
Iceberg	Iceberg	Témpano de hielo	Ghiacciaio	Ledenjak
Incendie	Fire (conflagration)	Incendio (fuego)	Incendio (fuoco)	Požar
Inondation	Flood	Inundación	Inondazione	Poplava
Invasion	Invasion	Invasión	Invasione	Invazija
Lac	Lake	Lago	Lago	Jezero
Lave	Lava	Lava	Lava	Lava
Mer	Sea	Mar	Mare	More
Mine	Mine	Mina	Mina	Mina
Mine marine (mine sous-marine)	Naval mine	Mina marina	Mina navale	Morska mina
Mine terrestre	Land mine	Mina terrestre	Mina terrestre	Kopnena mina
Montagne	Mountain	Montaña	Montagna	Planina
Naufrage du navire	Sinking of a ship	Hundimiento de un barco	Affondamento della nave	Potonuće broda
Navire	Ship	Barco	Nave	Brod
Neige	Snow	Nieve (zapada)	Neve	Snijeg
Neurotoxine	Neurotoxin	Neurotoxina	Neurotossina	Živčani otrov (neurotoksin)
Noyade	Drowning	Ahogamiento	Annegamento	Utapanje
Noyé	Drowned person	Ahogado	Annegato	Utopljenik
Onde de marée	Tidal wave	Ola de marea	Onda di marea	Plimni val
Otage	Hostage	Rehén	Ostaggio	Taoc (talac)
Ouragan	Hurricane	Huracán	Uragano	Uragan
Pandémie	Pandemic	Pandemia	Pandemia	Pandemija
Parachute	Parachute	Paracáidas	Paracadute	Padobran
Pirate	Pirate	Pirata	Pirata	Gusar
Plutonium	Plutonium	Plutonio	Plutonio	Plutonij
Pollution chimique	Chemical pollution	Polución química	Inquinamento chimico	Kemijsko zagađenje
Rayonnement	Radiation	Radiación	Radiazione	Zračenje
Recherche	Search	Búsqueda	Ricerca	Potraga
Réfugié	Refugee	Refugiado	Rifugiato	Izbjeglica
Rivière	River	Río	Fiume	Rijeka
Roche	Rock	Roca	Roccia	Stijena
Ruine	Ruins	Ruinas	Macerie (rovine)	Ruševine
Sauvetage	Salvage	Salvamento	Salvataggio	Spašavanje
Sauvetage en mer	Marine salvage	Salvamento marítimo	Salvataggio navale	Spašavanje broda
Sauveur	Rescuer	Salvador (rescatador)	Salvatore	Spasilac
Sécurité civile	Civil defense	Protección civil	Difesa civile	Civilna zaštita
Séisme (tremblement de terre)	Earthquake	Terremoto	Terremoto	Potres
Shrapnel	Shrapnel	Metralla	Shrapnel	Šrapnel
Signal d'alarme	Alarm signal	Señal de alarma	Segnale di allarme	Znak za uzbunu
Suicide	Suicide	Suicidio	Suicidio	Samoubojstvo
Tempête	Storm	Tormenta (tempestad)	Tempesta	Nevrijeme (oluja)
Tempête de neige	Snow storm	Nevasca (ventisca de nieve)	Bufera di neve (nevicata)	Snježna mećava
Tempête de sable	Sandstorm	Tormenta de arena	Tempesta di sabbia	Pješćana oluja
Terre	Land	Tierra	Terra	Kopno
Terroriste	Terrorist	Terrorista	Terrorista	Terorist
Trafic d'êtres humains	Human trafficking	Trata de personas	Traffico di esseri umani	Trgovina ljudima
Trombe marine	Waterspout	Managa de agua (tromba marina)	Tromba marina	Morska pijavica
Tsunami (raz-de-marée)	Tsunami	Tsunami (maremoto)	Tsunami	Tsunami
Typhon	Typhoon	Tifón	Tifone	Tajfun
Uranium	Uranium	Uranio	Uranio	Uranij
Uranium enrichi	Enriched uranium	Uranio einriquecido	Uranio arricchito	Obogaćeni uranij
Victime	Victim	Víctima	Vittima	Žrtva

Français	Anglais	Espagnol	Italien	Croate
Viol	Rape (violation)	Violación	Violenza sessuale	Silovanje
Virus	Virus	Virus	Virus	Virus
Vol	Robbery	Robo	Rapina	Pljačka
PARTIES DU CORPS HUMAIN:	**PARTS OF THE HUMAN BODY :**	**PARTES DEL CUERPO HUMANO:**	**PARTI DEL CORPO UMANO:**	**DIJELOVI LJUDSKOG TIJELA:**
Abdomen	Belly (abdomen)	Abdomen (panza)	Addome (ventre, pancia)	Trbuh (abdomen)
Acetabulum	Acetabulum	Acetábulo	Cotile (acetabolo)	Čašica zdjelične kosti (acetabulum)
Acétylcholine	Acetylcholine	Acetilcolina	Acetilcolina	Acetilkolin
Acide aminé	Amino acid	Aminoácido	Amminoacido	Aminokiselina
Acide désoxyribonucléique	Deoxyribonucleic acid (DNA)	Ácido desoxirribonucleico	Acido desossiribonucleico (DNA)	Dezoksiribonukleinska kiselina (DNK)
Acide gastrique	Gastric acid	Ácido gástrico	Acido gastrico	Želučana kiselina
Acide ribonucléique (ARN)	Ribonucleic acid	Ácido ribonucleico (ARN)	Acido ribonucleico (ARN)	Ribonukleinska kiselina
Adénohypophyse	Adenohypophysis	Adenohipófisis	Adenoipofisi	Adenohipofiza
Adrénaline	Adrenalin (adrenaline)	Adrenalina	Adrenalina	Adrenalin
Agglutinine	Agglutinin	Aglutinina	Agglutinina	Aglutinin
Agglutinogène	Agglutinogen	Aglutinógeno	Agglutinogeno	Aglutinogen
Aine	Groin	Ingle	Inguine	Prepona
Aisselle	Armpit (axilla, underarm)	Sobaco (axila)	Ascella	Pazuh (aksila)
Albumine	Albumin	Albúmina	Albumina	Albumin
Aldostérone	Aldosterone	Aldosterona	Aldosterone	Aldosteron
Alvéole	Alveolus	Alvéolo	Alveolo	Alveola
Ammoniac	Ammonia	Amoníaco	Ammoniaca	Amonijak
Annulaire	Ring finger	Dedo anular	Anulare	Prstenjak
Anus	Anus	Ano	Ano	Čmar (anus)
Aorte	Aorta	Aorta	Aorta	Aorta
Aorte abdominale	Abdominal aorta	Aorta abdominal	Aorta addominale	Abdominalna aorta
Aorte thoracique	Thoracic aorta	Aorta torácica	Aorta toracica	Torakalna aorta
Aponévrose	Aponeurosis	Aponeurosis	Aponeurosi	Široka plosnata tetiva (aponeuroza)
Appendice iléo-caecal (appendice, appendice vermiforme)	Vermiform appendix (cecal appaendix)	Apéndice vermiforme (apéndice cecal, apéndice)	Appendice vermiforme	Slijepo crijevo (crvuljak)
Arachnoïde	Arachnoid mater	Aracnoides	Aracnoide	Paučinasta ovojnica (arachnoidea)
Artère	Artery	Arteria	Arteria	Arterija
Artère coronaire	Coronary artery	Arteria coronaria	Arteria coronaria	Koronarna arterija
Artère pulmonaire	Pulmonary artery	Arteria pulmonar (tronco pulmonar, tronco de las pulmonares)	Arteria polmonare	Plućna arterija
Artériole	Arteriole	Arteriola	Arteriola	Arteriola
Articulation	Joint	Articulación	Articolazione	Zglob
Articulation oléacranienne	Elbow joint	Articulación del codo	Articolazione del gomito	Lakatni zglob
Astrocyte	Astrocyte	Astrocito	Astrocita	Astrocit
Auriculaire (petit doigt)	Little finger (pinky)	Dedo meñique	Mignolo	Mali prst
Avant-bras	Forearm	Antebrazo	Avambraccio	Podlaktica
Base du crâne	Skull base	Base del cráneo	Base del cranio	Baza lubanje
Bassin osseux	Innominate bone (pelvis)	Pelvis	Bacino	Zdjelica
Bile	Gall (bile)	Bilis	Bile	Žuč
Bilirubine	Bilirubin	Bilirrubina	Bilirubina	Bilirubin
Bouche	Mouth	Boca	Bocca	Usta
Bourse séreuse	Synovial bursa	Bursa (bolsa sinovial)	Borsa sierosa	Sluzna vreća (bursa)
Bras	Arm	Brazo	Braccio	Ruka
Bronche	Bronchus	Bronquio	Bronco	Dušnica (bronh)
Bronchiole	Bronchiole	Bronquiolo	Bronchiolo	Bronhiola
Cage thoracique	Rib cage	Caja torácica	Gabbia toracica	Grudni koš
Calcanéus (calcanéum)	Calcaneus	Calcáneo	Calcagno	Petna kost (kalkaneus)
Calcitonine	Calcitonin	Calcitonina	Calcitonina	Kalcitonin
Canal de Schlemm	Canal of Schlemm	Canal de Schlemm	Canale di Schlemm	Schlemmov kanal
Canal éjaculateur	Ejaculatory duct	Conducto eyaculador	Dotto eiaculatore	Sjemenovod
Canal lacrymonasal (canal lacrimal, canal des larmes)	Nasolacrimal duct (tear duct)	Conducto nasolagrimal	Canale naso-lacrimale	Suzno-nosni kanal
Canine	Canine tooth	Canino (diente colmillo)	Canino	Očnjak (kanin)
Capillaire	Capillary	Capilar	Capillare	Kapilara
Capsule articulaire	Articular capsule (joint capsule)	Cápsula articular	Capsula articolare	Zglobna čahura
Carpe	Carpus	Carpo	Carpo	Zapešče
Cartilage	Cartilage	Cartílago	Cartilagine	Hrskavica
Cartilage articulaire	Joint cartilage	Cartílago articular	Cartilagine articolare	Zglobna hrskavica
Cartilage cricoïde	Cartilage ring	Cartílago circoides	Anello cartilagineo	Hrskavični prsten
Catécholamine	Catecholamine	Catecolamina	Catecolamina	Katekolamin
Cavité buccale	Mouth cavity (oral cavity)	Cavidad bucal (cavidad oral)	Cavità orale	Usna šupljina
Cavité tympanique	Tympanic cavity	Cavidad timpánica	Cassa del timpano	Bubnjište
Cellule	Cell	Célula	Cellula	Stanica
Cément	Cementum	Cemento dental	Cemento	Zubni cement

Français	Anglais	Espagnol	Italien	Croate
Cerveau	Brain	Cerebro	Cervello	Mozak
Cervelet	Cerebellum	Cerebelo	Cervelletto	Mali mozak
Cheveu	Hair	Cabello	Capelli	Kosa
Cheville (cou-de pied)	Ankle joint	Tobillo	Caviglia	Skočni zglob (gležanj)
Cholestérol	Cholesterol	Colesterol	Colesterolo	Kolesterol
Choroïde	Choroid	Coroides	Coroide	Žilnica
Cil	Eyelash	Pestaña	Ciglia	Trepavica
Cire de l'oreille (cérumen)	Earwax (cerumen)	Cerumen (cerilla)	Cerume	Ušna mast (ušna smola, cerumen)
Clavicule	Collarbone (clavicle)	Clavícula	Clavicola	Ključna kost (klavikula)
Clitoris	Clitoris	Clítoris	Clitoride	Dražica (klitoris)
Coccyx	Tailbone (coccyx)	Cóccix (coxis)	Coccige	Trtica
Cochlée	Cochlea	Cóclea (caracol)	Coclea	Pužnica
Coeur	Heart	Corazón	Cuore	Srce
Collagène	Collagen	Colágeno	Collagene	Kolagen
Côlon sigmoïde	Sigmoid colon	Colon sigmoide	Sigma (colon sigmoideo)	Sigmoidni dio debelog crijeva
Colonne vertébrale (rachis)	Spine (spinal column, backbone)	Columna vertebral	Colonna vertebrale	Kralježnica
Complexe articulaire de l'épaule	Shoulder joint	Articulación del hombro	Articolazione della spalla	Rameni zglob
Conduit auditif externe (canal auriculaire)	Auditory canal (ear canal)	Conducto auditivo externo	Meato acustico esterno	Slušni kanal
Corde vocale	Vocal chord	Cuerda vocal	Corda vocale	Glasnica
Cornée	Cornea	Córnea	Cornea	Rožnica
Corps jaune	Corpus luteum	Cuerpo lúteo (cuerpo amarillo)	Corpo luteo	Žuto tijelo
Cortex cérébral (écorce cérébrale)	Cerebral cortex	Corteza cerebral	Corteccia cerebrale	Moždana kora
Corticostéroïde	Corticosteroid	Corticosteroide	Corticosteroide	Kortikosteroid
Corticostérone	Corticosterone	Corticosterona	Corticosterone	Kortikosteron
Cortisol (hydro-cortisone)	Cortisol	Cortisol (hidrocortisona)	Cortisolo	Kortizol
Cortisone	Cortisone	Cortisona	Cortisone	Kortizon
Côte	Rib	Costilla	Costola (costa)	Rebro
Cou	Neck	Cuello	Collo	Vrat
Articulation oléacranienne	Elbow joint	Articulación del codo	Articolazione del gomito	Lakatni zglob
Couronne de la dent	Crown of a tooth	Corona del diente	Corona del dente	Kruna zuba
Crâne	Skull	Calavera (cráneo)	Cranio	Lubanja
Cristallin	Lens	Cristalino	Cristallino	Leća
Cuir chevelu	Scalp	Cuero cabelludo (capa capilar)	Cuoio capelluto	Vlasište
Cuisse	Thigh	Muslo (región femoral)	Coscia	Natkoljenica (bedro)
Dendrite	Dendrite	Dendrita	Dendrite	Dendrit
Dent	Tooth	Diente	Dente	Zub
Dent temporaire	Milk tooth	Diente de leche	Dente da latte	Mliječni zub
Dentine (ivoire)	Dentin	Dentina	Dentina	Zubni dentin
Diaphragme	Diaphragm	Diafragma	Muscolo diaframma	Ošit (dijafragma)
Diencéphale	Diencephalon	Diencéfalo	Diencefalo	Međumozak
Disque intervertébral	Intervertebral disc	Disco intervertebral	Disco intervertebrale	Međukralježnični disk
Doigt	Finger	Dedo de la mano	Dito della mano	Ručni prst
Dos	Back	Espalda	Schiena (dorso)	Leđa
Duodénum	Duodenum	Duodeno	Duodeno	Dvanaesnik (duodenum)
Dure-mère	Dura mater	Duramadre	Dura madre (pachimeninge)	Tvrda moždana ovojnica
Élastine	Elastin	Elastina	Elastina	Elastin
Électrolyte	Electrolyte	Electrolito	Elettrolita	Elektrolit
Émail dentaire	Tooth enamel	Esmalte dental	Smalto	Zubna caklina
Enclume	Anvil (incus)	Yunque	Incudine	Nakovanj
Éosinophile	Eosinophil	Eosinófilo	Eosinofilo	Eozinofil
Épaule	Shoulder	Hombro	Spalla	Rame
Épididyme	Epididymis	Epidídimo	Epididimo	Pasjemenik
Érythrocyte (hématie, globule rouge)	Erythrocyte (red blood cell)	Eritrocito (glóbulo rojo)	Eritrocita (globulo rosso)	Eritrocit (crveno krvno tjelešce)
Estomac	Stomach	Estómago	Stomaco	Želudac
Estradiol	Estradiol	Estradiol	Estradiolo	Folikulin (estradiol)
Estrogène	Estrogen	Estrógeno	Estrogeno	Estrogen
Étrier	Stirrup (stapes)	Estribo	Staffa (columella)	Stremen
Face de la cavité abdominale	Abdominal wall	Pared abdominal	Parete addominale	Trbušna stijenka
Faisceau de His	Bundle of His	Haz de His	Fascio di His	Hisov snopić
Fascia musculaire (périmysium)	Muscular fascia	Fascia profunda	Fascia muscolare	Mišićna fascija
Fèces	Stool (feces)	Excrementos (heces)	Feci	Stolica (feces, izmet)
Fibrine	Fibrin	Fibrina	Fibrina	Fibrin
Fibrinogène	Fibrinogen	Fibrinógeno	Fibrinogeno	Fibrinogen
Fibroblaste	Fibroblast	Fibroblasto (célula fija)	Fibroblasto	Fibroblast
Fibula (péroné)	Fibula (calf bone)	Peroné (fibula)	Perone (fibula)	Lisna kost (fibula)
Fluide corporel	Body fluid	Fluido corporal	Fluido corporale	Tjelesna tekućina

Français	Anglais	Espagnol	Italien	Croate
Foie	Liver	Hígado	Fegato	Jetra
Front	Forehead	Frente	Fronte	Čelo
Ganglion lymphatique (noeud lymphatique)	Lymph gland (lymph node)	Ganglio linfático	Linfonodo	Limfna žlijezda
Gaz	Gas	Gas	Gas	Plin
Gencive	Gums (gingiva)	Encía	Gengiva	Desni
Rotule (patella)	Kneecap (patella)	Rótula (patela)	Rotula (patella)	Iver (patela)
Gland	Glans	Glande	Glande	Glavić
Glande	Gland	Glándula	Ghiandola	Žlijezda
Glande de Bartholin	Bartholin's gland	Glándula de Bartolino	Ghiandola di Bartolini	Bartolinova žlijezda
Glande de Cowper (glande bulbo-uretrale)	Bulbourethral gland (Cowper's gland)	Glándula bulbouretral (glándula de Cowper)	Ghiandola bulbouretrale (ghiandola di Cowper)	Bulbouretralna žlijezda (Cowperova žlijezda)
Glande lacrymale	Lachrymal gland	Glándula lagrimal	Ghiandola lacrimale	Suzna žlijezda
Glande pinéale (épiphyse)	Pineal body (pineal gland, epiphysis)	Glándula pineal (epífisis)	Ghiandola pineale (epifisi)	Pinealna žlijezda (epifiza)
Glande salivaire	Salivary gland	Glándula salival	Ghiandola salivare	Žlijezda slinovnica
Glande sébacée	Sebaceous gland	Glándula sebácea	Ghiandola sebacea	Žlijezda lojnica
Glande sudoripare (sudorale)	Sweat gland	Glándula sudorípara	Ghiandola sudoripara	Žlijezda znojnica
Glande surrénale	Adrenal gland	Glándula suprarrenal	Surrene	Nadbubrežna žlijezda
Globe oculaire	Eyeball	Globo ocular	Bulbo oculare	Očna jabučica
Globuline	Globulin	Globulina	Globulina	Globulin
Glomérule	Glomerulus	Glomérulo	Glomerulo	Glomerul
Glucagon	Glucagon	Glucagón	Glucagone	Glukagon
Glucocorticoïde	Glucocorticoid	Glucocorticoide	Glucocorticoide	Glukokortikoid
Glucose	Glucose	Glucosa	Glucosio	Glukoza
Glycogène	Glycogen	Glucógeno	Glicogeno	Glikogen
Gonade	Sex gland (gonad)	Gónada	Gonade	Spolna žlijezda
Gonadotrophine	Gonadotrophin	Gonadotropina	Gonadotropina	Gonadotropin
Gorge	Throat	Garganta	Gola	Grlo
Granulocyte (polynucléaire)	Granulocyte	Granulocito	Granulocita	Granulocit
Granulocyte basophile	Basophil granulocyte	Basófilo	Granulocita basofilo	Bazofilni granulocit
Gros intestin (côlon)	Large intestine (colon)	Intestino grueso (colon)	Intestino crasso (colon)	Debelo crijevo
Groupe sanguin	Blood group	Grupo sanguíneo	Gruppo sanguigno	Krvna grupa
Groupe sanguin A	Blood group A	Grupo sanguíneoA	Gruppo sanguigno A	Krvna grupa A
Groupe sanguin AB	Blood group AB	Grupo sanguíneo AB	Gruppo sanguigno AB	Krvna grupa AB
Groupe sanguin B	Blood group B	Grupo sanguíneo B	Gruppo sanguigno B	Krvna grupa B
Groupe sanguin 0	Blood group 0	Grupo sanguíneo 0	Gruppo sanguigno 0	Krvna grupa 0
Hanche	Hip joint	Articulación de la cadera	Articolazione dell'anca	Kuk (zglob kuka)
Hémoglobine	Hemoglobin	Hemoglobina	Emoglobina	Hemoglobin
Hidrate de carbone (glucide)	Carbohydrate	Carbohidrato	Carboidrato (glucide)	Ugljikohidrat
Hormne lutéinisante	Luteinising hormone	Hormona luteinizante (lutropina)	Ormone luteinizzante	Luteinizirajući hormon
Hormone	Hormone	Hormona	Ormone	Hormon
Hormone antidiurétique (vasopressine)	Antidiuretic hormone (vasopressin)	Hormona anidiurética (arginina vasopresina)	Ormone antidiuretico (vasopressina)	Antidiuretski hormon (vazopresin)
Hormone corticotrope (adrenocorticotropic hormone, ACTH)	Corticotropin (adrenocorticotropic hormone)	Hormona adrenocorticotropa (corticotropina, corticotrofina)	Corticotropina (ormone adrenocorticotropo)	Kortikotropin
Hormone de croissance (somatotropine)	Growth hormone (somatotrophin)	Hormona de crecimiento somatotropa	Somatotropina	Hormon rasta (somatotropin)
Hormone mélanotrope (mélanocortine, mélanotropine)	Melanotropin	Melanotropina	Ormone melanotropo	Melanotropin
Humérus	Upper arm bone (humerus)	Húmero	Omero	Nadlaktična kost (humerus)
Hymen	Hymen	Himen	Imene	Djevičnjak (himen)
Hypophyse (glande pituitaire)	Hypophysis (pituitary gland)	Hipófisis (glándula pituitaria)	Ipòfisi (ghiandola pituitaria)	Hipofiza
Hypothalamus	Hypothalamus	Hipotálamo	Ipotalamo	Hipotalamus
Iléon (ileum)	Ileum	Íleon	Ileo	Ileum
Ilion (ilium)	Ilium	Ilion	Osso iliaco	Crijevna kost
Immunoglobuline	Immunoglobulin	Inmunoglobulina	Immunoglobulina	Imunoglobulin
Incisive	Incisor	Incisivo	Incisivo	Sjekutić (inciziv)
Index	Forefinger	Dedo índice	Dito indice	Kažiprst
Insuline	Insulin	Insulina	Insulina	Inzulin
Intestin	Intestine	Intestin	Intestino	Crijevo
Intestin grêle	Small intestine	Intestino delgado	Intestino tenue (piccolo intestino)	Tanko crijevo
Iris	Iris	Iris	Iride	Šarenica
Ischium	Ischium	Isquión	Ischio	Sjedna kost
Jambe	Lower leg	Pierna	Gamba	Potkoljenica
Jéjunum	Jejunum	Yeyuno	Digiuno	Jejunum
Joue	Cheek	Mejilla (carrillo)	Guancia	Obraz
Kératine	Keratin	Queratina	Cheratina	Keratin

Français	Anglais	Espagnol	Italien	Croate
Langue	Tongue	Lengua	Lingua	Jezik
Larme	Tear	Lágrima	Lacrima	Suza
Larynx	Larynx	Laringe	Laringe	Grkljan
Leucocyte	Leukocyte	Leucocito	Leucocita	Leukocit
Lèvre	Lip	Labio	Labbro	Usna
Ligament	Ligament	Ligamento	Legamento	Ligament
Liquide cérébro-spinal	Cerebrospinal fluid	Líquido cefalorraquídeo (líquido cerebrospinal)	Liquido cefalorachi-diano (liquor, liquido cerebrospinale)	Moždana tekućina (likvor)
Liquide interstitiel	Interstitial fluid	Líquido intersticial (líquido tisular)	Liquido extracellulare	Međustanična tekućina
Liquide synovial	Synovial fluid (synovia)	Líquido sinovial	Liquido sinoviale (sinovia)	Zglobna tekućina (sinovijalna tekućina)
Lombes	Loin	Espalda baja	Lombo	Križa
Lymphe	Lymph	Linfa	Linfa	Limfa
Lymphocyte	Lymphocyte	Linfocito	Linfocita	Limfocit
Mâchoire	Jaw	Quijada	Scheletro della bocca	Čeljust
Main	Hand	Mano	Mano	Šaka
Majeur	Middle finger	Dedo corazón	Dito medio	Srednji prst
Mamelon (papille)	Nipple	Pezón	Capezzolo	Bradavica
Mandibule	Lower jaw (mandible)	Mandíbula	Mandibola	Donja čeljust (mandibula)
Marteau (malléus)	Hammer (malleus)	Martillo (malleus)	Martello	Čekić (malleus)
Matière grasse	Fat	Grasa	Lipidi	Mast
Mélanine	Melanin	Melanina	Melanina	Melanin
Mélatonine (hormone du sommeil)	Melatonin	Melatonina	Melatonina	Melatonin
Membrane synoviale	Synovial membrane	Membrana sinovial	Membrana sinoviale	Sinovijalna opna
Membre inférieur	Leg	Miembro inferior	Arto inferiore	Noga
Méninge	Meninx	Meninge	Meninge	Moždana ovojnica
Ménisque	Meniscus	Menisco	Menisco	Zglobni menisk
Menton	Chin	Barbilla (mentón)	Mento	Brada
Métacarpe	Metacarpus	Metacarpo	Metacarpo	Pest (metakarpus)
Métatarse	Metatarsus	Metatarso	Metatarso	Donožje (metatarzus)
Minéralcorticoïde	Mineralcorticoid	Mineralocorticoide	Mineralcorticoide	Mineralkortikoid (Na-hormon)
Moelle allongée (medulla oblongata, bulbe rachidien, myélencéphale)	Medulla oblongata	Bulbo raquídeo (médula oblongada, miencéfalo)	Bulbo (midollo allungato, encefalo)	Produžena moždina
Moelle du cerveau	Brain marrow	Médula cerebral	Midollo cerebrale	Moždana srž
Moelle épinière (moelle spinale)	Spinal cord	Médula espinal	Midollo spinale	Kralježnična moždina
Moelle osseuse	Bone marrow	Médula ósea	Midollo osseo	Koštana srž
Molaire	Molar	Molar	Molare	Kutnjak (molar)
Mollet	Calf	Pantorrilla	Polpaccio	List
Monocyte	Monocyte	Monocito	Monocita	Monocit
Mucus	Mucus	Moco	Muco	Sluz
Muqueuse	Mucous membrane	Mucosa	Membrana mucosa	Sluznica
Muqueuse gastrique	Gastric mucous membrane	Mucosa estomacal	Mucosa gastrica	Želučana sluznica
Muscle	Muscle	Músculo	Muscolo	Mišić
Muscle adducteur	Adductor muscle	Músculo aductor	Muscolo adduttore	Mišić primicač
Muscle biceps brachial	Biceps brachii muscle	Músculo bíceps braquial	Muscolo bicipite brachiale	Dvoglavi mišić nadlaktice
Muscle biceps fémoral	Biceps femoris muscle	Músculo bíceps crural	Bicipite femorale	Dvoglavi bedreni mišić
Muscle brachial	Brachialis muscle	Braquial anterior	Muscolo brachiale	Nadlaktični mišić
Muscle ciliaire	Ciliary muscle	Músculo ciliar	Muscolo ciliare	Cilijarni mišić
Muscle couturier (muscle sartorius)	Tailor's muscle (sartorius muscle)	Músculo sartorio	Muscolo sartorio	Krojački mišić
Muscle deltoïde	Deltoid muscle	Músculo deltoides	Muscolo deltoide	Rameni mišić (deltoideus)
Muscle droit de l'abdomen	Rectus abdominis muscle	Músculo recto mayor del abdomen	Muscolo retto dell'addome	Ravni trbušni mišić
Muscle glutéal	Gluteal muscle	Músculo glúteo	Muscolo gluteo	Sjedni mišić
Muscle grand pectoral	Pectoralis major muscle	Músculo pectoral mayor	Muscolo grande pettorale	Veliki prsni mišić
Muscle intercostal	Intercostal muscle	Músculo intercostal	Muscolo intercostale	Međurebreni mišić
Muscle lisse	Smooth muscle	Músculo liso	Tessuto muscolare liscio	Glatki mišić
Muscle masséter	Masseter muscle	Músculo masetero	Muscolo massetere	Žvakaći mišić
Muscle oblique de l'abdomen	Abdominal oblique muscle	Músculo oblicuo del abdomen	Musculo obliquo dell'addome	Kosi trbušni mišić
Muscle petit pectoral	Pectoralis minor muscle	Músculo pectoral menor	Muscolo piccolo pettorale	Mali prsni mišić
Muscle quadriceps fémoral	Quadriceps femoris muscle	Músculo cuádriceps crural	Muscolo quadricipite femorale	Četveroglavi bedreni mišić
Muscle rhomboïde	Rhomboid muscle	Músculo romboides	Muscolo romboide	Romboidni mišić
Muscle semi-membraneux	Semimembranosus muscle	Músculo semimembranoso	Muscolo semimembranoso	Poluopnasti mišić
Muscle semi-tendineux	Semitendinosus muscle	Músculo semitendinoso	Muscolo semitendinoso	Polutetivni mišić
Muscle strié	Striated muscle	Músculo estriado	Muscolo striato	Poprečno-prugasti mišić
Muscle trapèze	Trapezius muscle	Músculo trapecio	Muscolo trapezio	Trapezni mišić
Muscle triceps brachial	Triceps brachii muscle	Músculo tríceps braquial	Muscolo tricipite del braccio	Troglavi mišić nadlaktice
Muscle triceps sural	Triceps surae muscle	Músculo tríceps sural	Muscolo tricipite della sura	Troglavi mišić potkoljenice

Français	Anglais	Espagnol	Italien	Croate
Myocarde	Cardiac muscle (myocardium)	Miocardio	Miocardio	Srčani mišić (miokard)
Narine	Nostril	Narina	Narice	Nosnica
Nerf	Nerve	Nervio	Nervo	Živac
Nerf crânien	Cranial nerve	Nervio craneal	Nervo cranico	Moždani živac
Nerf optique	Optic nerve	Nervio óptico	Nervo ottico	Vidni živac
Nerf spinal	Spinal nerve	Nervio espinal	Nervo spinale	Spinalni živac
Nerf vestibulocochléaire (nerf auditif)	Acoustic nerve (vestibulocochlear nerve)	Nervio auditivo (nervio vestibulococlear, nervio estatoacústico)	Nervo vestibolocochleare (nervo stato-acustico)	Slušni živac
Nez	Nose	Nariz	Naso	Nos
Noeud atrio-ventriculaire	Atrioventricular node	Nódulo auriculoventricular	Nodo atrioventricolare	Atrioventrikularni čvor
Noradrénaline	Noradrenaline	Noradrenalina	Noradrenalina	Noradrenalin
Nuque	Nape (occiput)	Nuca	Nuca	Zatiljak
Ocytocine (oxytocine)	Oxytocin	Oxitocina	Ossitocina	Oksitocin
Oeil	Eye	Ojo	Occhio	Oko
Oesophage	Gullet (oesophagus)	Esófago	Esofago	Jednjak
Ombilic (nombril)	Navel (belly button)	Ombligo (pupo)	Ombelico	Pupak
Omoplate (scapula)	Shoulder blade (scapula)	Omóplato (escápula)	Scapola (omoplata)	Lopatica (skapula)
Ongle	Nail	Uña	Unghia	Nokat
Orbite de l'oeil	Eye orbit	Órbita	Orbita oculare	Očna šupljina
Oreille	Ear	Óido	Orecchio	Uho
Oreille moyenne	Middle ear	Oído medio	Orecchio medio	Srednje uho
Oreillette	Cardiac atrium	Aurícula cardíaca (atrio)	Atrio	Srčana pretklijetka (atrij)
Organe	Organ	Órgano	Organo	Organ
Orteil	Toe	Dedo del pie	Dito del piede	Nožni prst
Os	Bone	Hueso	Osso	Kost
Os coxal	Hip bone	Hueso coxal	Osso dell'anca	Kost kuka
Os de la cuisse (fémur)	Thighbone (femur)	Fémur	Femore	Bedrena kost (femur)
Os du carpe	Wrist bone (carpal bone)	Hueso del carpo	Osso carpale	Kost zapešća (karpalna kost)
Os du métatarse	Metatarsal bone	Hueso del metatarso	Osso metatarsale	Kost donožja (metatarzalna kost)
Os du tarse	Tarsal bone	Hueso del tarso	Osso tarsale	Kost zastoplja (kost tarzusa)
Os ethmoïde	Ethmoid bone	Hueso etmoides	Osso etmoide	Sitasta kost (etmoidna kost)
Os frontal	Frontal bone	Hueso frontal	Osso frontale	Čeona kost
Os hyoïde (os lingual)	Hyoid bone (lingual bone)	Hueso hioides	Osso ioide	Podjezična kost
Os lacrymal (unguis)	Lachrymal bone	Unguis (hueso lacrimal)	Osso lacrimale	Suzna kost
Os maxillaire	Upper jaw (maxilla)	Hueso maxilar superior (maxila)	Osso mascellare	Gornja čeljust (maksila)
Os métacarpe	Metacarpal bone	Hueso del metacarpo	Osso metacarpale	Kost pesti (metakarpalna kost)
Os nasal	Nasal bone	Hueso proprio de la nariz (hueso nasal)	Osso nasale	Nosna kost
Os occipital	Occipital bone	Hueso occipital	Osso occipitale	Zatiljna kost
Os palatin	Palatine bone	Hueso palatino	Osso palatino	Nepčana kost
Os pariétal	Parietal bone	Hueso parietal	Osso parietale	Tjemena kost
Os pubien	Pubis (pubic bone)	Pubis	Pube (osso pubico)	Stidna kost
Os sésamoïde	Sesamoid bone	Hueso sesamoide	Osso sesamoide	Sezamska kost
Os sphénoïde	Sphenoid bone	Hueso esfenoides	Osso sfenoide	Klinasta kost (leptirasta kost)
Os temporal	Temporal bone	Hueso temporal	Osso temporale	Sljepoočna kost
Os zygomatique (zygoma)	Zygoma (cheekbone, malar bone)	Hueso cigomático (malar)	Osso zigomatico	Sponična kost
Ovaire	Ovary	Ovario	Ovaia	Jajnik
Ovule	Ovum	Óvulo	Uovo	Jajašce
Palais osseux	Hard palate	Paladar óseo	Palato duro (volta palatina)	Tvrdo nepce
Palaise	Palate	Paladar	Palato	Nepce
Pancréas	Pancreas	Páncreas	Pancreas	Gušterača
Papille gustative	Taste bud	Papila gustativa	Papilla gustativa	Okusni pupoljak
Parathormone (hormone parathyroïdienne)	Parathyroid hormone	Parathormona (hormona paratiroidea, paratirina)	Paratormone (ormone paratiroideo)	Paratireoidni hormon
Parathyroïde	Parathyroid gland	Glándula paratiroides	Paratiroide	Doštitnjača
Parti supérieur du dos	Upper back	Espalda superior	Schiena alto	Gornji dio leđa
Partie supérieure du bras	Upper arm	Parte superior del brazo	Barccio	Nadlaktica
Paume	Palm	Palma	Palmo	Dlan
Paupière	Eyelid	Párpado	Palpebra	Kapak
Pavillon auriculaire	Pinna (auricle)	Pabellón auricular (aurícula)	Padiglione auricolare	Ušna školjka
Peau	Skin	Piel	Pelle (cute)	Koža
Pénis	Penis	Pene (falo)	Pene	Penis
Péricarde	Pericardium	Pericardio	Pericardio	Osrčje (perikard)
Périnée	Perineum	Periné (perineo)	Perineo	Međica (perineum)
Péritoine	Peritoneum	Peritoneo	Peritoneo	Potrbušnica (peritoneum)
Phalange	Phalanx bone	Falange	Falange	Kost prsta (falanga)
Pharynx	Pharynx (gullet, gorge)	Faringe	Faringe	Ždrijelo
Phospholipide	Phospholipid	Fosfolípido	Fosfolipide	Fosfolipid

Français	Anglais	Espagnol	Italien	Croate
Pie-mère	Pia mater	Piamadre	Pia madre	Meka moždana ovojnica
Pied	Foot	Pie	Piede	Stopalo
Plante	Sole	Planta del pie	Pianta del piede	Taban
Plasma sanguin	Plasma	Plasma sanguíneo	Plasma	Plazma
Plèvre	Pleura	Pleura	Pleura (pleure)	Pleura
Plèvre pariétale	Parietal pleura	Pleura parietal	Pleura parietale	Porebrica (parijetalna pleura)
Plèvre viscérale	Visceral pleura	Pleura visceral	Pleura viscerale	Poplućnica (visceralna pleura)
Poignet	Wrist	Muñeca	Polso	Ručni zglob
Cheveu	Hair	Cabello	Capelli	Kosa
Pomme d' Adam	Adam's apple	Nuez de Adán	Pomo d'Adamo	Adamova jabučica
Pore	Pore	Poro	Poro	Pora
Pouce	Thumb	Dedo pulgar (pólice)	Pollice	Palac
Poumon	Lung	Pulmón	Polmone	Plućno krilo
Poumons	Lungs	Pulmones	Polmoni	Pluća
Prémolaire	Premolar	Premolar	Premolare	Pretkutnjak (premolar)
Prépuce	Foreskin (prepuce)	Prepucio	Prepuzio	Prepucij
Progestérone	Progesterone	Progesterona	Progesterone	Progesteron
Prostate	Prostate	Próstata	Prostata	Prostata
Protéine	Protein	Proteína	Proteina	Bjelančevina (protein)
Pulpe dentaire	Dental pulp	Pulpa dentaria	Polpa dentaria	Središte zuba (pulpa)
Pupille	Pupil	Pupila	Pupilla	Zjenica
Racine dentaire	Root of a tooth	Raíz del diente	Radice del dente	Korijen zuba
Radius	Radius	Radio	Radio	Palčana kost
Rate	Spleen	Bazo	Milza	Slezena
Rein	Kidney	Riñón	Rene	Bubreg
Rétine	Retina	Retina	Rètina	Mrežnica (retina)
Rotule (patella)	Kneecap (patella)	Rótula (patela)	Rotula (patella)	Iver (patela)
Salive	Saliva (spit, slobber)	Saliva	Saliva	Slina (pljuvačka)
Sang	Blood	Sangre	Sangue	Krv
Sclère	Sclera	Eclerótica	Sclera	Bjeloočnica
Sébum	Sebum	Sebo cutáneo	Sebo	Loj
Sein	Breast	Mama	Mammella	Dojka
Sinus	Sinus	Seno	Seno	Sinus
Sourcils	Eyebrow	Ceja	Sopracciglio	Obrva
Spermatozoïde	Sperm (spermatozoon)	Espermatozoide	Spermatozoo	Spermij
Sperme	Semen	Semen (esperma)	Sperma	Sperma
Sphincter	Sphincter	Esfinter	Sfintere	Kružni mišić (sfinkter)
Squelette	Skeleton	Esqueleto	Scheletro	Kostur
Sternum	Breastbone (sternum)	Esternón	Sterno	Prsna kost (sternum)
Suc gastrique	Gastric juice	Jugo gástrico	Succo gastrico	Želučani sok
Suc intestinal	Intestinal juice	Jugo intestinal	Succo intestinale	Crijevni sok
Suc pancréatique	Pancreatic juice	Jugo pancreático	Succo pancreatico	Sok gušterače
Sueur	Sweat	Sudor	Sudore	Znoj
Synapse	Synapse	Sinapsis	Sinapsi (bottone sinaptico)	Sinapsa
Système nerveux orthosympathique (système nerveux sympathique)	Sympathetic nervous system	Sistema nervioso simpático	Sistema nervoso simpatico	Simpatikus
Système nerveux parasympatique (système vagal)	Parasympathetic nervous system	Sistema nervioso parasimpático	Sistema nervoso parasimpatico	Parasimpatikus
Système Rhésus négatif	Rh factor negative	Factor Rh negativo	Fattore Rh negativo	Negativan Rh faktor
Système Rhésus positif	Rh factor positive	Factor Rh positivo	Fattore Rh positivo	Pozitivan Rh faktor
Talon	Heel	Talón (calcañar)	Tallone	Peta
Tarse	Tarsus	Tarso	Tarso	Zastoplje
Télencéphale (cerveau)	Cerebrum (telencephalon)	Telencéfalo	Telencefalo (cervello)	Veliki mozak (telencefalon)
Tempe	Temple	Sien	Tempia	Sljepoočnica
Tendon	Tendon (sinew)	Tendón	Tendine	Tetiva
Testicule	Testicle	Testículo	Testicolo	Jaje (mudo, testis)
Testostérone	Testosterone	Testosterona	Testosterone	Testosteron
Tête	Head	Cabeza	Testa	Glava
Thalamus	Thalamus	Tálamo	Talamo	Talamus
Thrombocyte	Thrombocyte	Plaqueta (trombocito)	Trombocita (piastrina)	Trombocit
Thymus	Thymus	Timo	Timo	Grudna žlijezda (timus)
Thyréostimuline (thyréotropine)	Thyroid-stimulating hormone (TSH, thyrotropin)	Tirotropina (TSH, hormona estimulante de la tiroides)	Tirotropina (ormone tireostimolante)	Tireotropin (TSH)
Thyroïde	Thyroid	Tiroides	Tiroide	Štitnjača
Thyroxine	Thyroxine	Tiroxina (tetrayodotironina, T4)	Tiroxina	Tiroksin
Tibia	Shinbone (tibia)	Tibia	Tibia	Goljenica (tibija)
Tissu	Tissue	Tejido	Tessuto	Tkivo
Tissu adipeux (masse grasse)	Fat tissue	Tejido graso (tejido adiposo)	Tessuto adiposo	Masno tkivo
Tonsille	Tonsil	Amígdala	Tonsille	Krajnik
Torse	Chest	Pecho	Torace	Grudište (prsa)

Français	Anglais	Espagnol	Italien	Croate
Trachée	Windpipe (trachea)	Tráquea	Trachea	Dušnik
Triglycéride	Triglyceride	Triglicérido	Trigliceride	Triglicerid
Triiodothyronine	Triiodothyronine	Triiodotironina	Triiodotironina	Trijodtironin
Trompe de Fallope	Fallopian tube (oviduct)	Trompa de Falopio (tuba uterina, oviducto)	Tuba di Falloppio	Jajovod
Tronc	Trunk (torso)	Tronco	Tronco	Trup (torzo)
Tronc cérébral	Brain stem	Tronco del encéfalo	Tronco encefalico	Moždano stablo
Tympan	Eardrum (tympanic membrane)	Tímpano	Timpano (membrana timpanica)	Bubnjić
Ulna (cubitus)	Ulna	Cúbito (ulna)	Ulna (cubito)	Lakatna kost (ulna)
Urée (carbamide)	Urea	Urea	Urea	Mokraćevina (urea, ureja)
Uretère	Ureter	Uréter	Uretere	Mokraćovod (ureter)
Urètre	Urethra	Uretra	Uretra	Vanjska mokraćna cijev (uretra)
Urine	Urine	Orina	Urina	Mokraća (urin)
Utérus	Womb (uterus)	Matriz (útero, seno materno)	Utero	Maternica (uterus)
Vagin	Vagina	Vagina (colpos)	Vagina	Rodnica (vagina)
Vaisseau lymphatique	Lymph vessel	Vaso linfático	Vaso linfatico	Limfna žila
Vaisseau sanguin	Blood vessel	Vaso sanguíneo	Vaso sanguigno	Krvna žila
Valve	Valve (valvula)	Válvula	Valvola	Zalistak
Valve aortique	Aortic valve	Válvula sigmoidea aórtica	Valvola semilunare aortica	Polumjesečasti aortni zalistak
Valve cardiaque	Heart valve (cardiac valve)	Válvula cardiaca (válvula de corazón)	Valvola cardiaca	Srčani zalistak
Valve mitrale (valve bicuspide)	Mitral valve (bicuspid valve)	Válvula bicúspide (válvula mitral)	Valvola mitrale (valvola bicuspide)	Mitralni zalistak (bikuspidalni zalistak)
Valve tricuspide	Tricuspid valve	Válvula tricúspide	Valvola tricuspide	Trolisni zalistak
Veine	Vein	Vena	Vena	Vena
Veine cave inférieure	Inferior vena cava	Vena cava inferior	Vena cava inferiore	Donja šuplja vena
Veine cave supérieure	Superior vena cava	Vena cava superior	Vena cava superiore	Gornja šuplja vena
Veine porte	Portal vein	Vena porta	Vena porta	Portalna vena
Veinule (vénule)	Venule	Vénula	Venula	Venula
Ventricule	Ventricle	Ventrículo	Ventricolo	Klijetka
Ventricule cardiaque	Cardiac ventricle	Ventrículo cardíaco	Ventricolo cardiaco	Srčana klijetka
Ventricule cérébral	Brain ventricle	Ventrículo cerebral	Ventricolo cerebrale	Moždana klijetka
Vertèbre	Vertebra	Vértebra	Vertebra	Kralježak
Vertèbre coccygienne	Coccygeal vertebra	Vértebra coccígea	Vertebra coccigea	Trtični kralježak
Vertèbre lombale	Lumbar vertebra	Vértebra lumbar	Vertebra lombare	Slabinski kralježak (lumbalni kralježak)
Vertèbre sacrale	Sacral vertebra	Vértebra sacra	Vertebra sacrale	Krstačni kralježak (sakralni kralježak)
Vertèbre thoracique	Thoracic vertebra	Vértebra torácica	Vertebra toracica	Leđni kralježak (grudni ili torakalni kralježak)
Vertex	Vertex (crown of head)	Vértice craneal	Vertice della testa	Tjeme
Vésicule biliare (cholécyste)	Gall bladder	Vesícula biliar	Cistifellea	Žućni mjehur
Vésicule séminale (glande vésiculeuse)	Seminal vesicle	Vesícula seminal	Vescicola seminale	Sjemena vrećica
Vessie	Urinary bladder	Vejiga urinaria	Vescica urinaria	Mokraćni mjehur
Vestibule	Vestibule	Vestíbulo	Vestibolo	Predvorje (vestibulum)
Villosité intestinale	Intestinal villus	Vellosidad intestinal	Villo intestinale	Crijevna resica
Visage	Face	Cara (faz)	Viso	Lice
Voie biliaire	Bile duct	Vía biliar	Coledoco	Žučovod
Voile du palais	Soft palate	Úvula	Palato molle	Meko nepce
Vomer	Vomer	Vómer	Vomere	Raonik (vomer)
Vulve	Vulva	Vulva	Vulva	Stidnica

LES SYMPTÔMES, BLESSURES ET MALADIES:	SYMPTOMS, INJURIES AND DISEASES:	SÍNTOMAS, HERIDAS Y ENFERMEDADES:	I SINTOMI, FERITE E MALATTIE:	SIMPTOMI, OZLJEDE I BOLESTI:
Abaissement de la paupière supérieure (blépharoptose)	Drooping of the upper eyelid (blepharoptosis)	Despredimiento del párpado superior (blefaroptosis)	Spostamento della palpebra (palpebra calante, blefaroptosi)	Spušteni kapak (blefaroptoza)
Abcès	Abscess	Absceso	Ascesso	Apsces
Abcès anale	Anal abscess	Absceso anal	Ascesso anale	Analni apsces
Abcès cérébral	Brain abscess	Absceso cerebral	Ascesso cerebrale	Apsces mozga
Abcès de Brodie	Brodie abscess	Absceso de Brodie	Ascesso di Brodie	Brodijev apsces
Abcès hépatique	Liver abscess	Absceso hepático	Ascesso epatico	Apsces jetre
Abcès périamygdalien	Quinsy (peritonsillar abscess)	Absceso peritonsilar	Ascesso peritonsillare	Gnojna upala krajnika
Abcès périanal	Perianal abscess	Absceso perianal	Ascesso perianale	Perianalni apsces
Abcès périnéphrique	Perinephric abscess	Absceso perinéfrico	Ascesso perinefrico	Paranefritički apsces
Abcès pulmonaire	Lung abscess	Absceso pulmonar	Ascesso polmonare	Apsces pluća
Abdomen aigu	Acute abdomen	Abdomen agudo	Addome acuto	Akutni abdomen

Français	Anglais	Espagnol	Italien	Croate
Aboulie	Aboulia (disorder of diminished motivation)	Abulia	Abulia	Abulija (poremećaj umanjene motivacije)
Absence de descente des testicules	Undescended testicle	Descenso incompleto de testículo	Mancata discesa del testicolo	Nespušteni testis
Absence de la conscience	Unconsciousness	Inconsciencia	Incoscienza (stato di incoscienza)	Nesvjestica
Absence de pouls	Absence of pulse	Pérdida de pulso	Perdita di polso	Gubitak pulsa
Absence des règles (aménorrhée)	Absence of menstrual period (amenorrhea)	Ausencia de la menstruación (amenorrea)	Assenza di mestruazioni (amenorrea)	Izostanak mjesečnice (amenoreja)
Acariase	Acariasis	Acariasis	Acariasi	Akarijaza
Accident thromboembolique	Thromboembolism	Tromboembolismo	Tromboembolia	Tromboembolija
Achlorhydrie	Achlorhydria	Aclorhidria	Acloridria	Aklorhidrija
Achondroplasie	Achondroplasia	Acondroplasia	Acondroplasia	Ahondroplazija
Acidose	Acidosis	Acidosis	Acidosi	Acidoza
Acidose métabolique	Metabolic acidosis	Acidosis metabólica	Acidosi metabolica	Metabolička acidoza
Acidose tubulaire rénale	Renal tubular acidosis	Acidosis tubular renal	Acidosi renale tubulare	Renalna tubularna acidoza
Acné	Acne	Acné	Acne	Akne
Acné papulo-pustuleuse	Acne vulgaris	Acné común (acne vulgaris)	Acne volgare (acne)	Vulgarne akne
Acouphène	Ringing in ears (tinnitus)	Pitidos en el oído (acúfeno, tinnitus)	Ronzio auricolare (acufene, tinnito)	Zujanje u ušima (tinitus)
Acrocyanose	Acrocyanosis	Acrocianosis	Acrocianosi	Akrocijanoza
Acromégalie	Acromegaly	Acromegalia	Acromegalia	Akromegalija
Acrophobie (peur des hauteurs)	Acrophobia (fear of heights)	Acrofobia (miedo a las alturas)	Acrofobia (paura dei luoghi elevati)	Akrofobija (strah od visine)
Actinomycose	Actinomycosis	Actinomicosis	Actinomicosi	Aktinomikoza
Adénocarcinome	Adenocarcinoma	Adenocarcinoma	Adenocarcinoma	Adenokarcinom
Adénome	Adenoma	Adenoma	Adenoma	Adenom
Adénome hépatocellulaire	Hepatocellular adenoma	Adenoma hepático (adenoma hepatocelular)	Adenoma epatocellulare	Hepatocelularni adenom
Adénome tubulaire	Tubular adenoma	Adenoma tubular	Adenoma tubulare	Tubularni adenom
Adénopathie	Adenopathy	Adenopatía	Adenopatia	Adenopatija
Adénose sclérosante	Sclerosing adenosis	Adenosis esclerosante	Adenosi sclerosante	Sklerozirajuća adenoza
Aerophobie (peur de l'avion)	Aviophobia (fear of flying)	Aerofobia (miedo a volar)	Aviofobia (paura di volare)	Aerofobija (strah od letenja)
Affaiblissement de l'organisme (asthénie)	Loss of strenght (asthenia)	Pérdida de fuerza muscular (astenia)	Riduzione della forza muscolare (astenia)	Gubitak mišićne snage (astenija)
Agénésie	Agenesis (absence of an organ)	Agenesia (ausencia de un órgano)	Agenesia (mancanza di un organo)	Agenezija (nedostatak jednog organa)
Agénésie rénale	Renal agenesis	Agenesia renal	Agenesia renale	Agenezija bubrega
Angiome	Angioma	Angioma	Angioma	Angiom
Agranulocytose	Agranulocytosis	Agranulocitosis	Agranulocitosi	Agranulocitoza
Albinisme	Albinism	Albinismo	Albinismo	Albinizam
Albuminurie	Albuminuria	Albuminuria	Albuminuria	Albuminurija
Alcalose	Alkalosis	Alcalosis	Alcalosi	Alkaloza
Alcalose respiratoire	Respiratory alkalosis	Alcalosis respiratoria	Alcalosi respiratoria	Respiratorna alkaloza
Alcoolisme	Alcoholism	Alcoholismo	Alcolismo	Alkoholizam
Algie vasculaire de la face	Cluster headache	Cefalea en racimos	Cefalea a grappolo	Cluster glavobolja
Algodystrophie	Algodystrophy	Algodistrofia	Algodistrofia	Algodistrofija
Allergie	Allergy	Alergia	Allergia	Alergija
Allergie à la poussière	Dust allergy	Alergia al polvo	Allergia a polvere	Alergija na prašinu
Allergie alimentaire	Food allergy	Alergia a alimentos	Allergia alimentare	Alergija na hranu
Allergie au pollen	Pollen allergy	Alergia al polen	Allergia da poline	Alergija na pelud
Allergie aux animaux à poils	Fur allergy	Alergia al pelo de los animales	Allergia a pello di animali	Alergija na životinjsku dlaku
Allergie aux médicaments	Drug allergy	Alergia al medicamento	Allergia a farmaci	Alergija na lijekove
Allergie aux plumes	Feather allergy	Alergia a las plumas	Allergia alle piume	Alergija na perje
Alopécie	Alopecia	Alopecia	Alopecia	Ćelavost
Alopécie areata	Alopecia areata	Alopecia areata	Alopecia areata	Alopecia areata
Alopécie universalis	Alopecia universalis	Alopecia areata universal	Alopecia universale	Opća alopecija
Altération d'origine chimique	Chemical injuries	Lesiones químicas	Ferita chimica	Kemijske ozljede
Amaigrissement	Weight loss (weight reduction)	Pérdida de peso	Dimagramento	Mršavljenje
Amibiase (dysenterie amibienne)	Amebiasis (amebic dysentery)	Disentería amebiana (amebiasis)	Amebiasi	Amebijaza
Amnésie	Amnesia	Amnesia	Amnesia	Amnezija
Amputation	Amputation	Amputación	Amputazione	Amputacija
Amylose (amyloïdose, maladie orpheline)	Amyloidosis	Amiloidosis	Amiloidosi	Amiloidoza
Analgésie	Analgesia (loss of pain sensation)	Analgesia	Analgesia	Analgezija (neosjetljivost na bol)
Androblastome (tumeur à cellule de Sertoli et Leydig)	Androblastoma (Sertoli-Leydig cell tumor)	Tumor de células de Sertoli-Leydig (arrenoblastoma)	Androblastoma	Androblastom (tumor Sertoli-Leydigovih stanica)
Anémie	Anemia	Anemia	Anemia	Slabokrvnost (anemija)
Anémie aplasique	Aplastic anemia	Anemia aplásica	Anemia aplastica	Aplastična anemija

Français	Anglais	Espagnol	Italien	Croate
Anémie des maladies chroniques	Anemia of chronic disease	Anemia de enfermedades crónicas	Anemia da malattia cronica	Anemija kronične bolesti
Anémie ferriprive	Iron deficiency anemia (sideropenic anemia)	Anemia ferropénica	Anemia da carenza di ferro	Anemija radi deficita željeza (sideropenična anemija)
Anémie hémolytique	Hemolytic anemia	Anemia hemolítica	Anemia emolitica	Hemolitična anemija
Anémie hypochrome	Hypochromic anemia	Anemia hipocrómica	Anemia ipocromica	Hipokromna anemija
Anémie mégaloblastique	Megaloblastic anemia	Anemia megaloblástica	Anemia megaloblastica	Megaloblastična anemija (anemija radi deficita vitamina)
Anémie pernicieuse	Pernicious anemia	Anemia perniciosa	Anemia perniciosa	Perniciozna anemija
Anencéphalie	Anencephaly	Anencefalia	Anencefalia	Anencefalija
Anévrisme (anévrysme)	Aneurysm (aneurism)	Aneurisma	Aneurisma	Aneurizma
Anévrisme aortique thoracique	Thoracic aortic aneurysm	Aneurisma de aorta torácica	Aneurisma dell'aorta toracica	Aneurizma torakalne aorte
Anévrisme congénital de l'artère à la base du cerveau	Congenital aneurysm of arteries at the base of the brain	Aneurisma congénito arterial de la base del cerebro	Aneurisma arteriosa congenita alla base dell'encefalo	Urođena aneurizma arterija baze mozga
Anévrisme de l'aorte	Aortic aneurysm	Aneurisma de aorta	Aneurisma aortico	Aneurizma aorte
Anévrisme de l'aorte abdominale	Abdominal aortic aneurysm	Aneurisma de aorta abdominal	Aneurisma dell'aorta abdominale	Aneurizma abdominalne aorte
Anévrisme intra-crânien	Cerebral aneurysm	Aneurisma cerebral	Aneurisma cerebrale	Cerebralna aneurizma
Anévrisme intracrânien en forme de sac	Ball-shaped aneurysm of the brain artery	Aneurisma cerebral arterial sacular	Aneurisma cerebrale sferica	Kuglasta aneurizma arterije mozga
Angine	Angina	Angina	Angina	Angina
Angine de poitrine (angor)	Angina pectoris	Angina de pecho (angor, angor pectoris)	Angina pectoris	Angina pektoris
Angine de Prinzmetal	Prinzmetal's angina	Angina de Prinzmetal	Angina di Prinzmetal	Prinzmetalova angina
Angiome	Angioma	Angioma	Angioma	Angiom
Angiome stellaire	Spider angioma (spider nevus)	Angioma en araña (angioma aracnoideo)	Angioma a ragno	Paukoliki angiom (spider nevus)
Angiosarcome	Angiosarcoma	Angiosarcoma	Angiosarcoma	Angiosarkom
Anisakiase	Anisakiasis	Anisakiasis (anisakidosis)	Anisakidosi	Anisakijaza
Ankylose	Ankylosis (joint stiffness)	Anquilosis	Anchilosi	Ankiloza (ukočenje zgloba)
Ankylostomose	Ancylostomiasis	Anquilostomiasis	Anchilostomiasi	Ankilostomijaza
Anomalie cérébrovasculaire	Cerebrovascular anomaly	Malformación arteriovenosa cerebral	Anomalia cerebrovascolare	Anomalija moždanih krvnih žila
Anomalie de Sprengel	Sprengel's deformity	Deformidad de Sprengel	Deformità di Sprengel	Sprengelova bolest (scapula alta)
Anomalie du développement cérébral	Brain development anomaly	Malformación del desarrollo cerebral	Anomalia di sviluppo del sistema nervoso	Anomalija u razvoju mozga
Anomalies de développement	Development anomalies	Anomalías del desarrollo	Anomalie di sviluppo	Razvojne anomalije
Anorexie	Anorexia	Anorexia	Anoressia	Anoreksija
Anthracose	Anthracosis	Antracosis	Antracosi	Antrakoza
Anthrax	Carbuncle	Ántrax (carbunco)	Carbonchio (pustola)	Karbunkul
Anurie (volume urinaire < 100 ml par 24 heures)	Anuria (passage of urine < 100 ml in 24 hours)	Anuria (menos de 100ml de orina en 24h)	Anuria (produzione di urina < 100 ml nelle 24 ore)	Anurija (lučenje urina < 100 ml u 24 sata)
Anxiété	Anxiety	Ansiedad	Ansia (ansietà)	Nemir (anksioznost)
Aphte (ulcère de la muqueuse buccale)	Aphtha (mouth ulcer)	Afta (úlcera en la mucosa oral)	Afta (ulcera all'interno della cavità orale)	Afte (ulceracija sluznice usta)
Aplasie	Aplasia	Aplasia	Aplasia	Aplazija
Apnée du sommeil	Sleep apnea	Apnea del sueño	Sindrome delle apnee nel sonno	Noćna desaturacija
Apoplexie (attaque d'apoplexie)	Apoplexy	Apoplejía (golpe apoplético)	Apoplessia	Moždano krvarenje (apopleksija)
Appendicite aiguë	Acute appendicitis	Apendicitis aguda	Appendicite acuta	Akutna upala crvuljka
Appétit	Appetite	Apetito	Appetito	Apetit
Aquaphobie	Aquaphobia	Acuafobia	Idrofobia	Hidrofobija
Arrêt cardiaque (arrêt ventilatoire, arrêt cardio-respiratoire)	Cardiac arrest (cardiopulmonary arrest)	Paro cardiaco (parada cardiorrespiratoria)	Arresto cardiaco	Zastoj srca (srčani arest)
Arrêt de la sécrétion d'urine	Nonpassage of urine	Supresión de la secreción de orina	Soppressione della secrezione di urina	Prestanak lučenja urina
Arrêt du développement d'un organe (aplasie d'un organe)	Absence in development of an organ (aplasia of an organ)	Desarrollo detenido de un órgano (aplasia de un órgano)	Mancato sviluppo di un organo (aplasia di un organo)	Nerazvijenost organa (aplazija organa)
Arrêt respiratoire (apnée)	Suspension of external breathing (apnea)	Falta de respiración (apnea)	Assenza di respirazione (apnea)	Zastoj disanja (apnea)
Artérite giganto-cellulaire (maladie de Horton, artérite temporale)	Giant cell arteritis (temporal arteritis)	Arteritis de células gigantes (arteritis de la temporal)	Arterite temporale (arterite di Horton)	Arteritis divovskih stanica (temporalni arteritis)
Artériosclérose	Arteriosclerosis	Arteriosclerosis	Arteriosclerosi	Arterioskleroza
Arthrite chronique juvénile	Juvenile rheumatoid arthritis	Artritis juvenil	Artrite idiopatica giovanile	Mladenački reumatoidni artritis (juvenilni reumatoidni artritis)
Arthrite psoriatique	Psoriatic arthritis	Artritis psoriásica	Artrite psoriasica	Psorijatični artritis

Français	Anglais	Espagnol	Italien	Croate
Arthrite réactive (syndrome de Reiter)	Reactive arthritis (Reiter's syndrome)	Síndrome de Reiter (artritis reactiva)	Sindrome di Reiter	Reiterov sindrom
Arthrite rhumatoïde	Rheumatoid arthritis	Artritis reumatoide	Artrite reumatoide	Reumatoidni artritis
Arthrite septique	Infectious arthritis (septic arthritis)	Artritis infecciosa (artritis séptica)	Artrite settica	Infekcijski artritis (septički artritis)
Arthrite tuberculeuse	Tuberculous arthritis	Artritis tuberculosa	Artrite tubercolare	Tuberkulozni artritis
Arthrogrypose	Arthrogryposis	Artrogriposis	Artrogriposi	Artrogripoza
Arthropathie	Arthropathy	Artropatía	Artropatia	Artropatija
Arthropathie hémophile	Hemophiliac arthropathy	Artropatía hemofilíca	Artropatia emofilica	Hemofilična artropatija
Arthrose (arthropathie chronique dégénérative)	Arthrosis (osteoarthritis, degenerative arthritis)	Artrosis	Artrosi	Artroza (osteoartritis, degenerativni artritis)
Arthrose de cheville	Ankle arthrosis	Artrosis de tobillo	Artrosi di caviglia	Artroza skočnog zgloba
Arthrose de hanche (coxarthrose)	Hip arthrosis	Artrosis de cadera (coxartrosis)	Artrosi di anca	Artroza kuka (koksartroza)
Arthrose de l'épaule	Shoulder arthrosis	Artrosis del hombro	Artrosi gleno-omerale	Artroza ramena
Arthrose de le main	Hand arthrosis	Artrosis de mano	Artrosi della mano	Artroza šake
Arthrose du coude	Elbow arthrosis	Artrosis de codo	Artrosi di gomito	Artroza lakta
Arthrose du disque intervertébral	Discarthrosis (degenerative disc disease)	Discartrosis	Discarthrosi (discopatia degenerativa)	Diskartroza
Arthrose du genou (gonarthrose)	Knee arthrosis	Artrosis de rodilla (gonartrosis)	Artrosi di ginocchio	Artroza koljena (gonartroza)
Arthrose du pied	Foot arthrosis	Artrosis del pie	Artrosi al piede	Artroza stopala
Arthrose du poignet	Wrist arthrosis	Artrosis de muñeca	Artrosi di polso	Artroza ručnog zgloba
Arythmie	Arrhythmia	Arrítmia	Aritmia	Aritmija
Arythmie cardiaque	Cardiac arrhythmia	Arrítmia cardíaca	Aritmia cardiaca	Srčana aritmija
Asbestose (amiantose)	Asbestosis	Asbestosis	Asbestosi	Azbestoza
Ascaridiose	Ascaridosis	Ascaridiasis	Ascaridiasi	Askaridijaza
Ascite	Ascites	Ascitis	Ascite	Ascites
Aspergillome	Aspergilloma (mycetoma, fungus ball)	Aspergiloma (micetoma)	Aspergilloma (micetoma)	Aspergilom
Aspergillose	Aspergillose	Aspergilosis	Aspergillosi	Aspergiloza
Asphyxie	Asphyxia	Asfixia	Asfissia	Asfiksija
Asthme	Asthma	Asma	Asma	Astma
Astigmatisme	Astigmatism	Astigmatismo	Astigmatismo	Astigmatizam
Astrocytome	Astrocytoma	Astrocitoma	Astrocitoma	Astrocitom
Ataxie héréditaire	Hereditary ataxia	Ataxia de Friidreich (ataxia hereditaria)	Atassia ereditaria	Heredoataksija
Atélectasie pulmonaire	Pulmonary atelectasis	Atelectasia pulmonar	Atelectasia polmonare	Atelektaza pluća
Athérosclérose	Atherosclerosis	Ateroesclerosis	Aterosclerosi	Ateroskleroza
Athétose	Athetosis	Atetosis	Atetosi	Atetoza
Atonie	Atony (atonia)	Atonía	Atonia muscolare	Atonija
Atrésie anale	Anal atresia	Atresia anal	Atresia anale	Atrezija anusa
Atrésie biliare	Bile duct atresia	Atresia biliar	Atresia biliare	Atrezija žučnih vodova
Atrésie de l'oesophage	Esophageal atresia	Atresia esofágica	Atresia esofagea	Atrezija jednjaka
Atrésie duodénale	Duodenal atresia	Atresia duodenal	Atresia duodenale	Atrezija dvanaesnika
Atrésie intestinale	Intestinal atresia	Atresia intestinal	Atresia intestinale	Crijevna atrezija
Atrophie	Atrophy	Atrofia	Atrofia	Atrofija
Atrophie de Sudeck	Sudeck's atrophy	Atrofia de Sudeck	Atrofia di Sudeck	Sudeckova distrofija
Atrophie multisystématisée	Multiple system atrophy	Atrofia multisistémica	Atrofia multi-sistemica	Multipla sistemska atrofija
Attaque cérébrale (accident vasculaire cérébral)	Stroke (cerebrovascular accident)	Derrame cerebral (accidente cerebrovascular)	Colpo apoplettico	Moždani udar
Augmentation d'un ganglion lymphatique (lymphadénopathie)	Enlarged lymph nodes (lymphadenopathy)	Aumento de volumen de los ganglios linfáticos (linfadenopatía)	Ingrossamento dei linfonodi (linfoadenopatia)	Povećanje limfnih čvorova (limfadenopatija)
Augmentation de la langue (macroglossie)	Enlarged tongue (macroglossia)	Lengua más grande de lo normal (macroglosia)	Eccessiva crescita della lingua (macroglossia)	Uvećani jezik (makroglosija)
Augmentation du foie (hépatomégalie)	Enlarged liver (hepatomegaly)	Aumento del tamaño del hígado (hepatomegalia)	Aumento di volume del fegato (epatomegalia)	Povećanje jetre (hepatomegalija)
Autisme	Autism	Autismo	Autolesionismo	Autizam
Automutilation	Self-harm	Autolesión (automutilación)	Autolesionismo	Samoozljeđivanje
Aversion pour la nourriture	Food aversion	Aversión por la comida	Ripugnanza al cibo	Gađenje prema hrani
Avitaminose	Avitaminosis	Avitaminosis	Avitaminosi	Avitamonoza
Bactériémie	Bacteremia	Bacteriemia (bacteremia)	Batteriemia	Bakterijemija
Bactériurie	Bacteriuria	Bacteriuria	Batteriuria	Bakteriurija
Bâillement	Yawn	Bostezo	Sbadiglio	Zijevanje
Baisse de la pression artérielle (hypotension artérielle)	Low blood pressure (hypotension)	Presión sanguínea baja (hipotensión)	Bassa pressione arteriosa (ipotensione)	Nizak krvni tlak (hipotenzija)
Ballonnements et vesse (flatulence)	Bloating and gases (flatulence)	Hinchazón y gases (flatulencia, ventosidad)	Gonfiezza e venti (flatulenza)	Nadutost i vjetrovi
Barotraumatisme	Barotrauma	Barotraumatismo (barotrauma)	Barotrauma	Barotrauma
Bartonellose	Bartonellosis	Bartonelosis	Bartonellosi	Bartoneloza
Basophilie	Basophilia	Basofilia	Basofilia	Bazofilija

79

Français	Anglais	Espagnol	Italien	Croate
Blastome	Blastoma	Blastoma	Blastoma	Blastom
Blastomycose	Blastomycosis	Blastomicosis	Blastomicosi	Blastomikoza
Blépharite	Blepharitis	Blefaritis	Blefarite	Blefaritis
Blessure de sportif	Sports injury	Lesión deportiva	Trauma sportivo	Sportska ozljeda
Blessure par balle	Gunshot wound	Herida de bala	Ferita da arma da fuoco	Prostrijelna rana
Blessure par explosion	Explosive wound	Lesión por explosión	Ferita esplosiva	Eksplozivna rana
Blessure par morsure	Bite wound	Herida por mordedura	Ferita da morso	Ugrizna rana
Blessure thermique	Thermal wound	Herida térmica	Ferita termica	Termička rana
Blessures à la tête et blessures du cerveau	Head and brain injuries	Lesiones de la cabeza y del cerebro	Lesioni della testa e del cervello	Ozljede glave i mozga
Bloc auriculo-ventriculaire	Atrioventricular block (AV block)	Bloqueo auriculoventricular	Blocco atrioventricolare	Atrijskoventrikularni blok
Bloc de branche	Bundle branch block	Bloqueo de rama	Blocco di branca	Blok grane Hisovog snopića
Bloc trifasciculaire	Trifascicular block	Bloqueo trifascicular	Blocco trifascicolare	Trifascikularni blok
Boitillement	Limping	Cojera	Zoppicamento	Šepanje
Borréliose	Borreliosis	Borreliosis	Borreliosi	Borelioza
Bossu	Hunchback	Joroba	Gibbo (gobba, gibbosità)	Grba
Botulisme	Botulism	Botulismo	Botulismo	Botulizam
Bouchon de cérumen	Impacted cerumen	Tapón de cerumen	Tappo di cerume	Ceruminozni čep
Bouffée de chaleur	Hot flushes	Sofocos	Vampata di calore	Valovi vrućine (valunzi)
Boulimie	Bulimia	Bulimia	Bulimia	Bulimija
Brachialgie	Brachial syndrome	Síndrome braquial	Brachialgia	Brahijalni sindrom bolne nadlaktice
Bronchectasie (dilatation des bronches)	Bronchiectasis	Bronquiectasia	Bronchiectasia	Bronhiektazije
Broncho-pneumopathie chronique obstructive	Chronic obstructive pulmonary disease	Enfermedad pulmonar obstructiva crónica	Bronchite cronica	Kronična opstruktivna plućna bolest
Bronchopneumonie	Bronchopneumonia	Neumonía bronquial	Broncopolmonite	Bronhopneumonija
Bronchospasme	Bronchospasm	Broncoespasmo	Broncospasmo	Bronhospazam
Brucellose (fièvre de Malte, fièvre méditerranéenne)	Brucellosis	Brucelosis	Brucellosi	Bruceloza (malteška ili sredozemna groznica, Bangova bolest)
Bruit anormal émis lors de la respiration (stridor)	Breathing sound due to blockage in the airway (stridor)	Estridor	Rumore durante la respirazione (stridore)	Glasno otežano disanje (stridor)
Brûlure	Burn	Quemadura	Ustione	Opeklina
Brûlure de l'estomac (pyrosis)	Heartburn	Ardor de estómago (acidez, pirosis)	Bruciore di stomaco (pirosi)	Žgaravica
Brûlure de méduse	Jellyfish sting burn	Quemadura de medusa	Ustione da medusa	Opeklina od meduze
Brûlure électrique	Electric shock burn	Quemadura eléctrica	Ustione da corrente elettrica	Opeklina od strujnog udara
Brûlures à la miction	Urinary burning	Ardor al orinar	Bruciore urinario	Pečenje za vrijeme mokrenja
Byssinose	Byssinosis (Monday fever)	Bisinosis (fiebre del lunes)	Bissinosi	Bisinoza
Cachexie	Cachexia	Caquexia	Cachessia	Kaheksija
Caillot sanguin (thrombus)	Blood clot (thrombus)	Coágulo sanguíneo (trombo)	Trombo	Krvni ugrušak (tromb)
Calcification	Calcification	Calcificación	Calcificazione	Ovapnjenje (kalcifikacija)
Calcul biliaire (cholélithiase)	Gallstone (cholelithiasis)	Cálculo biliar (litiasis biliar)	Calcolo biliare	Žučni kamenac (holelitijaza)
Calcul dans l'uretère	Ureteral stone (ureterolithiasis)	Cálculo en el uréter (ureterolitiasis)	Calcolo ureterale	Ureteralni kamenac (ureterolitijaza)
Calcul rénal (néphrolithiase, lithiase urinaire)	Kidney stone (nephrolithiasis)	Piedra en el riñon (cálculo renal, litiasis renal)	Calcolosi renale (nefrolitiasi)	Bubrežni kamenac (nefrolitijaza)
Calcul urinaire (urolithiase)	Bladder stone (urolithiasis)	Cálculo en el tracto urinario (urolitiasis)	Calcolo urinario (urolitiasi)	Kamenac mokraćnog mjehura
Callosité	Callosity (thickening)	Callosidad (callo)	Callosità (callo)	Zadebljanje kože
Canal artériel	Ductus arteriosus (ductus Botalli shunt)	Ductus arteriosus (conducto arterioso de Botal)	Dotto arterioso di Botallo	Ductus Botalli
Cancer de l'estomac	Stomach cancer (gastric cancer)	Cáncer de estómago (cáncer gástrico)	Cancro dello stomaco (cancro gastrico)	Rak želuca
Cancer de la prostate	Prostate cancer	Cáncer de próstata	Cancro della prostata	Rak prostate
Cancer du col utérin	Cervical cancer	Cáncer del cuello uterino (cáncer cervical)	Cancro della cervice uterina	Rak grlića maternice
Cancer du sein	Breast cancer	Cáncer de mama	Cancro della mammella	Rak dojke
Candidiase	Candidiasis (thrush)	Candidiasis	Candidosi (candidiasi)	Kandidijaza
Candidose orale	Thrush (oral candidiasis)	Candidiasis oral (muguet oral)	Mughetto (moniliasi orale)	Sor (oralna kandidijaza)
Capacité de mouvement	Movement ability	Capacidad de movimiento	Abilità di muoversi	Sposobnost kretanja
Carcinoïde	Carcinoid	Carcinoide	Carcinoide	Karcinoid
Carcinoïde bronchiale	Bronchial carcinoid	Carcinoide bronquial	Carcinoide bronchiale	Karcinoid bronha
Carcinome	Carcinoma	Carcinoma	Carcinoma	Karcinom
Carcinome à cellules rénales	Renal cell carcinoma (hypernephroma)	Carcinoma de células renales	Carcinoma a cellule renali	Hipernefrom
Carcinome à cellules de transition	Transitional cell carcinoma	Carcinoma de células transicionales	Carcinoma transizionale	Tranzicionalni karcinom
Carcinome anaplastique	Anaplastic carcinoma	Carcinoma anaplásico	Carcinoma anaplastico	Anaplastični karcinom

Français	Anglais	Espagnol	Italien	Croate
Carcinome basocellulaire	Basal cell carcinoma	Carcinoma de células basales (basilioma)	Basalioma (carcinoma basocellulare)	Karcinom bazalnih stanica (bazaliom)
Carcinome bronchique	Bronchial carcinoma	Carcinoma bronquial	Carcinoma bronchiale	Karcinom bronha
Carcinome de l'endomètre	Endometrial carcinoma	Carcinoma de endometrio	Carcinoma endometriale	Karcinom endometrija
Carcinome de l'estomac	Gastric carcinoma	Carcinoma gástrico	Carcinoma gastrico	Karcinom želuca
Carcinome de la prostate	Prostate carcinoma	Carcinoma de próstata	Carcinoma della prostata	Karcinom prostate
Carcinome du col utérin	Cervical carcinoma	Carcinoma del cuello uterino	Carcinoma della cervice uterina	Karcinom grlića maternice
Carcinome du sein	Breast carcinoma	Carcinoma de mama	Carcinoma mammario	Karcinom dojke
Carcinome embryonnaire	Embryonal carcinoma	Carcinoma embrional	Carcinoma embrionale	Embrionalni karcinom
Carcinome épithélial	Epithelial carcinoma	Carcinoma epitelial	Carcinoma epiteliale	Karcinom pokrovnog epitela
Carcinome hépatocellulaire	Hepatocellular carcinoma	Carcinoma hepatocelular	Carcinoma epatocellulare	Hepatocelularni karcinom
Carcinome médullaire	Medullary carcinoma	Carcinoma medular	Carcinoma midollare	Medularni karcinom
Carcinome papillaire	Papillary carcinoma	Carcinoma papilar	Carcinoma papillare	Papilarni karcinom
Carcinome spinocellulaire	Squamous cell carcino-ma (planocellular carcinoma)	Carcinoma de células escamosas	Carcinoma a cellule squamose	Planocelularni karcinom
Carcinose	Carcinosis	Carcinosis	Carcinosi (carcino-matosi, cancerosi)	Karcinoza
Carcinose péricardique	Pericardial carcinosis	Carcinosis pericárdica	Carcinosi pericardiale	Karcinoza perikarda
Carcinose péritonéale	Peritoneal carcinosis	Carcinosis peritoneal	Carcinosi peritoneale	Karcinoza peritoneuma
Carcinose pleurale	Pleural carcinosis	Carcinosis pleural	Carcinosi pleurica	Karcinoza pleure
Cardiomyopathie	Cardiomyopathy	Miocardiopatía	Cardiomiopatia	Kardiomiopatija
Cardiomyopathie alcoolique	Alcoholic cardiomyopathy	Miocardiopatía alcohólica	Miocardiopatia alcolica	Alkoholna kardiomiopatja
Cardiomyopathie dilatée	Dilated cardiomyopathy	Miocardiopatía dilatada	Cardiomiopatia dilatativa	Dilatacijska kardiomiopatija
Cardiomyopathie hypertrophique	Hypertrophic cardiomyopathy	Miocardiopatía hipertrófica	Cardiomiopatia ipertrofica	Hipertrofijska kardiomiopatija
Cardiomyopathie restrictive	Restrictive cardiomyopathy	Cardiomiopatía restrictiva	Cardiomiopatia restrittiva	Restriktivna kardiomiopatija
Cardiopathie congénitale	Congenital heart disease (congenital cardiopathy)	Cardiopatía congénita	Cardiopatia congenita	Urođena srčana bolest (kongenitalna kardiopatija)
Cardiotoxicité	Cardiotoxicity	Cardiotoxicidad	Cardiomiopatia tossica	Toksična kardiomiopatija
Cardite rhumatismale	Rheumatic heart disease	Cardiopatía reumática	Cardiopatia reumatica	Reumatska bolest srca
Carence en vitamine	Vitamin deficiency	Carencia de vitamina	Carenza di vitamine	Manjak vitamina
Carence en vitamine A	Vitamin A deficiency	Carencia de vitamina A	Carenza di vitamina A	Manjak vitamina A
Carence en vitamine B1	Vitamin B1 deficiency	Carencia de vitamina B1	Carenza di vitamina B1	Manjak vitamina B1
Carence en vitamine B2	Vitamin B2 deficiency	Carencia de vitamina B2	Carenza di vitamina B2	Manjak vitamina B2
Carence en vitamine B3	Vitamin B3 deficiency	Carencia de vitamina B3	Carenza di vitamina B3	Manjak vitamina B3
Carence en vitamine B12	Vitamin B12 deficiency	Carencia de vitamina B12	Carenza di vitamina B12	Manjak vitamina B12
Carence en vitamine C	Vitamin C deficiency	Carencia de vitamina C	Carenza de vitamina C	Manjak vitamina C
Carence en vitamine D	Vitamin D deficiency	Carencia de vitamina D	Carenza de vitamina D	Manjak vitamina D
Carence en vitamine K	Vitamin K deficiency	Carencia de vitamina K	Carenza de vitamina K	Manjak vitamina K
Carence oestrogénique	Estrogen deficiency	Deficiencia de estrógenos	Carenza di estrogeno	Manjak estrogena
Carie dentaire	Dental caries	Caries	Carie dentaria	Zubni karijes
Catalepsie	Catalepsy	Catalepsia	Catalessia	Katalepsija
Cataplexie	Cataplexy	Cataplexia (cataplejía)	Cataplessia	Katapleksija
Cataracte	Cataract	Catarata	Cataratta	Mrena (katarakta)
Catarrhe	Catarrh	Catarro	Catarro	Katar
Cavernome (angiome caverneux)	Cavernous hemangioma	Hemangioma cavernoso	Emangioma cavernoso	Kavernozni hemangiom
Cécité	Blindness	Ceguera	Cecità	Sljepoća
Cécité nocturne (héméralopie)	Night blindness (nyctalopia)	Ceguera nocturna (nictalopia)	Cecità notturna (nictalopia)	Noćno sljepilo
Cellulite	Cellulitis	Celulitis	Cellulite	Celulitis
Cellulite orbitale	Orbital cellulitis	Celulitis orbital	Cellulite orbitale	Celulitis orbite
Céphalée de tension	Tension headache	Cefalea tensional	Cefalea di tipo tensivo	Tenzijska glavobolja
Céphalée post-traumatique	Post-traumatic headache	Cefalea postraumática	Cefalea post-traumatica	Posttraumatska glavobolja
Céphalocèle	Cephalocele	Cefalocele	Cefalocèle	Cefalokela
Cercaire	Cercaria	Cercaria	Cercaria	Cerkarija
Cétoacidose diabétique	Diabetic ketoacidosis	Cetoacidosis diabética	Chetoacidosi diabetica	Dijabetična ketoacidoza
Chalazion	Stye (chalazion)	Orzuelo	Calazio	Ječmenac
Chalicose	Chalicosis	Calicosis	Calicosi	Kalikoza
Chancre	Chancre	Chancro	Sifiloma	Čankir
Chancre mou (chancrelle)	Chancroid (soft chancre)	Chancroide (chancro blando)	Ulcera venerea (cancroide)	Meki čankir
Changement de la muqueuse	Changes in mucous membrane	Cambios en la membrana mucosa	Cambiamenti della mucosa	Promjene na sluznici
Changements d'appétit	Appetite changes	Cambios en el apetito	Cambiamenti nell'appetito	Promjene apetita
Changements dans la forme des os	Changes in shape of bones	Cambios en la forma de los huesos	Cambiamenti nella forma delle ossa	Promjene oblika kosti
Changements dans les grains de beauté	Changes in moles	Cambios en los lunares	Cambiamenti di nevi	Promjene na madežima
Changements de conscience	Changes in consciousness	Cambios en la conciencia	Alterazione della conoscenza	Promjene stanja svijesti

Français	Anglais	Espagnol	Italien	Croate
Changements de couleur de la peau	Skin color changes	Cambios en el color de la piel	Cambiamento di colore della pelle	Promjene boje kože
Changements de personnalité	Personality changes	Cambios de personalidad	Cambiamenti di personalità	Promjene osobnosti
Changements de sensation de goût	Changes in taste sensation	Cambios en la sensación de sabores	Cambiamenti nelle sensazioni del gusto	Promjene osjeta okusa
Changements de voix	Voice changes	Cambios en la voz	Cambiamento di voce	Promjene glasa
Changements des sensations olfactives	Changes in olfactory sensation	Cambios en la sensibilidad olfatoria	Cambiamenti delle sensazoni olfattive	Promjene osjeta mirisa
Changements des sensations tactiles	Changes in tactile sensation	Cambios en la sensibilidad táctil	Cambiamenti della sensazione tattile	Promjene osjeta dodira
Changements psychiques	Psychic changes	Cambios psíquicos	Alterazioni dello stato psishico	Psihičke promjene
Charbon	Anthrax	Carbunco (ántrax)	Antrace	Antraks (bedrenica, crni prišt)
Chéloïde	Keloid	Queloide	Cheloide	Keloid
Chikungunya	Chikungunya	Chikungunya	Chikungunya	Chikungunya virusna bolest
Chleuasme (chloasma)	Melasma (chloasma faciei)	Melasma (cloasma)	Melasma	Kloazma (melazma)
Choc	Shock	Choque (shock)	Collaso circolatorio (shock)	Šok
Choc anaphylactique	Anaphylactic shock	Choque anafiláctico	Anafilassi	Anafilaktični šok
Choc cardiogénique	Cardiogenic shock	Choque cardiogénico	Shock cardiogeno	Kardiogeni šok
Choc endotoxique	Endotoxic shock	Choque endotoxico	Shock endotossico	Endotoksični šok
Choc hypovolémique	Hypovolemic shock	Choque hipovolémico	Shock ipovolemico	Hipovolemički šok
Choc neurogénique	Neurogenic shock	Choque neurogénico	Shock neurogeno	Neurogeni šok
Choc obstructive	Obstructive shock	Choque obstructivo	Shock ostruttivo	Opstruktivni šok
Choc post-opératoire	Surgical shock (postoperative shock)	Choque quirúrgico	Shock chirurgico	Kirurški šok
Choc septique	Septic shock	Choque séptico	Shock settico	Septički šok
Choc spinal	Spinal shock	Choque espinal	Shock spinale	Spinalni šok
Choc traumatique	Traumatic shock	Choque traumático	Shock traumatico	Traumatski šok
Cholangiocarcinome	Cholangiocellular carcinoma	Carcinoma de las vías biliares (colangiocarcinoma)	Colangiocarcinoma (carcinoma colangiocellulare)	Kolangiocelularni karcinom
Choléra	Cholera	Cólera	Colera	Kolera
Cholésterol sanguin élevée (hypercholestérolémie)	High blood cholesterol (hypercholesterolemia)	Colesterol elevado de la sangre (hipercolesterolemia)	Eccesso di colesterolo nel sangue (ipercolesterolemia)	Povišeni kolesterol u krvi (hiperkolesterolemija)
Chondroblastome	Chondroblastoma	Condroblastoma	Condroblastoma	Hondroblastom
Chondromalacie rotulienne	Chondromalacia patellae (runner's knee, patello-femoral pain syndrome)	Chondromalacia rotuliana (síndrome patelo-femoral)	Sindrome del dolore patello-femorale (ginocchio del corridore)	Hondromalacija patele (trkačko koljeno, sindrom patelofemoralne boli)
Chondrome	Chondroma	Condroma	Condroma	Hondrom
Chondrosarcome	Chondrosarcoma	Condrosarcoma	Condrosarcoma	Hondrosarkom
Chorée de Huntington (maladie de Huntington)	Huntington's chorea (Huntington's disease)	Enfermedad de Huntington (corea de Huntington)	Malattia di Huntington	Huntingtonova koreja
Choréoathétose	Choreoathetosis	Coreoatetosis	Coreoatetosi	Koreoatetoza
Choriocarcinome	Choriocarcinoma	Coriocarcinoma	Coriocarcinoma	Koriokarcinom
Chorioméningite lymphocytaire	Lymphocytic choriomeningitis	Coriomeningitis linfocítica	Coriomeningite linfocitaria	Limfocitni koriomeningitis
Chromomycose	Chromoblastomycosis (chromomycosis, Pedroso's disease)	Cromomicosis (cromoblastomicosis)	Cromomicosi (cromoblastomicosi)	Kromomikoza
Chylothorax	Chylothorax	Quilotórax	Chilotorace	Hilotoraks
Cicatrice	Scar	Cicatriz	Cicatrice (sfregio)	Ožiljak
Cirrhose alcoolique	Alcoholic cirrhosis	Cirrosis alcohólica	Cirrosi alcolica	Alkoholna ciroza
Cirrhose biliaire	Biliary cirrhosis	Cirrosis biliar	Cirrosi biliare	Bilijarna ciroza
Cirrhose cryptogénique	Cryptogenic cirrhosis	Cirrosis criptogénica	Cirrosi criptogenica	Kriptogena ciroza
Cirrhose hépatique	Liver cirrhosis	Cirrosis hepática	Cirrosi	Ciroza jetre
Cirrhose postnecrotique	Post-necrotic cirrhosis	Cirrosis postnecrótica	Cirrosi post-necrotica	Postnekrotična ciroza
Claudication intermittente	Intermittent claudication	Claudicación intermitente	Claudicatio intermittens	Intermitentna klaudikacija
Claustrophobie	Claustrophobia (fear of closed space)	Claustrofobia (miedo a los espacios cerrados)	Claustrofobia (paura di luoghi chiusi)	Klaustrofobija (strah od zatvorenog prostora)
Cleptomanie	Kleptomania	Cleptomanía	Cleptomania	Kleptomanija
Clonorchiase	Clonorchiasis	Clonorquiasis (clonorquiosis)	Clonorchiasi	Klonorkijaza
Coagulation intravasculaire disséminée	Disseminated intravascular coagulation	Coagulación intravascular diseminada	Coagulazione intravascolare disseminata	Diseminirana intravaskularna koagulacija
Coarctation de l'aorte	Coarctation of the aorta	Coartación de la aorta	Coartazione dell'aorta	Koarktacija aorte
Coccidioïmycose (fièvre de la vallée de San Joaquin, fièvre du désert)	Coccidioidomycosis (San Joaquin Valley fever)	Coccidioidomicosis	Coccidiomicosi	Kokcidioidomikoza (San Joaquin Valley vrućica)
Coccygodynie (douleur coccygienne)	Coccygodynia	Coccigodinia (dolor de coxis)	Coccigodinia	Kokcigodinija
Coeur pulmonaire	Pulmonary heart disease	Enfermedad cardíaca pulmonar (cor pulmonale)	Cuore polmonare	Plućno srce
Coeur pulmonaire aigu	Acute pulmonary heart	Cor pulmonale agudo	Cuore polmonare acuto	Akutno plućno srce
Colique	Colic	Cólico	Colica	Kolika

Français	Anglais	Espagnol	Italien	Croate
Colique abdominale	Abdominal colic	Cólico abdominal	Colica addominale	Trbušna kolika (abdominalna kolika)
Colique biliaire	Biliary colic	Cólico biliar	Colica biliare	Žučna kolika
Colique néphrétique	Renal colic	Cólico nefrítico (cólico renal)	Colica renale	Bubrežna kolika (renalna kolika)
Coliques de bébé	Baby colic	Cólico del recién nacido	Coliche del neonato	Novorođenačke kolike
Colite ulcéreuse	Ulcerative colitis	Colitis ulcerosa	Rettocolite ulcerosa	Ulcerozni kolitis
Collapsus	Collapse	Colapso	Collasso	Kolaps
Collection de sang dans la trompe de Fallope (hématosalpinx)	Bleeding into the fallopian tube (hematosalpinx)	Colección de sangre en la trompa de Falopio (hematosalpinx)	Flusso di sangue nella tuba di Falloppio	Krvarenje u jajovod (hematosalpinks)
Côlon irritable (côlon spastique)	Irritable bowel syndrome (spastic colon)	Síndrome de intestino irritable (colon irritable, colon espástico)	Sindrome del colon irritabile (colon spastico)	Sindrom iritabilnog crijeva (spastični kolon)
Côlon transverse	Transverse colon	Colon transverso	Colon trasverso	Poprečno debelo crijevo
Coma	Coma	Coma	Coma	Koma
Coma diabétique	Diabetic coma	Coma diabético	Coma diabetico	Dijabetična koma
Commotion cérébrale	Brain concussion	Conmoción cerebral	Commozione cerebrale	Potres mozga
Communication inter -auriculaire	Atrial septal defect	Comunicación interauricular	Difetto del setto interatriale	Atrijski septalni defekt
Communication inter -ventriculaire	Ventricular septal defect	Comunicación interventricular	Difetto del setto ventricolare	Ventrikularni septalni defekt
Compression cérébrale	Brain compression	Compresión cerebral	Compressione cerebrale	Kompresija mozga
Compression du nerf	Nerve compression (pinched nerve)	Compresión del nérvio	Compressone del nervo	Kompresija živca (ukliješten živac)
Conflit antérieur de la cheville	Ankle impingement syndrome	Pinzamiento anterolateral del tobillo	Sindrome da impingement della caviglia	Prednji sindrom sraza gornjeg nožnog zgloba
Conflit postérieur de la cheville	Posterior ankle impingement syndrome	Síndrome de pinzamiento posterior del tobillo	Sindrome da impingement posteriore di caviglia	Sindrom sraza stražnjeg nožnog zgloba
Confusion	Confusion	Confusión	Confusione (disordine)	Smetenost
Congestion nasale	Nasal congestion (stuffy nose)	Congestión nasal	Congestione nasale	Začepljeni nos
Congestion pulmonaire	Pulmonary congestion	Congestión pulmonar	Congestione polmonare	Plućna kongestija
Conjonctivite allergique	Allergic conjunctivitis	Conjuntivitis alérgica	Congiuntivite allergica	Alergijski konjuktivitis
Conjonctivite bactérienne	Bacterial conjunctivitis	Conjuntivitis bacteriana	Congiuntivite batterica	Bakterijski konjuktivitis
Conjonctivite chimique	Chemical conjunctivitis	Conjuntivitis química	Congiuntivite irritativa da agenti chimici	Kemijski konjuktivitis
Conjonctivite due à un corps étranger	Conjunctival foreign body	Conjuntivitis por cuerpo extraño	Congiuntivite irritativa da corpi estranei	Konjuktivitis izazvan stranim tijelom
Conjonctivite virale	Viral conjuctivitis	Conjuntivitis viral	Congiuntivite virale	Virusni konjuktivitis
Constipation	Constipation (obstipation)	Estreñimiento	Stitichezza (costipazione)	Zatvor (opstipacija)
Contracture	Contracture	Contractura	Contrattura	Kontraktura
Contracture articulaire	Joint contracture	Contractura articular	Contrattura articolare	Kontraktura zgloba
Contracture de Dupuytren	Dupuytren's contracture	Contractura de Dupuytren	Malattia di Dupuytren	Dupuytrenova kontraktura
Contracture musculaire	Muscular contracture	Contractura muscular	Contrattura muscolare	Kontraktura mišića
Contracture sur les muscles extenseurs de sorte que le corps est incurvé en arrière (opisthotonos)	Spastic arching position (opisthotonus)	Contracción del cuerpo entero de tal manera que se mantiene encorvado hacia atrás (opistótonos)	Iperestensione della regione posteriore del tronco (opistotono)	Izvijanje misića vrata i leđa u luk (opistotonus)
Contusion	Contusion	Contusión	Contusione	Nagnječenje (zgnječenje, kontuzija)
Contusion cérébrale	Cerebral contusion	Contusión cerebral	Contusione cerebrale	Nagnječenje mozga
Convulsion hyperthermique	Febrile convulsions	Convulsiones febriles	Convulsioni febbrili	Febrilne konvulzije
Convulsions	Convulsions	Convulsiones	Convulsioni	Konvulzije
Coqueluche	Whooping cough (pertussis)	Tos ferina (coqueluche)	Pertosse	Hripavac (pasji kašalj, pertussis)
Cor (cal)	Blister (corn)	Ampolla (callo)	Callo (vescica, bolla)	Žulj (plik, kurje oko)
Corps étranger dans l'oreille	Foreign body in ear	Cuerpo extraño en el oído	Corpo estraneo nell'orecchio	Strano tijelo u uhu
Corps étranger dans le nez	Foreign body in nose	Cuerpo extraño en la nariz	Corpo estraneo nel naso	Strano tijelo u nosu
Côte cervicale	Cervical rib	Costilla cervical	Costa cervicale	Vratno rebro
Coup de couteau	Stab wound	Estocada	Ferita da punta	Ubodna rana
Coup de soleil (insolation)	Sunstroke (heat stroke)	Insolación	Insolazione (colpo di sole)	Sunčanica
Crachat purulent	Pus in sputum	Esputo que contiene pus	Presenza di pus nello sputo	Gnojni ispljuvak
Crachat spumeux	Foamy sputum	Esputo espumoso	Sputo schiumoso	Pjenušavi ispljuvak
Crampe musculaire (spasme)	Muscular cramp (spasm)	Espasmo muscular (calambre)	Spasmo muscolare	Mišićni grč (spazam)
Crampes nocturnes des jambes	Nocturnal leg cramps	Calambres nocturnos en las piernas	Crampo notturno alle gambe	Noćni grčevi u nogama
Crépitation	Crepitation	Crepitación	Crepitazione	Krepitacija
Crise de panique	Panic attack	Ataque de pánico	Attaco di panico	Napadaj panike
Crise tonico-clonique	Tonic-clonic seizure	Crisis tónico-clónica	Crisi tonico-clonica	Toničko-klonički napadaj
Croup (laryngotrachéo-bronchite)	Croup (acute obstructive laryngitis)	Crup (laringotraqueo-bronquitis)	Croup (laringite acuta ostruttiva)	Krup (akutni opstruktivni laringitis)
Croûte	Crust (scab)	Costra	Crosta (escara)	Krasta

Français	Anglais	Espagnol	Italien	Croate
Cryptococcose	Cryptococcosis	Criptococcosis	Criptococcosi	Kriptokokoza
Cryptorchidie	Cryptorchidism	Criptorquidismo	Criptorchidismo	Retencija testisa (kriptorhizam)
Cyanose	Cyanosis	Cianosis	Cianosi	Cijanoza
Cycle menstruel anormalement excessice (ménorragie)	Abnormally heavy menstrual period (menorrhagia)	Pérdida de sangre mayor durante la menstruación (menorragia)	Anormale perdita di sangue durante il ciclo mestruale(menorragia)	Abnormalno velik gubitak krvi tijekom mjesečnice (menoragija)
Cypho-scoliose	Kyphoscoliosis	Cifoescoliosis	Cifoscoliosi	Kifoskolioza
Cyphose	Kyphosis	Cifosis	Cifosi	Kifoza
Cystadénocarcinome	Cystadenocarcinoma	Cistadenocarcinoma	Cistadenocarcinoma	Cistadenokarcinom
Cystadénofibrome	Cystadenofibroma	Cistadenofibroma	Cistadenofibroma	Cistadenofibrom
Cystadénome	Cystadenoma	Cistadenoma	Cistadenoma	Cistadenom
Cysticercose	Cysticercosis	Cisticercosis	Cisticercosi	Cisticerkoza
Daltonisme	Daltonism	Daltonismo	Daltonismo	Daltonizam
Déboîtement (luxation)	Dislocation (luxation)	Luxación (lujación, dislocación)	Lussazione	Iščašenje (dislokacija, luksacija)
Déchirure	Strain (sprain, pull)	Desgarro	Stiramento	Istegnuće
Déchirure au tendon	Tendon strain	Desgarro de tendón	Stiramento del tendine	Istegnuće tetive (distenzija tetive)
Déchirure ligamentaire	Ligament strain	Desgarro de ligamento	Stiramento del legamento	Istegnuće ligamenta
Déchirure musculaire (claquage)	Muscle strain (muscle pull)	Desgarro muscular	Strappo muscolare	Istegnuće mišića (distenzija mišića)
Décollement de la rétine	Retinal ablation (retinal detachment)	Desprendimiento de retina	Distacco di retina	Odvajanje mrežnice (ablacija retine)
Décompensation cardiaque	Cardiac decompensation	Descompensación cardíaca	Decompensazione cardiaca	Srčana dekompenzacija
Déficit en facteur de la coagulation	Coagulation factor deficiency	Deficiencia de factor de coagulación	Carenza di fattore di coagulazione	Manjak faktora koagulacije
Déformation de Madelung	Madelung's deformity	Deformidad de Madelung	Deformità di Madelung	Madelungov deformitet
Dégénérescence maculaire	Macular degeneration	Degeneración macular	Degenerazione maculare	Degeneracija makule
Dégénérescence de la rétine	Retinal degeneration	Degeneración retinal	Degenerazione della retina	Degeneracija mrežnice
Déglutition douloureuse (odynophagie)	Painful swallowing (odynophagia)	Dolor al tragar (odinofagia)	Deglutizione dolorosa (odinofagia)	Bolno gutanje (odinofagija)
Delirium	Delirium	Delirio	Delirio	Delirij
Démarche traînante	Shuffling gait	Marcha arrastrando los pies	Barcollamento	Teturav nesiguran hod
Démence	Dementia	Demencia	Demenza	Demencija
Déminéralisation	Demineralization	Desmineralización	Demineralizzazione	Demineralizacija
Dengue (grippe tropicale, dengue hémorragique)	Dengue fever	Dengue	Dengue	Dengue groznica
Dent pourri	Rotten tooth	Diente podrido	Dente guasto	Pokvareni zub
Dépendance (addiction)	Addiction	Adicción (dependencia)	Dipendenza	Ovisnost
Dépression	Depression	Depresión	Depressione	Depresija
Dermatite atopique	Atopic dermatitis	Dermatitis atópica	Neurodermite (dermatite atopica)	Atopijski dermatitis
Dermatite herpétiforme	Dermatitis herpetiformis (Duhring's disease)	Dermatitis herpetiforme (enfermedad de Duhring)	Dermatite erpetiforme di Duhring	Duhringova bolest (dermatitis herpetiformis)
Dermatite nummulaire	Nummular dermatitis	Dermatitis numular	Dermatite nummulare	Numularni dermatitis
Dermatomycose	Dermatomycosis	Dermatomicosis	Dermatomicosi	Dermatomikoza
Dermatomyosite	Dermatomyositis	Dermatomiositis	Dermatomiosite	Dermatomiozitis
Dermite de contact	Contact dermatitis	Dermatitis de contacto	Dermatite da contatto	Kontaktni dermatitis
Dermite de contact allergique	Allergic contact dermatitis	Dermatitis alérgica de contacto	Dermatite allergica	Alergijski kontaktni dermatitis
Dermite de contact irritative	Irritant contact dermatitis	Dermatitis irritante de contacto	Dermatite irritativo da contatto	Iritantni kontaktni dermatitis
Dermite séborrhéique infantile	Cradle cap (infantile seborrhoeic dermatitis)	Dermatitis seborreica infantil	Dermatite seborroica infantile	Tjemenica (dojenačka seboreja)
Déshydratation	Dehydration	Deshidratación	Disidratazione	Dehidracija
Désorientation	Disorientation	Desorientación	Disorientamento	Dezorijentiranost
Desquamation	Shedding of the skin (desquamation)	Desquamación	Perdita dello strato superiore della pelle (desquamazione)	Ljuštenje kože (deskvamacija)
Développement sexuel prématuré du même sexe	Premature sexual development of the same sex	Desarrollo sexual prematuro del mismo sexo	Prematuro sviluppo sessuale dello stesso sesso	Prerano splono fizičko sazrijevanje istog spola
Développement sexuel prématuré du sexe opposé	Premature sexual development of the opposite sex	Desarrollo sexual prematuro del sexo opuesto	Prematuro sviluppo sessuale del sesso opposto	Prerano spolno fizičko sazrijevanje suprotnog spola
Déviation du septum nasal	Nasal septum deviation	Desviación del tabique nasal	Deviazione del setto nasale	Devijacija nosnog septuma
Diabète	Diabetes	Diabetes	Diabete	Dijabetes
Diabète insipide	Diabetes insipidus	Diabetes insípida	Diabete insipido	Dijabetes insipidus
Diabète sucré	Diabetes mellitus	Diabetes mellitus (diabetes sacarina)	Diabete mellito	Dijabetes melitus
Diabète sucré de type 1 (diabète insulino-dépendant)	Diabetes mellitus type 1	Diabetes mellitus tipo 1	Diabete mellito di tipo 1	Dijabetes melitus tip 1
Diabète sucré de type 2 (diabète insulinorésistant)	Diabetes mellitus type 2	Diabetes mellitus tipo 2	Diabete mellito di tipo 2	Dijabetes melitus tip 2
Diarrhée	Diarrhea	Diarrea	Diarrea	Proljev (dijarea)

Français	Anglais	Espagnol	Italien	Croate
Différence de taille entres les pupilles (anisocorie)	Unequal size of pupils (anisocoria)	Asimetría del tamaño de las pupilas (anisocoria)	Diseguaglianza del diametro delle pupille (anisocoria)	Nejednaka veličina zjenica (anizokorija)
Difficulté à déféquer (ténesme)	Difficult defecation (tenesmus)	Dificultad para la defecación (tenesmo rectal)	Difficoltà a defecare (tenesmo)	Otežano pražnjenje crijeva (otežana defekacija)
Difficulté à uriner (dysurie)	Difficult urination (dysuria)	Dificultad al orinar (disuria)	Emissione di urine con difficoltà (disuria)	Otežano usporeno mokrenje (dizurija)
Difficulté de deglutition (dysphagie)	Difficult swallowing (dysphagia)	Dificultad para tragar (disfagia)	Difficoltà a deglutire (disfagia)	Otežano gutanje (disfagija)
Difficulté de respiration	Breathing difficulty	Dificultad de respiración	Respirazione difficoltosa	Otežano disanje
Difficulté respiratoire (dyspnée)	Shortness of breath (dyspnea)	Falta de aire (disnea)	Fame d'aria (dispnea, respirazione difficoltosa)	Zaduha (nedostatak daha, dispneja)
Difformité du pied	Foot deformity	Deformidad del pie	Difetto del piede	Deformacija stopala
Difformité spinale	Spinal deformity	Deformidad vertebral	Degenerazione spinale	Deformacija kralježnice
Dilatation aiguë de l'estomac	Acute gastric dilatation	Dilatación aguda del estómago	Dilatazione gastrica acuta	Akutna dilatacija želuca
Diphtérie	Diphtheria	Difteria	Difterite	Difterija
Dissection aortique	Aortic dissection	Disección aórtica	Dissecazione aortica	Disekcija aorte
Distorsion articulaire	Joint distortion	Distorsión articular	Distorsione	Uganuće zgloba (distorzija zgloba)
Distorsion de la cheville	Ankle distortion	Distorsión del tobillo	Distorsione alla caviglia	Uganuće skočnog zgloba
Diverticule	Diverticulum	Divertículo	Diverticolo	Divertikul
Diverticule de Meckel	Small intestine diverticulum	Divertículo de Meckel	Diverticolo di Meckel	Divertikul tankog crijeva
Diverticule du côlon	Colon diverticulum	Divertículo del colon	Diverticolo del colon	Divertikul na debelom crijevu
Diverticule duodenal	Duodenal diverticulum	Divertículo duodenal	Diverticolo duodenale	Divertikul na dvanaesniku
Diverticulite	Diverticulitis	Diverticulitis	Diverticolite	Divertikulitis
Diverticulose	Diverticulosis	Enfermedad diverticular	Diverticolosi	Divertikuloza
Douleur	Pain	Dolor	Dolore	Bol
Douleur abdominale	Abdominal pain	Dolor abdominal	Dolore addominale	Bol u trbuhu
Douleur aiguë	Acute pain	Dolor agudo	Dolore acuto	Akutna bol
Douleur articulaire (arthralgie)	Joint pain (arthralgia)	Dolor en articulación (artralgia)	Articolazione doloroso (artralgia)	Bol u zglobu (artralgija)
Douleur au sein (mastodynie)	Breast pain (mastalgia)	Dolor en la mama (mastalgia)	Dolore al seno (mastalgia)	Bol u dojci (mastalgija)
Douleur chronique	Chronic pain	Dolor crónico	Dolore cronico	Kronična bol
Douleur des sinus (sinusite)	Sinus headache	Dolor de cabeza por sinusitis	Sinusite	Sinusna glavobolja
Douleur du membre fantôme	Phantom pain	Dolor del miembro fantasma	Dolore fantomatico	Fantomska bol
Douleur épigastrique	Epigastric pain	Dolor epigástrico	Gastralgia	Bol u epigastriju
Douleur lors du rapport sexuel (dyspareunie)	Painful sexual intercourse (dyspareunia)	Relación sexual dolorosa (coitalgia, dispareunia)	Dolore durante rapporto sessuale (dispareunia)	Bol pri snošaju
Douleur musculaire (myalgie)	Muscle pain (myalgia)	Dolor muscular (mialgia)	Dolore muscolare (mialgia)	Bol u mišiću (mijalgija)
Douleur pulsatile	Pulsing pain	Dolor pulsante	Dolore pulsante	Pulsirajuća bol
Douleur sourde	Dull pain	Dolor sordo	Dolore ottuso	Tupa bol
Douleur thoracique	Chest pain	Dolor torácico	Dolore toracico	Bol u prsištu
Douleur tranchante	Sharp pain	Dolor afilado	Dolore tagliente	Oštra bol
Douleurs ovulatoires (mittelschmerz)	Ovulation pain (mittelschmerz)	Ovulación dolorosa	Dolore ovulatorio (mittelschmerz)	Bolna ovulacija (mittelschmerz)
Dracunculose	Dracunculiasis	Dracunculiasis	Dracunculiasi	Drakunkulijaza
Drépanocytose (anémie à cellules falciformes)	Sickle-cell disease (sickle-cell anemia)	Anemia falciforme (anemia drepanocítica)	Anemia drepanocitica	Anemija srpastih stanica
Dyschondroplasie	Dyschondroplasia	Discondroplasia	Discondroplasia	Dishondroplazija
Dysenterie	Dysentery (flux)	Disentería	Dissenteria	Dizenterija
Dysgénésie testiculaire	Testicular dysgenesis	Disgénesis testicular	Disgenesia gonadica	Testikularna disgeneza
Dysgerminome	Dysgerminoma	Disgerminoma	Disgerminoma	Disgerminom
Dyshidrose	Dyshidrosis	Eczema dishidrótico	Disidrosi	Dishidroza
Dyslexie	Dyslexia	Dislexia	Dislessia	Disleksija
Dyspepsie	Dyspepsia (upset stomach)	Dispepsia (indigestión)	Dispepsia	Dispepsija (nervozni želudac)
Dysplasie du col de l'utérus	Cervical dysplasia	Displasia del cuello uterino	Displasia cervicale	Cervikalna displazija
Dysplasie fibreuse	Fibrous dysplasia	Displasia fibrosa	Displasia fibrosa	Fibrozna displazija
Dysplasie ventriculair droite arythmogène	Arrhytmogenic right ventricular dysplasia	Displasia arritmogénica ventricular derecha	Displasia ventricolare destra aritmogena	Aritmogena displazija desne klijetke
Dyspnée chez un cardiaque	Cardiac asthma (paroxysmal nocturnal dyspnea)	Disnea paroxística nocturna	Dispnea parossistica notturna	Srčana astma (paroksizmalna dispneja)
Dystonie	Dystonia	Distonía	Distonia	Distonija
Dystrophie	Dystrophy	Distrofia	Distrofia	Distrofija
Dystrophie musculaire	Muscular dystrophy	Distrofia muscular	Distrofia muscolare	Mišićna distrofija
Dystrophie musculaire progressive	Progressive muscular dystrophy	Distrofia muscular progresiva	Distrofia muscolare progressiva	Progresivna mišićna distrofija
Ecchymose	Bruise (ecchymosis)	Moretón (equimosis)	Ammaccatura (ecchimosi)	Modrica (ekhimoza)
Échinococcose	Echinococcosis (hydatid disease)	Hidatidosis (equinococosis)	Echinococcosi (idatidosi)	Ehinokokoza
Échinococcose hépatique	Hepatic echinococcosis	Hidatidosis hepática	Echinococcosi epatica	Ehinokokoza jetre
Échinococcose pulmonaire	Pulmonary echinococcosis	Hidatidosis pulmonar	Echinococcosi polmonare	Ehinokokoza pluća

Français	Anglais	Espagnol	Italien	Croate
Écholalie	Echolalia	Ecolalia	Ecolalia	Eholalija
Échopraxie (tendance spontanée à répéter les mouvements d'une autre personne)	Echopraxia (involuntary repetition of the observed movements of another)	Ecopraxia (repetición de los movimientos de otra persona)	Ecoprassia (imitazione spontanea di movimenti osservati)	Ehopraksija (nevoljno ponavljanje tuđih pokreta)
Écorchure	Abrasion	Abrasión (escoriación)	Abrasione (escoriazione)	Ojedina (abrazija)
Écoulement de liquide cérébrospinal par l'oreille (otoliquorrhée)	Leakage of cerebrospinal fluid through the ear	Salida de líquido cerebroespinal por el oído (otoliquorrea)	Perdita di liquido cerebrospinale dall'orechio (otoliquorrea)	Curenje likvora na uho (cerebrospinalna otoreja)
Écoulement de liquide cérébrospinal par le nez (rhinoliquorrhée)	Leakage of cerebrospinal fluid through the nose	Salida de líquido cerebroespinal por la nariz (rinoliquorrea)	Perdita di liquido cerebrospinale dal naso (rinoliquorrea)	Curenje likvora na nos (cerebrospinalna rinoreja)
Écoulement par le nez (rhinorrhée)	Runny nose (rinorrhea)	Goteo nasal (rinorrea)	Naso che cola (rinorrea)	Curenje iz nosa (rinoreja)
Eczéma	Eczema	Eccema (eczema)	Eczema	Ekcem
Eczéma marginé de hebra	Crotch itch (tinea cruris)	Tiña crural (tinea cruris)	Tinea cruris	Gljivična infekcija prepona (tinea cruris)
Égratignure	Scratch	Rasguño	Graffio (graffiatura)	Ogrebotina
Éjaculation précoce	Premature ejaculation	Eyaculación precoz	Eiaculazione precoce	Prijevremena ejakulacija
Élancement	Twinging pain	Dolor tipo punzada	Dolore pungente	Probadajuća bol
Élargissement de la distance des organes (hypertélorisme)	Increased distance between two organs or parts of the body (hypertelorism)	Aumento de la separación de los organos (hipertelorismo)	Aumento della distanza fra due parti del corpo (ipertelorismo)	Povećan razmak izmedu dva organa ili dijela tijela (hipertelorizam)
Électrisation	Electrical injuries (electric shock)	Lesiones por corriente eléctrica	Folgorazione (elettrocuzione)	Ozljede električnom strujom (strujni udar)
Élévation de la température du corps	Elevated body temperature	Aumento en la temperatura corporal	Temperatura corporea elevata	Povišena tjelesna temperatura
Embolie	Embolism	Embolia	Embolismo (embolia)	Embolija
Embolie artérielle	Arterial embolism	Embolia arterial	Embolia dell'arteria	Arterijska embolija
Embolie de cholestérol	Fat embolism	Embolismo graso	Embolia adiposa	Masna embolija
Embolie gazeuse	Air embolism (gas embolism)	Embolia gaseosa	Embolia gassosa	Zračna embolija
Embolie pulmonaire	Pulmonary embolism	Embolia pulmonar	Embolia polmonare	Plućna embolija
Emphisème sous-cutané	Subcutaneous emphysema	Enfisema subcutáneo	Enfisema sottocutaneo	Potkožni emfizem
Emphysème	Emphysema	Enfisema	Enfisema	Emfizem
Empoisonnement (toxicité)	Poisoning (toxication)	Envenenamiento (intoxicación)	Avvelenamento (intossicazione)	Trovanje
Empoisonnement à l'arsenic	Arsenic poisoning	Envenenamiento por arsénico	Avvelenamento da arsenico	Trovanje arsenom
Empoisonnement alimentaires	Food poisoning	Intoxicación alimentaria	Avvelenamento da cibo	Trovanje hranom
Empoisonnement au cadmium	Cadmium poisoning	Envenenamiento por cadmio	Avvelenamento da cadmio	Trovanje kadmijem
Empoisonnement au cyanure	Cyanide poisoning	Envenenamiento por cianuro	Avvelenamento da cianuro	Trovanje cijanidom
Empoisonnement au fer	Iron poisoning	Intoxicación por hierro	Avvelenamento da ferro	Trovanje željezom
Empoisonnement au gaz	Gas poisoning	Envenenamiento por gas	Avvelenamento da gas	Trovanje plinom
Empoisonnement au insecticide	Insecticide poisoning	Envenenamiento por insecticidas	Avvelenamento da insetticidi	Trovanje insekticidima
Empoisonnement au lithium	Lithium poisoning	Intoxicación por litio	Avvelenamento da litio	Trovanje litijem
Empoisonnement au mercure	Mercury poisoning	Envenenamiento por mercurio	Avvelenamento da mercurio	Trovanje živom
Empoisonnement au méthanol	Methanol poisoning	Intoxicación por metanol	Avvelenamento da metanolo	Trovanje metanolom
Empoisonnement au monoxyde de carbone	Carbon monoxide poisoning	Intoxicación por monóxido de carbono	Avvelenamento da monossido di carbonio	Trovanje ugljičnim monoksidom
Empoisonnement au plomb	Lead poisoning	Envenenamiento por plomo	Avvelenamento da piombo (saturnismo)	Trovanje olovom
Empoisonnement au salicylate	Salicylate poisoning	Intoxicación por salicilatos	Avvelenamento da salicilati	Trovanje salicilatima
Empoisonnement au thallium	Thallium poisoning	Envenenamiento por talio	Avvelenamento da tallio	Trovanje talijem
Empoisonnement aux métaux lourds	Heavy metal poisoning	Envenenamiento por metales pesados	Intossicazione da metalli pesanti	Trovanje teškim metalima
Empoisonnement du poisson	Fish poisoning	Intoxicación por pescado	Avvelenamento da pesci	Trovanje ribom
Empoisonnement par alcalis	Alkali poisoning	Intoxicación por álcalis	Avvelenamento da alcali	Trovanje alkalima
Empoisonnement par des champignons	Mushroom poisoning	Envenenamiento por setas	Avvelenamento da funghi	Trovanje gljivama
Empoisonnement par l'alcool	Alcohol poisoning	Intoxicación por alcohol	Avvelenamento da alcool	Trovanje alkoholom
Empoisonnement par l'amiante	Asbestos poisoning	Envenenamiento por asbesto	Avvelenamento da amianto	Trovanje azbestom
Empoisonnement par radiations	Radiation poisoning	Envenenamiento por radiación	Avvelenamento da radiazione	Trovanje zračenjem

Français	Anglais	Espagnol	Italien	Croate
Empyème	Empyema	Empiema	Empiema	Empijem
Encéphalocèle	Encephalocele	Encefalocele	Encefalocele	Encefalokela
Encéphalopathie	Encephalopathy	Encefalopatía	Encefalopatia	Encefalopatija
Enchondrome	Enchondroma	Encondroma	Encondroma	Enhondrom
Encoprésie	Encopresis	Encopresis	Enconpresi	Enkopreza
Endocardite bactérienne	Bacterial endocarditis	Endocarditis bacteriana	Endocardite batterica	Bakterijski endokarditis
Endométriose	Endometriosis	Endometriosis	Endometriosi	Endometrioza
Engelure	Chilblain (perniosis)	Sabañón	Perniosi	Smrzotina
Engourdissements dans les membres (paresthésie)	Numbness in limbs	Adormecimiento de las extremidades	Parestesie delle estremità	Utrnulost udova
Enrouement	Hoarseness	Ronquera	Raucedine	Promuklost
Enthésiopathie	Enthesopathy	Entesopatía	Entesopatia	Entezopatija
Envie de l'ongle	Agnail (hangnail)	Padrastro	Pipita	Zanoktica
Envie de vomir	Urge to vomit	Ganas de vomitar	Impulso a vomitare	Podražaj na povraćanje
Éosinophilie	Eosinophilia	Eosinofilia	Eosinofilia	Eozinofilija
Épanchement de sang à l'intérieur d'une articulation (hémarthrose)	Bleeding into joint space (hemarthrosis)	Sangrado interno de las articulaciones (hemartrosis)	Emartro	Krvarenje u zglob (hemartroza)
Épanchement péricardique	Pericardial effusion (hydropericard)	Derrame pericárdico	Idropericardio	Hidroperikard
Épaule bloquée (périarthrite scapulo-humérale)	Frozen shoulder (adhesive capsulitis of shoulder)	Capsulitis adhesiva del hombro	Capsulite adesiva	Sindrom bolnog ramena (adhezivni kapsulitis ramena, smrznuto rame)
Épendymome	Ependymoma	Ependimoma	Ependimoma	Ependimom
Éperon de talon (epine calcaneenne)	Heel spur (calcaneal spur)	Espuela de talón (espuela calcánea)	Spina nel calcagno (spina calcaneare)	Petni trn
Épicondylite latérale	Tennis elbow	Codo del tenista (epicondilitis lateral)	Gomito del tennista (epicondilite)	Teniski lakat
Épilepsie	Epilepsy	Epilepsia	Epilessia	Epilepsija
Épiphysiolyse de l'extrémité supérieure du fémur	Epiphyseolysis capitis femoris	Epifisario de la cabeza femoral (epifisiolisis capitis femoris)	Epifisiolisi della testa femorale	Epifizeoliza glave bedrene kosti
Épispadias	Epispadias	Epispadia	Epispadia	Epispadija
Érection persistente douloureuse (priapisme)	Long-lasting painful erection (priapism)	Erección sostenida y dolorosa (priapismo)	Erezione persistente dolorosa (priapismo)	Dugotrajna bolna erekcija (prijapizam)
Érosion du col de l'utérus	Cervical erosion	Erosión cervical	Erosione cervicale	Cervikalna erozija
Érysipèle (érésipèle)	Erysipelas (Ignis sacer, St. Anthony's fire)	Erisipela	Erisipela	Crveni vjetar (vrbanac, erizipel)
Erysipéloïde	Erysipeloid	Erisipeloide	Erisipeloide	Erizipeloid
Érythème (rougeur de la peau)	Redness of the skin (erythema)	Enrojecimiento de la piel (eritema)	Eritema	Crvenilo kože (eritem)
Érythème infectieux (cinquième maladie)	Infectious erythema (fifth disease)	Eritema infeccioso (quinta enfermedad)	Eritema infettivo (quinta malattia)	Infektivni eritem (peta bolest)
Érythromelalgie	Erythromelalgia (acromelalgia)	Eritromelalgia	Eritromelalgia	Eritromelalgija
Érythroplasie	Erythroplakia (erythroplasia)	Eritroplasia	Eritroplachia (eritroplasia)	Eritroplazija
Érythroplasie de Queyrat	Erythroplasia of Queyrat	Eritroplasia de Queyrat	Eritroplasia di Queyrat	Eritroplazija Queyrat
Escarre (plaie de lit, ulcère de décubitus)	Bedsore (decubitus ulcer)	Úlcera de decúbito	Piaga da decubito (decubito)	Dekubitus
Éternuement	Sneezing	Estornudo	Starnuto	Kihanje
Exanthème	Exanthem	Exantema	Esantema	Egzantem
Exaspération (irritation)	Exasperation	Exasperación	Esasperazione (irritazione)	Razdražljivost
Excrétion urinaire à prédominance nocturne (nycturie)	Frequent urination at night (nocturia)	Emisión excesiva de orina durante la noche (nicturia)	Urinazione notturna (nicturia)	Noćno mokrenje (nokturija)
Exophtalmie (proptose)	Bulging eyes (exophthalmos)	Exoftalmos	Esoftalmo	Izbuljene oči (egzoftalmus)
Exostose	Exostosis	Exostosis	Esostosi	Egzostoza
Faiblesse	Weakness	Debilidad	Debolezza	Slabost
Faim	Hunger	Hambre	Fame	Glad
Faim excessive (polyphagie)	Excessive hunger (polyphagia)	Aumento anormal de la necesidad de comer (polifagia)	Aumento incontrollato dell'appetito (polifagia)	Neumjerena glad
Famine	Starvation	Inanición	Inedia	Izgladnjelost
Fasciculation musculaire	Muscle twitch (fasciculation)	Crispar del músculo (fasciculación)	Scossa muscolare (fasciciolazione)	Trzanje mišića
Fasciite de la main (fasciite palmaire)	Hand fibrositis	Fibrositis de la mano	Fibrosite di mano	Fibrozitis šake
Fasciite nécrosante	Necrotizing fasciitis	Fascitis necrotizante	Fascite necrotizzante	Nekrotizirajući fasciitis
Français	Anglais	Espagnol	Italien	Croate
Fasciite plantaire	Plantar fasciitis	Fascitis plantar	Fasciosi plantare	Plantarni fasciitis
Fatigue (affaiblissement)	Fatigue (exhaustion, lethargy)	Cansancio (fatiga, letargo, astenia)	Stanchezza (fatica, astenia)	Iscrpljenost (umor, fatigo)
Favus	Favus	Tiña favosa (favus, tinea favosa)	Tinea favosa	Tinea favosa (favus)

Français	Anglais	Espagnol	Italien	Croate
Fente labiale et fente palatine	Cleft lip and palate	Labio leporino (fisura labial)	Labbro leporino	Rascjep usne i nepca
Fibrillation auriculaire	Atrial fibrillation	Fibrilación auricular	Fibrillazione atriale	Atrijska fibrilacija
Fibrillation ventriculaire	Ventricular fibrillation	Fibrilación ventricular	Fibrillazione ventricolare	Ventrikularna fibrilacija
Fibroadénome	Fibroadenoma	Fibroadenoma	Fibroadenoma	Fibroadenom
Fibroélastose endocardique	Endocardial fibroelastosis	Fibroelastosis endocardial	Fibroelastosi endocardica	Fibroelastoza endokarda
Fibrome	Fibroma	Fibroma	Fibroma	Fibrom
Fibrome chondromyxoïde	Chondromyxoid fibroma	Fibroma condromixoide	Fibroma condromixoide	Hondromiksoidni fibrom
Fibromyalgie	Fibromyalgia	Fibromialgia	Fibromialgia	Fibromialgija
Fibrosarcome	Fibrosarcoma (fibroblastic sarcoma)	Fibrosarcoma	Fibrosarcoma	Fibrosarkom
Fibrose	Fibrosis	Fibrosis	Fibrosi	Fibroza
Fibrose pulmonaire idiopathique	Idiopathic pulmonary fibrosis	Fibrosis pulmonar idiopática	Fibrosi polmonare idiopatica	Plućna idiopatska fibroza
Fibrose rétropéritonéale (maladie d'Ormond)	Retroperitoneal fibrosis (Ormond's disease)	Fibrosis retroperitoneal	Fibrosi retroperitoneale	Retroperitonealna fibroza (Ormondova bolest)
Fibrosite du tendon	Tendinous fibrositis	Fibrositis de tendón	Fibrosi tendinea	Fibrozitis tetive
Fibrosite musculaire	Muscular fibrositis	Fibrositis (reumatismo muscular)	Fibrosite muscolare	Fibrozitis mišića
Fièvre	Fever	Fiebre	Febbre	Groznica (vrućica)
Fièvre à tiques du Colorado (fièvre à tiques des montagnes)	Colorado tick fever (mountain tick fever)	Fiebre del Colorado por garrapatas (fiebre de montaña americana por garrapatas)	Febbre da zecca del Colorado	Groznica planinskog krpelja
Fièvre d'Oroya (maladie de Carrion)	Oroya fever (Carrion's disease)	Fiebre de la Oroya (enfermedad de Carrión, verruga peruana)	Febbre di Oroya	Oroya groznica (Carrionova bolest)
Fièvre de la morsure de rat	Rat-bite fever	Fiebre por mordedura de rata	Febbre da morso di ratto	Groznica štakorskog ugriza
Fièvre de la vallée du Rift	Rift Valley fever	Fiebre de Rift Valley	Febbre della Rift Valley	Rift Valley groznica
Fièvre de Lassa	Lassa fever	Fiebre de Lassa	Febbre di Lassa	Groznica Lassa
Fièvre des métaux	Metal fume fever	Fiebre de los vapores metálicos	Febbre da inalazione di fumi metallici	Metalna groznica
Fièvre du Nil occidental	West Nile fever	Fiebre del Nilo Occidental	Febbre del Nilo occidentale	Groznica zapadnog Nila
Fièvre Ébola	Ebola hemorrhagic fever	Fiebre hemorrágica viral de Ébola	Febbre del Nilo occidentale Ebola	Groznica Ebola
Fièvre fluviale du Japon (typhus à chiques)	Scrub typhus (Japanese river fever, Tsutsugamushi fever)	Tsutsugamushi (fiebre fluvial japonesa, tifus de los matorrales)	Tsutsugamushi (tifo fluviale giapponese)	Japanska riječna gro-znica (Tsutsugamushi groznica)
Fièvre hémorragique avec syndrome rénal (fièvre hémorragique de Corée)	Hemorrhagic fever with renal syndrome (Korean hemorrhagic fever)	Fiebre hemorrágica con síndrome renal (fiebre hemorrágica coreana)	Febbre emorragica con sindrome renale (febbre emorragica coreana)	Hemoragijska groznica s renalnim sindromom (korejska hemoragijska groznica)
Fièvre hémorragique de Congo-Crimée	Crimean-Congo hemorrhagic fever	Fiebre hemorrágica de Crimea-Congo	Febbre emorragica Crimean-Congo	Krimska hemoragijska groznica
Fièvre hémorragique de Marbourg	Marburg hemorrhagic fever	Fiebre hemorrágica de Marburgo	Febbre emorragica di Marburg	Marburška hemoragijska groznica
Fièvre hémorragique virale	Viral hemorrhagic fever	Fiebre hemorrágica viral	Febbre emorragica	Virusna hemoragijska groznica
Fièvre jaune	Yellow fever	Fiebre amarilla	Febbre gialla	Žuta groznica
Fièvre méditerranéenne familiale	Familial Mediterranean fever	Fiebre mediterránea familiar	Febbre mediterranea familiare	Obiteljska mediteranska groznica
Fièvre pappataci (fièvre à phlébotomes)	Pappataci fever (phlebotomus fever, sandfly fever)	Fiebre pappataci	Febbre da pappataci (febbre da Flebotomi)	Papatači-groznica
Fièvre paratyphoïde	Paratyphoid fever	Fiebre paratifoidea	Febbre paratifoide	Trbušni paratifus
Fièvre Q	Q fever	Fiebre Q	Febbre Q	Q-groznica
Fièvre récurrente	Relapsing fever	Fiebre reincidente	Febbre ricorrente	Povratna groznica
Fièvre typhoïde (typhus abdominal)	Typhoid fever (typhoid)	Fiebre tifoidea (fiebre entérica)	Febbre tifoide (tifo)	Tifusna groznica (tifus)
Fièvre Zika	Zika fever	Fiebre del Zika	Febbre Zika	Zika groznica
Filariose	Filariasis	Filariasis	Filariasi	Filarijaza
Fissure anale	Anal fissure	Fisura anal	Fissura anale	Analna fisura
Fistule	Fistula	Fístula	Fistola	Fistula
Fistule anale	Anal fistula	Fístula anal	Fistola anale	Analna fistula
Fistule bronchopleurale	Bronchopleural fistula	Fístula bronco-pleural	Fistola broncopleurica	Bronhopleuralna fistula
Flexibilité anormale	Abnormal flexibility	Flexibilidad anormal	Movimento anormale	Abnormalna gibljivost
Folliculite	Folliculitis	Foliculitis	Follicolite	Folikulitis
Fourmillement	Tingling	Hormigueo	Intormentire	Trnjenje
Fracture à déplacement	Fracture with displacement	Fractura-dislocación	Frattura con dislocazione	Prijelom kosti s pomakom
Fracture comminutive	Comminuted fracture	Fractura cominuta	Frattura comminuta	Kominutivni prijelom kosti
Fracture de côte	Broken rib (rib fracture)	Fractura de costilla	Frattura della costola	Prijelom rebra
Fracture de fatigue	Stress fracture	Fractura por estrés	Frattura da stress	Prijelom zamora
Fracture de fatigue du tibia	Tibia stress fracture	Fractura por estrés de la tibia	Frattura da stress della tibia	Prijelom zamora goljenične kosti

Français	Anglais	Espagnol	Italien	Croate
Fracture de l'extrémité inferieure du radius (fracture de Pouteau-Colles)	Distal radial fracture	Fractura distal del radio	Frattura di Pouteau-Colles (frattura delle metafisi radiali distali)	Prijelom palčane kosti loco typico
Fracture de l'humérus	Broken upper arm (humerus fracture)	Fractura del húmero	Frattura dell'omero	Prijelom nadlaktice
Fracture de l'olécrâne	Broken elbow (olecranon fracture)	Fractura de olécranon	Frattura dell'olecrano	Prijelom lakatnog vrha (prijelom olekranona)
Fracture de l'ulna	Broken ulna (ulna fracture)	Fractura de cúbito	Frattura dell'ulna	Prijelom lakatne kosti
Fracture de la base du crâne	Base of skull fracture (basal skull fracture)	Fractura de la base del cráneo	Frattura della base del cranio	Prijelom baze lubanje
Fracture de la cheville	Broken ankle (ankle fracture)	Fractura de tobillo	Frattura della caviglia	Prijelom gležnja
Fracture de la clavicule	Broken collarbone (clavicle fracture)	Fractura de clavícula	Frattura della clavicola	Prijelom ključne kosti
Fracture de la diaphyse fémorale	Diaphyseal tightbone fracture	Fractura de la diáfisis del fémur	Frattura della diafisi femorale	Prijelom dijafize bedrene kosti
Fracture de la fibula	Broken fibula (fibula fracture)	Fractura del peroné	Frattura della fibula	Prijelom lisne kosti
Fracture de la scapula	Broken shoulder blade (scapula fracture)	Fractura de escápula	Frattura della scapola	Prijelom lopatice
Fracture de la tête radiale	Radial head fracture (radial capitulum fracture)	Fractura de la cabeza del radio	Frattura del capitello radiale	Prijelom glavice palčane kosti
Fracture de rotule	Broken knee cap (patellar fracture)	Fractura de la rótula	Frattura della rotula	Prijelom ivera (prijelom patele)
Fracture des os	Broken bone (bone fracture)	Fractura de hueso	Frattura	Prijelom kosti (fraktura kosti)
Fracture diaphysaire de l'humérus	Diaphyseal humeral fracture	Fractura diafisaria del húmero	Frattura diafisaria dell'omero	Prijelom nadlaktice u području dijafize
Fracture du bassin	Broken pelvis (pelvis fracture)	Fractura de pelvis	Frattura del bacino	Prijelom zdjelice
Fracture du calcanéus	Broken heel bone (calcaneus fracture)	Fractura del calcáneo	Frattura del calcagno	Prijelom petne kosti
Fracture du col de l'humérus	Humeral neck fracture	Fractura de cuello del húmero	Frattura del collo dell'omero	Prijelom vrata nadlaktične kosti
Fracture du col du fémur	Femoral neck fracture	Fractura de cuello del fémur	Frattura del collo del femore	Prijelom vrata bedrene kosti
Fracture du condyle huméral	Epicondylar elbow fracture	Fractura de epicóndilo humeral	Frattura dell'epicondilo omerale	Prijelom kondila nadlaktične kosti
Fracture du doigt	Broken finger (finger fracture)	Fractura de falange del dedo	Frattura della falange del dito	Prijelom članka prsta
Fracture du fémur	Broken thighbone (femur fracture)	Fractura de fémur	Frattura del femore	Prijelom bedrene kosti
Fracture du gros orteil	Broken big toe (fractured hallux)	Fractura de los huesos del dedo gordo del pie	Frattura dell'alluce	Prijelom falange nožnog palca
Fracture du maxillaire et/ou de la mandibule	Upper and/or lower jaw fracture (broken upper/lower jaw)	Fractura de maxilar y/o mandíbula	Frattura della mascella e/o della mandibola	Prijelom gornje i/ili donje čeljusti
Fracture du plateau vertébral	Broken vertebral body (vertebral corpus fracture)	Fractura de cuerpo vertebral	Frattura del corpo vertebrale	Prijelom trupa kralješka
Fracture du radius	Radius fracture	Fractura del radio	Frattura del radio	Prijelom palčane kosti
Fracture du radius et du cubitus	Broken forearm (frac-tured ulna and radius)	Fractura de radio y cúbito	Frattura di radio e ulna	Prijelom obje podlaktične kosti
Fracture du scaphoïde	Broken navicular bone (navicular fracture)	Fractura de escafoides (fractura navicular)	Frattura dell'osso navicolare	Prijelom navikularne kosti
Fracture du tibia	Broken shinbone (tibia fracture)	Fractura de tibia	Frattura della tibia	Prijelom goljenične kosti
Fracture du tibia et de la fibula	Broken lower leg bones (fractured tibia and fibula)	Fractura de tibia y peroné	Frattura di tibia e perone	Prijelom obje kosti potkoljenice
Fracture en bois vert	Greenstick fracture	Fractura en rama verde	Frattura a legno verde	Prijelom mlade kosti
Fracture en spirale	Spiral fracture	Fractura espiral	Frattura a spirale	Spiralni prijelom kosti
Fracture incomplète	Incomplete fracture	Fractura incompleta	Frattura incompleta (infrazione)	Nepotpuni prijelom kosti (napuknuće kosti)
Fracture métatarsienne	Broken foot (metatarsal fracture)	Fractura de metatarso	Frattura del metatarso	Prijelom kosti stopala
Fracture oblique	Oblique fracture	Fractura obliqua	Frattura obliqua	Kosi prijelom kosti
Fracture ouverte	Open fracture (compound fracture)	Fractura abierta	Frattura aperta (frattura esposta)	Otvoreni prijelom kosti
Fracture répétée	Refracturing (repeated fracture)	Fractura repetida	Frattura ripetuta	Opetovani prijelom kosti
Fracture simple	Simple bone fracture	Fractura simple	Frattura semplice	Jednostavni prijelom kosti
Fracture supracondylienne de l'humérus	Supracondylar humerus fracture	Fractura supracondilar del húmero	Frattura sovracondiloidea di omero	Suprakondilarni prijelom nadlaktice
Fracture supracondylienne du fémur	Supracondylar femoral fracture	Fractura supracondilar del fémur	Frattura sovracondiloidea del femore	Suprakondilarni prijelom bedrene kosti
Fracture tibia péroné sus-malléolaire	Supramaleolar fracture of tibia and fibula	Fractura supramaleolar de tibia y peroné	Frattura del terzo distale di tibia e perone	Supramaleolarni prijelom potkoljenice
Fracture transversale	Transverse fracture	Fractura transversal	Frattura trasversale	Poprečni prijelom kosti

Français	Anglais	Espagnol	Italien	Croate
Fractures spontanées	Spontaneous fractures	Fracturas espontáneas	Fratture spontanee	Spontane frakture
Fragments deboîtées	Dislocated fragments	Dislocación de los fragmentos	Dislocazione dei frammenti	Dislokacija ulomaka
Fréquence du pouls accélérée	Accelerated pulse rate	Pulso acelerado	Polso accelerato	Ubrzani puls
Frigidité	Frigidity	Frigidez	Frigidità	Frigidnost
Frissonnement	Shivering	Escalofrío (tiritón)	Brivido	Zimica (tresavica)
Furoncle	Furuncle (boil)	Forúnculo (furúnculo)	Foruncolo	Furunkul (čir na koži)
Fusion congénitale de vertèbres cervicales (Syndrome de Klippel-Feil)	Congenital fusion of cervical vertebrae (Klippel-Feil syndrome)	Fusión congenita de vértebras cervicales (síndrome de Klippel-Feil)	Fusione di vertebre cervicali (Sindrome di Klippel Feil)	Srašteni vrat (sindrom Klippel-Feil)
Galactorrhée	Galactorrhea	Galactorrea	Galattorrea	Galaktoreja
Gale (mal de Sainte-Marie)	Scabies (the itch)	Arador de la sarna (escabiosis)	Scabbia (rogna)	Svrab (skabijes)
Gangrène	Gangrene	Gangrena	Cancrena	Gangrena
Gangrène de Fournier	Fournier gangrene	Gangrena de Fournier	Gangrena di Fournier	Fournierova gangrena
Gangrène gazeuse	Gas gangrene	Gangrena gaseosa	Gangrene gassosa	Plinska gangrena
Gangrène humide	Wet gangrene	Gangrena húmeda	Gangrena umida	Vlažna gangrena
Gangrène sèche	Dry gangrene	Gangrena seca	Gangrena secca	Suha gangrena
Gargouillements (borborygme)	Stomach growling (borborygmus)	Sonidos de tripas (borborigmo)	Borborigmo	Kruljenje u želucu
Gastroentérite	Gastroenteritis	Gastroenteritis	Gastroenterite	Gastroenteritis
Gelure	Frostbite	Congelamiento	Congelamento	Ozeblina
Genou cagneux (genu valgum, genou en X)	Knock knees (genu valgum)	Genu valgo	Ginocchio valgo	Genu valgum
Genou du sauteur (tendinite rotulienne)	Irritated knee (jumper's knee, patellar tendinopathy)	Rodilla de saltador (tendinopatía rotuliana)	Peritendite rotulea (ginocchio del saltatore)	Podraženo koljeno (skakačko koljeno)
Genu varum	Bow legs (genu varum)	Genu varum	Ginocchio varo (genu varum)	Genu varum
Gigantisme	Gigantism	Gigantismo	Gigantismo	Divovski stas
Glaucome	Glaucoma	Glaucoma	Glaucoma	Glaukom
Glioblastome	Glioblastoma	Glioblastoma	Glioblastoma	Glioblastom
Gliome	Glioma	Glioma	Glioma	Gliom
Gliose	Gliosis	Gliosis	Gliosi	Glioza
Glomérulonéphrite	Glomerulonephritis	Glomerulonefritis	Glomerulonefrite	Glomerulonefritis
Goitre	Goiter	Bocio (coto)	Gozzo	Guša (struma)
Goitre multinodulaire	Nodular goiter	Bocio nodular	Gozzo multinodulare	Čvorasta guša (nodularna struma)
Gonadoblastome	Gonadoblastoma	Gonadoblastoma	Gonadoblastoma	Gonadoblastom
Gonflement (enflure)	Swelling	Hinchazón	Gonfiore	Oteklina
Gonorrhée (blennorragie, chaude-pisse)	Gonorrhea	Gonorrea (blenorragia, blenorrea)	Gonorrea (blenorragia)	Gonoreja (kapavac, triper)
Goutte	Gout (gouty arthritis)	Gota (enfermedad gotosa)	Gotta	Ulozi (giht)
Grain de beauté (naevus)	Birthmark (nevus)	Nevus (nevo)	Voglia (neo, nevo)	Madež (nevus)
Gripe porcine	Pig flu (swine influenza, influenzavirus A subtype H1N1)	Gripe porcina (influenza porcina, gripe del cerdo)	Influenza suina	Svinjska gripa
Grippe (influenza)	Flu (influenza)	Gripe (gripa, influenza)	Influenza	Gripa (influenca)
Grippe aviaire (influenza virus A sous-type H5N1)	Bird flu (influenzavirus A subtype H5N1)	Gripe aviar H5N1	Influenza aviaria H5N1	Ptičja gripa podtip H5N1
Grippe espagnole	Spanish flu	Gripe española	Influenza spagnola	Španjolska gripa
Grossesse extra-utérine	Ectopic pregnancy (extrauterine pregnancy)	Embarazo ectópico	Gravidanza ectopica	Izvanmaternična trudnoća (ektopična trudnoća)
Grossissement	Gaining weight	Engorde (ganar peso)	Ingrossamento (divenire grosso)	Debljanje
Gynécomastie	Gynecomastia	Ginecomastia	Ginecomastia	Ginekomastija
Hallucination	Hallucination	Alucinación	Allucinazione	Halucinacija
Hallux valgus	Bunion	Bunión (hallux valgus)	Alluce valgo	Čukalj
Hamstring syndrome	Tight hamstrings syndrome	Síndrome de isquiosurales cortos	Sindrome degli ischio-crurali (sindrome dell'hamstring)	Sindrom stražnje lože natkoljenice (sindrom hamstringsa)
Hémangioendothéliome	Hemangioendothelioma	Hemangioendotelioma	Emangioendotelioma	Hemangioendoteliom
Hémangiome	Hemangioma	Hemangioma	Emangioma	Hemangiom
Hémangiome capillaire	Capillary hemangioma (infantile hemangioma, strawberry hemangioma)	Hemangioma capilar (marca de fresa)	Emangioma capillare	Kapilarni hemangiom
Hématome	Hematoma	Hematoma	Ematoma	Hematom
Hématome épidural	Epidural hematoma	Hematoma epidural	Ematoma epidurale	Epiduralni hematom
Hématome intracérébral	Intracerebral hematoma	Hematoma intracerebral	Ematoma cerebrale	Intracerebralni hematom
Hématome subdural	Subdural hematoma	Hematoma subdural	Ematoma subdurale	Subduralni hematom
Héméralopie	Day blindness (hemeralopia)	Falta de visión en luz brillante (hemeralopia)	Emeralopia	Kokošje sljepilo (hemeralopija)
Hémicrânie paroxystique chronique	Chronic paroxysmal hemicrania (Sjaastad syndrome)	Hemicránea crónica paroxismal	Emicrania cronica parossistica	Kronična paroksi-zmalna hemikranija (Sjaastadov sindrom)
Hémivertèbre	Hemivertebrae	Hemivértebra	Emivertebra	Hemivertebra
Hémochromatose	Hemochromatosis	Hemocromatosis	Emocromatosi	Hemokromatoza

Français	Anglais	Espagnol	Italien	Croate
Hémoglobine dans l'urine (hémoglobinurie)	Hemoglobin in urine (hemoglobinuria)	Hemoglobina en orina (hemoglobinuria)	Presenza di emoglobina nelle urine (emoglobinuria)	Hemoglobin u urinu (hemoglobinurija)
Hémophilie	Hemophilia	Hemofilia	Emofilia	Hemofilija
Hémopneumothorax	Hemopneumothorax	Hemoneumotórax	Emopneumotorace	Hemopneumotoraks
Hémorragie artérielle	Arterial bleeding	Hemorragia arterial	Emorragia arteriosa	Arterijsko krvarenje
Hémorragie épidurale	Epidural bleeding	Hemorragia epidural	Emorragia epidurale	Epiduralno krvarenje
Hémorragie intracérébrale	Intracerebral hemorrhage	Hemorragia intracerebral	Emorragia cerebrale	Intracerebralno krvarenje
Hémorragie sous arachnoïdienne	Subarachnoid hemorrhage	Hemorragia subaracnoidea	Emorragia subaracnoidea	Subarahnoidalno krvarenje
Hémorragie subdural	Subdural hemorrhage	Hemorragia subdural	Emorragia subdurale	Subduralno krvarenje
Hémorroïdes	Hemorrhoids	Hemorroides	Emorroidi	Hemoroidi
Hémosidérose	Hemosiderosis	Hemosiderosis	Emosiderosi	Hemosideroza
Hémothorax	Hemothorax	Hemotórax	Emotorace	Hemotoraks
Hépatite A	Hepatitis A	Hepatitis A	Epatite virale A	Hepatitis A
Hépatite B	Hepatitis B	Hepatitis B	Epatite virale B	Hepatitis B
Hépatite C	Hepatitis C	Hepatitis C	Epatite virale C	Hepatitis C
Hépatite D	Hepatitis D	Hepatitis D	Epatite virale D	Hepatitis D
Hépatite E	Hepatitis E	Hepatitis E	Epatite virale E	Hepatitis E
Hépatite virale	Viral hepatitis	Hepatitis viral	Epatite virale	Virusni hepatitis
Hermaphrodisme	Hermaphroditism	Hermafroditismo	Ermafroditismo	Dvospolnost
Hernie	Hernia	Hernia	Ernia	Kila (bruh, hernija)
Hernie de la paroi abdominale (hernie abdominale externe)	External abdominal wall hernia	Hernia de la pared abdominal	Ernia esterna addominale	Kila vanjske trbušne stijenke
Hernie diaphragmatique	Diaphragmatic hernia	Hernia diafragmática	Ernia diaframmatica	Dijafragmalna kila
Hernie discale	Spinal disc herniation	Hernia discal	Ernia del disco	Hernija intervertebralnog diska
Hernie hiatale	Hiatus hernia	Hernia de hiato	Ernia iatale	Hijatusna kila
Hernie inguinale	Inguinal hernia	Hernia inguinal	Ernia inguinale	Preponska kila
Hernie ombilicale	Umbilical hernia	Hernia umbilical	Ernia ombelicale	Pupčana kila (umbilikalna hernija)
Herpangine	Herpangina (mouth blisters)	Herpangina	Erpangina (faringite vescicolare)	Herpangina
Herpès (infection herpétique)	Herpes simplex	Herpes simple	Herpes simplex	Herpes simpleks
Herpès génital	Genital herpes	Herpes genital	Herpes genitalis	Genitalni herpes
Hippocratisme digital (doigts en baguettes de tambour)	Finger clubbing (digital clubbing)	Acropaquia (hipocratismo digital)	Dita ippocratiche (dita a bacchetta di tamburo)	Batićasti prsti
Hirsutisme	Hirsutism	Hirsutismo	Irsutismo	Hirzutizam
Histiocytome fibreux	Fibrous histiocytoma	Histiocitoma fibroso	Fibroistiocitoma benigno	Fibrozni histiocitom
Histoplasmose	Histoplasmosis (Darling's disease)	Histoplasmosis	Istoplasmosi	Histoplazmoza
Hoquet	Hiccup	Hipo	Singhiozzo	Štucavica
Hydrémie	Hydremia	Hidremia	Idremia	Hidremija
Hydrocèle	Hydrocele	Hidrocele	Idrocele	Hidrokela
Hydrocéphalie	Hydrocephalus	Hidrocefalia	Idrocefalo	Hidrocefalus
Hydronéphrose	Hydronephrosis	Hidronefrosis	Idronefrosi	Hidronefroza
Hydrops	Hydrops	Hidrops	Idrope	Hidrops
Hydrops de la vésicule biliaire	Gallbladder hydrops	Hidrops vesicular	Idrope della colecisti	Hidrops žučnog mjehura
Hydrothorax	Hydrothorax	Hidrotórax	Idrotorace	Hidrotoraks
Hygroma	Hygroma	Higroma	Igroma	Higrom
Hyperactivité	Hyperactivity	Hiperactividad	Iperattività	Hiperaktivnost
Hyperaldostéronisme	Aldosteronism (hyperaldosteronism)	Aldosteronismo (hiperaldosteronismo)	Iperaldosteronismo	Aldosteronizam
Hypercalcémie	Hypercalcemia	Hipercalcemia	Ipercalcemia	Hiperkalcijemija
Hyperinsulinisme	Hyperinsulinism	Hiperinsulinismo	Iperinsulinismo	Povišen inzulin u krvi (hiperinzulinizam)
Hyperkaliémie	Hyperkalemia	Hiperpotasemia (hipercalemia)	Iperkaliemia	Hiperkalijemija
Hypermétropie	Farsightedness (hyperopia)	Hipermetropía	Ipermetropia	Dalekovidnost
Hyperparathyroïdie	Hyperparathyroidism	Hiperparatiroidismo	Iperparatiroidismo	Hiperparatireoidizam
Hyperpituitarisme	Hyperpituitarism	Hiperpituitarismo	Iperpituitarismo	Hiperpituitarizam
Hyperplasie endométriale	Endometrial hyperplasia	Hiperplasia endometrial	Iperplasia endometriale	Hiperplazija endometrija
Hyperplasie pseudo-épithéliomateuse	Pseudoepitheliomatous hyperplasia	Hiperplasia pseudoepiteliomatosa	Iperplasia pseudoepiteliomatosa	Pseudoepiteliematozna hiperplazija
Hypersensibilité aux stimuli extérieurs (hyperesthésie)	Increased sensitivity to stimuli of the senses (hyperesthesia)	Sensación exagerada de los estímulos táctiles (hiperestesia)	Ippersensibilità ai normali stimoli esterni (iperestesia)	Preosjetljivost na podražaj (hiperestezija)
Hypersialorrhée (ptyalisme)	Drooling (ptyalism, sialorrhea, slobbering)	Sialorrea (ptialismo)	Sbavando (ptialismo, scialorrea)	Slinjenje
Hypertension artérielle essentielle	Essential hypertension	Hipertensión esencial	Ipertensione arteriosa essenziale	Esencijalna hipertenzija
Hypertension artérielle maligne	Malignant hypertension	Hipertensión maligna	Ipertensione maligna	Maligna hipertenzija

Français	Anglais	Espagnol	Italien	Croate
Hypertension artérielle pulmonaire	Pulmonary hypertension	Hipertensión arterial pulmonar	Ipertensione arteriosa polmonare	Plućna hipertenzija
Hypertension intra-crânienne	Intracranial hypertension	Hipertensión intracraneal	Elevata pressione intracranica	Intrakranijalna hipertenzija
Hypertension portale	Portal hypertension	Hipertensión portal	Ipertensione portale	Portalna hipertenzija
Hypertension rénovasculaire	Renovacsular hypertension	Hipertensión renovascular	Ipertensione renale	Renovaskularna hipertenzija
Hypertension secondaire	Secondary hyperten-sion (inessential hypertension)	Hipertensión secundaria	Ipertensione arteriosa secondaria	Sekundarna hipertenzija
Hyperthermie	Hyperthermia	Hipertermia	Ipertermia	Hipertermija
Hyperthyroïdie	Hyperthyroidism	Hipertiroidismo	Ipertiroidismo	Hipertireoza
Hypertrophie	Hypertrophy	Hipertrofia	Ipertrofia	Hipertrofija
Hypertrophie bénigne dela prostate	Benign prostatic hyperthroph	Hiperplasia benigna de próstata	Ipertrofia prostatica benigna	Benigna hipertrofija prostate
Hypertrophie cardiaque du sportif (coeur d'athlète)	Athlete's heart (cardiac hypertrophy)	Corazón de atleta (hipertrofia del corazón del deportista)	Cuore dell'atleta (ipertrofia cardiaca da sport)	Sportsko srce
Hypertrophie ventriculaire	Ventricular hypertrophy	Hipertrofia ventricular	Ipertrofia ventricolare	Ventrikularna hipertrofija
Hyperuricémie	Hyperuricemia	Hiperuricemia	Iperuricemia	Hiperurikemija
Hyperventilation	Hyperventilation	Hiperventilación	Iperventilazione	Hiperventilacija
Hypervitaminose	Hypervitaminosis	Hipervitaminosis	Ipervitaminosi	Hipervitaminoza
Hypervolémie (augmentation du volume de sang dans les vaisseaux)	Hypervolemia (increased level of fluid in the blood)	Hipervolemia (aumento del volumen de sangre en la circulación)	Ipervolemia (aumento del volume ematico circolante)	Hipervolemija (porast volumena krvi u optoku)
Hyphème	Hyphema	Hipema	Ifema	Hifema
Hypoalbuminémie	Hypoalbuminemia	Hipoalbuminemia	Ipoalbuminemia	Hipoalbuminemija
Hypocalcémie	Hypocalcemia	Hipocalcemia	Ipocalcemia	Hipokalcijemija
Hypocondrie	Hypochondria	Hipocondría	Ipocondria	Hipohondrija
Hypoglycémie	Hypoglycemia	Hipoglicemia	Ipoglicemia	Hipoglikemija
Hypoinsulinisme	Hypoinsulinism	Hipoinsulinismo	Ipoinsulinemia	Hipoinzulinizam
Hypokaliémie	Hypokalemia	Hipocaliemia	Ipokaliemia	Hipokalijemija
Hypoparathyroïdie	Hypoparathyroidism	Hipoparatiroidismo	Ipoparatiroidismo	Hipoparatireodizam
Hypopituitarisme	Hypopituitarism	Hipopituitarismo	Ipopituitarismo	Hipopituitarizam
Hypoplasie pulmonaire	Pulmonary hypoplasia	Hipoplasia pulmonar	Ipoplasia del tronco polmonare	Hipoplazija plućnog režnja
Hypospadias	Hypospadias	Hipospadias	Ipospadia	Hipospadija
Hypotension et syncope	Hypotension and syncope	Hipotensión y síncope	Ipotensione e sincope	Hipotenzija i sinkope
Hypothermie	Hypothermia	Hipotermia	Ipotermia	Pothlađenost (hipotermija)
Hypothyroïdie	Hypothyroidism	Hipotiroidismo	Ipotiroidismo	Hipotireoza
Hypotonie	Hypotonia	Hipotonía	Ipotonia	Hipotonija
Hypotonie musculaire	Muscular hypotonia	Hipotonía muscular	Ipotonia muscolare	Mišićna hipotonija
Hypoxie	Hypoxia	Hipoxia	Ipossia	Hipoksija
Hystérie	Hysteria	Histeria	Isteria (isterismo)	Histerija
Ictère (jaunisse)	Jaundice (icterus)	Ictericia	Ittero (itterizia)	Žutica (ikterus)
Ictère néonatal	Neonatal jaundice	Ictericia del recién nacido	Ittero neonatale	Novorođenačka žutica
Ictère par obstruction des voies biliaires	Mechanic icterus (bile duct obstruction)	Ictericia obstructiva	Ittero ostruttivo	Mehanički ikterus
Iléus	Ileus	Íleo	Ileo	Ileus
Imbécillité	Imbecility	Imbecilidad	Imbecillità	Slaboumnost
Immunodéficience	Immunodeficiency	Inmunodeficiencia	Immunodeficienza	Sniženi imunitet
Impétigo	Impetigo	Impétigo	Impetigine	Impetigo
Impotence	Impotency	Impotencia	Impotenza	Impotencija
Incapacité d'uriner	Inability to urinate	Incapacidad para orinar	Mancata secrezione di urina	Nemogućnost mokrenja
Incapacité de se mouvoir	Movement inability	Incapacidad de movimiento	Mancanza di movimento	Nemogućnost kretanja
Incontinence	Incontinence	Incontinencia	Incontinenza	Inkontinencija
Incontinence urinarie d'effort	Stress urinary incontinence	Incontinencia urinaria por estrés	Incontinenza urinaria da sforzo	Stres-inkontinencija urina
Incontinence urinaire	Urinary incontinence	Incontinencia urinaria	Incontinenza urinaria	Urinarna inkotinencija
Indigestion	Indigestion	Indigestión	Indigestione	Probavne smetnje
Infarctus	Infarct	Infarto	Infarto	Infarkt
Infarctus cérébral hémorragique	Hemorrhagic brain infarction	Infarto cerebral hemorrágico	Ictus emorragico	Hemoragijski infarkt mozga
Infarctus du myocarde	Heart attack (myocardial infarction)	Infarto de miocardio	Infarto miocardico acuto	Infarkt miokarda
Infarctus pulmonaire	Pulmonary infarction	Infarto pulmonar	Infarto polmonare	Infarkt pluća
Infection	Infection	Infección	Infezione (malattia infettiva)	Infekcija
Infection à Chlamydia	Chlamydia infection	Infección por clamidia	Infezione da clamidia	Klamidijska infekcija
Infection bactérienne	Bacterial infection	Infección bacteriana	Infezione batterica	Bakterijska infekcija
Infection fongique	Fungal infection	Infección por hongos	Infezione fungina	Gljivična infekcija
Infection osseuse ou de la moelle osseuse (ostéomyélite)	Infection of the bone or bone marrow (osteomyelitis)	Infección del hueso o médula ósea (osteomielitis)	Infezione dell'apparato osteo-articolare (osteomielite)	Infekcija kosti ili koštane srži (osteomijelitis)
Infection par le virus du papillome humain (VPH)	Human papilloma virus (HPV) infection	Infeccion por el virus del papilom humano (VPH)	Infezione da Papilloma Virus Umano (HPV)	Infekcija humanim papiloma virusom (HPV)
Infection respiratoire haute	Upper respiratory tract infection	Infección respiratoria alta	Infezione del tratto respiratorio superiore	Infekcija gornjih dišnih puteva
Infection virale	Viral infection	Infección viral	Infezione virale	Virusna infekcija

Français	Anglais	Espagnol	Italien	Croate
Infertilité (stérilité)	Infertility (sterility)	Infertilidad	Sterilità (infecondità)	Neplodnost (sterilitet)
Infestation par des poux (pédiculose)	Infestation with head lice (pediculosis)	Infestación por piojos (pediculosis)	Infestazione da pidocchi (pediculosi)	Infestacija ušima (ušljivost, pedikuloza)
Infestation par des poux du pubic (phtiriase)	Infestation with pubic lice (phthiriasis)	Infestación por ladilla (ftiriasis)	Infestazione da pidocchi del pube (ftiriasi)	Infestacija stidnim ušima (iftirijaza)
Infestation par des vers parasites intestinaux (helminthiase)	Infestation with intestinal parasitic warms (helminthiasis)	Infestación de gusanos (helmintiasis)	Infestazione da vermi (elmintiasi)	Infestacija crijevnim parazitima (helmintijaza)
Infirmité motorice cérébrale	Cerebral palsy	Parálisis cerebral	Paralisi cerebrale infantile	Cerebralna paraliza
Inflammation	Inflammation	Inflamación	Infiammazione (flogosi)	Upala
Inflammation d'un tendon (tendinite)	Inflammation of the tendon (tendinitis, tendonitis)	Inflamación de un tendón (tendinitis)	Infiammazione del tendine (tendinite)	Upala tetive (tendinitis)
Inflammation d'un tendon et de sa gaine synoviale (ténosynovite)	Inflammation of the synovium and tendon (tenosynovitis)	Inflamación de un tendón y de su vaina (tenosinovitis)	Infiammazione di tendine e di guaina tendinea (tenosinovite)	Upala tetive s ovojnicom (tenosinovitis)
Inflammation de l'appendice iléo-caecal (appendicite)	Inflammation of the appendix (appendicitis)	Inflamación del apéndice (apendicitis)	Infiammazione dell'appendice vermiforme (appendicite)	Upala slijepog crijeva (apendicitis)
Inflammation de l'endocarde (endocardite)	Inflammation of the endocardium (endocarditis)	Inflamación del endocardio (endocarditis)	Infiammazione dell'endocardio (endocardite)	Upala srčane ovojnice (endokarditis)
Inflammation de l'endomètre (endométrite)	Inflammation of the endometrium (endometritis)	Inflamación del endometrio (endometritis)	Infiammazione dell'endometrio (endometrite)	Upala endometrija maternice (endometritis)
Inflammation de l'enthèse (enthésite)	Inflammation of the entheses (enthesitis)	Inflamación de la zona de inserción de un músculo (entesitis)	Infiammazione dell'inserzione di muscolo (entesite)	Upala hvatišta mišića (entezitis)
Inflammation de l'épididyme (épididymite)	Inflammation of the epididymis (epididymitis)	Inflamación del epidídimo (epididimitis)	Infiammazione dell'epididimo (epididimite)	Upala pasjemenika (epididimitis)
Inflammation de l'épiglotte (épiglottite)	Inflammation of the epiglottis (epiglottitis)	Inflamación de la epiglotis (epiglotitis)	Infiammazione del'epiglottide (epiglottite)	Upala epiglotisa (epiglotitis)
Inflammation de l'oreille interne (labyrinthite, otite interne)	Inflammation of the inner ear (labyrinthitis)	Inflamación del laberinto del oído interno (laberintitis)	Infiammazione di labirinto nell'orecchio interno (labirintite)	Upala labirinta u unutarnjem uhu (labirintitis)
Inflammation de l'urètre (urétrite)	Inflammation of the urethra (urethritis)	Inflamación de la uretra (uretritis)	Infiammazione dell'uretra (uretrite)	Upala sluznice mokraćne cijevi (uretritis)
Inflammation de l'uvée (uvéite)	Inflammation of the middle layer of the eye (uveitis)	Inflamación de la lámina intermedia del ojo (uveítis)	Infiammazione della tunica media dell'occhio (uveite)	Upala srednje ovojnice oka (uveitis)
Inflammation de la bourse séreuse articulaire (hygroma, bursite)	Inflammation of the synovial fluid sac (bursitis)	Inflamación de la bursa (bursitis)	Infiammazione della borsa sierosa di un'articolazione (borsite)	Upala sluzne vreće (burzitis)
Inflammation de la conjonctive (conjonctivite)	Inflammation of the conjunctiva (conjunctivitis)	Inflamación de la conjuntiva (conjuntivitis)	Infiammazione della congiuntiva (congiuntivite)	Upala sluznice oka (konjuktivitis)
Inflammation de la conjonctive et de la cornée (kératoconjonctivite)	Inflammation of the cornea and conjunctiva (keratoconjunctivitis)	Inflamación de la córnea y de la conjuntiva (queratoconjuntivitis)	Infiammazione della cornea e della congiutiva (cheratocongiuntivite)	Upala rožnice i sluznice oka (keratokonjuktivitis)
Inflammation de la cornée (kératite)	Inflammation of the cornea (keratitis)	Inflamación de la córnea (queratitis)	Infiammazione della cornea (cheratite)	Upala rožnice (keratitis)
Inflammation de la gaine synoviale (synovite)	Inflammation of the synovial membrane (synovitis)	Inflamación de la membrana sinovial (sinovitis)	Infiammazione della membrana sinoviale (sinovite)	Upala tetivne ovojnice (sinovitis)
Inflammation de la gencive (gingivite)	Inflammation of the gums (gingivitis)	Inflamación de las encías (gingivitis)	Infiammazione dei tessuti gengivali (gengivite)	Upala desni (gingivitis)
Inflammation de la glande thyroïde (thyroïdite)	Inflammation of the thyroid gland (thyroiditis)	Inflamación de la glándula tiroides (tiroiditis)	Infiammazione della tiroide (tiroidite)	Upala štitnjače (tireoiditis)
Inflammation de la mamelle (mastite)	Inflammation of the breast (mastitis)	Inflamación del seno (mastitis)	Infiammazione della mammella (mastite)	Upala dojke (mastitis)
Inflammation de la muqueuse buccale (stomatite)	Inflammation of the mouth mucous lining (stomatitis)	Inflamación de la mucosa bucal (estomatitis)	Infiammazione delle mucose della bocca (stomatite)	Upala sluznice usta (stomatitis)
Inflammation de la paroi de l'estomac (gastrite)	Inflammation of the stomach lining (gastritis)	Inflamación de la mucosa gástrica (gastritis)	Infiammazione della mucosa gastrica (gastrite)	Upala želučane sluznice (gastritis)
Inflammation de la plèvre (pleurésie)	Inflammation of the pleura (pleuritis)	Inflamación de la pleura (pleuritis, pleuresía)	Infiammazione della pleura (pleurite)	Upala plućne ovojnice (pleuritis)
Inflammation de la prostate (prostatite)	Inflammation of the prostate gland (prostatitis)	Inflamación de la próstata (prostatitis)	Infiammazione della ghiandola prostatica (prostatite)	Upala prostate (prostatitis)
Inflammation de la rétine (rétinite)	Inflammation of the retina (retinitis)	Inflamación de la retina (retinitis)	Infiammazione della retina (retinite)	Upala mrežnice (retinitis)
Inflammation de la trachée (trachéite)	Inflammation of the windpipe (tracheitis)	Inflamación de la tráquea (traqueitis)	Infiammazione della trachea (tracheite)	Upala dušnika (traheitis)
Inflammation de la vésicule biliaire (cholécystite)	Inflammation of the gall bladder (cholecystitis)	Inflamación de la vesícula biliar (colecistitis)	Infiammazione della colecisti (colecistite)	Upala žučnog mjehura (holecistitis)

Français	Anglais	Espagnol	Italien	Croate
Inflammation de la vessie (cystite)	Inflammation of the urinary bladder (cystitis)	Inflamación de la vejiga urinaria (cistitis)	Infiammazione della vescica urinaria (cistite)	Upala mokraćnog mjehura (cistitis)
Inflammation de la vulve (vulvite)	Inflammation of the vulva (vulvitis)	Inflamación de la vulva (vulvitis)	Infiammazione della vulva (vulvite)	Upala stidnice (vulvitis)
Inflammation des articulations (arthrite)	Inflammation of the joint (arthritis)	Inflamación de una articulación (artritis)	Infiammazione articolare (artrite)	Upala zgloba (artritis)
Inflammation des bronches des poumons (bronchite)	Inflammation of the bronchi (bronchitis)	Inflamación de los bronquios (bronquitis)	Infiammazione dei bronchi (bronchite)	Upala bronhija (bronhitis)
Inflammation des ganglions (adénite, lymphadénite)	Inflammation of the lymph node (lymphadenitis)	Inflamación de los ganglios linfáticos (linfadenitis)	Infiammazione delle ghiandole linfatiche (linfoadenite)	Upala limfnog čvora (limfadenitis)
Inflammation des glandes salivaires (sialoadénite)	Inflammation of the salivary gland (sialadenitis)	Inflamación de las glándulas salivales (sialadenitis)	Infiammazione delle ghiandole salivari (sialoadenite)	Upala žlijezda slinovnica (sialadenitis)
Inflammation des méninges (méningite)	Inflammation of the meninges (meningitis)	Inflamación de las meninges (meningitis)	Infiammazione delle meningi (meningite)	Upala moždanih ovojnica (meningitis)
Inflammation des parois des artères (artérite)	Inflammation of the arterial walls (arteritis)	Inflamación de las arterias (arteritis)	Infiammazione delle arterie (arterite)	Upala stijenke arterije (arteritis)
Inflammation des petites bronches (bronchiolite)	Inflammation of the bronchioles (bronchiolitis)	Inflamación de los bronquiolos (bronquiolitis)	Infiammazione dei bronchioli (bronchiolite)	Upala bronhiola (bronhiolitis)
Inflammation des poumons (pneumonie)	Inflammation of the lung (pneumonia)	Inflamación de los pulmones (neumonía, pulmonía, neumonitis)	Infiammazione dei polmoni (polmonite)	Upala pluća (pneumonija)
Inflammation des testicules (orchite)	Inflammation of the testes (orchitis)	Inflamación del testículo (orquitis)	Infiammazione dei testicoli (orchite)	Upala testisa (orhitis)
Inflammation des tonsilles (tonsillite)	Inflammation of the tonsils (tonsillitis)	Inflamación de las amígdalas palatinas (amigdalitis)	Infiammazione delle tonsille (tonsillite)	Upala krajnika (tonzilitis)
Inflammation des veines (phlébite)	Inflammation of the vein (phlebitis)	Inflamación de las venas (flebitis)	Infiammazione delle vene (flebite)	Upala vena (flebitis)
Inflammation du cerveau (encéphalite)	Inflammation of the brain (encephalitis)	Inflamación del encéfalo (encefalitis)	Infiammazione del cervello (encefalite)	Upala mozga (encefalitis)
Inflammation du fascia (fasciite)	Inflammation of the fascia (fasciitis)	Inflamación de la fascia (fascitis)	Infiammazione della fascia (fascite)	Upala fascije (fasciitis)
Inflammation du foie (hépatite)	Inflammation of the liver (hepatitis)	Inflamación del hígado (hepatitis)	Infiammazione del fegato (epatite)	Upala jetre (hepatitis)
Inflammation du gland du pénis (balanite)	Inflammation of the glans penis (balanitis)	Inflamación del glande del pene (balanitis)	Infiammazione della testa del glande (balanite)	Upala glavića penisa (balanitis)
Inflammation du larynx (laryngite)	Inflammation of the larynx (laryngitis)	Inflamación de la laringe (laringitis)	Infiammazione della laringe (laringite)	Upala glasnica (laringitis)
Inflammation du myocarde (myocardite)	Inflammation of the heart muscle (myocarditis)	Inflamación del miocardio (miocarditis)	Infiammazione del miocardio (miocardite)	Upala srčanog mišića (miokarditis)
Inflammation du nerf (névrite)	Inflammation of the nerve (neuritis)	Inflamación del nervio (neuritis)	Infiammazione del nervo (neurite, nevrite)	Upala živca (neuritis)
Inflammation du pancréas (pancréatite)	Inflammation of the pancreas (pancreatitis)	Inflamación del páncreas (pancreatitis)	Infiammazione del pancreas (pancreatite)	Upala gušterače (pankreatitis)
Inflammation du paramètre (paramétrite)	Inflammation of the parametrium (parametritis)	Inflamación del parametrio (parametritis)	Infiammazione del parametrio (parametrite)	Upala parametrija (parametritis)
Inflammation du péricarde (péricardite)	Inflammation of the pericardium (pericarditis)	Inflamación del pericardio (pericarditis)	Infiammazione del pericardio (pericardite)	Upala osrčja (perikarditis)
Inflammation du péritoine (péritonite)	Inflammation of the peritoneum (peritonitis)	Inflamación del peritoneo (peritonitis)	Infiammazione dela sierosa peritoneale (peritonite)	Upala potrbušnice (peritonitis)
Inflammation du rein (néphrite)	Inflammation of the kidney (nephritis)	Inflamación del riñón (nefritis)	Infiammazione dei reni (nefrite)	Upala bubrega (nefritis)
Inflammation du sinus (sinusite)	Inflammation of the paranasal sinuses (sinusitis)	Inflamación de los senos paranasales (sinusitis)	Infiammazione dei seni paranasali (sinusite)	Upala sinusa (sinusitis)
Inflammation du thymus	Inflammation of the thymus (thymitis)	Inflamación del timo (timitis)	Infiammazione del timo	Upala prsne žlijezde (timitis)
Inflammation du tissu musculaire (myosite)	Inflammation of the muscles (myositis)	Inflamación del músculo esquelético (miositis)	Infiammazione del tessuto muscolare (miosite)	Upala mišića (miozitis)
Inflammation du vagin (vaginite)	Inflammation of the vagina (vaginitis)	Inflamación de la vagina (vaginitis)	Infiammazione della vagina (vaginite)	Upala rodnice (vaginitis)
Inflammation granulomateuse	Granulomatous inflammation	Inflamación granulomatosa	Infiammazione granulomatosa	Granulomatozna upala (granulom)
Inflammaton de la peau (dermatite)	Inflammation of the skin (dermatitis)	Inflamación de la piel (dermatitis)	Infiammazione della pelle (dermatite)	Upala kože (dermatitis)
Insomnie	Insomnia	Insomnio	Insomnia	Nesanica
Insuffisance hépatique	Liver insufficiency	Fallo hepático (insuficiencia hepática)	Insufficienza epatica	Zatajenje jetre
Insuffisance rénale	Kidney failure (renal insufficiency)	Fallo renal (insuficiencia renal)	Insufficienza renale	Zatajenje bubrega (insuficijencija bubrega)
Insuffisance rénale aiguë	Acute kidney failure	Insuficiencia renal aguda	Insufficienza renale acuta	Akutno zatajenje bubrega
Insuffisance rénale chronique	Chronic renal failure	Insuficiencia renal crónica	Insufficienza renale cronica	Kronično zatajenje bubrega
Insuffisance veineuse cérébro-spinale chronique	Chronic cerebrospinal venous insufficiency	Insuficiencia venosa cerebro-espinal crónica	Insufficienza venosa cronica cerebrospinale	Kronična cerebrospinalna venozna insuficijencija
Intolérance au gluten	Gluten intolerance	Intolerancia al gluten	Intolleranza al glutine	Nepodnošenje glutena

Français	Anglais	Espagnol	Italien	Croate
Intolérance au lactose	Lactose intolerance	Intolerancia a la lactosa	Intolleranza al lattosio	Nepodnošenje laktoze (netolerancija laktoze)
Intoxcation par arme chimique	Chemical warfare poisoning	Intoxicación por armas químicas	Avvelenamento da armi chimiche	Trovanje kemijskim oružjem
Intoxication alimentaire staphylococcique	Staphylococcal food poisoning	Intoxicación alimentaria por estafilococo dorado	Intossicazione alimentare da stafilococco	Stafilokokno trovanje hranom
Intoxication par des coquillages	Shellfish poisoning	Intoxicación por mariscos	Avvelenamento da molluschi	Trovanje školjkašima
Intoxication par gaz de combat	Warfare gases poisoning	Intoxicación por armas gaseosas	Avvelenamento da gas tossico	Trovanje bojnim otrovima
Intoxication par le paracétamol	Paracetamol poisoning	Intoxicación por paracetamol	Avvelenamento da paracetamolo	Trovanje paracetamolom
Iridodialyse	Iridodialysis (coredialysis)	Iridodiálisis	Iridodialisi	Iridodijaliza
Iritis	Iritis	Iritis	Irite	Iritis
Irradiation ionisante	Ionising irradiation	Exposición a las radiaciones ionizantes	Esposizione alle radiazioni ionizzanti	Ionizirajuća ozračenost
Irradiation non-ionisante	Non-ionising irradiation	Irradiación no-ionizante	Irradiazione non ionizzante	Neionizirajuća ozračenost
Irradiation par rayons radioactifs (contamination radioactive)	Radioactive irradiation	Irradiación radioactiva	Irradiazione radioattiva	Radioaktivna ozračenost
Ischémie	Ischemia	Isquemia	Ischemia	Ishemija
Ischémie des membres	Ischemic limbs	Isquemia de miembros	Ischemia degli arti	Ishemični udovi
Ischémie myocardique	Ischemic heart disease	Isquemia miocárdica (angina de pecho)	Ischemia miocardica	Ishemijska bolest srca
Isosporose	Isosporiasis	Isosporiasis	Isosporiasi	Izosporijaza
Jeu pathologique (jeu compulsif)	Gambling addiction (ludomania)	Adicción a jugar (ludopatía, ludomanía)	Giocco d'azzardo patologico	Ovisnost o kockanju (ludopatija)
Kala azar (fièvre noire)	Kala-azar (black fever)	Kala azar (fiebre negra)	Kala-azar (febbre d'Assam, splenomegalia infantile)	Kala-azar
Kératose (kératodermie)	Keratosis	Keratosis	Cheratosi	Keratoza
Kératose actinique	Actinic keratosis	Queratosis actínica	Cheratosi solare	Aktinička keratoza
Kératose séborrhéïque	Seborrheic keratosis	Queratosis seborreica	Cheratosi seborroica	Seboreična keratoza
Kernictère	Kernicterus	Kernicterus (encefalopatía neonatal bilirrubínica)	Kernittero (encefalopatia bilirubinica)	Žutica moždanih jezgri
Kuru	Kuru	Kuru (muerte de la risa)	Kuru	Kuru (smrtni smijeh)
Kyste	Cyst	Quiste	Cisti (ciste)	Cista
Kyste dermoïde	Dermoid cyst	Quiste dermoide	Cisti dermoide	Dermoidna cista
Kyste du canal thyréoglosse	Thyroglossal duct cyst	Quiste tirogloso	Cisti del dotto tirogloso	Cista na tireoglosnom vodu
Kyste du pancréas	Pancreatic cyst	Quiste de páncreas	Cisti pancreatica	Cista na gušterači
Kyste ovarien	Ovarian cyst	Quiste ovárico	Cisti ovarica	Cista na jajniku
Kyste pilonidal	Pilonidal cyst	Quiste pilonidal	Cisti pilonidale	Pilonidalna cista
Kyste rénal	Renal cyst	Quiste de riñón	Cisti renale	Cista na bubregu
Kyste sébacé	Sebaceous cyst (wen)	Quiste sebáceo	Cisti sebacea	Lojna cista
Kyste thyroïdien	Thyroid cyst	Quiste de tiroides	Cisti tiroidea	Cista na štitnjači
Kystome	Cystoma	Cistoma	Cistoma	Cistom
Lacération	Laceration (tear)	Laceración	Lacerazione (strappo)	Razderotina
Lacération cérébrale	Brain laceration	Laceración cerebral	Lacerazione cerebrale	Laceracija mozga
Lambliase (giardiase)	Lambliasis (giardiasis)	Giardiasis (lambliasis)	Giardiasi (lambliasi)	Lamblijaza (giardijaza)
Laryngospasme	Laryngospasm	Laringoespasmo	Laringospasmo	Laringospazam
Léiomyome	Leiomyoma	Leiomioma	Leiomioma	Lejomiom
Leiomyosarcome	Leiomyosarcoma	Leiomiosarcoma	Leiomiosarcoma	Lejomiosarkom
Leishmaniose	Leishmaniasis	Leishmaniasis	Leishmaniosi	Lišmenijaza
Leishmaniose cutanée (bouton d'Orient)	Cutaneous leishmaniasis (Oriental sore)	Leishmaniasis cutánea (uta)	Leishmaniosi cutanea	Orijentalni ulkus (kožna lišmenijaza)
Lèpre	Leprosy	Lepra	Lebbra	Lepra (guba)
Leptospirose	Leptospirosis	Leptospirosis	Leptospirosi	Leptospiroza
Lésion du nerf	Nerve lesion	Lesión de nervio	Lesione del nervo	Oštećenje živca (lezija živca)
Lésion du nerf périphérique	Peripheral nerve lesion	Lesión de nervio periférico	Lesione del nervo periferico	Oštećenje perifernog živca
Lésion due à un surmenage répétitif	Repetitive strain injury (cumulative trauma disorder)	Síndrome de sobreuso	R.S.I (Repetitive Strain Injury)	Sindrom prenaprezanja
Lésion obstructive de l'intestin grêle	Obstructive lesion of the small intestine	Lesión obstructiva del intestino delgado	Lesione ostruttiva dell'intestino tenue	Opstruktivna lezija tankog crijeva
Lésions mécaniques	Mechanical injuries	Lesiones mecánicas	Lesioni meccaniche	Mehaničke ozljede
Lésions provoquées par une explosion thermonucléaire	Thermonuclear injuries	Lesiones por una explosión termonuclear	Ferite provocate da esplosioni termonucleari	Termonuklearne ozljede
Lésions thermiques	Thermal injuries	Lesiones térmicas	Lesioni termiche	Termičke ozljede
Leucémie	Leukemia	Leucemia	Leucemia	Leukemija
Leucémie aiguë myéloblastique	Acute myeloid leukemia (AML)	Leucemia mieloide aguda	Leucemia mieloide acuta	Akutna mijeloična leukemija
Leucémie lymphoblastique aiguë	Acute lymphoblastic leukemia	Leucemia linfoblástica aguda	Leucemia acuta linfoblastica	Akutna limfatična leukemija
Leucémie lymphoïde	Lymphatic leukemia	Leucemia linfática	Leucemia linfatica	Limfatična leukemija

Français	Anglais	Espagnol	Italien	Croate
Leucémie lymphoïde chronique	Chronic lymphocytic leukemia	Leucemia linfocítica crónica	Leucemia linfatica cronica	Kronična limfocitna leukemija
Leucémie monocytique	Monocytic leukemia	Leucemia monocítica	Leucemia monocitica	Monocitična leukemija
Leucémie myéloïde	Myeloid leukemia	Leucemia mieloide	Leucemia mieloide	Mijeloična leukemija
Leucémie myéloïde chronique	Chronic myeloid leukemia	Leucemia mieloide crónica	Leucemia mieloide cronica	Kronična mijeloična leukemija
Leucocytose	Leukocytosis	Leucocitosis	Leucocitosi	Leukocitoza
Leucodystrophie	Leukodystrophy	Leucodistrofia	Leucodistrofia	Leukodistrofija
Leucoplasie	Leukoplakia	Leucoplaquia	Leucoplachia	Leukoplakija
Leucorrhée	Leukorrhea	Leucorrea	Leucorea	Bijelo pranje
Lichen plan	Lichen planus	Liquen plano	Lichen planus	Lišaj (lichen planus)
Lipodystrophie	Lipodystrophy	Lipodistrofia	Lipodistrofia	Lipodistrofija
Lipomatose du pancréas	Pancreatic lipomatosis	Lipomatosis pancreática (reemplazo graso del páncreas)	Lipomatosi pancreatica	Lipomatoza gušterače (masna infiltracija gusterače)
Lipome	Lipoma	Lipoma	Lipoma	Lipom
Liposarcome	Liposarcoma	Liposarcoma	Liposarcoma	Liposarkom
Listériose	Listeriosis	Listeriosis	Listeriosi	Listerioza
Lombalgie	Low back pain (lumbago, lumbosacral syndrome)	Dolor de espalda baja (lumbalgia)	Lombaggine	Križobolja (lumbosakralni sindrom)
Lombalgie du gymnaste	Gymnastics lower back pain	Espalda del gimnasta	Lombalgia dell'atleta	Gimnastičarska bolna križa
Lombalgie posturale	Postural back pain	Dolor de espalda postural	Mal di schiena su base posturale	Posturalna križobolja
Lordose	Lordosis	Lordosis	Lordosi	Lordoza
Lupus érythémateux	Lupus erythematosus	Lupus eritematoso sistémico	Lupus eritematoso sistemico	Sistemski lupus eritematozus
Luxation acromio-claviculaire	Separated shoulder (acromioclavicular dislocation)	Luxación de la articulación acromioclavicular	Lussazione acromio-clavicolare	Iščašenje akromio-klavikularnog zgloba
Luxation congénitale de la hanche	Congenital dysplasia of the hip (congenital hip dislocation)	Displasia congénita de la cadera (luxación congénita de cadera)	Lussazione congenita dell'anca (displasia dell'anca)	Urođeno iščašenje kuka (kongenitalna displazija kuka)
Luxation de l'épaule	Dislocated shoulder	Luxación del hombro	Lussazione della spalla	Iščašenje ramena
Luxation de la cheville	Dislocated ankle joint	Luxación del tobillo	Lussazione della caviglia	Iščašenje skočnog zgloba
Luxation de la hanche	Dislocation of a hip	Luxación de la cadera	Lussazione dell'anca	Iščašenje kuka
Luxation de la rotule	Luxating patella (trick knee, floating patella)	Luxación de la rótula	Lussazione della rotula	Iščašenje čašice
Luxation des doigts et du poignet	Hand and finger joints dislocation	Luxaciones de la mano y los dedos	Lussazioni delle atricolazioni della mano e delle dita	Iščašenje zglobova šake i prstiju
Luxation du coude	Elbow dislocation (luxation of the elbow)	Luxación del codo	Lussazione del gomito	Iščašenje lakta
Luxation du genou	Knee dislocation (luxation of the knee)	Luxación de la rodilla	Lussazione del ginocchio	Iščašenje koljena
Luxation incomplète (subluxation)	Partial dislocation (subluxation)	Desplazamiento de una articulación (subluxación)	Lussazione incompleta (sublussazione)	Djelomična dislokacija (subluksacija)
Luxation temporo-mandibulaire	Mandibular dislocation	Dislocación de la mandíbula	Lussazione della mandibola	Iščašenje vilice
Lymphadénite tuberculeuse	Tuberculous lymphadenitis	Tuberculosis ganglionar (linfadenitis tubercular)	Linfadenite tubercolare	Tuberkuloza limfnih čvorova
Lymphangiome	Lymphangioma	Linfangioma	Linfangioma	Limfangiom
Lymphangiosarcome	Lymphangiosarcoma	Linfangiosarcoma	Linfangiosarcoma	Limfangiosarkom
Lymphoedème	Lymphedema	Linfedema	Linfedema	Limfedem (zastoj limfe)
Lymphome	Lymphoma	Linfoma	Linfoma	Limfom
Lymphome non-Hodgkinien	Non-Hodgkin's lymphoma	Linfoma no-Hodgkin	Linfoma non Hodgkin	Non-Hodgkinov limfom
Mal à l'oreille (otalgie)	Ear pain (otalgia)	Dolor en oído (otalgia)	Dolore auricolare (otalgia)	Bol u uhu (otalgija)
Mal à la gorge (inflammattion du pharinx, pharingite)	Sore throat (inflammation of the throat, pharyngitis)	Mal de garganta (inflamación de la faringe, faringitis)	Mal di gola (inflammazione della faringe, faringite)	Upala grla (grlobolja, faringitis)
Mal aigu des montagnes	Altitude sickness (acute mountain sickness)	Mal de montaña (mal de altura)	Mal di montagna	Visinska bolest
Mal de dents	Toothache	Dolor de muelas	Mal di denti	Zubobolja
Mal de dos (dorsalgie)	Back pain (dorsalgia)	Dolor de espalda (dorsalgia)	Mal di schiena (dorsopatia)	Bol u leđima (dorzopatija)
Mal de mer	Seasickness	Mal de mar	Mal di mare	Morska bolest
Mal de Pott (tuberculose vertébrale)	Tuberculous spondylitis (Pott disease)	Espondilitis tuberculosa	Spondilite tubercolare (morbo di Pott)	Tuberkulozni spondilitis (Pottova bolest)
Mal de tête (céphalée)	Headache	Dolor de cabeza	Mal di testa	Glavobolja
Mal-voyance (amblyopie)	Lazy eye (amblyopia)	Ojo vago (ambliopía)	Ambliopia	Slabovidnost
Malabsorption	Malabsorption	Malabsorción	Malassorbimento	Malapsorpcija
Maladie auto-immune	Autoimmune disease	Enfermedad autoinmune	Malattia autoimmunitaria	Autoimunološka bolest
Maladie cardiaque (cardiopathie)	Heart disease (cardiopathy)	Enfermedad del corazón (cardiopatía)	Malattia del cuore (cardiopatia)	Srčana bolest (kardiopatija)
Maladie coeliaque	Coeliac disease (celiac disease)	Celiaquía (enfermedad celíaca)	Celiachia (malattia caliacha)	Celijakija
Maladie coronarienne	Coronary disease	Enfermedad coronaria	Coronaropatia	Koronarna bolest (koronaropatija)

Français	Anglais	Espagnol	Italien	Croate
Maladie d'Addison	Addison's disease	Enfermedad de Addison	Morbo di Addison	Addisonova bolest
Maladie d'Alzheimer	Alzheimer's diesase	Enfermedad de Alzheimer	Morbo di Alzheimer	Alzheimerova bolest
Maladie d'Osgood-Schlatter	Osgood-Schlatter disease (rugby knee)	Enfermedad de Osgood-Schlatter	Sindrome di Osgood-Schlatter	Osgood-Schlatterova bolest
Maladie de Basedow	Basedow Graves disease	Enfermedad de Graves Basedow	Morbo di Basedow-Graves	Basedowljeva bolest
Maladie de Behçet	Behçet's disease	Síndrome de Behçet	Sindrome di Behçet	Behçetova bolest
Maladie de Blount	Blount's disease	Enfermedad de Blount (tibia vara)	Sindrome di Blount	Blountova bolest
Maladie de Bornholm (myalgie épidémique)	Bornholm disease (epidemic myalgia)	Enfermedad de Bornholm (mialgia epidémica)	Malattia di Bornholm (mialgia epidemica)	Bornholmska bolest (epidemijska mialgija)
Maladie de Bowen	Bowen's disease (squamous cell carcinoma in situ)	Enfermedad de Bowen	Morbo di Bowen	Bowenova bolest
Maladie de Brill-Zinserr (typhus résurgent)	Brill's disease	Enfermedad de Brill	Malattia di Brill-Zinsser	Brillova bolest (Brill-Zinsserova bolest)
Maladie de Buerger (thromboangéite oblitérante)	Buerger's disease (thromboangiitis obliterans)	Enfermedad de Buerger (tromboangeítis obliterante)	Morbo di Buerger	Buergerova bolest
Maladie de Chagas (trypanosomiase américaine)	Chagas disease (American trypanosomiasis)	Enfermedad de Chagas (tripanosomiasis americana)	Malattia di Chagas	Chagasova bolest (americka tripanosomijaza)
Maladie de Charcot-Marie- Tooth	Charcot-Marie-Tooth disease	Enfermedad de Charcot-Marie Tooth	Malattia di Charcot-Marie-Tooth	Bolest Charcot-Marie-Tooth
Maladie de Creutzfeldt-Jakob	Creutzfeldt-Jakob disease (so called "mad cow disease")	Enfermedad de Creutzfeldt-Jakob	Malattia di Creutzfeldt-Jakob (cosiddetta "malattia della mucca pazza")	Creutzfeldt-Jakobova bolest (tzv. "kravlje ludilo")
Maladie de Crohn	Crohn's disease	Enfermedad de Crohn	Malattia di Crohn	Crohnova bolest
Maladie de décompression (maladie des plongeurs, maladie des caissons)	Decompression sickness (diver's disease, caisson disease)	Síndrome de decompresión (enfermedad de los buzos, mal de presión)	Malattia di decompressione (sindrome di Caisson)	Dekompresijska bolest (kesonska bolest)
Maladie de Freiberg	Freiberg's disease	Enfermedad de Freiberg	Malattia di Freiberg	Freibergova bolest
Maladie de Haglund	Haglund's disease	Enfermedad de Haglund (deformidad de Haglund)	Malattia di Haglund (deformità di Haglund)	Haglundova bolest
Maladie de Hirschsprung (mégacolôn)	Hirschsprung's disease (congenital aganglionic megacolon)	Enfermedad de Hirschsprung (megacolon agangliónico)	Malattia di Hirschsprung (malattia di Mya)	Hirschsprungova bolest (kongenitalni aganglionarni megakolon)
Maladie de Hodgkin	Hodgkin's disease	Enfermedad de Hodgkin	Linfoma di Hodgkin	Hodgkinova bolest
Maladie de Hoffa	Hoffa's disease	Enfermedad de Hoffa	Sindrome di Hoffa	Morbus Hoffa
Maladie de Kawasaki	Kawasaki disease	Enfermedad de Kawasaki	Sindrome di Kawasaki	Kawasakijeva bolest (mukokutani limfo-glandularni sindrom)
Maladie de Kienböck	Kienböck's disease	Enfermedad de Kienböck	Morbo di Kienböck	Kienböckova bolest
Maladie de Köhler	Köhler disease	Enfermedad de Köhler	Malattia di Köhler	Köhlerova bolest
Maladie de La Peyronie	Peyronie's disease (induratio penis plastica)	Enfermedad de La Peyronie (induración plástica del pene)	Induratio penis plastica (malattia di Peyronie)	Plastična induracija penisa
Maladie de Legg-Calvé-Perthes (ostéochondrite primitive de hanche)	Legg-Calvé-Perthes disease	Síndrome de Legg-Calvé-Perthes	Malattia di Legg-Perthes-Calvé	Legg-Calvé-Perthesova bolest
Maladie de Lyme	Lyme disease (lyme borreliosis)	Enfermedad de Lyme (borreliosis de Lyme)	Malattia di Lyme (borreliosi di Lyme)	Lajmska bolest (Lajmska borelioza)
Maladie de Menière	Meniere's disease	Enfermedad de Menière	Sindrome di Menière	Menierova bolest
Maladie de Morquio (mucopolysaccharidose type IV)	Morquio's syndrome (mucopolysaccharidosis IV)	Enfermedad de Morquio (mucopolisacaridosis tipo IV)	Malattia di Morquio (mucopolisaccaridosi IV)	Sindrom Morquio (mukopolisaharidoza tip IV)
Maladie de Paget	Paget's disease	Enfermedad de Paget	Morbo di Paget	Pagetova bolest
Maladie de Panner	Panner's disease	Enfermedad de Panner	Malattia di Panner	Pannerova bolest
Maladie de Parkinson	Parkinson's disease	Enfermedad de Parkinson	Morbo di Parkinson	Parkinsonova bolest
Maladie de Pellegrini-Stieda	Pellegrini-Stieda disease	Enfermedad de Pellegrini-Stieda	Malattia di Pellegrini-Stieda	Bolest Pellegrini-Stieda
Maladie de Preiser	Preiser disease	Enfermedad de Preiser	Sindrome di Preiser	Morbus Preiser
Maladie de Raynaud	Raynaud's disease	Enfermedad de Raynaud	Sindrome di Raynaud	Raynaudova bolest
Maladie de Sever	Sever's disease	Enfermedad de Sever	Malattia di Sever	Severova bolest
Maladie de Van Neck-Odelberg	Van Neck disease	Enfermedad de Van Neck	Malattia di Van Neck	Morbus Van Neck
Maladie de Whipple	Whipple's disease	Enfermedad de Whipple	Morbo di Whipple	Whippleova bolest
Maladie des exostoses multiples	Hereditary multiple exostoses	Exostosis múltiple hereditaria	Esostosi multipla ereditaria	Multiple egzostoze
Maladie des membranes hyalines (détresse respiratoire néonatale)	Hyaline membrane disease (infant respiratory distress syndrome)	Enfermedad de la membrana hialina (síndrome de distrés respiratorio)	Sindrome da distress respiratorio del neonato (malattia da membrane ialine polmonari)	Bolest hijaline membrane (respiratorni sindrom novorođenčeta)
Maladie des ouvriers des silos	Silo-filler's disease	Enfermedad de los ensiladores	Malattia dei riempitori dei silos	Silosna pluća
Maladie des vibrations	Vibration disease	Enfermedad de las vibraciones	Malattia da vibrazioni	Vibracijska bolest

Français	Anglais	Espagnol	Italien	Croate
Maladie du cri du chat (syndrome de Lejeune)	Cat cry syndrome (5p minus syndrome, Lejeune's syndrome)	Síndrome del maullido del gato (síndrome de Lejeune)	Sindrome del grido di gatto	Sindrom mačjeg krika
Maladie du motoneurone	Motor neurone disease	Enfermedad de la motoneurona	Malattia del motoneurone	Bolest motornog neurona
Maladie du poumon de fermier	Farmer's lung	Pulmón de granjero	Febbre da fieno	Farmerska pluća
Maladie du sommeil (trypanosomiase africaine)	African trypanosomiasis (sleeping sickness)	Tripanosomiasis africana (enfermedad del sueño)	Tripanosomiasi africana (malattia del sonno)	Afrička tripanosomijaza (bolest spavanja)
Maladie hémolytique du nouveau-né	Rh incompatibility (hemolytic disease of the newborn)	Enfermedad hemolítica del recién nacido (incompatibilidad Rh)	Eritroblastosi fetale (malattia emolitica del neonato)	Rh-inkompatibilnost (hemolitička bolest novorođenčeta)
Maladie occlusive aorto-iliaque	Aortoiliac occlusive disease (Leriche's syndrome)	Síndrome de Leriche	Sindrome di Leriche	Lericheov sindrom
Maladie parasitique (parasitose)	Parasitic disease (parasitosis)	Enfermedad parasitaria (parasitosis)	Malattia parassitaria (parassitosi)	Parazitarna bolest (parazitoza)
Maladie pelvienne inflammatoire	Pelvic inflammatory disease	Enfermedad pélvica inflamatoria	Malattia infiammatoria pelvica	Upalna bolest zdjelice
Maladie professionnelle	Occupational disease	Enfermedad profesional	Malattia professionale	Profesionalno oboljenje
Maladie pulmonaire interstitielle	Interstitial lung disease	Enfermedad pulmonar intersticial	Pneumopatia interstiziale	Intersticijska bolest pluća
Maladie vénérienne	Sexually transmitted disease	Enfermedad de transmisión sexual	Malattia sessualmente trasmissibile	Spolno prenosiva bolest
Maladies de l'aorte	Diseases of the aorta	Enfermedades de la aorta	Malattie dell'aorta	Bolesti aorte
Maladies des vaisseaux sanguins	Blood vessel diseases	Enfermedades de los vasos sanguíneos	Malattie dei vasi sanguigni	Bolesti krvnih žila
Maladies des valves cardiaques	Heart valve diseases	Enfermedades de las válvulas del corazón	Malattie delle valvole cardiache	Bolesti srčanih zalistaka
Maladies infectieuses des enfants	Childhood infectious diseases	Enfermedades infantiles contagiosas	Malattie infettive dei bambini	Dječje zarazne bolesti
Malaria	Malaria	Malaria (paludismo)	Malaria	Malarija
Malformation congénitale du coeur	Congenital heart defect	Malformación cardiaca congénita	Difetto cardiaco congenito	Urođena srčana greška
Malnutrition	Underfedness (malnutrition)	Desnutrición	Sottopeso (grave magrezza)	Neuhranjenost
Manie	Mania	Manía	Mania	Manija
Mastopathie	Mastopathy	Mastopatía	Mastopatia	Mastopatija
Mastopathie fibrocystique	Fibrocystic breast disease	Mastitis quística crónica (enfermedad fibroquística)	Mastopatia fibrocistica	Fibrocistična bolest dojke
Mauvaise heleine (halitose)	Bad breath (halitosis)	Mal aliento (halitosis)	Odore sgradevole dell'alito (alitosi, bromopnea)	Zadah iz usta (halitoza)
Mauvaise vision de près liée à l'âge (presbytie)	Age-related long-sightedness (presbyopia)	Vista cansada por la edad (presbiopía)	Presbiopia (presbitismo)	Staračka dalekovidnost (prezbiopija)
Médulloblastome	Medulloblastoma	Meduloblastoma	Medulloblastoma	Meduloblastom
Mégacolôn	Megacolon	Megacolon	Megacolon	Megakolon
Mélanome	Melanoma	Melanoma	Melanoma	Melanom
Mélioïdose	Melioidosis (Whitmore disease)	Melioidosis	Melioidosi	Melioidoza
Membres sourds	Dullness in limbs	Torpeza en las extremidades	Ottusità alle estremità	Tupost u udovima
Méningiome	Meningioma	Meningioma	Meningioma	Meningeom
Méningo-encéphalite amibienne primaire	Primary amoebic meningoencephalitis	Meningoencefalitis amebiana primaria	Meningoencefalite amebica primaria	Primarni amebni meningoencefalitis
Méningocèle	Meningocele	Meningocele	Meningocele	Meningokela
Méningoencéphalite à tique	Tick-borne meningoencephalitis	Meningoencefalitis de garrapata	Encefalite trasmessa da zecche	Krpeljni meningoencefalitis
Méningoencphalocèle	Meningoencephalocele	Meningoencefalocele	Meningoencefalocele	Meningoencefalokela
Meniscopathie	Meniscal disease	Meniscopatia	Meniscopatia	Meniskopatija
Ménopause	Menopause	Menopausia	Menopausa	Menopauza (klimakterij)
Mésothéliome	Mesothelioma	Mesotélioma	Mesotelioma	Mezoteliom
Mésothéliome sarcomatoïde	Sarcomatoid mesothelioma	Mesotélioma sarcomatoide	Mesotelioma sarcomatoide	Mezoteliosarkom
Métabolisme basal diminué	Slow basal metabolism	Metabolismo basal lento	Basso metabolismo basale	Usporen bazalni metabolizam
Metabolisme de base accéléré	Accelerated basal metabolism	Metabolismo basal acelerado	Metabolismo basale accelerato	Ubrzan bazalni metabolizam
Métastase	Metastasis	Metástasis	Metastasi	Metastaza
Métatarsalgie	Metatarsalgia (Morton's neuroma)	Metatarsalgia	Metatarsalgia	Metatarzalgija (Mortonova metatarzalgija)
Météoropathie	Meteoropathy	Meteoropatía	Meteoropatia	Meteoropatija
Miction fréquente	Frequent urination	Micción frecuente	Urinazione frequente (pollachiuria)	Učestalo mokrenje
Migraine	Migraine	Migraña (jaqueca)	Emicrania	Migrena
Miliarie rouge	Miliaria rubra (sweat rash)	Miliaria rubra (sarpullido por el calor)	Miliaria rubra	Milijarija rubra
Milium (grutum, acné miliaire)	Milia (milk spots)	Milium (milia)	Acne miliare	Milije (dječje akne)
Mobilité atriculaire limitée	Limited joint mobility	Rango de movimiento articular limitado	Ridotta mobilità articolare	Ograničena pokretljivost zgloba

Français	Anglais	Espagnol	Italien	Croate
Molluscum contagiosum	Molluscum contagiosum	Molusco contagioso	Mollusco contagioso	Molusk
Molluscum pendulum (acrochordon)	Soft fibroma (fibroma molle, acrochordon)	Fibroma blando (fibroma molle)	Mollusco pendule (fibroma molle)	Kožni privjesak (mekani fibrom)
Mononucléose infectieuse (maladie du baiser, maladie des amoureux)	Infectious mononucleosis (Pfeiffer's disease, kissing disease, glandular fever)	Mononucleosis infecciosa (fiebre glandular, enfermedad de Pfeiffer)	Mononucleosi infettiva (malattia del bacio)	Mononukleoza (bolest poljupca)
Morsure	Bite	Mordedura	Morsicatura	Ugriz
Morsure d'un animal infecté par le virus de la rage	Bite by rabies infected animal	Mordedura de un animal enfermo de rabia	Morsicatura di animale rabbioso	Ugriz bijesne životinje
Morsure de chat	Cat bite	Mordedura de gato	Morsicatura di gatto	Ugriz mačke
Morsure de chien	Dog bite	Mordedura de perro	Morsicatura di cane	Ugriz psa
Morsure de rat	Rat bite	Mordedura de rata	Morsicatura di ratto	Ugriz štakora
Morsure de veuve noire	Black widow bite	Mordedura de viuda negra	Morso della vedova nera	Ugriz crne udovice
Morsure de vipère	Snake bite	Mordedura de víbora	Morsicatura di serpenti	Ugriz zmije
Morsure humaine	Human bite	Mordedura humana	Morsicatura di uomo	Ugriz čovjeka (ljudski ugriz)
Mort	Death	Muerte	Morte	Smrt
Mort naturelle	Natural death	Muerte natural	Morte naturale	Prirodna smrt
Mort violente	Violent death	Muerte violenta	Morte violenta	Nasilna smrt
Morve	Glanders	Muermo	Morva umana	Sakagija
Mouvements involontaires anarchiques des globes oculaires (opsoclonus)	Uncontrolled eye movement (opsoclonus)	Movimientos involuntarios y rápidos de los ojos (opsoclonus)	Movimenti incontrollati degli occhi (opsoclono)	Nekontrirani pokreti očiju (opsoklonus)
Mucocèle	Mucocele	Mucocele	Mucocele	Mukocela
Mucopolysaccharidose	Mucopolysaccharidosis	Mucopolisacaridosis	Mucopolisaccaridosi	Mukopolisaharidoza
Mucoviscidose (fibrose kystique)	Cystic fibrosis	Fibrosis quística (mucoviscidosis)	Fibrosi cistica	Cistična fibroza
Mucus dans les selles	Mucus in stool	Moco en las heces	Muco nelle feci	Sluzava stolica
Mucus nasal	Nasal secretion (mucus)	Moco (mucus) nasal	Muco nasale	Sekrecija iz nosa
Muscle flasque (hypotonie musculaire)	Flaccid muscle (untoned muscle)	Músculo flácido	Muscolo flaccido	Mlohavi mišić
Myalgie cervicale	Neck myalgia	Mialgia cervical	Mialgia cervicale	Mijalgični sindrom vrata
Myasthénie grave	Myasthenia gravis	Miastenia gravis	Miastenia gravis	Miastenija gravis
Mycétome	Mycetoma	Micetoma	Micetoma	Micetoma
Mycose	Mycosis	Micosis	Micosi	Mikoza
Myéloméningocèle	Meningomyelocele	Mielomeningocele	Mielomeningocele	Meningomijelokela
Myoclonie	Myoclonic twitches (myoclonus)	Mioclono	Mioclono	Miokloničko trzanje (mioklonus)
Myogélose	Myogelosis	Miogelosis	Miogelosi	Miogeloza
Myome	Myoma	Mioma	Mioma	Miom
Myopathie de Duchenne	Duchenne muscular dystrophy	Distrofia muscular de Duchenne	Distrofia di Duchenne	Duchenneova mišićna distrofija
Myopie	Shortsightedness (myopia)	Miopía	Miopia	Kratkovidnost
Myosarcome	Myosarcoma	Miosarcoma	Miosarcoma	Miosarkom
Myosite ossifiante	Myositis ossificans	Miositis osificante	Miosite ossificante	Osificirajući miozitis
Myosite ossifiante progressive	Myositis ossificans progressiva	Miositis osificante progresiva	Miosite ossificante progressiva	Progresivno okoštavanje mišića
Myxoedème	Myxedema	Mixedema	Mixedema	Miksedem
Myxome	Myxoma	Mixoma	Mixoma	Miksom
Myxosarcome	Myxosarcoma	Mixosarcoma	Mixosarcoma	Miksosarkom
Nanisme	Dwarfism (nanism)	Enanismo	Nanismo	Patuljasti rast (nanizam)
Narcolepsie (maladie de Gélineau)	Narcolepsy	Narcolepsia (síndrome de Gelineau, epilepsia del sueño)	Narcolessia	Narkolepsija
Nausée	Nausea	Náusea	Nausea	Mučnina
Nécrose	Necrosis	Necrosis	Necrosi	Nekroza
Nécrose fibrinoïde	Fibrinoid necrosis	Necrosis fibrinoide	Necrosi fibrinoide	Fibrinoidna nekroza
Néphrite interstitielle	Interstitial nephritis	Nefritis intersticial	Nefrite interstiziale	Intersticijska upala bubrega
Néphropathie diabétique	Diabetic nephropathy	Nefropatía diabética	Nefropatia diabetica	Dijabetična nefropatija
Néphrose	Nephrosis	Nefrosis	Nefrosi	Nefroza
Neurasthénie	Neurasthenia	Neurastenia	Nevrastenia	Neurastenija
Neurinome	Neurinoma	Neurinoma	Neurinoma (Schwannoma)	Neurinom
Neuroblastome	Neuroblastoma	Neuroblastoma	Neuroblastoma	Neuroblastom
Neuroborréliose	Neuroborreliosis	Neuroborreliosis	Neuroborreliosi	Neuroborelioza
Neurofibromatose de type 1 (maladie de Von Recklinghausen)	Neurofibromatosis type1 (Von Recklinghausen's disease)	Neurofibromatosis de tipo 1 (enfermedad de Von Recklinghausen)	Neurofibromatosi di tipo1 (malattia di von Recklinghausen)	Von Recklinghausenova bolest
Neurome	Neuroma	Neuroma	Neuroma	Neurom
Neurome acoustique	Acoustic neuroma	Neuroma acústico	Neuroma dell'acustico	Neurom slušnog živca
Neuropathie	Neuropathy	Neuropatía	Neuropatia	Neuropatija
Neuropathie diabétique	Diabetic neuropathy	Neuropatía diabética	Neuropatia diabetica	Dijabetična neuropatija
Névralgie	Neuralgia	Neuralgia	Nevralgia	Neuralgija
Névralgie des nerfs crâniens	Cranial neuralgia	Neuralgia craneal	Nevralgia del nervo cranico	Neuralgija moždanih živaca
Névralgie du trijumeau (névralgie trigéminale)	Trigeminal neuralgia	Neuralgia del trigémino	Nevralgia del trigemino	Neuralgija trigeminusa

Français	Anglais	Espagnol	Italien	Croate
Nèvralgie occipitale	Occipital neuralgia (Arnold's neuralgia)	Síndrome occipital (neuralgia occipital)	Nevralgia occipitale (nevralgia di Arnold)	Okcipitalna neuralgija
Névrose (neurose)	Neurosis	Neurosis	Nevrosi	Neuroza
Nodule	Knot (lump)	Nudo	Nodo (nodulo)	Kvržica
Nodule de Soeur Marie Joseph (métastase cutanée ombilicale)	Sister Mary Joseph nodule	Nódulo de la hermana María José	Nodulo di Suor Maria Giuseppa	Čvor sestre Mary Joseph (umbilikalna metastaza)
Nodules d'Heberden	Heberden's nodes	Nódulos de Heberden	Noduli di Heberden	Heberdenovi čvorići
Nodules de Bouchard	Bouchard's nodes	Nudosidades de Bouchard	Noduli di Bouchard	Bouchardovi čvorići
Noyade	Drowning	Ahogamiento	Affogamento	Utapanje
Nystagmus	Nystagmus	Nistagmo	Nistagmo	Nistagmus
Obésité	Obesity	Obesidad	Obesità	Debljina (gojaznost)
Occlusion de l'artère de la rétine	Retinal artery occlusion	Oclusión de la arteria de la retina	Occlusione arteria retinica	Blokada mrežnične arterije
Oedème	Edema	Edema (hidropesía)	Edema	Edem
Oedème cérébral	Cerebral edema	Edema cerebral	Edema cerebrale	Edem mozga
Oedème de Quincke (angio-oedème)	Angioedema (angioneurotic edema)	Angioedema (edema de Quincke)	Angioedema (edema di Quincke, edema angioneurotico)	Angioedem (Quinckeov edem, angioneurotski edem)
Oedème du nerf optique	Optic nerve edema	Edema del nervio óptico	Papilledema (edema del nervo ottico)	Otok očnog živca (zastojna papila)
Oedème généralisé (anasarque)	Generalized edema (anasarca)	Anasarca	Edema diffuso (anasarca)	Generalizirani edem (anasarka)
Oedème postural	Postural edema	Edema postural	Edema posturale	Posturalni edem (statički edem)
Oedème pulmonaire	Pulmonary edema	Edema pulmonar	Edema polmonare	Plućni edem
Oeil sec (kératoconjonctivite sèche)	Dry eyes (keratoconjunctivitis sicca)	Sequedad de los ojos (xeroftalmia)	Occhi secchi (xeroftalmia)	Suhe oči (kseroftalmija)
Oligodendrocytome	Oligodendroglioma	Oligodendroglioma	Oligodendroglioma	Oligodendrogliom
Oligoménorrhée	Oligomenorrhea	Oligomenorrea	Oligomenorrea	Oligomenoreja
Onchocercose (cécité des rivières)	Onchocerciasis (river blindness)	Oncocercosis	Oncocercosi (cecità fluviale)	Onkocerkijaza (riječno sljepilo)
Ongle incarné (onychocryptose)	Ingrown nail (onychocryptosis, unguis incarnatus)	Uña encarnada (onicocriptosis)	Unghia incarnita (onicocriptosi)	Urasli nokat (ungvis inkarnatus)
Oreillons (parotidite virale)	Mumps (epidemic parotitis)	Paperas (parotiditis)	Parotite (orecchioni)	Zaušnjaci (mumps, parotitis)
Ostéite fibrokystique	Osteitis fibrosa cystica	Ostéitis fibrosa quística	Osteitis fibrosa cistica	Fibrozna cistična upala kosti
Ostéo-arthropathie hypertrophiante de Pierre Marie (syndrome de Marie-Bamberger)	Hyperthropic osteoarthropaty (Pierre Marie-Bamberger syndrome)	Osteoartropatía hipertrófica (enfermedad de Bamberger-Marie)	Osteoartropatia ipertrofizzante (sindrome di Pierre Marie-Bamberger)	Osteoartropatija hipertrofika Pierre Marie
Ostéochondrome	Osteochondroma	Osteocondroma	Osteocondroma	Osteohondrom
Ostéochondrose juvénile	Juvenile osteochondrosis	Osteocondrosis juvenil	Osteocondrite dissecante	Juvenilna osteohondroza
Ostéogenèse imparfaite	Osteogenesis imperfecta (brittle bone disease)	Osteogénesis imperfecta (huesos de cristal)	Osteogenesi imperfetta	Osteogeneza imperfekta (staklaste kosti)
Ostéomalacie	Osteomalacia	Osteomalacia	Osteomalacia	Osteomalacija
Ostéome	Osteoma	Osteoma	Osteoma	Osteom
Ostéomyélite fongique	Fungal osteomyelitis	Osteomielitis micótica	Osteomielite fungale	Gljivični osteomijelitis
Ostéomyélite syphilitique	Luetic osteomyelitis	Osteomielitis luética	Osteomielite luetica	Luetični osteomijelitis
Ostéopétrose (os de marbre)	Osteopetrosis (marble bone disease)	Osteopetrosis (enfermedad de los huesos de marmol)	Osteopetrosi (malattia delle ossa di marmo)	Osteopetroza (zadebljane kosti, bolest mramornih kostiju)
Ostéoporose	Osteoporosis	Osteoporosis	Osteoporosi	Osteoporoza
Ostéosarcome	Osteosarcoma	Osteosarcoma	Osteosarcoma	Osteosarkom
Ostéosclérose	Osteosclerosis	Osteosclerosis	Osteosclerosi	Osteoskleroza
Pâleur	Paleness (pallor)	Palidez	Pallore	Bljedilo
Palpitation	Palpitation	Palpitación	Cardiopalmo (palpitazione)	Lupanje srca (palpitacije)
Panaris	Whitlow (felon)	Panadizo	Patereccio	Panaricij
Pancréas aberrant	Aberrant pancreas	Pancreas aberrante	Pancraes aberrante	Aberantni pankreas
Papillome	Papilloma	Papiloma	Papilloma	Papilom
Paracoccidioidose brésilienne	Paracoccidioidomycosis (Brazilian blastomycosis)	Paracoccidioidomicosis	Paracoccidioidimicosi (blastomicosi sudamericana)	Parakokcidioidomikoza (brazilska blastomikoza)
Paragonimiase humaine	Paragonimiasis	Paragonimosis (paragonimiasis)	Paragonimiasi	Paragonimijaza
Paralysie	Paralysis	Parálisis	Paralisi	Paraliza (oduzetost, kljenut)
Paralysie de Bell	Bell's palsy	Parálisis de Bell	Paralisi di Bell	Bellova paraliza
Paralysie de la moitié du corps (hémiplégie)	Paralysis of one half of a body (hemiplegia)	Parálisis de una mitad lateral de cuerpo (hemiplejía)	Paralisi di una metà del corpo (emiplegia)	Oduzetost jedne polovine tijela (hemiplegija)
Paralysie des membres inférieurs (paraplégie)	Paralysis of lower extremities (paraplegia)	Parálisis de la parte inferior del cuerpo (paraplejía)	Paralisi di parte inferiore del corpo (paraplegia)	Oduzetost donjih ekstremiteta (paraplegija)
Paralysie des quatre membres (tétraplégie)	Paralysis of all limbs and torso (quadriplegia, tetraplegia)	Parálisis en brazos y piernas (tetraplejía, cuadriplejía)	Paralisi dei arti superiori e inferiori(quadriplegia)	Oduzetost gornjih i donjih ekstremiteta i torza(kvadriplegija, tetraplegija)

Français	Anglais	Espagnol	Italien	Croate
Paralysie des régions symétriques du corps (diplégie)	Paralysis of symmetrical parts of the body (diplegia)	Parálisis de partes simétricas del cuerpo (diplejía)	Paralisi di una parte di corpo simmetrica (diplegia)	Oduzetost simetričnih dijelova tijela (diplegija)
Paranoïa	Paranoia	Paranoia	Paranoia	Paranoja
Paraphimosis	Paraphimosis	Parafimosis	Parafimosi	Parafimoza
Parésie	Paresis	Paresis	Paresi	Pareza
Parodontite	Periodontitis	Periodontitis (piorrea)	Parodontite	Parodontoza
Paronychie	Paronychia	Paroniquia	Paronichia	Paronihija
Paumes des mains chaudes et humides	Warm sweaty palms	Palmas de las manos calientes y mojadas	Palmi delle mani caldi e sudati	Topli i vlažni dlanovi
Pectus carinatum	Pigeon chest (pectus carinatum)	Pectus carinatum	Petto carenato	Kokošja prsa
Pellicule	Dandruff	Caspa	Forfora	Perut
Pemphigus	Pemphigus	Pénfigo	Pemfigo	Pemfigus
Perforation d'ulcère	Perforated ulcer	Úlcera perforada	Ulcera perforata	Puknuće čira (perforacija ulkusa)
Perforation du tympan	Perforated eardrum (tympanorrhexis)	Perforación del tímpano	Perforazione del timpano	Puknuće bubnjića (perforacija bubnjića, timpanoreksija)
Périostite tibiale	Shin splints	Dolor en las espinillas	Sindrome da stress tibiale mediale	Trkačka potkoljenica
Persistance du canal artériel	Patent ductus arteriosus (persistent ductus arteriosus)	Ductus arterioso persistente (conducto arterioso persistente)	Dotto arterioso persistente (ductus arteriosus persistente)	Otvoreni ductus arteriosus (Ductus arteriosus persistens)
Personnalité borderline	Borderline personality disorder	Trastorno límite de la personalidad	Disturbo borderline di personalità	Granični poremećaj osobnosti
Perte d'appétit	Loss of appetite	Pérdida de apetito	Mancanza dell'appetito	Gubitak apetita
Perte d'habileté d'expression du langage (mutisme, aphasie)	Loss of language ability (aphasia)	Pérdida de capacidad de producir lenguaje (afasia)	Perdita di abilità di produzione del linguaggio verbale (afasia)	Gubitak sposobnosti govora (afazija)
Perte d'ouïe	Hearing loss	Pérdida de la capacidad auditiva	Perdita di udito	Gubitak sluha
Perte de cheveux excessive	Increased hair loss	Aumento de la cáida del cabello	Aumento di perdita di capelli	Pojačano opadanje kose
Perte de l'audition liée à l'age (presbyacousie)	Age-related hearing loss (presbycusis)	Trastorno de la capacidad para oír de las personas envejecen (presbiacusia)	Perdita dell'udito dovuta all'avanzamento dell'età (presbiacusia)	Staračka nagluhost (prezbiakuzija)
Perte de la sensibilité aux odeurs (anosmie)	Loss of olfaction (anosmia)	Pérdida del sentido del olfato (anosmia)	Incapacità di percipire gli odori (disosmia)	Gubitak osjeta mirisa
Perte de la vue dans une moitié du champ visuel (hémianopsie)	Loss of half of a field of vision (hemianopsia)	Pérdida de la mitad del campo visual (hemianopsia)	Perdita di metà di campo visivo (emianopsia)	Gubitak polovice vidnog polja (hemianopsija)
Perte de mémoire	Memory loss	Pérdida de la memoria	Perdita di memoria	Gubitak pamćenja
Perte du sens du goût (agueusie)	Loss of the sense of taste (ageusia)	Pérdida del sentido del gusto (ageusia)	Incapacità di percipire i sapori (ageusia)	Gubitak osjeta okusa
Perte du sens du toucher	Loss of the sense of touch	Pérdida del sentido del tacto	Perdita di senso di tocco	Gubitak osjeta dodoira
Pertes vaginales	Vaginal discharge	Flujo vaginal	Fuoriuscita vaginale	Vaginalni iscjedak
Peste	Plague (pest)	Peste	Peste (pestilenza)	Kuga
Pet (flatulence, vesse)	Passing gas (flatulence, farting)	Tener gases (flatulencia)	Miscela di gas (flatulenza)	Puštanje vjetra (flatulencija, plinovi)
Pétéchie	Petechia	Petequia	Petecchia	Petehije
Pharyngite streptococcique	Streptococcal pharyngitis	Faringitis por estreptococo	Faringite streptococcica	Streptokokna angina
Phase prodromique	Early symptom (prodrome)	Síndrome prodrómico	Sindrome prodromica	Predsimptom bolesti prije nego se bolest razvije
Phénomène de Bell	Bell's phenomenon	Fenómeno de Bell	Fenomeno di Bell	Bellov fenomen
Phénylcétonurie	Phenylketonuria	Fenilcetonuria	Fenilchetonuria	Fenilketonurija
Phéochromocytome	Pheochromocytoma	Feocromocitoma	Feocromocitoma	Feokromocitom (tumor srži nadbubrežne žlijezde)
Phimosis	Phimosis	Fimosis	Fimosi	Fimoza
Phlébothrombose	Phlebothrombosis	Flebotrombosis	Flebotrombosi	Flebotromboza
Phlegmon	Phlegmon	Flegmón	Flemmone	Flegmona
Phlyctène (ampoule, cloque)	Blister	Ampolla	Vescichetta (bolla)	Plik
Phobie	Phobia	Fobia	Fobia	Fobija
Photophobie (crainte de la lumière)	Photophobia (fear of light)	Fotofobia (intolerancia a la luz)	Fotofobia	Fotofobija (strah od svjetla)
Pian	Yaws (pian)	Pian (frambesia)	Framboesia	Frambezija
Pied calcanéus	Pes calcaneus	Pie calcáneo	Piede calcaneo	Petno stopalo
Pied creux	High arches (pes cavus)	Pie cavo (pes cavus)	Piede cavo (pes cavus)	Izdubljeno stopalo (pes excavatus)
Pied d'athlète (tinea pedis)	Athlete's foot (tinea pedis)	Tiña del pie (pie de atleta, tinea pedis)	Piede d'atleta (tinea pedis)	Atletsko stopalo (gljivična infekcija stopala, tinea pedis)
Pied-bot (pied-bot équin)	Club foot (talipes equinovarus)	Pie equinovaro (talipes equinovarus, pie bot, pie retorcido)	Piede equino (talipes equinovarus)	Čopavo stopalo (uvrnuto stopalo, pes equinovarus)

Français	Anglais	Espagnol	Italien	Croate
Pied equin	Dancer's foot (pes equinus)	Pie equino	Piede equino	Balerinsko stopalo (pes equinus)
Pied plat (pes planus)	Flat foot (pes planus)	Pie plano (pes planus, arcos vencidos)	Piede piatto (pes planus)	Spušteno stopalo (pes planus)
Pied valgus	Pes valgus	Pie valgo	Piede piatto valgo (pes valgus)	Izvrnuto stopalo (pes valgus)
Pilosité excessive (hypertrichose)	Increased hairiness (hypertrichosis)	Exceso de cabello (hipertricosis)	Aumento della pelosità (ipertricosi)	Pojačana dlakavost
Pince de homard (aplasie digitale, ectrodactylie)	Split foot (lobster claw foot, ectrodactyly)	Ectrodactilia en pie	Lobster-claw deformità di piede	Lobster Claw stopalo
Pinta	Pinta	Pinta	Pinta	Pinta
Piqûre d'araignée	Spider bite	Picadura de araña	Morsicatura di ragno	Ugriz pauka
Piqûre de fourmi	Ant sting	Picadura de hormiga	Puntura di formiche	Ugriz mrava
Piqûre de moustique infecté	Infected mosquito bite	Picadura de mosquito infectado	Puntura di zanzara infetta	Ugriz zaraženog komarca
Piqûre de scorpion	Scorpion sting	Picadura de escorpión	Puntura di scorpione	Ugriz škorpiona
Piqûre de tique infectée	Infected tick bite	Picadura de garrapata infectada	Morsicatura di zecca infetta	Ugriz zaraženog krpelja
Pityriasis versicolor	Tinea versicolor (pityriasis versicolor, haole rot)	Tiña versicolor (pitiriasis versicolor)	Pitiriasi versicolor (tinea versicolor)	Pitirijaza (svjetlije mrlje na osunčanoj koži, Tinea versicolor)
Plaie	Wound (injury, lesion)	Herida	Ferita	Rana
Plaie par objet tranchant	Cut wound	Herida por corte	Ferita da taglio	Rezna rana (posjekotina)
Plaque dentaire	Dental plaque (dental tartar)	Placa dental	Placca (tartaro)	Zubni kamenac
Plasmocytome (myélome multiple)	Plasmacytoma (multiple myeloma)	Plasmacitoma (mieloma múltiple)	Mieloma multiplo	Plazmocitom (multipli mijelom)
Pneumoconiose	Pneumoconiosis	Neumoconiosis	Pneumoconiosi	Pneumokonioza
Pneumocystose	Pneumocystis pneumonia (pneumocystosis)	Neumonía por Pneumocystis	Polmonite da Pneumocisti	Pneumocistična upala pluća
Pneumonie atypique	Atypical pneumonia	Neumonía atípica	Polmonite atipica	Atipična upala pluća
Pneumonie bactérienne	Bacterial pneumonia	Neumonía bacteriana	Polmonite batterica	Bakterijska upala pluća
Pneumonie virale	Viral pneumonia	Neumonía viral	Polmonite virale	Virusna upala pluća
Pneumothorax	Pneumothorax	Neumotórax	Pneumotorace	Pneumotoraks
Poliomyélite (polio, paralysie spinale infantile)	Poliomyelitis (polio, infantile paralysis)	Poliomielitis (parálisis infantil)	Poliomielite (polio, paralisi infantile)	Dječja paraliza (polio, poliomijelitis)
Polycythémie	Polycythemia	Policitemia	Policitemia	Policitemija
Polydactylie	Polydactyly	Polidactilia	Polidattilia	Polidaktilija
Polymyalgia rheumatica	Polymyalgia rheumatica	Polimialgia reumática	Polimialgia reumatica	Reumatska polimialgija
Polymyosite	Polymyositis	Polimiositis	Polimiosite	Polimiozitis
Polynucléose	Granulocytosis	Granulocitosis	Granulocitosi	Granulocitoza
Polype	Polyp	Pólipo	Polipo	Polip
Polype au col de l'utérus	Cervical polyp	Pólipo cervical	Polipo cervicale	Polip na grliću maternice
Polype des cordes vocales	Vocal chords polyp	Pólipo de las cuerdas vocales	Polipo della corda vocale	Polip na glasnicama
Polype du côlon	Colon polyp	Pólipo de colon	Polipo del colon	Polip na debelom crijevu
Polype nasal	Nasal polyp	Pólipo nasal	Polipo nasale	Polip u nosu (nosni polip)
Polype utérin	Endometrial polyp (uterine polyp)	Pólipo endometrial	Polipo endometriale	Polip maternice
Porphyrie	Porphyria	Porfiria	Porfiria	Porfirija
Première période de menstruations (ménarche)	First menstrual cycle (menarche)	Primera menstruación (menarquia)	Primo flusso mestruale (menarca)	Prva mjesečnica (menarha)
Présence de pus dans l'urine (pyurie)	Pus in urine (pyuria)	Presencia de pus en la orina (piuria)	Presenza di pus nelle urine (piuria)	Gnoj u urinu (piurija)
Présence de spermatozoïdes en quantité faible (oligospermie)	Low semen volume (oligospermia)	Bajo volumen de semen (oligospermia)	Produzione di pochi spermatozoi (oligospermia)	Manjak sperme (oligospermija)
Pression artérielle effondrée	Blood pressure fall	Caída de la presión arterial	Abbassamento della pressione del sangue	Pad krvnog tlaka
Pression artérielle élevée (hypertension artérielle)	High blood pressure (hypertension)	Incremento de la presión sanguínea (hipertensión)	Ipertensione arteriosa sistemica	Visoki krvni tlak (hipertenzija)
Prise excessive d'aliments (hyperphagie)	Abnormally large intake of food (hyperphagia)	Ingestas descontroladas de alimentos (hiperfagia)	Aumento incontrollato di assunzione di cibo (iperfagia)	Prekomjerno jedenje (hiperfagija)
Proctite	Proctitis	Proctitis	Proctite	Proktitis
Prolapsus de l'utérus	Uterine prolapse (fallen womb)	Prolapso del útero	Prolasso uterino	Prolaps maternice (spuštena maternica)
Prolapsus rectal	Rectal prolapse	Prolapso rectal	Prolasso del retto	Prolaps rektuma
Protéinose alvéolaire pulmonaire	Pulmonary alveolar proteinosis	Proteinosis alveolar pulmonar	Proteinosi alveolare polmonare	Alveolarna proteinoza pluća
Protéinurie (excès de protéines dans l'urine)	Proteinuria (presence of proteins in urine)	Proteinuria	Proteinuria	Bjelančevine u urinu (proteinurija)
Prurit	Itching	Prurito (picazón, comezón, rasquiña)	Prurito (pizzicore)	Svrbež
Psittacose	Psittacosis (parrot fever)	Psitacosis (fiebre del loro)	Psittacosi (psittacornitosi)	Psitakoza
Psoriasis	Psoriasis	Psoriasis	Psoriasi	Psorijaza
Psychonévrose	Psychoneurosis	Psiconeurosis	Psiconevrosi (nevrosi)	Psihoneuroza
Psychopathie	Psychopathy	Psicopatía	Psicopatia	Psihopatija

Français	Anglais	Espagnol	Italien	Croate
Psychose	Psychosis	Psicosis	Psicosi	Psihoza
Pubalgie du sportif	Groin pain syndrome	Síndrome de dolor inguinal	Pubalgia dello sportivo	Sindrom bolnih prepona
Puberté précoce	Precocious puberty (premature puberty)	Pubertad precoz	Pubertà precoce (pubertà prematura)	Preuranjeni pubertet
Puberté tardive	Delayed puberty	Retraso de la pubertad	Pubertà tardiva	Zakašnjeli pubertet
Pupilles dilatées	Enlarged pupils	Pupilas dilatadas	Pupille dilatate	Proširene zjenice
Pupilles diminuées	Small pupils	Pupilas pequeñas	Pupille costrette	Sužene zjenice
Purpura	Purpura	Púrpura	Porpora	Purpura
Purpura thrombotique thrombocytopénique	Thrombotic thrombocytopenic purpura	Púrpura trombocitopénica trombótica	Porpora trombotica trombocitopenica	Trombotska trombocitopenična purpura
Pus	Pus	Pus	Pus	Gnoj
Pustule	Pustule	Pústula	Pustola	Gnojni mjehurić
Pyélonéphrite (infection bactérienne des voies urinaires hautes)	Pyelonephritis (kidney infection)	Pielonefritis (infección urinaria alta)	Pielonefrite	Pijelonefritis (infekcija bubrega)
Pyonéphrose (pus dans le rein)	Pyonephrosis	Pionefrosis	Pionefrosi	Pionefroza
Pyromanie	Pyromania	Piromanía	Piromania	Piromanija
Rachitisme	Rickets (rachitis)	Raquitismo	Rachitismo	Rahitis
Rachitisme rénal	Renal rickets	Raquitismo renal	Rachitismo renale	Bubrežni rahitis
Rage	Rabies	Rabia	Rabbia	Bjesnoća (rabies)
Raideur	Stiffness	Agarrotamiento	Rigidità	Ukočenost
Raideur articulaire	Joint stiffness	Rigidez de las articulaciones	Rigidità dell'articolazione	Zakočenost zgloba
Raideur de nuque (raideur méningée)	Nuchal rigidity (stiff neck)	Rigidez de nuca (cuello rígido)	Rigidità nucale	Kočenje šije (ukočeni vrat)
Raréfaction du volume des urines (oligurie)	Decreased production of urine (oliguria)	Disminución de producción de orina (oliguria)	Diminuita escrezione urinaria (oliguria)	Smanjeno izlučivanje urina (oligurija)
Rash (eczéma)	Rash (eruption, eczema)	Sarpullido (erupción, eccema)	Sfogo (eruzione cutanea)	Osip
Règle douloureuse (dysménorrhée)	Painful menstruation (dysmenorrhea)	Menstruación dolorosa (dismenorrea)	Mestruazione dolorosa (dismenorrea)	Bolna menstruacija (dismenoreja)
Rein en fer à cheval	Horseshoe kidney (renal fusion)	Riñón de herradura (fusión en los riñones)	Rene a ferro di cavallo (fusione renale)	Potkovičasti bubreg
Rein polykystique	Polycystic kidney disease	Enfermedad poliquística renal	Rene policistico	Policistični bubreg
Rejet de sang issu des voies aériennes (hémoptysie)	Expectoration of blood (hemoptysis)	Expectoración de sangre (hemoptisis)	Espettorazione di sangue (emottisi)	Iskašljavanje krvi (hemoptiza, hemoptoja)
Renifler	Sniffing (sniffle)	Sorberse la nariz (moqueo)	Tirare su col naso	Šmrcanje
Réponses psychophysiologiques lentes	Slow psychophysiolo-gical responses	Respuestas psicofisiológicas lentas	Lentezza psicofisica	Psihofizička usporenost
Respiration accélérée (tachypnée)	Rapid breathing (tachypnea)	Respiración rápida (taquipnea)	Aumento del ritmo respiratorio (tachipnea)	Ubrzano disanje (tahipnea)
Respiration Cheynes-Stokes	Periodic breathing (Cheyne-Stokes respiration)	Respiración periódica (respiración de Cheynes-Stokes)	Respiro di Cheyne-Stokes	Periodično disanje (Cheyne-Stokesovo disanje)
Respiration de Biot	Biot's respiration	Respiración de Biot	Respiro di Biot	Biotovo disanje
Respiration de type Kussmaul	Kussmaul breathing	Respiración de Kussmaul	Respiro di Kussmaul	Kussmaulovo disanje
Respiration ralentie (bradypnée)	Slow breathing rate (bradypnea)	Descenso de la frecuencia respiratoria (bradipnea)	Riduzione della frequenza respiratoria (bradipnea)	Usporeno disanje (bradipneja)
Respiration superficielle	Shallow breathing	Respiración superficial	Respirazione superficiale	Površinsko plitko disanje
Retard mental (handicap mental)	Mental retardation	Retraso mental	Ritardo mentale	Mentalna retardacija
Rétention d'urine	Urinary retention (ischuria)	Retención de orina	Ritenzione urinaria	Zastoj urina (urinarna retencija)
Rétinite pigmentaire	Retinitis pigmentosa (retinal pigment epithelium dystrophy)	Retinitis pigmentosa	Retinite pigmentosa	Pigmentna distrofija mrežnice
Rétinopathie diabétique	Diabetic retinopathy	Retinopatía diabética	Retinopatia diabetica	Dijabetična retinopatija
Rétinopathie du prématuré	Retinopathy of prematurity (retrolental fibroplasia)	Retinopatía de la prematuridad	Retinopatia del prematuro	Retrolentalna fibroplazija
Retour à la bouche du contenu de l'estomac (régurgitation)	Expulsion of undigested food from stomack to the mouth (regurgitation)	Regreso del contenido alimentario a través del esófago (regurgitación)	Risalita di alimenti dallo stomaco alla bocca (rigurgito)	Vraćanje hrane iz želuca u usta (regurgitacija)
Rhabdomyome	Rhabdomyoma	Rabdomioma	Rabdomioma	Rabdomiom
Rhabdomyome granocellulaire	Myoblastoma	Mioblastoma	Mioblastoma	Mioblastom
Rhabdomyosarcome	Rhabdomyosarcoma	Rabdomiosarcoma	Rabdomiosarcoma	Rabdomiosarkom
Rhinite	Rhinitis	Rinitis	Rinite	Rinitis
Rhinite allergique	Allergic rhinitis	Rinitis alérgica	Rinite allergica	Alergijski rinitis
Rhinite vasomotrice	Vasomotor rhinitis	Rinitis vasomotora	Rinite vasomotoria	Vazomotorni rinitis
Rhizarthrose	Thumb joint arthritis	Rizartrosis	Rizartrosi (artrosi dell'articolazione alla base del police)	Rizartroza

Français	Anglais	Espagnol	Italien	Croate
Rhumatisme articulaire aigu (maladie de Bouillaud)	Rheumatic fever	Fiebre reumática	Febbre reumatica	Reumatska groznica
Rhumatisme extraarticulaire	Extrajoint rheumatism	Reumatismo extraarticular	Reumatismo extra-articolare	Izvanzglobni reumatizam
Rhume	Common cold	Resfriado común (resfrío)	Infreddatura (raffreddore)	Prehlada (hunjavica)
Rickettsiose	Rickettsiosis	Rickettsiosis	Rickettsiosi	Rikecioza
Ride	Wrinkle	Arruga	Ruga	Bora
Rosacée (couperose)	Rosacea	Rosácea	Rosacea	Rozacea
Roséole (exanthème subit, sixième maladie)	Exanthema subitum (roseola infantum, sixth disease)	Roséola (exantema súbito)	Sesta malattia (roseola infantum, esantema subitum)	Rozeola infantum (egzantema subitum, šesta bolest)
Rot (renvoi, éructation)	Burping (belching)	Eructo	Eruttazione	Podrigivanje
Rougeole (1re maladie)	Measles	Sarampión	Morbillo	Ospice (morbili)
Rubéole	German measles (rubella)	Rubéola	Rosolia	Rubeola (crljenac)
Rupture	Rupture	Ruptura (rotura)	Rottura	Prsnuće (puknuće, razdor, ruptura)
Rupture d'anévrisme	Aneurysm rupture	Ruptura del aneurisma	Rottura di aneurisma	Prsnuće aneurizme
Rupture de la coiffe des rotateurs	Rotator cuff rupture (rotator cuff tear)	Ruptura del manguito rotador	Rottura della cuffia dei rotatori	Razdor rotatorne manžete ramenog zgloba
Rupture de la rate	Ruptured spleen	Ruptura del bazo	Rottura della milza	Ruptura slezene
Rupture de la vessie	Rupture of urinary bladder	Ruptura de la vejiga urinaria	Rottura della vescica urinaria	Rascjep mokraćnog mjehura
Rupture du ligament croisé antéro-externe (rupture du LCA)	Anterior cruciate ligament rupture (ACL rupture)	Ruptura de ligamento cruzado anterior	Rottura del legamento crociato anteriore del ginocchio	Razdor prednje ukrižene sveze koljenskog zgloba
Rupture du ménisque	Meniscus rupture (meniscus tear)	Ruptura de menisco	Rottura del menisco	Razdor meniskusa
Rupture du tendon	Tendon rupture (torn tendon)	Ruptura del tendón	Rottura del tendine	Puknuće tetive
Rupture du tendon d'Achille	Achilles tendon rupture	Ruptura del tendón de Aquiles	Rottura del tendine di Achille	Puknuće Ahilove tetive
Rupture ligamentaire	Ligament rupture (torn ligament)	Ruptura de ligamento	Rottura del legamento	Puknuće ligamenta
Rupture musculaire	Muscle rupture	Ruptura muscular	Rottura muscolare	Rastrgnuće mišića (ruptura mišića)
Rythme cardiaque bas (bradycardie)	Slow pulse rate (bradycardia)	Descenso de la frecuencia cardiaca (bradicardia)	Riduzione della frequenza cardiaca (bradicardia)	Usporen puls (bradikardija)
Sac herniaire	Hernia sack	Saco de hernia (saco herniario)	Sacco dell'ernia	Kilna vreća
Saignement (hémorragie)	Bleeding (haemorrhage)	Desangramiento (hemorragia)	Emorragia	Krvarenje (hemoragija)
Saignement anal (rectorragie)	Anal bleeding	Pérdida de sangre a través del ano (rectorragia)	Perdita di sangue dall'ano (rettoragia, proctorragia)	Krvarenje iz analnog otvora
Saignement de l'oreille	Ear bleeding	Hemorragia de oído (otorragia)	Fuoriuscita di sangue dall'orecchio (otorragia)	Krvarenje iz uha
Saignement de l'utérus (métrorragie)	Uterine bleeding (metrorrhagia)	Pérdida de sangre uterina (metrorragia)	Perdita di sangue al di fuori della mestruazione (metrorragia)	Krvarenje iz maternice (metroragija)
Saignement de nez (épistaxis)	Nose bleeding (epistaxis)	Pérdida de sangre por la nariz (epistaxis)	Epistassi (rinorragia)	Krvarenje iz nosa (epistaksa)
Saignement externe (hémorragie externe)	External bleeding	Sangrado externo (hemorragia externa)	Emorragia esterna	Vanjsko krvarenje
Saignement interne (hémorragie interne)	Internal bleeding	Sangrado interno (hemorragia interna)	Emorragia interna	Unutarnje krvarenje
Saignement veineux	Venous bleeding	Sangrado venoso (hemorragia venosa)	Emorragia venosa	Vensko krvarenje
Salmonellose	Salmonellosis	Salmonelosis	Salmonellosi	Salmoneloza
Sang dans l'expectoration (hémoptysie)	Blood in sputum (hemoptysis)	Sangre en el esputo (hemoptisis)	Sangue nello sputo (emottisi)	Krvavi iskašljaj (hemoptiza)
Sang dans le liquide cérébro-spinal	Blood in cerebrospinal fluid	Sangre en el líquido cefalorraquídeo	Sangue al liquido cerebrospinale	Krv u likvoru
Sang dans les selles (hématochézie)	Blood in stool (hematochezia)	Sangre en las heces (hematochezia)	Sangue nelle feci (ematochezia)	Krv u stolici (hematohezija)
Sang dans les urines (hématurie)	Blood in urine (hematuria)	Sangre en la orina (hematuria)	Ematuria	Krv u urinu (hematurija)
Sarcoïdose (maladie de Besnier-Boeck-Schaumann)	Sarcoidosis (sarcoid, Besnier-Boeck disease)	Sarcoidosis (enfermedad de Besnier-Boeck)	Sarcoidosi	Sarkoidoza
Sarcome	Sarcoma	Sarcoma	Sarcoma	Sarkom
Sarcome botryoïde	Botryoid sarcoma	Sarcoma botrioide	Sarcoma botrioide	Botrioidni sarkom
Sarcome d'Ewing	Ewing's sarcoma	Sarcoma de Ewing	Sarcoma di Ewing	Ewing sarkom (endoteliosarkom)
Sarcome de Kaposi	Kaposi's sarcoma	Sarcoma de Kaposi	Sarcoma di Kaposi	Kaposijev sarkom (endoteliosarkom)

Français	Anglais	Espagnol	Italien	Croate
Sarcome réticuloendothélial	Reticuloendothelial sarcoma	Reticulosarcoma (sarcoma reticuloendotelial)	Reticoloendotelioma (reticolosarcoma)	Retikuloendotelijalni sarkom
Sarcome synovial	Synovial sarcoma	Sarcoma sinovial	Sarcoma sinoviale	Sinovijalni sarkom
Sarcopénie	Sarcopenia	Sarcopenia	Sarcopenia	Sarkopenija
Sarcopsyllose	Tungiasis (nigua, pique)	Tungiasis	Tungiasi (tunga penetrans)	Tungijaza
SARM	MRSA	SARM	MSSA (MRSA)	MRSA
Saute d'humeur	Mood swing	Oscilaciones del humor	Cambiamento d'umore	Promjene raspoloženja
Scarlatine (fièvre écarlate)	Scarlet fever	Escarlatina (fiebre escarlata)	Scarlattina	Šarlah (skarlatina)
Schistosomiase (bilharziose)	Schistosomiasis (snail fever)	Esquistosomiasis (bilharziasis)	Schistosomiasi	Šistosomijaza
Schizophrénie	Schizophrenia	Esquizofrenia	Schizofrenia	Šizofrenija
Sciatique	Sciatica	Ciática	Sciatica	Išijas
Sclérodermie	Scleroderma	Esclerodermia	Sclerodermia	Sklerodermija
Sclérose en plaques	Multiple sclerosis	Esclerosis múltiple	Sclerosi multipla	Multipla skleroza
Sclérose latérale amyotrophique (maladie de Charcot)	Amyotrophic lateral sclerosis	Esclerosis lateral amiotrófica	Sclerosi laterale amiotrofica	Amiotrofična lateralna skleroza
Scoliose	Scoliosis	Escoliosis	Scoliosi	Skolioza
Scorbut	Scurvy	Escorbuto	Scorbuto	Skorbut
Scotome	Scotoma	Escotoma	Scotoma	Skotom
Se ronger les ongles (onychophagie)	Nail biting (onychophagia)	Comerse las uñas (onicofagia)	Abitudine di mangiare le unghie (onicofagia)	Griženje noktiju (onikofagija)
Séborrhée	Seborrhea	Seborrea	Seborrea	Seboreja
Sècheresse de la bouche (xèrostomie)	Dry mouth (xerostomia)	Sequedad de la boca (xerostomía)	Scarsa secrezione salivare (xerostomia)	Suha sluznica usta
Sécrétion (suintement, écoulement)	Discharge	Flujo (descarga, secreción)	Fuoriuscita (scolo)	Iscjedak
Sécrétion d'urine en quantité abondante (polyurie)	Passage of large volumes of urine (polyuria)	Gasto urinario excesivo (poliuria)	Aumentata emissione di urina (poliuria)	Učestalo mokrenje velikih količina mokraće (poliurija)
Sécrétion de la salive excessive	Excessive secretion of saliva (hypersalivation)	Excesiva producción de saliva (hipersalivación)	Produzione di saliva eccessiva (ipersalivazione)	Pojačano lučenje sline (hipersalivacija)
Selles aqueuses	Watery stool	Heces acuosas	Consistenza acquosa delle feci	Vodenasta stolica
Selles jaunes	Yellow stool	Heces amarillas	Feci gialle	Žuta stolica
Selles noir (melanea, méléna)	Black stool (melena)	Heces negras (melena)	Feci picee (melena)	Crna stolica (melena)
Selles rouges	Red colored stool	Heces de color rojo	Feci di colore rosso	Crvena stolica
Selles vertes	Green stool	Heces verdes	Feci di colore verde	Zelenkasta stolica
Semi-coma	Semicoma	Semicoma	Semi-coma	Semikoma
Sensation cuisante	Burning sensation	Sensación de ardor	Sensazione bruciante	Pećenje (žarenje)
Sensation de peur	Sensation of fear	Sensación de miedo	Senso della paura	Osjećaj straha
Sensation des chaussures très serré	"Tight shoes" sensation	Sensación de "zapatos apretados"	Senso delle scarpe troppo strette	Osjećaj "tijesnih cipela"
Sensibilité à la douleur (algésie)	Sensitivity to pain (algesia)	Sensibilidad al dolor (algesia)	Sensibilità al dolore (algesia)	Osjetljivost na bol (algezija)
Sensibilité éléctromagnétique	Electromagnetic hypersensitivity	Hipersensibilidad electromagnética	Elettrosensibilità	Elektromagnetska hipersenzibilnost
Sepsis	Sepsis	Sepsis	Sepsi	Sepsa
Septicémie	Septicemia	Septicemia	Setticemia	Septikemija
Sevrage	Withdrawal	Síndrome de abstinencia	Crisi d'astinenza	Apstinencijska kriza
Sexualité compulsive	Sexual addiction	Adicción sexual	Dipendenza sessuale	Ovisnost o seksu
Shigellose	Shigellosis (bacillary dysentery)	Shigelosis	Shigellosi	Šigeloza
SIDA (syndrome d'immunodéficience acquise)	AIDS (acquired immune deficiency syndrome)	SIDA (síndrome de inmunodeficiencia adquirida)	SIDA (sindrome da ImmunoDeficienza Acquisita, AIDS)	SIDA (sindrom stečene imunodeficijencije, AIDS)
Sidérose	Siderosis	Siderosis	Siderosi	Sideroza
Signe de Koplik	Koplik's spots	Manchas de Koplik	Macchie di Koplik	Koplikove pjege
Silicose	Silicosis	Silicosis	Silicosi	Silikoza
Soif	Thirst	Sed	Sete	Žeđ
Soif excessive (polydipsie)	Increased thirst senasation (polydipsia)	Aumento anormal de la sed (polidipsia)	Aumento del senso della sete (polidipsia)	Pojačan osjećaj žeđi (polidipsija)
Somnabulisme	Sleepwalking (somnambulism)	Sonambulismo (noctambulismo)	Sonnambulismo	Mjesečarenje (somnambulizam)
Somnolence	Somnolence	Somnolencia	Sonnolenza	Pospanost (somnolencija)
Sopor	Sopor	Sopor	Stupor	Sopor
Souffle cardiaque	Heart murmur	Soplo del corazón	Soffio cardiaco	Šum na srcu
Spasme (crampe)	Spasm (cramp)	Espasmo (calambre)	Spasmo (contrazione involuntaria)	Grč (spazam)
Spasme du pylore	Pylorospasm	Pilorospasmo	Pilorospasmo	Pilorospazam
Spasme facial	Facial spasm	Espasmo facial	Spasmo facciale	Grč mišića lica
Spasme vaginal (vaginisme)	Vaginal spasm (vaginismus)	Espasmo vaginal (vaginismo)	Spasmo di vagina (vaginismo)	Grč rodnice (vaginizam)
Spermatocèle	Spermatocele	Espermatocele	Spermatocele (cisti spermatica)	Spermatokela (cista epididimisa)
Spina bifida	Spina bifida	Espina bifida	Spina bifida	Spina bifida

Français	Anglais	Espagnol	Italien	Croate
Splénomégalie	Splenomegaly	Esplenomegalia	Splenomegalia	Splenomegalija
Spondilite	Spondylitis	Espondilitis	Spondilite	Spondilitis
Spondylarthrite ankylosante (morbus Bechterew)	Ankylosing spondylitis (Bechterew's syndrome)	Espondilitis anquilosante (morbus Bechterew)	Spondilite anchilosante	Ankilozantni spondilitis (Bechterewov sindrom)
Spondylolisthésis	Spondylolisthesis	Espondilolistesis	Spondilolistesi	Spondilolisteza
Spondylose	Spondylosis	Espondilosis	Spondilosi	Spondiloza
Sporotrichose	Sporotrichosis	Esporotricosis	Sporotricosi	Sporotrihoza
Stéatose hépatique	Fatty liver metamorphosis	Metamorfosis grasa del hígado	Metamorfosi grassa del fegato	Masna metamorfoza jetre
Sténose congénitale du pylore	Congenital pyloric stenosis	Estenosis congénita del píloro	Stenosi pilorica congenita	Urođena stenoza pilorusa
Sténose de l'artère pulmonaire	Stenosis of pulmonary artery	Estenosis de la arteria pulmonar	Stenosi dell'arteria polmonare	Stenoza plućne arterije
Sténose de la valve pulmonaire	Pulmonary valve stenosis	Estenosis de la válvula pulmonar	Stenosi polmonare	Stenoza plućnog ušća (pulmonalna stenoza)
Sténose du pylore	Pyloric stenosis	Estenosis del píloro	Stenosi pilorica	Stenoza pilorusa (pilorostenoza)
Sténose hypertrophique du pylore	Hypertrophic pyloric stenosis	Estenosis pilórica hipertrófica	Stenosi ipertrofica del piloro	Hipertrofijska stenoza pilorusa
Sténose mitrale	Mitral stenosis	Estenosis mitral	Stenosi mitralica	Stenoza mitralnog ušća
Sténose oesophagienne	Esophageal stenosis	Estenosis esofágica	Stenosi esofagea	Stenoza jednjaka
Sténose valvulaire aortique	Aortic valve stenosis	Estenosis de la válvula aórtica	Stenosi aortica	Stenoza aortnog ušća
Strabisme	Strabismus	Estrabismo	Strabismo	Razrokost (strabizam)
Strangulation (étranglement)	Strangulation	Estrangulamiento	Strangolamento (strozzamento)	Davljenje
Stupeur	Stupor	Estupor	Stupore	Stupor
Sucre dans les urines (glycosurie)	Glucose in urine (glycosuria)	Azúcar en orina (glucosuria)	Glicosuria (mellituria)	Šećer u urinu (glikozurija)
Sudation	Sweating	Transpiración (sudación)	Sudorazione (traspirazione)	Znojenje
Sudation excessive (hyperhidrose)	Excessive sweating (hyperhidrosis)	Excesiva producción de sudor (hiperhidrosis)	Aumento della sudorazione (iperidrosi)	Prekomjerno znojenje (hiperhidroza)
Sueurs nocturnes	Night sweats	Sudor nocturno	Sudore notturno	Noćno znojenje
Suffocation	Choking (suffocation)	Atragantamiento	Soffocamento (soffocazione, asfissia)	Gušenje
Surdité	Deafness	Sordera	Sordità	Gluhoća
Surdité partielle	Hard of hearing	Corto de oído (parcialmente sordo)	Sordità parziale	Nagluhost
Surdose de drogue	Drug overdose	Sobredosis por droga	Overdose di droga	Predoziranje drogom
Surdose du médicament	Medication overdose	Sobredosis de medicamentos	Overdose di farmaci	Predoziranje lijekom
Syncope	Syncope	Síncope	Sincope	Sinkopa
Syndactylie	Syndactyly	Sindactilia	Sindattilia	Sindaktilija
Syndrome carcinoïde	Carcinoid syndrome	Síndrome carcinoide	Sindrome da carcinoide	Karcinoidni sindrom
Syndrome cervical	Cervicocephal syndrome	Síndrome cervical	Sindrome cervicale	Cervikocefalni sindrom
Syndrome cervico-brachial	Cervicobrachial syndrome	Síndrome cérvico-braquial	Sindrome cervico-brachiale (sindrome spalla-mano)	Sindrom vrat-rame (cervikobrahijalni sindrom)
Syndrome d'alcoolisation foetale	Fetal alcohol syndrome	Síndrome de alcoholismo fetal	Sindrome alcolica fetale	Fetusni alkoholni sindrom
Syndrome d'écrasement	Crush-syndrome	Síndrome de aplastami-ento (síndrome de crush)	Sindrome da schiacciamento	Crush-sindrom
Syndrome d'Edwards (trisomie 18)	Edwards syndrome (trisomy 18)	Síndrome de Edwards (trisomía del 18)	Sindrome di Edwards	Trisomija 18D (Edwardsov sindrom)
Syndrome d'Eisenmenger	Eisenmenger's syndrome	Síndrome de Eisenmenger	Sindrome di Eisenmenger	Eisenmengerov sindrom
Syndrome de blast	Blast-syndrome	Síndrome por explosion	Lesioni da scoppio (blast-syndrome)	Blast-sindrom
Syndrome de Cushing (hypercorticisme)	Cushing's syndrome (hypercorticism)	Síndrome de Cushing (hipercortisolismo)	Sindrome di Cushing (ipercortisolismo)	Cushingov sindrom (hiperkortikolizam)
Syndrome de DeQuervain (ténosynovite de DeQuervain)	DeQuervain syndrome	Síndrome de DeQuervain	Sindrome di De Quervain	Sindrom bubnjarskog palca (Morbus DeQuervain)
Syndrome de détresse respiratoire	Respiratory distress syndrome	Síndrome de distrés respiratorio	Sindrome da distress respiratorio	Respiratorni distres sindrom
Syndrome de douleur	Pain syndrome	Síndrome doloroso	Sindrome dolorosa	Bolni sindrom
Syndrome de Down	Down syndrome	Síndrome de Down	Sindrome di Down	Downov sindrom (mongoloidizam)
Syndrome de fatigue chronique	Chronic fatigue syndrome	Síndrome de fatiga crónica	Sindrome da fatica cronica	Sindrom kroničnog umora
Syndrome de Goodpasture (maladie des anticorps anti-membrane basale glomérulaire)	Goodpasture's syndrome	Síndrome de Goodpasture	Sindrome di Goodpasture	Goodpastureov sindrom
Syndrome de Guillain-Barré	Guillain-Barré syndrome	Síndrome de Guillain-Barré	Sindrome di Guillain-Barré	Guillain-Barréov sindrom

Français	Anglais	Espagnol	Italien	Croate
Syndrome de la bandelette iliotibiale (syndrome de l'essuie glace)	Iliotibial band friction syndrome	Síndrome de fricción de la banda iliotibial	Sindrome della benderella ileotibiale	Sindrom trenja iliotibijalnog traktusa
Syndrome de Marfan	Marfan syndrome	Síndrome de Marfan	Sindrome di Marfan	Marfanov sindrom
Syndrome de McCune-Albright	McCune-Albright syndrome	Síndrome de McCune-Albright	Sindrome di McCune-Albright-Sternberg	Albrightov sindrom
Syndrome de mort subite du nourrisson	Sudden infant death syndrome (crib death, cot death)	Síndrome de muerte súbita del lactante (muerte en cuna)	Sindrome della morte improvvisa del lattante	Sindrom iznenadne smrti dojenčeta
Syndrome de Patau (trisomie 13)	Patau syndrome (trisomy 13)	Síndrome de Patau (trisomía en el par 13)	Sindrome di Patau	Trisomija 13D (Patauov sindrom)
Syndrome de Reye	Reye's syndrome	Síndrome de Reye	Sindrome di Reye	Reyeov sindrom
Syndrome de Sjögren	Sjögren's syndrome	Síndrome de Sjögren	Sindrome di Sjögren	Sjögrenov sindrom
Syndrome de Tourette	Tourette's syndrome	Síndrome de Tourette	Sindrome di Tourette	Touretteov sindrom
Syndrome de traversée thoraco-cervico-brachiale	Thoracic outlet syndrome	Síndrome del estrecho torácico	Sindrome dello stretto toracico superiore	Torakalni sindrom
Syndrome de Turner	Turner syndrome	Síndrome de Turner	Sindrome di Turner	Turnerov sindrom
Syndrome de Volkmann	Volkmann's ischemic contracture	Contractura isquémica de Volkmann	Contrattura ischemica di Volkmann	Volkmannova ishemična kontraktura
Syndrome des loges	Compartment syndrome	Síndrome compartimental	Sindrome compartimentale	Sindrom fascijalnog prostora
Syndrome des vibrations du système main-bras	Hand-arm vibration syndrome (vibration white finger)	Vibraciones mano brazo (dedo blanco inducido por vibraciones)	Sindrome da vibrazioni mano-braccio	Vibracijski sindrom šaka-ruka
Syndrome du bébé mou	Floppy infant syndrome	Síndrome de bebé flácido	Sindrome del bambino flaccido	Sindrom mlohavog djeteta
Syndrome du brasseur aux genoux	Swimmer's knee	Rodilla de nadador de pecho (bursitis de la pata de ganso)	Ginocchio del nuotatore a rana (stiramento cronico del legamento mediale)	Plivačko koljeno
Syndrome du canal carpien	Carpal tunnel syndrome	Síndrome del túnel carpiano	Sindrome del tunnel carpale	Sindrom karpalnog tunela
Syndrome du canal tarsien	Tarsal tunnel syndrome	Síndrome del túnel tarsiano	Sindrome del tunnel tarsale	Sindrom tarzalnog kanala
Syndrome du conflit sous-acromial	Shoulder impingement syndrome (subacromial impingement syndrome)	Síndrome del conflicto subacromial	Sindrome da conflitto subacromiale (impingement sub-acromiale)	Sindrom sraza ramena (subakromijalni sindrom sraza)
Syndrome du rein flottant (néphroptose)	Floating kidney (nephroptosis, renal ptosis)	Riñón flotante (ptosis renal, nefroptosis)	Spostamento del rene (ptosi renale, nefroptosi)	Spušteni bubreg (putujući bubreg, nefroptoza)
Syndrome du tunnel cubital	Little league elbow syndrome (LLE syndrome)	Síndrome del túnel cubital	Sindrome del tunnel cubitale	Sindrom kopljaškog lakta
Syndrome hépato-rénal	Hepatorenal syndrome	Síndrome hepatorrenal	Sindrome epato-renale	Hepatorenalni sindrom
Syndrome myélodysplasique	Myelodysplastic syndrome	Síndrome mielodisplásico (preleucemia)	Sindrome mielodisplasica	Mijelodisplastični sindrom
Syndrome néphrotique	Nephrotic syndrome	Síndrome nefrótico	Sindrome nefrosica	Nefrotski sindrom
Syndrome poplité douloureux	Popliteus syndrome	Tendinitis poplítea	Tendinite del popliteo	Sindrom m. popliteusa
Syndrome post-thrombotique	Post-thrombotic syndrome	Síndrome postrombótico	Sindrome post trombotica	Posttrombotički sindrom
Syndrome prémenstruel (SPM)	Premenstrual syndrome (PMS)	Síndrome premenstrual	Sindrome premestruale	Predmenstruacijski sindrom (PMS)
Syndrome respiratoire aigu sévère (SRAS)	Severe acute respiratory syndrome (SARS)	Síndrome respiratorio agudo severo (SRAS, SARS)	SARS (Sindrome Acuta Respiratoria Severa)	Sindrom akutne respiratorne insuficijencije (SARS)
Syndrome tibial postérieur	Tibialis posterior syndrome	Síndrome del tibial posterior	Periostite tibiale (sindrome del muscolo tibiale posteriore)	Sindrom stražnjeg tibijalnog mišića
Synostose radio-ulnaire	Radioulnar synostosis	Sinostosis radiocubital	Sinostosi radio-ulnare	Radioulnarna sinostoza
Synoviome	Synovioma	Sinovioma	Sinovioma	Sinoviom
Syphilis (vérole)	Syphilis	Sífilis	Sifilide (lue)	Sifilis (lues)
Syringomyélie	Syringomyelia	Siringomielia	Siringomielia	Siringomijelija
Tachycardie	Tachycardia	Taquicardia	Tachicardia	Tahikardija
Tamponnade cardiaque	Pericardial tamponade (cardiac tamponade)	Tamponamiento cardíaco (tampona-miento pericárdiaco)	Tamponamento cardiaco	Tamponada perikarda
Taux de sucre dans le sang élevé (hyperglycémie)	High blood sugar (hyperglicemia)	Cantidad excesiva de glucosa en la sangre (hiperglucemia, hiperglicemia)	Eccesso di glucosio nel sangue (iperglicemia)	Povišeni šećer u krvi (hiperglikemija)
Teigne (tinea capitis)	Tinea capitis (scalp ringworm)	Tiña de la cabeza (tinea capitis)	Tigna (tinea capitis)	Gljivična infekcija vlasišta (tinea capitis)
Température corporelle basse (hypothermie)	Decreased body temperature (hypothermia)	Temperatura corporal baja (hipotermia)	Bassa temperatura corporea (ipotermia)	Snižena temperatura tijela (hipotermija)
Tendinite achilléenne chronique	Achilles tendon overuse injury	Tendinitis por sobreuso en el tendón de Aquiles	Tendinopatia Achille da overuse	Sindrom prenaprezanja Ahilove tetive
Tendinite de l'avant-bras	Forearm tendinitis	Tendinitis en el antebrazo	Tendinite dell'avambraccio	Veslačka podlaktica (tendinitis podlaktice)
Tendinite des danseurs (fléchisseur de l'hallux tendinite)	Dancer's tendinitis (flexor hallucis tendinitis)	Tendinitis del flexor hallucis longus	Tendinite del flessore lungo dell'alluce	Tendinitis plesača (tendinitis dugog pregibača palca)

Français	Anglais	Espagnol	Italien	Croate
Tendinite des extenseurs des orteils	Extensor tendinitis (inflammation of the extensor tendons of the toes)	Tendinitis de los extensores de los dedos	Tendinite dei estensori delle dita del piede	Tendinitis ekstenzora prstiju stopala
Tendinite du tendon d'Achille	Achillodynia (Achilles tendinitis)	Tendinitis de Aquiles	Tendinopatia achillea (achillodinia)	Ahilodinija (tendinitis Ahilove tetive)
Tendinopathie du tibial postérieur	Tibialis posterior tendinitis	Tendinopatía tibial posterior	Tendinite del muscolo tibiale posteriore	Tendinitis stražnjeg tibijalnog mišića
Tendinose	Tendinosis (chronic tendon injury)	Tendinosis (lesión crónica del tendón)	Tendinosi	Tendinoza (kronična ozljeda tetive)
Tension de la paroi stomacale	Abdominal wall tension	Tensión de la pared abdominal	Tensione di parete addominale	Napetost trbušne stijenke
Tératocarcinome	Teratocarcinoma	Teratocarcinoma	Teratocarcinoma	Teratokarcinom
Tératome	Teratoma	Teratoma	Teratoma	Teratom
Tétanie	Tetany	Tetania	Tetania	Tetanija
Tétanos	Tetanus	Tétanos (tétano)	Tetano	Tetanus (zli grč)
Téton ombiliqué	Inverted nipple	Pezón invertido	Capezzolo invertito	Uvučena bradavica
Tétralogie deFallot	Tetralogy of Fallot	Tetralogía de Fallot	Tetralogia di Fallot	Fallotova tetralogija
Thalassémie	Thalassemia	Talasemia	Talassemia	Talasemija
Thorax en entonnoir (pectus excavatum)	Pectus excavatum	Pecho hundido (pectus excavatum)	Torace a imbuto (petto escavato)	Udubljena prsa (ljevkasta prsa)
Thrombocytopénie	Thrombocytopenia	Trombocitopenia	Trombocitopenia	Trombocitopenija
Thrombophlébite	Thrombophlebitis	Tromboflebitis	Tromboflebite	Tromboflebitis
Thrombose	Thrombosis	Trombosis	Trombosi	Tromboza
Thrombose du voyageur	Traveller's thrombosis (economy class syndrome)	Síndrome de la clase turista	Sindrome della classe economica	Sindrom ekonomske klase
Thrombose veineuse	Venous thrombosis	Trombosis venosa	Trombosi venosa	Venska tromboza
Thyréotoxicose	Thyrotoxicosis	Tirotoxicosis	Tireotossicosi	Tireotoksikoza (tireotoksična oluja)
Thyroïdite de Hashimoto	Hashimoto's disease	Tiroiditis de Hashimoto	Tiroidite di Hashimoto	Hashimotov sindrom
Thyroïdite de Riedel	Riedel's thyroiditis	Tiroiditis de Riedel	Tiroidite di Riedel	Riedelov tireoiditis
Tic	Tic	Tic	Tic	Tik
Tic de langage à dire des mots vulgaires (coprolalie)	Involuntary swearing (coprolalia)	Expresión vocal involuntaria de obsceni dades (coprolalia)	Coprolalia	Nekontrolirano psovanje (koprolalija)
Tinea corporis	Tinea corporis	Tiña corporal (tinea corporis)	Tinea corporis	Tinea corporis
Torsion osseuse	Bone bending (bone torsion)	Torsión del hueso	Torsione dell'osso	Savijanje kosti
Torsion testiculaire	Testicular torsion	Torsión testicular	Torsione del testicolo	Torzija testisa
Torticolis	Wry neck (torticollis)	Tortícolis	Torcicollo	Krivi vrat (tortikolis)
Toux	Cough	Tos	Tosse	Kašalj
Toux productive	Productive cough	Tos productiva	Tosse produttiva	Produktivni kašalj
Toux sèche	Dry cough	Tos seca (tos perruna)	Tosse secca	Suhi kašalj
Toxi-infection à Clostridium perfringens	Clostridium perfringens toxic infection	Tóxico-infección por Clostridium perfringens	Tossinfezione da Clostridium perfringens	Toksična infekcija Clostridium perfringensom
Toxicomanie	Drug addiction	Adicción a las drogas (drogodependencia)	Tossicodipendenza (tossicomania)	Ovisnost o drogama
Toxocarose	Toxocariasis	Toxocariasis	Toxocariasi	Toksokarijaza
Toxoplasmose	Toxoplasmosis	Toxoplasmosis	Toxoplasmosi	Toksoplazmoza
Trachome	Trachoma	Tracoma	Tracoma	Trahom
Transplantation rénale	Kidney transplatation	Transplante de riñón	Trapianto renale	Transplantacija bubrega
Transposition de l'aorte	Transposition of aorta	Transposición de la aorta	Trasposizione dell'aorta	Transpozicija aorte
Transposition de l'artère pulmonaire	Transposition of pulmonary artery	Transposición de la arteria pulmonar	Trasposizione dell'arteria polmonare	Transpozicija plućne arterije
Transposition des gros vaisseaux	Transposition of the great vessels	Transposición de los grandes vasos	Trasposizione dei grossi vasi	Transpozicija velikih žila
Tremblement	Tremor	Temblor	Tremito (tremore)	Drhtanje (tremor)
Tremblement des mains	Hand tremor	Temblor en las manos	Tremore delle mani	Drhtanje ruku
Trichinose	Trichinosis (trichinellosis)	Triquinelosis (triquinosis)	Trichinosi	Trihinoza (trihineloza)
Trichomonas vaginalis	Trichomonas vaginalis	Trichomonas vaginalis	Trichomonas vaginalis	Trihomonazni vaginitis
Trichomoniase	Trichomoniasis	Trichomoniasis	Trichomoniasi	Trihomonijaza
Trouble bipolaire (psychose maniaco-dépressive)	Bipolar disorder (manic-depressive psychosis)	Trastorno bipolar (psicosis maníaco-depresiva)	Psicosi maniaco-depressiva	Bipolarni poremećaj (manično-depresivna psihoza)
Trouble de conduite alimentaire	Eating disorder	Trastorno alimentario	Disturbo del comporta-mento alimentare	Poremećaj ishrane
Trouble de coordination des mouvements musculaires (ataxie)	Lack of coordination of muscle movements (ataxia)	Descoordinación en el movimientos musculares (ataxia)	Disturbo della coordinazione muscolare (atassia)	Poremećaj koordinacije mišićnih pokreta (ataksija)
Trouble de l'apprentissage	Learning disability	Dificultad del aprendizaje	Disturbo di apprendimento	Poremećaj učenja
Trouble de l'apprentissage du langage (dysphasie)	Speech difficulty (dysphasia)	Trastorno del lenguaje (disfasia)	Disturbo del linguaggio verbale (afasia)	Otežan govor (disfazija)
Trouble de l'audition	Hearing disorder	Trastorno de la audición	Disturbo dell'udito	Poremećaj sluha
Trouble de l'équilibre	Balance disorder	Trastorno del equilibrio	Disturbo dell'equilibrio	Poremećaj ravnoteže
Trouble de la différenciation sexuelle	Sexual differentiation disorder	Trastorno de la diferenciación sexual	Disordine della differenziazione sessuale	Poremećaj spolne diferencijacije
Trouble de la miction	Urination disorder	Trastorno de la micción	Disturbo della minzione	Poremećaj mokrenja
Trouble de la personnalité	Personality disorder	Trastorno de personalidad	Disturbo di personalità	Poremećaj osobnosti

Français	Anglais	Espagnol	Italien	Croate
Trouble de la vue	Sight disorder	Trastorno de la visión	Disturbo della vista	Poremećaj vida
Trouble de stress post-traumatique	Posttraumatic stress disorder	Trastorno por estrés postraumático	Disturbo post traumatico da stress	Posttraumatski stresni poremećaj (PTSP)
Trouble déficit de l'attention	Attention deficit disorder	Trastorno por déficit de atención	Disturbo della concentrazione	Poremećaj koncentracije
Trouble du comportement	Behavioral disorder	Trastorno del comportamiento	Disturbo dell'umore	Poremećaj ponašanja
Trouble du mouvement	Movement disorder	Trastorno de movimiento	Disordine del movimento	Poremećaj kretanja
Trouble du sommeil	Sleeping disorder	Trastorno del sueño	Disturbo del sonno	Poremećaj spavanja
Troubles du cycle menstruel	Menstrual disorder	Trastorno menstrual	Disturbi mestruali	Menstrualne smetnje
Trypanosomiase	Trypanosomiasis	Tripanosomiasis	Tripanosomiasi	Tripanosomijaza
Tuberculose	Tuberculosis (TBC)	Tuberculosis (tisis, TBC)	Tubercolosi (tisi)	Tuberkuloza (sušica, TBC)
Tuberculose des os	Bone tuberculosis	Tuberculosis ósea	Tubercolosi delle ossa	Tuberkuloza kosti
Tuberculose hépatique	Hepatic tuberculosis	Tuberculosis hepática	Tubercolosi epatica	Tuberkuloza jetre
Tuberculose intestinale	Intestinal tuberculosis	Tuberculosis intestinal	Tubercolosi intestinale	Tuberkuloza crijeva
Tuberculose pulmonaire	Pulmonary tuberculosis	Tuberculosis pulmonar	Tubercolosi polmonare	Tuberkuloza pluća
Tuberculose rénale	Renal tuberculosis	Tuberculosis renal	Tubercolosi dei reni	Tuberkuloza bubrega
Tuberculose urogénitale	Urogenital tuberculosis	Tuberculosis urogenital	Tubercolosi urogenitale	Urogenitalna tuberkuloza
Tularémie	Tularemia (rabbit fever)	Tularemia (fiebre de los conejos)	Tularemia (febbre dei conigli)	Tularemija (zečja groznica)
Tumeur	Tumor (tumour)	Tumor	Tumore	Tumor
Tumeur à cellules géantes	Gigantocellular tumor (osteoclastoma)	Tumor de células gigantes (osteoclastoma)	Osteoclastoma (tumore a cellule giganti)	Gigantocelularni tumor (osteoklastom)
Tumeur bénigne	Benign tumor	Tumor benigno	Tumore benigno	Dobroćudni tumor (benigni tumor)
Tumeur de Brenner	Brenner tumour	Tumor de Brenner	Tumore di Brenner	Brennerov tumor
Tumeur de la granulosa	Granulosa cell tumor	Tumor de células de la granulosa (tumor de teca-granulosa)	Follicoloma	Granuloza tumor
Tumeur de Wilms (néphroblastome)	Wilm's tumor (nephroblastoma)	Tumor de Wilms (nefroblastoma)	Tumore di Wilms (nefroblastoma)	Wilmsov tumor (nefroblastom)
Tumeur du sac vitellin	Yolk sac tumor (endodermal sinus tumor)	Tumor de saco vitelino	Tumore del sacco vitellino	Tumor žumanjčane vreće (endodermalni sinus tumor)
Tumeur du système uro-génital	Urogenital neoplasm	Tumor urogenital	Neoplasie del tratto urogenitale	Urogenitalni tumor
Tumeur glomique (glomangiome)	Glomus tumor (glomangioma)	Tumor glómico (glomangioma)	Glomangioma (paraganglioma)	Glomus-tumor
Tumeur maligne (cancer)	Malignant tumor (cancer)	Tumor maligno (cáncer)	Tumore maligno	Zloćudni tumor (maligni tumor, rak)
Tumeur mixte	Mixed tumor	Tumor mixto	Tumore misto	Mješoviti tumor
Tumeur mixte malin	Malignant mixed tumor	Tumor mixto maligno	Tumore misto maligno	Mješoviti maligni tumor
Typhus épidémique (typhus à poux, typhus européen)	Epidemic typhus (louse-borne typhus)	Tifus exantemático epidémico	Tifo esantematico (tifo epidemico)	Trbušni tifus (epidemjski tifus, pjegavac)
Typhus murin	Murine typhus (endemic typhus)	Tifus endémico murino	Tifo murino (tifo endemico)	Štakorski pjegavac
Ulcère	Ulcer	Úlcera (llaga)	Ulcera (ulcerazione)	Čir (ulkus)
Ulcère de l'estomac	Gastric ulcer	Úlcera gástrica	Ulcera gastrica	Čir na želucu
Ulcère du doudénum	Duodenal ulcer	Úlcera duodenal	Ulcera duodenale	Čir na dvanaesniku
Ulcère ischémique	Ischemic ulceration	Úlcera isquémica	Ulcera ischemica	Ishemična ulceracija
Ulcère veineux	Venous ulcer (varicose ulcer)	Úlcera varicosa	Ulcera varicosa	Varikozni ulcer (venski ulcer)
Urémie (le taux de l'urée dans le sang)	Uremia (autointoxication due to kidney failure)	Uremia (acumulación en la sangre de los productos tóxicos por un fallo renal)	Uremia (accumulo nel sangue di sostanze azotate a causa dell'insufficienza renale)	Uremija (autointoksikacija radi nelučenja urina)
Urination douloureuse (strangurie)	Painful urination (strangury)	Micción dolorosa (angurria)	Minzione dolorosa (stranguria)	Bol pri mokrenju (strangurija)
Urine marron	Brown urine	Orina de color marrón	Urina marrone	Smeđi urin
Urine opaque	Unclear urine (foggy urine)	Orina turbia	Urine torbide	Mutni urin
Urine rouge	Red urine	Orina de color rojo	Urina di colore rosso	Crveni urin
Urticaire	Hives (urticaria)	Urticaria	Orticaria	Koprivnjača (urtikarija)
Utérus rétroversé	Retroverted uterus	Retroversión del útero	Retroflessione uterina	Retrovertirani uterus
Vaginose bactérienne	Bacterial vaginosis	Vaginosis bacteriana	Infezione della vagina batterica (vaginosi)	Bakterijska infekcija rodnice (bakterijska vaginoza)
Varice dans le cou	Neck varicose veins	Varices del cuello	Vene varicose del collo	Proširene vratne vene
Varicelle	Chicken-pox	Varicela	Varicella	Vodene kozice (varičela)
Varices	Varicose veins	Varices	Varicosi (varici, malattia varicosa)	Proširene vene
Varices des membres inférieurs	Leg varicose veins	Venas varicosas de las piernas	Varici degli arti inferiori	Proširene vene na nogama
Varices oesophagiennes	Esophageal varices	Varices esofágicas	Varici esofagee	Proširene vene jednjaka (flebektazije)
Varicocèle	Varicocele	Varicocele	Varicocele	Varikokela

Français	Anglais	Espagnol	Italien	Croate
Variole (petite vérole)	Smallpox	Viruela	Variola vera (vaiolo)	Velike boginje (crne boginje, variola vera)
Verrue	Wart	Verruga	Verruca	Bradavica (virusna bradavica)
Verrue génitale	Genital wart	Verruga genital (condiloma acuminata)	Condiloma	Genitalna bradavica (venerična bradavica)
Vertige	Dizziness (vertigo)	Vértigo	Capogiro (vertigine)	Vrtoglavica
Vertige paroxystique positionnel bénign	Benign positional vertigo	Vértigo posicional paroxístico benigno	Cupololitiasi (canalolitiasi)	Benigna pozicijska vrtoglavica
Vision double (diplopie)	Double vision (diplopia)	Visión doble (diplopía)	Visione doppia (diplopia)	Dvoslike
Vitiligo	Vitiligo	Vitíligo	Vitiligine	Vitiligo
Volvulus	Abnormal twisting of the intestines (volvulus)	Retorcimiento anormal del intestino (vólvulo)	Volvolo	Zapletaj crijeva
Vomissement	Vomiting	Vómito (emesis)	Vomito (emetismo)	Povraćanje
Vomissement de sang (hématémèse)	Vomiting of blood (hematemesis)	Vómito de sangre (hematemesis)	Emesi emorragica (ematemesi)	Povraćanje krvi (hematemeza)
Vomissement en fusée sans effort	Vomiting without nausea (cerebral vomiting)	Vómito sin náusea (vómito cerebral)	Vomito senza nausea (vomito a getto, vomito cerebrale)	Povraćanje bez mučnine (povraćanje u luku, cerebralno povraćanje)
Xanthelasma	Xanthelasma	Xantelasma	Xantelasma	Ksantelazma
Xanthome	Xanthoma	Xantoma	Xantoma	Ksantom
Yeux larmoyants	Watery eyes	Ojos llorosos	Occhi lacrimosi	Suzenje očiju
Zona	Herpes zoster	Herpes zóster (herpes zona)	Herpes zoster	Herpes zoster
Zoonose	Zoonosis	Zoonosis	Zoonosi	Zoonoza

PHARMACIE:	PHARMACY:	FARMACIA:	FARMACIA:	LJEKARNA:
À jeun	On an empty stomach (before the meal)	En ayunas	A digiuno	Na tašte
À midi	At noon	A mediodía	A mezzogiorno	U podne
Acide borique	Boric acid	Ácido bórico	Acido borico	Borova otopina
Acides gras oméga-3	Omega-3 fatty acid	Ácido graso omega 3	Omega-3 acidi grassi	Omega-3 masne kiseline
Adrénaline	Adrenaline	Adrenalina	Adrenalina	Adrenalin
Aérosol	Aerosol	Aerosol	Aerosol	Aerosol
Agent antiarythmique	Antiarrhythmic agent	Agente antiarrítmico	Farmaco antiaritmico	Antiaritmik
Aiguille	Needle	Aguja	Ago	Igla
Alcohol	Alcohol	Alcol	Alcool	Alkohol
Allergie à un médicament	Drug allergy	Alergia al medicamento	Allergia a medicamento	Alergija na lijek
Aminophylline	Aminophylline	Aminofilina	Aminofillina	Aminofilin
Ampicilline	Ampicillin	Ampicilina	Ampicillina	Ampicilin
Ampoule	Ampoule	Ampolla (recipiente)	Ampolla (fiala)	Ampula
Analgésique	Analgesic (painkiller)	Analgésico	Analgesico	Analgetik
Anesthésique	Anesthetic	Anestésico	Anestetico	Anestetik
Antihelminthique	Antihelminthic	Antihelmíntico	Antielmintici	Antihelmintik
Anti-inflammatoire	Anti-inflammatory	Antiinflamatorio (antiflogístico)	Antinfiammatorio	Protuupalno
Anti-inflammatoire non stéroïdien	Non-steroidal anti-inflammatory drug	Antiinflamatorio no esteroideo	Farmaco anti-infiammatore non steroide-FANS	Nesteroidni antireumatik
Antiacide	Antacid	Antiácido	Antiacido	Antacid
Antiallergique	Antiallergic drug	Antialérgico	Farmaco antiallergico	Antialergik
Antibiotique	Antibiotic	Antibiótico	Antibiotico	Antibiotik
Anticoagulant	Anticoagulant	Anticoagulante	Anticoagulante	Antikoagulans
Antidépresseur	Antidepressant	Antidepresivo	Antidepressivo	Antidepresiv
Antidote	Antidote	Antídoto	Antidoto	Antidot
Antiémétique	Antiemetic and motion sickness drug	Antiemético	Antiemetico	Lijek protiv mučnine i povraćanja
Antiépileptique (anticonvulsivant)	Anticonvulsant	Anticonvulsivo (antiepiléptico)	Anticonvulsante	Antiepileptik (antikonvulziv)
Antihistaminique	Antihistamine	Antihistamínico	Antistaminico	Antihistaminik
Antihypertenseur	Antihypertensive drug	Antihipertensivo	Farmaco antiipertensivo	Antihipertenziv
Antimalarique	Antimalarial drug	Antimalárico	Antimalarico	Antimalarik
Antimycosique	Antimycotic	Antimicótico (antifúngico)	Antimicotico	Antimikotik
Antioxydant	Antioxidant	Antioxidante	Antiossidante (sostanza antiossidante)	Antioksidans
Antipsychotique	Antipsychotic	Antipsicótico	Antipsicotico	Antipsihotik
Antipyrétique	Antipyretic	Antipirético	Antipiretico	Antipiretik
Antiseptique	Antiseptic	Antiséptico	Antisettico	Antiseptik
Antiseptique urinaire	Urinary antiseptic	Antiséptico de las vías urinarias	Antisettico urinario	Uroantiseptik
Antisérum	Antiserum	Antisuero	Antisiero	Antiserum
Antitoxine	Antitoxin	Antitoxina	Antitossina	Protuotrov
Antituberculeux	Antitubercular agent	Fármaco tuberculostático	Farmaco antitubercolare	Antituberkulotik
Après-repas	After meal	Después de una comida	Dopo il pasto	Nakon jela
Aspirine	Aspirin	Aspirina	Aspirina	Aspirin
Atropine	Atropine	Atropina	Atropina	Atropin
Balance	Scales	Balanza	Bilancia	Vaga
Bandage	Bandage	Venda	Bendaggio	Zavoj
Barbiturique	Barbiturate	Barbitúrico	Barbiturico	Barbiturat

Français	Anglais	Espagnol	Italien	Croate
Bouillotte	Hot water bottle	Bolsa de agua caliente (guatero)	Bouillotte (bouilloire)	Termofor
Bronchodilatateur	Bronchodilator	Broncodilatador	Broncodilatatore	Bronhodilatator
Caféine	Caffeine	Cafeína	Caffeina	Kofein
Calcium	Calcium	Calcio	Calcio	Kalcij
Camomille	Chamomile	Manzanilla	Camomilla	Kamilica
Cannabis médical	Medical cannabis	Cannabis medicinal	Cannabis terapeutica	Medicinski kanabis
Céphalosporine	Cephalosporin	Cefalosporina	Cefalosporina	Cefalosporin
Charbon actif	Activated carbon	Carbón activado	Carbone attivo	Aktivni ugljen
Chimiothérapie	Chemotherapy	Quimioterapia	Chemioterapia	Kemoterapija
Chloramphénicol	Chloramphenicol	Cloranfenicol	Cloramfenicolo	Kloramfenikol
Chlore	Chlorine	Cloro	Cloro	Klor
Clystère	Enema (clyster)	Enema (clisma)	Clistere	Klizma (klistir)
Cobalt	Cobalt	Cobalto	Cobalto	Kobalt
Codéine	Codeine	Codeína	Codeina	Kodein
Collyre (gouttes ophtalmiques)	Eye drops	Colirio	Collirio	Kapi za oči
Compresse	Compress	Compresa	Compressa	Oblog
Comprimé	Tablet	Comprimido	Compressa (pasticca, tavoletta)	Dražeja (tableta)
Comprimé effervescent	Water-soluble tablets	Solubilizantes (comprimidos dispersables en agua)	Compresse solubili	Šumeće tablete
Contraceptif	Contraceptive	Anticonceptivo	Contraccettivo	Kontraceptiv
Contraception orale	Contraceptive pill (oral contraceptive)	Pildora anticonceptiva	Pillola anticoncezionale	Kontracepcijska pilula
Corticostéroïde	Corticosteroid	Corticosteroide	Corticosteroide	Kortikosteroid
Crème	Skin cream	Crema	Crema	Krema
Crème solaire	Sunscreen (sunblock)	Protector solar	Filtro solare (crema solare ad alta protezione)	Sredstvo za zaštitu od sunca
Cuillère	Spoon	Cuchara	Cucchiaio	Žlica
Cuivre	Copper	Cobre	Rame	Bakar
Cytostatique	Cytostatic	Citostático	Citostatico	Citostatik
Dentifrice	Tooth paste	Pasta de dientes (dentífrico)	Dentifricio	Pasta za zube
Déodorant	Antiperspirant	Desodorante	Antidiaforetico	Antiperspirant
Diaphragme	Diaphragm (Dutch cap)	Diafragma	Diaframma	Dijafragma
Diurétique	Diuretic	Diurético	Diuretico	Diuretik
Dose	Dose	Dosis	Dose	Doza
Eau dentifrice	Mouthwash liquid	Enjuague bucal (colutorio)	Collutorio	Tekućina za ispiranje usne šupljine
Édulcorant	Sugar substitute	Edulcorante artificial	Dolcificante artificiale	Umjetno sladilo
Effets indésirables d'un médicament	Drug side-effects	Reacción adversa a medicamento	Effetti indesiderati da farmaco	Nuspojave lijeka
Émulsion	Emulsion	Emulsión	Emulsione	Emulzija
Éponge contraceptive	Contraceptive sponge	Esponja anticonceptiva	Spugna contraccettiva	Kontracepcijska spužva
Érythromycine	Erythromycin	Eritromicina	Eritromicina	Eritromicin
Expectorant	Expectorant	Expectorante	Espettorante	Sredstvo za iskašljavanje
Fentanyl	Fentanyl	Fentanilo	Fentanyl	Fentanil
Fer	Iron	Hierro (fierro)	Ferro	Željezo
Fil dentaire	Dental floss	Seda dental (hilo dental)	Filo interdentale	Zubni konac
Fiole	Vial	Frasquito	Bottiglietta (boccetta)	Bočica
Gaze	Gauze sponge	Gasa	Garza	Gaza
Gel	Gel	Gel	Gel	Gel
Gélule	Capsule	Cápsula	Capsula	Kapsula
Gentamicine	Gentamicin	Gentamicina	Gentamicina	Gentamicin
Glucose	Glucose	Glucosa	Glucosio	Glukoza
Gomme à la nicotine	Nicotine gum	Goma de mascar de nicotina	Gomma da masticare antifumo	Nikotinska guma za žvakanje
Gouttes	Drops	Gotas	Gocce	Kapi (kapljice)
Gouttes auriculaires	Ear drops	Gotas óticas	Gocce per il mal di orecchi	Kapi za uši
Gouttes nasales	Nasal drops	Gotas nasales	Gocce nasali	Kapi za nos
Gramme	Gram (gramme)	Gramo	Grammo	Gram
Hémostatique	Antihemorrhagic (hemostatic)	Hemostático	Emostatico	Hemostatik
Héparine	Heparin	Heparina	Eparina	Heparin
Hormonothérapie de substitution	Hormone replacement therapy	Terapia de sustitución hormonal	Terapia ormonale sostitutiva	Hormonalna nadomjesna terapija
Huile d'amande	Almond oil	Aceite de almendras dulces	Olio di mandorla	Bademovo ulje
Huile de jojoba	Jojoba oil	Aceite de jojoba	Olio di jojoba	Jojobino ulje
Huile de ricin	Castor oil	Aceite de ricino	Olio di ricino	Ricinusovo ulje
Huile essentielle	Essential oil	Aceite esencial	Olio essenziale (olio eterico)	Eterično ulje
Huile minérale	Mineral oil	Aceite mineral	Olio minerale	Mineralno ulje
Hypnotique (somnifère)	Hypnotic (soporific)	Hipnótico	Ipnotico	Hipnotik
Immunoglobuline	Immunoglobulin	Inmunoglobulina	Immunoglobulina	Imunoglobulin
Immunosuppresseur	Immunosuppressive	Inmunosupresor	Immunosoppressivo	Imunosupresiv

Français	Anglais	Espagnol	Italien	Croate
Inhalation	Inhalation	Inhalación	Inalazione (farmaco per inalazioni)	Inhalacija
Insuline	Insulin	Insulina	Insulina	Inzulin
Interféron	Interferon	Interferón	Interferone	Interferon
Injection	Injection	Inyección	Iniezione	Injekcija
Iode	Iodine	Yodo (iodo)	Iodio (tintura di iodio)	Jod
Laxatif	Laxative	Laxante	Lassativo	Laksativ
Le matin	In the morning	Por la mañana	Di mattina	U jutro
Le soir	In the evening	Por la noche	La sera	Na večer
Lentille de contact rigide	Hard contact lens	Lente de contacto duro	Lente a contatto rigida	Tvrda kontaktna leća
Lentille de contact souple	Soft contact lens	Lente de contacto blanda	Lente a contatto morbida	Meka kontaktna leća
Lentilles de contact	Contact lenses	Lentes de contacto (lentillas, pupilentes)	Lenti a contatto	Kontaktne leće
Litre	Litre	Litro	Litro	Litra
Lotion	Lotion	Loción	Lozione	Losion
Lubrifiant	Lubricant	Lubricante	Lubrificante	Lubrikant
Lunettes de vue	Glasses	Gafas	Occhiali	Naočale
Magnésium	Magnesium	Magnesio	Magnesio	Magnezij
Manganèse	Manganese	Manganeso	Manganese	Mangan
Médicament	Medication (remedy, drug)	Medicamento (fármaco)	Medicamento (farmaco, rimedio)	Lijek
Médicament anti-obésité	Anti-obesity medication	Fármaco antiobesidad	Dimagrante (farmaco antiobesità)	Dijetetsko sredstvo
Médicament antianémique	Antianemic	Antianémico	Farmaco antianemico	Antianemik
Médicament antidiabétique	Anti-diabetic drug	Antidiabético	Antidiabetico	Antidiabetik
Médicament antidiarrhéique	Antidiarrhoeal drug	Antidiarréico	Antidiarroici	Antidiaroik
Médicament antiprotozoal	Antiprotozoal agent	Antiprotozoario	Farmaco antiprotozoico	Antiprotozoik
Médicament antirhumatismal	Antirheumatic drug	Antireumático	Antireumatico	Antireumatik
Médicament antiviral	Antiviral drug	Fármaco antiviral	Farmaco antivirale	Antivirusni lijek
Médicament cardiotonique	Cardiotonic agent	Cardiotónico	Cardiotonico	Kardiotonik
Médicament contre la dépendance à l'alcool	Antialcoholic drug	Fármaco antialcohólico	Farmaco anti-alcol	Antialkoholik
Médicament digestif	Digestive	Digestivo	Digestivo	Digestiv
Méthadone	Methadone	Metadona	Metadone	Metadon
Microgramme	Microgram	Microgramo	Microgrammo	Mikrogram
Milligramme	Milligram (milligramme)	Miligramo	Milligrammo	Miligram
Millilitre	Millilitre	Mililitro	Millilitro	Mililitar
Minéral	Mineral	Mineral	Minerale	Mineral
Molybdène	Molybdenum	Molibdeno	Molibdeno	Molibden
Morceau	Piece	Pieza	Pezzo (porzione)	Komad
Morphine	Morphine	Morfina	Morfina	Morfin
Mousse	Foam	Espuma	Schiuma (spuma)	Pjena
Mousse contraceptive	Contraceptive foam	Espuma anticonceptiva	Schiuma anticoncezionale	Kontracepcijska pjena
Mucolytique	Mucolytic	Mucolítico	Mucolitico	Mukolitik
Myorelaxant	Muscle relaxant	Relajante muscular (miorrelajante)	Miorilassante	Miorelaksator
Nutriment (élément nutritif)	Nutrient	Nutrimento (nutriente)	Sostanza nutriente (sostanza nutritiva)	Nutritiv
Nystatine	Nystatin	Nistatina	Nistatina	Nistatin
Opioïde	Opioid	Opioide	Oppioide	Opijat (opioid)
Ordonnance médicale	Prescription	Receta	Prescrizione (rimedio prescritto)	Recept
Ouate (coton hydrophile)	Cotton-wool	Algodón hidrófilo	Ovatta	Vata
Ovule (suppositoire vaginal)	Vaginal suppository	Supositorio vaginal	Candelette	Vaginaleta
Oxycodone	Oxycodone	Oxicodona	Ossicodone	Oksikodon
Pansement	Plaster (adhesive strip)	Tira adhesiva sanitaria	Cerotto	Flaster
Par voie orale	Orally	Por vía oral	Oralmente (per via orale, per bocca)	Na usta
Paracétamol	Paracetamol	Paracetamol	Paracetamolo	Paracetamol
Paraffine	Paraffin	Parafina	Paraffina	Parafin
Pastille	Pastille (lozenge)	Pastilla	Pasticca (pastiglia)	Tableta za sisanje (pastila)
Pâte	Paste	Pasta	Pasta	Pasta
Pénicilline	Penicillin	Penicilina	Penicillina	Penicilin
Pharmacien	Pharmacist	Farmacéutico	Farmacista	Ljekarnik
Phosphore	Phosphorus	Fósforo	Fosforo	Fosfor
Phytothérapie	Phytotherapy	Fitoterapia	Fitoterapia	Fitoterapija
Pilule du lendemain (contraception postcoïtale, contraception d'urgence)	'Morning-after' pill (postcoital contraception, emergency contraception)	Anticonceptivo de emergencia (contracepción poscoital)	Pillola del "giorno doppo" (contraccezione postcoitale, contraccezione di emergenza)	Pilula za "dan poslije" (postkoitalna kontracepcija, hitna kontracepcija)
Poison	Poison	Veneno	Veleno	Otrov
Pommade	Ointment (fat)	Ungüento (pomada)	Pomata (unguento)	Pomada (mast)

Français	Anglais	Espagnol	Italien	Croate
Pommade à l'oxyde de zinc	Zinc ointment	Pasta de óxido de zinc	Zinco pasta	Cinkova pasta
Potassium	Potassium	Potasio	Potassio	Kalij
Potion	Potion	Poción	Pozione	Ljekoviti napitak
Poudre	Powder	Polvo	Polverina (polvere)	Prašak (puder)
Poudre fluide	Liquid powder	Polvo líquido	Polvere liquido	Tekući puder
Pour l'application externe	For external application	De uso externo	Per l'applicazione esterna	Za vanjsku primjenu
Préservatif	Condom	Preservativo (condón, profiláctico)	Preservativo (profilattico, condom)	Prezervativ (kondom)
Psychostimulant	Psychostimulant	Psicoestimulante	Psicostimulanti	Psihostimulans
Purgatif	Purgative	Purgante (purgativo)	Purgante (purga)	Purgativ
Rectal	Rectal	Rectal	Rettale	Rektalno
Répulsif antimoustiques	Mosquito repellent	Repelente de mosquitos	Repellente antizanzare	Sredstvo protiv komaraca
Répulsif d'insectes	Insect repellent	Repelente de insectos	Insettifugo	Sredstvo protiv insekata
Rinçage	Rinsing	Lavado	Sciacquatra (risciacquatura)	Ispiranje
Salicylate	Salicylate	Salicilato	Salicilato	Salicilat
Savon	Soap	Jabón	Sapone	Sapun
Sédatif	Sedative	Sedativo	Sedativo (calmante)	Sedativ
Seringue	Syringe	Jeringa	Siringa per iniezioni	Šprica
Sérum	Serum	Suero	Siero	Serum
Serviette hygiénique (protège-slip)	Sanitary pads (sanitary napkins)	Toalla sanitaria (com-presa, pantiprotector)	Assorbenti igienici	Higijenski ulošci
Sirop	Syrup	Jarabe	Sciroppo	Sirup
Slip d'incontinence	Incontinence pads (adult diapers)	Pañal para adultos	Assorbenti per l'incontinenza	Pelene za inkontinenciju
Sodium	Sodium	Sodio	Sodio	Natrij
Solution	Solution	Soluto	Soluzione	Otopina
Solution nettoyante pour lentilles	Contact lenses cleaning solution	Solución limpiadora de lentes de contacto	Soluzione per pulizia lenti a contatto	Tekućina za čišćenje kontaktnih leća
Solution nettoyante pour les prothèses	Denture cleaning solution	Solución limpiadora de dentadura	Soluzione per pulizia dentiera	Tekućina za čišćenje umjetnog zubala
Solution physiologique	Saline solution	Suero fisiológico	Soluzione fisiologica	Fiziološka otopina
Soufre	Sulphur	Azufre	Zolfo	Sumpor
Spasmolytique	Spasmolytic	Espasmolítico	Spasmolitico	Spazmolitik
Spermicide	Spermicide	Espermicida	Spermicida	Spermicid
Spray	Spray	Rociada	Spruzzo (vaporizzato)	Sprej
Sublingual	Sublingual administration	Vía sublingual	Sublinguale	Pod jezik
Sulfamidé	Sulphonamide	Sulfonamida	Sulfamidici (sulfonamidici)	Sulfonamid
Suppositoire	Suppository	Supositorio	Supposta	Čepić
Surdose	Overdose	Sobredosis	Sovradosaggio	Predoziranje
Système international d'unités	International System of Units	Sistema Internacional de Unidades	Sistema internazionale di unità di misura	Sustav međunarodnih mjernih jedinica
Tampon hygiénique	Tampon	Tampón	Tampone	Tampon
Teinture	Tincture	Tintura	Tintura	Tinktura
Tensiomètre (sphygmomanomètre)	Blood pressure meter (sphygmomanometer)	Tensiómetro (esfigmomanómetro)	Misuratore di pressione (sfigmomanometro)	Tlakomjer
Test de grossesse	Home pregnancy test	Prueba de embarazo	Test di gravidanza ad uso domiciliare	Kućni test za trudnoću
Tétracycline	Tetracycline	Tetraciclina	Tetraciclina	Tetraciklin
Thermomètre	Thermometer	Termómetro	Termometro	Toplomjer
Timbre à la nicotine	Nicotine patch	Parche de nicotina	Cerotto antifumo	Nikotinski flaster
Tisane	Herbal tea	Tisana (infusión de hierbas)	Tisana (infuso di erbe)	Biljni čaj
Tonique	Tonic	Tónico	Tonico (ricostituente)	Tonik
Tramadol	Tramadol	Tramadol	Tramadolo	Tramal
Tube de soin pour lèvres	Lip balm	Bálsamo de labios	Burrocacao	Grožđana mast
Vaccin	Vaccine	Vacuna	Vaccino	Cjepivo
Vasodilatateur	Vasodilator	Vasodilatador	Vasodilatatore	Vazodilatator
Viagra (citrate de sildénafil)	Viagra (sildenafil citrate)	Viagra	Viagra (citrato di sildenafil)	Viagra
Vitamine	Vitamin	Vitamina	Vitamina	Vitamin
Vitamine A (rétinol)	Vitamin A (retinol)	Vitamina A (retinol)	Vitamina A (retinolo)	Vitamin A (retinol)
Vitamine B1 (thiamine)	Vitamin B1 (thiamin)	Vitamina B1 (tiamina)	Vitamina B1 (tiamina)	Vitamin B1 (tiamin)
Vitamine B2 (riboflavine)	Vitamin B2 (riboflavin)	Vitamina B2 (riboflavina)	Vitamina B2 (riboflavina)	Vitamin B2 (riboflavin)
Vitamine B3 (nicotinamide, PP)	Vitamin B3 (niacin)	Vitamina B3 (niacina, vitamina PP)	Vitamina B3 (niacina, vitamina PP)	Vitamin B3 (niacin)
Vitamine B4 (adénine)	Vitamin B4 (adenine)	Vitamina B4 (adenina)	Vitamina B4 (adenina)	Vitamin B4 (adenin)
Vitamine B5 (acide pantothénique)	Vitamin B5 (pantothenic acid)	Vitamina B5 (ácido pantoténico)	Vitamina B5 (acido pantotenico, vitamina W)	Vitamin B5 (pantotenska kiselina)
Vitamine B6 (pyridoxine)	Vitamin B6 (pyridoxine)	Vitamina B6 (piridoxina)	Vitamina B6 (piridossina)	Vitamin B6 (piridoksin)
Vitamine B7 (inositol)	Vitamin B7 (inositol)	Vitamina B7 (inositol)	Vitamina B7 (inositolo)	Vitamin B7 (inozitol)
Vitamine B8 (biotine)	Vitamin B8 (biotin)	Vitamina B8 (biotina)	Vitamina B8 (biotina)	Vitamin B8 (biotin)
Vitamine B9 (acide folique)	Vitamin B9 (folic acid)	Vitamina B9 (ácido fólico)	Vitamina B9 (acido folico)	Vitamin B9 (folna kiselina)
Vitamine B10 (vitamine R)	Vitamin B10 (factor-R)	Vitamina B10 (vitamina R)	Vitamina B10 (vitamina R)	Vitamin B10 (faktor-R)
Vitamine B11 (carnitine)	Vitamin B11 (factor-S)	Vitamina B11 (vitamina S)	Vitamina B11 (vitamina S)	Vitamin B11 (faktor-S)
Vitamine B12 (cobalamine)	Vitamin B12 (cobalamin)	Vitamina B12 (ciancobalamina)	Vitamina B12 (cobalamina)	Vitamin B12 (kobalamin)

Français	Anglais	Espagnol	Italien	Croate
Vitamine C (acide ascorbique)	Vitamin C (L-ascorbic acid)	Vitamine C (enantióme-ro L de ácido ascórbico)	Vitamina C (acido L-ascorbico)	Vitamin C (L-askorbinska kiselina)
Vitamine D2 (ergocalciférol)	Vitamin D2 (ergocalciferol)	Vitamina D2 (ergocalciferol)	Vitamina D2 (ergocalciferolo)	Vitamin D2 (ergokalciferol)
Vitamine D3 (cholécalciférol)	Vitamin D3 (cholecalciferol)	Vitamina D3 (colecalciferol)	Vitamina D3 (colecalciferolo)	Vitamin D3 (kolekalciferol)
Vitamine D4	Vitamin D4	Vitamina D4	Vitamina D4 (diidroergocalciferolo)	Vitamin D4
Vitamine D5 (sitocalciférol)	Vitamin D5 (sitocalciferol)	Vitamina D5 (sitocalciferol)	Vitamina D5 (sitocalciferolo)	Vitamin D5 (sitokalciferol)
Vitamine E (tocophérol)	Vitamin E (tocopherol)	Vitamina E (alfatocoferol)	Vitamina E (tocoferolo)	Vitamin E (tokoferol)
Vitamine F (acide linoléique)	Vitamin F (linoleic acid)	Ácido linoleico	Vitamina F (acido linoleico)	Vitamin F (linoleična kiselina)
Vitamine J (choline)	Vitamin J (choline)	Vitamina J (colina)	Vitamina J (colina)	Vitamin J (kolin)
Vitamine K (phylloquinone)	Vitamin K (phylloquinone)	Vitamina K (filoquinona)	Vitamina K (fillochinone)	Vitamin K (filokinon)
Vitamine L1 (acide anthranilique)	Vitamin L1 (anthranilic acid)	Vitamina L1 (ácido antranílico)	Vitamina L1 (acido antranilico)	Vitamin L1 (antranilna kiselina)
Vitamine P (flavonoïde)	Vitamin P (flavonoids)	Vitamina P (flavonoide)	Vitamina P (flavonoidi)	Vitamin P (flavonoidi)
Zinc	Zinc	Zinc (cinc)	Zinco	Cink

ÉTABLISSEMENTS MÉDICAUX, PROCÉDURES ET SOINS:	MEDICAL FACILITIES, PROCEDURES AND CARE:	FACILIDADES MÉDICAS, PROCEDIMIENTOS Y ASISTENCIA MÉDICA:	ISTITUZIONI, PROCEDURE E CURE DI MEDICINA:	MEDICINSKE USTANOVE, ZAHVATI I NJEGA:
Ablation chirurgicale d'un lobe d'organe (lobectomie)	Surgical removal of a lobe of some organ (lobectomy)	Extirpación quirúrgica de un lóbulo de un órgano (lobectomía)	Asportazione chirurgica di struttura lobale di un organo (lobectomia)	Kirurško odstranjenje režnja nekog organa (lobektomija)
Ablation chirurgicale d'une ou des deux glandes surrénales (adrenalectomie)	Surgical removal of one or both adrenal glands (adrenalectomy)	Extirpación quirúrgica de una glándula suprarrenal (adrenalectomía)	Asportazione chirurgica di uno o etrambi surreni(surrenectomia, adrenalectomia)	Kirurško odstranjenje nadbubrežne žlijezde (adrenalektomija)
Ablation chirurgicale d'une partie du thalamus (thalamotomie)	Surgical procedure on the thalamus (thalamotomy)	Cirugía del tálamo (talamotomía)	Intervento chirurgico delle connessioni talamiche (talamotomia)	Kirurški zahvat na talamusu (talamotomija)
Ablation chirurgicale de l'appendice iléo-caecal (appendicectomie)	Surgical removal of the vermiform appendix (appendectomy)	Extirpación quirúrgica del apéndice cecal (apendicectomía)	Asportazione chirurgica dell'appendice (appendicectomia)	Kirurško odstranjenje slijepog crijeva (apendektomija)
Ablation chirurgicale de l'estomac (gastrectomie)	Surgical removal of the stomach (gastrectomy)	Extirpación quirúrgica del estómago (gastrectomía)	Asportazione chirurgica dello stomaco (gastrectomia)	Kirurško odstranjenje želuca (gastrektomija)
Ablation chirurgicale de l'étrier (stapédectomie)	Surgical procedure on the middle ear (stapedectomy)	Cirugía del oído medio (stapedectomía)	Intervento chirurgico dell'orecchio medio (stapedectomia)	Kirurški zahvat na srednjem uhu (stapedektomija)
Ablation chirurgicale de la prostate (prostatectomie)	Surgical removal of the prostate gland (prostatectomy)	Extirpación quirúrgica de la próstata (prostatectomía)	Asportazione chirurgica della prostata (prostatectomia)	Kirurško odstranjenje prostate (prostatektomija)
Ablation chirurgicale de la rate (splénectomie)	Surgical removal of the spleen (splenectomy)	Extirpación quirúrgica del bazo (esplenectomía)	Asportazione chirurgica della milza (splenectomia)	Kirurško odstranjenje slezene (splenektomija)
Ablation chirurgicale de la thyroïde (thyroïdectomie, isthmectomie)	Surgical removal of the thyroid gland (thyroidectomy)	Extirpación quirúrgica de la glándula tiroides (tiroidectomía)	Asportazione chirurgica della tiroide (tiroidectomia)	Kirurško odstranjenje štitne žlijezde (tiroidektomija)
Ablation chirurgicale des amygdales palatines (amygdalectomie, tonsillectomie)	Surgical removal of tonsils (tonsillectomy)	Extracción quirúrgica de las amígdalas (tonsilectomía)	Asportazione chirurgica delle tonsille (tonsillectomia)	Kirurško odstranjenje krajnika (tonzilektomija)
Ablation chirurgicale des fibromes utérins (myomectomie)	Surgical removal of ute-rine myomas (myome-ctomy, fibroidectomy)	Extirpación quirúrgica de los fibromas uterinos (miomectomía)	Asportazione chirurgica di fibromi nell'utero (miomectomia)	Kirurško odstranjenje mioma u maternici (miomektomija)
Ablation chirurgicale des hémorroïdes (hémorroïdectomie)	Surgical removal of a hemorrhoid (hemorrhoidectomy)	Extirpación quirúrgica de las hemorroides (hemorroidectomía)	Asportazione chirurgica delle emorroidi (emorroidectomia)	Kirurško odstranjenje hemeroida (hemoroidektomija)
Ablation chirurgicale des végétations adénoïdes (adénoïdectomie)	Surgical removal of adenoids (adenoidectomy)	Extirpación quirúrgica de las adenoides (adenoidectomía)	Asportazione chirurgica delle adenoidi (adenoidectomia)	Kirurško odstranjenje trećeg krajnika (adenoidektomija)
Ablation chirurgicale du larynx (laryngectomie)	Surgical removal of the larynx (laryngectomy)	Extirpación quirúrgica de la laringe (laringectomía)	Asportazione chirurgica della laringe (laringectomia)	Kirurško odstranjenje grkljana (laringektomija)
Ablation chirurgicale du pancréas (pancréatectomie)	Surgical removal of the pancreas (pancreatectomy)	Extirpación quirúrgica del páncreas (pancreatectomía)	Asportazione chirurgica del pancreas (pancreatectomia)	Kirurško odstranjenje gušterače (pankreatektomija)
Ablation chirurgicale du thymus (thymectomie)	Surgical removal of the thymus (thymectomy)	Extirpación quirúrgica del timo (timectomía)	Asportazione chirurgica del timo (timectomia)	Kirurško odstranjenje prsne žlijezde (timektomija)
Administration des médicaments	Administration of drugs	Administración de fármacos	Somministrazione dei farmaci	Davanje lijekova
Aide médicale urgente	Emergency medical services	Servicios médicos de emergencia	Servizio di urgenza ed emergenza medica	Hitna služba
Alarme	Alarm	Alarma	Allarme	Uzbuna (alarm)

Français	Anglais	Espagnol	Italien	Croate
Aller aux toilettes	Using a toilet	Ir al servicio	Uso del gabinetto	Obaviti nuždu
Ambulance	Ambulance	Ambulancia	Autoambulanza	Kola hitne pomoći
Amputation	Amputation	Amputación	Amputazione	Amputacija
Amputation chirurgicale d'un ou des deux testicules (orchidectomie, orchiectomie)	Surgical removal of a testicle (orchidectomy)	Extirpación quirúrgica del testículo (orquidectomía)	Asportazione chirurgica del testicolo (orchiectomia)	Kirurško odstranjenje testisa (orhidektomija)
Anesthésie	Anesthesia	Anestesia	Anestesia	Anestezija (narkoza)
Anesthésie générale	General anesthesia	Anestesia general	Anestesia generale	Opća anestezija
Anesthésie locale	Local anesthesia	Anestesia local	Anestesia locale	Lokalna anestezija
Angioplastie coronaire (dilatation transluminale)	Percutaneous coronary intervention (coronary angioplasty)	Intervención coronaria percutánea	Angioplastica coronarica	Perkutana koronarna angioplastika
Appareil à succion	Suction unit (aspirator)	Aspirador	Aspiratore di secreti	Aspirator
Appareil acoustique	Hearing assist device	Audífono	Apparecchio acustico	Slušni aparat
Appareil respiratoire	Respirator	Aparato respiratorio	Respiratore	Aparat za disanje (respirator)
Armoire	Wardrobe (cupboard, cabinet)	Armario	Armadio (credenza)	Ormar
Arthrodèse	Arthrodesis	Artrodesis	Artrodesi	Artrodeza
Ascenseur	Elevator	Elevador	Ascensore	Dizalo
Assurance maladie	Health insurance	Seguro de salud	Assicurazione sanitaria	Zdravstveno osiguranje
Autopsie	Autopsy	Autopsia	Autopsia	Obdukcija
Béquille	Crutch	Muleta	Gruccia (stampella)	Štaka
Blanchisserie	Laundry	Lavandería	Lavanderia	Vešeraj
Bloc opératoire	Operating room	Quirófano	Sala operatoria	Operacijska sala
Blouse de protection	Protection gown	Gabacha desechable	Camicia protettiva	Zaštitna navlaka za odjeću
Brassard du manomètre	Manometer cuff	Manguito de presión arterial	Manicotto di sfigmomanometro	Manšeta tlakomjera
Brucelles	Tweezers	Pinzas	Pinzette	Pinceta
Bureau du médecin	Doctor's office	Consultorio de médico	Ufficio del medico	Liječnička ambulanta
Cadavre	Corpse	Cadáver	Cadavere (salma)	Leš
Calendrier des vaccinations	Vaccination schedule	Calendario de vacunación	Calendario vaccinale	Kalendar cijepljenja
Canule	Airway (cannula)	Cánula	Cannula	Kanila
Canule de Guedel	Oropharyngeal airway	Cánula orofaríngea (tubo de Mayo, cánula de Guédel)	Cannula oro-faringea	Orofaringealna kanila
Canule nasale	Nasal cannula	Cánula nasal	Cannula nasale	Nosna kanila
Cardiologie	Cardiology	Cardiología	Cardiologia	Kardiologija
Cathéter	Catheter	Catéter	Catetere	Kateter
Cathéter à succion	Suction catheter	Catéter de succión	Tubo d'aspirazione	Usisni kateter
Cathéter urologique	Urological catheter	Catéter urinario	Catetere vescicale	Urinarni kateter
Cause de la mort	Cause of death	Causa de muerte	Causa di morte	Uzrok smrti
Cautérisation	Cauterization	Cauterización	Cauterizzazione	Kauterizacija
Centre médical	Medical center	Centro médico	Centro di medicina	Medicinski centar
Chaise d'évacuation	Escape chair	Silla de evacuación	Sedia portantina	Sjedalica za evakuaciju
Chambre de malade	Patient's room	Cuarto del paciente	Camera di malato	Bolesnička soba
Chariot	Hospital trolley	Camilla	Carrello	Kolica
Charlotte à usage unique	Protection cap	Gorra desechable	Cuffietta protettiva	Zaštitna kapa
Chausson	Slippers	Pantuflas	Ciabatte	Šlape
Chemise de nuit	Nightgown	Camisón	Camicia da notte	Spavačica
Chimiothérapie	Chemotherapy	Quimioterapia	Chemioterapia	Kemoterapija
Chirurgie	Surgery	Cirugía	Chirurgia	Kirurgija
Circoncision	Circumcision	Circuncisión	Circoncisione	Obrezivanje
Ciseau	Scissors	Tijeras	Forbici	Škare
Civière	Stretcher	Camilla enrollable	Barella (lettiga)	Nosila
Composite dentaire	Dental filling	Empaste (emplomadura)	Otturazione odontoiatrica	Zubna plomba
Contagieux /contagieuse	Contagious	Contagioso	Contagioso (infettivo)	Zarazno
Couronne	Dental crown	Corona	Corona	Zubna krunica
Coussin de positionnement	Body positioner	Almohada de posicionamiento	Posizionatore	Udlaga za pozicioniranje
Couverture	Cover	Cubrecama (colcha, manta)	Coperta	Pokrivač
Couverture	Blanket	Manta (cobija)	Schiavina	Deka
Cracher	Spit	Escupir	Sputare	Pljunuti
Cryo-extraction	Cryoextraction	Crío-extracción	Crioestrazione	Krioekstrakcija
Cuvette	Wash basin	Palangana (ajofaina)	Secchia	Lavor
Cytologie	Cytology	Citología	Citologia	Citologija
Déambulateur (cadre de marche, gadot)	Walker (walking frame)	Andador	Deambulatore (tutore per disabili)	Hodalica
Débris	Debris	Materia de desperdicio	Rottami	Otpad (otpadni proizvod)
Défécation	Defecation	Defecación	Defecazione	Pražnjenje stolice (defekacija)
Défibrillateur	Defibrillator	Desfibrilador	Defibrillatore	Defibrilator
Défibrillateur manuel	Manual defibrillator	Desfibrilador manual	Defibrillatore manuale	Ručni defibrilator
Défibrillation	Defibrillation	Desfibrilación	Defibrillazione	Defibrilacija
Déjeuner	Lunch	Almuerzo	Pranzo	Ručak
Dentier	Dentures	Prótesis dental	Protesi dentale	Umjetno zubalo

Français	Anglais	Espagnol	Italien	Croate
Dentiste	Dentist	Dentista	Dentista	Stomatolog (zubar)
Dermatologie	Dermatology	Dermatología	Dermatologia	Dermatologija
Détermination de l'heure de la mort	Calling of the time of death	Determinación del tiempo de muerte	Proclamazione del tempo della morte	Proglašenje vremena smrti
Diagnostic	Diagnosis	Diagnóstico	Diagnosi	Dijagnoza
Dialyse	Dialysis	Diálisis	Dialisi	Dijaliza
Dialyse hépatique	Liver dialysis	Diálisis de hígado	Dialisi epatica	Dijaliza jetre
Dialyse rénale	Renal dialysis	Diálisis renal	Dialisi renale	Dijaliza bubrega
Digestion	Digestion	Digestión	Digestione	Probava
Dîner (souper)	Dinner (supper)	Cena	Cena	Večera
Don de sang	Blood donation	Donación de sangre	Donazione del sangue	Darovanje krvi (donacija krvi)
Donneur	Donor	Donante	Donatore/donatrice	Davalac (donator)
Drain	Drain tube	Sonda de drenaje	Tubo di drenaggio	Dren
Drainage	Drainage	Drenaje	Drenaggio	Drenaža
Drainage postural	Postural drainage	Drenaje postural	Drenaggio posturale	Drenažni položaj
Drap	Sheet	Sábana	Lenzuolo	Plahta
Dynamomètre	Dynamometer	Dinamómetro	Dinamometro	Dinamometar
Eau	Water	Agua	Acqua	Voda
Électrochirurgie	Electrosurgery	Electrocirugía	Elettrochirurgia	Elektrokirurgija
Électrode	Electrode	Electrodo	Elettrodo	Elektroda
Électrothérapie	Electrotherapy	Electroterapia	Elettroterapia	Elektroterapija
Enlèvement chirurgical d'un sein (mastectomie)	Surgical removal of a breast (mastectomy)	Remoción quirúrgica de seno (mastectomía)	Asportazione chirur-gica della mammella (mastectomia)	Kirurško odstranjenje dojke (mastektomija)
Enlèvement chirurgical de l'uterus (hystérectomie)	Surgical removal of the uterus (hysterectomy)	Extracción quirúrgica del útero (histerectomía)	Asportazione chirurgica dell'utero (isterectomia)	Kirurško odstranjenje maternice (histerektomija)
Enlèvement chirurgical de la vésicule biliaire (cholécystectomie)	Surgical removal of the gallbladder (cholecystectomy)	Extracción quirúrgica de la vesícula biliar (colecistectomía)	Asportazione chirurgica della colecisti (colecistectomia)	Kirurško odstranjenje žučnog mjehura (kolecistektomija)
Entraînement de l'equilibre	Balance training	Entrenamiento del equilibrio	Esercizi di equilibrio	Trening ravnoteže
Éponge	Sponge	Esponja	Spugna	Spužva
Ergothérapeute	Occupational therapist	Terapeuta ocupacional	Terapista occupazionale	Radni terapeut
Exercice	Exercise	Ejercicio	Esercizio	Vježbanje
Exercice de Kegel	Kegel exercise	Ejercicios de Kegel	Esercizi di Kegel	Kegelove vježbe
Exercice de respiration	Breathing exercises	Ejercicios de respiración	Esercizi di respirazione	Vježbe disanja
Extraction chirurgicale des pierres de la vessie (lithotomie)	Surgical removal of stones (lithotomy)	Extracción quirúrgica de los cálculos (litotomía)	Asportazione chirurgica di calcolo (litotomia)	Kirurško odstranjenje kamenca (litotomija)
Extraction dentaire	Dental extraction	Exodoncia dental	Estrazione del dente	Vađenje zuba
Fauteuil roulant (charriot, charrette)	Wheelchair	Silla de ruedas	Sedia a rotelle (carrozzella)	Invalidska kolica
Fenêtre	Window	Ventana	Finestra	Prozor
Fermer	Close	Cerrar	Chiudere	Zatvoriti
Formation chirurgicale de la stomie (colostomie)	Surgical procedure of formation of stoma (colostomy)	Exteriorización de una parte de intestino a tra-vés de la cavidad abdo-minal (colostomía)	Formazione chirurgica di stomia (colostomia)	Kirurški zahvat formiranja stome (kolostomija)
Gants à usage unique	Protect gloves	Guantes desechables	Guanti protettivi	Zaštitne rukavice
Gel électroconductif	Electrode conductive gel	Gel conductor	Gel elettro-conduttivo	Kontaktni gel za elektrode
Germes	Germs	Gérmenes	Germi	Klice
Gérontologie	Gerontology	Gerontología	Gerontologia	Gerontologija
Goniomètre	Goniometer	Goniómetro	Goniometro	Goniometar
Greffe (transplantation)	Transplantation	Trasplante	Trapianto	Presađivanje (transplantacija)
Guérison	Recovery	Recuperación	Guarigione (ristabilimento)	Oporavak
Gynécologie	Gynecology	Ginecología	Ginecologia	Ginekologija
Hôpital	Hospital	Hospital	Ospedale (policlinico)	Bolnica
Hydrothérapie	Hydrotherapy	Hidroterapia	Idroterapia	Hidroterapija
Immobiliseur de tête	Head immobilizer	Inmovilizador de cabeza	Fermacapo	Imobilizator glave
Immunologie	Immunology	Inmunología	Immunologia	Imunologija
Implant mammaire	Breast implant	Implante de mama	Protese mammaria	Umetak za dojku
Infirmerie	Ambulance (clinic)	Enfermería	Ambulanza	Ambulanta
Infirmier	Nurse	Enfermera	Infermiera/infermiere	Medicinska sestra
Intubation	Intubation	Intubación	Intubazione	Intubacija
Injection	Injection	Inyección	Iniezione	Injekcija
Laparoscopie (coelioscopie)	Laparoscopic surgery	Cirugía laparoscópica	Chirurgia laparoscopica	Laparoskopska operacija
Laryngoscope	Laryngoscope	Laringoscopio	Laringoscopio	Laringoskop
Lavage gastrique	Gastric lavage (stomach pumping)	Lavado gástrico	Lavanda gastrica	Ispiranje želuca
Laver	Bath (wash)	Darse un baño	Lavare (fare il bagno)	Kupati
Lifting facial (rhytidectomie, lissage, remodelage)	Facelift (rhytidectomy)	Estiramiento de la cara (ritidectomía)	Lift facciale (ritidectomia)	Lifting lica (ritidektomija)

Français	Anglais	Espagnol	Italien	Croate
Ligature des canaux déférents des testicules (vasectomie)	Surgical sterilization of a man (vasectomy)	Esterilización quirúrgica masculina (vasectomía)	Vasectomia	Kirurška sterilizacija muškarca (vazektomija)
Liposuccion	Liposuction	Liposucción	Liposuzione	Liposukcija
Lit	Bed	Cama	Letto	Krevet
Lobotomie	Lobotomy	Lobotomía	Lobotomia	Lobotomija
Lumière	Light	Luz	Luce	Svjetlo
Masque à oxygène	Oxygen mask	Máscara de oxígeno	Maschera dell'ossigeno	Maska za kisik
Masque de protection	Protection face mask	Mascarilla desechable	Mascherina di protezione	Zaštitna maska za lice
Masque de réanimation	CPR mask	Máscara de reanimación	Maschera per rianimazione	Maska za oživljavanje
Masque laryngé	Laryngeal mask airway	Máscara laríngea	Maschera laringea	Laringealna maska
Matelas	Mattress	Colchón	Materasso	Madrac
Matelas immobilisateur à dépression	Vacuum mattress	Colchón al vácio	Materassino a depressione	Vakumirani madrac
Médecin	Doctor (physician)	Médico	Dottore/dottoressa (medico)	Liječnik
Médecin généraliste (médecin omnipraticien)	General practitioner	Médico de cabecera	Medico di medicina generale (medico di famiglia)	Liječnik opće prakse
Médicine interne	Internal medicine	Medicina interna	Medicina interna	Interna medicina
Méthode de Heimlich	Heimlich maneuver (abdominal thrusts)	Maniobra de Heimlich	Manovra di Heimlich	Heimlichov zahvat
Miction	Urination (voiding)	Micción	Urinazione	Mokrenje (uriniranje)
Moniteur de signes vitaux	Vital signs monitor	Monitor de signos vitales	Monitor per parametri vitali	Monitor za praćenje vitalnih znakova
Mordre	Bite	Morder	Addentare	Zagristi
Morgue	Morgue (mortuary)	Depósito de cadáveres (morgue)	Obitorio (mortorio)	Mrtvačnica
Mourir	Die	Morir	Morire	Umrijeti
Neurologie	Neurology	Neurología	Neurologia	Neurologija
Oncologie (cancérologie)	Oncology	Oncología	Oncologia	Onkologija
Opération chirurgicale	Operation (surgery)	Operación quirúrgica	Operazione (intervento chirurgico)	Operacija
Opération de chirurgie esthétique de la paroi abdominale (abdominoplastie)	Plastic surgery of the abdomen ("tummy tuck", abdominoplasty)	Cirugía estética del abdomen (abdominoplastia)	Procedura di chirurgia plastica dell'addome (addominoplastica)	Plastična operacija trbuha (abdominoplastika)
Opération de chirurgie esthétique des paupières (blépharoplastie)	Plastic surgery of the eyelid (blepharoplasty)	Cirugía estética de los párpados (blefaroplastia)	Procedura di chirurgia plastica della palpebra (blefaroplastica)	Plastična operacija očnog kapka (blefaroplastika)
Opération de chirurgie esthétique des seins (mammoplastie)	Plastic surgery of the breasts (mammoplasty)	Cirugía estética de los senos (mamoplastia)	Procedura di chirurgia plastica del seno (mastoplastica)	Plastična operacija dojke (mastoplastika)
Opération de chirurgie esthétique du nez (rhinoplastie)	Plastic surgery of the nose (rhinoplasty)	Cirugía estética de la nariz (rinoplastia)	Procedura di chirurgia plastica del naso (rinoplastica)	Plastična operacija nosa (rinoplastika)
Oreiller	Pillow	Almohada	Cuscino	Jastuk
Orthopédie	Orthopedics	Ortopedia	Ortopedia	Ortopedija
Oto-rhino-laryngologie	Otorhinolaryngology	Otorrinolaringología	Otorinolaringoiatria	Uho-grlo-nos
Ouverture chirurgicale d'une articulation (arthrotomie)	Surgical procedure on a joint (arthrotomy)	Incisión quirúrgica de una articulación (artrotomía)	Apertura chirurgica di un articolazione (artrotomia)	Kirurški zahvat na zglobu (artrotomija)
Ouverture chirurgicale dans la trachée (trachéotomie)	Surgical opening of a direct airway on the neck (tracheostomy)	Incisión quirúrgica en la tráquea (traqueotomía)	Incisione chirurgica della trachea (tracheotomia)	Kirurško otvaranje dišnog puta (traheotomija)
Ouverture chirurgicale du crâne (craniotomie)	Surgical opnening of the cranium (craniotomy)	Abertura quirúrgica en el cráneo (craneotomía)	Apertura chirurgica del cranio (craniotomia)	Kirurški zahvat otvaranja lubanje (kraniotomija)
Ouvrir	Open	Abrir	Aprire	Otvoriti
Palpation	Palpation	Palpación	Palpazione	Pregled pipanjem (palpacija)
Pansement	Dressing	Apósito	Fasciatura (bendaggio)	Previjanje
Pathologie	Pathology	Patología	Patologia	Patologija
Patient (malade)	Patient	Paciente	Paziente (ammalato)	Bolesnik
Pédiatrie	Pediatrics	Pediatría	Pediatria	Pedijatrija
Perceuse	Drill	Taladro	Trapano (trivella)	Bušilica
Percussion	Percussion	Percusión	Percussione	Pregled kucanjem (perkusija)
Perfusion	Infusion	Infusión	Infusione	Infuzija
Pessaire (pessus)	Pessary	Pesario	Pessario	Pesar
Petit déjeuner	Breakfast	Desayuno	Colazione	Doručak
Physiothérapeute	Physiotherapist	Fisioterapeuta	Fisioterapista	Fizioterapeut
Physiothérapie	Physical therapy	Fisioterapia	Fisioterapia	Fizikalna terapija
Pied à perfusion	Infusion stand	Intravenoso poste	Piantana portaflebo	Stalak za infuziju
Plâtre pour immobilisation rigide	Plaster cast (immobilization plaster)	Escayola de inmovilización	Bendaggio gessato	Gipsana udlaga
Pontage	Bypass	By-pass	Bypass	Premosnica
Pontage (shunt)	Shunt	Shunt	Shunt	Spoj (skretnica)
Porte	Door	Puerta	Porta	Vrata

Français	Anglais	Espagnol	Italien	Croate
Position de Trendelenburg	Trendelenburg position	Posición de Trendelenburg	Posizione di Trendelenburg	Trendelenburgov položaj
Pot de chambre	Chamber-pot	Orinal	Vaso da notte (pitale)	Noćna posuda
Poubelle	Litter bin	Papelera	Pattumiera	Kanta za smeće
Premiers secours	First aid	Primeros auxilios	Primo soccorso	Prva pomoć
Protège-matelas	Incontinence pad	Sábana de hule para la incontinencia	Proteggi materasso cerato	Gumirano platno
Psychiatrie	Psychiatry	Psiquiatría	Psichiatria	Psihijatrija
Psychologue	Psychologist	Psicólogo	Psicologo	Psiholog
Purification	Cleansing	Purificación	Purificazione	Pročišćavanje
Pyjama	Pyjamas (pajamas)	Pijama (piyama)	Pigiama	Pidžama
Quarantaine	Quarantine	Cuarentena	Quarantena	Karantena
Radiation	Radiation	Radiación	Radiazione	Zračenje
Radiographie	Radiology	Radiología	Radiologia	Radiologija
Réanimation	Reanimation	Reanimación	Rianimazione	Oživljavanje (reanimacija)
Réception	Reception office	Mostrador de recepción	Accettazione	Prijemni ured
Receveur de greffe	Recipient of an organ	Receptor de un órgano	Ricevente di trapianto	Primatelj organa
Régime alimentaire	Diet	Régimen (dieta)	Dieta (regime dietetico)	Dijeta
Réhabilitation	Rehabilitation (rehab)	Rehabilitación	Riabilitazione	Rehabilitacija
Rémission	Remission	Fase de remisión	Remissione	Stadij mirovanja bolesti (remisija)
Repos au lit	Bed rest	Guardar cama	Riposo a letto	Mirovanje u krevetu
Résection chirurgicale d'une poche anévrismale (anevrismectomie)	Surgical removal of the aneurysm (aneurysmectomy)	Extirpación quirúrgica de un aneurisma (aneurismectomía)	Asportazione chirurgica della sacca aneurismatica (aneurismectomia)	Kirurško odstranjenje aneurizme (aneurizmektomija)
Résection chirurgicale des lames vertébrales (laminectomie)	Surgical procedure on the spine (laminectomy)	Extirpación quirúrgica de parte de una vértebra (laminectomía)	Asportazione chirurgica della lamina di vertebre (laminectomia)	Kirurški zahvat na kralježnici (laminektomija)
Résection transurétrale de la prostate	Transurethral resection of the prostate	Resección transuretral de la próstata	Resezione transuretrale della prostata	Transuretralna resekcija prostate
Réservoir d'oxygène	Oxygen storage tank	Tanque de oxígeno	Serbatoio di ossigeno	Boca s kisikom
Respirateur manuel type Ambu	Ambu bag valve mask	Bolsa Ambú de ventilación manual	Pallone autoespandibile	Ambu balon s maskom
Rhinologie	Rhinology	Rinología	Rinologia	Rinologija
Rincer	Rinse	Lavar	Sciacquare	Isprati
Salle	Ward	Sala (pabellón)	Padiglione (reparto)	Odjel
Salle à manger	Dining-room	Comedor	Sala da pranzo (cenàcolo)	Blagavaonica
Salle d'attente	Waiting-room	Sala de espera	Sala d'aspetto	Čekaonica
Salle d'ophtalmologie	Ophtalmology ward	Sala de oftalmología	Reparto di oftalmologia	Očni odjel
Salle de bains	Bathroom	Cuarto de baño	Bagno	Kupaonica
Salle de pneumologie	Pulmonary ward	Sala de neumología	Reparto polmonare	Plućni odjel
Salle maladies infectieuses	Infectious disease unit	Pabellón de enfermedades infecciosas	Reparto di malattie infettive	Zarazni odjel
Scalpel	Scalpel	Escalpelo	Scalpello	Skalpel
Se changer	Get changed	Cambiarse	Cambiarsi	Presvući se
Se remettre (se guérir)	Recover (heal)	Reponerse (recuperarse)	Sanare (guarire, recuperare)	Ozdraviti
Soins de santé	Nursing (care)	Asistencia (cuidado)	Assistenza infermieristica	Njega
Soins de santé primaire	Primary health care	Atención primaria de salud	Assistenza sanitaria primaria	Primarna zdravstvena zaštita
Soins intensifs	Intensive care	Cuidados intensivos	Terapia intensiva	Intenzivna njega
Soins semi-intensifs	Semi-intensive care	Cuidados semi-intensivos	Terapia semi-intensiva	Poluintenzivna njega
Sonde	Sonde	Sonda	Sonda	Sonda
Sonde d'alimentation	Feeding tube	Sonda de alimentación	Sonda gastrica per nutrizione	Sonda za hranjenje
Sonde d'intubation endotrachéale	Endotracheal tube	Sonda endotraqueal	Tubo endotracheale	Endotrahealna kanila
Stérile	Sterile (aseptic)	Estéril	Sterile	Sterilno
Stérilisation	Sterilization	Esterilización	Sterilizzazione	Sterilizacija
Stérilisation chirurgicale au femme (ligature des trompes)	Surgical sterilization of a woman (tubal ligation)	Esterilizatióm quirúrgica femenina (ligadura de trompas)	Chiusura delle tube	Kirurška sterilizacija žene (podvezivanje jajovoda)
Stéthoscope	Stethoscop	Estetoscopio	Stetofonendoscopio	Stetoskop
Stimulateur cardiaque (pacemaker, pile)	Pacemaker	Marcapasos	Cardiostimolatore (stimolatore cardiaco)	Električni stimulator srca
Stockage	Storage	Almacenaje	Deposito (magazzino)	Spremište
Support de cou	Neck immobilizer	Collar cervical	Collare cervicale	Imobilizator vrata
Sur-chaussures à usage unique	Protection shoe cover	Cubrezapatos	Sovrascarpe protettive	Zaštitna navlaka za obuću
Suture de la plaie	Wound stitching	Suturar la herida	Suturare la ferita	Šivanje rane
Table	Table (desk)	Mesa (escritorio)	Tavolo (scrivania)	Stol
Table de chevet (table de nuit)	Night table (bedside table)	Mesilla de noche	Comodino	Noćni ormarić
Table de lit	Overbed table	Mesa para cama	Carrello servitore	Stolić za serviranje hrane
Talonnières et coudières	Heel and elbow protectors	Protectores talón/codo antiescaras	Talloniere e gomitiere antidecubito	Zaštitnici za pete i laktove
Thé	Tea	Té	Tè	Čaj
Thérapie (traitement curatif)	Therapy	Tratamiento (terapia)	Terapia	Liječenje (terapija)

Français	Anglais	Espagnol	Italien	Croate
Toilette (cabinet)	Toilet (lavatory)	Servicio	Vaso sanitario	Nužnik
Traction	Traction	Tracción	Trazione	Trakcija
Transfusion	Transfusion	Transfusión	Trasfusione	Transfuzija
Trauma	Trauma	Trauma	Trauma	Trauma
Trousse de secours	First aid kit	Botiquín de primeros auxilios	Cassetta di pronto soccorso	Kutija prve pomoći
Tube à essai	Test tube	Tubo de ensayo	Provetta	Epruveta
Unité de soins intensifs	Intensive care unit	Unidad de cuidados intensivos	Stanza da terapia intensiva	Jedinica intenzivne njege
Urologie	Urology	Urología	Urologia	Urologija
Vaccination (inoculation)	Vaccination (inoculation)	Vacunación	Vaccinazione (inoculazione)	Cijepljenje
Ventilation artificielle	Artificial respiration	Respiración artificial	Respirazione artificiale	Umjetno disanje
Vernis à dents	Teeth polishing	Pulidor de los dientes	Pulitura dei denti	Poliranje zuba
Visite	Visit	Visita	Visita	Posjeta
Visiteur	Visitor	Visitante	Ospite (visitatore/visitatrice)	Posjetitelj

EXAMENS MÉDICAUX:	MEDICAL EXAMS:	EXÁMENES MÉDICOS:	ESAMI MEDICI:	MEDICINSKE PRETRAGE:
Albumine dans le sang	Serum albumin	Albúmina en la sangre	Seroalbumina	Albumin u serumu
Amniocentèse	Amniocentesis	Amniocentesis	Amniocentesi	Amniocenteza
Analyse chimique de l'urine	Urine chemical analysis	Análisis químico de orina	Analisi chimiche delle urine	Kemijska analiza urina
Analyse chimique du suc gastrique	Gastric juice chemical examination	Análisis químico del jugo gástrico	Esame chimico di succo gastrico	Kemijski pregled želučanog soka
Analyse de biochimie du sang	Biochemical blood tests	Exámenes bioquímicos de sangre	Test biochimici di sangue	Biokemijske pretrage krvi
Analyse de l'ADN	DNA analysis	Análisis de DNA	Analisi del DNA	DNK analiza
Analyse du liquide céphalo-rachidien	Cerebrospinal fluid analysis	Análisis del líquido cefalorraquídeo	Analisi del liquido cerebro-spinale	Pregled likvora
Analyse fécale de benzidine	Benzidine stool test	Prueba de la bencidina	Prova della benzidina	Benzidinski test stolice
Analyse médicale (examens de biologie médicale)	Laboratory tests	Pruebas de laboratorio	Esami di laboratorio	Laboratorijske pretrage
Analyse sérologique	Serology blood tests	Pruebas de serología	Esami sierologici	Serološke pretrage na antitijela
Angiographie	Angiography	Angiografía	Angiografia	Angiografija
Angiographie cérébrale	Cerebral angiography	Angiografía cerebral	Angiografia cerebrale	Cerebralna angiografija
Angiographie interventionnelle utilisant un cathéter	Catheter angiography	Angiografía por catéter	Angiografia con cateterismo	Kateterska angiografija
Angiographie numérique	Digital subtraction angiography	Angiografía de sustracción digital	Angiografia digitale a sottrazione	Digitalna supstrak-cijska angiografija
Angiographie pulmonaire	Pulmonary angiography	Angiografía pulmonar	Angiografia polmonare	Pulmonalna angiografija
Angiographie spinale	Spinal angiography	Angiografía espinal	Angiografia spinale	Spinalna angiografija
Antibiogramme	Antibiogram	Antibiograma	Antibiogramma	Antibiogram
Antigène carcino-embryonnaire (ACE)	Carcinoembryonic antigen (CEA)	Antígeno carcinoembrionario	Antigene carcino-embrionario (CEA)	Karcinoembrionski antigen (CEA)
Antigène de cancer CA 19-9 (antigène d'hydrate de carbone)	CA 19-9 (carbohydrate antigen)	CA 19-9 (antígeno carbohidrato 19-9)	CA 19-9 (antigene carboidratico)	CA 19-9 (karbohidratni antigen)
Antigène de cancer CA 125	CA 125 (cancer antigen 125)	Marcador tumoral CA 125	CA 125 (antigene di carcinoma 125)	CA 125 (karcinomski antigen 125)
Antigène HbsAg (antigène de surface du virus de l'hépatite B)	HbsAg (Hepatitis B surface antigen)	HbsAg (antígeno de superficie de la hepatitis B)	HbsAg (antigene di superficie dell'epatite B)	HbsAg (hepatitis B površinski antigen)
Antigène prostatique spécifique	Prostate specific antigen	Antígeno prostático específico	Semenogelasi (antigene prostatico specifico)	Prostatični specifični antigen (PSA)
Anuscopie	Anoscopy	Anoscopía	Anoscopia	Anoskopija
Aortographie	Aortography	Aortografía	Aortografia	Aortografija
Artériographie	Arteriography	Arteriografía	Arteriografia	Arteriografija
Arthrographie	Joint X-ray (arthrography)	Artrografía	Artrografia	Rendgensko snimanje zgloba
Arthroscopie	Arthroscopy	Artroscopia	Artroscopia	Artroskopija
Aspartate transaminase (SGOT)	Aspartate transaminase (SGOT)	Aspartato aminotransferasa (AST, transaminasa glutámico-oxalacética GOT)	Aspartato transaminasi (SGOT)	Transaminaze u serumu
Audiométrie	Audiometry	Audiometría	Audiometria	Audiometrija
Audiométrie vocale	Speech audiometry	Audiometría del habla	Audiometria di discorso	Govorna audiometrija
Azote d'urée dans le sang	Blood urea nitrogen test (BUN)	Nitrógeno ureico en sangre (BUN)	Azoto ureico nel sangue (BUN)	Ostatni dušik u krvi (urea nitrogen test)
Biligraphie intraveineuse	Intravenous biligraphy	Biligrafia intravenosa	Biligrafia venosa	Intravenozna biligrafija
Biomarqueur	Biomarker	Marcador biológico	Biomarcatore	Biomarker
Biopsie	Biopsy	Biopsia	Biopsia	Biopsija
Biopsie d'un ventricule cérébral	Brain ventricle biopsy	Biopsia cerebral	Biopsia cerebrale (biopsia dei ventricoli cerebrali)	Biopsija moždanih klijetki (ventrikulopunkcija)
Biopsie de peau	Skin biopsy	Biopsia de piel	Biopsia cutanea	Biopsija kože
Biopsie du foie	Liver biopsy	Biopsia hepática	Biopsia epatica	Biopsija jetre
Biopsie du ganglion lymphatoque	Lymph node biopsy	Biopsia de ganglio linfático	Biopsia del linfonodo	Biopsija limfnog čvora

Français	Anglais	Espagnol	Italien	Croate
Biopsie endométriale	Endometrial biopsy	Biopsia endometrial	Biopsia endometriale	Biopsija endometrija
Biopsie ostéomédullaire	Bone marrow biopsy	Biopsia de médula ósea	Biopsia del midollo osseo	Biopsija koštane srži
Biopsie pleurale	Pleural biopsy	Biopsia pleural	Biopsia pleurica	Biopsija pleure
Biopsie rénale	Kidney biopsy	Biopsia renal	Biopsia renale	Biopsija bubrega
Biopsie stéréotaxique	Stereotactic biopsy	Biopsia estereotáctica	Biopsia stereotassica	Stereotaktična biopsija
Biopsie thyroïdienne	Thyroid biopsy	Biopsia de tiroides	Biopsia della tiroide	Biopsija štitnjače
Bronchographie	Bronchography	Broncografía	Broncografia	Bronhografija
Bronchoscopie	Bronchoscopy	Broncoscopia	Broncoscopia	Bronhoskopija
Cardiotocographie	Cardiotocography	Cardiotocografía	Cardiotocografia	Kardiotokografija
Caryotype	Karyotype	Cariotipo	Cariotipo	Kariotip
Cathétérisme cardiaque	Cardiac catheterization (heart cath, angiocardiography)	Cateterismo cardíaco	Cateterismo cardiaco (angiocardiografia)	Kateterizacija srca (angiokardiografija)
Céphalométrie	Cephalometry	Cefalometría	Cefalometria	Cefalometrija
Cholangiographie	Cholangiography	Colangiografía	Colangiografia	Kolangiografija
Cholangiopancréato graphie rétrograde endoscopique	Endoscopic retrograde cholangiopancreatography (ERCP)	Colangiopancreatografía retrógrada endoscópica	Colangio-pancreatografia endoscopica retrograda	Endoskopska retrogradna kolangiopankreatografija (ERCP)
Cholécystographie orale	Oral cholecystography	Colecistografía oral	Colecistografia orale	Rendgensko snimanje žučnog mjehura s kontrastom (peroralna kolecistografija)
Colonoscopie	Colonoscopy	Colonoscopia	Colonscopia	Kolonoskopija
Colposcopie	Colposcopy	Colposcopia	Colposcopia	Kolposkopija
Conisation	Cervical conization	Conización	Conizzazione	Konizacija
Coronarographie	Coronary catheterization (coronarography)	Coronariografía	Coronarografia	Koronarografija
Craniographie	Skull X-ray (craniography)	Craneografía	Craniografia	Rendgensko snimanje lubanje
Culture de crachat	Sputum culture	Cultivo de esputo	Coltura di sputo	Mikrobiološki pregled ispljuvka
Culture de gorge avec le coton-tige	Throat swab culture	Exudado faríngeo	Coltura di gola	Mikrobiološki pregled brisa grla
Culture du liquide cérébro-spinal	Cerebrospinal fluid culture	Cultivo de líquido cefalorraquídeo	Coltura del liquor	Mikrobiološki pregled likvora
Culture microbiologique	Microbiological culture	Cultivo	Coltura di microrganismi	Mikrobiološki pregled (kultura)
Culture vaginale	Vaginal swab culture	Cultivo vaginal	Coltura vaginale	Mikrobiološki pregled brisa rodnice
Cystographie	Cystography	Cistografía	Cistografia	Cistografija
Cystoscopie	Cystoscopy	Cistoscopia	Cistoscopia	Cistoskopija
Défécographie	Defecography	Defecografía	Defecografia	Defekografija
Dermatoscopie (dermoscopie)	Dermatoscopy (dermoscopy)	Dermatoscopia	Dermatoscopia (dermoscopia)	Dermatoskopija (dermoskopija)
Diagnostic différentiel	Differential diagnosis	Diagnóstico diferencial	Diagnosi differenziale	Diferencijalna dijagnoza
Diagnostic différentiel pour bilirubine sérique	Serum bilirubin	Análisis de bilirrubina sérica	Test della bilirubina	Bilirubin u serumu
Dilatation des pupilles provoquée par les médicaments	Drug induced pupillary dilatation	Dilatación pupilar inducida por fármacos	Dilatazione delle pupille provocando con tropicamide	Širenje zjenica potaknuto lijekovima
Échelle de Glasgow	Glasgow coma scale	Escala de coma de Glasgow	Punteggio del coma di Glasgow	Glasgowska skala kome
Échocardiographie	Cardiac ultrasound (echocardiography)	Ecocardiografía	Ecocardiografia	Ultrazvuk srca (ehokardiografija)
Échocardiographie doppler	Doppler echocardiography	Ecocardiografía doppler	Ecocardiografia doppler	Ultrazvuk srca s dopplerom
Échoencéphalographie	Echoencephalography	Ecoencefalografía	Ecoencefalografia	Ehoencefalografija
Échographie	Ultrasound (medical ultrasonography)	Ultrasonografía (ecografía)	Ecografia	Ultrazvuk
Échographie abdominale	Abdominal ultrasound	Ecografía abdominal (ultrasonido abdominal)	Ecografia addominale	Ultrazvuk abdomena
Échographie du foie (échographie hépatique)	Liver ultrasound	Ecografía hepática (ultrasonido hepático)	Ecografia epatica	Ultrazvuk jetre
Échographie du pancréas	Pancreas ultrasound	Ecografía de páncreas (ultrasonido de páncreas)	Ecografia pancreatica	Ultrazvuk gušterače
Échographie la vésicule biliaire et les voies biliaires	Ultrasound of the gallbladder and bile ducts	Ecografía de vesícula y vías biliares	Ecografia colecisti e vie biliari	Ultrazvuk žuči i žučnih vodova
Échographie mammaire	Breast ultrasound	Ecografia de mama (ultrasonido de mama)	Ecografia mammaria	Ultrazvuk dojke
Échographie rénale	Renal ultrasound	Ecografía renal (ultrasonido renal)	Ecografia renale	Ultrazvuk bubrega
Échographie thyroïdienne	Thyroid ultrasound	Ecografía de la tiroides (ultrasonido de la tiroides)	Ecografia della tiroide	Ultrazvuk štitnjače
Électro-encéphalographie (EEG)	Electroencephalography (EEG)	Electroencefalografía	Elettroencefalografia	Elektroencefalografija (EEG)
Électrocardiographie (ECG)	Electrocardiography (ECG)	Electrocardiografía (ECG, EKG)	Elettrocardiografia	Elektrokardiografija (EKG)

Français	Anglais	Espagnol	Italien	Croate
Électromyographie	Electromyography (EMG)	Electromiografía	Elettromiografia	Elektromiografija (EMG)
Électroneurographie	Electroneurography	Electroneurografia	Elettroneurografia	Elektroneurografija
Électrophorèse des protéines	Serum protein electrophoresis	Electroforesis de proteínas séricas	Elettroforesi delle sieroproteine	Elektroforeza proteina u serumu
Électrorétinographie	Electroretinography	Electrorretinografia	Elettroretinografia	Elektroretinografija
Encéphalographie gazeuse	Pneumoencephalography	Neumoencefalografia	Pneumoencefalografia	Pneumoencefalografija
Endoscopie	Endoscopy	Endoscopia	Endoscopia	Endoskopija
Endoscopie oeso-gastro-duodénale	Esophagogastroduodenoscopy	Esofagogastroduodenoscopia	Esofagogastroduodenoscopia	Ezofagogastroduodenoskopija
Entéroscopie	Enteroscopy	Enteroscopia	Enteroscopia	Enteroskopija
Épruve à la phénosulfonphtaléine	Phenolsulfonphthalein test (PSP test)	Prueba de la fenolsulfonftaleína	Test alla fenolsulfonftaleina	Fenolsulfoftaleinski test (PSP-test)
Épruve d'élimination de l'urée sanguine	Urea clearance test	Prueba de aclaramiento de urea sanguínea	Urea clearance (clearance dell'urea)	Urea klirens
Ergométrie	Ergometry test	Ergometría	Ergometria (ECG sotto sforzo)	Test opterećenja (ergometrija)
Examen du sein	Breast examination	Exploración física de mama	Esame della mammella	Pregled dojke
Examen gynécologique	Gynecological examination	Examen ginecológico	Esame ginecologico	Ginekološki pregled
Explorations fonctionnelles hépatiques	Liver function tests	Pruebas de función hepática	Test di funzionalità epatica	Funkcionalne pretrage jetre
Fixation thyroïdienne de l'iode 131	Iodine-131 thyroid test	Captación tiroidea de 131yodo	Test di captazione tiroidea dello iodio 131	Test štitnjače na provodljivost radioaktivnog joda 131
Fluoroscopie	Fluoroscopy	Fluoroscopia	Fluoroscopia	Fluoroskopija
Fond d'oeil	Dilated fundus examination	Exámen dilatado de fundus	Esame del fundus oculi	Pregled očnog fundusa
Forage-biopsie	Fine needle aspiration biopsy	Punción aspiración con aguja fina	Agoaspirato (biopsia mediante ago sottile)	Punkcijsko-aspiracijska biopsija
Gastroscopie	Gastroscopy	Gastroscopia	Gastroscopia	Gastroskopija
Gonioscopie	Gonioscopy	Gonioscopia	Gonioscopia	Gonioskopija
Hématocrite	Hematocrit	Hematocrito	Ematocrito	Hematokrit
Hémoculture	Blood culture	Hemocultivo	Emocoltura	Mikrobiološki pregled krvi (hemokultura)
Hémogramme (numération formule sanguine)	Complete blood count	Hemograma (conteo sanguíneo completo)	Emocromo (analisi del sangue, esame emocromocitometrico)	Kompletna krvna slika
Hystérosalpingographie	Hysterosalpingography	Histerosalpingografia	Isterosalpingografia	Rendgensko snimanje maternice i jajovoda
Hystéroscopie	Hysterescopy	Histeroscopia	Isteroscopia	Histeroskopija
Imagerie par résonance magnétique (IRM)	Magnetic resonance imaging (MRI)	Imagen por resonancia magnética (IRM)	Imaging a risonanza magnetica (risonanza magnetica tomografica)	Magnetska rezonancija (MR)
Imagerie par résonance magnétique fonctionnelle (IRMf)	Functional magnetic resonance imaging (functional MRI)	Imagen por resonancia magnética funcional (IRMf)	Risonanza magnetica funzionale	Funkcionalna magnetska rezonancija (FMR)
Laboratoire	Laboratory (lab)	Laboratorio	Laboratorio	Laboratorij
Laparoscopie	Laparoscopy	Laparoscopia	Laparoscopia	Laparoskopija
Laryngoscopie	Laryngoscopy	Laringoscopia	Laringoscopia	Laringoskopija
Lavement baryté	Barium enema	Enema de bario con doble contraste	Indagini radiologiche del colon con clisma opaco a doppio contrasto	Rendgensko snimanje debelog crijeva i rektuma s kontrastom barija
Lymphographie	Lymphography (lymphangiography)	Linfografia	Linfangiografia (linfografia)	Limfografija
Magnétoencéphalographie	Magnetoencephalography (MEG)	Magnetoencefalografia	Magnetoencefalografia	Magnetoencefalografija (MEG)
Mammographie	Mammography	Mamografia	Mammografia (mastografia)	Mamografija
Manométrie oesophagienne	Esophageal manometry	Manometría esofágica	Manometria esofagea	Manometrija jednjaka
Marqueur tumoral	Tumor marker	Marcador tumoral	Marker tumorale	Tumorski marker
Médiastinoscopie	Mediastinoscopy	Mediastinoscopia	Mediastinoscopia	Medijastinoskopija
Médicine nucléaire	Radioisotope scanning (nuclear medicine)	Medicina nuclear	Medicina nucleare	Radioizotopna dijagnostika
Monitoring de la pression artérielle	Blood pressure monitoring	Monitorización de la presión arterial	Misurazione della pressione arteriosa	Mjerenje krvnog pritiska
Myélographie	Myelography	Mielografia	Mielografia	Mijelografija
Myélographie lombaire	Lumbar myelography	Mielografia lumbar	Mielografia lombare	Lumbalna mijelografija
Myélographie sous-occipitale	Suboccipital myelography	Mielografia cervical suboccipital	Mielografia sotto-occipitale	Subokcipitalna mijelografija
Ophtalmoscopie	Ophtalmoscopy	Oftalmoscopia	Oftalmoscopia	Oftalmoskopija
Ostéodensitométrie	Bone densitometry (dual energy X-ray absorpriometry)	Densitometría ósea	Densità minerale ossea	Denzitometrija kostiju (apsorpciometrija kostiju)
Otoscopie	Otoscopy	Otoscopía	Otoscopia	Otoskopija
Patch test	Patch test	Prueba de emplasto (prueba del parche)	Patch test	Kožni alergološki test flasterom
Pelvigraphie	Pelvigraphy	Pelvigrafia	Pelvigrafia	Rendgensko snimanje zdjelice i porođajnog kanala
Pelvimétrie	Pelvimetry	Pelvimetria	Pelvimetria	Pelvimetrija
Périmétrie	Perimetry	Campimetría (perimetría)	Perimetria	Perimetrija

Français	Anglais	Espagnol	Italien	Croate
Phlébographie	Phlebography	Flebografía	Flebografia	Venografija (flebografija)
Phosphatase alcaline	Alkaline phosphatase	Fosfatasa alcalina	Fosfatasi alcalina totale	Alkalna fosfataza
Pléthysmographie	Plethysmography	Pletismografía	Pletismografia	Pletizmografija
Poids spécifique de l'urine	Urine specific gravity	Gravedad específica de la orina	Esame delle urine peso specifico	Specifična težina urina
Polysomnographie (polygraphie du sommeil)	Polysomnography (sleep study)	Polisomnografía	Polisonnografia	Polisomnografija (viseparametarski test u pracenju procesa sna)
Ponction lombaire (rachicentèse)	Lumbar puncture	Punción lumbar	Puntura lombare (rachicentesi)	Lumbalna punkcija
Ponction sous-occipitale	Suboccipital puncture	Punción suboccipital	Puntura suboccipitale	Subokcipitalna punkcija
Ponction transthoracique percutanée à l'aiguille fine	Transthoracic percutaneous fine needle aspiration	Punción transtorácica aspi.-rativa con aguja ultrafina	Agoaspirato polmonare percutaneo transtoracico	Perkutana transtorakalna punkcija pluća
Prélèvement des gaz du sang	Blood gas test	Prueba de gases en la sangre	Analisi dei gas nel sangue (emogas analisi)	Analiza plinova u krvi
Pression veineuse centrale	Central venous pressure (CVP)	Presión venosa central	Pressione venosa centrale	Centralni venozni pritisak (CVP)
Prise de pouls	Pulse monitoring	Comprobación del pulso	Misurazione del polso	Mjerenje pulsa
Produit de contraste	Contrast medium	Medio de contraste	Mezzo di contrasto	Kontrast
Protéines dans les urines	Urine protein test	Proteínas en la orina	Proteine nelle urine	Bjelančevine u urinu
Radiographie	X-ray (radiography)	Radiografía	Radiografia	Rendgen
Radiographie de l'abdomen en bouillie de sulfate de baryum	Barium meal (upper gastrointestinal series)	Radiografía de esófago, estómago y duodeno tomada con comida baritada	Radiografia gastroduodenale con pasto baritato	Rendgensko snimanje želuca i dvanaesnika barijevom kašom
Radiographie de la colonne vertébrale	Spine X-ray (spine radiography)	Radiografía de la columna vertebral (radiografía vertebral)	Radiografia della colonna vertebrale	Rendgensko snimanje kralježnice
Radiographie de thorax	Chest X-ray	Radiografía de tórax	Radiografia del torace	Rendgensko snimanje srca i pluća
Radiographie dentaire	Dental X-ray	Radiografía dental	Radiografia dentale	Rendgensko snimanje zuba
Radiographie des os	Bone X-ray (bone radiography)	Radiografía de hueso (radiografía ósea)	Radiografia ossea	Rendgensko snimanje kostiju
Réaction de Coombs indirecte	Indirect Coombs test	Prueba de Coombs indirecta	Test di Coombs indiretto	Indirektni Coombsov test
Réaction de Waaler Rose	Rose Waaler test	Test de Waaler-Rose	Rose Waaler test	Rose Waaler test
Rectoscopie	Rectoscopy	Rectoscopia	Rettoscopia	Rektoskopija
Réflexe rotulien	Patellar reflex	Reflejo patelar	Riflesso patellare	Patelarni refleks
Réfractométrie	Refractometry	Refractomería	Rifrattometria	Ispitivanje refrakcije
Scintigraphie hépato-biliaire au Technétium 99m	Hepatobiliary scintigraphy with technetium -99m	Gammagrafía hepatobiliar con tecnecio 99m	Scintigrafia epatobiliare con tecnezio -99m	Scintigrafija jetre i žučnih vodova radioaktivnim izotopima
Scintigraphie osseuse	Bone scintigraphy	Gammagrafía ósea	Scintigrafia ossea	Scintigrafija kostiju
Scintigraphie pulmonaire	Lung scintigraphy	Gammagrafía pulmonar	Scintigrafia polmonare	Scintigrafija pluća
Scintigraphie rénale	Renal scintigraphy	Gammagrafía renal	Scintigrafia renale	Scintigrafija bubrega
Scintigraphie splénique au Technétium 99m	Spleen scintigraphy with technetium -99m	Gammagrafía de bazo con tecnecio 99m	Scintigrafia splenica con tecnezio -99m	Scintigrafija slezene radioaktivnim izotopima
Scintigraphie thyroïdienne	Thyroid scintigraphy	Gammagrafía tiroidea	Scintigrafia tiroidea	Scintigrafija štitnjače
Sialographie	Sialography	Sialografía	Sialografia (scialografia)	Sijalografija
Sigmoïdoscopie	Sigmoidoscopy	Sigmoidoscopia	Sigmoidoscopia	Sigmoidoskopija
Spermogramme	Semen analysis	Espermiograma	Spermiogramma	Spermogram
Spirométrie	Spirometry (vital capacity test)	Espirometría	Spirometria (pneumometria)	Spirometrija (mjerenje vitalnog kapaciteta)
Taux d'hormones thyroïdiennes dans le sang	Thyroid blood tests	Concetración de hormonas tiroideas en sangre	Test di ormoni tiroidei nel sangue	Test na hormone štitnjače u krvi
Taux de la glycémie	Blood sugar concetration (glucose level)	Concentración de glucosa en sangre	Concentrazione del glucosio nel plasma	Šećer u krvi
Taux de prothrombine	Prothrombin time	Tiempo de protrombina	Tempo di protrombina	Protrombinski indeks
Temps de céphaline activée (TCA)	Partial thromboplastin time (PTT)	Tiempo de tromboplastina parcial activado	Tempo di tromboplastina parziale	Parcijalno tromboplastinsko vrijeme (PTT)
Test d'agglutination	Agglutination tests	Análisis de aglutinación	Test di agglutinazione	Test aglutinacije
Test d'alpha-foetoprotéine	Alpha-fetoprotein test (AFP test)	Prueba de alfa-fetoproteína	Test alfa-fetoproteina	Alfafetoproteinski test (AFP)
Test de diagnostic rapide du streptocoque	Rapid strep test	Prueba rápida para estreptococo	Test rapido dello streptococco	Brzi test na streptokok (strep-test)
Test de grossesse	Pregnancy test	Pruebas de embarazo	Test di gravidanza	Test na trudnoću
Test de la bromesulfonephtaléine	Bromsulphalein liver function test	Prueba de la función hepática con bromosulfaleína	Test dela bromosulfaleina di funzionalità epatica	Brom-sulfalein test funkcije jetre
Test de la piqûre	Skin allergy testing (prick test)	Test cutaneos de alergia (prick)	Test cutaneo per le allergie "prick test"	Alergološko testiranje kože (prick test)
Test de tolérance orale au glucose (TTOG)	Oral glucose tolerance test (OGTT)	Test de tolerancia oral a la glucosa	Test orale di tolleranca al glucosio (OGTT, curva da carico orale di glucosio)	Oralni test tolerancije na glukozu (OGTT)
Test de Weber	Weber test	Prueba de Weber	Prova di Weber	Weberov test
Test du sucre dans les urines	Glucose urine test	Examen de glucosa en orina	Glucosio nelle urine	Šećer u urinu
Test Mantoux (test PPD)	Mantoux test (PPD test)	Test de Mantoux (PPD)	Mantoux test	Tuberkulinski kožni test

Français	Anglais	Espagnol	Italien	Croate
Test PAP	Papanicolau test (Pap test)	Prueba de Papanicolau	Test di Papanicolaou (Pap test)	Papa-test (Papanicolaouova klasifikacija)
Test respiratoire à l'urée	Urea breath test	Prueba del aliento con urea	Test del respiro (urea breath test)	Urea izdisajni test
Thoracoscopie	Thoracoscopy	Toracoscopia	Toracoscopia	Torakoskopija
Tomodensitométrie (TDM)	Computed tomography (CT)	Tomografía computada	Tomografia computerizzata (TC)	Kompjuterizirana tomografija (CT)
Tomographie	Tomography	Tomografía	Tomografia	Tomografija
Tomographie par émission de positrons	Positron emission tomography	Tomografía por emisión de positrones	Tomografia ad emissione di positroni	Pozitronska emisijska tomografija (PET)
Tonométrie oculaire	Tonometry	Tonometría	Tonometria	Tonometrija oka
Toucher rectal	Rectal examination	Tacto rectal	Esplorazione rettale	Rektalni pregled
Tympanocentese	Tympanocentesis	Tímpanocentesis	Timpanocentesi	Timpanocenteza
Tympanométrie	Tympanometry	Timpanometría	Timpanometria	Timpanometrija
Ultrasons focalisés de haute intensité	High intensity focused ultrasound	Ultrasonido focalizado de alta intensidad (HIFU)	Ultrasuono ad alta intensità focalizzato	Fokusirani ultrazvuk visokog intenziteta
Urétéro-pyélographie rétrograde	Retrograde pyelography	Pielografía retrógrada	Pielografia retrograda	Retrogradna pijelografija
Urétéroscopie	Ureteroscopy	Ureteroscopía	Ureteroscopia	Ureteroskopija
Urétrographie	Urethrography	Uretrografía	Uretrografia	Uretrografija
Urobilinogène dans les urines	Urobilinogen in urine	Urobilinógeno en orina	Urobilinogeno nelle urine	Urobilinogen u urinu
Uroculture	Urine culture	Urocultivo	Urinocoltura	Mikrobiološki pregled mokraće (urinokultura)
Urographie	Pyelography	Urografía	Urografia	Pijelografija (urografija)
Urographie intra-veineuse	Intravenous pyelography	Urografía intravenosa	Urografia intravenosa (pielografia intravenosa)	Intravenozna pijelografija (i.v. Urografija)
Ventriculographie	Ventriculography	Ventriculografía	Ventricolografia	Ventrikulografija
Vitesse de sédimentation	Erythrocyte sedimentation rate	Velocidad de sedimentación globular	Velocità di eritrosedimentazione	Sedimentacija eritrocita
Volume urinaire résiduel	Post-void residual urine volume	Volumen residual de orina	Volume urinario residuo	Ostatni urin (rezidualni urin)

GROSSESSE ET OBSTÉTRIQUE:	PREGNANCY AND OBSTETRICS:	EMBARAZO Y OBSTETRICIA:	GRAVIDANZA ED OSTETRICIA:	TRUDNOĆA I PORODNIŠTVO:
Abruption placentaire (rupture placentaire)	Placental abruption	Desprendimiento prematuro de placenta	Distacco di placenta (abruptio placentae)	Abrupcija posteljice
Absence des règles (aménorrhée)	Absence of menstrual period (amenorrhea)	Ausencia de la menstruación (amenorrea)	Assenza di mestru-azioni (amenorrea)	Izostanak mjesečnice (amenoreja)
Accouchement (naissance)	Childbirth	Parto	Parto	Porod
Accouchement à terme	Full term birth	Parto a término	Parto a termine	Ročni porod
Accouchement dans l'eau	Water birth	Parto en agua	Parto nell'acqua	Porod u vodi
Accouchement pathologique	Pathological birth	Parto patológico	Parto patologico	Patološki porod
Accouchement prolongé	Prolonged birth	Parto prolongado	Parto prolungato	Produljeni porod
Amniocentèse	Amniocentesis	Amniocentesis	Amniocentesi	Amniocenteza
Amnios (sac amniotique)	Amniotic sac	Saco amniótico	Amnios	Vodenjak
Amnioscopie	Amnioscopy	Amnioscopia	Amnioscopia	Amnioskopija
Anomalies foetales	Fetal anomalies (fetal abnormalities)	Anomalías fetales	Anomalie di sviluppo fetale (anomalie fetali)	Anomalije fetusa
Avortement	Abortion (pregnancy termination)	Aborto inducido	Interruzione di gravidanza (aborto)	Prekid trudnoće (abortus)
Avortement à répétition	Habitual abortion (recurrent miscarriage)	Aborto habitual	Aborto abituale	Habitualni pobačaj
Baby blues	Maternity blues (baby blues)	Baby blues (leve depresión post parto)	Sindrome del terzo giorno (baby blues)	Labilno psihičko raspoloženje (baby blues)
Banque du sperme	Sperm bank	Banco de semen	Banca del seme	Banka sperme
Bassin contracté	Contracted pelvis	Pelvis contraída	Pelvi ristretto	Sužena zdjelica
Blastocyste	Blastocyst	Blastocisto	Blastocisti	Blastocista
Canal galactophore	Lactiferous duct	Conducto mamario (conducto galactóforo)	Dotto galattoforo	Mliječni vod
Canal utérin	Birth canal	Canal del parto	Canale del parto	Porodni kanal
Cardiotocographie	Cardiotocography	Cardiotocografía	Cardiotocografia	Kardiotokografija
Césarienne	Cesarean section (C-section)	Cesárea	Taglio cesareo	Carski rez
Chorioamnionite	Inflammation of the fetal membranes (chorioamnionitis)	Infección de las membranas placentarias (corioamnionitis)	Inflammazione del sacco amniotico (corioamniosite)	Upala plodovih ovoja (korioamnionitis)
Choriocarcinome	Choriocarcinoma	Coriocarcinoma	Coriocarcinoma	Koriokarcinom
Choriocentèse	Chorionic villus sampling	Muestra de vellosidades coriónicas	Villocentesi	Uzorak korionskih resica
Chorion	Chorion	Corion	Corion (corio)	Korion
Clarté nucale	Nuchal scan (nuchal translucency)	Traslucencia nucal	Translucenza nucale	Nuhalna translucencija
Conception (fécondation)	Conception	Fecundación (fertilización)	Concezione	Začeće (oplodnja)
Contractions utérines du travail	Labor contractions	Contracciones del trabajo de parto (contracciones uterinas)	Contrazioni del travaglio	Trudovi

Français	Anglais	Espagnol	Italien	Croate
Cordocentèse	Cordocentesis	Cordocentesis	Cordocentesi	Kordocenteza
Cordon ombilical	Umbilical cord	Cordón umbilical	Funicolo ombelicale	Pupkovina (pupčana vrpca)
Cou	Neck	Cuello	Collo	Vrat
Couche -culotte	Diaper	Pañal	Pannolino	Pelena
Couper	Cut	Cortar	Tagliare (intersecare)	Presjeći
Couveuse (incubateur)	Incubator	Incubadora	Incubatrice	Inkubator
Curetage	Curettage	Legrado	Raschiamento (curetage)	Kiretaža
Cycle menstruel	Menstrual cycle	Ciclo menstrual	Ciclo mestruale	Menstruacijski ciklus
Dépression post-natale (dépression post-partum)	Postnatal depression (postpartum depression)	Depresión postparto (depresión postnatal)	Depressione post-partum	Postporođajna depresija
Diabète gestationnel	Gestational diabetes	Diabetes gestacional	Diabete gestazionale	Gestacijski dijabetes
Dilatation cervicale	Cervical dilation	Dilatación del cuello uterino	Dilatazione della cervice uterina	Otvaranje ušća maternice
Donneuse d'ovule	Egg donation	Donación de ovocitos	Ovodonazione	Donacija jajašca
Durée de la contraction utérine	Duration of contraction	Duración de las contracciones uterinas	Durata di contrazioni	Trajanje truda
Durée de la grossesse	Duration of pregnancy	Duración del embarazo	Durata della gravidanza	Trajanje trudnoće
Échographie	Ultrasound (medical ultrasonography)	Ultrasonografía (ecografía)	Ecografia	Ultrazvuk
Éclampsie	Eclampsia	Eclampsia	Eclampsia	Eklampsija
Éjaculation	Ejaculation	Eyaculación	Eiaculazione	Ejakulat
Embryon	Embryo	Embrión	Embrione	Embrij (zametak)
Enlèvement chirurgical de l'uterus (hystérectomie)	Surgical removal of the uterus (hysterectomy)	Extracción quirúrgica del útero (histerectomía)	Asportazione chirurgica dell'utero (isterectomia)	Kirurško odstranjenje maternice (histerektomija)
Épisiotomie	Episiotomy	Episiotomía	Episiotomia	Kirurško proširenje porođajnog kanala (epiziotomija)
Expulsion du bébé	Expulsion of the baby	Expulsión del producto	Espulsione del feto	Istiskivanje ploda
Expulsion du placenta	Expulsion of placenta	Expulsión de la placenta	Espulsione della placenta	Istiskivanje posteljice i ovoja
Facteurs de risque de la grossesse	Pregnancy risk factors	Agentes teratogénicos	Rischio teratogenico	Teratogeni faktori rizika
Fausse contraction (contraction de Braxton Hicks)	Braxton Hicks contractons	Contracción de Braxton Hicks	False contrazioni (contrazioni di Braxton Hicks)	Lažni trudovi
Fausse couche	Spontaneous abortion (miscarriage)	Aborto espontáneo	Aborto spontaneo	Spontani pobačaj
Fécondation in vitro	In vitro fertilisation	Fecundación in vitro	Fertilizzazione in vitro	Oplodnja in vitro
Fièvre puerpérale	Puerperal fever	Fiebre puerperal	Febbre puerperale	Puerperalna groznica (babinja groznica)
Foetoscopie	Fetoscopy	Fetoscopia	Fetoscopia	Fetoskopija
Foetus	Fetus	Feto	Feto	Fetus
Follicule de Graaf	Graafian follicle	Folículo de Graaf	Follicolo di Graaf	Graafov folikul
Forceps	Forceps	Fórceps	Forcipe	Forceps (kliješta)
Fréquence des contractions utérines	Labor contraction frequency	Frecuencia de las contracciones uterinas	Frequenza di contrazioni uterine	Frekvencija trudova
Géniteur	Parent	Padre (primario)	Genitore	Roditelj
Gonadotrophine chorionique	Chorion-gonadotrophin	Gonadotropina coriónica	Gonadotropina corionica	Korion-gonadotropin
Grossesse	Pregnancy	Embarazo	Gravidanza (gestazione)	Trudnoća
Grossesse extra-utérine	Ectopic pregnancy (extrauterine pregnancy)	Embarazo ectópico	Gravidanza ectopica	Izvanmaternična trudno-ća (ektopična trudnoća)
Grossesse multiple	Multiple pregnancy	Embarazo múltiple	Gravidanza gemellare	Blizanačka trudnoća
Gynécologie	Gynecology	Ginecología	Ginecologia	Ginekologija
Hymen	Hymen	Himen	Imene	Djevičnjak (himen)
Hyperhémie ovarienne	Ovarian hyperemia	Hiperemia del ovario	Iperemia dell'ovaio	Hiperemija jajnika
Hyperplasie endométriale	Endometrial hyperplasia	Hiperplasia endometrial	Iperplasia endometriale	Hiperplazija maternice
Hypertrophie de l'utérus	Hypertrophy of uterus	Hipertrofia del útero	Ipertrofia dell'utero	Hipertrofija maternice
Hypotrophie foetale	Fetal hypotrophy	Hipotrofia fetal	Ipotrofia fetale	Fetalna hipotrofija
Iléus méconial	Meconium ileus	Enfermedad de Hirschsprung (megacolon agangliónico)	Malattia di Hirschsprung (ostruzione del colon congenita)	Mekonijalni ileus
Implantation	Implantation	Implatación	Impianto	Implantacija (usađivanje)
Incontinence urinaire	Urinary incontinence	Incontinencia urinaria	Incontinenza urinaria	Urinarna inkotinencija
Infection	Infection	Infección	Infezione	Infekcija
Infections TORCH	TORCH infections	Infecciones TORCH	Complesso TORCH	TORCH infekcije
Inflammation de la vessie (cystite)	Inflammation of the urinary bladder (cystitis)	Inflamación de la vejiga urinaria (cistitis)	Infiammazione della vescica urinaria (cistite)	Upala mokraćnog mjehura (cistitis)
Insémination artificielle	Artificial insemination	Inseminación artificial	Fecondazione assistita (fecondazione artificiale)	Umjetna oplodnja
Intensité des contractions utérines	Intensity of contractions	Intensidad de contracciones uterinas	Intensità di contrazione	Snaga trudova
Injection intra-cytoplasmique de spermatozoïdes	Intracytoplasmatic sperm injection	Inyección intracitoplasmática de espermatozoides	Iniezione intracitoplasmatica dello spermatozoo	Intracitoplazmatska spermalna injekcija
Jumeaux	Twins	Gemelos	Gemelli	Blizanci
Jumeaux dizygotes	Dizygotic twins (biovular twins)	Gemelos dicigóticos (mellizos)	Gemelli fraterni (gemelli dizigoti)	Dvojajčani blizanci

Français	Anglais	Espagnol	Italien	Croate
Jumeaux monozygotes	Monozygotic twins (identical twins)	Gemelos monocigóticos	Gemelli identici (gemelli monozigoti)	Jednojajčani blizanci
Lactation	Lactation	Lactancia	Lattazione	Dojenje (laktacija)
Liquide amniotique	Amniotic fluid	Líquido amniótico	Liquido amniotico	Plodna voda (amnijska tekućina)
Lithopédion (enfant pétrifié)	Lithopedion (stone baby)	Litopedion	Lithopedion	Litopedion (okamenjeno dijete)
Lochies	Lochia	Loquios	Lochi	Lohija (iscjedak u babinjama)
Macrosomie foetale	Macrosomia (big baby syndrome)	Macrosomía fetal	Macrosomia fetale	Fetalna hipertrofija
Maladie hémolytique du nouveau-né	Hemolytic disease of the newborn	Enfermedad hemolítica del recién nacido (eritroblastosis fetal)	Eritroblastosi fetale (malattia emolitica del neonato)	Hemolitička bolest novorođenčeta
Malformations utérines	Uterine anomalies	Malformaciones uterinas	Anomalie uterine	Anomalije maternice
Mamelon (papille)	Nipple	Pezón	Capezzolo	Bradavica
Mammite puerpérale	Puerperal mastitis	Mastitis puerperal	Mastite puerperale	Puerperalni mastitis
Maternité	Maternity hospital	Hospital de maternidad	Clinica ostetrica	Rodilište
Méconium	Meconium	Meconio	Meconio	Mekonij
Médicament pour interrompre le déclenchement du travail (tocolytique)	Medication that suppresses premature labor (tocolytic)	Fármaco utilizado para suprimir el trabajo de parto prematuro (tocolítico)	Farmaco con lo scopo di arrestare le contrazioni uterine (tocolisi)	Lijek za sprečavanje trudova (tokolitik)
Médicaments abortifs	Abortifacients	Fármacos abortivos	Farmaci abortivi	Abortivni lijekovi
Ménopause	Menopause	Menopausia	Menopausa	Menopauza (klimakterij)
Mère	Mother	Madre	Madre	Majka
Mère porteuse	Surrogate mother (womb mother)	Madre de alquiler	Surrogazione di maternità	Surogat majka (zamjenska majka)
Microcéphalie	Microcephaly	Microcefalia	Microcefalia	Mikrocefalija (sitnoglavost)
Mifépristone	Mifepristone	Mifepristona	Mifepristone	Mifepriston
Mort-né	Stillborn	Nacido muerto	Nato morto	Mrtvorođenče
Morula	Morula	Mórula	Morula	Morula
Multipare	Multigravida	Multigrávida	Pluripara	Višerotkinja
Muqueuse utérine (endomètre)	Inner membrane of the uterus (endometrium)	Mucosa interior del útero (endometrio)	Mucosa interna dell'utero (endometrio)	Sluznica maternice (endometrij)
Naissance après terme	Postmature birth	Parto postérmino	Parto post-termine	Poslijeročni porod
Nausée	Nausea	Náusea	Nausea	Mučnina
Néonatologie	Neonatology	Neonatología	Neonatologia	Neonatologija
Nouveau-né	Newborn (infant)	Neonato(recién nacido)	Neonato	Novorođenče
Nouveau-né prématuré	Preterm newborn	Recién nacido pre-término	Neonato pretermine	Nedonošče
Obstétricien	Obstetrician	Tocólogo (obstetra)	Ostetrico	Porodničar (opstetičar)
Obstétrique	Obstetrics	Obstetricia	Ostetricia	Porodništvo
Oedème	Edema	Edema (hidropesía)	Edema	Edem
Oestrogène placentaire	Placental estrogen	Estrógeno de la placenta	Estrogeno placentare	Estrogen placente
Ombilic (nombril)	Navel (belly button)	Ombligo (pupo)	Ombelico	Pupak
Ovaire	Ovary	Ovario	Ovaia (ovario)	Jajnik
Ovogenèse	Oogenesis	Ovogénesis	Ovogenesi	Ovogeneza (oogeneza)
Ovulation	Ovulation	Ovulación	Ovulazione	Ovulacija
Ovule	Ovum	Óvulo	Uovo	Jajašce
Parent biologique	Biological parent	Padre biológico	Genitore biologico	Biološki roditelj
Pelvimétrie	Pelvimetry	Pelvimetría	Pelvimetria	Pelvimetrija
Père	Father	Padre	Padre	Otac
Péritonite méconiale	Meconium peritonitis	Peritonitis meconial	Peritonite da meconio	Mekonijalni peritonitis
pH-métrie foetale	Fetal pH-metry	pH-metría fetal	pH-metria fetale	Fetalna pH-metrija
Placenta	Placenta	Placenta	Placenta	Posteljica (placenta)
Placenta accreta	Placenta accreta	Placenta accreta	Placenta accreta	Prirasla posteljica (placenta accreta)
Placenta praevia	Placenta previa	Placenta previa	Placenta previa	Placenta previja
Plagiocéphalie	Plagiocephaly	Plagiocefalia	Plagiocefalia	Plagiocefalija
Poids de naissance	Fetal weight (birth mass)	Peso al nacer	Peso di neonato	Težina ploda (porođajna težina)
Position transversale du foetus	Transverse fetal position	Feto posición transversal	Posizione del feto trasversale	Kosi položaj ploda
Post-partum	Postnatal (postpartum period, puerperium)	Puerperio	Puerperio	Babinje (puerperij)
Pousser	Push	Empujar	Spingere	Tiskati
Pré-éclampsie	EPH gestosis (preeclampsia)	Preeclampsia	Preeclampsia (gestosi)	EPH-gestoze (preeklampsija)
Prématurité	Premature birth	Parto pretérmino	Parto pretermine	Prijevremeni porod
Présentation podalique (présentation du siège)	Breech position	Posición de nalgas	Posizione podalica del feto	Stav zatkom
Pression artérielle élevée (hypertension artérielle)	High blood pressure (hypertension)	Incremento de la presión sanguínea (hipertensión)	Ipertensione arteriosa sistemica	Visoki krvni tlak (hipertenzija)
Primigeste	Primigravida	Primigesta	Primipara	Prvorotkinja
Procréation médicalement assistée	Medically assisted procreation	Reproducción asistida	Procreazione assistita	Medicinski potpomognuta oplodnja

Français	Anglais	Espagnol	Italien	Croate
Profil biophysique foetal	Biophysical profile of the fetus	Perfil biofisico fetal	Profilo biofisico fetale	Biofizikalni profil fetusa
Progestérone	Progesterone	Progesterona	Progesterone	Progesteron
Progestérone placentaire	Placental progesterone	Progesterona de placenta	Progesterone placentare	Progesteron placente
Prolactine	Prolactin	Prolactina	Prolattina	Prolaktin
Prolapsus du cordon ombilical	Umbilical cord prolapse	Prolapso del cordón umbilical	Prolasso del funicolo ombelicale	Ispala pupkovina (prolaps pupkovine)
Psychose puerpérale	Postpartum psychosis	Psicosis postparto	Psicosi post-partum	Puerperalna psihoza
Pyélonéphrite	Pyelonephritis	Pielonefritis	Pielonefrite	Pijelonefritis
Quadruplés	Quadruplets	Cuatrillizos	Quattro gemelli	Četvorci
Règle (menstruation)	Menstruation	Menstruación (período)	Mestruazione	Menstruacija
Respiration	Breathing	Respiración	Respirazione	Disanje
Rétention d'urine	Urinary retention (ischuria)	Retención de orina	Ritenzione urinaria	Zastoj urina (urinarna retencija)
Rupture des membranes	Rupture of membranes	Ruptura de membrana	Rottura delle membrane	Prsnuće vodenjaka
Rupture prématurée des membranes	Premature rupture of membranes	Ruptura prematura de membrana	Rottura precoce delle membrane	Prijevremeno prsnuće vodenjaka
Sage-femme	Midwife	Matrona (matrón)	Ostetrica (levatrice)	Babica
Saignement (hémorragie)	Bleeding (haemorrhage)	Desangramiento (hemorragia)	Emorragia	Krvarenje (hemoragija)
Salle d'accouchement	Delivery room	Sala de partos	Sala parto	Rađaona
Sécrétion de la salive excessive	Excessive secretion of saliva (hypersalivation)	Excesiva producción de saliva (hipersalivación)	Produzione di saliva eccessiva (ipersalivazione)	Pojačano lučenje sline (hipersalivacija)
Sein	Breast	Mama	Mammella	Dojka
Septicémie puerpérale	Puerperal sepsis	Sepsis puerperal	Sepsi puerperale	Puerperalna sepsa
Siège	Breech	Nalga	Culatta (deretano)	Zadak
Signe de Chadwick	Chadwick's sign	Signo de Chadwick	Segno del Chadwick (tinta bluastra alla vagina)	Hiperemična sluznica rodnice (Chadwickov znak)
Spermatozoïde	Spermatozoon (sperm cell)	Espermatozoide	Spermatozoo	Spermij
Sperme	Semen (sperm)	Semen (esperma)	Seme (sperma)	Sjemena tekućina (sperma)
Stade du travail	Stage of birth	Etapas del parto	Fase del parto	Porodno doba
Stérilité	Infertility	Infertilidad	Sterilità	Neplodnost (sterilitet)
Succion	Suckling	Succión	Suzione	Sisanje
Syndrome d'aspiration méconiale	Meconium aspiration syndrome	Síndrome de aspiración de meconio	Sindrome da aspirazione di meconio	Mekonijalni aspiracijski sindrom
Taille corporelle du nouveau-né	Body length of a newborn	Talla de un neonato	Lunghezza di neonato	Dužina novorođenčeta
Tête	Head	Cabeza	Testa	Glavica
Tire-lait	Breast pump	Sacaleches	Pompa tiralatte	Pumpica za izdajanje
Trompes de Fallope	Fallopian tube (oviduct)	Trompa de Falopio (tuba uterina, oviducto)	Ovidotto (ovidutto)	Jajovod
Utérus	Womb (uterus)	Útero (matriz, seno materno)	Utero	Maternica (uterus)
Vacuum extractor	Vacuum extractor (ventouse)	Aspirador al vacío	Aspiratore a vuoto	Vakuumski ekstraktor
Vagin	Vagina	Vagina	Vagina	Rodnica
Varices des membres inférieurs	Leg varicose veins	Venas varicosas de las piernas	Varici degli arti inferiori	Proširene vene na nogama
Viabilité du sperme	Sperm viability	Viabilidad de espermatozoides	Sopravvivenza di spermatozoo	Životna sposobnost spermija
Villosités choriales	Chorionic villi	Vellosidades coriónicas	Villi coriali	Korionske resice
Vomissement	Vomiting	Vómito (emesis)	Vomito (emetismo)	Povraćanje

DICCIONARIO MULTILINGÜE DE EMERGENCIAS MÉDICAS

Español-Inglés-Francés-Italiano-Croata

Español	Inglés	Francés	Italiano	Croata
NÚMEROS:	**NUMBERS:**	**NUMÉROS:**	**NUMERI:**	**BROJEVI:**
Cero	Zero	Zéro	Zero	Nula
Uno	One	Un	Uno	Jedan
Dos	Two	Deux	Due	Dva
Tres	Three	Trois	Tre	Tri
Cuatro	Four	Quatre	Quattro	Četiri
Cinco	Five	Cinq	Cinque	Pet
Seis	Six	Six	Sei	Šest
Siete	Seven	Sept	Sette	Sedam
Ocho	Eight	Huit	Otto	Osam
Nueve	Nine	Neuf	Nove	Devet
Diez	Ten	Dix	Dieci	Deset
Once	Eleven	Onze	Undici	Jedanaest
Doce	Twelve	Douze	Dodici	Dvanaest
Trece	Thirteen	Treize	Tredici	Trinaest
Catorce	Fourteen	Quatorze	Quattordici	Četrnaest
Quince	Fifteen	Quinze	Quindici	Petnaest
Dieciséis	Sixteen	Seize	Sedici	Šesnaest
Diecisiete	Seventeen	Dix-sept	Diciassette	Sedamnaest
Dieciocho	Eighteen	Dix-huit	Diciotto	Osamnaest
Diecinueve	Nineteen	Dix-neuf	Diciannove	Devetnaest
Veinte	Twenty	Vingt	Venti	Dvadeset
Veintiuno	Twenty-one	Vingt et un	Ventuno	Dvadest i jedan
Veintidós	Twenty-two	Vingt-deux	Ventidue	Dvadeset i dva
Treinta	Thirty	Trente	Trenta	Trideset
Cuarenta	Forty	Quarante	Quaranta	Četrdeset
Cincuenta	Fifty	Cinquante	Cinquanta	Pedeset
Sesenta	Sixty	Soixante	Sessanta	Šezdeset
Setenta	Seventy	Soixante-dix	Settanta	Sedamdeset
Ochenta	Eighty	Quatre-vingts	Ottanta	Osamdeset
Noventa	Ninety	Quatre-vingt-dix	Novanta	Devedeset
Cien	Hundred	Cent	Cento	Sto
Ciento uno	One hundred and one	Cent un	Centouno	Sto jedan
Ciento veintitrés	One hundred and twenty-three	Cent vingt-trois	Centoventitre	Sto dvadeset i tri
Doscientos	Two hundred	Deux cents	Duecento	Dvjesto
Trescientos	Three hundred	Trois cents	Trecento	Tristo
Cuatrocientos	Four hundred	Quatre cents	Quattrocento	Četristo
Quinientos	Five hundred	Cinq cents	Cinquecento	Petsto
Seiscientos	Six hundred	Six cents	Seicento	Šesto
Setecientos	Seven hundred	Sept cents	Settecento	Sedamsto
Ochocientos	Eight hundred	Huit cents	Ottocento	Osamsto
Novecientos	Nine hundred	Neuf cents	Novecento	Devetsto
Mil	Thousand	Mille	Mille	Tisuća
Dos mil	Two thousand	Deux mille	Duemila	Dvije tisuće
Millón	Million	Million	Un milione	Milijun
Mil millones (miliarda)	Milliard (billion)	Milliard	Un miliardo	Milijarda
ORIENTACIÓN EN EL TIEMPO:	**ORIENTATION IN TIME:**	**ORIENTATION DANS LE TEMPS:**	**ORIENTAMENTO NEL TEMPO:**	**ORIJENTACIJA U VREMENU:**
Ayer	Yesterday	Hier	Ieri	Jučer
Hoy	Today	Aujourd'hui	Oggi	Danas
Día de mañana	Tomorrow	Demain	Domani	Sutra
Año	Year	Année	Anno	Godina
Mes	Month	Mois	Mese	Mjesec
Semana	Week	Semaine	Settimana	Tjedan
Día	Day	Jour	Giorno	Dan
Hora	Hour	Heure	Ora	Sat
Minuto	Minute	Minute	Minuto	Minuta
Segundo	Second	Seconde	Secondo	Sekunda
Mañana	Morning	Matin	Mattina	Jutro (prijepodne)
Tarde	Afternoon	Après-midi	Pomeriggio	Poslijepodne
Anochecer	Evening	Soir	Sera	Večer
Noche	Night	Nuit	Notte	Noć
ORIENTACIÓN EN EL ESPACIO:	**ORIENTATION IN SPACE:**	**ORIENTATION DANS L'ESPACE:**	**ORIENTAMENTO NELLO SPAZIO:**	**ORIJENTACIJA U PROSTORU:**
Arriba	Up (above)	En haut (au-dessus)	Su	Gore (iznad)
Abajo	Down (below)	En bas (au-dessous)	In basso	Dolje (ispod)
Izquierda	Left	Gauche	Sinistra	Lijevo
Derecha	Right	Droite	Destra	Desno
Enfrente	In front	Devant	Davanti	Ispred
Detrás	Behind	Derrière	Dietro	Iza
Dentro	Inside	Dedans	Dentro	Unutra
Fuera	Outside	Dehors	Fuori	Vani

Español ACCIDENTES, CATÁSTROFES Y ANGUSTIA:	Inglés ACCIDENTS, CATASTROPHES AND DISTRESS:	Francés LES ACCIDENTS, CATASTROPHES ET DÉTRESSE:	Italiano GLI ACCIDENTI, CATASTROFI E ANGOSCIA:	Croata NESREĆE, KATASTROFE I POGIBELJNE SITUACIJE:
Abrigo	Shelter	Abri	Rifugio	Sklonište
Accidente automovilístico (siniestro de tráfico)	Car accident	Accident automobile (accident de la route)	Incidente stradale	Automobilska nesreća
Accidente de aviación	Airplane crash	Accident aérien	Incidente aereo	Pad aviona
Accidente de tráfico	Traffic accident	Accident sur la voie publique	Incidente di traffico	Prometna nesreća
Accidente doméstico	Domestic accident	Accident domestique	Infortunio domestico	Nesreća u kući
Accidente laboral	Occupational accident	Accident du travail	Infortunio sul lavoro	Nesreća na radu
Accidente nuclear	Nuclear accident	Accident nucléaire	Accidente nucleare	Nuklearna nesreća
Agua	Water	Eau	Acqua	Voda
Ahogado	Drowned person	Noyé	Annegato	Utopljenik
Ahogamiento	Drowning	Noyade	Annegamento	Utapanje
Alarma	Alarm	Alarme	Allarme	Uzbuna
Arma	Weapon	Arme	Arma	Oružje
Arma atómica	Atomic weapons	Arme atomique	Arma atomica	Atomsko oružje
Arma biológica	Biological weapon	Arme biologique	Arma biologica	Biološko oružje
Arma blanca	Cold weapon	Arme de contact	Arma bianca	Hladno oružje
Arma convencional	Conventional weapon	Arme conventionnelle	Arma convenzionale	Konvencionalno oružje
Arma de fuego	Firearm	Arme à feu	Arma da fuoco	Vatreno oružje
Arma láser	Laser weapon	Arme de laser	Armi laser	Lasersko oružje
Arma nuclear	Nuclear weapon	Arme nucléaire	Arma nucleare	Nuklearno oružje
Arma nuclear estratégica	Strategic nuclear weapon	Arme nucléaire stratégique	Arma nucleare strategica	Strateško nuklearno oružje
Arma nuclear táctica	Tactical nuclear weapon	Arme nucléaire tactique (mini-nuke)	Arma nucleare tattica	Taktičko nuklearno oružje
Arma química	Chemical weapon	Arme chimique	Arma chimica	Kemijsko oružje
Armas atómicas, biológicas y químicas (ABQ)	ABC weapons	Arme nucléaire, biologique et chimique (NBC)	Armi nucleari, biologiche e chimiche (NBC)	Atomsko biološko i kemijsko oružje
Armas de destrucción masiva	Weapon of mass destruction	Arme de destruction massive	Arma di distruzione di massa	Oružje za masovno uništavanje
Asalto físico	Physical assault	Attaque physique	Attacco fisico	Tjelesni napad
Ataque	Attack	Attaque	Attaco	Napad
Ataque aéreo	Air attack	Attaque aérienne	Incursione area	Zračni napad
Ataque de piratas	Pirate attack	Attaque de pirates	Attacco dei pirati	Gusarski napad
Ataque de tiburón	Shark attack	Attaque de requin	Attacco di squalo	Napad morskog psa
Ataque terrorista	Terrorist attack	Attaque terroriste	Attentato terroristico	Teroristički napad
Avalancha	Avalanche	Avalanche	Valanga	Lavina
Bacteria	Bacteria	Bacteria	Batterio	Bakterija
Bala	Bullet	Balle	Pallottola	Metak
Banquisa (hielo marino)	Sea ice	Banquise	Banchisa (ghiaccio marino; banchiglia)	Santa leda
Barco	Ship	Navire	Nave	Brod
Bomba	Bomb	Bombe	Bomba	Bomba
Bomba atómica (bomba A)	Atomic bomb (A-bomb)	Bombe atomique (bombe A)	Bomba atomica (bomba A)	Atomska bomba
Bomba de cobalto	Cobalt bomb	Bombe salée	Bomba al cobalto (bomba gamma, bomba G)	Kobaltna bomba
Bomba de hidrógeno (bomba H)	Hidrogen bomb (H-bomb)	Bombe à hydrogène (bombe H)	Bomba all'idrogeno (bomba H)	Hidrogenska bomba
Bomba de neutrones (bomba N)	Neutron bomb	Bombe à neutrons	Bomba al neutrone (bomba N)	Neutronska bomba
Bomba sucia	Dirty bomb	Bombe radiologique (bombe sale)	Bomba sporca	Prljava bomba
Bote salvavidas	Lifeboat	Canot de secours	Scialuppa	Čamac za spašavanje
Boya salvavidas	Lifebelt (lifebuoy)	Bouée couronne	Boa di salvataggio	Pojas za spašavanje
Buque naufragado	Ship wreck	Épave de navire	Relitto	Olupina broda
Búsqueda	Search	Recherche	Ricerca	Potraga
Caída	Fall	Chute	Cadutta (cascata)	Pad
Campamento para refugiados	Refugee camp	Camp de réfugiés	Campo per rifugiati	Izbjeglički logor
Campo minero	Mine field	Champ de mines	Campo minato	Minsko polje
Célula terrorista	Terrorist cell	Cellule terroriste (cellule dormante)	Cellula terroristica	Teroristička ćelija
Chaleco salvavidas	Lifejacket (life vest)	Gilet de sauvetage	Giubbotto di salvataggio	Prsluk za spašavanje
Choque eléctrico	Electric shock	Électrisation (électrocution)	Folgorazione (elettrocuzione)	Strujni udar
Colisión	Collision	Collision	Collisione	Sudar
Cuerda	Rope	Corde	Cordone	Uže
Cueva	Cave	Grotte	Grotta	Špilja
Desechos nucleares	Nuclear waste (radioactive waste)	Déchet radioactif (déchet nucléaire)	Scoria nucleare (scoria radioattiva)	Nuklearni otpad (radioaktivni otpad)
Desminado (eliminación de minas)	Mine clearance (demining)	Déminage	Eliminazione di mine (sminamento)	Razminiranje
Encallamiento de barco	Stranding of a ship	Échouage du navire	Incaglio di nave	Nasukavanje broda

Español	Inglés	Francés	Italiano	Croata
Epidemia	Epidemic	Épidémie	Epidemia	Epidemija
Equipo de búsqueda y rescate	Search and rescue team	Équpie de recherche et sauvetage	Squadra di ricerca e salvataggio	Ekipa za traganje i spašavanje
Erupción volcánica	Volcanic eruption	Éruption volcanique	Eruzione vulcanica	Erupcija vulkana
Esclavitud	Slavery	Esclavage	Schiavitù (prigionia)	Ropstvo
Explosión	Explosion	Explosion	Esplosione	Eksplozija
Explosivo	Explosive	Explosif	Esplosivo	Eksploziv
Fuego	Fire	Feu	Fuoco	Vatra
Gas tóxico	Poison gas	Gaz toxique	Gas tossico	Bojni otrov (otrovni plin)
Golpe	Stroke (hit, blow)	Coup	Colpo (botta)	Udarac
Golpe de calor	Heat stroke	Coup de chaleur	Colpo di calore	Toplotni udar
Guerra	War	Guerre	Guerra	Rat
Helicóptero	Helicopter (chopper)	Hélicoptère	Elicottero	Helikopter
Hielo	Ice	Glace	Ghiaccio	Led
Homicidio (asesinato)	Homicide (murder)	Homicide (assassinat)	Omicidio (uccisione)	Ubojstvo
Hundimiento de un barco	Sinking of a ship	Naufrage du navire	Affondamento della nave	Potonuće broda
Huracán	Hurricane	Ouragan	Uragano	Uragan
Incendio (fuego)	Fire (conflagration)	Incendie	Incendio (fuoco)	Požar
Inundación	Flood	Inondation	Inondazione	Poplava
Invasión	Invasion	Invasion	Invasione	Invazija
Lago	Lake	Lac	Lago	Jezero
Lava	Lava	Lave	Lava	Lava
Llamada de socorro	Call for help	Appel à l'aide	Chiamata di aiuto	Poziv u pomoć
Llamada de SOS	SOS call	Appel SOS	SOS richiesta	SOS poziv
Managa de agua (tromba marina)	Waterspout	Trombe marine	Tromba marina	Morska pijavica
Mar	Sea	Mer	Mare	More
Metralla	Shrapnel	Shrapnel	Shrapnel	Šrapnel
Mina	Mine	Mine	Mina	Mina
Mina marina	Naval mine	Mine marine (mine sous-marine)	Mina navale	Morska mina
Mina terrestre	Land mine	Mine terrestre	Mina terrestre	Kopnena mina
Montaña	Mountain	Montagne	Montagna	Planina
Neurotoxina	Neurotoxin	Neurotoxine	Neurotossina	Živčani otrov (neurotoksin)
Nevasca (ventisca de nieve)	Snow storm	Tempête de neige	Bufera di neve (nevicata)	Snježna mećava
Nieve (zapada)	Snow	Neige	Neve	Snijeg
Ola de marea	Tidal wave	Onde de marée	Onda di marea	Plimni val
Pandemia	Pandemic	Pandémie	Pandemia	Pandemija
Paracáidas	Parachute	Parachute	Paracadute	Padobran
Pelea	Fight	Combat	Combattimento	Tučnjava
Perro de búsqueda y rescate	Search and rescue dog	Chien de sauvetage	Cane da ricerca e salvataggio	Pas za traganje i spašavanje
Pirata	Pirate	Pirate	Pirata	Gusar
Plutonio	Plutonium	Plutonium	Plutonio	Plutonij
Polución química	Chemical pollution	Pollution chimique	Inquinamento chimico	Kemijsko zagađenje
Protección civil	Civil defense	Sécurité civile	Difesa civile	Civilna zaštita
Prueba nuclear (ensayo nuclear)	Nuclear weapons testing	Essai nucléaire	Test nucleare	Nuklearni pokus
Radiación	Radiation	Rayonnement	Radiazione	Zračenje
Refugiado	Refugee	Réfugié	Rifugiato	Izbjeglica
Rehén	Hostage	Otage	Ostaggio	Taoc (talac)
Río	River	Rivière	Fiume	Rijeka
Robo	Robbery	Vol	Rapina	Pljačka
Roca	Rock	Roche	Roccia	Stijena
Rompehielos	Icebreaker	Brise-glace	Rompighiaccio	Ledolomac
Ruinas	Ruins	Ruine	Macerie (rovine)	Ruševine
Salvador (rescatador)	Rescuer	Sauveur	Salvatore	Spasilac
Salvamento	Salvage	Sauvetage	Salvataggio	Spašavanje
Salvamento marítimo	Marine salvage	Sauvetage en mer	Salvataggio navale	Spašavanje broda
Secuestro	Kidnapping	Enlèvement (rapt)	Rapimento	Otmica
Señal de alarma	Alarm signal	Signal d'alarme	Segnale di allarme	Znak za uzbunu
"¡Socorro!"	"Help!"	"Aide!"	"Aiuto!"	"U pomoć!"
Suicidio	Suicide	Suicide	Suicidio	Samoubojstvo
Témpano de hielo	Iceberg	Iceberg	Ghiacciaio	Ledenjak
Terremoto	Earthquake	Séisme (tremblement de terre)	Terremoto	Potres
Terrorista	Terrorist	Terroriste	Terrorista	Terorist
Tierra	Land	Terre	Terra	Kopno
Tifón	Typhoon	Typhon	Tifone	Tajfun
Tormenta (tempestad)	Storm	Tempête	Tempesta	Nevrijeme (oluja)
Tormenta de arena	Sandstorm	Tempête de sable	Tempesta di sabbia	Pješćana oluja
Trata de personas	Human trafficking	Trafic d'êtres humains	Traffico di esseri umani	Trgovina ljudima
Trueno	Thunderclap	Foudre	Percossa dal fulmine	Udar groma
Tsunami (maremoto)	Tsunami	Tsunami (raz-de-marée)	Tsunami	Tsunami
Uranio	Uranium	Uranium	Uranio	Uranij
Uranio einriquecido	Enriched uranium	Uranium enrichi	Uranio arricchito	Obogaćeni uranij

Español	Inglés	Francés	Italiano	Croata
Víctima	Victim	Victime	Vittima	Žrtva
Violación	Rape (violation)	Viol	Violenza sessuale	Silovanje
Virus	Virus	Virus	Virus	Virus
PARTES DEL CUERPO HUMANO:	PARTS OF THE HUMAN BODY :	PARTIES DU CORPS HUMAIN:	PARTI DEL CORPO UMANO:	DIJELOVI LJUDSKOG TIJELA:
Abdomen (panza)	Belly (abdomen)	Abdomen	Addome (ventre, pancia)	Trbuh (abdomen)
Acetábulo	Acetabulum	Acetabulum	Cotile (acetabolo)	Čašica zdjelične kosti (acetabulum)
Acetilcolina	Acetylcholine	Acétylcholine	Acetilcolina	Acetilkolin
Ácido desoxirribonucleico	Deoxyribonucleic acid (DNA)	Acide désoxyribonucléique	Acido desossiribonucleico (DNA)	Dezoksiribonukleinska kiselina (DNK)
Ácido gástrico	Gastric acid	Acide gastrique	Acido gastrico	Želučana kiselina
Ácido ribonucleico (ARN)	Ribonucleic acid	Acide ribonucléique (ARN)	Acido ribonucleico (ARN)	Ribonukleinska kiselina
Adenohipófisis	Adenohypophysis	Adénohypophyse	Adenoipofisi	Adenohipofiza
Adrenalina	Adrenalin (adrenaline)	Adrénaline	Adrenalina	Adrenalin
Aglutinina	Agglutinin	Agglutinine	Agglutinine	Aglutinin
Aglutinógeno	Agglutinogen	Agglutinogène	Agglutinogeno	Aglutinogen
Albúmina	Albumin	Albumine	Albumina	Albumin
Aldosterona	Aldosterone	Aldostérone	Aldosterone	Aldosteron
Alvéolo	Alveolus	Alvéole	Alveolo	Alveola
Amígdala	Tonsil	Tonsille	Tonsille	Krajnik
Aminoácido	Amino acid	Acide aminé	Amminoacido	Aminokiselina
Amoníaco	Ammonia	Ammoniac	Ammoniaca	Amonijak
Ano	Anus	Anus	Ano	Čmar (anus)
Antebrazo	Forearm	Avant-bras	Avambraccio	Podlaktica
Aorta	Aorta	Aorte	Aorta	Aorta
Aorta abdominal	Abdominal aorta	Aorte abdominale	Aorta addominale	Abdominalna aorta
Aorta torácica	Thoracic aorta	Aorte thoracique	Aorta toracica	Torakalna aorta
Apéndice vermiforme (apéndice cecal, apéndice)	Vermiform appendix (cecal appaendix)	Appendice iléo-caecal (appendice, appendice vermiforme)	Appendice vermiforme	Slijepo crijevo (crvuljak)
Aponeurosis	Aponeurosis	Aponévrose	Aponeurosi	Široka plosnata tetiva (aponeuroza)
Aracnoides	Arachnoid mater	Arachnoïde	Aracnoide	Paučinasta ovojnica (arachnoidea)
Arteria	Artery	Artère	Arteria	Arterija
Arteria coronaria	Coronary artery	Artère coronaire	Arteria coronaria	Koronarna arterija
Arteria pulmonar (tronco pulmonar, tronco de las pulmonares)	Pulmonary artery	Artère pulmonaire	Arteria polmonare	Plućna arterija
Arteriola	Arteriole	Artériole	Arteriola	Arteriola
Articulación	Joint	Articulation	Articolazione	Zglob
Articulación de la cadera	Hip joint	Hanche	Articolazione dell'anca	Kuk (zglob kuka)
Articulación del codo	Elbow joint	Articulation oléacranienne	Articolazione del gomito	Lakatni zglob
Articulación del hombro	Shoulder joint	Complexe articulaire de l'épaule	Articolazione della spalla	Rameni zglob
Astrocito	Astrocyte	Astrocyte	Astrocita	Astrocit
Aurícula cardíaca (atrio)	Cardiac atrium	Oreillette	Atrio	Srčana pretklijetka (atrij)
Barbilla (mentón)	Chin	Menton	Mento	Brada
Base del cráneo	Skull base	Base du crâne	Base del cranio	Baza lubanje
Basófilo	Basophil granulocyte	Granulocyte basophile	Granulocita basofilo	Bazofilni granulocit
Bazo	Spleen	Rate	Milza	Slezena
Bilirrubina	Bilirubin	Bilirubine	Bilirubina	Bilirubin
Bilis	Gall (bile)	Bile	Bile	Žuč
Boca	Mouth	Bouche	Bocca	Usta
Braquial anterior	Brachialis muscle	Muscle brachial	Muscolo brachiale	Nadlaktični mišić
Brazo	Arm	Bras	Braccio	Ruka
Bronquio	Bronchus	Bronche	Bronco	Dušnica (bronh)
Bronquiolo	Bronchiole	Bronchiole	Bronchiolo	Bronhiola
Bulbo raquídeo (médula oblongada, miencéfalo)	Medulla oblongata	Moelle allongée (medulla oblongata, bulbe rachidien, myélencéphale)	Bulbo (midollo allungato, encefalo)	Produžena moždina
Bursa (bolsa sinovial)	Synovial bursa	Bourse séreuse	Borsa sierosa	Sluzna vreća (bursa)
Cabello	Hair	Cheveu	Capelli	Kosa
Cabeza	Head	Tête	Testa	Glava
Caja torácica	Rib cage	Cage thoracique	Gabbia toracica	Grudni koš
Calavera (cráneo)	Skull	Crâne	Cranio	Lubanja
Calcáneo	Calcaneus	Calcanéus (calcanéum)	Calcagno	Petna kost (kalkaneus)
Calcitonina	Calcitonin	Calcitonine	Calcitonina	Kalcitonin
Canal de Schlemm	Canal of Schlemm	Canal de Schlemm	Canale di Schlemm	Schlemmov kanal
Canino (diente colmillo)	Canine tooth	Canine	Canino	Očnjak (kanin)
Capilar	Capillary	Capillaire	Capillare	Kapilara
Cápsula articular	Articular capsule (joint capsule)	Capsule articulaire	Capsula articolare	Zglobna čahura
Cara (faz)	Face	Visage	Viso	Lice
Carbohidrato	Carbohydrate	Hidrate de carbone (glucide)	Carboidrato (glucide)	Ugljikohidrat
Carpo	Carpus	Carpe	Carpo	Zapešće

Español	Inglés	Francés	Italiano	Croata
Cartílago	Cartilage	Cartilage	Cartilagine	Hrskavica
Cartílago articular	Joint cartilage	Cartilage articulaire	Cartilagine articolare	Zglobna hrskavica
Cartílago circoides	Cartilage ring	Cartilage cricoïde	Anello cartilagineo	Hrskavični prsten
Catecolamina	Catecholamine	Catécholamine	Catecolamina	Katekolamin
Cavidad bucal (cavidad oral)	Mouth cavity (oral cavity)	Cavité buccale	Cavità orale	Usna šupljina
Cavidad timpánica	Tympanic cavity	Cavité tympanique	Cassa del timpano	Bubnjište
Ceja	Eyebrow	Sourcils	Sopracciglio	Obrva
Célula	Cell	Cellule	Cellula	Stanica
Cemento dental	Cementum	Cément	Cemento	Zubni cement
Cerebelo	Cerebellum	Cervelet	Cervelletto	Mali mozak
Cerebro	Brain	Cerveau	Cervello	Mozak
Cerumen (cerilla)	Earwax (cerumen)	Cire de l'oreille (cérumen)	Cerume	Ušna mast (ušna smola, cerumen)
Clavícula	Collarbone (clavicle)	Clavicule	Clavicola	Ključna kost (klavikula)
Clítoris	Clitoris	Clitoris	Clitoride	Dražica (klitoris)
Cóccix (coxis)	Tailbone (coccyx)	Coccyx	Coccige	Trtica
Cóclea (caracol)	Cochlea	Cochlée	Coclea	Pužnica
Codo	Elbow	Coude	Gomito	Lakat
Colágeno	Collagen	Collagène	Collagene	Kolagen
Colesterol	Cholesterol	Cholestérol	Colesterolo	Kolesterol
Colon sigmoide	Sigmoid colon	Côlon sigmoïde	Sigma (colon sigmoideo)	Sigmoidni dio debelog crijeva
Columna vertebral	Spine (spinal column, backbone)	Colonne vertébrale (rachis)	Colonna vertebrale	Kralježnica
Conducto auditivo externo	Auditory canal (ear canal)	Conduit auditif externe (canal auriculaire)	Meato acustico esterno	Slušni kanal
Conducto eyaculador	Ejaculatory duct	Canal éjaculateur	Dotto eiaculatore	Sjemenovod
Conducto nasolagrimal	Nasolacrimal duct (tear duct)	Canal lacrymonasal (canal lacrimal, canal des larmes)	Canale naso-lacrimale	Suzno-nosni kanal
Corazón	Heart	Coeur	Cuore	Srce
Córnea	Cornea	Cornée	Cornea	Rožnica
Coroides	Choroid	Choroïde	Coroide	Žilnica
Corona del diente	Crown of a tooth	Couronne de la dent	Corona del dente	Kruna zuba
Corteza cerebral	Cerebral cortex	Cortex cérébral (écorce cérébrale)	Corteccia cerebrale	Moždana kora
Corticosteroide	Corticosteroid	Corticostéroïde	Corticosteroide	Kortikosteroid
Corticosterona	Corticosterone	Corticostérone	Corticosterone	Kortikosteron
Cortisol (hidrocortisona)	Cortisol	Cortisol (hydro-cortisone)	Cortisolo	Kortizol
Cortisona	Cortisone	Cortisone	Cortisone	Kortizon
Costilla	Rib	Côte	Costola (costa)	Rebro
Cristalino	Lens	Cristallin	Cristallino	Leća
Cúbito (ulna)	Ulna	Ulna (cubitus)	Ulna (cubito)	Lakatna kost (ulna)
Cuello	Neck	Cou	Collo	Vrat
Cuerda vocal	Vocal chord	Corde vocale	Corda vocale	Glasnica
Cuero cabelludo (capa capilar)	Scalp	Cuir chevelu	Cuoio capelluto	Vlasište
Cuerpo lúteo (cuerpo amarillo)	Corpus luteum	Corps jaune	Corpo luteo	Žuto tijelo
Dedo anular	Ring finger	Annulaire	Anulare	Prstenjak
Dedo corazón	Middle finger	Majeur	Dito medio	Srednji prst
Dedo de la mano	Finger	Doigt	Dito della mano	Ručni prst
Dedo del pie	Toe	Orteil	Dito del piede	Nožni prst
Dedo índice	Forefinger	Index	Dito indice	Kažiprst
Dedo meñique	Little finger (pinky)	Auriculaire (petit doigt)	Mignolo	Mali prst
Dedo pulgar (pólice)	Thumb	Pouce	Pollice	Palac
Dendrita	Dendrite	Dendrite	Dendrite	Dendrit
Dentina	Dentin	Dentine (ivoire)	Dentina	Zubni dentin
Diafragma	Diaphragm	Diaphragme	Muscolo diaframma	Ošit (dijafragma)
Diencéfalo	Diencephalon	Diencéphale	Diencefalo	Međumozak
Diente	Tooth	Dent	Dente	Zub
Diente de leche	Milk tooth	Dent temporaire	Dente da latte	Mliječni zub
Disco intervertebral	Intervertebral disc	Disque intervertébral	Disco intervertebrale	Međukralježnični disk
Duodeno	Duodenum	Duodénum	Duodeno	Dvanaesnik (duodenum)
Dura madre	Dura mater	Dure-mère	Dura madre (pachimeninge)	Tvrda moždana ovojnica
Eclerótica	Sclera	Sclère	Sclera	Bjeloočnica
Elastina	Elastin	Élastine	Elastina	Elastin
Electrolito	Electrolyte	Électrolyte	Elettrolita	Elektrolit
Encía	Gums (gingiva)	Gencive	Gengiva	Desni
Eosinófilo	Eosinophil	Éosinophile	Eosinofilo	Eozinofil
Epidídimo	Epididymis	Épididyme	Epididimo	Pasjemenik
Eritocito (glóbulo rojo)	Erythrocyte (red blood cell)	Érythrocyte (hématie, globule rouge)	Eritrocita (globulo rosso)	Eritrocit (crveno krvno tjelešce)
Esfínter	Sphincter	Sphincter	Sfintere	Kružni mišić (sfinkter)
Esmalte dental	Tooth enamel	Émail dentaire	Smalto	Zubna caklina
Esófago	Gullet (oesophagus)	Oesophage	Esofago	Jednjak

Español	Inglés	Francés	Italiano	Croata
Espalda	Back	Dos	Schiena (dorso)	Leđa
Espalda baja	Loin	Lombes	Lombo	Križa
Espalda superior	Upper back	Parti supérieur du dos	Schiena alto	Gornji dio leđa
Espermatozoide	Sperm (spermatozoon)	Spermatozoïde	Spermatozoo	Spermij
Esqueleto	Skeleton	Squelette	Scheletro	Kostur
Esternón	Breastbone (sternum)	Sternum	Sterno	Prsna kost (sternum)
Estómago	Stomach	Estomac	Stomaco	Želudac
Estradiol	Estradiol	Estradiol	Estradiolo	Folikulin (estradiol)
Estribo	Stirrup (stapes)	Étrier	Staffa (columella)	Stremen
Estrógeno	Estrogen	Estrogène	Estrogeno	Estrogen
Excrementos (heces)	Stool (feces)	Fèces	Feci	Stolica (feces, izmet)
Factor Rh negativo	Rh factor negative	Système Rhésus négatif	Fattore Rh negativo	Negativan Rh faktor
Factor Rh positivo	Rh factor positive	Système Rhésus positif	Fattore Rh positivo	Pozitivan Rh faktor
Falange	Phalanx bone	Phalange	Falange	Kost prsta (falanga)
Faringe	Pharynx (gullet, gorge)	Pharynx	Faringe	Ždrijelo
Fascia profunda	Muscular fascia	Fascia musculaire (périmysium)	Fascia muscolare	Mišićna fascija
Fémur	Thighbone (femur)	Os de la cuisse (fémur)	Femore	Bedrena kost (femur)
Fibrina	Fibrin	Fibrine	Fibrina	Fibrin
Fibrinógeno	Fibrinogen	Fibrinogène	Fibrinogeno	Fibrinogen
Fibroblasto (célula fija)	Fibroblast	Fibroblaste	Fibroblasto	Fibroblast
Fluido corporal	Body fluid	Fluide corporel	Fluido corporale	Tjelesna tekućina
Fosfolípido	Phospholipid	Phospholipide	Fosfolipide	Fosfolipid
Frente	Forehead	Front	Fronte	Čelo
Ganglio linfático	Lymph gland (lymph node)	Ganglion lymphatique (noeud lymphatique)	Linfonodo	Limfna žlijezda
Garganta	Throat	Gorge	Gola	Grlo
Gas	Gas	Gaz	Gas	Plin
Glande	Glans	Gland	Glande	Glavić
Glándula	Gland	Glande	Ghiandola	Žlijezda
Glándula bulbo-uretral (glándula de Cowper)	Bulbourethral gland (Cowper's gland)	Glande de Cowper (glande bulbo-uretrale)	Ghiandola bulbouretrale (ghiandola di Cowper)	Bulbouretralna žlijezda (Cowperova žlijezda)
Glándula de Bartolino	Bartholin's gland	Glande de Bartholin	Ghiandola di Bartolini	Bartolinova žlijezda
Glándula lagrimal	Lachrymal gland	Glande lacrymale	Ghiandola lacrimale	Suzna žlijezda
Glándula paratiroides	Parathyroid gland	Parathyroïde	Paratiroide	Doštitnjača
Glándula pineal (epífisis)	Pineal body (pineal gland, epiphysis)	Glande pinéale (épiphyse)	Ghiandola pineale (epifisi)	Pinealna žlijezda (epifiza)
Glándula salival	Salivary gland	Glande salivaire	Ghiandola salivare	Žlijezda slinovnica
Glándula sebácea	Sebaceous gland	Glande sébacée	Ghiandola sebacea	Žlijezda lojnica
Glándula sudorípara	Sweat gland	Glande sudoripare (sudorale)	Ghiandola sudoripara	Žlijezda znojnica
Glándula suprarrenal	Adrenal gland	Glande surrénale	Surrene	Nadbubrežna žlijezda
Globo ocular	Eyeball	Globe oculaire	Bulbo oculare	Očna jabučica
Globulina	Globulin	Globuline	Globulina	Globulin
Glomérulo	Glomerulus	Glomérule	Glomerulo	Glomerul
Glucagón	Glucagon	Glucagon	Glucagone	Glukagon
Glucocorticoide	Glucocorticoid	Glucocorticoïde	Glucocorticoide	Glukokortikoid
Glucógeno	Glycogen	Glycogène	Glicogeno	Glikogen
Glucosa	Glucose	Glucose	Glucosio	Glukoza
Gónada	Sex gland (gonad)	Gonade	Gonade	Spolna žlijezda
Gonadotropina	Gonadotrophin	Gonadotrophine	Gonadotropina	Gonadotropin
Granulocito	Granulocyte	Granulocyte (polynucléaire)	Granulocita	Granulocit
Grasa	Fat	Matière grasse	Lipidi	Mast
Grupo sanguíneo	Blood group	Groupe sanguin	Gruppo sanguigno	Krvna grupa
Grupo sanguíneo A	Blood group A	Groupe sanguin A	Gruppo sanguigno A	Krvna grupa A
Grupo sanguíneo AB	Blood group AB	Groupe sanguin AB	Gruppo sanguigno AB	Krvna grupa AB
Grupo sanguíneo B	Blood group B	Groupe sanguin B	Gruppo sanguigno B	Krvna grupa B
Grupo sanguíneo 0	Blood group 0	Groupe sanguin 0	Gruppo sanguigno 0	Krvna grupa 0
Haz de His	Bundle of His	Faisceau de His	Fascio di His	Hisov snopić
Hemoglobina	Hemoglobin	Hémoglobine	Emoglobina	Hemoglobin
Hígado	Liver	Foie	Fegato	Jetra
Himen	Hymen	Hymen	Imene	Djevičnjak (himen)
Hipófisis (glándula pituitaria)	Hypophysis (pituitary gland)	Hypophyse (glande pituitaire)	Ipòfisi (ghiandola pituitaria)	Hipofiza
Hipotálamo	Hypothalamus	Hypothalamus	Ipotalamo	Hipotalamus
Hombro	Shoulder	Épaule	Spalla	Rame
Hormona	Hormone	Hormone	Ormone	Hormon
Hormona adrenocorticotropa (corticotropina, corticotrofina)	Corticotropin (adrenocorticotropic hormone)	Hormone corticotrope (adrenocorticotropic hormone, ACTH)	Corticotropina (ormone adrenocorticotropo)	Kortikotropin
Hormona anidiurética (arginina vasopresina)	Antidiuretic hormone (vasopressin)	Hormone antidiurétique (vasopressine)	Ormone antidiuretico (vasopressina)	Antidiuretski hormon (vazopresin)
Hormona de crecimiento somatotropa	Growth hormone (somatotrophin)	Hormone de croissance (somatotropine)	Somatotropina	Hormon rasta (somatotropin)
Hormona luteinizante (lutropina)	Luteinising hormone	Hormne lutéinisante	Ormone luteinizzante	Luteinizirajući hormon

Español	Inglés	Francés	Italiano	Croata
Hueso	Bone	Os	Osso	Kost
Hueso cigomático (malar)	Zygoma (cheekbone, malar bone)	Os zygomatique (zygoma)	Osso zigomatico	Sponična kost
Hueso coxal	Hip bone	Os coxal	Osso dell'anca	Kost kuka
Hueso del carpo	Wrist bone (carpal bone)	Os du carpe	Osso carpale	Kost zapešča (karpalna kost)
Hueso del metacarpo	Metacarpal bone	Os métacarpe	Osso metacarpale	Kost pesti (metakarpalna kost)
Hueso del metatarso	Metatarsal bone	Os du métatarse	Osso metatarsale	Kost donožja (metatarzalna kost)
Hueso del tarso	Tarsal bone	Os du tarse	Osso tarsale	Kost zastoplja (kost tarzusa)
Hueso esfenoides	Sphenoid bone	Os sphénoïde	Osso sfenoide	Klinasta kost (leptirasta kost)
Hueso etmoides	Ethmoid bone	Os ethmoïde	Osso etmoide	Sitasta kost (etmoidna kost)
Hueso frontal	Frontal bone	Os frontal	Osso frontale	Čeona kost
Hueso hioides	Hyoid bone (lingual bone)	Os hyoïde (os lingual)	Osso ioide	Podjezična kost
Hueso maxilar superior (maxila)	Upper jaw (maxilla)	Os maxillaire	Osso mascellare	Gornja čeljust (maksila)
Hueso occipital	Occipital bone	Os occipital	Osso occipitale	Zatiljna kost
Hueso palatino	Palatine bone	Os palatin	Osso palatino	Nepčana kost
Hueso parietal	Parietal bone	Os pariétal	Osso parietale	Tjemena kost
Hueso proprio de la nariz (hueso nasal)	Nasal bone	Os nasal	Osso nasale	Nosna kost
Hueso sesamoide	Sesamoid bone	Os sésamoïde	Osso sesamoide	Sezamska kost
Hueso temporal	Temporal bone	Os temporal	Osso temporale	Sljepoočna kost
Húmero	Upper arm bone (humerus)	Humérus	Omero	Nadlaktična kost (humerus)
Íleon	Ileum	Iléon (ileum)	Ileo	Ileum
Ilion	Ilium	Ilion (ilium)	Osso iliaco	Crijevna kost
Incisivo	Incisor	Incisive	Incisivo	Sjekutić (inciziv)
Ingle	Groin	Aine	Inguine	Prepona
Inmunoglobulina	Immunoglobulin	Immunoglobuline	Immunoglobulina	Imunoglobulin
Insulina	Insulin	Insuline	Insulina	Inzulin
Intestin	Intestine	Intestin	Intestino	Crijevo
Intestino delgado	Small intestine	Intestin grêle	Intestino tenue (piccolo intestino)	Tanko crijevo
Intestino grueso (colon)	Large intestine (colon)	Gros intestin (côlon)	Intestino crasso (colon)	Debelo crijevo
Iris	Iris	Iris	Iride	Šarenica
Isquión	Ischium	Ischium	Ischio	Sjedna kost
Jugo gástrico	Gastric juice	Suc gastrique	Succo gastrico	Želučani sok
Jugo intestinal	Intestinal juice	Suc intestinal	Succo intestinale	Crijevni sok
Jugo pancreático	Pancreatic juice	Suc pancréatique	Succo pancreatico	Sok gušterače
Labio	Lip	Lèvre	Labbro	Usna
Lágrima	Tear	Larme	Lacrima	Suza
Laringe	Larynx	Larynx	Laringe	Grkljan
Lengua	Tongue	Langue	Lingua	Jezik
Leucocito	Leukocyte	Leucocyte	Leucocita	Leukocit
Ligamento	Ligament	Ligament	Legamento	Ligament
Linfa	Lymph	Lymphe	Linfa	Limfa
Linfocito	Lymphocyte	Lymphocyte	Linfocita	Limfocit
Líquido cefalorraquídeo (líquido cerebrospinal)	Cerebrospinal fluid	Liquide cérébro-spinal	Liquido cefalorachidiano (liquor, liquido cerebrospinale)	Moždana tekućina (likvor)
Líquido intersticial (líquido tisular)	Interstitial fluid	Liquide interstitiel	Liquido extracellulare	Međustanična tekućina
Líquido sinovial	Synovial fluid (synovia)	Liquide synovial	Liquido sinoviale (sinovia)	Zglobna tekućina (sinovijalna tekućina)
Mama	Breast	Sein	Mammella	Dojka
Mandíbula	Lower jaw (mandible)	Mandibule	Mandibola	Donja čeljust (mandibula)
Mano	Hand	Main	Mano	Šaka
Martillo (malleus)	Hammer (malleus)	Marteau (malléus)	Martello	Čekić (malleus)
Matriz (útero, seno materno)	Womb (uterus)	Utérus	Utero	Maternica (uterus)
Médula cerebral	Brain marrow	Moelle du cerveau	Midollo cerebrale	Moždana srž
Médula espinal	Spinal cord	Moelle épinière (moelle spinale)	Midollo spinale	Kralježnična moždina
Médula ósea	Bone marrow	Moelle osseuse	Midollo osseo	Koštana srž
Mejilla (carrillo)	Cheek	Joue	Guancia	Obraz
Melanina	Melanin	Mélanine	Melanina	Melanin
Melanotropina	Melanotropin	Hormone mélanotrope (mélanocortine, mélanotropine)	Ormone melanotropo	Melanotropin
Melatonina	Melatonin	Mélatonine (hormone du sommeil)	Melatonina	Melatonin
Membrana sinovial	Synovial membrane	Membrane synoviale	Membrana sinoviale	Sinovijalna opna
Meninge	Meninx	Méninge	Meninge	Moždana ovojnica
Menisco	Meniscus	Ménisque	Menisco	Zglobni menisk
Metacarpo	Metacarpus	Métacarpe	Metacarpo	Pest (metakarpus)

Español	Inglés	Francés	Italiano	Croata
Metatarso	Metatarsus	Métatarse	Metatarso	Donožje (metatarzus)
Miembro inferior	Leg	Membre inférieur	Arto inferiore	Noga
Mineralo corticoide	Mineralcorticoid	Minéralcorticoïde	Mineralcorticoide	Mineralkortikoid (Na-hormon)
Miocardio	Cardiac muscle (myocardium)	Myocarde	Miocardio	Srčani mišić (miokard)
Moco	Mucus	Mucus	Muco	Sluz
Molar	Molar	Molaire	Molare	Kutnjak (molar)
Monocito	Monocyte	Monocyte	Monocita	Monocit
Mucosa	Mucous membrane	Muqueuse	Membrana mucosa	Sluznica
Mucosa estomacal	Gastric mucous membrane	Muqueuse gastrique	Mucosa gastrica	Želučana sluznica
Muñeca	Wrist	Poignet	Polso	Ručni zglob
Músculo	Muscle	Muscle	Muscolo	Mišić
Músculo aductor	Adductor muscle	Muscle adducteur	Muscolo adduttore	Mišić primicač
Músculo bíceps braquial	Biceps brachii muscle	Muscle biceps brachial	Muscolo bicipite brachiale	Dvoglavi mišić nadlaktice
Músculo bíceps crural	Biceps femoris muscle	Muscle biceps fémoral	Bicipite femorale	Dvoglavi bedreni mišić
Músculo ciliar	Ciliary muscle	Muscle ciliaire	Muscolo ciliare	Cilijarni mišić
Músculo cuádriceps crural	Quadriceps femoris muscle	Muscle quadriceps fémoral	Muscolo quadricipite femorale	Četveroglavi bedreni mišić
Músculo deltoides	Deltoid muscle	Muscle deltoïde	Muscolo deltoide	Rameni mišić (deltoideus)
Músculo estriado	Striated muscle	Muscle strié	Muscolo striato	Poprečno-prugasti mišić
Músculo glúteo	Gluteal muscle	Muscle glutéal	Muscolo gluteo	Sjedni mišić
Músculo intercostal	Intercostal muscle	Muscle intercostal	Muscolo intercostale	Međurebreni mišić
Múscolo liso	Smooth muscle	Muscle lisse	Tessuto muscolare liscio	Glatki mišić
Músculo masetero	Masseter muscle	Muscle masséter	Muscolo massetere	Žvakaći mišić
Músculo oblicuo del abdomen	Abdominal oblique muscle	Muscle oblique de l'abdomen	Musculo obliquo dell'addome	Kosi trbušni mišić
Músculo pectoral mayor	Pectoralis major muscle	Muscle grand pectoral	Muscolo grande pettorale	Veliki prsni mišić
Músculo pectoral menor	Pectoralis minor muscle	Muscle petit pectoral	Muscolo piccolo pettorale	Mali prsni mišić
Músculo recto mayor del abdomen	Rectus abdominis muscle	Muscle droit de l'abdomen	Muscolo retto dell'addome	Ravni trbušni mišić
Músculo romboides	Rhomboid muscle	Muscle rhomboïde	Muscolo romboide	Romboidni mišić
Músculo sartorio	Tailor's muscle (sartorius muscle)	Muscle couturier (muscle sartorius)	Muscolo sartorio	Krojački mišić
Músculo semimembranoso	Semimembranosus muscle	Muscle semi-membraneux	Muscolo semimembranoso	Poluopnasti mišić
Músculo semitendinoso	Semitendinosus muscle	Muscle semi-tendineux	Muscolo semitendinoso	Polutetivni mišić
Músculo trapecio	Trapezius muscle	Muscle trapèze	Muscolo trapezio	Trapezni mišić
Músculo tríceps braquial	Triceps brachii muscle	Muscle triceps brachial	Muscolo tricipite del braccio	Troglavi mišić nadlaktice
Músculo tríceps sural	Triceps surae muscle	Muscle triceps sural	Muscolo tricipite della sura	Troglavi mišić potkoljenice
Muslo (región femoral)	Thigh	Cuisse	Coscia	Natkoljenica (bedro)
Narina	Nostril	Narine	Narice	Nosnica
Nariz	Nose	Nez	Naso	Nos
Nervio	Nerve	Nerf	Nervo	Živac
Nervio auditivo (nervio vestibulococlear, nervio estatoacústico)	Acoustic nerve (vestibulocochlear nerve)	Nerf vestibulocochléaire (nerf auditif)	Nervo vestibolococleare (nervo stato-acustico)	Slušni živac
Nervio craneal	Cranial nerve	Nerf crânien	Nervo cranico	Moždani živac
Nervio espinal	Spinal nerve	Nerf spinal	Nervo spinale	Spinalni živac
Nervio óptico	Optic nerve	Nerf optique	Nervo ottico	Vidni živac
Nódulo auriculoventricular	Atrioventricular node	Noeud atrio-ventriculaire	Nodo atrioventricolare	Atrioventrikularni čvor
Noradrenalina	Noradrenaline	Noradrénaline	Noradrenalina	Noradrenalin
Nuca	Nape (occiput)	Nuque	Nuca	Zatiljak
Nuez de Adán	Adam's apple	Pomme d'Adam	Pomo d'Adamo	Adamova jabučica
Óido	Ear	Oreille	Orecchio	Uho
Óido medio	Middle ear	Oreille moyenne	Orecchio medio	Srednje uho
Ojo	Eye	Oeil	Occhio	Oko
Ombligo (pupo)	Navel (belly button)	Ombilic (nombril)	Ombelico	Pupak
Omóplato (escápula)	Shoulder blade (scapula)	Omoplate (scapula)	Scapola (omoplata)	Lopatica (skapula)
Órbita	Eye orbit	Orbite de l'oeil	Orbita oculare	Očna šupljina
Órgano	Organ	Organe	Organo	Organ
Orina	Urine	Urine	Urina	Mokraća (urin)
Ovario	Ovary	Ovaire	Ovaia	Jajnik
Óvulo	Ovum	Ovule	Uovo	Jajašce
Oxitocina	Oxytocin	Ocytocine (oxytocine)	Ossitocina	Oksitocin
Pabellón auricular (aurícula)	Pinna (auricle)	Pavillon auriculaire	Padiglione auricolare	Ušna školjka
Paladar	Palate	Palaise	Palato	Nepce
Paladar óseo	Hard palate	Palais osseux	Palato duro (volta palatina)	Tvrdo nepce
Palma	Palm	Paume	Palmo	Dlan
Páncreas	Pancreas	Pancréas	Pancreas	Gušterača
Pantorrilla	Calf	Mollet	Polpaccio	List
Papila gustativa	Taste bud	Papille gustative	Papilla gustativa	Okusni pupoljak
Parathormona (hormona paratiroidea, paratirina)	Parathyroid hormone	Parathormone (hormone parathyroïdienne)	Paratormone (ormone paratiroideo)	Paratireoidni hormon
Pared abdominal	Abdominal wall	Face de la cavité abdominale	Parete addominale	Trbušna stijenka

Español	Inglés	Francés	Italiano	Croata
Párpado	Eyelid	Paupière	Palpebra	Kapak
Parte superior del brazo	Upper arm	Partie supérieure du bras	Barccio	Nadlaktica
Pecho	Chest	Torse	Torace	Grudište (prsa)
Pelo	Hair	Poil	Pelo	Dlaka
Pelvis	Innominate bone (pelvis)	Bassin osseux	Bacino	Zdjelica
Pene (falo)	Penis	Pénis	Pene	Penis
Pericardio	Pericardium	Péricarde	Pericardio	Osrčje (perikard)
Periné (perineo)	Perineum	Périnée	Perineo	Međica (perineum)
Peritoneo	Peritoneum	Péritoine	Peritoneo	Potrbušnica (peritoneum)
Peroné (fíbula)	Fibula (calf bone)	Fibula (péroné)	Perone (fibula)	Lisna kost (fibula)
Pestaña	Eyelash	Cil	Ciglia	Trepavica
Pezón	Nipple	Mamelon (papille)	Capezzolo	Bradavica
Pia madre	Pia mater	Pie-mère	Pia madre	Meka moždana ovojnica
Pie	Foot	Pied	Piede	Stopalo
Piel	Skin	Peau	Pelle (cute)	Koža
Pierna	Lower leg	Jambe	Gamba	Potkoljenica
Planta del pie	Sole	Plante	Pianta del piede	Taban
Plaqueta (trombocito)	Thrombocyte	Thrombocyte	Trombocita (piastrina)	Trombocit
Plasma sanguíneo	Plasma	Plasma sanguin	Plasma	Plazma
Pleura	Pleura	Plèvre	Pleura (pleure)	Pleura
Pleura parietal	Parietal pleura	Plèvre pariétale	Pleura parietale	Porebrica (parijetalna pleura)
Pleura visceral	Visceral pleura	Plèvre viscérale	Pleura viscerale	Poplućnica (visceralna pleura)
Poro	Pore	Pore	Poro	Pora
Premolar	Premolar	Prémolaire	Premolare	Pretkutnjak (premolar)
Prepucio	Foreskin (prepuce)	Prépuce	Prepuzio	Prepucij
Progesterona	Progesterone	Progestérone	Progesterone	Progesteron
Próstata	Prostate	Prostate	Prostata	Prostata
Proteína	Protein	Protéine	Proteina	Bjelančevina (protein)
Pubis	Pubis (pubic bone)	Os pubien	Pube (osso pubico)	Stidna kost
Pulmón	Lung	Poumon	Polmone	Plućno krilo
Pulmones	Lungs	Poumons	Polmoni	Pluća
Pulpa dentaria	Dental pulp	Pulpe dentaire	Polpa dentaria	Središte zuba (pulpa)
Pupila	Pupil	Pupille	Pupilla	Zjenica
Queratina	Keratin	Kératine	Cheratina	Keratin
Quijada	Jaw	Mâchoire	Scheletro della bocca	Čeljust
Radio	Radius	Radius	Radio	Palčana kost
Raíz del diente	Root of a tooth	Racine dentaire	Radice del dente	Korijen zuba
Retina	Retina	Rétine	Rètina	Mrežnica (retina)
Riñón	Kidney	Rein	Rene	Bubreg
Rodilla	Knee	Genou	Ginocchio	Koljeno
Rótula (patela)	Kneecap (patella)	Rotule (patella)	Rotula (patella)	Iver (patela)
Saliva	Saliva (spit, slobber)	Salive	Saliva	Slina (pljuvačka)
Sangre	Blood	Sang	Sangue	Krv
Sebo cutáneo	Sebum	Sébum	Sebo	Loj
Semen (esperma)	Semen	Sperme	Sperma	Sperma
Seno	Sinus	Sinus	Seno	Sinus
Sien	Temple	Tempe	Tempia	Sljepoočnica
Sinapsis	Synapse	Synapse	Sinapsi (bottone sinaptico)	Sinapsa
Sistema nervioso parasimpático	Parasympathetic nervous system	Système nerveux parasympatique (système vagal)	Sistema nervoso parasimpatico	Parasimpatikus
Sistema nervioso simpático	Sympathetic nervous system	Système nerveux orthosympathique (système nerveux sympathique)	Sistema nervoso simpatico	Simpatikus
Sobaco (axila)	Armpit (axilla, underarm)	Aisselle	Ascella	Pazuh (aksila)
Sudor	Sweat	Sueur	Sudore	Znoj
Tálamo	Thalamus	Thalamus	Talamo	Talamus
Talón (calcañar)	Heel	Talon	Tallone	Peta
Tarso	Tarsus	Tarse	Tarso	Zastoplje
Tejido	Tissue	Tissu	Tessuto	Tkivo
Tejido graso (tejido adiposo)	Fat tissue	Tissu adipeux (masse grasse)	Tessuto adiposo	Masno tkivo
Telencéfalo	Cerebrum (telencephalon)	Télencéphale (cerveau)	Telencefalo (cervello)	Veliki mozak (telencefalon)
Tendón	Tendon (sinew)	Tendon	Tendine	Tetiva
Testículo	Testicle	Testicule	Testicolo	Jaje (mudo, testis)
Testosterona	Testosterone	Testostérone	Testosterone	Testosteron
Tibia	Shinbone (tibia)	Tibia	Tibia	Goljenica (tibija)
Timo	Thymus	Thymus	Timo	Grudna žlijezda (timus)
Tímpano	Eardrum (tympanic membrane)	Tympan	Timpano (membrana timpanica)	Bubnjić
Tiroides	Thyroid	Thyroïde	Tiroide	Štitnjača
Tirotropina (TSH, hormona estimulante de la tiroides)	Thyroid-stimulating hormone (TSH, thyrotropin)	Thyréostimuline (thyréotropine)	Tirotropina (ormone tireostimolante)	Tireotropin (TSH)
Tiroxina (tetrayodotironina, T4)	Thyroxine	Thyroxine	Tiroxina	Tiroksin

Español	Inglés	Francés	Italiano	Croata
Tobillo	Ankle joint	Cheville (cou-de pied)	Caviglia	Skočni zglob (gležanj)
Tráquea	Windpipe (trachea)	Trachée	Trachea	Dušnik
Triglicérido	Triglyceride	Triglycéride	Trigliceride	Triglicerid
Triiodotironina	Triiodothyronine	Triiodothyronine	Triiodotironina	Trijodtironin
Trompa de Falopio (tuba uterina, oviducto)	Fallopian tube (oviduct)	Trompe de Fallope	Tuba di Falloppio	Jajovod
Tronco	Trunk (torso)	Tronc	Tronco	Trup (torzo)
Tronco del encéfalo	Brain stem	Tronc cérébral	Tronco encefalico	Moždano stablo
Uña	Nail	Ongle	Unghia	Nokat
Unguis (hueso lacrimal)	Lachrymal bone	Os lacrymal (unguis)	Osso lacrimale	Suzna kost
Urea	Urea	Urée (carbamide)	Urea	Mokraćevina (urea, ureja)
Uréter	Ureter	Uretère	Uretere	Mokraćovod (ureter)
Uretra	Urethra	Urètre	Uretra	Vanjska mokraćna cijev (uretra)
Úvula	Soft palate	Voile du palais	Palato molle	Meko nepce
Vagina (colpos)	Vagina	Vagin	Vagina	Rodnica (vagina)
Válvula	Valve (valvula)	Valve	Valvola	Zalistak
Válvula bicúspide (válvula mitral)	Mitral valve (bicuspid valve)	Valve mitrale (valve bicuspide)	Valvola mitrale (valvola bicuspide)	Mitralni zalistak (bikuspidalni zalistak)
Válvula cardiaca (válvula de corazón)	Heart valve (cardiac valve)	Valve cardiaque	Valvola cardiaca	Srčani zalistak
Válvula sigmoidea aórtica	Aortic valve	Valve aortique	Valvola semilunare aortica	Polumjesečasti aortni zalistak
Válvula tricúspide	Tricuspid valve	Valve tricuspide	Valvola tricuspide	Trolisni zalistak
Vaso linfático	Lymph vessel	Vaisseau lymphatique	Vaso linfatico	Limfna žila
Vaso sanguíneo	Blood vessel	Vaisseau sanguin	Vaso sanguigno	Krvna žila
Vejiga urinaria	Urinary bladder	Vessie	Vescica urinaria	Mokraćni mjehur
Vellosidad intestinal	Intestinal villus	Villosité intestinale	Villo intestinale	Crijevna resica
Vena	Vein	Veine	Vena	Vena
Vena cava inferior	Inferior vena cava	Veine cave inférieure	Vena cava inferiore	Donja šuplja vena
Vena cava superior	Superior vena cava	Veine cave supérieure	Vena cava superiore	Gornja šuplja vena
Vena porta	Portal vein	Veine porte	Vena porta	Portalna vena
Ventrículo	Ventricle	Ventricule	Ventricolo	Klijetka
Ventrículo cardíaco	Cardiac ventricle	Ventricule cardiaque	Ventricolo cardiaco	Srčana klijetka
Ventrículo cerebral	Brain ventricle	Ventricule cérébral	Ventricolo cerebrale	Moždana klijetka
Vénula	Venule	Veinule (vénule)	Venula	Venula
Vértebra	Vertebra	Vertèbre	Vertebra	Kralježak
Vértebra coccígea	Coccygeal vertebra	Vertèbre coccygienne	Vertebra coccigea	Trtični kralježak
Vértebra lumbar	Lumbar vertebra	Vertèbre lombale	Vertebra lombare	Slabinski kralježak (lumbalni kralježak)
Vértebra sacra	Sacral vertebra	Vertèbre sacrale	Vertebra sacrale	Krstačni kralježak (sakralni kralježak)
Vértebra torácica	Thoracic vertebra	Vertèbre thoracique	Vertebra toracica	Leđni kralježak (grudni ili torakalni kralježak)
Vértice craneal	Vertex (crown of head)	Vertex	Vertice della testa	Tjeme
Vesícula biliar	Gall bladder	Vésicule biliare (cholécyste)	Cistifellea	Žućni mjehur
Vesícula seminal	Seminal vesicle	Vésicule séminale (glande vésiculeuse)	Vescicola seminale	Sjemena vrećica
Vestíbulo	Vestibule	Vestibule	Vestibolo	Predvorje (vestibulum)
Vía biliar	Bile duct	Voie biliaire	Coledoco	Žučovod
Vómer	Vomer	Vomer	Vomere	Raonik (vomer)
Vulva	Vulva	Vulve	Vulva	Stidnica
Yeyuno	Jejunum	Jéjunum	Digiuno	Jejunum
Yunque	Anvil (incus)	Enclume	Incudine	Nakovanj
SÍNTOMAS, HERIDAS Y ENFERMEDADES:	SYMPTOMS, INJURIES AND DISEASES:	LES SYMPTÔMES, BLESSURES ET MALADIES:	I SINTOMI, FERITE E MALATTIE:	SIMPTOMI, OZLJEDE I BOLESTI:
Abdomen agudo	Acute abdomen	Abdomen aigu	Addome acuto	Akutni abdomen
Abrasión (escoriación)	Abrasion	Écorchure	Abrasione (escoriazione)	Ojedina (abrazija)
Absceso	Abscess	Abcès	Ascesso	Apsces
Absceso anal	Anal abscess	Abcès anale	Ascesso anale	Analni apsces
Absceso cerebral	Brain abscess	Abcès cérébral	Ascesso cerebrale	Apsces mozga
Absceso de Brodie	Brodie abscess	Abcès de Brodie	Ascesso di Brodie	Brodijev apsces
Absceso hepático	Liver abscess	Abcès hépatique	Ascesso epatico	Apsces jetre
Absceso perianal	Perianal abscess	Abcès périanal	Ascesso perianale	Perianalni apsces
Absceso perinéfrico	Perinephric abscess	Abcès périnéphrique	Ascesso perinefrico	Paranefritički apsces
Absceso peritonsilar	Quinsy (peritonsillar abscess)	Abcès périamygdalien	Ascesso peritonsillare	Gnojna upala krajnika
Absceso pulmonar	Lung abscess	Abcès pulmonaire	Ascesso polmonare	Apsces pluća
Abulia	Aboulia (disorder of diminished motivation)	Aboulie	Abulia	Abulija (poremećaj umanjene motivacije)
Acariasis	Acariasis	Acariase	Acariasi	Akarijaza
Acidosis	Acidosis	Acidose	Acidosi	Acidoza
Acidosis metabólica	Metabolic acidosis	Acidose métabolique	Acidosi metabolica	Metabolička acidoza
Acidosis tubular renal	Renal tubular acidosis	Acidose tubulaire rénale	Acidosi renale tubulare	Renalna tubularna acidoza
Aclorhidria	Achlorhydria	Achlorhydrie	Acloridria	Aklorhidrija
Acné	Acne	Acné	Acne	Akne

Español	Inglés	Francés	Italiano	Croata
Acné común (acne vulgaris)	Acne vulgaris	Acné papulo-pustuleuse	Acne volgare (acne)	Vulgarne akne
Acondroplasia	Achondroplasia	Achondroplasie	Acondroplasia	Ahondroplazija
Acrocianosis	Acrocyanosis	Acrocyanose	Acrocianosi	Akrocijanoza
Acrofobia (miedo a las alturas)	Acrophobia (fear of heights)	Acrophobie (peur des hauteurs)	Acrofobia (paura dei luoghi elevati)	Akrofobija (strah od visine)
Acromegalia	Acromegaly	Acromégalie	Acromegalia	Akromegalija
Acropaquia (hipocratismo digital)	Finger clubbing (digital clubbing)	Hippocratisme digital (doigts en baguettes de tambour)	Dita ippocratiche (dita a bacchetta di tamburo)	Batićasti prsti
Actinomicosis	Actinomycosis	Actinomycose	Actinomicosi	Aktinomikoza
Acuafobia	Aquaphobia	Aquaphobie	Idrofobia	Hidrofobija
Adenocarcinoma	Adenocarcinoma	Adénocarcinome	Adenocarcinoma	Adenokarcinom
Adenoma	Adenoma	Adénome	Adenoma	Adenom
Adenoma hepático (adenoma hepatocelular)	Hepatocellular adenoma	Adénome hépatocellulaire	Adenoma epatocellulare	Hepatocelularni adenom
Adenoma tubular	Tubular adenoma	Adénome tubulaire	Adenoma tubulare	Tubularni adenom
Adenopatía	Adenopathy	Adénopathie	Adenopatia	Adenopatija
Adenosis esclerosante	Sclerosing adenosis	Adénose sclérosante	Adenosi sclerosante	Sklerozirajuća adenoza
Adicción (dependencia)	Addiction	Dépendance (addiction)	Dipendenza	Ovisnost
Adicción a jugar (ludopatía, ludomanía)	Gambling addiction (ludomania)	Jeu pathologique (jeu compulsif)	Giocco d'azzardo patologico	Ovisnost o kockanju (ludopatija)
Adicción a las drogas (drogodependencia)	Drug addiction	Toxicomanie	Tossicodipendenza (tossicomania)	Ovisnost o drogama
Adicción sexual	Sexual addiction	Sexualité compulsive	Dipendenza sessuale	Ovisnost o seksu
Adormecimiento de las extremidades	Numbness in limbs	Engourdissements dans les membres (paresthésie)	Parestesie delle estremità	Utrnulost udova
Aerofobia (miedo a volar)	Aviophobia (fear of flying)	Aerophobie (peur de l'avion)	Aviofobia (paura di volare)	Aerofobija (strah od letenja)
Afta (úlcera en la mucosa oral)	Aphtha (mouth ulcer)	Aphte (ulcère de la muqueuse buccale)	Afta (ulcera all'interno della cavità orale)	Afte (ulceracija sluznice usta)
Agarrotamiento	Stiffness	Raideur	Rigidità	Ukočenost
Agenesia (ausencia de un órgano)	Agenesis (absence of an organ)	Agénésie	Agenesia (mancanza di un organo)	Agenezija (nedostatak jednog organa)
Agenesia renal	Renal agenesis	Agénésie rénale	Agenesia renale	Agenezija bubrega
Agranulocitosis	Agranulocytosis	Agranulocytose	Agranulocitosi	Agranulocitoza
Ahogamiento	Drowning	Noyade	Affogamento	Utapanje
Albinismo	Albinism	Albinisme	Albinismo	Albinizam
Albuminuria	Albuminuria	Albuminurie	Albuminuria	Albuminurija
Alcalosis	Alkalosis	Alcalose	Alcalosi	Alkaloza
Alcalosis respiratoria	Respiratory alkalosis	Alcalose respiratoire	Alcalosi respiratoria	Respiratorna alkaloza
Alcoholismo	Alcoholism	Alcoolisme	Alcolismo	Alkoholizam
Aldosteronismo (hiperaldosteronismo)	Aldosteronism (hyperaldosteronism)	Hyperaldostéronisme	Iperaldosteronismo	Aldosteronizam
Alergia	Allergy	Allergie	Allergia	Alergija
Alergia a alimentos	Food allergy	Allergie alimentaire	Allergia alimentare	Alergija na hranu
Alergia a las plumas	Feather allergy	Allergie aux plumes	Allergia alle piume	Alergija na perje
Alergia al medicamento	Drug allergy	Allergie aux médicaments	Allergia a farmaci	Alergija na lijekove
Alergia al pelo de los animales	Fur allergy	Allergie aux animaux à poils	Allergia a pello di animali	Alergija na životinjsku dlaku
Alergia al polen	Pollen allergy	Allergie au pollen	Allergia da poline	Alergija na pelud
Alergia al polvo	Dust allergy	Allergie à la poussière	Allergia a polvere	Alergija na prašinu
Algodistrofia	Algodystrophy	Algodystrophie	Algodistrofia	Algodistrofija
Alopecia	Alopecia	Alopécie	Alopecia	Ćelavost
Alopecia areata	Alopecia areata	Alopécie areata	Alopecia areata	Alopecia areata
Alopecia areata universal	Alopecia universalis	Alopécie universalis	Alopecia universale	Opća alopecija
Alucinación	Hallucination	Hallucination	Allucinazione	Halucinacija
Amiloidosis	Amyloidosis	Amylose (amyloïdose, maladie orpheline)	Amiloidosi	Amiloidoza
Amnesia	Amnesia	Amnésie	Amnesia	Amnezija
Ampolla	Blister	Phlyctène (ampoule, cloque)	Vescichetta (bolla)	Plik
Ampolla (callo)	Blister (corn)	Cor (cal)	Callo (vescica, bolla)	Žulj (plik, kurje oko)
Amputación	Amputation	Amputation	Amputazione	Amputacija
Analgesia	Analgesia (loss of pain sensation)	Analgésie	Analgesia	Analgezija (neosjetljivost na bol)
Anasarca	Generalized edema (anasarca)	Oedème généralisé (anasarque)	Edema diffuso (anasarca)	Generalizirani edem (anasarka)
Anemia	Anemia	Anémie	Anemia	Slabokrvnost (anemija)
Anemia aplásica	Aplastic anemia	Anémie aplasique	Anemia aplastica	Aplastična anemija
Anemia de enfermedades crónicas	Anemia of chronic disease	Anémie des maladies chroniques	Anemia da malattia cronica	Anemija kronične bolesti
Anemia falciforme (anemia drepanocítica)	Sickle-cell disease (sickle-cell anemia)	Drépanocytose (anémie à cellules falciformes)	Anemia drepanocitica	Anemija srpastih stanica
Anemia ferropénica	Iron deficiency anemia (sideropenic anemia)	Anémie ferriprive	Anemia da carenza di ferro	Anemija radi deficita željeza (sideropenična anemija)

Español	Inglés	Francés	Italiano	Croata
Anemia hemolítica	Hemolytic anemia	Anémie hémolytique	Anemia emolitica	Hemolitična anemija
Anemia hipocrómica	Hypochromic anemia	Anémie hypochrome	Anemia ipocromica	Hipokromna anemija
Anemia megaloblástica	Megaloblastic anemia	Anémie mégaloblastique	Anemia megaloblastica	Megaloblastična anemija (anemija radi deficita vitamina)
Anemia perniciosa	Pernicious anemia	Anémie pernicieuse	Anemia perniciosa	Perniciozna anemija
Anencefalia	Anencephaly	Anencéphalie	Anencefalia	Anencefalija
Aneurisma	Aneurysm (aneurism)	Anévrisme (anévrysme)	Aneurisma	Aneurizma
Aneurisma cerebral	Cerebral aneurysm	Anévrisme intra-crânien	Aneurisma cerebrale	Cerebralna aneurizma
Aneurisma cerebral arterial sacular	Ball-shaped aneurysm of the brain artery	Anévrisme intra-crânien en forme de sac	Aneurisma cerebrale sferica	Kuglasta aneurizma arterije mozga
Aneurisma congénito arterial de la base del cerebro	Congenital aneurysm of arteries at the base of the brain	Anévrisme congénital de l'artère à la base du cerveau	Aneurisma arteriosa congenita alla base dell'encefalo	Urođena aneurizma arterija baze mozga
Aneurisma de aorta	Aortic aneurysm	Anévrisme de l'aorte	Aneurisma aortico	Aneurizma aorte
Aneurisma de aorta abdominal	Abdominal aortic aneurysm	Anévrisme de l'aorte abdominale	Aneurisma dell'aorta addominale	Aneurizma abdominalne aorte
Aneurisma de aorta torácica	Thoracic aortic aneurysm	Anévrisme aortique thoracique	Aneurisma dell'aorta toracica	Aneurizma torakalne aorte
Angina	Angina	Angine	Angina	Angina
Angina de pecho (angor, angor pectoris)	Angina pectoris	Angine de poitrine (angor)	Angina pectoris	Angina pektoris
Angina de Prinzmetal	Prinzmetal's angina	Angine de Prinzmetal	Angina di Prinzmetal	Prinzmetalova angina
Angioedema (edema de Quincke)	Angioedema (angioneurotic edema)	Oedème de Quincke (angio-oedème)	Angioedema (edema di Quincke, edema angioneurotico)	Angioedem (Quinckeov edem, angioneurotski edem)
Angioma	Angioma	Angiome	Angioma	Angiom
Angioma en araña (angioma aracnoideo)	Spider angioma (spider nevus)	Angiome stellaire	Angioma a ragno	Paukoliki angiom (spider nevus)
Angiosarcoma	Angiosarcoma	Angiosarcome	Angiosarcoma	Angiosarkom
Anisakiasis (anisakidosis)	Anisakiasis	Anisakiase	Anisakidosi	Anisakijaza
Anomalías del desarrollo	Development anomalies	Anomalies de développement	Anomalie di sviluppo	Razvojne anomalije
Anorexia	Anorexia	Anorexie	Anoressia	Anoreksija
Anquilosis	Ankylosis (joint stiffness)	Ankylose	Anchilosi	Ankiloza (ukočenje zgloba)
Anquilostomiasis	Ancylostomiasis	Ankylostomose	Anchilostomiasi	Ankilostomijaza
Ansiedad	Anxiety	Anxiété	Ansia (ansietà)	Nemir (anksioznost)
Antracosis	Anthracosis	Anthracose	Antracosi	Antrakoza
Ántrax (carbunco)	Carbuncle	Anthrax	Carbonchio (pustola)	Karbunkul
Anuria (menos de 100 ml de orina en 24h)	Anuria (passage of urine < 100 ml in 24 hours)	Anurie (volume urinaire < 100 ml par 24 heures)	Anuria (produzione di urina < 100 ml nelle 24 ore)	Anurija (lučenje urina < 100 ml u 24 sata)
Apendicitis aguda	Acute appendicitis	Appendicite aiguë	Appendicite acuta	Akutna upala crvuljka
Apetito	Appetite	Appétit	Appetito	Apetit
Aplasia	Aplasia	Aplasie	Aplasia	Aplazija
Apnea del sueño	Sleep apnea	Apnée du sommeil	Sindrome delle apnee nel sonno	Noćna desaturacija
Apoplejía (golpe apoplético)	Apoplexy	Apoplexie (attaque d'apoplexie)	Apoplessia	Moždano krvarenje (apopleksija)
Arador de la sarna (escabiosis)	Scabies (the itch)	Gale (mal de Sainte-Marie)	Scabbia (rogna)	Svrab (skabijes)
Ardor al orinar	Urinary burning	Brûlures à la miction	Bruciore urinario	Pečenje za vrijeme mokrenja
Ardor de estómago (acidez, pirosis)	Heartburn	Brûlure de l'estomac (pyrosis)	Bruciore di stomaco (pirosi)	Žgaravica
Arrítmia	Arrhythmia	Arythmie	Aritmia	Aritmija
Arrítmia cardíaca	Cardiac arrhythmia	Arythmie cardiaque	Aritmia cardiaca	Srčana aritmija
Arruga	Wrinkle	Ride	Ruga	Bora
Arteriosclerosis	Arteriosclerosis	Artérosclérose	Arteriosclerosi	Arterioskleroza
Arteritis de células gigantes (arteritis de la temporal)	Giant cell arteritis (temporal arteritis)	Artérite gigantocellu-laire (maladie de Hor-ton, artérite temporale)	Arterite temporale (arterite di Horton)	Arteritis divovskih stanica (temporalni arteritis)
Artritis infecciosa (artritis séptica)	Infectious arthritis (septic arthritis)	Arthrite septique	Artrite settica	Infekcijski artritis (septički artritis)
Artritis juvenil	Juvenile rheumatoid arthritis	Arthrite chronique juvénile	Artrite idiopatica giovanile	Mladenački reumatoidni artritis (juvenilni reumatoidni artritis)
Artritis psoriásica	Psoriatic arthritis	Arthrite psoriatique	Artrite psoriasica	Psorijatični artritis
Artritis reumatoide	Rheumatoid arthritis	Arthrite rhumatoïde	Artrite reumatoide	Reumatoidni artritis
Artritis tuberculosa	Tuberculous arthritis	Arthrite tuberculeuse	Artrite tubercolare	Tuberkulozni artritis
Artrogriposis	Arthrogryposis	Arthrogrypose	Artrogriposi	Artrogripoza
Artropatía	Arthropathy	Arthropathie	Artropatia	Artropatija
Artropatía hemofilíca	Hemophiliac arthropathy	Arthropathie hémophile	Artropatia emofilica	Hemofilična artropatija
Artrosis	Arthrosis (osteoarthritis, degenerative arthritis)	Arthrose (arthropathie chronique dégénérative)	Artrosi	Artroza (osteoartritis, degenerativni artritis)
Artrosis de cadera (coxartrosis)	Hip arthrosis	Arthrose de hanche (coxarthrose)	Artrosi di anca	Artroza kuka (koksartroza)
Artrosis de codo	Elbow arthrosis	Arthrose du coude	Artrosi di gomito	Artroza lakta

Español	Inglés	Francés	Italiano	Croata
Artrosis de mano	Hand arthrosis	Arthrose de le main	Artrosi della mano	Artroza šake
Artrosis de muñeca	Wrist arthrosis	Arthrose du poignet	Artrosi di polso	Artroza ručnog zgloba
Artrosis de rodilla (gonartrosis)	Knee arthrosis	Arthrose du genou (gonarthrose)	Artrosi di ginocchio	Artroza koljena (gonartroza)
Artrosis de tobillo	Ankle arthrosis	Arthrose de cheville	Artrosi di caviglia	Artroza skočnog zgloba
Artrosis del hombro	Shoulder arthrosis	Arthrose de l'épaule	Artrosi gleno-omerale	Artroza ramena
Artrosis del pie	Foot arthrosis	Arthrose du pied	Artrosi al piede	Artroza stopala
Asbestosis	Asbestosis	Asbestose (amiantose)	Asbestosi	Azbestoza
Ascaridiasis	Ascaridosis	Ascaridiose	Ascaridiasi	Askaridijaza
Ascitis	Ascites	Ascite	Ascite	Ascites
Asfixia	Asphyxia	Asphyxie	Asfissia	Asfiksija
Asimetría del tamaño de las pupilas (anisocoria)	Unequal size of pupils (anisocoria)	Différence de taille entres les pupilles (anisocorie)	Diseguaglianza del diametro delle pupille (anisocoria)	Nejednaka veličina zjenica (anizokorija)
Asma	Asthma	Asthme	Asma	Astma
Aspergiloma (micetoma)	Aspergilloma (mycetoma, fungus ball)	Aspergillome	Aspergilloma (micetoma)	Aspergilom
Aspergilosis	Aspergillosis	Aspergillose	Aspergillosi	Aspergiloza
Astigmatismo	Astigmatism	Astigmatisme	Astigmatismo	Astigmatizam
Astrocitoma	Astrocytoma	Astrocytome	Astrocitoma	Astrocitom
Ataque de pánico	Panic attack	Crise de panique	Attaco di panico	Napadaj panike
Ataxia de Friidreich (ataxia hereditaria)	Hereditary ataxia	Ataxie héréditaire	Atassia ereditaria	Heredoataksija
Atelectasia pulmonar	Pulmonary atelectasis	Atélectasie pulmonaire	Atelectasia polmonare	Atelektaza pluća
Ateroesclerosis	Atherosclerosis	Athérosclérose	Aterosclerosi	Ateroskleroza
Atetosis	Athetosis	Athétose	Atetosi	Atetoza
Atonía	Atony (atonia)	Atonie	Atonia muscolare	Atonija
Atragantamiento	Choking (suffocation)	Suffocation	Soffocamento (soffocazione, asfissia)	Gušenje
Atresia anal	Anal atresia	Atrésie anale	Atresia anale	Atrezija anusa
Atresia biliar	Bile duct atresia	Atrésie biliare	Atresia biliare	Atrezija žučnih vodova
Atresia duodenal	Duodenal atresia	Atrésie duodénale	Atresia duodenale	Atrezija dvanaesnika
Atresia esofágica	Esophageal atresia	Atrésie de l'oesophage	Atresia esofagea	Atrezija jednjaka
Atresia intestinal	Intestinal atresia	Atrésie intestinale	Atresia intestinale	Crijevna atrezija
Atrofia	Atrophy	Atrophie	Atrofia	Atrofija
Atrofia de Sudeck	Sudeck's atrophy	Atrophie de Sudeck	Atrofia di Sudeck	Sudeckova distrofija
Atrofia multisistémica	Multiple system atrophy	Atrophie multisystématisée	Atrofia multi-sistemica	Multipla sistemska atrofija
Aumento anormal de la necesidad de comer (polifagia)	Excessive hunger (polyphagia)	Faim excessive (polyphagie)	Aumento incontrollato dell'appetito (polifagia)	Neumjerena glad
Aumento anormal de la sed (polidipsia)	Increased thirst senasation (polydipsia)	Soif excessive (polydipsie)	Aumento del senso della sete (polidipsia)	Pojačan osjećaj žeđi (polidipsija)
Aumento de la cáida del cabello	Increased hair loss	Perte de cheveux excessive	Aumento di perdita di capelli	Pojačano opadanje kose
Aumento de la separación de los organos (hipertelorismo)	Increased distance between two organs or parts of the body (hypertelorism)	Élargissement de la distance des organes (hypertélorisme)	Aumento della distanza fra due parti del corpo (ipertelorismo)	Povećan razmak izmedu dva organa ili dijela tijela (hipertelorizam)
Aumento de volumen de los ganglios linfáticos (linfadenopatía)	Enlarged lymph nodes (lymphadenopathy)	Augmentation d'un ganglion lymphatique (lymphadénopathie)	Ingrossamento dei linfonodi (linfoadenopatia)	Povećanje limfnih čvorova (limfadenopatija)
Aumento del tamaño del hígado (hepatomegalia)	Enlarged liver (hepatomegaly)	Augmentation du foie (hépatomégalie)	Aumento di volume del fegato (epatomegalia)	Povećanje jetre (hepatomegalija)
Aumento en la temperatura corporal	Elevated body temperature	Élévation de la température du corps	Temperatura corporea elevata	Povišena tjelesna temperatura
Ausencia de la menstruación (amenorrea)	Absence of menstrual period (amenorrhea)	Absence des règles (aménorrhée)	Assenza di mestruazioni (amenorrea)	Izostanak mjesečnice (amenoreja)
Autismo	Autism	Autisme	Autismo	Autizam
Autolesión (automutilación)	Self-harm	Automutilation	Autolesionismo	Samoozljeđivanje
Aversión por la comida	Food aversion	Aversion pour la nourriture	Ripugnanza al cibo	Gađenje prema hrani
Avitaminosis	Avitaminosis	Avitaminose	Avitaminosi	Avitamonoza
Azúcar en orina (glucosuria)	Glucose in urine (glycosuria)	Sucre dans les urines (glycosurie)	Glicosuria (mellituria)	Šećer u urinu (glikozurija)
Bacteriemia (bacteremia)	Bacteremia	Bactériémie	Batteriemia	Bakterijemija
Bacteriuria	Bacteriuria	Bactériurie	Batteriuria	Bakteriurija
Bajo volumen de semen (oligospermia)	Low semen volume (oligospermia)	Présence de spermatozoïdes en quantité faible (oligospermie)	Produzione di pochi spermatozoi (oligospermia)	Manjak sperme (oligospermija)
Barotraumatismo (barotrauma)	Barotrauma	Barotraumatisme	Barotrauma	Barotrauma
Bartonelosis	Bartonellosis	Bartonellose	Bartonellosi	Bartoneloza
Basofilia	Basophilia	Basophilie	Basofilia	Bazofilija
Bisinosis (fiebre del lunes)	Byssinosis (Monday fever)	Byssinose	Bissinosi	Bisinoza
Blastoma	Blastoma	Blastome	Blastoma	Blastom
Blastomicosis	Blastomycosis	Blastomycose	Blastomicosi	Blastomikoza
Blefaritis	Blepharitis	Blépharite	Blefarite	Blefaritis
Bloqueo auriculoventricular	Atrioventricular block (AV block)	Bloc auriculo-ventriculaire	Blocco atrioventricolare	Atrijskoventrikularni blok

Español	Inglés	Francés	Italiano	Croata
Bloqueo de rama	Bundle branch block	Bloc de branche	Blocco di branca	Blok grane Hisovog snopića
Bloqueo trifascicular	Trifascicular block	Bloc trifasciculaire	Blocco trifascicolare	Trifascikularni blok
Bocio (coto)	Goiter	Goitre	Gozzo	Guša (struma)
Bocio nodular	Nodular goiter	Goitre multinodulaire	Gozzo multinodulare	Čvorasta guša (nodularna struma)
Borreliosis	Borreliosis	Borréliose	Borreliosi	Borelioza
Bostezo	Yawn	Bâillement	Sbadiglio	Zijevanje
Botulismo	Botulism	Botulisme	Botulismo	Botulizam
Broncoespasmo	Bronchospasm	Bronchospasme	Broncospasmo	Bronhospazam
Bronquiectasia	Bronchiectasis	Bronchectasie (dilatation des bronches)	Bronchiectasia	Bronhiektazije
Brucelosis	Brucellosis	Brucellose (fièvre de Malte, fièvre méditerranéenne)	Brucellosi	Bruceloza (malteška ili sredozemna groznica, Bangova bolest)
Bulimia	Bulimia	Boulimie	Bulimia	Bulimija
Bunión (hallux valgus)	Bunion	Hallux valgus	Alluce valgo	Čukalj
Caída de la presión arterial	Blood pressure fall	Pression artérielle effondrée	Abbassamento della pressione del sangue	Pad krvnog tlaka
Calambres nocturnos en las piernas	Nocturnal leg cramps	Crampes nocturnes des jambes	Crampo notturno alle gambe	Noćni grčevi u nogama
Calcificación	Calcification	Calcification	Calcificazione	Ovapnjenje (kalcifikacija)
Cálculo en el tracto urinario (urolitiasis)	Bladder stone (urolithiasis)	Calcul urinaire (urolithiase)	Calcolo urinario (urolitiasi)	Kamenac mokraćnog mjehura
Cálculo biliar (litiasis biliar)	Gallstone (cholelithiasis)	Calcul biliaire (cholélithiase)	Calcolo biliare	Žučni kamenac (holelitijaza)
Cálculo en el uréter (ureterolitiasis)	Ureteral stone (ureterolithiasis)	Calcul dans l'uretère	Calcolo ureterale	Ureteralni kamenac (ureterolitijaza)
Calicosis	Chalicosis	Chalicose	Calicosi	Kalikoza
Callosidad (callo)	Callosity (thickening)	Callosité	Callosità (callo)	Zadebljanje kože
Cambios de personalidad	Personality changes	Changements de personnalité	Cambiamenti di personalità	Promjene osobnosti
Cambios en el apetito	Appetite changes	Changements d'appétit	Cambiamenti nell'appetito	Promjene apetita
Cambios en el color de la piel	Skin color changes	Changements de couleur de la peau	Cambiamento di colore della pelle	Promjene boje kože
Cambios en la conciencia	Changes in consciousness	Changements de conscience	Alterazione della conoscenza	Promjene stanja svijesti
Cambios en la forma de los huesos	Changes in shape of bones	Changements dans la forme des os	Cambiamenti nella forma delle ossa	Promjene oblika kosti
Cambios en la membrana mucosa	Changes in mucous membrane	Changement de la muqueuse	Cambiamenti della mucosa	Promjene na sluznici
Cambios en la sensación de sabores	Changes in taste sensation	Changements de sensation de goût	Cambiamenti nelle sensazioni del gusto	Promjene osjeta okusa
Cambios en la sensibilidad olfatoria	Changes in olfactory sensation	Changements des sensations olfactives	Cambiamenti delle sensazoni olfattive	Promjene osjeta mirisa
Cambios en la sensibilidad táctil	Changes in tactile sensation	Changements des sensations tactiles	Cambiamenti della sensazione tattile	Promjene osjeta dodira
Cambios en la voz	Voice changes	Changements de voix	Cambiamento di voce	Promjene glasa
Cambios en los lunares	Changes in moles	Changements dans les grains de beauté	Cambiamenti di nevi	Promjene na madežima
Cambios psíquicos	Psychic changes	Changements psychiques	Alterazioni dello stato psishico	Psihičke promjene
Cáncer de estómago (cáncer gástrico)	Stomach cancer (gastric cancer)	Cancer de l'estomac	Cancro dello stomaco (cancro gastrico)	Rak želuca
Cáncer de mama	Breast cancer	Cancer du sein	Cancro della mammella	Rak dojke
Cáncer de próstata	Prostate cancer	Cancer de la prostate	Cancro della prostata	Rak prostate
Cáncer del cuello uterino (cáncer cervical)	Cervical cancer	Cancer du col utérin	Cancro della cervice uterina	Rak grlića maternice
Candidiasis	Candidiasis (thrush)	Candidiase	Candidosi (candidiasi)	Kandidijaza
Candidiasis oral (muguet oral)	Thrush (oral candidiasis)	Candidose orale	Mughetto (moniliasi orale)	Sor (oralna kandidijaza)
Cansancio (fatiga, letargo, astenia)	Fatigue (exhaustion, lethargy)	Fatigue (affaiblissement)	Stanchezza (fatica, astenia)	Iscrpljenost (umor, fatigo)
Cantidad excesiva de glucosa en la sangre (hiperglucemia, hiperglicemia)	High blood sugar (hyperglicemia)	Taux de sucre dans le sang élevé (hyperglycémie)	Eccesso di glucosio nel sangue (iperglicemia)	Povišeni šećer u krvi (hiperglikemija)
Capacidad de movimiento	Movement ability	Capacité de mouvement	Abilità di muoversi	Sposobnost kretanja
Capsulitis adhesiva del hombro	Frozen shoulder (adhesive capsulitis of shoulder)	Épaule bloquée (périarthrite scapulo-humérale)	Capsulite adesiva	Sindrom bolnog ramena (adhezivni kapsulitis ramena, smrznuto rame)
Caquexia	Cachexia	Cachexie	Cachessia	Kaheksija
Carbunco (ántrax)	Anthrax	Charbon	Antrace	Antraks (bedrenica, crni prišt)
Carcinoide	Carcinoid	Carcinoïde	Carcinoide	Karcinoid
Carcinoide bronquial	Bronchial carcinoid	Carcinoïde bronchiale	Carcinoide bronchiale	Karcinoid bronha
Carcinoma	Carcinoma	Carcinome	Carcinoma	Karcinom
Carcinoma anaplásico	Anaplastic carcinoma	Carcinome anaplastique	Carcinoma anaplastico	Anaplastični karcinom

Español	Inglés	Francés	Italiano	Croata
Carcinoma bronquial	Bronchial carcinoma	Carcinome bronchique	Carcinoma bronchiale	Karcinom bronha
Carcinoma de células basales (basilioma)	Basal cell carcinoma	Carcinome basocellulaire	Basalioma (carcinoma basocellulare)	Karcinom bazalnih stanica (bazaliom)
Carcinoma de células escamosas	Squamous cell carcino-ma (planocellular carcinoma)	Carcinome spinocellulaire	Carcinoma a cellule squamose	Planocelularni karcinom
Carcinoma de células renales	Renal cell carcinoma (hypernephroma)	Carcinome à cellules rénales	Carcinoma a cellule renali	Hipernefrom
Carcinoma de células transicionales	Transitional cell carcinoma	Carcinome à cellules de transition	Carcinoma transizionale	Tranzicionalni karcinom
Carcinoma de endometrio	Endometrial carcinoma	Carcinome de l'endomètre	Carcinoma endometriale	Karcinom endometrija
Carcinoma de las vías biliares (colangiocarcinoma)	Cholangiocellular carcinoma	Cholangiocarcinome	Colangiocarcinoma (carcinoma colangiocellulare)	Kolangiocelularni karcinom
Carcinoma de mama	Breast carcinoma	Carcinome du sein	Carcinoma mammario	Karcinom dojke
Carcinoma de próstata	Prostate carcinoma	Carcinome de la prostate	Carcinoma della prostata	Karcinom prostate
Carcinoma del cuello uterino	Cervical carcinoma	Carcinome du col utérin	Carcinoma della cervice uterina	Karcinom grlića maternice
Carcinoma embrional	Embryonal carcinoma	Carcinome embryonnaire	Carcinoma embrionale	Embrionalni karcinom
Carcinoma epitelial	Epithelial carcinoma	Carcinome épithélial	Carcinoma epiteliale	Karcinom pokrovnog epitela
Carcinoma gástrico	Gastric carcinoma	Carcinome de l'estomac	Carcinoma gastrico	Karcinom želuca
Carcinoma hepatocelular	Hepatocellular carcinoma	Carcinome hépatocellulaire	Carcinoma epatocellulare	Hepatocelularni karcinom
Carcinoma medular	Medullary carcinoma	Carcinome médullaire	Carcinoma midollare	Medularni karcinom
Carcinoma papilar	Papillary carcinoma	Carcinome papillaire	Carcinoma papillare	Papilarni karcinom
Carcinosis	Carcinosis	Carcinose	Carcinosi (carcinomatosi, cancerosi)	Karcinoza
Carcinosis pericárdica	Pericardial carcinosis	Carcinose péricardique	Carcinosi pericardiale	Karcinoza perikarda
Carcinosis peritoneal	Peritoneal carcinosis	Carcinose péritonéale	Carcinosi peritoneale	Karcinoza peritoneuma
Carcinosis pleural	Pleural carcinosis	Carcinose pleurale	Carcinosi pleurica	Karcinoza pleure
Cardiomiopatía restrictiva	Restrictive cardiomyopathy	Cardiomyopathie restrictive	Cardiomiopatia restrittiva	Restriktivna kardiomiopatija
Cardiopatía congénita	Congenital heart disease (congenital cardiopathy)	Cardiopathie congénitale	Cardiopatia congenita	Urođena srčana bolest (kongenitalna kardiopatija)
Cardiopatía reumática	Rheumatic heart disease	Cardite rhumatismale	Cardiopatia reumatica	Reumatska bolest srca
Cardiotoxicidad	Cardiotoxicity	Cardiotoxicité	Cardiomiopatia tossica	Toksična kardiomiopatija
Carencia de vitamina	Vitamin deficiency	Carence en vitamine	Carenza di vitamine	Manjak vitamina
Carencia de vitamina A	Vitamin A deficiency	Carence en vitamine A	Carenza di vitamina A	Manjak vitamina A
Carencia de vitamina B1	Vitamin B1 deficiency	Carence en vitamine B1	Carenza di vitamina B1	Manjak vitamina B1
Carencia de vitamina B2	Vitamin B2 deficiency	Carence en vitamine B2	Carenza di vitamina B2	Manjak vitamina B2
Carencia de vitamina B3	Vitamin B3 deficiency	Carence en vitamine B3	Carenza di vitamina B3	Manjak vitamina B3
Carencia de vitamina B12	Vitamin B12 deficiency	Carence en vitamine B12	Carenza di vitamina B12	Manjak vitamina B12
Carencia de vitamina C	Vitamin C deficiency	Carence en vitamine C	Carenza de vitamina C	Manjak vitamina C
Carencia de vitamina D	Vitamin D deficiency	Carence en vitamine D	Carenza de vitamina D	Manjak vitamina D
Carencia de vitamina K	Vitamin K deficiency	Carence en vitamine K	Carenza de vitamina K	Manjak vitamina K
Caries	Dental caries	Carie dentaire	Carie dentaria	Zubni karijes
Caspa	Dandruff	Pellicule	Forfora	Perut
Catalepsia	Catalepsy	Catalepsie	Catalessia	Katalepsija
Cataplexia (cataplejía)	Cataplexy	Cataplexie	Cataplessia	Katapleksija
Catarata	Cataract	Cataracte	Cataratta	Mrena (katarakta)
Catarro	Catarrh	Catarrhe	Catarro	Katar
Cefalea en racimos	Cluster headache	Algie vasculaire de la face	Cefalea a grappolo	Cluster glavobolja
Cefalea postraumática	Post-traumatic headache	Céphalée post-traumatique	Cefalea post-traumatica	Posttraumatska glavobolja
Cefalea tensional	Tension headache	Céphalée de tension	Cefalea di tipo tensivo	Tenzijska glavobolja
Cefalocele	Cephalocele	Céphalocèle	Cefalocèle	Cefalokela
Ceguera	Blindness	Cécité	Cecità	Sljepoća
Ceguera nocturna (nictalopia)	Night blindness (nyctalopia)	Cécité nocturne (héméralopie)	Cecità notturna (nictalopia)	Noćno sljepilo
Celiaquía (enfermedad celíaca)	Coeliac disease (celiac disease)	Maladie coeliaque	Celiachia (malattia caliacha)	Celijakija
Celulitis	Cellulitis	Cellulite	Cellulite	Celulitis
Celulitis orbital	Orbital cellulitis	Cellulite orbitale	Cellulite orbitale	Celulitis orbite
Cercaria	Cercaria	Cercaire	Cercaria	Cerkarija
Cetoacidosis diabética	Diabetic ketoacidosis	Cétoacidose diabétique	Chetoacidosi diabetica	Dijabetična ketoacidoza
Chancro	Chancre	Chancre	Sifiloma	Čankir
Chancroide (chancro blando)	Chancroid (soft chancre)	Chancre mou (chancrelle)	Ulcera venerea (cancroide)	Meki čankir
Chikungunya	Chikungunya	Chikungunya	Chikungunya	Chikungunya virusna bolest
Chondromalacia rotuliana (síndrome patelo-femoral)	Chondromalacia patellae (runner's knee, patello-femoral pain syndrome)	Chondromalacie rotulienne	Sindrome del dolore patello-femorale (ginocchio del corridore)	Hondromalacija patele (trkačko koljeno, sindrom patelofemoralne boli)
Choque (shock)	Shock	Choc	Collaso circolatorio (shock)	Šok
Choque anafiláctico	Anaphylactic shock	Choc anaphylactique	Anafilassi	Anafilaktični šok
Choque cardiogénico	Cardiogenic shock	Choc cardiogénique	Shock cardiogeno	Kardiogeni šok
Choque endotoxico	Endotoxic shock	Choc endotoxique	Shock endotossico	Endotoksični šok
Choque espinal	Spinal shock	Choc spinal	Shock spinale	Spinalni šok
Choque hipovolémico	Hypovolemic shock	Choc hypovolémique	Shock ipovolemico	Hipovolemički šok
Choque neurogénico	Neurogenic shock	Choc neurogénique	Shock neurogeno	Neurogeni šok
Choque obstructivo	Obstructive shock	Choc obstructive	Shock ostruttivo	Opstruktivni šok

Español	Inglés	Francés	Italiano	Croata
Choque quirúrgico	Surgical shock (postoperative shock)	Choc post-opératoire	Shock chirurgico	Kirurški šok
Choque séptico	Septic shock	Choc septique	Shock settico	Septički šok
Choque traumático	Traumatic shock	Choc traumatique	Shock traumatico	Traumatski šok
Cianosis	Cyanosis	Cyanose	Cianosi	Cijanoza
Ciática	Sciatica	Sciatique	Sciatica	Išijas
Cicatriz	Scar	Cicatrice	Cicatrice (sfregio)	Ožiljak
Cifoescoliosis	Kyphoscoliosis	Cypho-scoliose	Cifoscoliosi	Kifoskolioza
Cifosis	Kyphosis	Cyphose	Cifosi	Kifoza
Cirrosis alcohólica	Alcoholic cirrhosis	Cirrhose alcoolique	Cirrosi alcolica	Alkoholna ciroza
Cirrosis biliar	Biliary cirrhosis	Cirrhose biliaire	Cirrosi biliare	Bilijarna ciroza
Cirrosis criptogénica	Cryptogenic cirrhosis	Cirrhose cryptogénique	Cirrosi criptogenica	Kriptogena ciroza
Cirrosis hepática	Liver cirrhosis	Cirrhose hépatique	Cirrosi	Ciroza jetre
Cirrosis postnecrótica	Post-necrotic cirrhosis	Cirrhose postnecrotique	Cirrosi post-necrotica	Postnekrotična ciroza
Cistadenocarcinoma	Cystadenocarcinoma	Cystadénocarcinome	Cistadenocarcinoma	Cistadenokarcinom
Cistadenofibroma	Cystadenofibroma	Cystadénofibrome	Cistadenofibroma	Cistadenofibrom
Cistadenoma	Cystadenoma	Cystadénome	Cistadenoma	Cistadenom
Cisticercosis	Cysticercosis	Cysticercose	Cisticercosi	Cisticerkoza
Cistoma	Cystoma	Kystome	Cistoma	Cistom
Claudicación intermitente	Intermittent claudication	Claudication intermittente	Claudicatio intermittens	Intermitentna klaudikacija
Claustrofobia (miedo a los espacios cerrados)	Claustrophobia (fear of closed space)	Claustrophobie	Claustrofobia (paura di luoghi chiusi)	Klaustrofobija (strah od zatvorenog prostora)
Cleptomanía	Kleptomania	Cleptomanie	Cleptomania	Kleptomanija
Clonorquiasis (clonorquiosis)	Clonorchiasis	Clonorchiase	Clonorchiasi	Klonorkijaza
Coagulación intravascular diseminada	Disseminated intravascular coagulation	Coagulation intravasculaire disséminée	Coagulazione intravascolare disseminata	Diseminirana intravaskularna koagulacija
Coágulo sanguíneo (trombo)	Blood clot (thrombus)	Caillot sanguin (thrombus)	Trombo	Krvni ugrušak (tromb)
Coartación de la aorta	Coarctation of the aorta	Coarctation de l'aorte	Coartazione dell'aorta	Koarktacija aorte
Coccidioidomicosis	Coccidioidomycosis (San Joaquin Valley fever)	Coccidioïmycose (fièvre de la vallée de San Joaquin, fièvre du désert)	Coccidiomicosi	Kokcidioidomikoza (San Joaquin Valley vrućica)
Coccigodinia (dolor de coxis)	Coccygodynia	Coccygodynie (douleur coccygienne)	Coccigodinia	Kokcigodinija
Codo del tenista (epicondilitis lateral)	Tennis elbow	Épicondylite latérale	Gomito del tennista (epicondilite)	Teniski lakat
Cojera	Limping	Boitillement	Zoppicamento	Šepanje
Colapso	Collapse	Collapsus	Collasso	Kolaps
Colección de sangre en la trompa de Falopio (hematosalpinx)	Bleeding into the fallopian tube (hematosalpinx)	Collection de sang dans la trompe de Fallope (hématosalpinx)	Flusso di sangue nella tuba di Falloppio	Krvarenje u jajovod (hematosalpinks)
Cólera	Cholera	Choléra	Colera	Kolera
Colesterol elevado de la sangre (hipercolesterolemia)	High blood cholesterol (hypercholesterolemia)	Cholésterol sanguin élevée (hypercholestérolémie)	Eccesso di colesterolo nel sangue (ipercolesterolemia)	Povišeni kolesterol u krvi (hiperkolesterolemija)
Cólico	Colic	Colique	Colica	Kolika
Cólico abdominal	Abdominal colic	Colique abdominale	Colica addominale	Trbušna kolika (abdominalna kolika)
Cólico biliar	Biliary colic	Colique biliaire	Colica biliare	Žučna kolika
Cólico del recién nacido	Baby colic	Coliques de bébé	Coliche del neonato	Novorođenačke kolike
Cólico nefrítico (cólico renal)	Renal colic	Colique néphrétique	Colica renale	Bubrežna kolika (renalna kolika)
Colitis ulcerosa	Ulcerative colitis	Colite ulcéreuse	Rettocolite ulcerosa	Ulcerozni kolitis
Colon transverso	Transverse colon	Côlon transverse	Colon trasverso	Poprečno debelo crijevo
Coma	Coma	Coma	Coma	Koma
Coma diabético	Diabetic coma	Coma diabétique	Coma diabetico	Dijabetična koma
Comerse las uñas (onicofagia)	Nail biting (onychophagia)	Se ronger les ongles (onychophagie)	Abitudine di mangiare le unghie (onicofagia)	Griženje noktiju (onikofagija)
Compresión cerebral	Brain compression	Compression cérébrale	Compressione cerebrale	Kompresija mozga
Compresión del nérvio	Nerve compression (pinched nerve)	Compression du nerf	Compressone del nervo	Kompresija živca (uklješten živac)
Comunicación interauricular	Atrial septal defect	Communication inter-auriculaire	Difetto del setto interatriale	Atrijski septalni defekt
Comunicación interventricular	Ventricular septal defect	Communication inter-ventriculaire	Difetto del setto ventricolare	Ventrikularni septalni defekt
Condroblastoma	Chondroblastoma	Chondroblastome	Condroblastoma	Hondroblastom
Condroma	Chondroma	Chondrome	Condroma	Hondrom
Condrosarcoma	Chondrosarcoma	Chondrosarcome	Condrosarcoma	Hondrosarkom
Confusión	Confusion	Confusion	Confusione (disordine)	Smetenost
Congelamiento	Frostbite	Gelure	Congelamento	Ozeblina
Congestión nasal	Nasal congestion (stuffy nose)	Congestion nasale	Congestione nasale	Začepljeni nos
Congestión pulmonar	Pulmonary congestion	Congestion pulmonaire	Congestione polmonare	Plućna kongestija
Conjuntivitis alérgica	Allergic conjunctivitis	Conjonctive allergique	Congiuntivite allergica	Alergijski konjuktivitis
Conjuntivitis bacteriana	Bacterial conjunctivitis	Conjonctivite bactérienne	Congiuntivite batterica	Bakterijski konjuktivitis

Español	Inglés	Francés	Italiano	Croata
Conjuntivitis por cuerpo extraño	Conjunctival foreign body	Conjonctivite due à un corps étranger	Congiuntivite irritativa da corpi estranei	Konjuktivitis izazvan stranim tijelom
Conjuntivitis química	Chemical conjunctivitis	Conjonctivite chimique	Congiuntivite irritativa da agenti chimici	Kemijski konjuktivitis
Conjuntivitis viral	Viral conjuctivitis	Conjonctivite virale	Congiuntivite virale	Virusni konjuktivitis
Conmoción cerebral	Brain concussion	Commotion cérébrale	Commozione cerebrale	Potres mozga
Contracción del cuerpo entero de tal manera que se mantiene encorvado hacia atrás (opistótonos)	Spastic arching position (opisthotonus)	Contracture sur les muscles extenseurs de sorte que le corps est incurvé en arrière (opisthotonos)	Iperestenzione della regione posteriore del tronco (opistotono)	Izvijanje mišića vrata i leđa u luk (opistotonus)
Contractura	Contracture	Contracture	Contrattura	Kontraktura
Contractura articular	Joint contracture	Contracture articulaire	Contrattura articolare	Kontraktura zgloba
Contractura de Dupuytren	Dupuytren's contracture	Contracture de Dupuytren	Malattia di Dupuytren	Dupuytrenova kontraktura
Contractura isquémica de Volkmann	Volkmann's ischemic contracture	Syndrome de Volkmann	Contrattura ischemica di Volkmann	Volkmannova ishemična kontraktura
Contractura muscular	Muscular contracture	Contracture musculaire	Contrattura muscolare	Kontraktura mišića
Contusión	Contusion	Contusion	Contusione	Nagnječenje (zgnječenje, kontuzija)
Contusión cerebral	Cerebral contusion	Contusion cérébrale	Contusione cerebrale	Nagnječenje mozga
Convulsiones	Convulsions	Convulsions	Convulsioni	Konvulzije
Convulsiones febriles	Febrile convulsions	Convulsion hyperthermique	Convulsioni febbrili	Febrilne konvulzije
Cor pulmonale agudo	Acute pulmonary heart	Coeur pulmonaire aigu	Cuore polmonare acuto	Akutno plućno srce
Corazón de atleta (hipertrofia del corazón del deportista)	Athlete's heart (cardiac hypertrophy)	Hypertrophie cardiaque du sportif (coeur d'athlète)	Cuore dell'atleta (ipertrofia cardiaca da sport)	Sportsko srce
Coreoatetosis	Choreoathetosis	Choréoathétose	Coreoatetosi	Koreoatetoza
Coriocarcinoma	Choriocarcinoma	Choriocarcinome	Coriocarcinoma	Koriokarcinom
Coriomeningitis linfocítica	Lymphocytic choriomeningitis	Choriomeningite lymphocytaire	Coriomeningite linfocitaria	Limfocitni koriomeningitis
Corto de oído (parcialmente sordo)	Hard of hearing	Surdité partielle	Sordità parziale	Nagluhost
Costilla cervical	Cervical rib	Côte cervicale	Costa cervicale	Vratno rebro
Costra	Crust (scab)	Croûte	Crosta (escara)	Krasta
Crepitación	Crepitation	Crépitation	Crepitazione	Krepitacija
Criptococcosis	Cryptococcosis	Cryptococcose	Criptococcosi	Kriptokokoza
Criptorquidismo	Cryptorchidism	Cryptorchidie	Criptorchidismo	Retencija testisa (kriptorhizam)
Crisis tónico-clónica	Tonic-clonic seizure	Crise tonico-clonique	Crisi tonico-clonica	Toničko-klonički napadaj
Crispar del músculo (fasciculación)	Muscle twitch (fasciculation)	Fasciculation musculaire	Scossa muscolare (fasciciolazione)	Trzanje mišića
Cromomicosis (cromoblastomicosis)	Chromoblastomycosis (chromomycosis, Pedroso's disease)	Chromomycose	Cromomicosi (cromoblastomicosi)	Kromomikoza
Crup (laringotraqueo-bronquitis)	Croup (acute obstructive laryngitis)	Croup (laryngotrachéo-bronchite)	Croup (laringite acuta ostruttiva)	Krup (akutni opstruktivni laringitis)
Cuerpo extraño en el oído	Foreign body in ear	Corps étranger dans l'oreille	Corpo estraneo nell'orecchio	Strano tijelo u uhu
Cuerpo extraño en la nariz	Foreign body in nose	Corps étranger dans le nez	Corpo estraneo nel naso	Strano tijelo u nosu
Daltonismo	Daltonism	Daltonisme	Daltonismo	Daltonizam
Debilidad	Weakness	Faiblesse	Debolezza	Slabost
Deficiencia de estrógenos	Estrogen deficiency	Carence oestrogénique	Carenza di estrogeno	Manjak estrogena
Deficiencia de factor de coagulación	Coagulation factor deficiency	Déficit en facteur de la coagulation	Carenza di fattore di coagulazione	Manjak faktora koagulacije
Deformidad de Madelung	Madelung's deformity	Déformation de Madelung	Deformità di Madelung	Madelungov deformitet
Deformidad de Sprengel	Sprengel's deformity	Anomalie de Sprengel	Deformità di Sprengel	Sprengelova bolest (scapula alta)
Deformidad del pie	Foot deformity	Difformité du pied	Difetto del piede	Deformacija stopala
Deformidad vertebral	Spinal deformity	Difformité spinale	Degenerazione spinale	Deformacija kralježnice
Degeneración macular	Macular degeneration	Dégénérescence maculaire	Degenerazione maculare	Degeneracija makule
Degeneración retinal	Retinal degeneration	Dégénérescence de la rétine	Degenerazione della retina	Degeneracija mrežnice
Delirio	Delirium	Delirium	Delirio	Delirij
Demencia	Dementia	Démence	Demenza	Demencija
Dengue	Dengue fever	Dengue (grippe tropicale, dengue hémorragique)	Dengue	Dengue groznica
Depresión	Depression	Dépression	Depressione	Depresija
Dermatitis alérgica de contacto	Allergic contact dermatitis	Dermite de contact allergique	Dermatite allergica	Alergijski kontaktni dermatitis
Dermatitis atópica	Atopic dermatitis	Dermatite atopique	Neurodermite (dermatite atopica)	Atopijski dermatitis
Dermatitis de contacto	Contact dermatitis	Dermite de contact	Dermatite da contatto	Kontaktni dermatitis
Dermatitis herpetiforme (enfermedad de Duhring)	Dermatitis herpetiformis (Duhring's disease)	Dermite herpétiforme	Dermatite erpetiforme di Duhring	Duhringova bolest (dermatitis herpetiformis)
Dermatitis irritante de contacto	Irritant contact dermatitis	Dermite de contact irritative	Dermatite irritativo da contatto	Iritantni kontaktni dermatitis
Dermatitis numular	Nummular dermatitis	Dermatite nummulaire	Dermatite nummulare	Numularni dermatitis

Español	Inglés	Francés	Italiano	Croata
Dermatitis seborreica infantil	Cradle cap (infantile seborrhoeic dermatitis)	Dermite séborrhéique infantile	Dermatite seborroica infantile	Tjemenica (dojenačka seboreja)
Dermatomicosis	Dermatomycosis	Dermatomycose	Dermatomicosi	Dermatomikoza
Dermatomiositis	Dermatomyositis	Dermatomyosite	Dermatomiosite	Dermatomiozitis
Derrame cerebral (accidente cerebrovascular)	Stroke (cerebrovascular accident)	Attaque cérébrale (accident vasculaire cérébral)	Colpo apoplettico	Moždani udar
Derrame pericárdico	Pericardial effusion (hydropericard)	Épanchement péricardique	Idropericardio	Hidroperikard
Desangramiento (hemorragia)	Bleeding (haemorrhage)	Saignement (hémorragie)	Emorragia	Krvarenje (hemoragija)
Desarrollo de tenido de un órgano (aplasia de un órgano)	Absence in development of an organ (aplasia of an organ)	Arrêt du développement d'un organe (aplasie d'un organe)	Mancato sviluppo di un organo (aplasia di un organo)	Nerazvijenost organa (aplazija organa)
Desarrollo sexual prematuro del mismo sexo	Premature sexual development of the same sex	Développement sexuel prématuré du même sexe	Prematuro sviluppo sessuale dello stesso sesso	Prerano splono fizičko sazrijevanje istog spola
Desarrollo sexual prematuro del sexo opuesto	Premature sexual development of the opposite sex	Développement sexuel prématuré du sexe opposé	Prematuro sviluppo sessuale del sesso opposto	Prerano spolno fizičko sazrijevanje suprotnog spola
Descenso de la frecuencia cardiaca (bradicardia)	Slow pulse rate (bradycardia)	Rythme cardiaque bas (bradycardie)	Riduzione della frequenza cardiaca (bradicardia)	Usporen puls (bradikardija)
Descenso de la frecuencia respiratoria (bradipnea)	Slow breathing rate (bradypnea)	Respiration ralentie (bradypnée)	Riduzione della frequenza respiratoria (bradipnea)	Usporeno disanje (bradipneja)
Descenso incompleto de testículo	Undescended testicle	Absence de descente des testicules	Mancata discesa del testicolo	Nespušteni testis
Descompensación cardíaca	Cardiac decompensation	Décompensation cardiaque	Decompensazione cardiaca	Srčana dekompenzacija
Descoordinación en los movimientos musculares (ataxia)	Lack of coordination of muscle movements (ataxia)	Trouble de coordination des mouvements musculaires (ataxie)	Disturbo della coordinazione muscolare (atassia)	Poremećaj koordinacije mišićnih pokreta (ataksija)
Desgarro	Strain (sprain, pull)	Déchirure	Stiramento	Istegnuće
Desgarro de ligamento	Ligament sprain	Déchirure ligamentaire	Stiramento del legamento	Istegnuće ligamenta
Desgarro de tendón	Tendon strain	Déchirure au tendon	Stiramento del tendine	Istegnuće tetive (distenzija tetive)
Desgarro muscular	Muscle strain (muscle pull)	Déchirure musculaire (claquage)	Strappo muscolare	Istegnuće mišića (distenzija mišića)
Deshidratación	Dehydration	Déshydratation	Disidratazione	Dehidracija
Desmineralización	Demineralization	Déminéralisation	Demineralizzazione	Demineralizacija
Desnutrición	Underfedness (malnutrition)	Malnutrition	Sottopeso (grave magrezza)	Neuhranjenost
Desorientación	Disorientation	Désorientation	Disorientamento	Dezorijentiranost
Desplazamiento de una articulación (subluxación)	Partial dislocation (subluxation)	Luxation incomplète (subluxation)	Lussazione incompleta (sublussazione)	Djelomična dislokacija (subluksacija)
Despredimiento del párpado superior (blefaroptosis)	Drooping of the upper eyelid (blepharoptosis)	Abaissement de la paupière supérieure (blépharoptose)	Spostamento della palpebra (palpebra calante, blefaroptosi)	Spušteni kapak (blefaroptoza)
Desprendimiento de retina	Retinal ablation (retinal detachment)	Décollement de la rétine	Distacco di retina	Odvajanje mrežnice (ablacija retine)
Desquamación	Shedding of the skin (desquamation)	Desquamation	Perdita dello strato superiore della pelle (desquamazione)	Ljuštenje kože (deskvamacija)
Desviación del tabique nasal	Nasal septum deviation	Déviation du septum nasal	Deviazione del setto nasale	Devijacija nosnog septuma
Diabetes	Diabetes	Diabète	Diabete	Dijabetes
Diabetes insípida	Diabetes insipidus	Diabète insipide	Diabete insipido	Dijabetes insipidus
Diabetes mellitus (diabetes sacarina)	Diabetes mellitus	Diabète sucré	Diabete mellito	Dijabetes melitus
Diabetes mellitus tipo 1	Diabetes mellitus type 1	Diabète sucré de type 1 (diabète insulino-dépendant)	Diabete mellito di tipo 1	Dijabetes melitus tip 1
Diabetes mellitus tipo 2	Diabetes mellitus type 2	Diabète sucré de type 2 (diabète insulinorésistant)	Diabete mellito di tipo 2	Dijabetes melitus tip 2
Diarrea	Diarrhea	Diarrhée	Diarrea	Proljev (dijarea)
Diente podrido	Rotten tooth	Dent pourri	Dente guasto	Pokvareni zub
Dificultad al orinar (disuria)	Difficult urination (dysuria)	Difficulté à uriner (dysurie)	Emissione di urine con difficoltà (disuria)	Otežano usporeno mokrenje (dizurija)
Dificultad de respiración	Breathing difficulty	Difficulté de respiration	Respirazione difficoltosa	Otežano disanje
Dificultad del aprendizaje	Learning disability	Trouble de l'apprentissage	Disturbo di apprendimento	Poremećaj učenja
Dificultad para la defecación (tenesmo rectal)	Difficult defecation (tenesmus)	Difficulté à déféquer (ténesme)	Difficoltà a defecare (tenesmo)	Otežano pražnjenje crijeva (otežana defekacija)
Dificultad para tragar (disfagia)	Difficult swallowing (dysphagia)	Difficulté de déglutition (dysphagie)	Difficoltà a deglutire (disfagia)	Otežano gutanje (disfagija)
Difteria	Diphtheria	Diphtérie	Difterite	Difterija
Dilatación aguda del estómago	Acute gastric dilatation	Dilatation aiguë de l'estomac	Dilatazione gastrica acuta	Akutna dilatacija želuca
Discartrosis	Discarthrosis (degenerative disc disease)	Arthrose du disque intervertébral	Discartrosi (discopatia degenerativa)	Diskartroza
Discondroplasia	Dyschondroplasia	Dyschondroplasie	Discondroplasia	Dishondroplazija

Español	Inglés	Francés	Italiano	Croata
Disección aórtica	Aortic dissection	Dissection aortique	Dissecazione aortica	Disekcija aorte
Disentería	Dysentery (flux)	Dysenterie	Dissenteria	Dizenterija
Disentería amebiana (amebiasis)	Amebiasis (amebic dysentery)	Amibiase (dysenterie amibienne)	Amebiasi	Amebijaza
Disgénesis testicular	Testicular dysgenesis	Dysgénésie testiculaire	Disgenesia gonadica	Testikularna disgeneza
Disgerminoma	Dysgerminoma	Dysgerminome	Disgerminoma	Disgerminom
Dislexia	Dyslexia	Dyslexie	Dislessia	Disleksija
Dislocación de la mandibula	Mandibular dislocation	Luxation temporo-mandibulaire	Lussazione della mandibola	Iščašenje vilice
Dislocación de los fragmentos	Dislocated fragments	Fragments deboîtées	Dislocazione dei frammenti	Dislokacija ulomaka
Disminución de producción de orina (oliguria)	Decreased production of urine (oliguria)	Raréfaction du volume des urines (oligurie)	Diminuita escrezione urinaria (oliguria)	Smanjeno izlučivanje urina (oligurija)
Disnea paroxística nocturna	Cardiac asthma (paroxysmal nocturnal dyspnea)	Dyspnée chez un cardiaque	Dispnea parossistica notturna	Srčana astma (paroksizmalna dispneja)
Dispepsia (indigestión)	Dyspepsia (upset stomach)	Dyspepsie	Dispepsia	Dispepsija (nervozni želudac)
Displasia arritmogénica ventricular derecha	Arrhytmogenic right ventricular dysplasia	Dysplasie ventriculair droite arythmogène	Displasia ventricolare destra aritmogena	Aritmogena displazija desne klijetke
Displasia congénita de la cadera (luxación congénita de cadera)	Congenital dysplasia of the hip (congenital hip dislocation)	Luxation congénitale de la hanche	Lussazione congenita dell'anca (displasia dell'anca)	Urođeno iščašenje kuka (kongenitalna displazija kuka)
Displasia del cuello uterino	Cervical dysplasia	Dysplasie du col de l'utérus	Displasia cervicale	Cervikalna displazija
Displasia fibrosa	Fibrous dysplasia	Dysplasie fibreuse	Displasia fibrosa	Fibrozna displazija
Distonía	Dystonia	Dystonie	Distonia	Distonija
Distorsión articular	Joint distortion	Distorsion articulaire	Distorsione	Uganuće zgloba (distorzija zgloba)
Distorsión del tobillo	Ankle distortion	Distorsion de la cheville	Distorsione alla caviglia	Uganuće skočnog zgloba
Distrofia	Dystrophy	Dystrophie	Distrofia	Distrofija
Distrofia muscular	Muscular dystrophy	Dystrophie musculaire	Distrofia muscolare	Mišićna distrofija
Distrofia muscular de Duchenne	Duchenne muscular dystrophy	Myopathie de Duchenne	Distrofia di Duchenne	Duchenneova mišićna distrofija
Distrofia muscular progresiva	Progressive muscular dystrophy	Dystrophie musculaire progressive	Distrofia muscolare progressiva	Progresivna mišićna distrofija
Diverticulitis	Diverticulitis	Diverticulite	Diverticolite	Divertikulitis
Divertículo	Diverticulum	Diverticule	Diverticolo	Divertikul
Divertículo de Meckel	Small intestine diverticulum	Diverticule de Meckel	Diverticolo di Meckel	Divertikul tankog crijeva
Divertículo del colon	Colon diverticulum	Diverticule du côlon	Diverticolo del colon	Divertikul na debelom crijevu
Divertículo duodenal	Duodenal diverticulum	Diverticule duodenal	Diverticolo duodenale	Divertikul na dvanaesniku
Dolor	Pain	Douleur	Dolore	Bol
Dolor abdominal	Abdominal pain	Douleur abdominale	Dolore addominale	Bol u trbuhu
Dolor afilado	Sharp pain	Douleur tranchante	Dolore tagliente	Oštra bol
Dolor agudo	Acute pain	Douleur aiguë	Dolore acuto	Akutna bol
Dolor al tragar (odinofagia)	Painful swallowing (odynophagia)	Déglutition douloureuse (odynophagie)	Deglutizione dolorosa (odinofagia)	Bolno gutanje (odinofagija)
Dolor crónico	Chronic pain	Douleur chronique	Dolore cronico	Kronična bol
Dolor de cabeza	Headache	Mal de tête (céphalée)	Mal di testa	Glavobolja
Dolor de cabeza por sinusitis	Sinus headache	Douleur des sinus (sinusite)	Sinusite	Sinusna glavobolja
Dolor de espalda (dorsalgia)	Back pain (dorsalgia)	Mal de dos (dorsalgie)	Mal di schiena (dorsopatia)	Bol u leđima (dorzopatija)
Dolor de espalda baja (lumbalgia)	Low back pain (lumbago, lumbosacral syndrome)	Lombalgie	Lombaggine	Križobolja (lumbosakralni sindrom)
Dolor de espalda postural	Postural back pain	Lombalgie posturale	Mal di schiena su base posturale	Posturalna križobolja
Dolor de muelas	Toothache	Mal de dents	Mal di denti	Zubobolja
Dolor del miembro fantasma	Phantom pain	Douleur du membre fantôme	Dolore fantomatico	Fantomska bol
Dolor en articulación (artralgia)	Joint pain (arthralgia)	Douleur articulaire (arthralgie)	Articolazione doloroso (artralgia)	Bol u zglobu (artralgija)
Dolor en la mama (mastalgia)	Breast pain (mastalgia)	Douleur au sein (mastodynie)	Dolore al seno (mastalgia)	Bol u dojci (mastalgija)
Dolor en las espinillas	Shin splints	Périostite tibiale	Sindrome da stress tibiale mediale	Trkačka potkoljenica
Dolor en oído (otalgia)	Ear pain (otalgia)	Mal à l'oreille (otalgie)	Dolore auricolare (otalgia)	Bol u uhu (otalgija)
Dolor epigástrico	Epigastric pain	Douleur épigastrique	Gastralgia	Bol u epigastriju
Dolor muscular (mialgia)	Muscle pain (myalgia)	Douleur musculaire (myalgie)	Dolore muscolare (mialgia)	Bol u mišiću (mijalgija)
Dolor pulsante	Pulsing pain	Douleur pulsatile	Dolore pulsante	Pulsirajuća bol
Dolor sordo	Dull pain	Douleur sourde	Dolore ottuso	Tupa bol
Dolor tipo punzada	Twinging pain	Élancement	Dolore pungente	Probadajuća bol
Dolor torácico	Chest pain	Douleur thoracique	Dolore toracico	Bol u prsištu
Dracunculiasis	Dracunculiasis	Dracunculose	Dracunculiasi	Drakunkulijaza

Español	Inglés	Francés	Italiano	Croata
Ductus arterioso persistente (conducto arterioso persistente)	Patent ductus arteriosus (persistent ductus arteriosus)	Persistance du canal artériel	Dotto arterioso persistente (ductus arteriosus persistente)	Otvoreni ductus arteriosus (Ductus arteriosus persistens)
Ductus arteriosus (conducto arterioso de Botal)	Ductus arteriosus (ductus Botalli shunt)	Canal artériel	Dotto arterioso di Botallo	Ductus Botalli
Eccema (eczema)	Eczema	Eczéma	Eczema	Ekcem
Ecolalia	Echolalia	Écholalie	Ecolalia	Eholalija
Ecopraxia (repetición de los movimientos de otra persona)	Echopraxia (involuntary repetition of the observed movements of another)	Échopraxie (tendance spontanée à répéter les mouvements d'une autre personne)	Ecoprassia (imitazione spontanea di movimenti osservati)	Ehopraksija (nevoljno ponavljanje tuđih pokreta)
Ectrodactilia en pie	Split foot (lobster claw foot, ectrodactyly)	Pince de homard (aplasie digitale, ectrodactylie)	Lobster-claw deformità di piede	Lobster Claw stopalo
Eczema dishidrótico	Dyshidrosis	Dyshidrose	Disidrosi	Dishidroza
Edema (hidropesía)	Edema	Oedème	Edema	Edem
Edema cerebral	Cerebral edema	Oedème cérébral	Edema cerebrale	Edem mozga
Edema del nervio óptico	Optic nerve edema	Oedème du nerf optique	Papilledema (edema del nervo ottico)	Otok očnog živca (zastojna papila)
Edema postural	Postural edema	Oedème postural	Edema posturale	Posturalni edem (statički edem)
Edema pulmonar	Pulmonary edema	Oedème pulmonaire	Edema polmonare	Plućni edem
Elefantiasis	Elephantiasis (lymphedema)	Éléphantiasis (filariose lymphatique)	Elefantiasi	Elefantijaza (limfedem)
Embarazo ectópico	Ectopic pregnancy (extrauterine pregnancy)	Grossesse extra-utérine	Gravidanza ectopica	Izvanmaternična trudnoća (ektopična trudnoća)
Embolia	Embolism	Embolie	Embolismo (embolia)	Embolija
Embolia arterial	Arterial embolism	Embolie artérielle	Embolia dell'arteria	Arterijska embolija
Embolia gaseosa	Air embolism (gas embolism)	Embolie gazeuse	Embolia gassosa	Zračna embolija
Embolia pulmonar	Pulmonary embolism	Embolie pulmonaire	Embolia polmonare	Plućna embolija
Embolismo graso	Fat embolism	Embolie de cholestérol	Embolia adiposa	Masna embolija
Emisión excesiva de orina durante la noche (nicturia)	Frequent urination at night (nocturia)	Excrétion urinaire à prédominance nocturne (nycturie)	Urinazione notturna (nicturia)	Noćno mokrenje (nokturija)
Empiema	Empyema	Empyème	Empiema	Empijem
Enanismo	Dwarfism (nanism)	Nanisme	Nanismo	Patuljasti rast (nanizam)
Encefalocele	Encephalocele	Encéphalocèle	Encefalocele	Encefalokela
Encefalopatía	Encephalopathy	Encéphalopathie	Encefalopatia	Encefalopatija
Encondroma	Enchondroma	Enchondrome	Encondroma	Enhondrom
Encopresis	Encopresis	Encoprésie	Enconpresi	Enkopreza
Endocarditis bacteriana	Bacterial endocarditis	Endocardite bactérienne	Endocardite batterica	Bakterijski endokarditis
Endometriosis	Endometriosis	Endométriose	Endometriosi	Endometrioza
Enfermedad autoinmune	Autoimmune disease	Maladie auto-immune	Malattia autoimmunitaria	Autoimunološka bolest
Enfermedad cardíaca pulmonar (cor pulmonale)	Pulmonary heart disease	Coeur pulmonaire	Cuore polmonare	Plućno srce
Enfermedad coronaria	Coronary disease	Maladie coronarienne	Coronaropatia	Koronarna bolest (koronaropatija)
Enfermedad de Addison	Addison's disease	Maladie d'Addison	Morbo di Addison	Addisonova bolest
Enfermedad de Alzheimer	Alzheimer's diesase	Maladie d'Alzheimer	Morbo di Alzheimer	Alzheimerova bolest
Enfermedad de Blount (tibia vara)	Blount's disease	Maladie de Blount	Sindrome di Blount	Blountova bolest
Enfermedad de Bornholm (mialgia epidémica)	Bornholm disease (epidemic myalgia)	Maladie de Bornholm (myalgie épidémique)	Malattia di Bornholm (mialgia epidemica)	Bornholmska bolest (epidemijska mialgija)
Enfermedad de Bowen	Bowen's disease (squamous cell carcinoma in situ)	Maladie de Bowen	Morbo di Bowen	Bowenova bolest
Enfermedad de Brill	Brill's disease	Maladie de Brill-Zinserr (typhus résurgent)	Malattia di Brill-Zinsser	Brillova bolest (Brill-Zinsserova bolest)
Enfermedad de Buerger (tromboangeítis obliterante)	Buerger's disease (thromboangiitis obliterans)	Maladie de Buerger (thromboangéite oblitérante)	Morbo di Buerger	Buergerova bolest
Enfermedad de Chagas (tripanosomiasis americana)	Chagas disease (American trypanosomiasis)	Maladie de Chagas (trypanosomiase américaine)	Malattia di Chagas	Chagasova bolest (americka tripanosomijaza)
Enfermedad de Charcot-Marie Tooth	Charcot-Marie-Tooth disease	Maladie de Charcot-Marie-Tooth	Malattia di Charcot-Marie-Tooth	Bolest Charcot-Marie-Tooth
Enfermedad de Creutzfeldt-Jakob	Creutzfeldt-Jakob disease (so called "mad cow disease")	Maladie de Creutzfeldt-Jakob	Malattia di Creutzfeldt-Jakob (cosiddetta "malattia della mucca pazza")	Creutzfeldt-Jakobova bolest (tzv. "kravlje ludilo")
Enfermedad de Crohn	Crohn's disease	Maladie de Crohn	Malattia di Crohn	Crohnova bolest
Enfermedad de Freiberg	Freiberg's disease	Maladie de Freiberg	Malattia di Freiberg	Freibergova bolest
Enfermedad de Graves Basedow	Basedow Graves disease	Maladie de Basedow	Morbo di Basedow-Graves	Basedowljeva bolest
Enfermedad de Haglund (deformidad de Haglund)	Haglund's disease	Maladie de Haglund	Malattia di Haglund (deformità di Haglund)	Haglundova bolest
Enfermedad de Hirschsprung (megacolon agangliónico)	Hirschsprung's disease (congenital aganglionic megacolon)	Maladie de Hirschsprung (mégacolôn)	Malattia di Hirschsprung (malattia di Mya)	Hirschsprungova bolest (kongenitalni aganglionarni megakolon)

Español	Inglés	Francés	Italiano	Croata
Enfermedad de Hodgkin	Hodgkin's disease	Maladie de Hodgkin	Linfoma di Hodgkin	Hodgkinova bolest
Enfermedad de Hoffa	Hoffa's disease	Maladie de Hoffa	Sindrome di Hoffa	Morbus Hoffa
Enfermedad de Huntington (corea de Huntington)	Huntington's chorea (Huntington's disease)	Chorée de Huntington (maladie de Huntington)	Malattia di Huntington	Huntingtonova koreja
Enfermedad de Kawasaki	Kawasaki disease	Maladie de Kawasaki	Sindrome di Kawasaki	Kawasakijeva bolest (mukokutani limfoglandularni sindrom)
Enfermedad de Kienböck	Kienböck's disease	Maladie de Kienböck	Morbo di Kienböck	Kienböckova bolest
Enfermedad de Köhler	Köhler disease	Maladie de Köhler	Malattia di Köhler	Köhlerova bolest
Enfermedad de la membrana hialina (síndrome de distrés respiratorio)	Hyaline membrane disease (infant respiratory distress syndrome)	Maladie des membranes hyalines (détresse respiratoire néonatale)	Sindrome da distress respiratorio del neonato (malattia da membrane ialine polmonari)	Bolest hijaline membrane (respiratorni sindrom novorođenćeta)
Enfermedad de la motoneurona	Motor neurone disease	Maladie du motoneurone	Malattia del motoneurone	Bolest motornog neurona
Enfermedad de La Peyronie (induración plástica del pene)	Peyronie's disease (induratio penis plastica)	Maladie de La Peyronie	Induratio penis plastica (malattia di Peyronie)	Plastična induracija penisa
Enfermedad de las vibraciones	Vibration disease	Maladie des vibrations	Malattia da vibrazioni	Vibracijska bolest
Enfermedad de los ensiladores	Silo-filler's disease	Maladie des ouvriers des silos	Malattia dei riempitori dei silos	Silosna pluća
Enfermedad de Lyme (borreliosis de Lyme)	Lyme disease (lyme borreliosis)	Maladie de Lyme	Malattia di Lyme (borreliosi di Lyme)	Lajmska bolest (Lajmska borelioza)
Enfermedad de Menière	Meniere's disease	Maladie de Menière	Sindrome di Menière	Menierova bolest
Enfermedad de Morquio (mucopolisacaridosis tipo IV)	Morquio's syndrome (mucopolysaccharidosis IV)	Maladie de Morquio (mucopolysaccharidose type IV)	Malattia di Morquio (mucopolisaccaridosi IV)	Sindrom Morquio (mukopolisaharidoza tip IV)
Enfermedad de Osgood-Schlatter	Osgood-Schlatter disease (rugby knee)	Maladie d'Osgood-Schlatter	Sindrome di Osgood-Schlatter	Osgood-Schlatterova bolest
Enfermedad de Paget	Paget's disease	Maladie de Paget	Morbo di Paget	Pagetova bolest
Enfermedad de Panner	Panner's disease	Maladie de Panner	Malattia di Panner	Pannerova bolest
Enfermedad de Parkinson	Parkinson's disease	Maladie de Parkinson	Morbo di Parkinson	Parkinsonova bolest
Enfermedad de Pellegrini-Stieda	Pellegrini-Stieda disease	Maladie de Pellegrini-Stieda	Malattia di Pellegrini-Stieda	Bolest Pellegrini-Stieda
Enfermedad de Preiser	Preiser disease	Maladie de Preiser	Sindrome di Preiser	Morbus Preiser
Enfermedad de Raynaud	Raynaud's disease	Maladie de Raynaud	Sindrome di Raynaud	Raynaudova bolest
Enfermedad de Sever	Sever's disease	Maladie de Sever	Malattia di Sever	Severova bolest
Enfermedad de transmisión sexual	Sexually transmitted disease	Maladie vénérienne	Malattia sessualmente trasmissibile	Spolno prenosiva bolest
Enfermedad de Van Neck	Van Neck disease	Maladie de Van Neck-Odelberg	Malattia di Van Neck	Morbus Van Neck
Enfermedad de Whipple	Whipple's disease	Maladie de Whipple	Morbo di Whipple	Whippleova bolest
Enfermedad del corazón (cardiopatía)	Heart disease (cardiopathy)	Maladie cardiaque (cardiopathie)	Malattia del cuore (cardiopatia)	Srčana bolest (kardiopatija)
Enfermedad diverticular	Diverticulosis	Diverticulose	Diverticolosi	Divertikuloza
Enfermedad hemolítica del recién nacido (incompatibilidad Rh)	Rh incompatibility (hemolytic disease of the newborn)	Maladie hémolytique du nouveau-né	Eritroblastosi fetale (malattia emolitica del neonato)	Rh-inkompatibilnost (hemolitička bolest novorođenćeta)
Enfermedad parasitaria (parasitosis)	Parasitic disease (parasitosis)	Maladie parasitique (parasitose)	Malattia parassitaria (parassitosi)	Parazitarna bolest (parazitoza)
Enfermedad pélvica inflamatoria	Pelvic inflammatory disease	Maladie pelvienne inflammatoire	Malattia infiammatoria pelvica	Upalna bolest zdjelice
Enfermedad poliquística renal	Polycystic kidney disease	Rein polykystique	Rene policistico	Policistični bubreg
Enfermedad profesional	Occupational disease	Maladie professionnelle	Malattia professionale	Profesionalno oboljenje
Enfermedad pulmonar intersticial	Interstitial lung disease	Maladie pulmonaire interstitielle	Pneumopatia interstiziale	Intersticijska bolest pluća
Enfermedad pulmonar obstructiva crónica	Chronic obstructive pulmonary disease	Broncho-pneumopathie chronique obstructive	Bronchite cronica	Kronična opstruktivna plućna bolest
Enfermedades de la aorta	Diseases of the aorta	Maladies de l'aorte	Malattie dell'aorta	Bolesti aorte
Enfermedades de las válvulas del corazón	Heart valve diseases	Maladies des valves cardiaques	Malattie delle valvole cardiache	Bolesti srčanih zalistaka
Enfermedades de los vasos sanguíneos	Blood vessel diseases	Maladies des vaisseaux sanguins	Malattie dei vasi sanguigni	Bolesti krvnih žila
Enfermedades infantiles contagiosas	Childhood infectious diseases	Maladies infectieuses des enfants	Malattie infettive dei bambini	Dječje zarazne bolesti
Enfisema	Emphysema	Emphysème	Enfisema	Emfizem
Enfisema subcutáneo	Subcutaneous emphysema	Emphisème sous-cutané	Enfisema sottocutaneo	Potkožni emfizem
Engorde (ganar peso)	Gaining weight	Grossissement	Ingrossamento (divenire grosso)	Debljanje
Enrojecimiento de la piel (eritema)	Redness of the skin (erythema)	Érythème (rougeur de la peau)	Eritema	Crvenilo kože (eritem)
Entesopatía	Enthesopathy	Enthésiopathie	Entesopatia	Entezopatija
Envenenamiento (intoxicación)	Poisoning (toxication)	Empoisonnement (toxicité)	Avvelenamento (intossicazione)	Trovanje

Español	Inglés	Francés	Italiano	Croata
Envenenamiento por arsénico	Arsenic poisoning	Empoisonnement à l'arsenic	Avvelenamento da arsenico	Trovanje arsenom
Envenenamiento por asbesto	Asbestos poisoning	Empoisonnement par l'amiante	Avvelenamento da amianto	Trovanje azbestom
Envenenamiento por cadmio	Cadmium poisoning	Empoisonnement au cadmium	Avvelenamento da cadmio	Trovanje kadmijem
Envenenamiento por cianuro	Cyanide poisoning	Empoisonnement au cyanure	Avvelenamento da cianuro	Trovanje cijanidom
Envenenamiento por gas	Gas poisoning	Empoisonnement au gaz	Avvelenamento da gas	Trovanje plinom
Envenenamiento por insecticidas	Insecticide poisoning	Empoisonnement au insecticide	Avvelenamento da insetticidi	Trovanje insekticidima
Envenenamiento por mercurio	Mercury poisoning	Empoisonnement au mercure	Avvelenamento da mercurio	Trovanje živom
Envenenamiento por metales pesados	Heavy metal poisoning	Empoisonnement aux métaux lourds	Intossicazione da metalli pesanti	Trovanje teškim metalima
Envenenamiento por plomo	Lead poisoning	Empoisonnement au plomb	Avvelenamento da piombo (saturnismo)	Trovanje olovom
Envenenamiento por radiación	Radiation poisoning	Empoisonnement par radiations	Avvelenamento da radiazione	Trovanje zračenjem
Envenenamiento por setas	Mushroom poisoning	Empoisonnement par des champignons	Avvelenamento da funghi	Trovanje gljivama
Envenenamiento por talio	Thallium poisoning	Empoisonnement au thallium	Avvelenamento da tallio	Trovanje talijem
Eosinofilia	Eosinophilia	Éosinophilie	Eosinofilia	Eozinofilija
Ependimoma	Ependymoma	Épendymome	Ependimoma	Ependimom
Epifisario de la cabeza femoral (epifisiolisis capitis femoris)	Epiphyseolysis capitis femoris	Épiphysiolyse de l'extrémité supérieure du fémur	Epifisiolisi della testa femorale	Epifizeoliza glave bedrene kosti
Epilepsia	Epilepsy	Épilepsie	Epilessia	Epilepsija
Epispadia	Epispadias	Épispadias	Epispadia	Epispadija
Erección sostenida y dolorosa (priapismo)	Long-lasting painful erection (priapism)	Érection persistente douloureuse (priapisme)	Erezione persistente dolorosa (priapismo)	Dugotrajna bolna erekcija (prijapizam)
Erisipela	Erysipelas (Ignis sacer, St. Anthony's fire)	Érysipèle (érésipèle)	Erisipela	Crveni vjetar (vrbanac, erizipel)
Erisipeloide	Erysipeloid	Érysipéloïde	Erisipeloide	Erizipeloid
Eritema infeccioso (quinta enfermedad)	Infectious erythema (fifth disease)	Érythème infectieux (cinquième maladie)	Eritema infettivo (quinta malattia)	Infektivni eritem (peta bolest)
Eritromelalgia	Erythromelalgia (acromelalgia)	Érythromelalgie	Eritromelalgia	Eritromelalgija
Eritroplasia	Erythroplakia (erythroplasia)	Érythroplasie	Eritroplachia (eritroplasia)	Eritroplazija
Eritroplasia de Queyrat	Erythroplasia of Queyrat	Érythroplasie de Queyrat	Eritroplasia di Queyrat	Eritroplazija Queyrat
Erosión cervical	Cervical erosion	Érosion du col de l'utérus	Erosione cervicale	Cervikalna erozija
Eructo	Burping (belching)	Rot (renvoi, éructation)	Eruttazione	Podrigivanje
Escalofrío (tiritón)	Shivering	Frissonnement	Brivido	Zimica (tresavica)
Escarlatina (fiebre escarlata)	Scarlet fever	Scarlatine (fièvre écarlate)	Scarlattina	Šarlah (skarlatina)
Esclerodermia	Scleroderma	Sclérodermie	Sclerodermia	Sklerodermija
Esclerosis lateral amiotrófica	Amyotrophic lateral sclerosis	Sclérose latérale amyotrophique (maladie de Charcot)	Sclerosi laterale amiotrofica	Amiotrofična lateralna skleroza
Esclerosis múltiple	Multiple sclerosis	Sclérose en plaques	Sclerosi multipla	Multipla skleroza
Escoliosis	Scoliosis	Scoliose	Scoliosi	Skolioza
Escorbuto	Scurvy	Scorbut	Scorbuto	Skorbut
Escotoma	Scotoma	Scotome	Scotoma	Skotom
Espalda del gimnasta	Gymnastics lower back pain	Lombalgie du gymnaste	Lombalgia dell'atleta	Gimnastičarska bolna križa
Espasmo (calambre)	Spasm (cramp)	Spasme (crampe)	Spasmo (contrazione involontaria)	Grč (spazam)
Espasmo facial	Facial spasm	Spasme facial	Spasmo facciale	Grč mišića lica
Espasmo muscular (calambre)	Muscular cramp (spasm)	Crampe musculaire (spasme)	Spasmo muscolare	Mišićni grč (spazam)
Espasmo vaginal (vaginismo)	Vaginal spasm (vaginismus)	Spasme vaginal (vaginisme)	Spasmo di vagina (vaginismo)	Grč rodnice (vaginizam)
Espermatocele	Spermatocele	Spermatocèle	Spermatocele (cisti spermatica)	Spermatokela (cista epididimisa)
Espina bífida	Spina bifida	Spina bifida	Spina bifida	Spina bifida
Esplenomegalia	Splenomegaly	Splénomégalie	Splenomegalia	Splenomegalija
Espondilitis	Spondylitis	Spondilite	Spondilite	Spondilitis
Espondilitis anquilosante (morbus Bechterew)	Ankylosing spondylitis (Bechterew's syndrome)	Spondylarthrite ankylosante (morbus Bechterew)	Spondilite anchilosante	Ankilozantni spondilitis (Bechterewov sindrom)
Espondilitis tuberculosa	Tuberculous spondylitis (Pott disease)	Mal de Pott (tuberculose vertébrale)	Spondilite tubercolare (morbo di Pott)	Tuberkulozni spondilitis (Pottova bolest)
Espondilolistesis	Spondylolisthesis	Spondylolisthésis	Spondilolistesi	Spondilolisteza
Espondilosis	Spondylosis	Spondylose	Spondilosi	Spondiloza
Esporotricosis	Sporotrichosis	Sporotrichose	Sporotricosi	Sporotrihoza
Espuela de talón (espuela calcánea)	Heel spur (calcaneal spur)	Éperon de talon (epine calcaneenne)	Spina nel calcagno (spina calcaneare)	Petni trn

Español	Inglés	Francés	Italiano	Croata
Esputo espumoso	Foamy sputum	Crachat spumeux	Sputo schiumoso	Pjenušavi ispljuvak
Esputo que contiene pus	Pus in sputum	Crachat purulent	Presenza di pus nello sputo	Gnojni ispljuvak
Esquistosomiasis (bilharziasis)	Schistosomiasis (snail fever)	Schistosomiase (bilharziose)	Schistosomiasi	Šistosomijaza
Esquizofrenia	Schizophrenia	Schizophrénie	Schizofrenia	Šizofrenija
Estenosis congénita del píloro	Congenital pyloric stenosis	Sténose congénitale du pylore	Stenosi pilorica congenita	Urođena stenoza pilorusa
Estenosis de la arteria pulmonar	Stenosis of pulmonary artery	Sténose de l'artère pulmonaire	Stenosi dell'arteria polmonare	Stenoza plućne arterije
Estenosis de la válvula aórtica	Aortic valve stenosis	Sténose valvulaire aortique	Stenosi aortica	Stenoza aortnog ušća
Estenosis de la válvula pulmonar	Pulmonary valve stenosis	Sténose de la valve pulmonaire	Stenosi polmonare	Stenoza plućnog ušća (pulmonalna stenoza)
Estenosis del píloro	Pyloric stenosis	Sténose du pylore	Stenosi pilorica	Stenoza pilorusa (pilorostenoza)
Estenosis esofágica	Esophageal stenosis	Sténose oesophagienne	Stenosi esofagea	Stenoza jednjaka
Estenosis mitral	Mitral stenosis	Sténose mitrale	Stenosi mitralica	Stenoza mitralnog ušća
Estenosis pilórica hipertrófica	Hypertrophic pyloric stenosis	Sténose hypertrophique du pylore	Stenosi ipertrofica del piloro	Hipertrofijska stenoza pilorusa
Estocada	Stab wound	Coup de couteau	Ferita da punta	Ubodna rana
Estornudo	Sneezing	Éternuement	Starnuto	Kihanje
Estrabismo	Strabismus	Strabisme	Strabismo	Razrokost (strabizam)
Estrangulamiento	Strangulation	Strangulation (étranglement)	Strangolamento (strozzamento)	Davljenje
Estreñimiento	Constipation (obstipation)	Constipation	Stitichezza (costipazione)	Zatvor (opstipacija)
Estridor	Breathing sound due to blockage in the airway (stridor)	Bruit anormal émis lors de la respiration (stridor)	Rumore durante la respirazione (stridore)	Glasno otežano disanje (stridor)
Estupor	Stupor	Stupeur	Stupore	Stupor
Exantema	Exanthem	Exanthème	Esantema	Egzantem
Exasperación	Exasperation	Exaspération (irritation)	Esasperazione (irritazione)	Razdražljivost
Excesiva producción de saliva (hipersalivación)	Excessive secretion of saliva (hypersalivation)	Sécrétion de la salive excessive	Produzione di saliva eccessiva (ipersalivazione)	Pojačano lučenje sline (hipersalivacija)
Excesiva producción de sudor (hiperhidrosis)	Excessive sweating (hyperhidrosis)	Sudation excessive (hyperhidrose)	Aumento della sudorazione (iperidrosi)	Prekomjerno znojenje (hiperhidroza)
Exceso de cabello (hipertricosis)	Increased hairiness (hypertrichosis)	Pilosité excessive (hypertrichose)	Aumento della pelosità (ipertricosi)	Pojačana dlakavost
Exoftalmos	Bulging eyes (exophthalmos)	Exophtalmie (proptose)	Esoftalmo	Izbuljene oči (egzoftalmus)
Exostosis	Exostosis	Exostose	Esostosi	Egzostoza
Exostosis múltiple hereditaria	Hereditary multiple exostoses	Maladie des exostoses multiples	Esostosi multipla ereditaria	Multiple egzostoze
Expectoración de sangre (hemoptisis)	Expectoration of blood (hemoptysis)	Rejet de sang issu des voies aériennes (hémoptysie)	Espettorazione di sangue (emottisi)	Iskašljavanje krvi (hemoptiza, hemoptoja)
Exposición a las radiaciones ionizantes	Ionising irradiation	Irradiation ionisante	Esposizione alle radiazioni ionizzanti	Ionizirajuća ozračenost
Expresión vocal involuntaria de obscenidades (coprolalia)	Involuntary swearing (coprolalia)	Tic de langage à dire des mots vulgaires (coprolalie)	Coprolalia	Nekontrolirano psovanje (koprolalija)
Eyaculación precoz	Premature ejaculation	Éjaculation précoce	Eiaculazione precoce	Prijevremena ejakulacija
Fallo hepático (insuficiencia hepática)	Liver insufficiency	Insuffisance hépatique	Insufficienza epatica	Zatajenje jetre
Fallo renal (insuficiencia renal)	Kidney failure (renal insufficiency)	Insuffisance rénale	Insufficienza renale	Zatajenje bubrega (insuficijencija bubrega)
Falta de aire (disnea)	Shortness of breath (dyspnea)	Difficulté respiratoire (dyspnée)	Fame d'aria (dispnea, respirazione difficoltosa)	Zaduha (nedostatak daha, dispneja)
Falta de respiración (apnea)	Suspension of external breathing (apnea)	Arrêt respiratoire (apnée)	Assenza di respirazione (apnea)	Zastoj disanja (apnea)
Falta de visión en luz brillante (hemeralopia)	Day blindness (hemeralopia)	Héméralopie	Emeralopia	Kokošje sljepilo (hemeralopija)
Faringitis por estreptococo	Streptococcal pharyngitis	Pharyngite streptococcique	Faringite streptococcica	Streptokokna angina
Fascitis necrotizante	Necrotizing fasciitis	Fasciite nécrosante	Fascite necrotizzante	Nekrotizirajući fasciitis
Fascitis plantar	Plantar fasciitis	Fasciite plantaire	Fasciosi plantare	Plantarni fasciitis
Fenilcetonuria	Phenylketonuria	Phénylcétonurie	Fenilchetonuria	Fenilketonurija
Fenómeno de Bell	Bell's phenomenon	Phénomène de Bell	Fenomeno di Bell	Bellov fenomen
Feocromocitoma	Pheochromocytoma	Phéochromocytome	Feocromocitoma	Feokromocitom (tumor srži nadbubrežne žljezde)
Fibrilación auricular	Atrial fibrillation	Fibrillation auriculaire	Fibrillazione atriale	Atrijska fibrilacija
Fibrilación ventricular	Ventricular fibrillation	Fibrillation ventriculaire	Fibrillazione ventricolare	Ventrikularna fibrilacija
Fibroadenoma	Fibroadenoma	Fibroadénome	Fibroadenoma	Fibroadenom
Fibroelastosis endocardial	Endocardial fibroelastosis	Fibroélastose endocardique	Fibroelastosi endocardica	Fibroelastoza endokarda
Fibroma	Fibroma	Fibrome	Fibroma	Fibrom
Fibroma blando (fibroma molle)	Soft fibroma (fibroma molle, acrochordon)	Molluscum pendulum (acrochordon)	Mollusco pendule (fibroma molle)	Kožni privjesak (mekani fibrom)
Fibroma condromixoide	Chondromyxoid fibroma	Fibrome chondromyxoïde	Fibroma condromixoide	Hondromiksoidni fibrom
Fibromialgia	Fibromyalgia	Fibromyalgie	Fibromialgia	Fibromialgija

Español	Inglés	Francés	Italiano	Croata
Fibrosarcoma	Fibrosarcoma (fibroblastic sarcoma)	Fibrosarcome	Fibrosarcoma	Fibrosarkom
Fibrosis	Fibrosis	Fibrose	Fibrosi	Fibroza
Fibrosis pulmonar idiopática	Idiopathic pulmonary fibrosis	Fibrose pulmonaire idiopathique	Fibrosi polmonare idiopatica	Plućna idiopatska fibroza
Fibrosis quística (mucoviscidosis)	Cystic fibrosis	Mucoviscidose (fibrose kystique)	Fibrosi cistica	Cistična fibroza
Fibrosis retroperitoneal	Retroperitoneal fibrosis (Ormond's disease)	Fibrose rétropéritonéale (maladie d'Ormond)	Fibrosi retroperitoneale	Retroperitonealna fibroza (Ormondova bolest)
Fibrositis (reuma-tismo muscular)	Muscular fibrositis	Fibrosite musculaire	Fibrosite muscolare	Fibrozitis mišića
Fibrositis de la mano	Hand fibrositis	Fasciite de la main (fasciite palmaire)	Fibrosite di mano	Fibrozitis šake
Fibrositis de tendón	Tendinous fibrositis	Fibrosite du tendon	Fibrosi tendinea	Fibrozitis tetive
Fiebre	Fever	Fièvre	Febbre	Groznica (vrućica)
Fiebre amarilla	Yellow fever	Fièvre jaune	Febbre gialla	Žuta groznica
Fiebre de la Oroya (enfermedad de Carrión, verruga peruana)	Oroya fever (Carrion's disease)	Fièvre d'Oroya (maladie de Carrion)	Febbre di Oroya	Oroya groznica (Carrionova bolest)
Fiebre de Lassa	Lassa fever	Fièvre de Lassa	Febbre di Lassa	Groznica Lassa
Fiebre de los vapores metálicos	Metal fume fever	Fièvre des métaux	Febbre da inalazione di fumi metallici	Metalna groznica
Fiebre de Rift Valley	Rift Valley fever	Fièvre de la vallée du Rift	Febbre della Rift Valley	Rift Valley groznica
Fiebre del Colorado por garrapatas (fiebre de montaña americana por garrapatas)	Colorado tick fever (mountain tick fever)	Fièvre à tiques du Colorado (fièvre à tiques des montagnes)	Febbre da zecca del Colorado	Groznica planinskog krpelja
Fiebre del Nilo Occidental	West Nile fever	Fièvre du Nil occidental	Febbre del Nilo occidentale	Groznica zapadnog Nila
Fiebre del Zika	Zika fever	Fièvre Zika	Febbre Zika	Zika groznica
Fiebre hemorrágica con síndrome renal (fiebre hemorrágica coreana)	Hemorrhagic fever with renal syndrome (Korean hemorrhagic fever)	Fièvre hémorragique avec syndrome rénal (fièvre hémorragique de Corée)	Febbre emorragica con sindrome renale (febbre emorragica coreana)	Hemoragijska groznica s renalnim sindromom (korejska hemoragijska groznica)
Fiebre hemorrágica de Crimea-Congo	Crimean-Congo hemorrhagic fever	Fièvre hémorragique de Congo-Crimée	Febbre emorragica Crimean-Congo	Krimska hemoragijska groznica
Fiebre hemorrágica de Marburgo	Marburg hemorrhagic fever	Fièvre hémorragique de Marbourg	Febbre emorragica di Marburg	Marburška hemoragijska groznica
Fiebre hemorrágica viral	Viral hemorrhagic fever	Fièvre hémorragique virale	Febbre emorragica	Virusna hemoragijska groznica
Fiebre hemorrágica viral de Ébola	Ebola hemorrhagic fever	Fièvre Ébola	Ebola	Groznica Ebola
Fiebre mediterránea familiar	Familial Mediterranean fever	Fièvre méditerranéenne familiale	Febbre mediterranea familiare	Obiteljska mediteranska groznica
Fiebre pappataci	Pappataci fever (phlebotomus fever, sandfly fever)	Fièvre pappataci (fièvre à phlébotomes)	Febbre da pappataci (febbre da Flebotomi)	Papatači-groznica
Fiebre paratifoidea	Paratyphoid fever	Fièvre paratyphoïde	Febbre paratifoide	Trbušni paratifus
Fiebre por mordedura de rata	Rat-bite fever	Fièvre de la morsure de rat	Febbre da morso di ratto	Groznica štakorskog ugriza
Fiebre Q	Q fever	Fièvre Q	Febbre Q	Q-groznica
Fiebre reincidente	Relapsing fever	Fièvre récurrente	Febbre ricorrente	Povratna groznica
Fiebre reumática	Rheumatic fever	Rhumatisme articulaire aigu (maladie de Bouillaud)	Febbre reumatica	Reumatska groznica
Fiebre tifoidea (fiebre entérica)	Typhoid fever (typhoid)	Fièvre typhoïde (typhus abdominal)	Febbre tifoide (tifo)	Tifusna groznica (tifus)
Filariasis	Filariasis	Filariose	Filariasi	Filarijaza
Fimosis	Phimosis	Phimosis	Fimosi	Fimoza
Fístula	Fistula	Fistule	Fistola	Fistula
Fístula anal	Anal fistula	Fistule anale	Fistola anale	Analna fistula
Fístula bronco-pleural	Bronchopleural fistula	Fistule bronchopleurale	Fistola broncopleurica	Bronhopleuralna fistula
Fisura anal	Anal fissure	Fissure anale	Fissura anale	Analna fisura
Flebotrombosis	Phlebothrombosis	Phlébothrombose	Flebotrombosi	Flebotromboza
Flegmón	Phlegmon	Phlegmon	Flemmone	Flegmona
Flexibilidad anormal	Abnormal flexibility	Flexibilité anormale	Movimento anormale	Abnormalna gibljivost
Flujo (descarga, secreción)	Discharge	Sécrétion (suintement, écoulement)	Fuoriuscita (scolo)	Iscjedak
Flujo vaginal	Vaginal discharge	Pertes vaginales	Fuoriuscita vaginale	Vaginalni iscjedak
Fobia	Phobia	Phobie	Fobia	Fobija
Foliculitis	Folliculitis	Folliculite	Follicolite	Folikulitis
Forúnculo (furúnculo)	Furuncle (boil)	Furoncle	Foruncolo	Furunkul (čir na koži)
Fotofobia (intolerancia a la luz)	Photophobia (fear of light)	Photophobie (crainte de la lumière)	Fotofobia	Fotofobija (strah od svjetla)
Fractura abierta	Open fracture (compound fracture)	Fracture ouverte	Frattura aperta (frattura esposta)	Otvoreni prijelom kosti
Fractura cominuta	Comminuted fracture	Fracture comminutive	Frattura comminuta	Kominutivni prijelom kosti
Fractura de clavícula	Broken collarbone (clavicle fracture)	Fracture de la clavicule	Frattura della clavicola	Prijelom ključne kosti

Español	Inglés	Francés	Italiano	Croata
Fractura de costilla	Broken rib (rib fracture)	Fracture de côte	Frattura della costola	Prijelom rebra
Fractura de cúbito	Broken ulna (ulna fracture)	Fracture de l'ulna	Frattura dell'ulna	Prijelom lakatne kosti
Fractura de cuello del fémur	Femoral neck fracture	Fracture du col du fémur	Frattura del collo del femore	Prijelom vrata bedrene kosti
Fractura de cuello del húmero	Humeral neck fracture	Fracture du col de l'humérus	Frattura del collo dell'omero	Prijelom vrata nadlaktične kosti
Fractura de cuerpo vertebral	Broken vertebral body (vertebral corpus fracture)	Fracture du plateau vertébral	Frattura del corpo vertebrale	Prijelom trupa kralješka
Fractura de epicóndilo humeral	Epicondylar elbow fracture	Fracture du condyle huméral	Frattura dell'epicondilo omerale	Prijelom kondila nadlaktične kosti
Fractura de escafoides (fractura navicular)	Broken navicular bone (navicular fracture)	Fracture du scaphoïde	Frattura dell'osso navicolare	Prijelom navikularne kosti
Fractura de escápula	Broken shoulder blade (scapula fracture)	Fracture de la scapula	Frattura della scapola	Prijelom lopatice
Fractura de falange del dedo	Broken finger (finger fracture)	Fracture du doigt	Frattura della falange del dito	Prijelom članka prsta
Fractura de fémur	Broken thighbone (femur fracture)	Fracture du fémur	Frattura del femore	Prijelom bedrene kosti
Fractura de hueso	Broken bone (bone fracture)	Fracture des os	Frattura	Prijelom kosti (fraktura kosti)
Fractura de la base del cráneo	Base of skull fracture (basal skull fracture)	Fracture de la base du crâne	Frattura della base del cranio	Prijelom baze lubanje
Fractura de la cabeza del radio	Radial head fracture (radial capitulum fracture)	Fracture de la tête radiale	Frattura del capitello radiale	Prijelom glavice palčane kosti
Fractura de la diáfisis del fémur	Diaphyseal tightbone fracture	Fracture de la diaphyse fémorale	Frattura della diafisi femorale	Prijelom dijafize bedrene kosti
Fractura de la rótula	Broken knee cap (patellar fracture)	Fracture de rotule	Frattura della rotula	Prijelom ivera (prijelom patele)
Fractura de los huesos del dedo gordo del pie	Broken big toe (fractured hallux)	Fracture du gros orteil	Frattura dell'alluce	Prijelom falange nožnog palca
Fractura de maxilar y/o mandíbula	Upper and/or lower jaw fracture (broken upper/lower jaw)	Fracture du maxillaire et/ou de la mandibule	Frattura della mascella e/o della mandibola	Prijelom gornje i/ili donje čeljusti
Fractura de metatarso	Broken foot (metatarsal fracture)	Fracture métatarsienne	Frattura del metatarso	Prijelom kosti stopala
Fractura de olécranon	Broken elbow (olecranon fracture)	Fracture de l'olécrâne	Frattura dell'olecrano	Prijelom lakatnog vrha (prijelom olekranona)
Fractura de pelvis	Broken pelvis (pelvis fracture)	Fracture du bassin	Frattura del bacino	Prijelom zdjelice
Fractura de radio y cúbito	Broken forearm (fractured ulna and radius)	Fracture du radius et du cubitus	Frattura di radio e ulna	Prijelom obje podlaktične kosti
Fractura de tibia	Broken shinbone (tibia fracture)	Fracture du tibia	Frattura della tibia	Prijelom goljenične kosti
Fractura de tibia y peroné	Broken lower leg bones (fractured tibia and fibula)	Fracture du tibia et de la fibula	Frattura di tibia e perone	Prijelom obje kosti potkoljenice
Fractura de tobillo	Broken ankle (ankle fracture)	Fracture de la cheville	Frattura della caviglia	Prijelom gležnja
Fractura del calcáneo	Broken heel bone (calcaneus fracture)	Fracture du calcanéus	Frattura del calcagno	Prijelom petne kosti
Fractura del húmero	Broken upper arm (humerus fracture)	Fracture de l'humérus	Frattura dell'omero	Prijelom nadlaktice
Fractura del peroné	Broken fibula (fibula fracture)	Fracture de la fíbula	Frattura della fibula	Prijelom lisne kosti
Fractura del radio	Radius fracture	Fracture du radius	Frattura del radio	Prijelom palčane kosti
Fractura diafisaria del húmero	Diaphyseal humeral fracture	Fracture diaphysaire de l'humérus	Frattura diafisaria dell'omero	Prijelom nadlaktice u području dijafize
Fractura distal del radio	Distal radial fracture	Fracture de l'extrémité inferieure du radius (fracture de Pouteau-Colles)	Frattura di Pouteau-Colles (frattura delle metafisi radiali distali)	Prijelom palčane kosti loco typico
Fractura en rama verde	Greenstick fracture	Fracture en bois vert	Frattura a legno verde	Prijelom mlade kosti
Fractura espiral	Spiral fracture	Fracture en spirale	Frattura a spirale	Spiralni prijelom kosti
Fractura incompleta	Incomplete fracture	Fracture incomplète	Frattura incompleta (infrazione)	Nepotpuni prijelom kosti (napuknuće kosti)
Fractura obliqua	Oblique fracture	Fracture oblique	Frattura obliqua	Kosi prijelom kosti
Fractura por estrés	Stress fracture	Fracture de fatigue	Frattura da stress	Prijelom zamora
Fractura por estrés de la tibia	Tibia stress fracture	Fracture de fatigue du tibia	Frattura da stress della tibia	Prijelom zamora goljenične kosti
Fractura repetida	Refracturing (repeated fracture)	Fracture répétée	Frattura ripetuta	Opetovani prijelom kosti
Fractura simple	Simple bone fracture	Fracture simple	Frattura semplice	Jednostavni prijelom kosti
Fractura supracondilar del fémur	Supracondylar femoral fracture	Fracture supracondylienne du fémur	Frattura sovracondiloidea del femore	Suprakondilarni prijelom bedrene kosti
Fractura supracondilar del húmero	Supracondylar humerus fracture	Fracture supracondylienne de l'humérus	Frattura sovracondiloidea di omero	Suprakondilarni prijelom nadlaktice
Fractura supramaleolar de tibia y peroné	Supramaleolar fracture of tibia and fibula	Fracture tibia péroné sus-malléolaire	Frattura del terzo distale di tibia e perone	Supramaleolarni prijelom potkoljenice

Español	Inglés	Francés	Italiano	Croata
Fractura transversal	Transverse fracture	Fracture transversale	Frattura trasversale	Poprečni prijelom kosti
Fractura-dislocación	Fracture with displacement	Fracture à déplacement	Frattura con dislocazione	Prijelom kosti s pomakom
Fracturas espontáneas	Spontaneous fractures	Fractures spontanées	Fratture spontanee	Spontane frakture
Frigidez	Frigidity	Frigidité	Frigidità	Frigidnost
Fusión congenita de vértebras cervicales (síndrome de Klippel-Feil)	Congenital fusion of cervical vertebrae (Klippel-Feil syndrome)	Fusion congénitale de vertèbres cervicales (Syndrome de Klippel-Feil)	Fusione di vertebre cervicali (Sindrome di Klippel Feil)	Srašteni vrat (sindrom Klippel-Feil)
Galactorrea	Galactorrhea	Galactorrhée	Galattorrea	Galaktoreja
Ganas de vomitar	Urge to vomit	Envie de vomir	Impulso a vomitare	Podražaj na povraćanje
Gangrena	Gangrene	Gangrène	Cancrena	Gangrena
Gangrena de Fournier	Fournier gangrene	Gangrène de Fournier	Gangrena di Fournier	Fournierova gangrena
Gangrena gaseosa	Gas gangrene	Gangrène gazeuse	Gangrene gassosa	Plinska gangrena
Gangrena húmeda	Wet gangrene	Gangrène humide	Gangrena umida	Vlažna gangrena
Gangrena seca	Dry gangrene	Gangrène sèche	Gangrena secca	Suha gangrena
Gasto urinario excesivo (poliuria)	Passage of large volumes of urine (polyuria)	Sécrétion d'urine en quantité abondante (polyurie)	Aumentata emissione di urina (poliuria)	Učestalo mokrenje velikih količina mokraće (poliurija)
Gastroenteritis	Gastroenteritis	Gastroentérite	Gastroenterite	Gastroenteritis
Genu valgo	Knock knees (genu valgum)	Genou cagneux (genu valgum, genou en X)	Ginocchio valgo	Genu valgum
Genu varum	Bow legs (genu varum)	Genu varum	Ginocchio varo (genu varum)	Genu varum
Giardiasis (lambliasis)	Lambliasis (giardiasis)	Lambliase (giardiase)	Giardiasi (lambliasi)	Lamblijaza (giardijaza)
Gigantismo	Gigantism	Gigantisme	Gigantismo	Divovski stas
Ginecomastia	Gynecomastia	Gynécomastie	Ginecomastia	Ginekomastija
Glaucoma	Glaucoma	Glaucome	Glaucoma	Glaukom
Glioblastoma	Glioblastoma	Glioblastome	Glioblastoma	Glioblastom
Glioma	Glioma	Gliome	Glioma	Gliom
Gliosis	Gliosis	Gliose	Gliosi	Glioza
Glomerulonefritis	Glomerulonephritis	Gloméluronéphrite	Glomerulonefrite	Glomerulonefritis
Gonadoblastoma	Gonadoblastoma	Gonadoblastome	Gonadoblastoma	Gonadoblastom
Gonorrea (blenorragia, blenorrea)	Gonorrhea	Gonorrhée (blennorragie, chaude-pisse)	Gonorrea (blenorragia)	Gonoreja (kapavac, triper)
Gota (enfermedad gotosa)	Gout (gouty arthritis)	Goutte	Gotta	Ulozi (giht)
Goteo nasal (rinorrea)	Runny nose (rinorrhea)	Écoulement par le nez (rhinorrhée)	Naso che cola (rinorrea)	Curenje iz nosa (rinoreja)
Granulocitosis	Granulocytosis	Polynucléose	Granulocitosi	Granulocitoza
Gripe (gripa, influenza)	Flu (influenza)	Grippe (influenza)	Influenza	Gripa (influenca)
Gripe aviar H5N1	Bird flu (influenzavirus A subtype H5N1)	Grippe aviaire (influenzavirus A sous-type H5N1)	Influenza aviaria H5N1	Ptičja gripa podtip H5N1
Gripe española	Spanish flu	Grippe espagnole	Influenza spagnola	Španjolska gripa
Gripe porcina (influenza porcina, gripe del cerdo)	Pig flu (swine influenza, influenzavirus A subtype H1N1)	Grippe porcine	Influenza suina	Svinjska gripa
Hambre	Hunger	Faim	Fame	Glad
Heces acuosas	Watery stool	Selles aqueuses	Consistenza acquosa delle feci	Vodenasta stolica
Heces amarillas	Yellow stool	Selles jaunes	Feci gialle	Žuta stolica
Heces de color rojo	Red colored stool	Selles rouges	Feci di colore rosso	Crvena stolica
Heces negras (melena)	Black stool (melena)	Selles noir (melanea, méléna)	Feci picee (melena)	Crna stolica (melena)
Heces verdes	Green stool	Selles vertes	Feci di colore verde	Zelenkasta stolica
Hemangioendotelioma	Hemangioendothelioma	Hémangio-endothéliome	Emangioendotelioma	Hemangioendoteliom
Hemangioma	Hemangioma	Hémangiome	Emangioma	Hemangiom
Hemangioma capilar (marca de fresa)	Capillary hemangioma (infantile hemangioma, strawberry hemangioma)	Hémangiome capillaire	Emangioma capillare	Kapilarni hemangiom
Hemangioma cavernoso	Cavernous hemangioma	Cavernome (angiome caverneux)	Emangioma cavernoso	Kavernozni hemangiom
Hematoma	Hematoma	Hématome	Ematoma	Hematom
Hematoma epidural	Epidural hematoma	Hématome épidural	Ematoma epidurale	Epiduralni hematom
Hematoma intracerebral	Intracerebral hematoma	Hématome intracérébral	Ematoma cerebrale	Intracerebralni hematom
Hematoma subdural	Subdural hematoma	Hématome subdural	Ematoma subdurale	Subduralni hematom
Hemicránea crónica paroxismal	Chronic paroxysmal hemicrania (Sjaastad syndrome)	Hémicrânie paroxystique chronique	Emicrania cronica parossistica	Kronična paroksizmalna hemikranija (Sjaastadov sindrom)
Hemivértebra	Hemivertebrae	Hémivertèbre	Emivertebra	Hemivertebra
Hemocromatosis	Hemochromatosis	Hémochromatose	Emocromatosi	Hemokromatoza
Hemofilia	Hemophilia	Hémophilie	Emofilia	Hemofilija
Hemoglobina en orina (hemoglobinuria)	Hemoglobin in urine (hemoglobinuria)	Hémoglobine dans l'urine (hémoglobinurie)	Presenza di emoglobina nelle urine (emoglobinuria)	Hemoglobin u urinu (hemoglobinurija)
Hemoneumotórax	Hemopneumothorax	Hémopneumothorax	Emopneumotorace	Hemopneumotoraks
Hemorragia arterial	Arterial bleeding	Hémorragie artérielle	Emorragia arteriosa	Arterijsko krvarenje
Hemorragia de oído (otorragia)	Ear bleeding	Saignement de l'oreille	Fuoriuscita di sangue dall'orecchio(otorragia)	Krvarenje iz uha
Hemorragia epidural	Epidural bleeding	Hémorragie épidurale	Emorragia epidurale	Epiduralno krvarenje
Hemorragia intracerebral	Intracerebral hemorrhage	Hémorragie intracérébrale	Emorragia cerebrale	Intracerebralno krvarenje

Español	Inglés	Francés	Italiano	Croata
Hemorragia subaracnoidea	Subarachnoid hemorrhage	Hémorragie sous arachnoïdienne	Emorragia subaracnoidea	Subarahnoidalno krvarenje
Hemorragia subdural	Subdural hemorrhage	Subdural hemorrhage	Emorragia subdurale	Subduralno krvarenje
Hemorroides	Hemorrhoids	Hémorroïdes	Emorroidi	Hemoroidi
Hemosiderosis	Hemosiderosis	Hémosidérose	Emosiderosi	Hemosideroza
Hemotórax	Hemothorax	Hémothorax	Emotorace	Hemotoraks
Hepatitis A	Hepatitis A	Hépatite A	Epatite virale A	Hepatitis A
Hepatitis B	Hepatitis B	Hépatite B	Epatite virale B	Hepatitis B
Hepatitis C	Hepatitis C	Hépatite C	Epatite virale C	Hepatitis C
Hepatitis D	Hepatitis D	Hépatite D	Epatite virale D	Hepatitis D
Hepatitis E	Hepatitis E	Hépatite E	Epatite virale E	Hepatitis E
Hepatitis viral	Viral hepatitis	Hépatite virale	Epatite virale	Virusni hepatitis
Herida	Wound (injury, lesion)	Plaie	Ferita	Rana
Herida de bala	Gunshot wound	Blessure par balle	Ferita da arma da fuoco	Prostrijelna rana
Herida por corte	Cut wound	Plaie par objet tranchant	Ferita da taglio	Rezna rana (posjekotina)
Herida por mordedura	Bite wound	Blessure par morsure	Ferita da morso	Ugrizna rana
Herida térmica	Thermal wound	Blessure thermique	Ferita termica	Termička rana
Hermafroditismo	Hermaphroditism	Hermaphrodisme	Ermafroditismo	Dvospolnost
Hernia	Hernia	Hernie	Ernia	Kila (bruh, hernija)
Hernia de hiato	Hiatus hernia	Hernie hiatale	Ernia iatale	Hijatusna kila
Hernia de la pared abdominal	External abdominal wall hernia	Hernie de la paroi abdominale (hernie abdominale externe)	Ernia esterna addominale	Kila vanjske trbušne stijenke
Hernia diafragmática	Diaphragmatic hernia	Hernie diaphragmatique	Ernia diaframmatica	Dijafragmalna kila
Hernia discale	Spinal disc herniation	Hernie discale	Ernia del disco	Hernija intervertrebralnog diska
Hernia inguinal	Inguinal hernia	Hernie inguinale	Ernia inguinale	Preponska kila
Hernia umbilical	Umbilical hernia	Hernie ombilicale	Ernia ombelicale	Pupčana kila (umbilikalna hernija)
Herpangina	Herpangina (mouth blisters)	Herpangine	Erpangina (faringite vescicolare)	Herpangina
Herpes genital	Genital herpes	Herpès génital	Herpes genitalis	Genitalni herpes
Herpes simple	Herpes simplex	Herpès (infection herpétique)	Herpes simplex	Herpes simpleks
Herpes zóster (herpes zona)	Herpes zoster	Zona	Herpes zoster	Herpes zoster
Hidatidosis (equinococosis)	Echinococcosis (hydatid disease)	Échinococcose	Echinococcosi (idatidosi)	Ehinokokoza
Hidatidosis hepática	Hepatic echinococcosis	Échinococcose hépatique	Echinococcosi epatica	Ehinokokoza jetre
Hidatidosis pulmonar	Pulmonary echinococcosis	Échinococcose pulmonaire	Echinococcosi polmonare	Ehinokokoza pluća
Hidremia	Hydremia	Hydrémie	Idremia	Hidremija
Hidrocefalia	Hydrocephalus	Hydrocéphalie	Idrocefalo	Hidrocefalus
Hidrocele	Hydrocele	Hydrocèle	Idrocele	Hidrokela
Hidronefrosis	Hydronephrosis	Hydronéphrose	Idronefrosi	Hidronefroza
Hidrops	Hydrops	Hydrops	Idrope	Hidrops
Hidrops vesicular	Gallbladder hydrops	Hydrops de la vésicule biliaire	Idrope della colecisti	Hidrops žučnog mjehura
Hidrotórax	Hydrothorax	Hydrothorax	Idrotorace	Hidrotoraks
Higroma	Hygroma	Hygroma	Igroma	Higrom
Hinchazón	Swelling	Gonflement (enflure)	Gonfiore	Oteklina
Hinchazón y gases (flatulencia, ventosidad)	Bloating and gases (flatulence)	Ballonnements et vesse (flatulence)	Gonfiezza e venti (flatulenza)	Nadutost i vjetrovi
Hipema	Hyphema	Hyphème	Ifema	Hifema
Hiperactividad	Hyperactivity	Hyperactivité	Iperattività	Hiperaktivnost
Hipercalcemia	Hypercalcemia	Hypercalcémie	Ipercalcemia	Hiperkalcijemija
Hiperinsulinismo	Hyperinsulinism	Hyperinsulinisme	Iperinsulinismo	Povišen inzulin u krvi (hiperinzulinizam)
Hipermetropía	Farsightedness (hyperopia)	Hypermétropie	Ipermetropia	Dalekovidnost
Hiperparatiroidismo	Hyperparathyroidism	Hyperparathyroïdie	Iperparatiroidismo	Hiperparatireoidizam
Hiperpituitarismo	Hyperpituitarism	Hyperpituitarisme	Iperpituitarismo	Hiperpituitarizam
Hiperplasia benigna de próstata	Benign prostatic hyperthroph	Hypertrophie bénigne de la prostate	Ipertrofia prostatica benigna	Benigna hipertrofija prostate
Hiperplasia endometrial	Endometrial hyperplasia	Hyperplasie endométriale	Iperplasia endometriale	Hiperplazija endometrija
Hiperplasia pseudoepiteliomatosa	Pseudoepitheliomatous hyperplasia	Hyperplasie pseudo-épithéliomateuse	Iperplasia pseudoepiteliomatosa	Pseudoepiteliematozna hiperplazija
Hiperpotasemia (hipercalemia)	Hyperkalemia	Hyperkaliémie	Iperkaliemia	Hiperkalijemija
Hipersensibilidad electromagnética	Electromagnetic hypersensitivity	Sensibilité électromagnétique	Elettrosensibilità	Elektromagnetska hipersenzibilnost
Hipertensión arterial pulmonar	Pulmonary hypertension	Hypertension artérielle pulmonaire	Ipertensione arteriosa polmonare	Plućna hipertenzija
Hipertensión esencial	Essential hypertension	Hypertension artérielle essentielle	Ipertensione arteriosa essenziale	Esencijalna hipertenzija
Hipertensión intracraneal	Intracranial hypertension	Hypertension intracrânienne	Elevata pressione intracranica	Intrakranijalna hipertenzija
Hipertensión maligna	Malignant hypertension	Hypertension artérielle maligne	Ipertensione maligna	Maligna hipertenzija

Español	Inglés	Francés	Italiano	Croata
Hipertensión portal	Portal hypertension	Hypertension portale	Ipertensione portale	Portalna hipertenzija
Hipertensión renovascular	Renovacsular hypertension	Hypertension rénovasculaire	Ipertensione renale	Renovaskularna hipertenzija
Hipertensión secundaria	Secondary hypertension (inessential hypertension)	Hypertension secondaire	Ipertensione arteriosa secondaria	Sekundarna hipertenzija
Hipertermia	Hyperthermia	Hyperthermie	Ipertermia	Hipertermija
Hipertiroidismo	Hyperthyroidism	Hyperthyroïdie	Ipertiroidismo	Hipertireoza
Hipertrofia	Hypertrophy	Hypertrophie	Ipertrofia	Hipertrofija
Hipertrofia ventricular	Ventricular hypertrophy	Hypertrophie ventriculaire	Ipertrofia ventricolare	Ventrikularna hipertrofija
Hiperuricemia	Hyperuricemia	Hyperuricémie	Iperuricemia	Hiperurikemija
Hiperventilación	Hyperventilation	Hyperventilation	Iperventilazione	Hiperventilacija
Hipervitaminosis	Hypervitaminosis	Hypervitaminose	Ipervitaminosi	Hipervitaminoza
Hipervolemia (aumento del volumen de sangre en la circulación)	Hypervolemia (increased level of fluid in the blood)	Hypervolémie (augmentation du volume de sang dans les vaisseaux)	Ipervolemia (aumento del volume ematico circolante)	Hipervolemija (porast volumena krvi u optoku)
Hipo	Hiccup	Hoquet	Singhiozzo	Štucavica
Hipoalbuminemia	Hypoalbuminemia	Hypoalbuminémie	Ipoalbuminemia	Hipoalbuminemija
Hipocalcemia	Hypocalcemia	Hypocalcemie	Ipocalcemia	Hipokalcijemija
Hipocaliemia	Hypokalemia	Hypokaliémie	Ipokaliemia	Hipokalijemija
Hipocondría	Hypochondria	Hypocondrie	Ipocondria	Hipohondrija
Hipoglicemia	Hypoglycemia	Hypoglycémie	Ipoglicemia	Hipoglikemija
Hipoinsulinismo	Hypoinsulinism	Hypoinsulinisme	Ipoinsulinemia	Hipoinzulinizam
Hipoparatiroidismo	Hypoparathyroidism	Hypoparathyroïdie	Ipoparatiroidismo	Hipoparatireodizam
Hipopituitarismo	Hypopituitarism	Hypopituitarisme	Ipopituitarismo	Hipopituitarizam
Hipoplasia pulmonar	Pulmonary hypoplasia	Hypoplasie pulmonaire	Ipoplasia del tronco polmonare	Hipoplazija plućnog režnja
Hipospadias	Hypospadias	Hypospadias	Ipospadia	Hipospadija
Hipotensión y síncope	Hypotension and syncope	Hypotension et syncope	Ipotensione e sincope	Hipotenzija i sinkope
Hipotermia	Hypothermia	Hypothermie	Ipotermia	Pothlađenost (hipotermija)
Hipotiroidismo	Hypothyroidism	Hypothyroïdie	Ipotiroidismo	Hipotireoza
Hipotonía	Hypotonia	Hypotonie	Ipotonia	Hipotonija
Hipotonía muscular	Muscular hypotonia	Hypotonie musculaire	Ipotonia muscolare	Mišićna hipotonija
Hipoxia	Hypoxia	Hypoxie	Ipossia	Hipoksija
Hirsutismo	Hirsutism	Hirsutisme	Irsutismo	Hirzutizam
Histeria	Hysteria	Hystérie	Isteria (isterismo)	Histerija
Histiocitoma fibroso	Fibrous histiocytoma	Histiocytome fibreux	Fibroistiocitoma benigno	Fibrozni histiocitom
Histoplasmosis	Histoplasmosis (Darling's disease)	Histoplasmose	Istoplasmosi	Histoplazmoza
Hormigueo	Tingling	Fourmillement	Intormentire	Trnjenje
Ictericia	Jaundice (icterus)	Ictère (jaunisse)	Ittero (itterizia)	Žutica (ikterus)
Ictericia del recién nacido	Neonatal jaundice	Ictère néonatal	Ittero neonatale	Novorođenačka žutica
Ictericia obstructiva	Mechanic icterus (bile duct obstruction)	Ictère par obstruction des voies biliaires	Ittero ostruttivo	Mehanički ikterus
Íleo	Ileus	Iléus	Ileo	Ileus
Imbecilidad	Imbecility	Imbécillité	Imbecillità	Slaboumnost
Impétigo	Impetigo	Impétigo	Impetigine	Impetigo
Impotencia	Impotency	Impotence	Impotenza	Impotencija
Inanición	Starvation	Famine	Inedia	Izgladnjelost
Incapacidad de movimiento	Movement inability	Incapacité de se mouvoir	Mancanza di movimento	Nemogućnost kretanja
Incapacidad para orinar	Inability to urinate	Incapacité d'uriner	Mancata secrezione di urina	Nemogućnost mokrenja
Inconsciencia	Unconsciousness	Absence de la conscience	Incoscienza (stato di incoscienza)	Nesvjestica
Incontinencia	Incontinence	Incontinence	Incontinenza	Inkontinencija
Incontinencia urinaria	Urinary incontinence	Incontinence urinaire	Incontinenza urinaria	Urinarna inkotinencija
Incontinencia urinaria por estrés	Stress urinary incontinence	Incontinence urinarie d'effort	Incontinenza urinaria da sforzo	Stres-inkontinencija urina
Incremento de la presión sanguínea (hipertensión)	High blood pressure (hypertension)	Pression artérielle élevée (hypertension artérielle)	Ipertensione arteriosa sistemica	Visoki krvni tlak (hipertenzija)
Indigestión	Indigestion	Indigestion	Indigestione	Probavne smetnje
Infarto	Infarct	Infarctus	Infarto	Infarkt
Infarto cerebral hemorrágico	Hemorrhagic brain infarction	Infarctus cérébral hémorragique	Ictus emorragico	Hemoragijski infarkt mozga
Infarto de miocardio	Heart attack (myocardial infarction)	Infarctus du myocarde	Infarto miocardico acuto	Infarkt miokarda
Infarto pulmonar	Pulmonary infarction	Infarctus pulmonaire	Infarto polmonare	Infarkt pluća
Infección	Infection	Infection	Infezione (malattia infettiva)	Infekcija
Infección bacteriana	Bacterial infection	Infection bactérienne	Infezione batterica	Bakterijska infekcija
Infección del hueso o médula ósea (osteomielitis)	Infection of the bone or bone marrow (osteomyelitis)	Infection osseuse ou de la moelle osseuse (ostéomyélite)	Infezione dell'apparato osteo-articolare (osteomielite)	Infekcija kosti ili koštane srži (osteomijelitis)
Infección por clamidia	Chlamydia infection	Infection à Chlamydia	Infezione da clamidia	Klamidijska infekcija
Infeccion por el virus del papilom humano (VPH)	Human papilloma virus (HPV) infection	Infection par le virus du papillome humain (VPH)	Infezione da Papilloma Virus Umano (HPV)	Infekcija humanim papiloma virusom (HPV)
Infección por hongos	Fungal infection	Infection fongique	Infezione fungina	Gljivična infekcija
Infección respiratoria alta	Upper respiratory tract infection	Infection respiratoire haute	Infezione del tratto respiratorio superiore	Infekcija gornjih dišnih puteva
Infección viral	Viral infection	Infection virale	Infezione virale	Virusna infekcija

Español	Inglés	Francés	Italiano	Croata
Infertilidad	Infertility (sterility)	Infertilité (stérilité)	Sterilità (infecondità)	Neplodnost (sterilitet)
Infestación de gusanos (helmintiasis)	Infestation with intestinal parasitic warms (helminthiasis)	Infestation par des vers parasites intestinaux (helminthiase)	Infestazione da vermi (elmintiasi)	Infestacija crijevnim parazitima (helmintijaza)
Infestación por ladilla (ftiriasis)	Infestation with pubic lice (phthiriasis)	Infestation par des poux du pubic (phtiriase)	Infestazione da pidocchi del pube (ftiriasi)	Infestacija stidnim ušima (iftirijaza)
Infestación por piojos (pediculosis)	Infestation with head lice (pediculosis)	Infestation par des poux (pédiculose)	Infestazione da pidocchi (pediculosi)	Infestacija ušima (ušljivost, pedikuloza)
Inflamación	Inflammation	Inflammation	Infiammazione (flogosi)	Upala
Inflamación de la bursa (bursitis)	Inflammation of the synovial fluid sac (bursitis)	Inflammation de la bo-urse séreuse articulaire (hygroma, bursite)	Infiammazione della borsa sierosa di un'ar-ticolazione (borsite)	Upala sluzne vreće (burzitis)
Inflamación de la conjuntiva (conjuntivitis)	Inflammation of the conjunctiva (conjunctivitis)	Inflammation de la conjonctive (conjonctivite)	Infiammazione della congiuntiva (congiuntivite)	Upala sluznice oka (konjuktivitis)
Inflamación de la córnea (queratitis)	Inflammation of the cornea (keratitis)	Inflammation de la cornée (kératite)	Infiammazione della cornea (cheratite)	Upala rožnice (keratitis)
Inflamación de la córnea y de la conjuntiva (queratoconjuntivitis)	Inflammation of the cornea and conjunctiva (keratoconjunctivitis)	Inflammation de la conjonctive et de la cornée (kératoconjonctivite)	Infiammazione della cornea e della congiutiva (cheratocongiuntivite)	Upala rožnice i sluznice oka (keratokonjuktivitis)
Inflamación de la epiglotis (epiglotitis)	Inflammation of the epiglottis (epiglottitis)	Inflammation de l'épiglotte (épiglottite)	Infiammazione del'epiglottide (epiglottite)	Upala epiglotisa (epiglotitis)
Inflamación de la fascia (fascitis)	Inflammation of the fascia (fasciitis)	Inflammation du fascia (fasciite)	Infiammazione della fascia (fascite)	Upala fascije (fasciitis)
Inflamación de la glándula tiroides (tiroiditis)	Inflammation of the thyroid gland (thyroiditis)	Inflammation de la glande thyroïde (thyroïdite)	Infiammazione della tiroide (tiroidite)	Upala štitnjače (tireoiditis)
Inflamación de la lámina intermedia del ojo (uveítis)	Inflammation of the middle layer of the eye (uveitis)	Inflammation de l'uvée (uvéite)	Infiammazione della tunica media dell'occhio (uveite)	Upala srednje ovojnice oka (uveitis)
Inflamación de la laringe (laringitis)	Inflammation of the larynx (laryngitis)	Inflammation du larynx (laryngite)	Infiammazione della laringe (laringite)	Upala glasnica (laringitis)
Inflamación de la membrana sinovial (sinovitis)	Inflammation of the synovial membrane (synovitis)	Inflammation de la gaine synoviale (synovite)	Infiammazione della membrana sinoviale (sinovite)	Upala tetivne ovojnice (sinovitis)
Inflamación de la mucosa bucal (estomatitis)	Inflammation of the mouth mucous lining (stomatitis)	Inflammation de la muqueuse buccale (stomatite)	Infiammazione delle mucose della bocca (stomatite)	Upala sluznice usta (stomatitis)
Inflamación de la mucosa gástrica (gastritis)	Inflammation of the stomach lining (gastritis)	Inflammation de la paroi de l'estomac (gastrite)	Infiammazione della mucosa gastrica (gastrite)	Upala želučane sluznice (gastritis)
Inflamación de la piel (dermatitis)	Inflammation of the skin (dermatitis)	Inflammaton de la peau (dermatite)	Infiammazione della pelle (dermatite)	Upala kože (dermatitis)
Inflamación de la pleura (pleuritis, pleuresía)	Inflammation of the pleura (pleuritis)	Inflammation de la plèvre (pleurésie)	Infiammazione della pleura (pleurite)	Upala plućne ovojnice (pleuritis)
Inflamación de la próstata (prostatitis)	Inflammation of the prostate gland (prostatitis)	Inflammation de la prostate (prostatite)	Infiammazione della ghian-dola prostatica (prostatite)	Upala prostate (prostatitis)
Inflamación de la retina (retinitis)	Inflammation of the retina (retinitis)	Inflammation de la rétine (rétinite)	Infiammazione della retina (retinite)	Upala mrežnice (retinitis)
Inflamación de la tráquea (traqueitis)	Inflammation of the windpipe (tracheitis)	Inflammation de la trachée (trachéite)	Infiammazione della trachea (tracheite)	Upala dušnika (traheitis)
Inflamación de la uretra (uretritis)	Inflammation of the urethra (urethritis)	Inflammation de l'urètre (urétrite)	Infiammazione dell'uretra (uretrite)	Upala sluznice mokra-ćne cijevi (uretritis)
Inflamación de la vagina (vaginitis)	Inflammation of the vagina (vaginitis)	Inflammation du vagin (vaginite)	Infiammazione della vagina (vaginite)	Upala rodnice (vaginitis)
Inflamación de la vejiga urinaria (cistitis)	Inflammation of the urinary bladder (cystitis)	Inflammation de la vessie (cystite)	Infiammazione della vescica urinaria (cistite)	Upala mokraćnog mjehura (cistitis)
Inflamación de la vesícula biliar (colecistitis)	Inflammation of the gall bladder (cholecystitis)	Inflammation de la vésicule biliaire (cholécystite)	Infiammazione della colecisti (colecistite)	Upala žučnog mjehura (holecistitis)
Inflamación de la vulva (vulvitis)	Inflammation of the vulva (vulvitis)	Inflammation de la vulve (vulvite)	Infiammazione della vulva (vulvite)	Upala stidnice (vulvitis)
Inflamación de la zona de inserción de un músculo (entesitis)	Inflammation of the entheses (enthesitis)	Inflammation de l'enthèse (enthésite)	Infiammazione dell'inserzione di muscolo (entesite)	Upala hvatišta mišića (entezitis)
Inflamación de las amígdalas palatinas (amigdalitis)	Inflammation of the tonsils (tonsillitis)	Inflammation des tonsilles (tonsillite)	Infiammazione delle tonsille (tonsillite)	Upala krajnika (tonzilitis)
Inflamación de las arterias (arteritis)	Inflammation of the arterial walls (arteritis)	Inflammation des paro-is des artères (artérite)	Infiammazione delle arterie (arterite)	Upala stijenke arterije (arteritis)
Inflamación de las encías (gingivitis)	Inflammation of the gums (gingivitis)	Inflammation de la gencive (gingivite)	Infiammazione dei tessuti gengivali (gengivite)	Upala desni (gingivitis)
Inflamación de las glándulas salivales (sialadenitis)	Inflammation of the salivary gland (sialadenitis)	Inflammation des glandes salivaires (sialoadénite)	Infiammazione delle ghiandole salivari (sialoadenite)	Upala žlijezda slinovnica (sialadenitis)
Inflamación de las meninges (meningitis)	Inflammation of the meninges (meningitis)	Inflammation des méninges (méningite)	Infiammazione delle meningi (meningite)	Upala moždanih ovojnica (meningitis)
Inflamación de las venas (flebitis)	Inflammation of the vein (phlebitis)	Inflammation des veines (phlébite)	Infiammazione delle vene (flebite)	Upala vena (flebitis)
Inflamación de los bronquiolos (bronquiolitis)	Inflammation of the bronchioles (bronchiolitis)	Inflammation des petites bronches (bronchiolite)	Infiammazione dei bronchioli (bronchiolite)	Upala bronhiola (bronhiolitis)

Español	Inglés	Francés	Italiano	Croata
Inflamación de los bronquios (bronquitis)	Inflammation of the bronchi (bronchitis)	Inflammation des bronches des poumons (bronchite)	Infiammazione dei bronchi (bronchite)	Upala bronhija (bronhitis)
Inflamación de los ganglios linfáticos (linfadenitis)	Inflammation of the lymph node (lymphadenitis)	Inflammation des ganglions (adénite, lymphadénite)	Infiammazione delle ghiandole linfatiche (linfoadenite)	Upala limfnog čvora (limfadenitis)
Inflamación de los pulmones (neumonía, pulmonía, neumonitis)	Inflammation of the lung (pneumonia)	Inflammation des poumons (pneumonie)	Infiammazione dei polmoni (polmonite)	Upala pluća (pneumonija)
Inflamación de los senos paranasales (sinusitis)	Inflammation of the paranasal sinuses (sinusitis)	Inflammation du sinus (sinusite)	Infiammazione dei seni paranasali (sinusite)	Upala sinusa (sinusitis)
Inflamación de un tendón (tendinitis)	Inflammation of the tendon (tendinitis, tendonitis)	Inflammation d'un tendon (tendinite)	Infiammazione del tendine (tendinite)	Upala tetive (tendinitis)
Inflamación de un tendón y de su vaina (tenosinovitis)	Inflammation of the synovium and tendon (tenosynovitis)	Inflammation d'un tendon et de sa gaine synoviale (ténosynovite)	Infiammazione di tendine e di guaina tendinea (tenosinovite)	Upala tetive s ovojnicom (tenosinovitis)
Inflamación de una articulación (artritis)	Inflammation of the joint (arthritis)	Inflammation des articulations (arthrite)	Infiammazione articolare (artrite)	Upala zgloba (artritis)
Inflamación del apéndice (apendicitis)	Inflammation of the appendix (appendicitis)	Inflammation de l'appendice iléo-caecal (appendicite)	Infiammazione dell'appendice vermiforme (appendicite)	Upala slijepog crijeva (apendicitis)
Inflamación del encéfalo (encefalitis)	Inflammation of the brain (encephalitis)	Inflammation du cerveau (encéphalite)	Infiammazione del cervello (encefalite)	Upala mozga (encefalitis)
Inflamación del endocardio (endocarditis)	Inflammation of the endocardium (endocarditis)	Inflammation de l'endocarde (endocardite)	Infiammazione dell'endocardio (endocardite)	Upala srčane ovojnice (endokarditis)
Inflamación del endometrio (endometritis)	Inflammation of the endometrium (endometritis)	Inflammation de l'endomètre (endométrite)	Infiammazione dell'endometrio (endometrite)	Upala endometrija maternice (endometritis)
Inflamación del epidídimo (epididimitis)	Inflammation of the epididymis (epididymitis)	Inflammation de l'épididyme (épididymite)	Infiammazione dell'epididimo (epididimite)	Upala pasjemenika (epididimitis)
Inflamación del glande del pene (balanitis)	Inflammation of the glans penis (balanitis)	Inflammation du gland du pénis (balanite)	Infiammazione della testa del glande (balanite)	Upala glavića penisa (balanitis)
Inflamación del hígado (hepatitis)	Inflammation of the liver (hepatitis)	Inflammation du foie (hépatite)	Infiammazione del fegato (epatite)	Upala jetre (hepatitis)
Inflamación del laberinto del oído interno (laberintitis)	Inflammation of the inner ear (labyrinthitis)	Inflammation de l'oreille interne (labyrinthite, otite interne)	Infiammazione di labirinto nell'orecchio interno (labirintite)	Upala labirinta u unutarnjem uhu (labirintitis)
Inflamación del miocardio (miocarditis)	Inflammation of the heart muscle (myocarditis)	Inflammation du myocarde (myocardite)	Infiammazione del miocardio (miocardite)	Upala srčanog mišića (miokarditis)
Inflamación del músculo esquelético (miositis)	Inflammation of the muscles (myositis)	Inflammation du tissu musculaire (myosite)	Infiammazione del tessuto muscolare (miosite)	Upala mišića (miozitis)
Inflamación del nervio (neuritis)	Inflammation of the nerve (neuritis)	Inflammation du nerf (névrite)	Infiammazione del nervo (neurite, nevrite)	Upala živca (neuritis)
Inflamación del páncreas (pancreatitis)	Inflammation of the pancreas (pancreatitis)	Inflammation du pancréas (pancréatite)	Infiammazione del pancreas (pancreatite)	Upala gušterače (pankreatitis)
Inflamación del parametrio (parametritis)	Inflammation of the parametrium (parametritis)	Inflammation du paramètre (paramétrite)	Infiammazione del parametrio (parametrite)	Upala parametrija (parametritis)
Inflamación del pericardio (pericarditis)	Inflammation of the pericardium (pericarditis)	Inflammation du péricarde (péricardite)	Infiammazione del pericardio (pericardite)	Upala osrčja (perikarditis)
Inflamación del peritoneo (peritonitis)	Inflammation of the peritoneum (peritonitis)	Inflammation du péritoine (péritonite)	Infiammazione dela sierosa peritoneale (peritonite)	Upala potrbušnice (peritonitis)
Inflamación del riñón (nefritis)	Inflammation of the kidney (nephritis)	Inflammation du rein (néphrite)	Infiammazione dei reni (nefrite)	Upala bubrega (nefritis)
Inflamación del seno (mastitis)	Inflammation of the breast (mastitis)	Inflammation de la mamelle (mastite)	Infiammazione della mammella (mastite)	Upala dojke (mastitis)
Inflamación del testículo (orquitis)	Inflammation of the testes (orchitis)	Inflammation des testicules (orchite)	Infiammazione dei testicoli (orchite)	Upala testisa (orhitis)
Inflamación del timo (timitis)	Inflammation of the thymus (thymitis)	Inflammation du thymus	Infiammazione del timo	Upala prsne žlijezde (timitis)
Inflamación granulomatosa	Granulomatous inflammation	Inflammation granulomateuse	Infiammazione granulomatosa	Granulomatozna upala (granulom)
Ingestas descontroladas de alimentos (hiperfagia)	Abnormally large intake of food (hyperphagia)	Prise excessive d'aliments (hyperphagie)	Aumento incontrollato di assunzione di cibo (iperfagia)	Prekomjerno jedenje (hiperfagija)
Inmunodeficiencia	Immunodeficiency	Immunodéficience	Immunodeficienza	Sniženi imunitet
Insolación	Sunstroke (heat stroke)	Coup de soleil (insolation)	Insolazione (colpo di sole)	Sunčanica
Insomnio	Insomnia	Insomnie	Insonnia	Nesanica
Insuficiencia renal aguda	Acute kidney failure	Insuffisance rénale aiguë	Insufficienza renale acuta	Akutno zatajenje bubrega
Insuficiencia renal crónica	Chronic renal failure	Insuffisance rénale chronique	Insufficienza renale cronica	Kronično zatajenje bubrega
Insuficiencia venosa cerebro-espinal crónica	Chronic cerebrospinal venous insufficiency	Insuffisance veineuse cérébro-spinale chronique	Insufficienza venosa cronica cerebrospinale	Kronična cerebrospinalna venozna insuficijencija
Intolerancia a la lactosa	Lactose intolerance	Intolérance au lactose	Intolleranza al lattosio	Nepodnošenje laktoze (netolerancija laktoze)
Intolerancia al gluten	Gluten intolerance	Intolérance au gluten	Intolleranza al glutine	Nepodnošenje glutena
Intoxicación alimentaria	Food poisoning	Empoisonnement alimentaires	Avvelenamento da cibo	Trovanje hranom

Español	Inglés	Francés	Italiano	Croata
Intoxicación alimentaria por estafilococo dorado	Staphylococcal food poisoning	Intoxication alimentaire staphylococcique	Intossicazione alimentare da stafilococco	Stafilokokno trovanje hranom
Intoxicación por álcalis	Alkali poisoning	Empoisonnement par alcalis	Avvelenamento da alcali	Trovanje alkalima
Intoxicación por alcohol	Alcohol poisoning	Empoisonnement par l'alcool	Avvelenamento da alcool	Trovanje alkoholom
Intoxicación por armas gaseosas	Warfare gases poisoning	Intoxication par gaz de combat	Avvelenamento da gas tossico	Trovanje bojnim otrovima
Intoxicación por armas químicas	Chemical warfare poisoning	Intoxcation par arme chimique	Avvelenamento da armi chimiche	Trovanje kemijskim oružjem
Intoxicación por hierro	Iron poisoning	Empoisonnement au fer	Avvelenamento da ferro	Trovanje željezom
Intoxicación por litio	Lithium poisoning	Empoisonnement au lithium	Avvelenamento da litio	Trovanje litijem
Intoxicación por mariscos	Shellfish poisoning	Intoxication par des coquillages	Avvelenamento da molluschi	Trovanje školjkašima
Intoxicación por metanol	Methanol poisoning	Empoisonnement au méthanol	Avvelenamento da metanolo	Trovanje metanolom
Intoxicación por monóxido de carbono	Carbon monoxide poisoning	Empoisonnement au monoxyde de carbone	Avvelenamento da monossido di carbonio	Trovanje ugljičnim monoksidom
Intoxicación por paracetamol	Paracetamol poisoning	Intoxication par le paracétamol	Avvelenamento da paracetamolo	Trovanje paracetamolom
Intoxicación por pescado	Fish poisoning	Empoisonnement du poisson	Avvelenamento da pesci	Trovanje ribom
Intoxicación por salicilatos	Salicylate poisoning	Empoisonnement au salicylate	Avvelenamento da salicilati	Trovanje salicilatima
Iridodiálisis	Iridodialysis (coredialysis)	Iridodialyse	Iridodialisi	Iridodijaliza
Iritis	Iritis	Iritis	Irite	Iritis
Irradiación no-ionizante	Non-ionising irradiation	Irradiation non-ionisante	Irradiazione non ionizzante	Neionizirajuća ozračenost
Irradiación radioactiva	Radioactive irradiation	Irradiation par rayons radioactifs (contamination radioactive)	Irradiazione radioattiva	Radioaktivna ozračenost
Isosporiasis	Isosporiasis	Isosporose	Isosporiasi	Izosporijaza
Isquemia	Ischemia	Ischémie	Ischemia	Ishemija
Isquemia de miembros	Ischemic limbs	Ischémie des membres	Ischemia degli arti	Ishemični udovi
Isquemia miocárdica (angina de pecho)	Ischemic heart disease	Ischémie myocardique	Ischemia miocardica	Ishemijska bolest srca
Joroba	Hunchback	Bossu	Gibbo (gobba, gibbosità)	Grba
Kala azar (fiebre negra)	Kala-azar (black fever)	Kala azar (fièvre noire)	Kala-azar (febbre d'Assam, splenomegalia infantile)	Kala-azar
Keratosis	Keratosis	Kératose (kératodermie)	Cheratosi	Keratoza
Kernicterus (encefalopatía neonatal bilirrubínica)	Kernicterus	Kernictère	Kernittero (encefalopatia bilirubinica)	Žutica moždanih jezgri
Kuru (muerte de la risa)	Kuru	Kuru	Kuru	Kuru (smrtni smijeh)
Labio leporino (fisura labial)	Cleft lip and palate	Fente labiale et fente palatine	Labbro leporino	Rascjep usne i nepca
Laceración	Laceration (tear)	Lacération	Lacerazione (strappo)	Razderotina
Laceración cerebral	Brain laceration	Lacération cérébrale	Lacerazione cerebrale	Laceracija mozga
Laringoespasmo	Laryngospasm	Laryngospasme	Laringospasmo	Laringospazam
Leiomioma	Leiomyoma	Léiomyome	Leiomioma	Lejomiom
Leiomiosarcoma	Leiomyosarcoma	Leiomyosarcome	Leiomiosarcoma	Lejomiosarkom
Leishmaniasis	Leishmaniasis	Leishmaniose	Leishmaniosi	Lišmenijaza
Leishmaniasis cutánea (uta)	Cutaneous leishmaniasis (Oriental sore)	Leishmaniose cutanée (bouton d'Orient)	Leishmaniosi cutanea	Orijentalni ulkus (kožna lišmenijaza)
Lengua más grande de lo normal (macroglosia)	Enlarged tongue (macroglossia)	Augmentation de la langue (macroglossie)	Eccessiva crescita della lingua (macroglossia)	Uvećani jezik (makroglosija)
Lepra	Leprosy	Lèpre	Lebbra	Lepra (guba)
Leptospirosis	Leptospirosis	Leptospirose	Leptospirosi	Leptospiroza
Lesión de nervio	Nerve lesion	Lésion du nerf	Lesione del nervo	Oštećenje živca (lezija živca)
Lesión de nervio periférico	Peripheral nerve lesion	Lésion du nerf périphérique	Lesione del nervo periferico	Oštećenje perifernog živca
Lesión deportiva	Sports injury	Blessure de sportif	Trauma sportivo	Sportska ozljeda
Lesión obstructiva del intestino delgado	Obstructive lesion of the small intestine	Lésion obstructive de l'intestin grêle	Lesione ostruttiva dell'intestino tenue	Opstruktivna lezija tankog crijeva
Lesión por explosión	Explosive wound	Blessure par explosion	Ferita esplosiva	Eksplozivna rana
Lesiones de la cabeza y del cerebro	Head and brain injuries	Blessures à la tête et blessures du cerveau	Lesioni della testa e del cervello	Ozljede glave i mozga
Lesiones mecánicas	Mechanical injuries	Lésions mécaniques	Lesioni meccaniche	Mehaničke ozljede
Lesiones por corriente eléctrica	Electrical injuries (electric shock)	Électrisation	Folgorazione (elettrocuzione)	Ozljede električnom strujom (strujni udar)
Lesiones por una explosión termonuclear	Thermonuclear injuries	Lésions provoquées par une explosion thermonucléaire	Ferite provocate da esplosioni termonucleari	Termonuklearne ozljede
Lesiones químicas	Chemical injuries	Altération d'origine chimique	Ferita chimica	Kemijske ozljede
Lesiones térmicas	Thermal injuries	Lésions thermiques	Lesioni termiche	Termičke ozljede
Leucemia	Leukemia	Leucémie	Leucemia	Leukemija
Leucemia linfática	Lymphatic leukemia	Leucémie lymphoïde	Leucemia linfatica	Limfatična leukemija
Leucemia linfoblástica aguda	Acute lymphoblastic leukemia	Leucémie lymphoblastique aiguë	Leucemia acuta linfoblastica	Akutna limfatična leukemija

Español	Inglés	Francés	Italiano	Croata
Leucemia linfocítica crónica	Chronic lymphocytic leukemia	Leucémie lymphoïde chronique	Leucemia linfatica cronica	Kronična limfocitna leukemija
Leucemia mieloide	Myeloid leukemia	Leucémie myéloïde	Leucemia mieloide	Mijeloična leukemija
Leucemia mieloide aguda	Acute myeloid leukemia (AML)	Leucémie aiguë myéloblastique	Leucemia mieloide acuta	Akutna mijeloična leukemija
Leucemia mieloide crónica	Chronic myeloid leukemia	Leucémie myéloïde chronique	Leucemia mieloide cronica	Kronična mijeloična leukemija
Leucemia monocítica	Monocytic leukemia	Leucémie monocytique	Leucemia monocitica	Monocitična leukemija
Leucocitosis	Leukocytosis	Leucocytose	Leucocitosi	Leukocitoza
Leucodistrofia	Leukodystrophy	Leucodystrophie	Leucodistrofia	Leukodistrofija
Leucoplaquia	Leukoplakia	Leucoplasie	Leucoplachia	Leukoplakija
Leucorrea	Leukorrhea	Leucorrhée	Leucorea	Bijelo pranje
Linfangioma	Lymphangioma	Lymphangiome	Linfangioma	Limfangiom
Linfangiosarcoma	Lymphangiosarcoma	Lymphangiosarcome	Linfangiosarcoma	Limfangiosarkom
Linfedema	Lymphedema	Lymphoedème	Linfedema	Limfedem (zastoj limfe)
Linfoma	Lymphoma	Lymphome	Linfoma	Limfom
Linfoma no-Hodgkin	Non-Hodgkin's lymphoma	Lymphome non-Hodgkinien	Linfoma non Hodgkin	Non-Hodgkinov limfom
Lipodistrofia	Lipodystrophy	Lipodystrophie	Lipodistrofia	Lipodistrofija
Lipoma	Lipoma	Lipome	Lipoma	Lipom
Lipomatosis pancreática (reemplazo graso del páncreas)	Pancreatic lipomatosis	Lipomatose du pancréas	Lipomatosi pancreatica	Lipomatoza gušterače (masna infiltracija gusterače)
Liposarcoma	Liposarcoma	Liposarcome	Liposarcoma	Liposarkom
Liquen plano	Lichen planus	Lichen plan	Lichen planus	Lišaj (lichen planus)
Listeriosis	Listeriosis	Listériose	Listeriosi	Listerioza
Lordosis	Lordosis	Lordose	Lordosi	Lordoza
Lupus eritematoso sistémico	Lupus erythematosus	Lupus érythémateux	Lupus eritematoso sistemico	Sistemski lupus eritematozus
Luxación (lujación, dislocación)	Dislocation (luxation)	Déboîtement (luxation)	Lussazione	Iščašenje (dislokacija, luksacija)
Luxación de la articulación acromioclavicular	Separated shoulder (acromioclavicular dislocation)	Luxation acromio-claviculaire	Lussazione acromio-clavicolare	Iščašenje akromio-klavikularnog zgloba
Luxación de la cadera	Dislocation of a hip	Luxation de la hanche	Lussazione dell'anca	Iščašenje kuka
Luxación de la rodilla	Knee dislocation (luxation of the knee)	Luxation du genou	Lussazione del ginocchio	Iščašenje koljena
Luxación de la rótula	Luxating patella (trick knee, floating patella)	Luxation de la rotule	Lussazione della rotula	Iščašenje čašice
Luxación del codo	Elbow dislocation (luxation of the elbow)	Luxation du coude	Lussazione del gomito	Iščašenje lakta
Luxación del hombro	Dislocated shoulder	Luxation de l'épaule	Lussazione della spalla	Iščašenje ramena
Luxación del tobillo	Dislocated ankle joint	Luxation de la cheville	Lussazione della caviglia	Iščašenje skočnog zgloba
Luxaciones de la mano y los dedos	Hand and finger joints dislocation	Luxation des doigts et du poignet	Lussazioni delle atricolazioni della mano e delle dita	Iščašenje zglobova šake i prstiju
Mal aliento (halitosis)	Bad breath (halitosis)	Mauvaise heleine (halitose)	Odore sgradevole dell'alito (alitosi, bromopnea)	Zadah iz usta (halitoza)
Mal de garganta (inflamación de la faringe, faringitis)	Sore throat (inflammation of the throat, pharyngitis)	Mal à la gorge (inflammattion du pharinx, pharingite)	Mal di gola (infiammazione della faringe, faringite)	Upala grla (grlobolja, faringitis)
Mal de mar	Seasickness	Mal de mer	Mal di mare	Morska bolest
Mal de montaña (mal de altura)	Altitude sickness (acute mountain sickness)	Mal aigu des montagnes	Mal di montagna	Visinska bolest
Malabsorción	Malabsorption	Malabsorption	Malassorbimento	Malapsorpcija
Malaria (paludismo)	Malaria	Malaria	Malaria	Malarija
Malformación arteriovenosa cerebral	Cerebrovascular anomaly	Anomalie cérébrovasculaire	Anomalia cerebrovascolare	Anomalija moždanih krvnih žila
Malformación cardiaca congénita	Congenital heart defect	Malformation congénitale du coeur	Difetto cardiaco congenito	Urođena srčana greška
Malformación del desarrollo cerebral	Brain development anomaly	Anomalie du développement cérébral	Anomalia di sviluppo del sistema nervoso	Anomalija u razvoju mozga
Manchas de Koplik	Koplik's spots	Signe de Koplik	Macchie di Koplik	Koplikove pjege
Manía	Mania	Manie	Mania	Manija
Marcha arrastrando los pies	Shuffling gait	Démarche traînante	Barcollamento	Teturav nesiguran hod
Mastitis quística crónica (enfermedad fibroquística)	Fibrocystic breast disease	Mastopathie fibrocystique	Mastopatia fibrocistica	Fibrocistična bolest dojke
Mastopatía	Mastopathy	Mastopathie	Mastopatia	Mastopatija
Meduloblastoma	Medulloblastoma	Médulloblastome	Medulloblastoma	Meduloblastom
Megacolon	Megacolon	Mégacolôn	Megacolon	Megakolon
Melanoma	Melanoma	Mélanome	Melanoma	Melanom
Melasma (cloasma)	Melasma (chloasma faciei)	Chleuasme (chloasma)	Melasma	Kloazma (melazma)
Melioidosis	Melioidosis (Whitmore disease)	Mélioïdose	Melioidosi	Melioidoza
Meningioma	Meningioma	Méningiome	Meningioma	Meningeom
Meningocele	Meningocele	Méningocèle	Meningocele	Meningokela

Español	Inglés	Francés	Italiano	Croata
Meningoencefalitis amebiana primaria	Primary amoebic meningoencephalitis	Méningo-encéphalite amibienne primaire	Meningoencefalite amebica primaria	Primarni amebni meningoencefalitis
Meningoencefalitis de garrapata	Tick-borne meningoencephalitis	Méningoencéphalite à tique	Encefalite trasmessa da zecche	Krpeljni meningoencefalitis
Meningoencefalocele	Meningoencephalocele	Méningoencphalocèle	Meningoencefalocele	Meningoencefalokela
Meniscopatia	Meniscal disease	Meniscopathie	Meniscopatia	Meniskopatija
Menopausia	Menopause	Ménopause	Menopausa	Menopauza (klimakterij)
Menstruación dolorosa (dismenorrea)	Painful menstruation (dysmenorrhea)	Règle douloureuse (dysménorrhée)	Mestruazione dolorosa (dismenorrea)	Bolna menstruacija (dismenoreja)
Mesotélioma	Mesothelioma	Mésothéliome	Mesotelioma	Mezoteliom
Mesotélioma sarcomatoide	Sarcomatoid mesothelioma	Mésothéliome sarcomatoïde	Mesotelioma sarcomatoide	Mezoteliosarkom
Metabolismo basal acelerado	Accelerated basal metabolism	Metabolisme de base accéléré	Metabolismo basale accelerato	Ubrzan bazalni metabolizam
Metabolismo basal lento	Slow basal metabolism	Métabolisme basal diminué	Basso metabolismo basale	Usporen bazalni metabolizam
Metamorfosis grasa del hígado	Fatty liver metamorphosis	Stéatose hépatique	Metamorfosi grassa del fegato	Masna metarmofoza jetre
Metástasis	Metastasis	Métastase	Metastasi	Metastaza
Metatarsalgia	Metatarsalgia (Morton's neuroma)	Métatarsalgie	Metatarsalgia	Metatarzalgija (Mortonova metatarzalgija)
Meteoropatía	Meteoropathy	Météoropathie	Meteoropatia	Meteoropatija
Mialgia cervical	Neck myalgia	Myalgie cervicale	Mialgia cervicale	Mijalgični sindrom vrata
Miastenia gravis	Myasthenia gravis	Myasthénie grave	Miastenia gravis	Miastenija gravis
Micción dolorosa (angurria)	Painful urination (strangury)	Urination douloureuse (strangurie)	Minzione dolorosa (stranguria)	Bol pri mokrenju (strangurija)
Micción frecuente	Frequent urination	Miction fréquente	Urinazione frequente (pollachiuria)	Učestalo mokrenje
Micetoma	Mycetoma	Mycétome	Micetoma	Micetoma
Micosis	Mycosis	Mycose	Micosi	Mikoza
Mielomeningocele	Meningomyelocele	Myéloméningocèle	Mielomeningocele	Meningomijelokela
Migraña (jaqueca)	Migraine	Migraine	Emicrania	Migrena
Miliaria rubra (sarpullido por el calor)	Miliaria rubra (sweat rash)	Miliarie rouge	Miliaria rubra	Milijarija rubra
Milium (milia)	Milia (milk spots)	Milium (grutum, acné miliaire)	Acne miliare	Milije (dječje akne)
Mioblastoma	Myoblastoma	Rhabdomyome granocellulaire	Mioblastoma	Mioblastom
Miocardiopatía	Cardiomyopathy	Cardiomyopathie	Cardiomiopatia	Kardiomiopatija
Miocardiopatía alcohólica	Alcoholic cardiomyopathy	Cardiomyopathie alcoolique	Miocardiopatia alcolica	Alkoholna kardiomiopatja
Miocardiopatía dilatada	Dilated cardiomyopathy	Cardiomyopathie dilatée	Cardiomiopatia dilatativa	Dilatacijska kardiomiopatija
Miocardiopatía hipertrófica	Hypertrophic cardiomyopathy	Cardiomyopathie hypertrophique	Cardiomiopatia ipertrofica	Hipertrofijska kardiomiopatija
Mioclono	Myoclonic twitches (myoclonus)	Myoclonie	Mioclono	Miokloničko trzanje (mioklonus)
Miogelosis	Myogelosis	Myogélose	Miogelosi	Miogeloza
Mioma	Myoma	Myome	Mioma	Miom
Miopía	Shortsightedness (myopia)	Myopie	Miopia	Kratkovidnost
Miosarcoma	Myosarcoma	Myosarcome	Miosarcoma	Miosarkom
Miositis osificante	Myositis ossificans	Myosite ossifiante	Miosite ossificante	Osificirajući miozitis
Miositis osificante progresiva	Myositis ossificans progressiva	Myosite ossifiante progressive	Miosite ossificante progressiva	Progresivno okoštavanje mišića
Mixedema	Myxedema	Myxoedème	Mixedema	Miksedem
Mixoma	Myxoma	Myxome	Mixoma	Miksom
Mixosarcoma	Myxosarcoma	Myxosarcome	Mixosarcoma	Miksosarkom
Moco (mucus) nasal	Nasal secretion (mucus)	Mucus nasal	Muco nasale	Sekrecija iz nosa
Moco en las heces	Mucus in stool	Mucus dans les selles	Muco nelle feci	Sluzava stolica
Molusco contagioso	Molluscum contagiosum	Molluscum contagiosum	Mollusco contagioso	Molusk
Mononucleosis infecciosa (fiebre glandular, enfermedad de Pfeiffer)	Infectious mononucleosis (Pfeiffer's disease, kissing disease, glandular fever)	Mononucléose infectieuse (maladie du baiser, maladie des amoureux)	Mononucleosi infettiva (malattia del bacio)	Mononukleoza (bolest poljupca)
Mordedura	Bite	Morsure	Morsicatura	Ugriz
Mordedura de gato	Cat bite	Morsure de chat	Morsicatura di gatto	Ugriz mačke
Mordedura de perro	Dog bite	Morsure de chien	Morsicatura di cane	Ugriz psa
Mordedura de rata	Rat bite	Morsure de rat	Morsicatura di ratto	Ugriz štakora
Mordedura de un animal enfermo de rabia	Bite by rabies infected animal	Morsure d'un animal infecté par le virus de la rage	Morsicatura di animale rabbioso	Ugriz bijesne životinje
Mordedura de víbora	Snake bite	Morsure de vipère	Morsicatura di serpenti	Ugriz zmije
Mordedura de viuda negra	Black widow bite	Morsure de veuve noire	Morso della vedova nera	Ugriz crne udovice
Mordedura humana	Human bite	Morsure humaine	Morsicatura di uomo	Ugriz čovjeka (ljudski ugriz)
Moretón (equimosis)	Bruise (ecchymosis)	Ecchymose	Ammaccatura (ecchimosi)	Modrica (ekhimoza)
Movimientos involuntarios y rápidos de los ojos (opsoclonus)	Uncontrolled eye movement (opsoclonus)	Mouvements involontaires anarchiques des globes oculaires (opsoclonus)	Movimenti incontrollati degli occhi (opsoclono)	Nekontrolirani pokreti očiju (opsoklonus)
Mucocele	Mucocele	Mucocèle	Mucocele	Mukocela
Mucopolisacaridosis	Mucopolysaccharidosis	Mucopolysaccharidose	Mucopolisaccaridosi	Mukopolisaharidoza

Español	Inglés	Francés	Italiano	Croata
Muermo	Glanders	Morve	Morva umana	Sakagija
Muerte	Death	Mort	Morte	Smrt
Muerte natural	Natural death	Mort naturelle	Morte naturale	Prirodna smrt
Muerte violenta	Violent death	Mort violente	Morte violenta	Nasilna smrt
Músculo flácido	Flaccid muscle (untoned muscle)	Muscle flasque (hypotonie musculaire)	Muscolo flaccido	Mlohavi mišić
Narcolepsia (síndrome de Gelineau, epilepsia del sueño)	Narcolepsy	Narcolepsie (maladie de Gélineau)	Narcolessia	Narkolepsija
Náusea	Nausea	Nausée	Nausea	Mučnina
Necrosis	Necrosis	Nécrose	Necrosi	Nekroza
Necrosis fibrinoide	Fibrinoid necrosis	Nécrose fibrinoïde	Necrosi fibrinoide	Fibrinoidna nekroza
Nefritis intersticial	Interstitial nephritis	Néphrite interstitielle	Nefrite interstiziale	Intersticijska upala bubrega
Nefropatía diabética	Diabetic nephropathy	Néphropathie diabétique	Nefropatia diabetica	Dijabetična nefropatija
Nefrosis	Nephrosis	Néphrose	Nefrosi	Nefroza
Neumoconiosis	Pneumoconiosis	Pneumoconiose	Pneumoconiosi	Pneumokonioza
Neumonía atípica	Atypical pneumonia	Pneumonie atypique	Polmonite atipica	Atipična upala pluća
Neumonía bacteriana	Bacterial pneumonia	Pneumonie bactérienne	Polmonite batterica	Bakterijska upala pluća
Neumonía bronquial	Bronchopneumonia	Bronchopneumonie	Broncopolmonite	Bronhopneumonija
Neumonía por Pneumocystis	Pneumocystis pneumonia (pneumocystosis)	Pneumocystose	Polmonite da Pneumocisti	Pneumocistična upala pluća
Neumonía viral	Viral pneumonia	Pneumonie virale	Polmonite virale	Virusna upala pluća
Neumotórax	Pneumothorax	Pneumothorax	Pneumotorace	Pneumotoraks
Neuralgia	Neuralgia	Névralgie	Nevralgia	Neuralgija
Neuralgia craneal	Cranial neuralgia	Névralgie des nerfs crâniens	Nevralgia del nervo cranico	Neuralgija moždanih živaca
Neuralgia del trigémino	Trigeminal neuralgia	Névralgie du trijumeau (névralgie trigéminale)	Nevralgia del trigemino	Neuralgija trigeminusa
Neurastenia	Neurasthenia	Neurasthénie	Nevrastenia	Neurastenija
Neurinoma	Neurinoma	Neurinome	Neurinoma (Schwannoma)	Neurinom
Neuroblastoma	Neuroblastoma	Neuroblastome	Neuroblastoma	Neuroblastom
Neuroborreliosis	Neuroborreliosis	Neuroborréliose	Neuroborreliosi	Neuroborelioza
Neurofibromatosis de tipo 1 (enfermedad de Von Recklinghausen)	Neurofibromatosis type1 (Von Recklinghausen's disease)	Neurofibromatose de type 1 (maladie de Von Recklinghausen)	Neurofibromatosi di tipo1 (malattia di von Recklinghausen)	Von Recklinghausenova bolest
Neuroma	Neuroma	Neurome	Neuroma	Neurom
Neuroma acústico	Acoustic neuroma	Neurome acoustique	Neuroma dell'acustico	Neurom slušnog živca
Neuropatía	Neuropathy	Neuropathie	Neuropatia	Neuropatija
Neuropatía diabética	Diabetic neuropathy	Neuropathie diabétique	Neuropatia diabetica	Dijabetična neuropatija
Neurosis	Neurosis	Névrose (neurose)	Nevrosi	Neuroza
Nevus (nevo)	Birthmark (nevus)	Grain de beauté (naevus)	Voglia (neo, nevo)	Madež (nevus)
Nistagmo	Nystagmus	Nystagmus	Nistagmo	Nistagmus
Nódulo de la hermana María José	Sister Mary Joseph nodule	Nodule de Soeur Marie Joseph (métastase cutanée ombilicale)	Nodulo di Suor Maria Giuseppa	Čvor sestre Mary Joseph (umbilikalna metastaza)
Nódulos de Heberden	Heberden's nodes	Nodules d'Heberden	Noduli di Heberden	Heberdenovi čvorići
Nudo	Knot (lump)	Nodule	Nodo (nodulo)	Kvržica
Nudosidades de Bouchard	Bouchard's nodes	Nodules de Bouchard	Noduli di Bouchard	Bouchardovi čvorići
Obesidad	Obesity	Obésité	Obesità	Debljina (gojaznost)
Oclusión de la arteria de la retina	Retinal artery occlusion	Occlusion de l'artère de la rétine	Occlusione arteria retinica	Blokada mrežnične arterije
Ojo vago (ambliopía)	Lazy eye (amblyopia)	Mal-voyance (amblyopie)	Ambliopia	Slabovidnost
Ojos llorosos	Watery eyes	Yeux larmoyants	Occhi lacrimosi	Suzenje očiju
Oligodendroglioma	Oligodendroglioma	Oligodendrocytome	Oligodendroglioma	Oligodendrogliom
Oligomenorrea	Oligomenorrhea	Oligoménorrhée	Oligomenorrea	Oligomenoreja
Oncocercosis	Onchocerciasis (river blindness)	Onchocercose (cécité des rivières)	Oncocercosi (cecità fluviale)	Onkocerkijaza (riječno sljepilo)
Orina de color marrón	Brown urine	Urine marron	Urina marrone	Smeđi urin
Orina de color rojo	Red urine	Urine rouge	Urina di colore rosso	Crveni urin
Orina turbia	Unclear urine (foggy urine)	Urine opaque	Urine torbide	Mutni urin
Orzuelo	Stye (chalazion)	Chalazion	Calazio	Ječmenac
Oscilaciones del humor	Mood swing	Saute d'humeur	Cambiamento d'umore	Promjene raspoloženja
Ostéitis fibrosa quística	Osteitis fibrosa cystica	Ostéite fibrokystique	Osteitis fibrosa cistica	Fibrozna cistična upala kosti
Osteoartropatía hipertrófica (enfermedad de Bamberger-Marie)	Hyperthropic osteoarthropaty (Pierre Marie-Bamberger syndrome)	Ostéo-arthropathie hypertrophiante de Pierre Marie (syndrome de Marie-Bamberger)	Osteoartropatia ipertrofizzante (sindrome di Pierre Marie-Bamberger)	Osteoartropatija hipertrofika Pierre Marie
Osteocondroma	Osteochondroma	Ostéochondrome	Osteocondroma	Osteohondrom
Osteocondrosis juvenil	Juvenile osteochondrosis	Ostéochondrose juvénile	Osteocondrite dissecante	Juvenilna osteohondroza
Osteogénesis imperfecta (huesos de cristal)	Osteogenesis imperfecta (brittle bone disease)	Ostéogenèse imparfaite	Osteogenesi imperfetta	Osteogeneza imperfekta (staklaste kosti)
Osteoma	Osteoma	Ostéome	Osteoma	Osteom
Osteomalacia	Osteomalacia	Ostéomalacie	Osteomalacia	Osteomalacija
Osteomielitis luética	Luetic osteomyelitis	Ostéomyélite syphilitique	Osteomielite luetica	Luetični osteomijelitis
Osteomielitis micótica	Fungal osteomyelitis	Ostéomyélite fongique	Osteomielite fungale	Gljivični osteomijelitis
Osteopetrosis (enfermedad de los huesos de marmol)	Osteopetrosis (marble bone disease)	Ostéopétrose (os de marbre)	Osteopetrosi (malattia delle ossa di marmo)	Osteopetroza (zadebljane kosti, bolest mramornih kostiju)

Español	Inglés	Francés	Italiano	Croata
Osteoporosis	Osteoporosis	Ostéoporose	Osteoporosi	Osteoporoza
Osteosarcoma	Osteosarcoma	Ostéosarcome	Osteosarcoma	Osteosarkom
Osteosclerosis	Osteosclerosis	Ostéosclérose	Osteosclerosi	Osteoskleroza
Ovulación dolorosa	Ovulation pain (mittelschmerz)	Douleurs ovulatoires (mittelschmerz)	Dolore ovulatorio (mittelschmerz)	Bolna ovulacija (mittelschmerz)
Padrastro	Agnail (hangnail)	Envie de l'ongle	Pipita	Zanoktica
Palidez	Paleness (pallor)	Pâleur	Pallore	Bljedilo
Palmas de las manos calientes y mojadas	Warm sweaty palms	Paumes des mains chaudes et humides	Palmi delle mani caldi e sudati	Topli i vlažni dlanovi
Palpitación	Palpitation	Palpitation	Cardiopalmo (palpitazione)	Lupanje srca (palpitacije)
Panadizo	Whitlow (felon)	Panaris	Patereccio	Panaricij
Pancreas aberrante	Aberrant pancreas	Pancréas aberrant	Pancraes aberrante	Aberantni pankreas
Paperas (parotiditis)	Mumps (epidemic parotitis)	Oreillons (parotidite virale)	Parotite (orecchioni)	Zaušnjaci (mumps, parotitis)
Papiloma	Papilloma	Papillome	Papilloma	Papilom
Paracoccidioidomicosis	Paracoccidioidomycosis (Brazilian blastomycosis)	Paracoccidioidose brésilienne	Paracoccidioidimicosi (blastomicosi sudamericana)	Parakokcidioidomikoza (brazilska blastomikoza)
Parafimosis	Paraphimosis	Paraphimosis	Parafimosi	Parafimoza
Paragonimosis (paragonimiasis)	Paragonimiasis	Paragonimiase humaine	Paragonimiasi	Paragonimijaza
Parálisis	Paralysis	Paralysie	Paralisi	Paraliza (oduzetost, kljenut)
Parálisis cerebral	Cerebral palsy	Infirmité motorice cérébrale	Paralisi cerebrale infantile	Cerebralna paraliza
Parálisis de Bell	Bell's palsy	Paralysie de Bell	Paralisi di Bell	Bellova paraliza
Parálisis de la parte inferior del cuerpo (paraplejía)	Paralysis of lower extremities (paraplegia)	Paralysie des membres inférieurs (paraplégie)	Paralisi di parte inferiore del corpo (paraplegia)	Oduzetost donjih ekstremiteta (paraplegija)
Parálisis de partes simétricas del cuerpo (diplejía)	Paralysis of symmetrical parts of the body (diplegia)	Paralysie des régions symétriques du corps (diplégie)	Paralisi di una parte di corpo simmetrica (diplegia)	Oduzetost simetričnih dijelova tijela (diplegija)
Parálisis de una mitad lateral de cuerpo (hemiplejía)	Paralysis of one half of a body (hemiplegia)	Paralysie de la moitié du corps (hémiplégie)	Paralisi di una metà del corpo (emiplegia)	Oduzetost jedne polovine tijela (hemiplegija)
Parálisis en brazos y piernas (tetraplejía, cuadriplejia)	Paralysis of all limbs and torso (quadriplegia, tetraplegia)	Paralysie des quatre membres (tétraplégie)	Paralisi dei arti superiori e inferiori(quadriplegia)	Oduzetost gornjih i donjih ekstremiteta i torza(kvadriplegija, tetraplegija)
Paranoia	Paranoia	Paranoïa	Paranoia	Paranoja
Paresis	Paresis	Parésie	Paresi	Pareza
Paro cardiaco (parada cardiorrespiratoria)	Cardiac arrest (cardiopulmonary arrest)	Arrêt cardiaque (arrêt ventilatoire, arrêt cardio-respiratoire)	Arresto cardiaco	Zastoj srca (srčani arest)
Paroniquia	Paronychia	Paronychie	Paronichia	Paronihija
Pecho hundido (pectus excavatum)	Pectus excavatum	Thorax en entonnoir (pectus excavatum)	Torace a imbuto (petto escavato)	Udubljena prsa (ljevkasta prsa)
Pectus carinatum	Pigeon chest (pectus carinatum)	Pectus carinatum	Petto carenato	Kokošja prsa
Pénfigo	Pemphigus	Pemphigus	Pemfigo	Pemfigus
Pérdida de capacidad de producir lenguaje (afasia)	Loss of language ability (aphasia)	Perte d'habileté d'expression du langage (mutisme, aphasie)	Perdita di abilità di produzione del linguaggio verbale (afasia)	Gubitak sposobnosti govora (afazija)
Pérdida de fuerza muscular (astenia)	Loss of strenght (asthenia)	Affaiblissement de l'organisme (asthénie)	Riduzione della forza muscolare (astenia)	Gubitak mišićne snage (astenija)
Pérdida de la capacidad auditiva	Hearing loss	Perte d'ouïe	Perdita di udito	Gubitak sluha
Pérdida de la memoria	Memory loss	Perte de mémoire	Perdita di memoria	Gubitak pamćenja
Pérdida de la mitad del campo visual (hemianopsia)	Loss of half of a field of vision (hemianopsia)	Perte de la vue dans une moitié du champ visuel (hémianopsie)	Perdita di metà di campo visivo (emianopsia)	Gubitak polovice vidnog polja (hemianopsija)
Pérdida de peso	Weight loss (weight reduction)	Amaigrissement	Dimagramento	Mršavljenje
Pérdida de pulso	Absence of pulse	Absence de pouls	Perdita di polso	Gubitak pulsa
Pérdida de sangre a través del ano (rectorragia)	Anal bleeding	Saignement anal (rectorragie)	Perdita di sangue dall'ano (rettoragia, proctorragia)	Krvarenje iz analnog otvora
Pérdida de sangre mayor durante la menstruación (menorragia)	Abnormally heavy menstrual period (menorrhagia)	Cycle menstruel anormalement excessice (ménorragie)	Anormale perdita di sangue durante il ciclo mestruale(menorragia)	Abnormalno velik gubitak krvi tijekom mjesečnice (menoragija)
Pérdida de sangre por la nariz (epistaxis)	Nose bleeding (epistaxis)	Saignement de nez (épistaxis)	Epistassi (rinorragia)	Krvarenje iz nosa (epistaksa)
Pérdida de sangre uterina (metrorragia)	Uterine bleeding (metrorrhagia)	Saignement de l'utérus (métrorragie)	Perdita di sangue al di fuori della mestruazione (metrorragia)	Krvarenje iz maternice (metroragija)
Pérdida del apetito	Loss of appetite	Perte d'appétit	Mancanza dell'appetito	Gubitak apetita
Pérdida del sentido del gusto (ageusia)	Loss of the sense of taste (ageusia)	Perte du sens du goût (agueusie)	Incapacità di percipire i sapori (ageusia)	Gubitak osjeta okusa
Pérdida del sentido del olfato (anosmia)	Loss of olfaction (anosmia)	Perte de la sensibilité aux odeurs (anosmie)	Incapacità di percipire gli odori (disosmia)	Gubitak osjeta mirisa

Español	Inglés	Francés	Italiano	Croata
Pérdida del sentido del tacto	Loss of the sense of touch	Perte du sens du toucher	Perdita di senso di tocco	Gubitak osjeta dodoira
Perforación del tímpano	Perforated eardrum (tympanorrhexis)	Perforation du tympan	Perforazione del timpano	Puknuće bubnjića (perforacija bubnjića, timpanoreksija)
Periodontitis (piorrea)	Periodontitis	Parodontite	Parodontite	Parodontoza
Peste	Plague (pest)	Peste	Peste (pestilenza)	Kuga
Petequia	Petechia	Pétéchie	Petecchia	Petehije
Pezón invertido	Inverted nipple	Téton ombiliqué	Capezzolo invertito	Uvučena bradavica
Pian (frambesia)	Yaws (pian)	Pian	Framboesia	Frambezija
Picadura de araña	Spider bite	Piqûre d'araignée	Morsicatura di ragno	Ugriz pauka
Picadura de escorpión	Scorpion sting	Piqûre de scorpion	Puntura di scorpione	Ugriz škorpiona
Picadura de garrapata infectada	Infected tick bite	Piqûre de tique infectée	Morsicatura di zecca infetta	Ugriz zaraženog krpelja
Picadura de hormiga	Ant sting	Piqûre de fourmi	Puntura di formiche	Ugriz mrava
Picadura de mosquito infectado	Infected mosquito bite	Piqûre de moustique infecté	Puntura di zanzara infetta	Ugriz zaraženog komarca
Pie calcáneo	Pes calcaneus	Pied calcanéus	Piede calcaneo	Petno stopalo
Pie cavo (pes cavus)	High arches (pes cavus)	Pied creux	Piede cavo (pes cavus)	Izdubljeno stopalo (pes excavatus)
Pie equino	Dancer's foot (pes equinus)	Pied equin	Piede equino	Balerinsko stopalo (pes equinus)
Pie quinovaro (talipes equinovarus, pie bot, pie retorcido)	Club foot (talipes equinovarus)	Pied-bot (pied-bot équin)	Piede equino (talipes equinovarus)	Čopavo stopalo (uvrnuto stopalo, pes equinovarus)
Pie plano (pes planus, arcos vencidos)	Flat foot (pes planus)	Pied plat (pes planus)	Piede piatto (pes planus)	Spušteno stopalo (pes planus)
Pie valgo	Pes valgus	Pied valgus	Piede piatto valgo (pes valgus)	Izvrnuto stopalo (pes valgus)
Piedra en el riñon (cálculo renal, litiasis renal)	Kidney stone (nephrolithiasis)	Calcul rénal (néphrolithiase, lithiase urinaire)	Calcolosi renale (nefrolitiasi)	Bubrežni kamenac (nefrolitijaza)
Pielonefritis (infección urinaria alta)	Pyelonephritis (kidney infection)	Pyélonéphrite (infection bactérienne des voies urinaires hautes)	Pielonefrite	Pijelonefritis (infekcija bubrega)
Pilorospasmo	Pylorospasm	Spasme du pylore	Pilorospasmo	Pilorospazam
Pinta	Pinta	Pinta	Pinta	Pinta
Pinzamiento anterolateral del tobillo	Ankle impingement syndrome	Conflit antérieur de la cheville	Sindrome da impingement della caviglia	Prednji sindrom sraza gornjeg nožnog zgloba
Pionefrosis	Pyonephrosis	Pyonéphrose (pus dans le rein)	Pionefrosi	Pionefroza
Piromanía	Pyromania	Pyromanie	Piromania	Piromanija
Pitidos en el oído (acúfeno, tinnitus)	Ringing in ears (tinnitus)	Acouphène	Ronzio auricolare (acufene, tinnito)	Zujanje u ušima (tinitus)
Placa dental	Dental plaque (dental tartar)	Plaque dentaire	Placca (tartaro)	Zubni kamenac
Plasmacitoma (mieloma múltiple)	Plasmacytoma (multiple myeloma)	Plasmocytome (myélome multiple)	Mieloma multiplo	Plazmocitom (multipli mijelom)
Policitemia	Polycythemia	Polycythémie	Policitemia	Policitemija
Polidactilia	Polydactyly	Polydactylie	Polidattilia	Polidaktilija
Polimialgia reumática	Polymyalgia rheumatica	Polymyalgia rheumatica	Polimialgia reumatica	Reumatska polimialgija
Polimiositis	Polymyositis	Polymyosite	Polimiosite	Polimiozitis
Poliomielitis (parálisis infantil)	Poliomyelitis (polio, infantile paralysis)	Poliomyélite (polio, paralysie spinale infantile)	Poliomielite (polio, paralisi infantile)	Dječja paraliza (polio, poliomijelitis)
Pólipo	Polyp	Polype	Polipo	Polip
Pólipo cervical	Cervical polyp	Polype au col de l'utérus	Polipo cervicale	Polip na grliću maternice
Pólipo de colon	Colon polyp	Polype du côlon	Polipo del colon	Polip na debelom crijevu
Pólipo de las cuerdas vocales	Vocal chords polyp	Polype des cordes vocales	Polipo della corda vocale	Polip na glasnicama
Pólipo endometrial	Endometrial polyp (uterine polyp)	Polype utérin	Polipo endometriale	Polip maternice
Pólipo nasal	Nasal polyp	Polype nasal	Polipo nasale	Polip u nosu (nosni polip)
Porfiria	Porphyria	Porphyrie	Porfiria	Porfirija
Presencia de pus en la orina (piuria)	Pus in urine (pyuria)	Présence de pus dans l'urine (pyurie)	Presenza di pus nelle urine (piuria)	Gnoj u urinu (piurija)
Presión sanguínea baja (hipotensión)	Low blood pressure (hypotension)	Baisse de la pression artérielle (hypotension artérielle)	Bassa pressione arteriosa (ipotensione)	Nizak krvni tlak (hipotenzija)
Primera menstruación (menarquia)	First menstrual cycle (menarche)	Première période de menstruations (ménarche)	Primo flusso mestruale (menarca)	Prva mjesečnica (menarha)
Proctitis	Proctitis	Proctite	Proctite	Proktitis
Prolapso del útero	Uterine prolapse (fallen womb)	Prolapsus de l'utérus	Prolasso uterino	Prolaps maternice (spuštena maternica)
Prolapso rectal	Rectal prolapse	Prolapsus rectal	Prolasso del retto	Prolaps rektuma
Proteinosis alveolar pulmonar	Pulmonary alveolar proteinosis	Protéinose alvéolaire pulmonaire	Proteinosi alveolare polmonare	Alveolarna proteinoza pluća
Proteinuria	Proteinuria (presence of proteins in urine)	Protéinurie (excès de protéines dans l'urine)	Proteinuria	Bjelančevine u urinu (proteinurija)
Prurito (picazón, comezón, rasquiña)	Itching	Prurit	Prurito (pizzicore)	Svrbež

Español	Inglés	Francés	Italiano	Croata
Psiconeurosis	Psychoneurosis	Psychonévrose	Psiconevrosi (nevrosi)	Psihoneuroza
Psicopatía	Psychopathy	Psychopathie	Psicopatia	Psihopatija
Psicosis	Psychosis	Psychose	Psicosi	Psihoza
Psitacosis (fiebre del loro)	Psittacosis (parrot fever)	Psittacose	Psittacosi (psittacornitosi)	Psitakoza
Psoriasis	Psoriasis	Psoriasis	Psoriasi	Psorijaza
Pubertad precoz	Precocious puberty (premature puberty)	Puberté précoce	Pubertà precoce (pubertà prematura)	Preuranjeni pubertet
Pulmón de granjero	Farmer's lung	Maladie du poumon de fermier	Febbre da fieno	Farmerska pluća
Pulso acelerado	Accelerated pulse rate	Fréquence du pouls accélérée	Polso accelerato	Ubrzani puls
Pupilas dilatadas	Enlarged pupils	Pupilles dilatées	Pupille dilatate	Proširene zjenice
Pupilas pequeñas	Small pupils	Pupilles diminuées	Pupille costrette	Sužene zjenice
Púrpura	Purpura	Purpura	Porpora	Purpura
Púrpura trombocitopénica trombótica	Thrombotic thrombocytopenic purpura	Purpura thrombotique thrombocytopénique	Porpora trombotica trombocitopenica	Trombotska trombocitopenična purpura
Pus	Pus	Pus	Pus	Gnoj
Pústula	Pustule	Pustule	Pustola	Gnojni mjehurić
Queloide	Keloid	Chéloïde	Cheloide	Keloid
Quemadura	Burn	Brûlure	Ustione	Opeklina
Quemadura de medusa	Jellyfish sting burn	Brûlure de méduse	Ustione da medusa	Opeklina od meduze
Quemadura eléctrica	Electric shock burn	Brûlure électrique	Ustione da corrente elettrica	Opeklina od strujnog udara
Queratosis actínica	Actinic keratosis	Kératose actinique	Cheratosi solare	Aktinička keratoza
Queratosis seborreica	Seborrheic keratosis	Kératose séborrhéïque	Cheratosi seborroica	Seboreična keratoza
Quilotórax	Chylothorax	Chylothorax	Chilotorace	Hilotoraks
Quiste	Cyst	Kyste	Cisti (ciste)	Cista
Quiste de páncreas	Pancreatic cyst	Kyste du pancréas	Cisti pancreatica	Cista na gušterači
Quiste de riñón	Renal cyst	Kyste rénal	Cisti renale	Cista na bubregu
Quiste de tiroides	Thyroid cyst	Kyste thyroïdien	Cisti tiroidea	Cista na štitnjači
Quiste dermoide	Dermoid cyst	Kyste dermoïde	Cisti dermoide	Dermoidna cista
Quiste ovárico	Ovarian cyst	Kyste ovarien	Cisti ovarica	Cista na jajniku
Quiste pilonidal	Pilonidal cyst	Kyste pilonidal	Cisti pilonidale	Pilonidalna cista
Quiste sebáceo	Sebaceous cyst (wen)	Kyste sébacé	Cisti sebacea	Lojna cista
Quiste tirogloso	Thyroglossal duct cyst	Kyste du canal thyréoglosse	Cisti del dotto tiroglosso	Cista na tireoglosnom vodu
Rabdomioma	Rhabdomyoma	Rhabdomyome	Rabdomioma	Rabdomiom
Rabdomiosarcoma	Rhabdomyosarcoma	Rhabdomyosarcome	Rabdomiosarcoma	Rabdomiosarkom
Rabia	Rabies	Rage	Rabbia	Bjesnoća (rabies)
Rango de movimiento articular limitado	Limited joint mobility	Mobilité atriculaire limitée	Ridotta mobilità articolare	Ograničena pokretljivost zgloba
Raquitismo	Rickets (rachitis)	Rachitisme	Rachitismo	Rahitis
Raquitismo renal	Renal rickets	Rachitisme rénal	Rachitismo renale	Bubrežni rahitis
Rasguño	Scratch	Égratignure	Graffio (graffiatura)	Ogrebotina
Regreso del contenido alimentario a través del esófago (regurgitación)	Expulsion of undigested food from the mouth (regurgitation)	Retour à la bouche du contenu de l'estomac (régurgitation)	Risalita di alimenti dallo stomaco alla bocca (rigurgito)	Vraćanje hrane iz želuca u usta (regurgitacija)
Relación sexual dolorosa (coitalgia, dispareunia)	Painful sexual intercourse (dyspareunia)	Douleur lors du rapport sexuel (dyspareunie)	Dolore durante rapporto sessuale (dispareunia)	Bol pri snošaju
Resfriado común (resfrío)	Common cold	Rhume	Infreddatura (raffreddore)	Prehlada (hunjavica)
Respiración de Biot	Biot's respiration	Respiration de Biot	Respiro di Biot	Biotovo disanje
Respiración de Kussmaul	Kussmaul breathing	Respiration de type Kussmaul	Respiro di Kussmaul	Kussmaulovo disanje
Respiración periódica (respiración de Cheynes-Stokes)	Periodic breathing (Cheyne-Stokes respiration)	Respiration Cheynes-Stokes	Respiro di Cheyne-Stokes	Periodično disanje (Cheyne-Stokesovo disanje)
Respiración rápida (taquipnea)	Rapid breathing (tachypnea)	Respiration accélérée (tachypnée)	Aumento del ritmo respiratorio (tachipnea)	Ubrzano disanje (tahipnea)
Respiración superficial	Shallow breathing	Respiration superficielle	Respirazione superficiale	Površinsko plitko disanje
Respuestas psicofisiológicas lentas	Slow psychophysiological responses	Réponses psychophysiologiques lentes	Lentezza psicofisica	Psihofizička usporenost
Retención de orina	Urinary retention (ischuria)	Rétention d'urine	Ritenzione urinaria	Zastoj urina (urinarna retencija)
Reticulosarcoma (sarcoma reticuloendotelial)	Reticuloendothelial sarcoma	Sarcome réticuloendothélial	Reticoloendotelioma (reticolosarcoma)	Retikuloendotelijalni sarkom
Retinitis pigmentosa	Retinitis pigmentosa (retinal pigment epithelium dystrophy)	Rétinite pigmentaire	Retinite pigmentosa	Pigmentna distrofija mrežnice
Retinopatía de la prematuridad	Retinopathy of prematurity (retrolental fibroplasia)	Rétinopathie du prématuré	Retinopatia del prematuro	Retrolentalna fibroplazija
Retinopatía diabética	Diabetic retinopathy	Rétinopathie diabétique	Retinopatia diabetica	Dijabetična retinopatija
Retorcimiento anormal del intestino (vólvulo)	Abnormal twisting of the intestines (volvulus)	Volvulus	Volvolo	Zapletaj crijeva
Retraso de la pubertad	Delayed puberty	Puberté tardive	Pubertà tardiva	Zakašnjeli pubertet
Retraso mental	Mental retardation	Retard mental (handicap mental)	Ritardo mentale	Mentalna retardacija
Retroversión del útero	Retroverted uterus	Utérus rétroversé	Retroflessione uterina	Retrovertirani uterus
Reumatismo extraarticular	Extrajoint rheumatism	Rhumatisme extraarticulaire	Reumatismo extra-articolare	Izvanzglobni reumatizam
Rickettsiosis	Rickettsiosis	Rickettsiose	Rickettsiosi	Rikecioza

Español	Inglés	Francés	Italiano	Croata
Rigidez de las articulaciones	Joint stiffness	Raideur articulaire	Rigidità dell'articolazione	Zakočenost zgloba
Rigidez de nuca (cuello rígido)	Nuchal rigidity (stiff neck)	Raideur de nuque (raideur méningée)	Rigidità nucale	Kočenje šije (ukočeni vrat)
Rinitis	Rhinitis	Rhinite	Rinite	Rinitis
Rinitis alérgica	Allergic rhinitis	Rhinite allergique	Rinite allergica	Alergijski rinitis
Rinitis vasomotora	Vasomotor rhinitis	Rhinite vasomotrice	Rinite vasomotoria	Vazomotorni rinitis
Riñón de herradura (fusión en los riñones)	Horseshoe kidney (renal fusion)	Rein en fer à cheval	Rene a ferro di cavallo (fusione renale)	Potkovičasti bubreg
Riñón flotante (ptosis renal, nefroptosis)	Floating kidney (nephroptosis, renal ptosis)	Syndrome du rein flottant (néphroptose)	Spostamento del rene (ptosi renale, nefroptosi)	Spušteni bubreg (putujući bubreg, nefroptoza)
Rizartrosis	Thumb joint arthritis	Rhizarthrose	Rizartrosi (artrosi dell'articolazione alla base del police)	Rizartroza
Rodilla de nadador de pecho (bursitis de la pata de ganso)	Swimmer's knee	Syndrome du brasseur aux genoux	Ginocchio del nuotatore a rana (stiramento cronico del legamento mediale)	Plivačko koljeno
Rodilla de saltador (tendinopatía rotuliana)	Irritated knee (jumper's knee, patellar tendinopathy)	Genou du sauteur (tendinite rotulienne)	Peritendite rotulea (ginocchio del saltatore)	Podraženo koljeno (skakačko koljeno)
Ronquera	Hoarseness	Enrouement	Raucedine	Promuklost
Rosácea	Rosacea	Rosacée (couperose)	Rosacea	Rozacea
Roséola (exantema súbito)	Exanthema subitum (roseola infantum, sixth disease)	Roséole (exanthème subit, sixième maladie)	Sesta malattia (roseola infantum, esantema subitum)	Rozeola infantum (egzantema subitum, šesta bolest)
Rubéola	German measles (rubella)	Rubéole	Rosolia	Rubeola (crljenac)
Ruptura (rotura)	Rupture	Rupture	Rottura	Prsnuće (puknuće, razdor, ruptura)
Ruptura de la vejiga urinaria	Rupture of urinary bladder	Rupture de la vessie	Rottura della vescica urinaria	Rascjep mokraćnog mjehura
Ruptura de ligamento	Ligament rupture (torn ligament)	Rupture ligamentaire	Rottura del legamento	Puknuće ligamenta
Ruptura de ligamento cruzado anterior	Anterior cruciate ligament rupture (ACL rupture)	Rupture du ligament croisé antéro-externe (rupture du LCA)	Rottura del legamento crociato anteriore del ginocchio	Razdor prednje ukrižene sveze koljenskog zgloba
Ruptura de menisco	Meniscus rupture (meniscus tear)	Rupture du ménisque	Rottura del menisco	Razdor meniskusa
Ruptura del aneurisma	Aneurysm rupture	Rupture d'anévrisme	Rottura di aneurisma	Prsnuće aneurizme
Ruptura del bazo	Ruptured spleen	Rupture de la rate	Rottura della milza	Ruptura slezene
Ruptura del manguito rotador	Rotator cuff rupture (rotator cuff tear)	Rupture de la coiffe des rotateurs	Rottura della cuffia dei rotatori	Razdor rotatorne manžete ramenog zgloba
Ruptura del tendón	Tendon rupture (torn tendon)	Rupture du tendon	Rottura del tendine	Puknuće tetive
Ruptura del tendón de Aquiles	Achilles tendon rupture	Rupture du tendon d'Achille	Rottura del tendine di Achille	Puknuće Ahilove tetive
Ruptura muscular	Muscle rupture	Rupture musculaire	Rottura muscolare	Rastrgnuće mišića (ruptura mišića)
Sabañón	Chilblain (perniosis)	Engelure	Perniosi	Smrzotina
Saco de hernia (saco herniario)	Hernia sack	Sac herniaire	Sacco dell'ernia	Kilna vreća
Salida de líquido cerebroespinal por el oído (otoliquorrea)	Leakage of cerebrospinal fluid through the ear	Écoulement de liquide cérébrospinal par l'oreille (otoliquorrhée)	Perdita di liquido cerebrospinale dall'orechio (otoliquorrea)	Curenje likvora na uho (cerebrospinalna otoreja)
Salida de líquido cerebroespinal por la nariz (rinoliquorrea)	Leakage of cerebrospinal fluid through the nose	Écoulement de liquide cérébrospinal par le nez (rhinoliquorrhée)	Perdita di liquido cerebrospinale dal naso (rinoliquorrea)	Curenje likvora na nos (cerebrospinalna rinoreja)
Salmonelosis	Salmonellosis	Salmonellose	Salmonellosi	Salmoneloza
Sangrado externo (hemorragia externa)	External bleeding	Saignement externe (hémorragie externe)	Emorragia esterna	Vanjsko krvarenje
Sangrado interno (hemorragia interna)	Internal bleeding	Saignement interne (hémorragie interne)	Emorragia interna	Unutarnje krvarenje
Sangrado interno de las articulaciones (hemartrosis)	Bleeding into joint space (hemarthrosis)	Épanchement de sang à l'intérieur d'une articulation (hémarthrose)	Emartro	Krvarenje u zglob (hemartroza)
Sangrado venoso (hemorragia venosa)	Venous bleeding	Saignement veineux	Emorragia venosa	Vensko krvarenje
Sangre en el esputo (hemoptisis)	Blood in sputum (hemoptysis)	Sang dans l'expectoration (hémoptysie)	Sangue nello sputo (emottisi)	Krvavi iskašljaj (hemoptiza)
Sangre en el líquido cefalorraquídeo	Blood in cerebrospinal fluid	Sang dans le liquide cérébro-spinal	Sangue al liquido cerebrospinale	Krv u likvoru
Sangre en la orina (hematuria)	Blood in urine (hematuria)	Sang dans les urines (hématurie)	Ematuria	Krv u urinu (hematurija)
Sangre en las heces (hematochezia)	Blood in stool (hematochezia)	Sang dans les selles (hématochézie)	Sangue nelle feci (ematochezia)	Krv u stolici (hematohezija)
Sarampión	Measles	Rougeole (1re maladie)	Morbillo	Ospice (morbili)
Sarcoidosis (enfermedad de Besnier-Boeck)	Sarcoidosis (sarcoid, Besnier-Boeck disease)	Sarcoïdose (maladie de Besnier-Boeck-Schaumann)	Sarcoidosi	Sarkoidoza
Sarcoma	Sarcoma	Sarcome	Sarcoma	Sarkom

Español	Inglés	Francés	Italiano	Croata
Sarcoma botrioide	Botryoid sarcoma	Sarcome botryoïde	Sarcoma botrioide	Botrioidni sarkom
Sarcoma de Ewing	Ewing's sarcoma	Sarcome d'Ewing	Sarcoma di Ewing	Ewing sarkom (endoteliosarkom)
Sarcoma de Kaposi	Kaposi's sarcoma	Sarcome de Kaposi	Sarcoma di Kaposi	Kaposijev sarkom (endoteliosarkom)
Sarcoma sinovial	Synovial sarcoma	Sarcome synovial	Sarcoma sinoviale	Sinovijalni sarkom
Sarcopenia	Sarcopenia	Sarcopénie	Sarcopenia	Sarkopenija
SARM	MRSA	SARM	MSSA (SARM)	SARM
Sarpullido (erupción, eccema)	Rash (eruption, eczema)	Rash (eczéma)	Sfogo (eruzione cutanea)	Osip
Seborrea	Seborrhea	Séborrhée	Seborrea	Seboreja
Sed	Thirst	Soif	Sete	Žed
Semicoma	Semicoma	Semi-coma	Semi-coma	Semikoma
Sensación de "zapatos apretados"	'Tight shoes' sensation	Sensation des chaussures très serré	Senso delle scarpe troppo strette	Osjećaj "tijesnih cipela"
Sensación de ardor	Burning sensation	Sensation cuisante	Sensazione bruciante	Pećenje (žarenje)
Sensación de miedo	Sensation of fear	Sensation de peur	Senso della paura	Osjećaj straha
Sensación exagerada de los estímulos táctiles (hiperestesia)	Increased sensitivity to stimuli of the senses (hyperesthesia)	Hypersensibilité aux stimuli extérieurs (hyperesthésie)	Ippersensibilità ai normali stimoli esterni (iperestesia)	Preosjetljivost na podražaj (hiperestezija)
Sensibilidad al dolor (algesia)	Sensitivity to pain (algesia)	Sensibilité à la douleur (algésie)	Sensibilità al dolore (algesia)	Osjetljivost na bol (algezija)
Sepsis	Sepsis	Sepsis	Sepsi	Sepsa
Septicemia	Septicemia	Septicémie	Setticemia	Septikemija
Sequedad de la boca (xerostomía)	Dry mouth (xerostomia)	Sècheresse de la bouche (xèrostomie)	Scarsa secrezione salivare (xerostomia)	Suha sluznica usta
Sequedad de los ojos (xeroftalmia)	Dry eyes (keratoconjuctivitis sicca)	Oeil sec (kérato-conjonctivite sèche)	Occhi secchi (xeroftalmia)	Suhe oči (kseroftalmija)
Shigelosis	Shigellosis (bacillary dysentery)	Shigellose	Shigellosi	Šigeloza
Sialorrea (ptialismo)	Drooling (ptyalism, sialorrhea, slobbering)	Hypersialorrhée (ptyalisme)	Sbavando (ptialismo, scialorrea)	Slinjenje
SIDA (síndrome de inmunodeficiencia adquirida)	AIDS (acquired immune deficiency syndrome)	SIDA (syndrome d'immunodéficience acquise)	SIDA (sindrome da ImmunoDeficienza Acquisita, AIDS)	SIDA (sindrom stečene imunodeficijencije, AIDS)
Siderosis	Siderosis	Sidérose	Siderosi	Sideroza
Sífilis	Syphilis	Syphilis (vérole)	Sifilide (lue)	Sifilis (lues)
Silicosis	Silicosis	Silicose	Silicosi	Silikoza
Síncope	Syncope	Syncope	Sincope	Sinkopa
Sindactilia	Syndactyly	Syndactylie	Sindattilia	Sindaktilija
Síndrome braquial	Brachial syndrome	Brachialgie	Brachialgia	Brahijalni sindrom bolne nadlaktice
Síndrome carcinoide	Carcinoid syndrome	Syndrome carcinoïde	Sindrome da carcinoide	Karcinoidni sindrom
Síndrome cervical	Cervicocephal syndrome	Syndrome cervical	Sindrome cervicale	Cervikocefalni sindrom
Síndrome cérvico-braquial	Cervicobrachial syndrome	Syndrome cervico-brachial	Sindrome cervico-brachiale (sindrome spalla-mano)	Sindrom vrat-rame (cervikobrahijalni sindrom)
Síndrome compartimental	Compartment syndrome	Syndrome des loges	Sindrome compartimentale	Sindrom fascijalnog prostora
Síndrome de abstinencia	Withdrawal	Sevrage	Crisi d'astinenza	Apstinencijska kriza
Síndrome de alcoholismo fetal	Fetal alcohol syndrome	Syndrome d'alcoolisation foetale	Sindrome alcolica fetale	Fetusni alkoholni sindrom
Síndrome de aplastamiento (síndrome de crush)	Crush-syndrome	Syndrome d'écrasement	Sindrome da schiacciamento	Crush-sindrom
Síndrome de bebé flácido	Floppy infant syndrome	Syndrome du bébé mou	Sindrome del bambino flaccido	Sindrom mlohavog djeteta
Síndrome de Behçet	Behçet's disease	Maladie de Behçet	Sindrome di Behçet	Behçetova bolest
Síndrome de Cushing (hipercortisolismo)	Cushing's syndrome (hypercorticism)	Syndrome de Cushing (hypercorticisme)	Sindrome di Cushing (ipercortisolismo)	Cushingov sindrom (hiperkortikolizam)
Síndrome de decompresión (enfermedad de los buzos, mal de presión)	Decompression sickness (diver's disease, caisson disease)	Maladie de décompression (maladie des plongeurs, maladie des caissons)	Malattia di decompressione (sindrome di Caisson)	Dekompresijska bolest (kesonska bolest)
Síndrome de DeQuervain	DeQuervain syndrome	Syndrome de DeQuervain (ténosynovite de DeQuervain)	Sindrome di De Quervain	Sindrom bubnjarskog palca (Morbus DeQuervain)
Síndrome de distrés respiratorio	Respiratory distress syndrome	Syndrome de détresse respiratoire	Sindrome da distress respiratorio	Respiratorni distres sindrom
Síndrome de dolor inguinal	Groin pain syndrome	Pubalgie du sportif	Pubalgia dello sportivo	Sindrom bolnih prepona
Síndrome de Down	Down syndrome	Syndrome de Down	Sindrome di Down	Downov sindrom (mongoloidizam)
Síndrome de Edwards (trisomía del 18)	Edwards syndrome (trisomy 18)	Syndrome d'Edwards (trisomie 18)	Sindrome di Edwards	Trisomija 18D (Edwardsov sindrom)
Síndrome de Eisenmenger	Eisenmenger's syndrome	Syndrome d'Eisenmenger	Sindrome di Eisenmenger	Eisenmengerov sindrom
Síndrome de fatiga crónica	Chronic fatigue syndrome	Syndrome de fatigue chronique	Sindrome da fatica cronica	Sindrom kroničnog umora

Español	Inglés	Francés	Italiano	Croata
Síndrome de fricción de la banda iliotibial	Iliotibial band friction syndrome	Syndrome de la bandelette iliotibiale (syndrome de l'essuie glace)	Sindrome della benderella ileotibiale	Sindrom trenja iliotibijalnog traktusa
Síndrome de Goodpasture	Goodpasture's syndrome	Syndrome de Goodpasture (maladie des anticorps anti-membrane basale glomérulaire)	Sindrome di Goodpasture	Goodpastureov sindrom
Síndrome de Guillain-Barré	Guillain-Barré syndrome	Syndrome de Guillain-Barré	Sindrome di Guillain-Barré	Guillain-Barréov sindrom
Síndrome de intestino irritable (colon irritable, colon espástico)	Irritable bowel syndrome (spastic colon)	Côlon irritable (côlon spastique)	Sindrome del colon irritabile (colon spastico)	Sindrom iritabilnog crijeva (spastični kolon)
Síndrome de isquiosurales cortos	Tight hamstrings syndrome	Hamstring syndrome	Sindrome degli ischio-crurali (sindrome dell'hamstring)	Sindrom stražnje lože natkoljenice (sindrom hamstringsa)
Síndrome de la clase turista	Traveller's thrombosis (economy class syndrome)	Thrombose du voyageur	Sindrome della classe economica	Sindrom ekonomske klase
Síndrome de Legg-Calvé-Perthes	Legg-Calvé-Perthes disease	Maladie de Legg-Calvé-Perthes (ostéochondrite primitive de hanche)	Malattia di Legg-Perthes-Calvé	Legg-Calvé-Perthesova bolest
Síndrome de Leriche	Aortoiliac occlusive disease (Leriche's syndrome)	Maladie occlusive aorto-iliaque	Sindrome di Leriche	Lericheov sindrom
Síndrome de Marfan	Marfan syndrome	Syndrome de Marfan	Sindrome di Marfan	Marfanov sindrom
Síndrome de McCune-Albright	McCune-Albright syndrome	Syndrome de McCune-Albright	Sindrome di McCune-Albright-Sternberg	Albrightov sindrom
Síndrome de muerte súbita del lactante (muerte en cuna)	Sudden infant death syndrome (crib death, cot death)	Syndrome de mort subite du nourrisson	Sindrome della morte improvvisa del lattante	Sindrom iznenadne smrti dojenčeta
Síndrome de Patau (trisomía en el par 13)	Patau syndrome (trisomy 13)	Syndrome de Patau (trisomie 13)	Sindrome di Patau	Trisomija 13D (Patauov sindrom)
Síndrome de pinzamiento posterior del tobillo	Posterior ankle impingement syndrome	Conflit postérieur de la cheville	Sindrome da impingement posteriore di caviglia	Sindrom sraza stražnjeg nožnog zgloba
Síndrome de Reiter (artritis reactiva)	Reactive arthritis (Reiter's syndrome)	Arthrite réactive (syndrome de Reiter)	Sindrome di Reiter	Reiterov sindrom
Síndrome de Reye	Reye's syndrome	Syndrome de Reye	Sindrome di Reye	Reyeov sindrom
Síndrome de Sjögren	Sjögren's syndrome	Syndrome de Sjögren	Sindrome di Sjögren	Sjögrenov sindrom
Síndrome de sobreuso	Repetitive strain injury (cumulative trauma disorder)	Lésion due à un surmenage répétitif	R.S.I (Repetitive Strain Injury)	Sindrom prenaprezanja
Síndrome de Tourette	Tourette's syndrome	Syndrome de Tourette	Sindrome di Tourette	Touretteov sindrom
Síndrome de Turner	Turner syndrome	Syndrome de Turner	Sindrome di Turner	Turnerov sindrom
Síndrome del conflicto subacromial	Shoulder impingement syndrome (subacromial impingement syndrome)	Syndrome du conflit sous-acromial	Sindrome da conflitto subacromiale (impingement sub-acromiale)	Sindrom sraza ramena (subakromijalni sindrom sraza)
Síndrome del estrecho torácico	Thoracic outlet syndrome	Syndrome de traversée thoraco-cervico-brachiale	Sindrome dello stretto toracico superiore	Torakalni sindrom
Síndrome del maullido del gato (síndrome de Lejeune)	Cat cry syndrome (5p minus syndrome, Lejeune's syndrome)	Maladie du cri du chat (syndrome de Lejeune)	Sindrome del grido di gatto	Sindrom mačjeg krika
Síndrome del tibial posterior	Tibialis posterior syndrome	Syndrome tibial postérieur	Periostite tibiale (sindrome del muscolo tibiale posteriore)	Sindrom stražnjeg tibijalnog mišića
Síndrome del túnel carpiano	Carpal tunnel syndrome	Syndrome du canal carpien	Sindrome del tunnel carpale	Sindrom karpalnog tunela
Síndrome del túnel cubital	Little league elbow syndrome (LLE syndrome)	Syndrome du tunnel cubital	Sindrome del tunnel cubitale	Sindrom kopljaškog lakta
Síndrome del túnel tarsiano	Tarsal tunnel syndrome	Syndrome du canal tarsien	Sindrome del tunnel tarsale	Sindrom tarzalnog kanala
Síndrome doloroso	Pain syndrome	Syndrome de douleur	Sindrome dolorosa	Bolni sindrom
Síndrome hepatorrenal	Hepatorenal syndrome	Syndrome hépato-rénal	Sindrome epato-renale	Hepatorenalni sindrom
Síndrome mielodisplásico (preleucemia)	Myelodysplastic syndrome	Syndrome myélodysplasique	Sindrome mielodisplasica	Mijelodisplastični sindrom
Síndrome nefrótico	Nephrotic syndrome	Syndrome néphrotique	Sindrome nefrosica	Nefrotski sindrom
Síndrome occipital (neuralgia occipital)	Occipital neuralgia (Arnold's neuralgia)	Nèvralgie occipitale	Nevralgia occipitale (nevralgia di Arnold)	Okcipitalna neuralgija
Síndrome por explosion	Blast-syndrome	Syndrome de blast	Lesioni da scoppio (blast-syndrome)	Blast-sindrom
Síndrome postrombótico	Post-thrombotic syndrome	Syndrome post-thrombotique	Sindrome post trombotica	Posttrombotički sindrom
Síndrome premenstrual	Premenstrual syndrome (PMS)	Syndrome prémenstruel (SPM)	Sindrome premestruale	Predmenstruacijski sindrom (PMS)
Síndrome prodrómico	Early symptom (prodrome)	Phase prodromique	Sindrome prodromica	Predsimptom bolesti prije nego se bolest razvije
Síndrome respiratorio agudo severo (SRAS, SARS)	Severe acute respiratory syndrome (SARS)	Syndrome respiratoire aigu sévère (SRAS)	SARS (Sindrome Acuta Respiratoria Severa)	Sindrom akutne respiratorne insuficijencije (SARS)
Sinostosis radiocubital	Radioulnar synostosis	Synostose radio-ulnaire	Sinostosi radio-ulnare	Radioulnarna sinostoza

Español	Inglés	Francés	Italiano	Croata
Sinovioma	Synovioma	Synoviome	Sinovioma	Sinoviom
Siringomielia	Syringomyelia	Syringomyélie	Siringomielia	Siringomijelija
Sobredosis de medicamentos	Medication overdose	Surdose du médicament	Overdose di farmaci	Predoziranje lijekom
Sobredosis por droga	Drug overdose	Surdose de drogue	Overdose di droga	Predoziranje drogom
Sofocos	Hot flushes	Bouffée de chaleur	Vampata di calore	Valovi vrućine (valunzi)
Somnolencia	Somnolence	Somnolence	Sonnolenza	Pospanost (somnolencija)
Sonambulismo (noctambulismo)	Sleepwalking (somnambulism)	Somnabulisme	Sonnambulismo	Mjesečarenje (somnambulizam)
Sonido de tripas (borborigmo)	Stomach growling (borborygmus)	Gargouillements (borborygme)	Borborigmo	Kruljenje u želucu
Soplo del corazón	Heart murmur	Souffle cardiaque	Soffio cardiaco	Šum na srcu
Sopor	Sopor	Sopor	Stupor	Sopor
Sorberse la nariz (moqueo)	Sniffing (sniffle)	Renifler	Tirare su col naso	Šmrcanje
Sordera	Deafness	Surdité	Sordità	Gluhoća
Sudor nocturno	Night sweats	Sueurs nocturnes	Sudore notturno	Noćno znojenje
Supresión de la secreción de orina	Nonpassage of urine	Arrêt de la sécrétion d'urine	Soppressione della secrezione di urina	Prestanak lučenja urina
Talasemia	Thalassemia	Thalassémie	Talassemia	Talasemija
Tamponamiento cardíaco (tamponamiento pericárdiaco)	Pericardial tamponade (cardiac tamponade)	Tamponnade cardiaque	Tamponamento cardiaco	Tamponada perikarda
Tapón de cerumen	Impacted cerumen	Bouchon de cérumen	Tappo di cerume	Ceruminozni čep
Taquicardia	Tachycardia	Tachycardie	Tachicardia	Tahikardija
Temblor	Tremor	Tremblement	Tremito (tremore)	Drhtanje (tremor)
Temblor en las manos	Hand tremor	Tremblement des mains	Tremore delle mani	Drhtanje ruku
Temperatura corporal baja (hipotermia)	Decreased body temperature (hypothermia)	Température corporelle basse (hypothermie)	Bassa temperatura corporea (ipotermia)	Snižena temperatura tijela (hipotermija)
Tendinitis de Aquiles	Achillodynia (Achilles tendinitis)	Tendinite du tendon d'Achille	Tendinopatia achillea (achillodinia)	Ahilodinija (tendinitis Ahilove tetive)
Tendinitis de los extensores de los dedos	Extensor tendinitis (inflammation of the extensor tendons of the toes)	Tendinite des extenseurs des orteils	Tendinite dei estensori delle dita del piede	Tendinitis ekstenzora prstiju stopala
Tendinitis del flexor hallucis longus	Dancer's tendinitis (flexor hallucis tendinitis)	Tendinite des danseurs (fléchisseur de l'hallux tendinite)	Tendinite del flessore lungo dell'alluce	Tendinitis plesača (tendinitis dugog pregibača palca)
Tendinitis en el antebrazo	Forearm tendinitis	Tendinite de l'avant-bras	Tendinite dell'avambraccio	Veslačka podlaktica (tendinitis podlaktice)
Tendinitis poplítea	Popliteus syndrome	Syndrome poplité douloureux	Tendinite del popliteo	Sindrom m. popliteusa
Tendinitis por sobreuso en el tendón de Aquiles	Achilles tendon overuse injury	Tendinite achilléenne chronique	Tendinopatia Achille da overuse	Sindrom prenaprezanja Ahilove tetive
Tendinopatía tibial posterior	Tibialis posterior tendinitis	Tendinopathie du tibial postérieur	Tendinite del muscolo tibiale posteriore	Tendinitis stražnjeg tibijalnog mišića
Tendinosis (lesión crónica del tendón)	Tendinosis (chronic tendon injury)	Tendinose	Tendinosi	Tendinoza (kronična ozljeda tetive)
Tener gases (flatulencia)	Passing gas (flatulence, farting)	Pet (flatulence, vesse)	Miscela di gas (flatulenza)	Puštanje vjetra (flatulencija, plinovi)
Tensión de la pared abdominal	Abdominal wall tension	Tension de la paroi stomacale	Tensione di parete addominale	Napetost trbušne stijenke
Teratocarcinoma	Teratocarcinoma	Tératocarcinome	Teratocarcinoma	Teratokarcinom
Teratoma	Teratoma	Tératome	Teratoma	Teratom
Tetania	Tetany	Tétanie	Tetania	Tetanija
Tétanos (tétano)	Tetanus	Tétanos	Tetano	Tetanus (zli grč)
Tetralogía de Fallot	Tetralogy of Fallot	Tétralogie de Fallot	Tetralogia di Fallot	Fallotova tetralogija
Tic	Tic	Tic	Tic	Tik
Tifus endémico murino	Murine typhus (endemic typhus)	Typhus murin	Tifo murino (tifo endemico)	Štakorski pjegavac
Tifus exantemático epidémico	Epidemic typhus (louse-borne typhus)	Typhus épidémique (typhus à poux, typhus européen)	Tifo esantematico (tifo epidemico)	Trbušni tifus (epidemjski tifus, pjegavac)
Tiña corporal (tinea corporis)	Tinea corporis	Tinea corporis	Tinea corporis	Tinea corporis
Tiña crural (tinea cruris)	Crotch itch (tinea cruris)	Eczéma marginé de hebra	Tinea cruris	Gljivična infekcija prepona (tinea cruris)
Tiña de la cabeza (tinea capitis)	Tinea capitis (scalp ringworm)	Teigne (tinea capitis)	Tigna (tinea capitis)	Gljivična infekcija vlasišta (tinea capitis)
Tiña del pie (pie de atleta, tinea pedis)	Athlete's foot (tinea pedis)	Pied d'athlète (tinea pedis)	Piede d'atleta (tinea pedis)	Atletsko stopalo (gljivična infekcija stopala, tinea pedis)
Tiña favosa (favus, tinea favosa)	Favus	Favus	Tinea favosa	Tinea favosa (favus)
Tiña versicolor (pitiriasis versicolor)	Tinea versicolor (pityriasis versicolor, haole rot)	Pityriasis versicolor	Pitiriasi versicolor (tinea versicolor)	Pitirijaza (svjetlije mrlje na osunčanoj koži, Tinea versicolor)
Tiroiditis de Hashimoto	Hashimoto's disease	Thyroïdite de Hashimoto	Tiroidite di Hashimoto	Hashimotov sindrom
Tiroiditis de Riedel	Riedel's thyroiditis	Thyroïdite de Riedel	Tiroidite di Riedel	Riedelov tireoiditis

Español	Inglés	Francés	Italiano	Croata
Tirotoxicosis	Thyrotoxicosis	Thyréotoxicose	Tireotossicosi	Tireotoksikoza (tireotoksična oluja)
Torpeza en las extremidades	Dullness in limbs	Membres sourds	Ottusità alle estremità	Tupost u udovima
Torsión del hueso	Bone bending (bone torsion)	Torsion osseuse	Torsione dell'osso	Savijanje kosti
Torsión testicular	Testicular torsion	Torsion testiculaire	Torsione del testicolo	Torzija testisa
Tortícolis	Wry neck (torticollis)	Torticolis	Torcicollo	Krivi vrat (tortikolis)
Tos	Cough	Toux	Tosse	Kašalj
Tos ferina (coqueluche)	Whooping cough (pertussis)	Coqueluche	Pertosse	Hripavac (pasji kašalj, pertussis)
Tos productiva	Productive cough	Toux productive	Tosse produttiva	Produktivni kašalj
Tos seca (tos perruna)	Dry cough	Toux sèche	Tosse secca	Suhi kašalj
Tóxico-infección por Clostridium perfringens	Clostridium perfringens toxic infection	Toxi-infection à Clostridium perfringens	Tossinfezione da Clostridium perfringens	Toksična infekcija Clostridium perfringensom
Toxocariasis	Toxocariasis	Toxocarose	Toxocariasi	Toksokarijaza
Toxoplasmosis	Toxoplasmosis	Toxoplasmose	Toxoplasmosi	Toksoplazmoza
Tracoma	Trachoma	Trachome	Tracoma	Trahom
Transpiración (sudación)	Sweating	Sudation	Sudorazione (traspirazione)	Znojenje
Transplante de riñón	Kidney transplatation	Transplantation rénale	Trapianto renale	Transplantacija bubrega
Transposición de la aorta	Transposition of aorta	Transposition de l'aorte	Trasposizione dell'aorta	Transpozicija aorte
Transposición de la arteria pulmonar	Transposition of pulmonary artery	Transposition de l'artère pulmonaire	Trasposizione dell'arteria polmonare	Transpozicija plućne arterije
Transposición de los grandes vasos	Transposition of the great vessels	Transposition des gros vaisseaux	Trasposizione dei grossi vasi	Transpozicija velikih žila
Trastorno alimentario	Eating disorder	Trouble de conduite alimentaire	Disturbo del comportamento alimentare	Poremećaj ishrane
Trastorno bipolar (psicosis maníaco-depresiva)	Bipolar disorder (manic-depressive psychosis)	Trouble bipolaire (psychose maniaco-dépressive)	Psicosi maniaco-depressiva	Bipolarni poremećaj (manično-depresivna psihoza)
Trastorno de la audición	Hearing disorder	Trouble de l'audition	Disturbo dell'udito	Poremećaj sluha
Trastorno de la capacidad para oír de las personas envejecen (presbiacusia)	Age-related hearing loss (presbycusis)	Perte de l'audition liée à l'age (presbyacousie)	Perdita dell'udito dovuta all'avanzamento dell'età (presbiacusia)	Staračka nagluhost (prezbiakuzija)
Trastorno de la diferenciación sexual	Sexual differentiation disorder	Trouble de la différenciation sexuelle	Disordine della differenziazione sessuale	Poremećaj spolne diferencijacije
Trastorno de la micción	Urination disorder	Trouble de la miction	Disturbo della minzione	Poremećaj mokrenja
Trastorno de la visión	Sight disorder	Trouble de la vue	Disturbo della vista	Poremećaj vida
Trastorno de movimiento	Movement disorder	Trouble du mouvement	Disordine del movimento	Poremećaj kretanja
Trastorno de personalidad	Personality disorder	Trouble de la personnalité	Disturbo di personalità	Poremećaj osobnosti
Trastorno del comportamiento	Behavioral disorder	Trouble du comportement	Disturbo dell'umore	Poremećaj ponašanja
Trastorno del equilibrio	Balance disorder	Trouble de l'équilibre	Disturbo dell'equilibrio	Poremećaj ravnoteže
Trastorno del lenguaje (disfasia)	Speech difficulty (dysphasia)	Trouble de l'apprentissage du langage (dysphasie)	Disturbo del linguaggio verbale (afasia)	Otežan govor (disfazija)
Trastorno del sueño	Sleeping disorder	Trouble du sommeil	Disturbo del sonno	Poremećaj spavanja
Trastorno límite de la personalidad	Borderline personality disorder	Personnalité borderline	Disturbo borderline di personalità	Granični poremećaj osobnosti
Trastorno menstrual	Menstrual disorder	Troubles du cycle menstruel	Disturbi mestruali	Menstrualne smetnje
Trastorno por déficit de atención	Attention deficit disorder	Trouble déficit de l'attention	Disturbo della concentrazione	Poremećaj koncentracije
Trastorno por estrés postraumático	Posttraumatic stress disorder	Trouble de stress post-traumatique	Disturbo post traumatico da stress	Posttraumatski stresni poremećaj (PTSP)
Trichomonas vaginalis	Trichomonas vaginalis	Trichomonas vaginalis	Trichomonas vaginalis	Trihomonazni vaginitis
Trichomoniasis	Trichomoniasis	Trichomoniase	Trichomoniasi	Trihomonijaza
Tripanosomiasis	Trypanosomiasis	Trypanosomiase	Tripanosomiasi	Tripanosomijaza
Tripanosomiasis africana (enfermedad del sueño)	African trypanosomiasis (sleeping sickness)	Maladie du sommeil (trypanosomiase africaine)	Tripanosomiasi africana (malattia del sonno)	Afrička tripanosomijaza (bolest spavanja)
Triquinelosis (triquinosis)	Trichinosis (trichinellosis)	Trichinose	Trichinosi	Trihinoza (trihineloza)
Trombocitopenia	Thrombocytopenia	Thrombocytopénie	Trombocitopenia	Trombocitopenija
Tromboembolismo	Thromboembolism	Accident thromboembolique	Tromboembolia	Tromboembolija
Tromboflebitis	Thrombophlebitis	Thrombophlébite	Tromboflebite	Tromboflebitis
Trombosis	Thrombosis	Thrombose	Trombosi	Tromboza
Trombosis venosa	Venous thrombosis	Thrombose veineuse	Trombosi venosa	Venska tromboza
Tsutsugamushi (fiebre fluvial japonesa, tifus de los matorrales)	Scrub typhus (Japanese river fever, Tsutsugamushi fever)	Fièvre fluviale du Japon (typhus à chiques)	Tsutsugamushi (tifo fluviale giapponese)	Japanska riječna groznica (Tsutsugamushi groznica)
Tuberculosis (tisis, TBC)	Tuberculosis (TBC)	Tuberculose	Tubercolosi (tisi)	Tuberkuloza (sušica, TBC)
Tuberculosis ganglionar (linfadenitis tubercular)	Tuberculous lymphadenitis	Lymphadénite tuberculeuse	Linfadenite tubercolare	Tuberkuloza limfnih čvorova
Tuberculosis hepática	Hepatic tuberculosis	Tuberculose hépatique	Tubercolosi epatica	Tuberkuloza jetre
Tuberculosis intestinal	Intestinal tuberculosis	Tuberculose intestinale	Tubercolosi intestinale	Tuberkuloza crijeva
Tuberculosis ósea	Bone tuberculosis	Tuberculose des os	Tubercolosi delle ossa	Tuberkuloza kosti
Tuberculosis pulmonar	Pulmonary tuberculosis	Tuberculose pulmonaire	Tubercolosi polmonare	Tuberkuloza pluća
Tuberculosis renal	Renal tuberculosis	Tuberculose rénale	Tubercolosi dei reni	Tuberkuloza bubrega
Tuberculosis urogenital	Urogenital tuberculosis	Tuberculose urogénitale	Tubercolosi urogenitale	Urogenitalna tuberkuloza
Tularemia (fiebre de los conejos)	Tularemia (rabbit fever)	Tularémie	Tularemia (febbre dei conigli)	Tularemija (zečja groznica)

Español	Inglés	Francés	Italiano	Croata
Tumor	Tumor (tumour)	Tumeur	Tumore	Tumor
Tumor benigno	Benign tumor	Tumeur bénigne	Tumore benigno	Dobroćudni tumor (benigni tumor)
Tumor de Brenner	Brenner tumour	Tumeur de Brenner	Tumore di Brenner	Brennerov tumor
Tumor de células de la granulosa (tumor de teca-granulosa)	Granulosa cell tumor	Tumeur de la granulosa	Follicoloma	Granuloza tumor
Tumor de células de Sertoli-Leydig (arrenoblastoma)	Androblastoma (Sertoli-Leydig cell tumor)	Androblastome (tumeur à cellule de Sertoli et Leydig)	Androblastoma	Androblastom (tumor Sertoli-Leydigovih stanica)
Tumor de células gigantes (osteoclastoma)	Gigantocellular tumor (osteoclastoma)	Tumeur à cellules géantes	Osteoclastoma (tumore a cellule giganti)	Gigantocelularni tumor (osteoklastom)
Tumor de saco vitelino	Yolk sac tumor (endodermal sinus tumor)	Tumeur du sac vitellin	Tumore del sacco vitellino	Tumor žumanjčane vreće (endodermalni sinus tumor)
Tumor de Wilms (nefroblastoma)	Wilm's tumor (nephroblastoma)	Tumeur de Wilms (néphroblastome)	Tumore di Wilms (nefroblastoma)	Wilmsov tumor (nefroblastom)
Tumor glómico (glomangioma)	Glomus tumor (glomangioma)	Tumeur glomique (glomangiome)	Glomangioma (paraganglioma)	Glomus-tumor
Tumor maligno (cáncer)	Malignant tumor (cancer)	Tumeur maligne (cancer)	Tumore maligno	Zloćudni tumor (maligni tumor, rak)
Tumor mixto	Mixed tumor	Tumeur mixte	Tumore misto	Mješoviti tumor
Tumor mixto maligno	Malignant mixed tumor	Tumeur mixte malin	Tumore misto maligno	Mješoviti maligni tumor
Tumor urogenital	Urogenital neoplasm	Tumeur du système uro-génital	Neoplasie del tratto urogenitale	Urogenitalni tumor
Tungiasis	Tungiasis (nigua, pique)	Sarcopsyllose	Tungiasi (tunga penetrans)	Tungijaza
Úlcera (llaga)	Ulcer	Ulcère	Ulcera (ulcerazione)	Čir (ulkus)
Úlcera de decúbito	Bedsore (decubitus ulcer)	Escarre (plaie de lit, ulcère de décubitus)	Piaga da decubito (decubito)	Dekubitus
Úlcera duodenal	Duodenal ulcer	Ulcère du doudénum	Ulcera duodenale	Čir na dvanaesniku
Úlcera gástrica	Gastric ulcer	Ulcère de l'estomac	Ulcera gastrica	Čir na želucu
Úlcera isquémica	Ischemic ulceration	Ulcère ischémique	Ulcera ischemica	Ishemična ulceracija
Úlcera perforada	Perforated ulcer	Perforation d'ulcère	Ulcera perforata	Puknuće čira (perforacija ulkusa)
Úlcera varicosa	Venous ulcer (varicose ulcer)	Ulcère veineux	Ulcera varicosa	Varikozni ulcer (venski ulcer)
Uña encarnada (onicocriptosis)	Ingrown nail (onychocryptosis, unguis incarnatus)	Ongle incarné (onychocryptose)	Unghia incarnita (onicocriptosi)	Urasli nokat (ungvis inkarnatus)
Uremia (acumulación en la sangre de los productos tóxicos por un fallo renal)	Uremia (autointoxication due to kidney failure)	Urémie (le taux de l'urée dans le sang)	Uremia (accumulo nel sangue di sostanze azotate a causa dell'insufficienza renale)	Uremija (autointoksikacija radi nelučenja urina)
Urticaria	Hives (urticaria)	Urticaire	Orticaria	Koprivnjača (urtikarija)
Vaginosis bacteriana	Bacterial vaginosis	Vaginose bactérienne	Infezione della vagina batterica (vaginosi)	Bakterijska infekcija rodnice (bakterijska vaginoza)
Varicela	Chicken-pox	Varicelle	Varicella	Vodene kozice (varičela)
Varices	Varicose veins	Varices	Varicosi (varici, malattia varicosa)	Proširene vene
Varices del cuello	Neck varicose veins	Varice dans le cou	Vene varicose del collo	Proširene vratne vene
Varices esofágicas	Esophageal varices	Varices oesophagiennes	Varici esofagee	Proširene vene jednjaka (flebektazije)
Varicocele	Varicocele	Varicocèle	Varicocele	Varikokela
Venas varicosas de las piernas	Leg varicose veins	Varices des membres inférieurs	Varici degli arti inferiori	Proširene vene na nogama
Verruga	Wart	Verrue	Verruca	Bradavica (virusna bradavica)
Verruga genital (condiloma acuminata)	Genital wart	Verrue génitale	Condiloma	Genitalna bradavica (venerična bradavica)
Vértigo	Dizziness (vertigo)	Vertige	Capogiro (vertigine)	Vrtoglavica
Vértigo posicional paroxístico benigno	Benign positional vertigo	Vertige paroxystique positionnel bénin	Cupololitiasi (canalolitiasi)	Benigna pozicijska vrtoglavica
Vibraciones mano brazo (dedo blanco inducido por vibraciones)	Hand-arm vibration syndrome (vibration white finger)	Syndrome des vibrations du système main-bras	Sindrome da vibrazioni mano-braccio	Vibracijski sindrom šaka-ruka
Viruela	Smallpox	Variole (petite vérole)	Variola vera (vaiolo)	Velike boginje (crne boginje, variola vera)
Visión doble (diplopía)	Double vision (diplopia)	Vision double (diplopie)	Visione doppia (diplopia)	Dvoslike
Vista cansada por la edad (presbiopía)	Age-related long-sightedness (presbyopia)	Mauvaise vision de près liée à l'âge (presbytie)	Presbiopia (presbitismo)	Staračka dalekovidnost (prezbiopija)
Vitíligo	Vitiligo	Vitiligo	Vitiligine	Vitiligo
Vómito (emesis)	Vomiting	Vomissement	Vomito (emetismo)	Povraćanje
Vómito de sangre (hematemesis)	Vomiting of blood (hematemesis)	Vomissement de sang (hématémèse)	Emesi emorragica (ematemesi)	Povraćanje krvi (hematemeza)
Vómito sin náusea (vómito cerebral)	Vomiting without nausea (cerebral vomiting)	Vomissement en fusée sans effort	Vomito senza nausea (vomito a getto, vomito cerebrale)	Povraćanje bez mučnine (povraćanje u luku, cerebralno povraćanje)

Español	Inglés	Francés	Italiano	Croata
Xantelasma	Xanthelasma	Xanthelasma	Xantelasma	Ksantelazma
Xantoma	Xanthoma	Xanthome	Xantoma	Ksantom
Zoonosis	Zoonosis	Zoonose	Zoonosi	Zoonoza
FARMACIA:	**PHARMACY:**	**PHARMACIE:**	**FARMACIA:**	**LJEKARNA:**
A mediodía	At noon	À midi	A mezzogiorno	U podne
Aceite de almendras dulces	Almond oil	Huile d'amande	Olio di mandorla	Bademovo ulje
Aceite de jojoba	Jojoba oil	Huile de jojoba	Olio di jojoba	Jojobino ulje
Aceite de ricino	Castor oil	Huile de ricin	Olio di ricino	Ricinusovo ulje
Aceite esencial	Essential oil	Huile essentielle	Olio essenziale (olio eterico)	Eterično ulje
Aceite mineral	Mineral oil	Huile minérale	Olio minerale	Mineralno ulje
Ácido bórico	Boric acid	Acide borique	Acido borico	Borova otopina
Ácido graso omega 3	Omega-3 fatty acid	Acides gras oméga-3	Omega-3 acidi grassi	Omega-3 masne kiseline
Adrenalina	Adrenaline	Adrénaline	Adrenalina	Adrenalin
Aerosol	Aerosol	Aérosol	Aerosol	Aerosol
Agente antiarrítmico	Antiarrhythmic agent	Agent antiarythmique	Farmaco antiaritmico	Antiaritmik
Aguja	Needle	Aiguille	Ago	Igla
Alcol	Alcohol	Alkohol	Alcool	Alcohol
Alergia al medicamento	Drug allergy	Allergie à un médicament	Allergia a medicamento	Alergija na lijek
Algodón hidrófilo	Cotton-wool	Ouate (coton hydrophile)	Ovatta	Vata
Aminofilina	Aminophylline	Aminophylline	Aminofillina	Aminofilin
Ampicilina	Ampicillin	Ampicilline	Ampicillina	Ampicilin
Ampolla (recipiente)	Ampoule	Ampoule	Ampolla (fiala)	Ampula
Analgésico	Analgesic (painkiller)	Analgésique	Analgesico	Analgetik
Anestésico	Anesthetic	Anesthésique	Anestetico	Anestetik
Antiácido	Antacid	Antiacide	Antiacido	Antacid
Antialérgico	Antiallergic drug	Antiallergique	Farmaco antiallergico	Antialergik
Antianémico	Antianemic	Médicament antianémique	Farmaco antianemico	Antianemik
Antibiótico	Antibiotic	Antibiotique	Antibiotico	Antibiotik
Anticoagulante	Anticoagulant	Anticoagulant	Anticoagulante	Antikoagulans
Anticonceptivo	Contraceptive	Contraceptif	Contraccettivo	Kontraceptiv
Anticonceptivo de emergencia (contracepción poscoital)	'Morning-after' pill (postcoital contraception, emergency contraception)	Pilule du lendemain (contraception postcoïtale, contraception d'urgence)	Pillola del "giorno do-ppo" (contraccezione post-coitale, contraccezione di emergenza)	Pilula za "dan poslije" (postkoitalna kontracepcija, hitna kontracepcija)
Anticonvulsivo (antiepiléptico)	Anticonvulsant	Antiépileptique (anticonvulsivant)	Anticonvulsante	Antiepileptik (antikonvulziv)
Antidepresivo	Antidepressant	Antidépresseur	Antidepressivo	Antidepresiv
Antidiabético	Anti-diabetic drug	Médicament antidiabétique	Antidiabetico	Antidiabetik
Antidiarréico	Antidiarrhoeal drug	Médicament antidiarrhéique	Antidiarroici	Antidiaroik
Antídoto	Antidote	Antidote	Antidoto	Antidot
Antiemético	Antiemetic and motion sickness drug	Antiémétique	Antiemetico	Lijek protiv mučnine i povraćanja
Antihelmíntico	Antihelminthic	Antihelminthique	Antielmintici	Antihelmintik
Antihipertensivo	Antihypertensive drug	Antihypertenseur	Farmaco antiipertensivo	Antihipertenziv
Antihistamínico	Antihistamine	Antihistaminique	Antistaminico	Antihistaminik
Antiinflamatorio (antiflogístico)	Anti-inflammatory	Anti-inflammatoire	Antinfiammatorio	Protuupalno
Antiinflamatorio no esteroideo	Non-steroidal anti-inflammatory drug	Anti-inflammatoire non stéroïdien	Farmaco anti-infiammatore non steroide-FANS	Nesteroidni antireumatik
Antimalárico	Antimalarial drug	Antimalarique	Antimalarico	Antimalarik
Antimicótico (antifúngico)	Antimycotic	Antimycosique	Antimicotico	Antimikotik
Antioxidante	Antioxidant	Antioxydant	Antiossidante (sostanza antiossidante)	Antioksidans
Antipirético	Antipyretic	Antipyrétique	Antipiretico	Antipiretik
Antiprotozoario	Antiprotozoal agent	Médicament antiprotozoal	Farmaco antiprotozoico	Antiprotozoik
Antipsicótico	Antipsychotic	Antipsychotique	Antipsicotico	Antipsihotik
Antireumático	Antirheumatic drug	Médicament antirhumatismal	Antireumatico	Antireumatik
Antiséptico	Antiseptic	Antiseptique	Antisettico	Antiseptik
Antiséptico de las vías urinarias	Urinary antiseptic	Antiseptique urinaire	Antisettico urinario	Uroantiseptik
Antisuero	Antiserum	Antisérum	Antisiero	Antiserum
Antitoxina	Antitoxin	Antitoxine	Antitossina	Protuotrov
Aspirina	Aspirin	Aspirine	Aspirina	Aspirin
Atropina	Atropine	Atropine	Atropina	Atropin
Azufre	Sulphur	Soufre	Zolfo	Sumpor
Balanza	Scales	Balance	Bilancia	Vaga
Bálsamo de labios	Lip balm	Tube de soin pour lèvres	Burrocacao	Grožđana mast
Barbitúrico	Barbiturate	Barbiturique	Barbiturico	Barbiturat
Bolsa de agua caliente (guatero)	Hot water bottle	Bouillotte	Bouillotte (bouilloire)	Termofor
Broncodilatador	Bronchodilator	Bronchodilatateur	Broncodilatatore	Bronhodilatator
Cafeína	Caffeine	Caféine	Caffeina	Kofein
Calcio	Calcium	Calcium	Calcio	Kalcij
Cannabis medicinal	Medical cannabis	Cannabis médical	Cannabis terapeutica	Medicinski kanabis

Español	Inglés	Francés	Italiano	Croata
Cápsula	Capsule	Gélule	Capsula	Kapsula
Carbón activado	Activated carbon	Charbon actif	Carbone attivo	Aktivni ugljen
Cardiotónico	Cardiotonic agent	Médicament cardiotonique	Cardiotonico	Kardiotonik
Cefalosporina	Cephalosporin	Céphalosporine	Cefalosporina	Cefalosporin
Citostático	Cytostatic	Cytostatique	Citostatico	Citostatik
Cloranfenicol	Chloramphenicol	Chloramphénicol	Cloramfenicolo	Kloramfenikol
Cloro	Chlorine	Chlore	Cloro	Klor
Cobalto	Cobalt	Cobalt	Cobalto	Kobalt
Cobre	Copper	Cuivre	Rame	Bakar
Codeína	Codeine	Codéine	Codeina	Kodein
Colirio	Eye drops	Collyre (gouttes ophtalmiques)	Collirio	Kapi za oči
Compresa	Compress	Compresse	Compressa	Oblog
Comprimido	Tablet	Comprimé	Compressa (pasticca, tavoletta)	Dražeja (tableta)
Corticosteroide	Corticosteroid	Corticostéroïde	Corticosteroide	Kortikosteroid
Crema	Skin cream	Crème	Crema	Krema
Cuchara	Spoon	Cuillère	Cucchiaio	Žlica
De uso externo	For external application	Pour l'application externe	Per l'applicazione esterna	Za vanjsku primjenu
Desodorante	Antiperspirant	Déodorant	Antidiaforetico	Antiperspirant
Después de una comida	After meal	Après-repas	Dopo il pasto	Nakon jela
Diafragma	Diaphragm (Dutch cap)	Diaphragme	Diaframma	Dijafragma
Digestivo	Digestive	Médicament digestif	Digestivo	Digestiv
Diurético	Diuretic	Diurétique	Diuretico	Diuretik
Dosis	Dose	Dose	Dose	Doza
Edulcorante artificial	Sugar substitute	Édulcorant	Dolcificante artificiale	Umjetno sladilo
Emulsión	Emulsion	Émulsion	Emulsione	Emulzija
En ayunas	On an empty stomach (before the meal)	À jeun	A digiuno	Na tašte
Enema (clisma)	Enema (clyster)	Clystère	Clistere	Klizma (klistir)
Enjuague bucal (colutorio)	Mouthwash liquid	Eau dentifrice	Collutorio	Tekućina za ispiranje usne šupljine
Eritromicina	Erythromycin	Érythromycine	Eritromicina	Eritromicin
Espasmolítico	Spasmolytic	Spasmolytique	Spasmolitico	Spazmolitik
Espermicida	Spermicide	Spermicide	Spermicida	Spermicid
Esponja anticonceptiva	Contraceptive sponge	Éponge contraceptive	Spugna contraccettiva	Kontracepcijska spužva
Espuma	Foam	Mousse	Schiuma (spuma)	Pjena
Espuma anticonceptiva	Contraceptive foam	Mousse contraceptive	Schiuma anticoncezionale	Kontracepcijska pjena
Expectorante	Expectorant	Expectorant	Espettorante	Sredstvo za iskašljavanje
Farmacéutico	Pharmacist	Pharmacien	Farmacista	Ljekarnik
Fármaco antialcohólico	Antialcoholic drug	Médicament contre la dépendance à l'alcool	Farmaco anti-alcol	Antialkoholik
Fármaco antiobesidad	Anti-obesity medication	Médicament anti-obésité	Dimagrante (farmaco antiobesità)	Dijetetsko sredstvo
Fármaco antiviral	Antiviral drug	Médicament antiviral	Farmaco antivirale	Antivirusni lijek
Fármaco tuberculostático	Antitubercular agent	Antituberculeux	Farmaco antitubercolare	Antituberkulotik
Fentanilo	Fentanyl	Fentanyl	Fentanyl	Fentanil
Fitoterapia	Phytotherapy	Phytothérapie	Fitoterapia	Fitoterapija
Fósforo	Phosphorus	Phosphore	Fosforo	Fosfor
Frasquito	Vial	Fiole	Bottiglietta (boccetta)	Bočica
Gafas	Glasses	Lunettes de vue	Occhiali	Naočale
Gasa	Gauze sponge	Gaze	Garza	Gaza
Gel	Gel	Gel	Gel	Gel
Gentamicina	Gentamicin	Gentamicine	Gentamicina	Gentamicin
Glucosa	Glucose	Glucose	Glucosio	Glukoza
Goma de mascar de nicotina	Nicotine gum	Gomme à la nicotine	Gomma da masticare antifumo	Nikotinska guma za žvakanje
Gotas	Drops	Gouttes	Gocce	Kapi (kapljice)
Gotas nasales	Nasal drops	Gouttes nasales	Gocce nasali	Kapi za nos
Gotas óticas	Ear drops	Gouttes auriculaires	Gocce per il mal di orecchi	Kapi za uši
Gramo	Gram (gramme)	Gramme	Grammo	Gram
Hemostático	Antihemorrhagic (hemostatic)	Hémostatique	Emostatico	Hemostatik
Heparina	Heparin	Héparine	Eparina	Heparin
Hierro (fierro)	Iron	Fer	Ferro	Željezo
Hipnótico	Hypnotic (soporific)	Hypnotique (somnifère)	Ipnotico	Hipnotik
Inhalación	Inhalation	Inhalation	Inalazione (farmaco per inalazioni)	Inhalacija
Inmunoglobulina	Immunoglobulin	Immunoglobuline	Immunoglobulina	Imunoglobulin
Inmunosupresor	Immunosuppressive	Immunosuppresseur	Immunosoppressivo	Imunosupresiv
Insulina	Insulin	Insuline	Insulina	Inzulin
Interferón	Interferon	Interféron	Interferone	Interferon
Inyección	Injection	Injection	Iniezione	Injekcija
Jabón	Soap	Savon	Sapone	Sapun
Jarabe	Syrup	Sirop	Sciroppo	Sirup
Jeringa	Syringe	Seringue	Siringa per iniezioni	Šprica
Lavado	Rinsing	Rinçage	Sciacquatra (risciacquatura)	Ispiranje

Español	Inglés	Francés	Italiano	Croata
Laxante	Laxative	Laxatif	Lassativo	Laksativ
Lente de contacto blanda	Soft contact lens	Lentille de contact souple	Lente a contatto morbida	Meka kontaktna leća
Lente de contacto duro	Hard contact lens	Lentille de contact rigide	Lente a contatto rigida	Tvrda kontaktna leća
Lentes de contacto (lentillas, pupilentes)	Contact lenses	Lentilles de contact	Lenti a contatto	Kontaktne leće
Litro	Litre	Litre	Litro	Litra
Loción	Lotion	Lotion	Lozione	Losion
Lubricante	Lubricant	Lubrifiant	Lubrificante	Lubrikant
Magnesio	Magnesium	Magnésium	Magnesio	Magnezij
Manganeso	Manganese	Manganèse	Manganese	Mangan
Manzanilla	Chamomile	Camomille	Camomilla	Kamilica
Medicamento (fármaco)	Medication (remedy, drug)	Médicament	Medicamento (farmaco, rimedio)	Lijek
Metadona	Methadone	Méthadone	Metadone	Metadon
Microgramo	Microgram	Microgramme	Microgrammo	Mikrogram
Miligramo	Milligram (milligramme)	Milligramme	Milligrammo	Miligram
Mililitro	Millilitre	Millilitre	Millilitro	Mililitar
Mineral	Mineral	Minéral	Minerale	Mineral
Molibdeno	Molybdenum	Molybdène	Molibdeno	Molibden
Español	**Inglés**	**Francés**	**Italiano**	**Croata**
Morfina	Morphine	Morphine	Morfina	Morfin
Mucolítico	Mucolytic	Mucolytique	Mucolitico	Mukolitik
Nistatina	Nystatin	Nystatine	Nistatina	Nistatin
Nutrimento (nutriente)	Nutrient	Nutriment (élément nutritif)	Sostanza nutriente (sostanza nutritiva)	Nutritiv
Opioide	Opioid	Opioïde	Oppioide	Opijat (opioid)
Oxicodona	Oxycodone	Oxycodone	Ossicodone	Oksikodon
Pañal para adultos	Incontinence pads (adult diapers)	Slip d'incontinence	Assorbenti per l'incontinenza	Pelene za inkontinenciju
Paracetamol	Paracetamol	Paracétamol	Paracetamolo	Paracetamol
Parafina	Paraffin	Paraffine	Paraffina	Parafin
Parche de nicotina	Nicotine patch	Timbre à la nicotine	Cerotto antifumo	Nikotinski flaster
Pasta	Paste	Pâte	Pasta	Pasta
Pasta de dientes (dentífrico)	Tooth paste	Dentifrice	Dentifricio	Pasta za zube
Pasta de óxido de zinc	Zinc ointment	Pommade à l'oxyde de zinc	Zinco pasta	Cinkova pasta
Pastilla	Pastille (lozenge)	Pastille	Pasticca (pastiglia)	Tableta za sisanje (pastila)
Penicilina	Penicillin	Pénicilline	Penicillina	Penicilin
Pieza	Piece	Morceau	Pezzo (porzione)	Komad
Píldora anticonceptiva	Contraceptive pill (oral contraceptive)	Contraception orale	Pillola anticoncezionale	Kontracepcijska pilula
Poción	Potion	Potion	Pozione	Ljekoviti napitak
Polvo	Powder	Poudre	Polverina (polvere)	Prašak (puder)
Polvo líquido	Liquid powder	Poudre fluide	Polvere liquido	Tekući puder
Por la mañana	In the morning	Le matin	Di mattina	U jutro
Por la noche	In the evening	Le soir	La sera	Na večer
Por vía oral	Orally	Par voie orale	Oralmente (per via orale, per bocca)	Na usta
Potasio	Potassium	Potassium	Potassio	Kalij
Preservativo (condón, profiláctico)	Condom	Préservatif	Preservativo (profilattico, condom)	Prezervativ (kondom)
Protector solar	Sunscreen (sunblock)	Crème solaire	Filtro solare (crema so-lare ad alta protezione)	Sredstvo za zaštitu od sunca
Prueba de embarazo	Home pregnancy test	Test de grossesse	Test di gravidanza ad uso domiciliare	Kućni test za trudnoću
Psicoestimulante	Psychostimulant	Psychostimulant	Psicostimulanti	Psihostimulans
Purgante (purgativo)	Purgative	Purgatif	Purgante (purga)	Purgativ
Quimioterapia	Chemotherapy	Chimiothérapie	Chemioterapia	Kemoterapija
Reacción adversa a medicamento	Drug side-effects	Effets indésirables d'un médicament	Effetti indesiderati da farmaco	Nuspojave lijeka
Receta	Prescription	Ordonnance médicale	Prescrizione (rimedio prescritto)	Recept
Rectal	Rectal	Rectal	Rettale	Rektalno
Relajante muscular (miorrelajante)	Muscle relaxant	Myorelaxant	Miorilassante	Miorelaksator
Repelente de insectos	Insect repellent	Répulsif d'insectes	Insettifugo	Sredstvo protiv insekata
Repelente de mosquitos	Mosquito repellent	Répulsif antimoustiques	Repellente antizanzare	Sredstvo protiv komaraca
Rociada	Spray	Spray	Spruzzo (vaporizzato)	Sprej
Salicilato	Salicylate	Salicylate	Salicilato	Salicilat
Seda dental (hilo dental)	Dental floss	Fil dentaire	Filo interdentale	Zubni konac
Sedativo	Sedative	Sédatif	Sedativo (calmante)	Sedativ
Sistema Internacional de Unidades	International System of Units	Système international d'unités	Sistema internazionale di unità di misura	Sustav međunarodnih mjernih jedinica
Sobredosis	Overdose	Surdose	Sovradosaggio	Predoziranje
Sodio	Sodium	Sodium	Sodio	Natrij

Español	Inglés	Francés	Italiano	Croata
Solubilizantes (comprimidos dispersables en agua)	Water-soluble tablets	Comprimé effervescent	Compresse solubili	Šumeće tablete
Solución limpiadora de dentadura	Denture cleaning solution	Solution nettoyante pour les prothèses	Soluzione per pulizia dentiera	Tekućina za čišćenje umjetnog zubala
Solución limpiadora de lentes de contacto	Contact lenses cleaning solution	Solution nettoyante pour lentilles	Soluzione per pulizia lenti a contatto	Tekućina za čišćenje kontaktnih leća
Soluto	Solution	Solution	Soluzione	Otopina
Suero	Serum	Sérum	Siero	Serum
Suero fisiológico	Saline solution	Solution physiologique	Soluzione fisiologica	Fiziološka otopina
Sulfonamida	Sulphonamide	Sulfamidé	Sulfamidici (sulfonamidici)	Sulfonamid
Supositorio	Suppository	Suppositoire	Supposta	Čepić
Supositorio vaginal	Vaginal suppository	Ovule (suppositoire vaginal)	Candelette	Vaginaleta
Tampón	Tampon	Tampon hygiénique	Tampone	Tampon
Tensiómetro (esfigmomanómetro)	Blood pressure meter (sphygmomanometer)	Tensiomètre (sphygmomanomètre)	Misuratore di pressione (sfigmomanometro)	Tlakomjer
Terapia de sustitución hormonal	Hormone replacement therapy	Hormonothérapie de substitution	Terapia ormonale sostitutiva	Hormonalna nadomjesna terapija
Termómetro	Thermometer	Thermomètre	Termometro	Toplomjer
Tetraciclina	Tetracycline	Tétracycline	Tetraciclina	Tetraciklin
Tintura	Tincture	Teinture	Tintura	Tinktura
Tira adhesiva sanitaria	Plaster (adhesive strip)	Pansement	Cerotto	Flaster
Tisana (infusión de hierbas)	Herbal tea	Tisane	Tisana (infuso di erbe)	Biljni čaj
Toalla sanitaria (compresa, pantiprotector)	Sanitary pads (sanitary napkins)	Serviette hygiénique (protège-slip)	Assorbenti igienici	Higijenski ulošci
Tónico	Tonic	Tonique	Tonico (ricostituente)	Tonik
Tramadol	Tramadol	Tramadol	Tramadolo	Tramal
Ungüento (pomada)	Ointment (fat)	Pommade	Pomata (unguento)	Pomada (mast)
Vacuna	Vaccine	Vaccin	Vaccino	Cjepivo
Vasodilatador	Vasodilatator	Vasodilatateur	Vasodilatatore	Vazodilatator
Venda	Bandage	Bandage	Bendaggio	Zavoj
Veneno	Poison	Poison	Veleno	Otrov
Vía sublingual	Sublingual administration	Sublingual	Sublinguale	Pod jezik
Viagra	Viagra (sildenafil citrate)	Viagra (citrate de sildénafil)	Viagra (citrato di sildenafil)	Viagra
Vitamina	Vitamin	Vitamine	Vitamina	Vitamin
Vitamina A (retinol)	Vitamin A (retinol)	Vitamine A (rétinol)	Vitamina A (retinolo)	Vitamin A (retinol)
Vitamina B1 (tiamina)	Vitamin B1 (thiamin)	Vitamine B1 (thiamine)	Vitamina B1 (tiamina)	Vitamin B1 (tiamin)
Vitamina B2 (riboflavina)	Vitamin B2 (riboflavin)	Vitamine B2 (riboflavine)	Vitamina B2 (riboflavina)	Vitamin B2 (riboflavin)
Vitamina B3 (niacina, vitamina PP)	Vitamin B3 (niacin)	Vitamine B3 (nicotinamide, PP)	Vitamina B3 (niacina, vitamina PP)	Vitamin B3 (niacin)
Vitamina B4 (adenina)	Vitamin B4 (adenine)	Vitamine B4 (adénine)	Vitamina B4 (adenina)	Vitamin B4 (adenin)
Vitamina B5 (ácido pantoténico)	Vitamin B5 (pantothenic acid)	Vitamine B5 (acide pantothénique)	Vitamina B5 (acido pantotenico, vitamina W)	Vitamin B5 (pantotenska kiselina)
Vitamina B6 (piridoxina)	Vitamin B6 (pyridoxine)	Vitamine B6 (pyridoxine)	Vitamina B6 (piridossina)	Vitamin B6 (piridoksin)
Vitamina B7 (inositol)	Vitamin B7 (inositol)	Vitamine B7 (inositol)	Vitamina B7 (inositolo)	Vitamin B7 (inozitol)
Vitamina B8 (biotina)	Vitamin B8 (biotin)	Vitamine B8 (biotine)	Vitamina B8 (biotina)	Vitamin B8 (biotin)
Vitamina B9 (ácido fólico)	Vitamin B9 (folic acid)	Vitamine B9 (acide folique)	Vitamina B9 (acido folico)	Vitamin B9 (folna kiselina)
Vitamina B10 (vitamina R)	Vitamin B10 (factor-R)	Vitamine B10 (vitamine R)	Vitamina B10 (vitamina R)	Vitamin B10 (faktor-R)
Vitamina B11 (vitamina S)	Vitamin B11 (factor-S)	Vitamine B11 (carnitine)	Vitamina B11 (vitamina S)	Vitamin B11 (faktor-S)
Vitamina B12 (ciancobalamina)	Vitamin B12 (cobalamin)	Vitamine B12 (cobalamine)	Vitamina B12 (cobalamina)	Vitamin B12 (kobalamin)
Vitamine C (enantiómero L de ácido ascórbico)	Vitamin C (L-ascorbic acid)	Vitamine C (acide ascorbique)	Vitamina C (acido L-ascorbico)	Vitamin C (L-askorbinska kiselina)
Vitamina D2 (ergocalciferol)	Vitamin D2 (ergocalciferol)	Vitamine D2 (ergocalciférol)	Vitamina D2 (ergocalciferolo)	Vitamin D2 (ergokalciferol)
Vitamina D3 (colecalciferol)	Vitamin D3 (cholecalciferol)	Vitamine D3 (cholécalciférol)	Vitamina D3 (colecalciferolo)	Vitamin D3 (kolekalciferol)
Vitamina D4	Vitamin D4	Vitamine D4	Vitamina D4 (diidroergocalciferolo)	Vitamin D4
Vitamina D5 (sitocalciferol)	Vitamin D5 (sitocalciferol)	Vitamine D5 (sitocalciférol)	Vitamina D5 (sitocalciferolo)	Vitamin D5 (sitokalciferol)
Vitamina E (alfatocoferol)	Vitamin E (tocopherol)	Vitamine E (tocophérol)	Vitamina E (tocoferolo)	Vitamin E (tokoferol)
Vitamina F (acido linoleico)	Vitamin F (linoleic acid)	Vitamine F (acide linoléique)	Vitamina F (acido linoleico)	Vitamin F (linoleična kiselina)
Vitamina J (colina)	Vitamin J (choline)	Vitamine J (choline)	Vitamina J (colina)	Vitamin J (kolin)
Vitamina K (filoquinona)	Vitamin K (phylloquinone)	Vitamine K (phylloquinone)	Vitamina K (fillochinone)	Vitamin K (filokinon)
Vitamina L1 (ácido antranílico)	Vitamin L1 (anthranilic acid)	Vitamine L1 (acide anthranilique)	Vitamina L1 (acido antranilico)	Vitamin L1 (antranilna kiselina)
Vitamina P (flavonoide)	Vitamin P (flavonoids)	Vitamine P (flavonoïde)	Vitamina P (flavonoidi)	Vitamin P (flavonoidi)
Yodo (iodo)	Iodine	Iode	Iodio (tintura di iodio)	Jod
Zinc (cinc)	Zinc	Zinc	Zinco	Cink

Español	Inglés	Francés	Italiano	Croata
FACILIDADES MÉDICAS, PROCEDIMIENTOS Y ASISTENCIA MÉDICA:	**MEDICAL FACILITIES, PROCEDURES AND CARE:**	**ÉTABLISSEMENTS MÉDICAUX, PROCÉDURES ET SOINS:**	**ISTITUZIONI, PROCEDURE E CURE DI MEDICINA:**	**MEDICINSKE USTANOVE, ZAHVATI I NJEGA:**
Abertura quirúrgica en el cráneo (craneotomía)	Surgical opnening of the cranium (craniotomy)	Ouverture chirurgicale du crâne (craniotomie)	Apertura chirurgica del cranio (craniotomia)	Kirurški zahvat otvaranja lubanje (kraniotomija)
Abrir	Open	Ouvrir	Aprire	Otvoriti
Administración de fármacos	Administration of drugs	Administration des médicaments	Somministrazione dei farmaci	Davanje lijekova
Agua	Water	Eau	Acqua	Voda
Alarma	Alarm	Alarme	Allarme	Uzbuna (alarm)
Almacenaje	Storage	Stockage	Deposito (magazzino)	Spremište
Almohada	Pillow	Oreiller	Cuscino	Jastuk
Almohada de posicionamiento	Body positioner	Coussin de positionnement	Posizionatore	Udlaga za pozicioniranje
Almuerzo	Lunch	Déjeuner	Pranzo	Ručak
Ambulancia	Ambulance	Ambulance	Autoambulanza	Kola hitne pomoći
Amputación	Amputation	Amputation	Amputazione	Amputacija
Andador	Walker (walking frame)	Déambulateur (cadre de marche, gadot)	Deambulatore (tutore per disabili)	Hodalica
Anestesia	Anesthesia	Anesthésie	Anestesia	Anestezija (narkoza)
Anestesia general	General anesthesia	Anesthésie générale	Anestesia generale	Opća anestezija
Anestesia local	Local anesthesia	Anesthésie locale	Anestesia locale	Lokalna anestezija
Aparato respiratorio	Respirator	Appareil respiratoire	Respiratore	Aparat za disanje (respirator)
Apósito	Dressing	Pansement	Fasciatura (bendaggio)	Previjanje
Armario	Wardrobe (cupboard, cabinet)	Armoire	Armadio (credenza)	Ormar
Artrodesis	Arthrodesis	Arthrodèse	Artrodesi	Artrodeza
Asistencia (cuidado)	Nursing (care)	Soins de santé	Assistenza infermieristica	Njega
Aspirador	Suction unit (aspirator)	Appareil à succion	Aspiratore di secreti	Aspirator
Atención primaria de salud	Primary health care	Soins de santé primaire	Assistenza sanitaria primaria	Primarna zdravstvena zaštita
Audífono	Hearing assist device	Appareil acoustique	Apparecchio acustico	Slušni aparat
Autopsia	Autopsy	Autopsie	Autopsia	Obdukcija
Bolsa Ambú de ventilación manual	Ambu bag valve mask	Respirateur manuel type Ambu	Pallone autoespandibile	Ambu balon s maskom
Botiquín de primeros auxilios	First aid kit	Trousse de secours	Cassetta di pronto soccorso	Kutija prve pomoći
By-pass	Bypass	Pontage	Bypass	Premosnica
Cadáver	Corpse	Cadavre	Cadavere (salma)	Leš
Calendario de vacunación	Vaccination schedule	Calendrier des vaccinations	Calendario vaccinale	Kalendar cijepljenja
Cama	Bed	Lit	Letto	Krevet
Cambiarse	Get changed	Se changer	Cambiarsi	Presvući se
Camilla	Hospital trolley	Chariot	Carrello	Kolica
Camilla enrollable	Stretcher	Civière	Barella (lettiga)	Nosila
Camisón	Nightgown	Chemise de nuit	Camicia da notte	Spavačica
Cánula	Airway (cannula)	Canule	Cannula	Kanila
Cánula nasal	Nasal cannula	Canule nasale	Cannula nasale	Nosna kanila
Cánula orofaríngea (tubo de Mayo, cánula de Guédel)	Oropharyngeal airway	Canule de Guedel	Cannula oro-faringea	Orofaringealna kanila
Cardiología	Cardiology	Cardiologie	Cardiologia	Kardiologija
Catéter	Catheter	Cathéter	Catetere	Kateter
Catéter de succión	Suction catheter	Cathéter à succion	Tubo d'aspirazione	Usisni kateter
Catéter urinario	Urological catheter	Cathéter urologique	Catetere vescicale	Urinarni kateter
Causa de muerte	Cause of death	Cause de la mort	Causa di morte	Uzrok smrti
Cauterización	Cauterization	Cautérisation	Cauterizzazione	Kauterizacija
Cena	Dinner (supper)	Dîner (souper)	Cena	Večera
Centro médico	Medical center	Centre médical	Centro di medicina	Medicinski centar
Cerrar	Close	Fermer	Chiudere	Zatvoriti
Circuncisión	Circumcision	Circoncision	Circoncisione	Obrezivanje
Cirugía	Surgery	Chirurgie	Chirurgia	Kirurgija
Cirugía del oído medio (stapedectomía)	Surgical procedure on the middle ear (stapedectomy)	Ablation chirurgicale de l'étrier (stapédectomie)	Intervento chirurgico dell'orecchio medio (stapedectomia)	Kirurški zahvat na srednjem uhu (stapedektomija)
Cirugía del tálamo (talamotomía)	Surgical procedure on the thalamus (thalamotomy)	Ablation chirurgicale d'une partie du thalamus (thalamotomie)	Intervento chirurgico delle connessioni talamiche (talamotomia)	Kirurški zahvat na talamusu (talamotomija)
Cirugía estética de la nariz (rinoplastia)	Plastic surgery of the nose (rhinoplasty)	Opération de chirurgie esthétique du nez (rhinoplastie)	Procedura di chirurgia plastica del naso (rinoplastica)	Plastična operacija nosa (rinoplastika)
Cirugía estética de los párpados (blefaroplastia)	Plastic surgery of the eyelid (blepharoplasty)	Opération de chirurgie esthétique des paupières (blépharoplastie)	Procedura di chirurgia plastica della palpebra (blefaroplastica)	Plastična operacija očnog kapka (blefaroplastika)

Español	Inglés	Francés	Italiano	Croata
Cirugía estética de los senos (mamoplastia)	Plastic surgery of the breasts (mammoplasty)	Opération de chirurgie esthétique des seins (mammoplastie)	Procedura di chirurgia plastica del seno (mastoplastica)	Plastična operacija dojke (mastoplastika)
Cirugía estética del abdomen (abdominoplastia)	Plastic surgery of the abdomen ("tummy tuck", abdominoplasty)	Opération de chirurgie esthétique de la paroi abdominale (abdominoplastie)	Procedura di chirurgia plastica dell'addome (addominoplastica)	Plastična operacija trbuha (abdominoplastika)
Cirugía laparoscópica	Laparoscopic surgery	Laparoscopie (coelioscopie)	Chirurgia laparoscopica	Laparoskopska operacija
Citología	Cytology	Cytologie	Citologia	Citologija
Colchón	Mattress	Matelas	Materasso	Madrac
Colchón al vácio	Vacuum mattress	Matelas immobili-sateur à dépression	Materassino a depressione	Vakumirani madrac
Collar cervical	Neck immobilizer	Support de cou	Collare cervicale	Imobilizator vrata
Comedor	Dining-room	Salle à manger	Sala da pranzo (cenàcolo)	Blagavaonica
Consultorio de médico	Doctor's office	Bureau du médecin	Ufficio del medico	Liječnička ambulanta
Contagioso	Contagious	Contagieux (contagieuse)	Contagioso (infettivo)	Zarazno
Corona	Dental crown	Couronne	Corona	Zubna krunica
Crío-extracción	Cryoextraction	Cryo-extraction	Crioestrazione	Krioekstrakcija
Cuarentena	Quarantine	Quarantaine	Quarantena	Karantena
Cuarto de baño	Bathroom	Salle de bains	Bagno	Kupaonica
Cuarto del paciente	Patient's room	Chambre de malade	Camera di malato	Bolesnička soba
Cubrecama (colcha, manta)	Cover	Couverture	Coperta	Pokrivač
Cubrezapatos	Protection shoe cover	Sur-chaussures à usage unique	Sovrascarpe protettive	Zaštitna navlaka za obuću
Cuidados intensivos	Intensive care	Soins intensifs	Terapia intensiva	Intenzivna njega
Cuidados semi-intensivos	Semi-intensive care	Soins semi-intensifs	Terapia semi-intensiva	Poluintenzivna njega
Darse un baño	Bath (wash)	Laver	Lavare (fare il bagno)	Kupati
Defecación	Defecation	Défécation	Defecazione	Pražnjenje stolice (defekacija)
Dentista	Dentist	Dentiste	Dentista	Stomatolog (zubar)
Depósito de cadáveres (morgue)	Morgue (mortuary)	Morgue	Obitorio (mortorio)	Mrtvačnica
Dermatología	Dermatology	Dermatologie	Dermatologia	Dermatologija
Desayuno	Breakfast	Petit déjeuner	Colazione	Doručak
Desfibrilación	Defibrillation	Défibrillation	Defibrillazione	Defibrilacija
Desfibrilador	Defibrillator	Défibrillateur	Defibrillatore	Defibrilator
Desfibrilador manual	Manual defibrillator	Défibrillateur manuel	Defibrillatore manuale	Ručni defibrilator
Determinación del tiempo de muerte	Calling of the time of death	Détermination de l'heure de la mort	Proclamazione del tempo della morte	Proglašenje vremena smrti
Diagnóstico	Diagnosis	Diagnostic	Diagnosi	Dijagnoza
Diálisis	Dialysis	Dialyse	Dialisi	Dijaliza
Diálisis de hígado	Liver dialysis	Dialyse hépatique	Dialisi epatica	Dijaliza jetre
Diálisis renal	Renal dialysis	Dialyse rénale	Dialisi renale	Dijaliza bubrega
Digestión	Digestion	Digestion	Digestione	Probava
Dinamómetro	Dynamometer	Dynamomètre	Dinamometro	Dinamometar
Donación de sangre	Blood donation	Don de sang	Donazione del sangue	Darovanje krvi (donacija krvi)
Donante	Donor	Donneur	Donatore/donatrice	Davalac (donator)
Drenaje	Drainage	Drainage	Drenaggio	Drenaža
Drenaje postural	Postural drainage	Drainage postural	Drenaggio posturale	Drenažni položaj
Ejercicio	Exercise	Exercice	Esercizio	Vježbanje
Ejercicios de Kegel	Kegel exercise	Exercice de Kegel	Esercizi di Kegel	Kegelove vježbe
Ejercicios de respiración	Breathing exercises	Exercice de respiration	Esercizi di respirazione	Vježbe disanja
Electrocirugía	Electrosurgery	Électrochirurgie	Elettrochirurgia	Elektrokirurgija
Electrodo	Electrode	Électrode	Elettrodo	Elektroda
Electroterapia	Electrotherapy	Électrothérapie	Elettroterapia	Elektroterapija
Elevador	Elevator	Ascenseur	Ascensore	Dizalo
Empaste (emplomadura)	Dental filling	Composite dentaire	Otturazione odontoiatrica	Zubna plomba
Enfermera	Nurse	Infirmier	Infermiera/infermiere	Medicinska sestra
Enfermería	Ambulance (clinic)	Infirmerie	Ambulanza	Ambulanta
Entrenamiento del equilibrio	Balance training	Entraînement de l'equilibre	Esercizi di equilibrio	Trening ravnoteže
Escalpelo	Scalpel	Scalpel	Scalpello	Skalpel
Escayola de inmovilización	Plaster cast (immobi-lization plaster)	Plâtre pour immobilisation rigide	Bendaggio gessato	Gipsana udlaga
Escupir	Spit	Cracher	Sputare	Pljunuti
Esponja	Sponge	Éponge	Spugna	Spužva
Estéril	Sterile (aseptic)	Stérile	Sterile	Sterilno
Esterilización	Sterilization	Stérilisation	Sterilizzazione	Sterilizacija
Esterilización quirúrgica masculina (vasectomía)	Surgical sterilization of a man (vasectomy)	Ligature des canaux déférents des testicules (vasectomie)	Vasectomia	Kirurška sterilizacija muškarca (vazektomija)
Esterilizatióm quirúrgica femenina (ligadura de trompas)	Surgical sterilization of a woman (tubal ligation)	Stérilisation chirurgicale au femme (ligature des trompes)	Chiusura delle tube	Kirurška sterilizacija žene (podvezivanje jajovoda)
Estetoscopio	Stethoscop	Stéthoscope	Stetofonendoscopio	Stetoskop

Español	Inglés	Francés	Italiano	Croata
Estiramiento de la cara (ritidectomía)	Facelift (rhytidectomy)	Lifting facial (rhytidectomie, lissage, remodelage)	Lift facciale (ritidectomia)	Lifting lica (ritidektomija)
Exodoncia dental	Dental extraction	Extraction dentaire	Estrazione del dente	Vađenje zuba
Exteriorización de una parte de intestino a través de la cavidad abdominal (colostomía)	Surgical procedure of formation of stoma (colostomy)	Formation chirurgicale de la stomie (colostomie)	Formazione chirurgica di stomia (colostomia)	Kirurški zahvat formiranja stome (kolostomija)
Extirpación quirúrgica de la glándula tiroides (tiroidectomía)	Surgical removal of the thyroid gland (thyroidectomy)	Ablation chirurgicale de la thyroïde (thyroïdectomie, isthmectomie)	Asportazione chirurgica della tiroide (tiroidectomia)	Kirurško odstranjenje štitne žlijezde (tiroidektomija)
Extirpación quirúrgica de la laringe (laringectomía)	Surgical removal of the larynx (laryngectomy)	Ablation chirurgicale du larynx (laryngectomie)	Asportazione chirurgica della laringe (laringectomia)	Kirurško odstranjenje grkljana (laringektomija)
Extirpación quirúrgica de la próstata (prostatectomía)	Surgical removal of the prostate gland (prostatectomy)	Ablation chirurgicale de la prostate (prostatectomie)	Asportazione chirurgica della prostata (prostatectomia)	Kirurško odstranjenje prostate (prostatektomija)
Extirpación quirúrgica de las adenoides (adenoidectomía)	Surgical removal of adenoids (adenoidectomy)	Ablation chirurgicale des végétations adénoïdes (adénoïdectomie)	Asportazione chirurgica delle adenoidi (adenoidectomia)	Kirurško odstranjenje trećeg krajnika (adenoidektomija)
Extirpación quirúrgica de las hemorroides (hemorroidectomía)	Surgical removal of a hemorrhoid (hemorrhoidectomy)	Ablation chirurgicale des hémorroïdes (hémorroïdectomie)	Asportazione chirurgica delle emorroidi (emorroidectomia)	Kirurško odstranjenje hemeroida (hemoroidektomija)
Extirpación quirúrgica de los fibromas uterinos (miomectomía)	Surgical removal of uterine myomas (myomectomy, fibroidectomy)	Ablation chirurgicale des fibromes utérins (myomectomie)	Asportazione chirurgica di fibromi nell'utero (miomectomia)	Kirurško odstranjenje mioma u maternici (miomektomija)
Extirpación quirúrgica de parte de una vértebra (laminectomía)	Surgical procedure on the spine (laminectomy)	Résection chirurgicale des lames vertébrales (laminectomie)	Asportazione chirurgica della lamina di vertebre (laminectomia)	Kirurški zahvat na kralježnici (laminektomija)
Extirpación quirúrgica de un aneurisma (aneurismectomía)	Surgical removal of the aneurysm (aneurysmectomy)	Résection chirurgicale d'une poche anévrismale (anevrismectomie)	Asportazione chirurgica della sacca aneurismatica (aneurismectomia)	Kirurško odstranjenje aneurizme (aneurizmektomija)
Extirpación quirúrgica de un lóbulo de un órgano (lobectomía)	Surgical removal of a lobe of some organ (lobectomy)	Ablation chirurgicale d'un lobe d'organe (lobectomie)	Asportazione chirurgica di struttura lobale di un organo (lobectomia)	Kirurško odstranjenje režnja nekog organa (lobektomija)
Extirpación quirúrgica de una glándula suprarrenal (adrenalectomía)	Surgical removal of one or both adrenal glands (adrenalectomy)	Ablation chirurgicale d'une ou des deux glandes surrénales (adrenalectomie)	Asportazione chirur-gica di uno o etrambi surreni(surrenectomia, adrenalectomia)	Kirurško odstranjenje nadbubrežne žlijezde (adrenalektomija)
Extirpación quirúrgica del apéndice cecal (apendicectomía)	Surgical removal of the vermiform appendix (appendectomy)	Ablation chirurgicale de l'appendice iléo-caecal (appendicectomie)	Asportazione chirurgica dell'appendice (appendicectomia)	Kirurško odstranjenje slijepog crijeva (apendektomija)
Extirpación quirúrgica del bazo (esplenectomía)	Surgical removal of the spleen (splenectomy)	Ablation chirurgicale de la rate (splénectomie)	Asportazione chirurgica della milza (splenectomia)	Kirurško odstranjenje slezene (splenektomija)
Extirpación quirúrgica del estómago (gastrectomía)	Surgical removal of the stomach (gastrectomy)	Ablation chirurgicale de l'estomac (gastrectomie)	Asportazione chirurgica dello stomaco (gastrectomia)	Kirurško odstranjenje želuca (gastrektomija)
Extirpación quirúrgica del páncreas (pancreatectomía)	Surgical removal of the pancreas (pancreatectomy)	Ablation chirurgicale du pancréas (pancréatectomie)	Asportazione chirurgica del pancreas (pancreatectomia)	Kirurško odstranjenje gušterače (pankreatektomija)
Extirpación quirúrgica del testículo (orquidectomía)	Surgical removal of a testicle (orchidectomy)	Amputation chirurgi-cale d'un ou des deux testicules (orchidectomie, orchiectomie)	Asportazione chirurgica del testicolo (orchiectomia)	Kirurško odstranjenje testisa (orhidektomija)
Extirpación quirúrgica del timo (timectomía)	Surgical removal of the thymus (thymectomy)	Ablation chirurgicale du thymus (thymectomie)	Asportazione chirurgica del timo (timectomia)	Kirurško odstranjenje prsne žlijezde (timektomija)
Extracción quirúrgica de la vesícula biliar (colecistectomía)	Surgical removal of the gallbladder (cholecystectomy)	Enlèvement chirurgical de la vésicule biliaire (cholécystectomie)	Asportazione chirurgica della colecisti (colecistectomia)	Kirurško odstranjenje žučnog mjehura (kolecistektomija)
Extracción quirúrgica de las amígdalas (tonsilectomía)	Surgical removal of tonsils (tonsillectomy)	Ablation chirurgicale des amygdales palatines (amygdalectomie, tonsillectomie)	Asportazione chirurgica delle tonsille (tonsillectomia)	Kirurško odstranjenje krajnika (tonzilektomija)
Extracción quirúrgica de los cálculos (litotomía)	Surgical removal of stones (lithotomy)	Extraction chirurgicale des pierres de la vessie (lithotomie)	Asportazione chirurgica di calcolo (litotomia)	Kirurško odstranjenje kamenca (litotomija)
Extracción quirúrgica del útero (histerectomía)	Surgical removal of the uterus (hysterectomy)	Enlèvement chirurgical de l'uterus (hystérectomie)	Asportazione chirurgica dell'utero (isterectomia)	Kirurško odstranjenje maternice (histerektomija)
Fase de remisión	Remission	Rémission	Remissione	Stadij mirovanja bolesti (remisija)
Fisioterapeuta	Physiotherapist	Physiothérapeute	Fisioterapista	Fizioterapeut
Fisioterapia	Physical therapy	Physiothérapie	Fisioterapia	Fizikalna terapija
Gabacha desechable	Protection gown	Blouse de protection	Camicia protettiva	Zaštitna navlaka za odjeću
Gel conductor	Electrode conductive gel	Gel électroconductif	Gel elettro-conduttivo	Kontaktni gel za elektrode
Gérmenes	Germs	Germes	Germi	Klice
Gerontología	Gerontology	Gérontologie	Gerontologia	Gerontologija
Ginecología	Gynecology	Gynécologie	Ginecologia	Ginekologija

Español	Inglés	Francés	Italiano	Croata
Goniómetro	Goniometer	Goniomètre	Goniometro	Goniometar
Gorra desechable	Protection cap	Charlotte à usage unique	Cuffietta protettiva	Zaštitna kapa
Guantes desechables	Protect gloves	Gants à usage unique	Guanti protettivi	Zaštitne rukavice
Guardar cama	Bed rest	Repos au lit	Riposo a letto	Mirovanje u krevetu
Hidroterapia	Hydrotherapy	Hydrothérapie	Idroterapia	Hidroterapija
Hospital	Hospital	Hôpital	Ospedale (policlinico)	Bolnica
Implante de mama	Breast implant	Implant mammaire	Protese mammaria	Umetak za dojku
Incisión quirúrgica de una articulación (artrotomía)	Surgical procedure on a joint (arthrotomy)	Ouverture chirurgicale d'une articulation (arthrotomie)	Apertura chirurgica di un articolazione (artrotomia)	Kirurški zahvat na zglobu (artrotomija)
Incisión quirúrgica en la tráquea (traqueotomía)	Surgical opening of a direct airway on the neck (tracheostomy)	Ouverture chirurgicale dans la trachée (trachéotomie)	Incisione chirurgica della trachea (tracheotomia)	Kirurško otvaranje dišnog puta (traheotomija)
Infusión	Infusion	Perfusion	Infusione	Infuzija
Inmovilizador de cabeza	Head immobilizer	Immobiliseur de tête	Fermacapo	Imobilizator glave
Inmunología	Immunology	Immunologie	Immunologia	Imunologija
Intervención coronaria percutánea	Percutaneous coronary intervention (coronary angioplasty)	Angioplastie coronaire (dilatation transluminale)	Angioplastica coronarica	Perkutana koronarna angioplastika
Intravenoso poste	Infusion stand	Pied à perfusion	Piantana portaflebo	Stalak za infuziju
Intubación	Intubation	Intubation	Intubazione	Intubacija
Inyección	Injection	Injection	Iniezione	Injekcija
Ir al servicio	Using a toilet	Aller aux toilettes	Uso del gabinetto	Obaviti nuždu
Laringoscopio	Laryngoscope	Laryngoscope	Laringoscopio	Laringoskop
Lavado gástrico	Gastric lavage (stomach pumping)	Lavage gastrique	Lavanda gastrica	Ispiranje želuca
Lavandería	Laundry	Blanchisserie	Lavanderia	Vešeraj
Lavar	Rinse	Rincer	Sciacquare	Isprati
Liposucción	Liposuction	Liposuccion	Liposuzione	Liposukcija
Lobotomía	Lobotomy	Lobotomie	Lobotomia	Lobotomija
Luz	Light	Lumière	Luce	Svjetlo
Manguito de presión arterial	Manometer cuff	Brassard du manomètre	Manicotto di sfigmomanometro	Manšeta tlakomjera
Maniobra de Heimlich	Heimlich maneuver (abdominal thrusts)	Méthode de Heimlich	Manovra di Heimlich	Heimlichov zahvat
Manta (cobija)	Blanket	Couverture	Schiavina	Deka
Marcapasos	Pacemaker	Stimulateur cardiaque (pacemaker, pile)	Cardiostimolatore (stimolatore cardiaco)	Električni stimulator srca
Máscara de oxígeno	Oxygen mask	Masque à oxygène	Maschera dell'ossigeno	Maska za kisik
Máscara de reanimación	CPR mask	Masque de réanimation	Maschera per rianimazione	Maska za oživljavanje
Máscara laríngea	Laryngeal mask airway	Masque laryngé	Maschera laringea	Laringealna maska
Mascarilla desechable	Protection face mask	Masque de protection	Mascherina di protezione	Zaštitna maska za lice
Materia de desperdicio	Debris	Débris	Rottami	Otpad (otpadni proizvod)
Medicina interna	Internal medicine	Médicine interne	Medicina interna	Interna medicina
Médico	Doctor (physician)	Médecin	Dottore/dottoressa (medico)	Liječnik
Médico de cabecera	General practitioner	Médecin généraliste (médecin omnipraticien)	Medico di medicina generale (medico di famiglia)	Liječnik opće prakse
Mesa (escritorio)	Table (desk)	Table	Tavolo (scrivania)	Stol
Mesa para cama	Overbed table	Table de lit	Carrello servitore	Stolić za serviranje hrane
Mesilla de noche	Night table (bedside table)	Table de chevet (table de nuit)	Comodino	Noćni ormarić
Micción	Urination (voiding)	Miction	Urinazione	Mokrenje (uriniranje)
Monitor de signos vitales	Vital signs monitor	Moniteur de signes vitaux	Monitor per parametri vitali	Monitor za praćenje vitalnih znakova
Morder	Bite	Mordre	Addentare	Zagristi
Morir	Die	Mourir	Morire	Umrijeti
Mostrador de recepción	Reception office	Réception	Accettazione	Prijemni ured
Muleta	Crutch	Béquille	Gruccia (stampella)	Štaka
Neurología	Neurology	Neurologie	Neurologia	Neurologija
Oncología	Oncology	Oncologie (cancérologie)	Oncologia	Onkologija
Operación quirúrgica	Operation (surgery)	Opération chirurgicale	Operazione (intervento chirurgico)	Operacija
Orinal	Chamber-pot	Pot de chambre	Vaso da notte (pitale)	Noćna posuda
Ortopedia	Orthopedics	Orthopédie	Ortopedia	Ortopedija
Otorrinolaringología	Otorhinolaryngology	Oto-rhino-laryngologie	Otorinolaringoiatria	Uho-grlo-nos
Pabellón de enfermedades infecciosas	Infectious disease unit	Salle maladies infectieuses	Reparto di malattie infettive	Zarazni odjel
Paciente	Patient	Patient (malade)	Paziente (ammalato)	Bolesnik
Palangana (ajofaina)	Wash basin	Cuvette	Secchia	Lavor
Palpación	Palpation	Palpation	Palpazione	Pregled pipanjem (palpacija)
Pantuflas	Slippers	Chausson	Ciabatte	Šlape
Papelera	Litter bin	Poubelle	Pattumiera	Kanta za smeće
Patología	Pathology	Pathologie	Patologia	Patologija
Pediatría	Pediatrics	Pédiatrie	Pediatria	Pedijatrija

Español	Inglés	Francés	Italiano	Croata
Percusión	Percussion	Percussion	Percussione	Pregled kucanjem (perkusija)
Pesario	Pessary	Pessaire (pessus)	Pessario	Pesar
Pijama (piyama)	Pyjamas (pajamas)	Pyjama	Pigiama	Pidžama
Pinzas	Tweezers	Brucelles	Pinzette	Pinceta
Posición de Trendelenburg	Trendelenburg position	Position de Trendelenburg	Posizione di Trendelenburg	Trendelenburgov položaj
Primeros auxilios	First aid	Premiers secours	Primo soccorso	Prva pomoć
Protectores talón/codo antiescaras	Heel and elbow protectors	Talonnières et coudières	Talloniere e gomitiere antidecubito	Zaštitnici za pete i laktove
Prótesis dental	Dentures	Dentier	Protesi dentale	Umjetno zubalo
Psicólogo	Psychologist	Psychologue	Psicologo	Psiholog
Psiquiatría	Psychiatry	Psychiatrie	Psichiatria	Psihijatrija
Puerta	Door	Porte	Porta	Vrata
Pulidor de los dientes	Teeth polishing	Vernis à dents	Pulitura dei denti	Poliranje zuba
Purificación	Cleansing	Purification	Purificazione	Pročišćavanje
Quimioterapia	Chemotherapy	Chimiothérapie	Chemioterapia	Kemoterapija
Quirófano	Operating room	Bloc opératoire	Sala operatoria	Operacijska sala
Radiación	Radiation	Radiation	Radiazione	Zračenje
Radiología	Radiology	Radiographie	Radiologia	Radiologija
Reanimación	Reanimation	Réanimation	Rianimazione	Oživljavanje (reanimacija)
Receptor de un órgano	Recipient of an organ	Receveur de greffe	Ricevente di trapianto	Primatelj organa
Recuperación	Recovery	Guérison	Guarigione (ristabilimento)	Oporavak
Régimen (dieta)	Diet	Régime alimentaire	Dieta (regime dietetico)	Dijeta
Rehabilitación	Rehabilitation (rehab)	Réhabilitation	Riabilitazione	Rehabilitacija
Remoción quirúrgica de seno (mastectomía)	Surgical removal of a breast (mastectomy)	Enlèvement chirurgical d'un sein (mastectomie)	Asportazione chirurgica della mammella (mastectomia)	Kirurško odstranjenje dojke (mastektomija)
Reponerse (recuperarse)	Recover (heal)	Se remettre (se guérir)	Sanare (guarire, recuperare)	Ozdraviti
Resección transuretral de la próstata	Transurethral resection of the prostate	Résection transurétrale de la prostate	Resezione transuretrale della prostata	Transuretralna resekcija prostate
Respiración artificial	Artificial respiration	Ventilation artificielle	Respirazione artificiale	Umjetno disanje
Rinología	Rhinology	Rhinologie	Rinologia	Rinologija
Sábana	Sheet	Drap	Lenzuolo	Plahta
Sábana de hule para la incontinencia	Incontinence pad	Protège-matelas	Proteggi materasso cerato	Gumirano platno
Sala (pabellón)	Ward	Salle	Padiglione (reparto)	Odjel
Sala de espera	Waiting-room	Salle d'attente	Sala d'aspetto	Čekaonica
Sala de neumología	Pulmonary ward	Salle de pneumologie	Reparto polmonare	Plućni odjel
Sala de oftalmología	Ophtalmology ward	Salle d'ophtalmologie	Reparto di oftalmologia	Očni odjel
Seguro de salud	Health insurance	Assurance maladie	Assicurazione sanitaria	Zdravstveno osiguranje
Servicio	Toilet (lavatory)	Toilette (cabinet)	Vaso sanitario	Nužnik
Servicios médicos de emergencia	Emergency medical services	Aide médicale urgente	Servizio di urgenza ed emergenza medica	Hitna služba
Shunt	Shunt	Pontage (shunt)	Shunt	Spoj (skretnica)
Silla de evacuación	Escape chair	Chaise d'évacuation	Sedia portantina	Sjedalica za evakuaciju
Silla de ruedas	Wheelchair	Fauteuil roulant (charriot, charrette)	Sedia a rotelle (carrozzella)	Invalidska kolica
Sonda	Sonde	Sonde	Sonda	Sonda
Sonda de alimentación	Feeding tube	Sonde d'alimentation	Sonda gastrica per nutrizione	Sonda za hranjenje
Sonda de drenaje	Drain tube	Drain	Tubo di drenaggio	Dren
Sonda endotraqueal	Endotracheal tube	Sonde d'intubation endotrachéale	Tubo endotracheale	Endotrahealna kanila
Suturar la herida	Wound stitching	Suture de la plaie	Suturare la ferita	Šivanje rane
Taladro	Drill	Perceuse	Trapano (trivella)	Bušilica
Tanque de oxígeno	Oxygen storage tank	Réservoir d'oxygène	Serbatoio di ossigeno	Boca s kisikom
Té	Tea	Thé	Tè	Čaj
Terapeuta ocupacional	Occupational therapist	Ergothérapeute	Terapista occupazionale	Radni terapeut
Tijeras	Scissors	Ciseau	Forbici	Škare
Tracción	Traction	Traction	Trazione	Trakcija
Transfusión	Transfusion	Transfusion	Trasfusione	Transfuzija
Trasplante	Transplantation	Greffe (transplantation)	Trapianto	Presađivanje (transplantacija)
Tratamiento (terapia)	Therapy	Thérapie (traitement curatif)	Terapia	Liječenje (terapija)
Trauma	Trauma	Trauma	Trauma	Trauma
Tubo de ensayo	Test tube	Tube à essai	Provetta	Epruveta
Unidad de cuidados intensivos	Intensive care unit	Unité de soins intensifs	Stanza da terapia intensiva	Jedinica intenzivne njege
Urología	Urology	Urologie	Urologia	Urologija
Vacunación	Vaccination (inoculation)	Vaccination (inoculation)	Vaccinazione (inoculazione)	Cijepljenje
Ventana	Window	Fenêtre	Finestra	Prozor
Visita	Visit	Visite	Visita	Posjeta
Visitante	Visitor	Visiteur	Ospite (visitatore/visitatrice)	Posjetitelj

Español EXÁMENES MÉDICOS:	Inglés MEDICAL EXAMS:	Francés EXAMENS MÉDICAUX:	Italiano ESAMI MEDICI:	Croata MEDICINSKE PRETRAGE:
Albúmina en la sangre	Serum albumin	Albumine dans le sang	Seroalbumina	Albumin u serumu
Amniocentesis	Amniocentesis	Amniocentèse	Amniocentesi	Amniocenteza
Análisis de aglutinación	Agglutination tests	Test d'agglutination	Test di agglutinazione	Test aglutinacije
Análisis de bilirrubina sérica	Serum bilirubin	Diagnostic différentiel pour bilirubine sérique	Test della bilirubina	Bilirubin u serumu
Análisis de DNA	DNA analysis	Analyse de l'ADN	Analisi del DNA	DNK analiza
Análisis del líquido cefalorraquídeo	Cerebrospinal fluid analysis	Analyse du liquide céphalo-rachidien	Analisi del liquido cerebro-spinale	Pregled likvora
Análisis químico del jugo gástrico	Gastric juice chemical examination	Analyse chimique du suc gastrique	Esame chimico di succo gastrico	Kemijski pregled želučanog soka
Angiografía	Angiography	Angiographie	Angiografia	Angiografija
Angiografía cerebral	Cerebral angiography	Angiographie cérébrale	Angiografia cerebrale	Cerebralna angiografija
Angiografía de sustracción digital	Digital subtraction angiography	Angiographie numérique	Angiografia digitale a sottrazione	Digitalna supstrakcijska angiografija
Angiografía espinal	Spinal angiography	Angiographie spinale	Angiografia spinale	Spinalna angiografija
Angiografía por catéter	Catheter angiography	Angiographie interventionnelle utilisant un cathéter	Angiografia con cateterismo	Kateterska angiografija
Angiografía pulmonar	Pulmonary angiography	Angiographie pulmonaire	Angiografia polmonare	Pulmonalna angiografija
Anoscopía	Anoscopy	Anuscopie	Anoscopia	Anoskopija
Antibiograma	Antibiogram	Antibiogramme	Antibiogramma	Antibiogram
Antígeno carcinoembrionario	Carcinoembryonic antigen (CEA)	Antigène carcino-embryonnaire (ACE)	Antigene carcino-embrionario (CEA)	Karcinoembrionski antigen (CEA)
Antígeno prostático específico	Prostate specific antigen	Antigène prostatique spécifique	Semenogelasi (antigene prostatico specifico)	Prostatični specifični antigen (PSA)
Aortografía	Aortography	Aortographie	Aortografia	Aortografija
Arteriografía	Arteriography	Artériographie	Arteriografia	Arteriografija
Artrografía	Joint X-ray (arthrography)	Arthrographie	Artrografia	Rendgensko snimanje zgloba
Artroscopia	Arthroscopy	Arthroscopie	Artroscopia	Artroskopija
Aspartato aminotransferasa (AST, transaminasa glutámico-oxalacética GOT)	Aspartate transaminase (SGOT)	Aspartate transaminase (SGOT)	Aspartato transaminasi (SGOT)	Transaminaze u serumu
Audiometría	Audiometry	Audiométrie	Audiometria	Audiometrija
Audiometría del habla	Speech audiometry	Audiométrie vocale	Audiometria di discorso	Govorna audiometrija
Biligrafia intravenosa	Intravenous biligraphy	Biligraphie intraveineuse	Biligrafia venosa	Intravenozna biligrafija
Biopsia	Biopsy	Biopsie	Biopsia	Biopsija
Biopsia cerebral	Brain ventricle biopsy	Biopsie d'un ventricule cérébral	Biopsia cerebrale (biopsia dei ventricoli cerebrali)	Biopsija moždanih klijetki (ventrikulopunkcija)
Biopsia de ganglio linfático	Lymph node biopsy	Biopsie du ganglion lymphatoque	Biopsia del linfonodo	Biopsija limfnog čvora
Biopsia de médula ósea	Bone marrow biopsy	Biopsie ostéomédullaire	Biopsia del midollo osseo	Biopsija koštane srži
Biopsia de piel	Skin biopsy	Biopsie de peau	Biopsia cutanea	Biopsija kože
Biopsia de tiroides	Thyroid biopsy	Biopsie thyroïdienne	Biopsia della tiroide	Biopsija štitnjače
Biopsia endometrial	Endometrial biopsy	Biopsie endométriale	Biopsia endometriale	Biopsija endometrija
Biopsia estereotáctica	Stereotactic biopsy	Biopsie stéréotaxique	Biopsia stereotassica	Stereotaktična biopsija
Biopsia hepática	Liver biopsy	Biopsie du foie	Biopsia epatica	Biopsija jetre
Biopsia pleural	Pleural biopsy	Biopsie pleurale	Biopsia pleurica	Biopsija pleure
Biopsia renal	Kidney biopsy	Biopsie rénale	Biopsia renale	Biopsija bubrega
Broncografía	Bronchography	Bronchographie	Broncografia	Bronhografija
Broncoscopia	Bronchoscopy	Bronchoscopie	Broncoscopia	Bronhoskopija
CA 19-9 (antígeno carbohidrato 19-9)	CA 19-9 (carbohydrate antigen)	Antigène de cancer CA 19-9 (antigène d'hydrate de carbone)	CA 19-9 (antigene carboidratico)	CA 19-9 (karbohidratni antigen)
Campimetría (perimetría)	Perimetry	Périmétrie	Perimetria	Perimetrija
Captación tiroidea de 131 yodo	Iodine-131 thyroid test	Fixation thyroïdienne de l'iode 131	Test di captazione tiroidea dello iodio 131	Test štitnjače na provodljivost radioaktivnog joda 131
Cardiotocografía	Cardiotocography	Cardiotocographie	Cardiotocografia	Kardiotokografija
Cariotipo	Karyotype	Caryotype	Cariotipo	Kariotip
Cateterismo cardíaco	Cardiac catheterization (heart cath, angiocardiography)	Cathétérisme cardiaque	Cateterismo cardiaco (angiocardiografia)	Kateterizacija srca (angiokardiografija)
Cefalometría	Cephalometry	Céphalométrie	Cefalometria	Cefalometrija
Cistografía	Cystography	Cystographie	Cistografia	Cistografija
Cistoscopia	Cystoscopy	Cystoscopie	Cistoscopia	Cistoskopija
Colangiografía	Cholangiography	Cholangiographie	Colangiografia	Kolangiografija
Colangiopancreatografía retrógrada endoscópica	Endoscopic retrograde cholangiopancreatography (ERCP)	Cholangiopancréatographie rétrograde endoscopique	Colangio-pancreatografia endoscopica retrograda	Endoskopska retrogradna kolangiopankreatografija (ERCP)
Colecistografía oral	Oral cholecystography	Cholécystographie orale	Colecistografia orale	Rendgensko snimanje žučnog mjehura s kontrastom (peroralna kolecistografija)

Español	Inglés	Francés	Italiano	Croata
Colonoscopia	Colonoscopy	Colonoscopie	Colonscopia	Kolonoskopija
Colposcopia	Colposcopy	Colposcopie	Colposcopia	Kolposkopija
Comprobación del pulso	Pulse monitoring	Prise de pouls	Misurazione del polso	Mjerenje pulsa
Concentración de glucosa en sangre	Blood sugar concetration (glucose level)	Taux de la glycémie	Concentrazione del glucosio nel plasma	Šećer u krvi
Concetración de hormonas tiroideas en sangre	Thyroid blood tests	Taux d'hormones thyroïdiennes dans le sang	Test di ormoni tiroidei nel sangue	Test na hormone štitnjače u krvi
Conización	Cervical conization	Conisation	Conizzazione	Konizacija
Coronariografía	Coronary catheteriza-tion (coronarography)	Coronarographie	Coronarografia	Koronarografija
Craneografía	Skull X-ray (craniography)	Craniographie	Craniografia	Rendgensko snimanje lubanje
Cultivo	Microbiological culture	Culture microbiologique	Coltura di microrganismi	Mikrobiološki pregled (kultura)
Cultivo de esputo	Sputum culture	Culture de crachat	Coltura di sputo	Mikrobiološki pregled ispljuvka
Cultivo de líquido cefalorraquídeo	Cerebrospinal fluid culture	Culture du liquide cérébro-spinal	Coltura del liquor	Mikrobiološki pregled likvora
Cultivo vaginal	Vaginal swab culture	Culture vaginale	Coltura vaginale	Mikrobiološki pregled brisa rodnice
Defecografía	Defecography	Défécographie	Defecografia	Defekografija
Densitometría ósea	Bone densitometry (dual energy X-ray absorpriometry)	Ostéodensitométrie	Densità minerale ossea	Denzitometrija kostiju (apsorpciometrija kostiju)
Dermatoscopia	Dermatoscopy (dermoscopy)	Dermatoscopie (dermoscopie)	Dermatoscopia (dermoscopia)	Dermatoskopija (dermoskopija)
Diagnóstico diferencial	Differential diagnosis	Diagnostic différentiel	Diagnosi differenziale	Diferencijalna dijagnoza
Dilatación pupilar inducida por fármacos	Drug induced pupillary dilatation	Dilatation des pupilles provoquée par les médicaments	Dilatazione delle pupille provocando con tropicamide	Širenje zjenica potaknuto lijekovima
Ecocardiografía	Cardiac ultrasound (echocardiography)	Échocardiographie	Ecocardiografia	Ultrazvuk srca (ehokardiografija)
Ecocardiografía doppler	Doppler echocardiography	Échocardiographie-doppler	Ecocardiografia doppler	Ultrazvuk srca s dopplerom
Ecoencefalografia	Echoencephalography	Échoencéphalographie	Ecoencefalografia	Ehoencefalografija
Ecografía abdominal (ultrasonido abdominal)	Abdominal ultrasound	Échographie abdominale	Ecografia addominale	Ultrazvuk abdomena
Ecografía de páncreas (ultrasonido de páncreas)	Pancreas ultrasound	Échographie du pancréas	Ecografia pancreatica	Ultrazvuk gušterače
Ecografía de la tiroides (ultrasonido de la tiroides)	Thyroid ultrasound	Échographie thyroïdienne	Ecografia della tiroide	Ultrazvuk štitnjače
Ecografía de mama (ultrasonido de mama)	Breast ultrasound	Échographie mammaire	Ecografia mammaria	Ultrazvuk dojke
Ecografía de vesícula y vías biliares	Ultrasound of the gallbladder and bile ducts	Échographie la vésicule biliaire et les voies biliaires	Ecografia colecisti e vie biliari	Ultrazvuk žuči i žučnih vodova
Ecografía hepática (ultrasonido hepático)	Liver ultrasound	Échographie du foie (échographie hépatique)	Ecografia epatica	Ultrazvuk jetre
Ecografía renal (ultrasonido renal)	Renal ultrasound	Échographie rénale	Ecografia renale	Ultrazvuk bubrega
Electrocardiografía (ECG, EKG)	Electrocardiography (ECG)	Électrocardiographie (ECG)	Elettrocardiografia	Elektrokardiografija (EKG)
Electroencefalografía	Electroencephalography (EEG)	Électro-encéphalographie (EEG)	Elettroencefalografia	Elektroencefalografija (EEG)
Electroforesis de proteínas séricas	Serum protein electrophoresis	Èlectrophorèse des protéines	Elettroforesi delle sieroproteine	Elektroforeza proteina u serumu
Electromiografía	Electromyography (EMG)	Électromyographie	Elettromiografia	Elektromiografija (EMG)
Electroneurografía	Electroneurography	Électroneurographie	Elettroneurografia	Elektroneurografija
Electrorretinografía	Electroretinography	Électrorétinographie	Elettroretinografia	Elektroretinografija
Endoscopia	Endoscopy	Endoscopie	Endoscopia	Endoskopija
Enema de bario con doble contraste	Barium enema	Lavement baryté	Indagini radiologiche del colon con clisma opaco a doppio contrasto	Rendgensko snimanje debelog crijeva i rektuma s kontrastom barija
Enteroscopia	Enteroscopy	Entéroscopie	Enteroscopia	Enteroskopija
Ergometría	Ergometry test	Ergométrie	Ergometria (ECG sotto sforzo)	Test opterećenja (ergometrija)
Escala de coma de Glasgow	Glasgow coma scale	Échelle de Glasgow	Punteggio del coma di Glasgow	Glasgowska skala kome
Esofagogastroduode-noscopia	Esophagogastroduo-denoscopy	Endoscopie oeso-gastro-duodénale	Esofagogastroduode-noscopia	Ezofagogastrodoude-noskopija
Espermiograma	Semen analysis	Spermogramme	Spermiogramma	Spermogram
Espirometría	Spirometry (vital capacity test)	Spirométrie	Spirometria (pneumometria)	Spirometrija (mjerenje vitalnog kapaciteta)
Examen de glucosa en orina	Glucose urine test	Test du sucre dans les urines	Glucosio nelle urine	Šećer u urinu
Exámen dilatado de fundus	Dilated fundus examination	Fond d'oeil	Esame del fundus oculi	Pregled očnog fundusa
Examen ginecológico	Gynecological examination	Examen gynécologique	Esame ginecologico	Ginekoliški pregled

Español	Inglés	Francés	Italiano	Croata
Exámenes bioquímicos de sangre	Biochemical blood tests	Analyse de biochimie du sang	Test biochimici di sangue	Biokemijske pretrage krvi
Exploración física de mama	Breast examination	Examen du sein	Esame della mammella	Pregled dojke
Exudado faríngeo	Throat swab culture	Culture de gorge avec le coton-tige	Coltura di gola	Mikrobiološki pregled brisa grla
Flebografía	Phlebography	Phlébographie	Flebografia	Venografija (flebografija)
Fluoroscopia	Fluoroscopy	Fluoroscopie	Fluoroscopia	Fluoroskopija
Fosfatasa alcalina	Alkaline phosphatase	Phosphatase alcaline	Fosfatasi alcalina totale	Alkalna fosfataza
Gammagrafía de bazo con tecnecio 99m	Spleen scintigraphy with technetium -99m	Scintigraphie splénique au Technétium 99m	Scintigrafia splenica con tecnezio -99m	Scintigrafija slezene radioaktivnim izotopima
Gammagrafía hepatobiliar con tecnecio 99m	Hepatobiliary scintigraphy with technetium -99m	Scintigraphie hépato-biliaire au Technétium 99m	Scintigrafia epatobiliare con tecnezio -99m	Scintigrafija jetre i žučnih vodova radioaktivnim izotopima
Gammagrafía ósea	Bone scintigraphy	Scintigraphie osseuse	Scintigrafia ossea	Scintigrafija kostiju
Gammagrafía pulmonar	Lung scintigraphy	Scintigraphie pulmonaire	Scintigrafia polmonare	Scintigrafija pluća
Gammagrafía renal	Renal scintigraphy	Scintigraphie rénale	Scintigrafia renale	Scintigrafija bubrega
Gammagrafía tiroidea	Thyroid scintigraphy	Scintigraphie thyroïdienne	Scintigrafia tiroidea	Scintigrafija štitnjače
Gastroscopia	Gastroscopy	Gastroscopie	Gastroscopia	Gastroskopija
Gonioscopia	Gonioscopy	Gonioscopie	Gonioscopia	Gonioskopija
Gravedad específica de la orina	Urine specific gravity	Poids spécifique de l'urine	Esame delle urine peso specifico	Specifična težina urina
HbsAg (antígeno de superficie de la hepatitis B)	HbsAg (Hepatitis B surface antigen)	Antigène HbsAg (antigène de surface du virus de l'hépatite B)	HbsAg (antigene di superficie dell'epatite B)	HbsAg (hepatitis B površinski antigen)
Hematocrito	Hematocrit	Hématocrite	Ematocrito	Hematokrit
Hemocultivo	Blood culture	Hémoculture	Emocoltura	Mikrobiološki pregled krvi (hemokultura)
Hemograma (conteo sanguíneo completo)	Complete blood count	Hémogramme (numération formule sanguine)	Emocromo (analisi del sangue, esame emocromocitometrico)	Kompletna krvna slika
Histerosalpingografía	Hysterosalpingography	Hystérosalpingographie	Isterosalpingografia	Rendgensko snimanje maternice i jajovoda
Histeroscopia	Hysterescopy	Hystéroscopie	Isteroscopia	Histeroskopija
Imagen por resonancia magnética (IRM)	Magnetic resonance imaging (MRI)	Imagerie par résonance magnétique (IRM)	Imaging a risonanza magnetica (risonanza magnetica tomografica)	Magnetska rezonancija (MR)
Imagen por resonancia magnética funcional (IRMf)	Functional magnetic resonance imaging (functional MRI)	Imagerie par résonance magnétique fonctionnelle (IRMf)	Risonanza magnetica funzionale	Funkcionalna magnetska rezonancija (FMR)
Laboratorio	Laboratory (lab)	Laboratoire	Laboratorio	Laboratorij
Laparoscopia	Laparoscopy	Laparoscopie	Laparoscopia	Laparoskopija
Laringoscopia	Laryngoscopy	Laryngoscopie	Laringoscopia	Laringoskopija
Linfografía	Lymphography (lymphangiography)	Lymphographie	Linfangiografia (linfografia)	Limfografija
Magnetoencefalografía	Magnetoencephalography (MEG)	Magnétoencéphalographie	Magnetoencefalografia	Magnetoencefalografija (MEG)
Mamografía	Mammography	Mammographie	Mammografia (mastografia)	Mamografija
Manometría esofágica	Esophageal manometry	Manométrie oesophagienne	Manometria esofagea	Manometrija jednjaka
Marcador biológico	Biomarker	Biomarqueur	Biomarcatore	Biomarker
Marcador tumoral	Tumor marker	Marqueur tumoral	Marker tumorale	Tumorski marker
Marcador tumoral CA 125	CA 125 (cancer antigen 125)	Antigène de cancer CA 125	CA 125 (antigene di carcinoma 125)	CA 125 (karcinomski antigen 125)
Mediastinoscopia	Mediastinoscopy	Médiastinoscopie	Mediastinoscopia	Medijastinoskopija
Medicina nuclear	Radioisotope scanning (nuclear medicine)	Médicine nucléaire	Medicina nucleare	Radioizotopna dijagnostika
Medio de contraste	Contrast medium	Produit de contraste	Mezzo di contrasto	Kontrast
Mielografía	Myelography	Myélographie	Mielografia	Mijelografija
Mielografía cervical suboccipital	Suboccipital myelography	Myélographie sous-occipitale	Mielografia sotto-occipitale	Subokcipitalna mijelografija
Mielografía lumbar	Lumbar myelography	Myélographie lombaire	Mielografia lombare	Lumbalna mijelografija
Monitorización de la presión arterial	Blood pressure monitoring	Monitoring de la pression artérielle	Misurazione della pressione arteriosa	Mjerenje krvnog pritiska
Neumoencefalografía	Pneumoencephalography	Encéphalographie gazeuse	Pneumoencefalografia	Pneumoencefalografija
Nitrógeno ureico en sangre (BUN)	Blood urea nitrogen test (BUN)	Azote d'urée dans le sang	Azoto ureico nel sangue (BUN)	Ostatni dušik u krvi (urea nitrogen test)
Oftalmoscopia	Ophtalmoscopy	Ophtalmoscopie	Oftalmoscopia	Oftalmoskopija
Otoscopia	Otoscopy	Otoscopie	Otoscopia	Otoskopija
Pelvigrafía	Pelvigraphy	Pelvigraphie	Pelvigrafia	Rendgensko snimanje zdjelice i porođajnog kanala
Pelvimetria	Pelvimetry	Pelvimétrie	Pelvimetria	Pelvimetrija
Pielografía retrógrada	Retrograde pyelography	Urétéro-pyélographie rétrograde	Pielografia retrograda	Retrogradna pijelografija
Pletismografía	Plethysmography	Pléthysmographie	Pletismografia	Pletizmografija
Polisomnografía	Polysomnography (sleep study)	Polysomnographie (polygraphie du sommeil)	Polisonnografia	Polisomnografija (viseparametarski test u pracenju procesa sna)

Español	Inglés	Francés	Italiano	Croata
Presión venosa central	Central venous pressure (CVP)	Pression veineuse centrale	Pressione venosa centrale	Centralni venozni pritisak (CVP)
Proteínas en la orina	Urine protein test	Protéines dans les urines	Proteine nelle urine	Bjelančevine u urinu
Prueba de aclaramiento de urea sanguínea	Urea clearance test	Épruve d'élimination de l'urée sanguine	Urea clearance (clearance dell'urea)	Urea klirens
Prueba de alfa-fetoproteína	Alpha-fetoprotein test (AFP test)	Test d'alpha-foetoprotéine	Test alfa-fetoproteina	Alfafetoproteinski test (AFP)
Prueba de Coombs indirecta	Indirect Coombs test	Réaction de Coombs indirecte	Test di Coombs indiretto	Indirektni Coombsov test
Prueba de gases en la sangre	Blood gas test	Prélèvement des gaz du sang	Analisi dei gas nel sangue (emogas analisi)	Analiza plinova u krvi
Prueba de la bencidina	Benzidine stool test	Analyse fécale de benzidine	Prova della benzidina	Benzidinski test stolice
Prueba de la fenolsulfonftaleína	Phenolsulfonphthalein test (PSP test)	Épruve à la phénosulfonphtaléine	Test alla fenolsulfonftaleina	Fenolsulfoftaleinski test (PSP-test)
Prueba de la función hepática con bromosulfaleína	Bromsulphalein liver function test	Test de la bromesulfonephtaléine	Test dela bromosulfaleina di funzionalità epatica	Brom-sulfalein test funkcije jetre
Prueba de Papanicolau	Papanicolau test (Pap test)	Test PAP	Test di Papanicolaou (Pap test)	Papa-test (Papanicola-ouova klasifikacija)
Prueba de Weber	Weber test	Test de Weber	Prova di Weber	Weberov test
Prueba del aliento con urea	Urea breath test	Test respiratoire à l'urée	Test del respiro (urea breath test)	Urea izdisajni test
Prueba rápida para estreptococo	Rapid strep test	Test de diagnostic rapide du streptocoque	Test rapido dello streptococco	Brzi test na streptokok (strep-test)
Pruebas de embarazo	Pregnancy test	Test de grossesse	Test di gravidanza	Test na trudnoću
Pruebas de función hepática	Liver function tests	Explorations fonctio-nnelles hépatiques	Test di funzionalità epatica	Funkcionalne pretrage jetre
Pruebas de laboratorio	Laboratory tests	Analyse médicale (examens de biologie médicale)	Esami di laboratorio	Laboratorijske pretrage
Pruebas de serología	Serology blood tests	Analyse sérologique	Esami sierologici	Serološke pretrage na antitijela
Punción aspiración con aguja fina	Fine needle aspiration biopsy	Forage-biopsie	Agoaspirato (biopsia mediante ago sottile)	Punkcijsko-aspiracijska biopsija
Punción lumbar	Lumbar puncture	Ponction lombaire (rachicentèse)	Puntura lombare (rachicentesi)	Lumbalna punkcija
Punción suboccipital	Suboccipital puncture	Ponction sous-occipitale	Puntura suboccipitale	Subokcipitalna punkcija
Punción transtorácica aspirativa con aguja ultrafina	Transthoracic percutaneous fine needle aspiration	Ponction transthora-cique percutanée à l'aiguille fine	Agoaspirato polmonare percutaneo transtoracico	Perkutana transtorakalna punkcija pluća
Radiografía	X-ray (radiography)	Radiographie	Radiografia	Rendgen
Radiografía de esófago, estómago y duodeno tomada con comida baritada	Barium meal (upper gastrointestinal series)	Radiographie de l'abdomen en bouillie de sulfate de baryum	Radiografia gastroduodenale con pasto baritato	Rendgensko snimanje želuca i dvanaesnika barijevom kašom
Radiografía de hueso (radiografía ósea)	Bone X-ray (bone radiography)	Radiographie des os	Radiografia ossea	Rendgensko snimanje kostiju
Radiografía de la columna vertebral (radiografía vertebral)	Spine X-ray (spine radiography)	Radiographie de la colonne vertébrale	Radiografia della colonna vertebrale	Rendgensko snimanje kralježnice
Radiografía de tórax	Chest X-ray	Radiographie de thorax	Radiografia del torace	Rendgensko snimanje srca i pluća
Radiografía dental	Dental X-ray	Radiographie dentaire	Radiografia dentale	Rendgensko snimanje zuba
Rectoscopia	Rectoscopy	Rectoscopie	Rettoscopia	Rektoskopija
Reflejo patelar	Patellar reflex	Réflexe rotulien	Riflesso patellare	Patelarni refleks
Refractomería	Refractometry	Réfractométrie	Rifrattometria	Ispitivanje refrakcije
Sialografía	Sialography	Sialographie	Sialografia (scialografia)	Sijalografija
Sigmoidoscopia	Sigmoidoscopy	Sigmoïdoscopie	Sigmoidoscopia	Sigmoidoskopija
Tacto rectal	Rectal examination	Toucher rectal	Esplorazione rettale	Rektalni pregled
Test cutaneos de alergia (prick)	Skin allergy testing (prick)	Test de la piqûre	Test cutaneo per le allergie "prick test"	Alergološko testiranje kože (prick test)
Test de Mantoux (PPD)	Mantoux test (PPD test)	Test Mantoux (test PPD)	Mantoux test	Tuberkulinski kožni test
Test de tolerancia oral a la glucosa	Oral glucose tolerance test (OGTT)	Test de tolérance orale au glucose (TTOG)	Test orale di tolleranca al glucosio (OGTT, curva da carico orale di glucosio)	Oralni test tolerancije na glukozu (OGTT)
Test de Waaler-Rose	Rose Waaler test	Réaction de Waaler Rose	Rose Waaler test	Rose Waaler test
Tiempo de protrombina	Prothrombin time	Taux de prothrombine	Tempo di protrombina	Protrombinski indeks
Tiempo de tromboplastina parcial activado	Partial thromboplastin time (PTT)	Temps de céphaline activée (TCA)	Tempo di tromboplastina parziale	Parcijalno trombopla-stinsko vrijeme (PTT)
Timpanocentesis	Tympanocentesis	Tympanocentese	Timpanocentesi	Timpanocenteza
Timpanometría	Tympanometry	Tympanométrie	Timpanometria	Timpanometrija
Tomografía	Tomography	Tomographie	Tomografia	Tomografija
Tomografía computada	Computed tomography (CT)	Tomodensitométrie (TDM)	Tomografia computerizzata (TC)	Kompjuterizirana tomografija (CT)
Tomografía por emisión de positrones	Positron emission tomography	Tomographie par émission de positrons	Tomografia ad emissione di positroni	Pozitronska emisijska tomografija (PET)
Tonometría	Tonometry	Tonométrie oculaire	Tonometria	Tonometrija oka
Toracoscopia	Thoracoscopy	Thoracoscopie	Toracoscopia	Torakoskopija

Español	Inglés	Francés	Italiano	Croata
Ultrasonido focalizado de alta intensidad (HIFU)	High intensity focused ultrasound	Ultrasons focalisés de haute intensité	Ultrasuono ad alta intensità focalizzato	Fokusirani ultrazvuk visokog intenziteta
Ultrasonografía (ecografía)	Ultrasound (medical ultrasonography)	Échographie	Ecografia	Ultrazvuk
Ureteroscopía	Ureteroscopy	Urétéroscopie	Ureteroscopia	Ureteroskopija
Uretrografía	Urethrography	Urétrographie	Uretrografia	Uretrografija
Urobilinógeno en orina	Urobilinogen in urine	Urobilinogène dans les urines	Urobilinogeno nelle urine	Urobilinogen u urinu
Urocultivo	Urine culture	Uroculture	Urinocoltura	Mikrobiološki pregled mokraće (urinokultura)
Urografía	Pyelography	Urographie	Urografia	Pijelografija (urografija)
Urografía intravenosa	Intravenous pyelography	Urographie intra-veineuse	Urografia intravenosa (pielografia intravenosa)	Intravenozna pijelogra-fija (i.v. Urografija)
Velocidad de sedimentación globular	Erythrocyte sedimentation rate	Vitesse de sédimentation	Velocità di eritrosedimentazione	Sedimentacija eritrocita
Ventriculografía	Ventriculography	Ventriculographie	Ventricolografia	Ventrikulografija
Volumen residual de orina	Post-void residual urine volume	Volume urinaire résiduel	Volume urinario residuo	Ostatni urin (rezidualni urin)
EMBARAZO Y OBSTETRICIA:	**PREGNANCY AND OBSTETRICS:**	**GROSSESSE ET OBSTÉTRIQUE:**	**GRAVIDANZA ED OSTETRICIA:**	**TRUDNOĆA I PORODNIŠTVO:**
Aborto espontáneo	Spontaneous abortion (miscarriage)	Fausse couche	Aborto spontaneo	Spontani pobačaj
Aborto habitual	Habitual abortion (recurrent miscarriage)	Avortement à répétition	Aborto abituale	Habitualni pobačaj
Aborto inducido	Abortion (pregnancy termination)	Avortement	Interruzione di gravidanza (aborto)	Prekid trudnoće (abortus)
Agentes teratogénicos	Pregnancy risk factors	Facteurs de risque de la grossesse	Rischio teratogenico	Teratogeni faktori rizika
Amniocentesis	Amniocentesis	Amniocentèse	Amniocentesi	Amniocenteza
Amnioscopia	Amnioscopy	Amnioscopie	Amnioscopia	Amnioskopija
Anomalías fetales	Fetal anomalies (fetal abnormalities)	Anomalies foetales	Anomalie di sviluppo fetale (anomalie fetali)	Anomalije fetusa
Aspirador al vacío	Vacuum extractor (ventouse)	Vacuum extractor	Aspiratore a vuoto	Vakuumski ekstraktor
Ausencia de la menstruación (amenorrea)	Absence of menstrual period (amenorrhea)	Absence des règles (aménorrhée)	Assenza di mestruazioni (amenorrea)	Izostanak mjesečnice (amenoreja)
Baby blues (leve depresión post parto)	Maternity blues (baby blues)	Baby blues	Sindrome del terzo giorno (baby blues)	Labilno psihičko raspo-loženje (baby blues)
Banco de semen	Sperm bank	Banque du sperme	Banca del seme	Banka sperme
Blastocisto	Blastocyst	Blastocyste	Blastocisti	Blastocista
Cabeza	Head	Tête	Testa	Glavica
Canal del parto	Birth canal	Canal utérin	Canale del parto	Porodni kanal
Cardiotocografía	Cardiotocography	Cardiotocographie	Cardiotocografia	Kardiotokografija
Cesárea	Cesarean section (C-section)	Césarienne	Taglio cesareo	Carski rez
Ciclo menstrual	Menstrual cycle	Cycle menstruel	Ciclo mestruale	Menstruacijski ciklus
Conducto mamario (conducto galactóforo)	Lactiferous duct	Canal galactophore	Dotto galattoforo	Mliječni vod
Contracción de Braxton Hicks	Braxton Hicks contractons	Fausse contraction (contraction de Braxton Hicks)	False contrazioni (contrazioni di Braxton Hicks)	Lažni trudovi
Contracciones del trabajo de parto (contracciones uterinas)	Labor contractions	Contractions utérines du travail	Contrazioni del travaglio	Trudovi
Cordocentesis	Cordocentesis	Cordocentèse	Cordocentesi	Kordocenteza
Cordón umbilical	Umbilical cord	Cordon ombilical	Funicolo ombelicale	Pupkovina (pupčana vrpca)
Coriocarcinoma	Choriocarcinoma	Choriocarcinome	Coriocarcinoma	Koriokarcinom
Corion	Chorion	Chorion	Corion (corio)	Korion
Cortar	Cut	Couper	Tagliare (intersecare)	Presjeći
Cuatrillizos	Quadruplets	Quadruplés	Quattro gemelli	Četvorci
Cuello	Neck	Cou	Collo	Vrat
Depresión postparto (depresión postnatal)	Postnatal depression (postpartum depression)	Dépression post-natale (dépression post-partum)	Depressione post-partum	Postporođajna depresija
Desangramiento (hemorragia)	Bleeding (haemorrhage)	Saignement (hémorragie)	Emorragia	Krvarenje (hemoragija)
Desprendimiento prematuro de placenta	Placental abruption	Abruption placentaire (rupture placentaire)	Distacco di placenta (abruptio placentae)	Abrupcija posteljice
Diabetes gestacional	Gestational diabetes	Diabète gestationnel	Diabete gestazionale	Gestacijski dijabetes
Dilatación del cuello uterino	Cervical dilation	Dilatation cervicale	Dilatazione della cervice uterina	Otvaranje ušća maternice
Donación de ovocitos	Egg donation	Donneuse d'ovule	Ovodonazione	Donacija jajašca
Duración de las contracciones uterinas	Duration of contraction	Durée de la contraction utérine	Durata di contrazioni	Trajanje truda
Duración del embarazo	Duration of pregnancy	Durée de la grossesse	Durata della gravidanza	Trajanje trudnoće
Eclampsia	Eclampsia	Éclampsie	Eclampsia	Eklampsija
Edema (hidropesía)	Edema	Oedème	Edema	Edem
Embarazo	Pregnancy	Grossesse	Gravidanza (gestazione)	Trudnoća

Español	Inglés	Francés	Italiano	Croata
Embarazo ectópico	Ectopic pregnancy (extrauterine pregnancy)	Grossesse extra-utérine	Gravidanza ectopica	Izvanmaternična trudnoća (ektopična trudnoća)
Embarazo múltiple	Multiple pregnancy	Grossesse multiple	Gravidanza gemellare	Blizanačka trudnoća
Embrión	Embryo	Embryon	Embrione	Embrij (zametak)
Empujar	Push	Pousser	Spingere	Tiskati
Enfermedad de Hirschsprung (megacolon aganglió nico)	Meconium ileus	Iléus méconial	Malattia di Hirschsprung (ostruzione del colon congenita)	Mekonijalni ileus
Enfermedad hemolítica del recién nacido (eritroblastosis fetal)	Hemolytic disease of the newborn	Maladie hémolytique du nouveau-né	Eritroblastosi fetale (malattia emolitica del neonato)	Hemolitička bolest novorođenčeta
Episiotomía	Episiotomy	Épisiotomie	Episiotomia	Kirurško proširenje porođajnog kanala (epiziotomija)
Espermatozoide	Spermatozoon (sperm cell)	Spermatozoïde	Spermatozoo	Spermij
Estrógeno de la placenta	Placental estrogen	Oestrogène placentaire	Estrogeno placentare	Estrogen placente
Etapas del parto	Stage of birth	Stade du travail	Fase del parto	Porodno doba
Excesiva producción de saliva (hipersalivación)	Excessive secretion of saliva (hypersalivation)	Sécrétion de la salive excessive	Produzione di saliva eccessiva (ipersalivazione)	Pojačano lučenje sline (hipersalivacija)
Expulsión de la placenta	Expulsion of placenta	Expulsion du placenta	Espulsione della placenta	Istiskivanje posteljice i ovoja
Expulsión del producto	Expulsion of the baby	Expulsion du bébé	Espulsione del feto	Istiskivanje ploda
Extracción quirúrgica del útero (histerectomía)	Surgical removal of the uterus (hysterectomy)	Enlèvement chirurgical de l'uterus (hystérectomie)	Asportazione chirurgica dell'utero (isterectomia)	Kirurško odstranjenje maternice (histerektomija)
Eyaculación	Ejaculation	Éjaculation	Eiaculazione	Ejakulat
Fármaco utilizado para suprimir el trabajo de parto prematuro (tocolítico)	Medication that suppresses premature labor (tocolytic)	Médicament pour interrompre le déclenchement du travail (tocolytique)	Farmaco con lo scopo di arrestare le contrazioni uterine (tocolisi)	Lijek za sprečavanje trudova (tokolitik)
Fármacos abortivos	Abortifacients	Médicaments abortifs	Farmaci abortivi	Abortivni lijekovi
Fecundación (fertilización)	Conception	Conception (fécondation)	Concezione	Začeće (oplodnja)
Fecundación in vitro	In vitro fertilisation	Fécondation in vitro	Fertilizzazione in vitro	Oplodnja in vitro
Feto	Fetus	Foetus	Feto	Fetus
Feto posición transversal	Transverse fetal position	Position transversale du foetus	Posizione del feto trasversale	Kosi položaj ploda
Fetoscopia	Fetoscopy	Foetoscopie	Fetoscopia	Fetoskopija
Fiebre puerperal	Puerperal fever	Fièvre puerpérale	Febbre puerperale	Puerperalna groznica (babinja groznica)
Folículo de Graaf	Graafian follicle	Follicule de Graaf	Follicolo di Graaf	Graafov folikul
Fórceps	Forceps	Forceps	Forcipe	Forceps (kliješta)
Frecuencia de las contracciones uterinas	Labor contraction frequency	Fréquence des contractions utérines	Frequenza di contrazioni uterine	Frekvencija trudova
Gemelos	Twins	Jumeaux	Gemelli	Blizanci
Gemelos dicigóticos (mellizos)	Dizygotic twins (biovular twins)	Jumeaux dizygotes	Gemelli fraterni (gemelli dizigoti)	Dvojajčani blizanci
Gemelos monocigóticos	Monozygotic twins (identical twins)	Jumeaux monozygotes	Gemelli identici (gemelli monozigoti)	Jednojajčani blizanci
Ginecología	Gynecology	Gynécologie	Ginecologia	Ginekologija
Gonadotropina coriónica	Chorion-gonadotrophin	Gonadotrophine chorionique	Gonadotropina corionica	Korion-gonadotropin
Himen	Hymen	Hymen	Imene	Djevičnjak (himen)
Hiperemia del ovario	Ovarian hyperemia	Hyperhémie ovarienne	Iperemia dell'ovaio	Hiperemija jajnika
Hiperplasia endometrial	Endometrial hyperplasia	Hyperplasie endométriale	Iperplasia endometriale	Hiperplazija maternice
Hipertrofia del útero	Hypertrophy of uterus	Hypertrophie de l'utérus	Ipertrofia dell'utero	Hipertrofija maternice
Hipotrofia fetal	Fetal hypotrophy	Hypotrophie foetale	Ipotrofia fetale	Fetalna hipotrofija
Hospital de maternidad	Maternity hospital	Maternité	Clinica ostetrica	Rodilište
Implatación	Implantation	Implantation	Impianto	Implantacija (usađivanje)
Incontinencia urinaria	Urinary incontinence	Incontinence urinaire	Incontinenza urinaria	Urinarna inkotinencija
Incremento de la presión sanguínea (hipertensión)	High blood pressure (hypertension)	Pression artérielle élevée (hypertension artérielle)	Ipertensione arteriosa sistemica	Visoki krvni tlak (hipertenzija)
Incubadora	Incubator	Couveuse (incubateur)	Incubatrice	Inkubator
Infección	Infection	Infection	Infezione	Infekcija
Infección de las membranas placentarias (corioamnionitis)	Inflammation of the fetal membranes (chorioamnionitis)	Chorioamnionite	Infiammazione del sacco amniotico (corioamniosite)	Upala plodovih ovoja (korioamnionitis)
Infecciones TORCH	TORCH infections	Infections TORCH	Complesso TORCH	TORCH infekcije
Infertilidad	Infertility	Stérilité	Sterilità	Neplodnost (sterilitet)
Inflamación de la vejiga urinaria (cistitis)	Inflammation of the urinary bladder (cystitis)	Inflammation de la vessie (cystite)	Infiammazione della vescica urinaria (cistite)	Upala mokraćnog mjehura (cistitis)
Inseminación artificial	Artificial insemination	Insémination artificielle	Fecondazione assistita (fecondazione artificiale)	Umjetna oplodnja
Intensidad de contracciones uterinas	Intensity of contractions	Intensité des contractions utérines	Intensità di contrazione	Snaga trudova
Inyección intracitoplasmática de espermatozoides	Intracytoplasmatic sperm injection	Injection intra-cytoplasmique de spermatozoïdes	Iniezione intracitoplasmatica dello spermatozoo	Intracitoplazmatska spermalna injekcija
Lactancia	Lactation	Lactation	Lattazione	Dojenje (laktacija)

Español	Inglés	Francés	Italiano	Croata
Legrado	Curettage	Curetage	Raschiamento (curetage)	Kiretaža
Líquido amniótico	Amniotic fluid	Liquide amniotique	Liquido amniotico	Plodna voda (amnijska tekućina)
Litopedion	Lithopedion (stone baby)	Lithopédion (enfant pétrifié)	Lithopedion	Litopedion (okamenjeno dijete)
Loquios	Lochia	Lochies	Lochi	Lohija (iscjedak u babinjama)
Macrosomía fetal	Macrosomia (big baby syndrome)	Macrosomie foetale	Macrosomia fetale	Fetalna hipertrofija
Madre	Mother	Mère	Madre	Majka
Madre de alquiler	Surrogate mother (womb mother)	Mère porteuse	Surrogazione di maternità	Surogat majka (zamjenska majka)
Malformaciones uterinas	Uterine anomalies	Malformations utérines	Anomalie uterine	Anomalije maternice
Mama	Breast	Sein	Mammella	Dojka
Mastitis puerperal	Puerperal mastitis	Mammite puerpérale	Mastite puerperale	Puerperalni mastitis
Matrona (matrón)	Midwife	Sage-femme	Ostetrica (levatrice)	Babica
Meconio	Meconium	Méconium	Meconio	Mekonij
Menopausia	Menopause	Ménopause	Menopausa	Menopauza (klimakterij)
Menstruación (período)	Menstruation	Règle (menstruation)	Mestruazione	Menstruacija
Microcefalia	Microcephaly	Microcéphalie	Microcefalia	Mikrocefalija(sitnoglavost)
Mifepristona	Mifepristone	Mifépristone	Mifepristone	Mifepriston
Mórula	Morula	Morula	Morula	Morula
Mucosa interior del útero (endometrio)	Inner membrane of the uterus (endometrium)	Muqueuse utérine (endomètre)	Mucosa interna dell'utero (endometrio)	Sluznica maternice (endometrij)
Muestra de vellosidades coriónicas	Chorionic villus sampling	Choriocentèse	Villocentesi	Uzorak korionskih resica
Multigrávida	Multigravida	Multipare	Pluripara	Višerotkinja
Nacido muerto	Stillborn	Mort-né	Nato morto	Mrtvorođenče
Nalga	Breech	Siège	Culatta (deretano)	Zadak
Náusea	Nausea	Nausée	Nausea	Mučnina
Neonato (recién nacido)	Newborn (infant)	Nouveau-né	Neonato	Novorođenče
Neonatología	Neonatology	Néonatologie	Neonatologia	Neonatologija
Obstetricia	Obstetrics	Obstétrique	Ostetricia	Porodništvo
Ombligo (pupo)	Navel (belly button)	Ombilic (nombril)	Ombelico	Pupak
Ovario	Ovary	Ovaire	Ovaia (ovario)	Jajnik
Ovogénesis	Oogenesis	Ovogenèse	Ovogenesi	Ovogeneza (oogeneza)
Ovulación	Ovulation	Ovulation	Ovulazione	Ovulacija
Óvulo	Ovum	Ovule	Uovo	Jajašce
Padre	Father	Père	Padre	Otac
Padre (primario)	Parent	Géniteur	Genitore	Roditelj
Padre biológico	Biological parent	Parent biologique	Genitore biologico	Biološki roditelj
Pañal	Diaper	Couche-culotte	Pannolino	Pelena
Parto	Childbirth	Accouchement (naissance)	Parto	Porod
Parto a término	Full term birth	Accouchement à terme	Parto a termine	Ročni porod
Parto en agua	Water birth	Accouchement dans l'eau	Parto nell'acqua	Porod u vodi
Parto patológico	Pathological birth	Accouchement pathologique	Parto patologico	Patološki porod
Parto postérmino	Postmature birth	Naissance après terme	Parto post-termine	Poslijeročni porod
Parto pretérmino	Premature birth	Prématurité	Parto pretermine	Prijevremeni porod
Parto prolongado	Prolonged birth	Accouchement prolongé	Parto prolungato	Produljeni porod
Pelvimetría	Pelvimetry	Pelvimétrie	Pelvimetria	Pelvimetrija
Pelvis contraída	Contracted pelvis	Bassin contracté	Pelvi ristretto	Sužena zdjelica
Perfil biofísico fetal	Biophysical profile of the fetus	Profil biophysique foetal	Profilo biofisico fetale	Biofizikalni profil fetusa
Peritonitis meconial	Meconium peritonitis	Péritonite méconiale	Peritonite da meconio	Mekonijalni peritonitis
Peso al nacer	Fetal weight (birth mass)	Poids de naissance	Peso di neonato	Težina ploda (porođajna težina)
Pezón	Nipple	Mamelon (papille)	Capezzolo	Bradavica
pH-metría fetal	Fetal pH-metry	pH-métrie foetale	pH-metria fetale	Fetalna pH-metrija
Pielonefritis	Pyelonephritis	Pyélonéphrite	Pielonefrite	Pijelonefritis
Placenta	Placenta	Placenta	Placenta	Posteljica (placenta)
Placenta accreta	Placenta accreta	Placenta accreta	Placenta accreta	Prirasla posteljica (placenta acreta)
Placenta previa	Placenta previa	Placenta praevia	Placenta previa	Placenta previja
Plagiocefalia	Plagiocephaly	Plagiocéphalie	Plagiocefalia	Plagiocefalija
Posición de nalgas	Breech position	Présentation podalique (présentation du siège)	Posizione podalica del feto	Stav zatkom
Preeclampsia	EPH gestosis (pre-eclampsia)	Pré-éclampsie	Preeclampsia (gestosi)	EPH-gestoze (preeklampsija)
Primigesta	Primigravida	Primigeste	Primipara	Prvorotkinja
Progesterona	Progesterone	Progestérone	Progesterone	Progesteron
Progesterona de placenta	Placental progesterone	Progestérone placentaire	Progesterone placentare	Progesteron placente
Prolactina	Prolactin	Prolactine	Prolattina	Prolaktin
Prolapso del cordón umbilical	Umbilical cord prolapse	Prolapsus du cordon ombilical	Prolasso del funicolo ombelicale	Ispala pupkovina (prolaps pupkovine)
Psicosis postparto	Postpartum psychosis	Psychose puerpérale	Psicosi post-partum	Puerperalna psihoza
Puerperio	Postnatal (postpartum period, puerperium)	Post-partum	Puerperio	Babinje (puerperij)

Español	Inglés	Francés	Italiano	Croata
Recién nacido pretérmino	Preterm newborn	Nouveau-né prématuré	Neonato pretermine	Nedonošče
Reproducción asistida	Medically assisted procreation	Procréation médicalement assistée	Procreazione assistita	Medicinski potpomognuta oplodnja
Respiración	Breathing	Respiration	Respirazione	Disanje
Retención de orina	Urinary retention (ischuria)	Rétention d'urine	Ritenzione urinaria	Zastoj urina (urinarna retencija)
Ruptura de membrana	Rupture of membranes	Rupture des membranes	Rottura delle membrane	Prsnuće vodenjaka
Ruptura prematura de membrana	Premature rupture of membranes	Rupture prématurée des membranes	Rottura precoce delle membrane	Prijevremeno prsnuće vodenjaka
Sacaleches	Breast pump	Tire-lait	Pompa tiralatte	Pumpica za izdajanje
Saco amniótico	Amniotic sac	Amnios (sac amniotique)	Amnios	Vodenjak
Sala de partos	Delivery room	Salle d'accouchement	Sala parto	Rađaona
Semen (esperma)	Semen (sperm)	Sperme	Seme (sperma)	Sjemena tekućina (sperma)
Sepsis puerperal	Puerperal sepsis	Septicémie puerpérale	Sepsi puerperale	Puerperalna sepsa
Signo de Chadwick	Chadwick's sign	Signe de Chadwick	Segno del Chadwick (tinta bluastra alla vagina)	Hiperemična sluznica rodnice (Chadwickov znak)
Síndrome de aspiración de meconio	Meconium aspiration syndrome	Syndrome d'aspiration méconiale	Sindrome da aspirazione di meconio	Mekonijalni aspiracijski sindrom
Succión	Suckling	Succion	Suzione	Sisanje
Talla de un neonato	Body length of a newborn	Taille corporelle du nouveau-né	Lunghezza di neonato	Dužina novorođenčeta
Tocólogo (obstetra)	Obstetrician	Obstétricien	Ostetrico	Porodničar (opstetičar)
Traslucencia nucal	Nuchal scan (nuchal translucency)	Clarté nucale	Translucenza nucale	Nuhalna translucencija
Trompa de Falopio (tuba uterina, oviducto)	Fallopian tube (oviduct)	Trompes de Fallope	Ovidotto (ovidutto)	Jajovod
Ultrasonografía (ecografía)	Ultrasound (medical ultrasonography)	Échographie	Ecografia	Ultrazvuk
Útero (matriz, seno materno)	Womb (uterus)	Utérus	Utero	Maternica (uterus)
Vagina	Vagina	Vagin	Vagina	Rodnica
Vellosidades coriónicas	Chorionic villi	Villosités choriales	Villi coriali	Korionske resice
Venas varicosas de las piernas	Leg varicose veins	Varices des membres inférieurs	Varici degli arti inferiori	Proširene vene na nogama
Viabilidad de espermatozoides	Sperm viability	Viabilité du sperme	Sopravvivenza di spermatozoo	Životna sposobnost spermija

DIZIONARIO MULTILINGUE DI EMERGENZE MEDICHE

Italiano-Inglese-Francese-Spagnolo-Croato

Italiano	Inglese	Francese	Spagnolo	Croato
NUMERI:	**NUMBERS:**	**NUMÉROS:**	**NÚMEROS:**	**BROJEVI:**
Zero	Zero	Zéro	Cero	Nula
Uno	One	Un	Uno	Jedan
Due	Two	Deux	Dos	Dva
Tre	Three	Trois	Tres	Tri
Quattro	Four	Quatre	Cuatro	Četiri
Cinque	Five	Cinq	Cinco	Pet
Sei	Six	Six	Seis	Šest
Sette	Seven	Sept	Siete	Sedam
Otto	Eight	Huit	Ocho	Osam
Nove	Nine	Neuf	Nueve	Devet
Dieci	Ten	Dix	Diez	Deset
Undici	Eleven	Onze	Once	Jedanaest
Dodici	Twelve	Douze	Doce	Dvanaest
Tredici	Thirteen	Treize	Trece	Trinaest
Quattordici	Fourteen	Quatorze	Catorce	Četrnaest
Quindici	Fifteen	Quinze	Quince	Petnaest
Sedici	Sixteen	Seize	Dieciséis	Šesnaest
Diciassette	Seventeen	Dix-sept	Diecisiete	Sedamnaest
Diciotto	Eighteen	Dix-huit	Dieciocho	Osamnaest
Diciannove	Nineteen	Dix-neuf	Diecinueve	Devetnaest
Venti	Twenty	Vingt	Veinte	Dvadeset
Ventuno	Twenty-one	Vingt et un	Veintiuno	Dvadest i jedan
Ventidue	Twenty-two	Vingt-deux	Veintidós	Dvadeset i dva
Trenta	Thirty	Trente	Treinta	Trideset
Quaranta	Forty	Quarante	Cuarenta	Četrdeset
Cinquanta	Fifty	Cinquante	Cincuenta	Pedeset
Sessanta	Sixty	Soixante	Sesenta	Šezdeset
Settanta	Seventy	Soixante-dix	Setenta	Sedamdeset
Ottanta	Eighty	Quatre-vingts	Ochenta	Osamdeset
Novanta	Ninety	Quatre-vingt-dix	Noventa	Devedeset
Cento	Hundred	Cent	Cien	Sto
Centouno	One hundred and one	Cent un	Ciento uno	Sto jedan
Centoventitre	One hundred and twenty-three	Cent vingt-trois	Ciento veintitrés	Sto dvadeset i tri
Duecento	Two hundred	Deux cents	Doscientos	Dvjesto
Trecento	Three hundred	Trois cents	Trescientos	Tristo
Quattrocento	Four hundred	Quatre cents	Cuatrocientos	Četristo
Cinquecento	Five hundred	Cinq cents	Quinientos	Petsto
Seicento	Six hundred	Six cents	Seiscientos	Šesto
Settecento	Seven hundred	Sept cents	Setecientos	Sedamsto
Ottocento	Eight hundred	Huit cents	Ochocientos	Osamsto
Novecento	Nine hundred	Neuf cents	Novecientos	Devetsto
Mille	Thousand	Mille	Mil	Tisuća
Duemila	Two thousand	Deux mille	Dos mil	Dvije tisuće
Un milione	Million	Million	Millón	Milijun
Un miliardo	Milliard (billion)	Milliard	Mil millones (miliarda)	Milijarda
ORIENTAMENTO NEL TEMPO:	**ORIENTATION IN TIME:**	**ORIENTATION DANS LE TEMPS:**	**ORIENTACIÓN EN EL TIEMPO:**	**ORIJENTACIJA U VREMENU:**
Ieri	Yesterday	Hier	Ayer	Jučer
Oggi	Today	Aujourd'hui	Hoy	Danas
Domani	Tomorrow	Demain	Día de mañana	Sutra
Anno	Year	Année	Año	Godina
Mese	Month	Mois	Mes	Mjesec
Settimana	Week	Semaine	Semana	Tjedan
Giorno	Day	Jour	Día	Dan
Ora	Hour	Heure	Hora	Sat
Minuto	Minute	Minute	Minuto	Minuta
Secondo	Second	Seconde	Segundo	Sekunda
Mattina	Morning	Matin	Mañana	Jutro (prijepodne)
Pomeriggio	Afternoon	Après-midi	Tarde	Poslijepodne
Sera	Evening	Soir	Anochecer	Večer
Notte	Night	Nuit	Noche	Noć
ORIENTAMENTO NELLO SPAZIO:	**ORIENTATION IN SPACE:**	**ORIENTATION DANS L'ESPACE:**	**ORIENTACIÓN EN EL ESPACIO:**	**ORIJENTACIJA U PROSTORU:**
Su	Up (above)	En haut (au-dessus)	Arriba	Gore (iznad)
In basso	Down (below)	En bas (au-dessous)	Abajo	Dolje (ispod)
Sinistra	Left	Gauche	Izquierda	Lijevo
Destra	Right	Droite	Derecha	Desno
Davanti	In front	Devant	Enfrente	Ispred
Dietro	Behind	Derrière	Detrás	Iza
Dentro	Inside	Dedans	Dentro	Unutra
Fuori	Outside	Dehors	Fuera	Vani

Italiano	Inglese	Francese	Spagnolo	Croato
GLI ACCIDENTI, CATASTROFI E ANGOSCIA:	**ACCIDENTS, CATASTROPHES AND DISTRESS:**	**LES ACCIDENTS, CATASTROPHES ET DÉTRESSE:**	**ACCIDENTES, CATÁSTROFES Y ANGUSTIA:**	**NESREĆE, KATASTROFE I POGIBELJNE SITUACIJE:**
Accidente nucleare	Nuclear accident	Accident nucléaire	Accidente nuclear	Nuklearna nesreća
Acqua	Water	Eau	Agua	Voda
Affondamento della nave	Sinking of a ship	Naufrage du navire	Hundimiento de un barco	Potonuće broda
"Aiuto!"	"Help!"	"Aide!"	"¡Socorro!"	"U pomoć!"
Allarme	Alarm	Alarme	Alarma	Uzbuna
Annegamento	Drowning	Noyade	Ahogamiento	Utapanje
Annegato	Drowned person	Noyé	Ahogado	Utopljenik
Arma	Weapon	Arme	Arma	Oružje
Arma atomica	Atomic weapons	Arme atomique	Arma atómica	Atomsko oružje
Arma bianca	Cold weapon	Arme de contact	Arma blanca	Hladno oružje
Arma biologica	Biological weapon	Arme biologique	Arma biológica	Biološko oružje
Arma chimica	Chemical weapon	Arme chimique	Arma química	Kemijsko oružje
Arma convenzionale	Conventional weapon	Arme conventionnelle	Arma convencional	Konvencionalno oružje
Arma da fuoco	Firearm	Arme à feu	Arma de fuego	Vatreno oružje
Arma di distruzione di massa	Weapon of mass destruction	Arme de destruction massive	Armas de destrucción masiva	Oružje za masovno uništavanje
Arma nucleare	Nuclear weapon	Arme nucléaire	Arma nuclear	Nuklearno oružje
Arma nucleare strategica	Strategic nuclear weapon	Arme nucléaire stratégique	Arma nuclear estratégica	Strateško nuklearno oružje
Arma nucleare tattica	Tactical nuclear weapon	Arme nucléaire tactique (mini-nuke)	Arma nuclear táctica	Taktičko nuklearno oružje
Armi laser	Laser weapon	Arme de laser	Arma láser	Lasersko oružje
Armi nucleari, biologiche e chimiche (NBC)	ABC weapons	Arme nucléaire, biologique et chimique (NBC)	Armas atómicas, biológicas y químicas (ABQ)	Atomsko biološko i kemijsko oružje
Attacco dei pirati	Pirate attack	Attaque de pirates	Ataque de piratas	Gusarski napad
Attacco di squalo	Shark attack	Attaque de requin	Ataque de tiburón	Napad morskog psa
Attacco fisico	Physical assault	Attaque physique	Asalto físico	Tjelesni napad
Attaco	Attack	Attaque	Ataque	Napad
Attentato terroristico	Terrorist attack	Attaque terroriste	Ataque terrorista	Teroristički napad
Banchisa (ghiaccio marino, banchiglia)	Sea ice	Banquise	Banquisa (hielo marino)	Santa leda
Batterio	Bacteria	Bacteria	Bacteria	Bakterija
Boa di salvataggio	Lifebelt (lifebuoy)	Bouée couronne	Boya salvavidas	Pojas za spašavanje
Bomba	Bomb	Bombe	Bomba	Bomba
Bomba al cobalto (bomba gamma, bomba G)	Cobalt bomb	Bombe salée	Bomba de cobalto	Kobaltna bomba
Bomba al neutrone (bomba N)	Neutron bomb	Bombe à neutrons	Bomba de neutrones (bomba N)	Neutronska bomba
Bomba all'idrogeno (bomba H)	Hidrogen bomb (H-bomb)	Bombe à hydrogène (bombe H)	Bomba de hidrógeno (bomba H)	Hidrogenska bomba
Bomba atomica (bomba A)	Atomic bomb (A-bomb)	Bombe atomique (bombe A)	Bomba atómica (bomba A)	Atomska bomba
Bomba sporca	Dirty bomb	Bombe radiologique (bombe sale)	Bomba sucia	Prljava bomba
Bufera di neve (nevicata)	Snow storm	Tempête de neige	Nevasca (ventisca de nieve)	Snježna mećava
Cadutta (cascata)	Fall	Chute	Caída	Pad
Campo minato	Mine field	Champ de mines	Campo minero	Minsko polje
Campo per rifugiati	Refugee camp	Camp de réfugiés	Campamento para refugiados	Izbjeglički logor
Cane da ricerca e salvataggio	Search and rescue dog	Chien de sauvetage	Perro de búsqueda y rescate	Pas za traganje i spašavanje
Cellula terroristica	Terrorist cell	Cellule terroriste (cellule dormante)	Célula terrorista	Teroristička ćelija
Chiamata di aiuto	Call for help	Appel à l'aide	Llamada de socorro	Poziv u pomoć
Collisione	Collision	Collision	Colisión	Sudar
Colpo (botta)	Stroke (hit, blow)	Coup	Golpe	Udarac
Colpo di calore	Heat stroke	Coup de chaleur	Golpe de calor	Toplotni udar
Combattimento	Fight	Combat	Pelea	Tučnjava
Cordone	Rope	Corde	Cuerda	Uže
Difesa civile	Civil defense	Sécurité civile	Protección civil	Civilna zaštita
Elicottero	Helicopter (chopper)	Hélicoptère	Helicóptero	Helikopter
Eliminazione di mine (sminamento)	Mine clearance (demining)	Déminage	Desminado (eliminación de minas)	Razminiranje
Epidemia	Epidemic	Épidémie	Epidemia	Epidemija
Eruzione vulcanica	Volcanic eruption	Éruption volcanique	Erupción volcánica	Erupcija vulkana
Esplosione	Explosion	Explosion	Explosión	Eksplozija
Esplosivo	Explosive	Explosif	Explosivo	Eksploziv
Fiume	River	Rivière	Río	Rijeka
Folgorazione (elettrocuzione)	Electric shock	Électrisation (électrocution)	Choque eléctrico	Strujni udar
Fuoco	Fire	Feu	Fuego	Vatra
Gas tossico	Poison gas	Gaz toxique	Gas tóxico	Bojni otrov (otrovni plin)
Ghiacciaio	Iceberg	Iceberg	Témpano de hielo	Ledenjak
Ghiaccio	Ice	Glace	Hielo	Led
Giubbotto di salvataggio	Lifejacket (life vest)	Gilet de sauvetage	Chaleco salvavidas	Prsluk za spašavanje

Italiano	Inglese	Francese	Spagnolo	Croato
Grotta	Cave	Grotte	Cueva	Špilja
Guerra	War	Guerre	Guerra	Rat
Incaglio di nave	Stranding of a ship	Échouage du navire	Encallamiento de barco	Nasukavanje broda
Incendio (fuoco)	Fire (conflagration)	Incendie	Incendio (fuego)	Požar
Incidente aereo	Airplane crash	Accident aérien	Accidente de aviación	Pad aviona
Incidente di traffico	Traffic accident	Accident sur la voie publique	Accidente de tráfico	Prometna nesreća
Incidente stradale	Car accident	Accident automobile (accident de la route)	Accidente automovilístico (siniestro de tráfico)	Automobilska nesreća
Incursione area	Air attack	Attaque aérienne	Ataque aéreo	Zračni napad
Infortunio domestico	Domestic accident	Accident domestique	Accidente doméstico	Nesreća u kući
Infortunio sul lavoro	Occupational accident	Accident du travail	Accidente laboral	Nesreća na radu
Inondazione	Flood	Inondation	Inundación	Poplava
Inquinamento chimico	Chemical pollution	Pollution chimique	Polución química	Kemijsko zagađenje
Invasione	Invasion	Invasion	Invasión	Invazija
Lago	Lake	Lac	Lago	Jezero
Lava	Lava	Lave	Lava	Lava
Macerie (rovine)	Ruins	Ruine	Ruinas	Ruševine
Mare	Sea	Mer	Mar	More
Mina	Mine	Mine	Mina	Mina
Mina navale	Naval mine	Mine marine (mine sous-marine)	Mina marina	Morska mina
Mina terrestre	Land mine	Mine terrestre	Mina terrestre	Kopnena mina
Montagna	Mountain	Montagne	Montaña	Planina
Nave	Ship	Navire	Barco	Brod
Neurotossina	Neurotoxin	Neurotoxine	Neurotoxina	Živčani otrov (neurotoksin)
Neve	Snow	Neige	Nieve (zapada)	Snijeg
Omicidio (uccisione)	Homicide (murder)	Homicide (assassinat)	Homicidio (asesinato)	Ubojstvo
Onda di marea	Tidal wave	Onde de marée	Ola de marea	Plimni val
Ostaggio	Hostage	Otage	Rehén	Taoc (talac)
Pallottola	Bullet	Balle	Bala	Metak
Pandemia	Pandemic	Pandémie	Pandemia	Pandemija
Paracadute	Parachute	Parachute	Paracáidas	Padobran
Percossa dal fulmine	Thunderclap	Foudre	Trueno	Udar groma
Pirata	Pirate	Pirate	Pirata	Gusar
Plutonio	Plutonium	Plutonium	Plutonio	Plutonij
Radiazione	Radiation	Rayonnement	Radiación	Zračenje
Rapimento	Kidnapping	Enlèvement (rapt)	Secuestro	Otmica
Rapina	Robbery	Vol	Robo	Pljačka
Relitto	Ship wreck	Épave de navire	Buque naufragado	Olupina broda
Ricerca	Search	Recherche	Búsqueda	Potraga
Rifugiato	Refugee	Réfugié	Refugiado	Izbjeglica
Rifugio	Shelter	Abri	Abrigo	Sklonište
Roccia	Rock	Roche	Roca	Stijena
Rompighiaccio	Icebreaker	Brise-glace	Rompehielos	Ledolomac
Salvataggio	Salvage	Sauvetage	Salvamento	Spašavanje
Salvataggio navale	Marine salvage	Sauvetage en mer	Salvamento marítimo	Spašavanje broda
Salvatore	Rescuer	Sauveur	Salvador (rescatador)	Spasilac
Schiavitù (prigionia)	Slavery	Esclavage	Esclavitud	Ropstvo
Scialuppa	Lifeboat	Canot de secours	Bote salvavidas	Čamac za spašavanje
Scoria nucleare (scoria radioattiva)	Nuclear waste (radioactive waste)	Déchet radioactif (déchet nucléaire)	Desechos nucleares	Nuklearni otpad (radioaktivni otpad)
Segnale di allarme	Alarm signal	Signal d'alarme	Señal de alarma	Znak za uzbunu
Shrapnel	Shrapnel	Shrapnel	Metralla	Šrapnel
SOS richiesta	SOS call	Appel SOS	Llamada de SOS	SOS poziv
Squadra di ricerca e salvataggio	Search and rescue team	Équipe de recherche et sauvetage	Equipo de búsqueda y rescate	Ekipa za traganje i spašavanje
Suicidio	Suicide	Suicide	Suicidio	Samoubojstvo
Tempesta	Storm	Tempête	Tormenta (tempestad)	Nevrijeme (oluja)
Tempesta di sabbia	Sandstorm	Tempête de sable	Tormenta de arena	Pješčana oluja
Terra	Land	Terre	Tierra	Kopno
Terremoto	Earthquake	Séisme (tremblement de terre)	Terremoto	Potres
Terrorista	Terrorist	Terroriste	Terrorista	Terorist
Test nucleare	Nuclear weapons testing	Essai nucléaire	Prueba nuclear (ensayo nuclear)	Nuklearni pokus
Tifone	Typhoon	Typhon	Tifón	Tajfun
Traffico di esseri umani	Human trafficking	Trafic d'êtres humains	Trata de personas	Trgovina ljudima
Tromba marina	Waterspout	Trombe marine	Managa de agua (tromba marina)	Morska pijavica
Tsunami	Tsunami	Tsunami (raz-de-marée)	Tsunami (maremoto)	Tsunami
Uragano	Hurricane	Ouragan	Huracán	Uragan
Uranio	Uranium	Uranium	Uranio	Uranij
Uranio arricchito	Enriched uranium	Uranium enrichi	Uranio einriquecido	Obogaćeni uranij
Valanga	Avalanche	Avalanche	Avalancha	Lavina
Violenza sessuale	Rape (violation)	Viol	Violación	Silovanje

Italiano	Inglese	Francese	Spagnolo	Croato
Virus	Virus	Virus	Virus	Virus
Vittima	Victim	Victime	Víctima	Žrtva
PARTI DEL CORPO UMANO:	**PARTS OF THE HUMAN BODY :**	**PARTIES DU CORPS HUMAIN:**	**PARTES DEL CUERPO HUMANO:**	**DIJELOVI LJUDSKOG TIJELA:**
Acetilcolina	Acetylcholine	Acétylcholine	Acetilcolina	Acetilkolin
Acido desossiribonucleico (DNA)	Deoxyribonucleic acid (DNA)	Acide désoxyribonucléique	Ácido desoxirribonucleico	Dezoksiribonukleinska kiselina (DNK)
Acido gastrico	Gastric acid	Acide gastrique	Ácido gástrico	Želučana kiselina
Acido ribonucleico (ARN)	Ribonucleic acid	Acide ribonucléique (ARN)	Ácido ribonucleico (ARN)	Ribonukleinska kiselina
Addome (ventre, pancia)	Belly (abdomen)	Abdomen	Abdomen (panza)	Trbuh (abdomen)
Adenoipofisi	Adenohypophysis	Adénohypophyse	Adenohipófisis	Adenohipofiza
Adrenalina	Adrenalin (adrenaline)	Adrénaline	Adrenalina	Adrenalin
Agglutinine	Agglutinin	Agglutinine	Aglutinina	Aglutinin
Agglutinogeno	Agglutinogen	Agglutinogène	Aglutinógeno	Aglutinogen
Albumina	Albumin	Albumine	Albúmina	Albumin
Aldosterone	Aldosterone	Aldostérone	Aldosterona	Aldosteron
Alveolo	Alveolus	Alvéole	Alvéolo	Alveola
Amminoacido	Amino acid	Acide aminé	Aminoácido	Aminokiselina
Ammoniaca	Ammonia	Ammoniac	Amoníaco	Amonijak
Anello cartilagineo	Cartilage ring	Cartilage cricoïde	Cartílago circoides	Hrskavični prsten
Ano	Anus	Anus	Ano	Čmar (anus)
Anulare	Ring finger	Annulaire	Dedo anular	Prstenjak
Aorta	Aorta	Aorte	Aorta	Aorta
Aorta addominale	Abdominal aorta	Aorte abdominale	Aorta abdominal	Abdominalna aorta
Aorta toracica	Thoracic aorta	Aorte thoracique	Aorta torácica	Torakalna aorta
Aponeurosi	Aponeurosis	Aponévrose	Aponeurosis	Široka plosnata tetiva (aponeuroza)
Appendice vermiforme	Vermiform appendix (cecal appaendix)	Appendice iléo-caecal (appendice, appendice vermiforme)	Apéndice vermiforme (apéndice cecal, apéndice)	Slijepo crijevo (crvuljak)
Aracnoide	Arachnoid mater	Arachnoïde	Aracnoides	Paučinasta ovojnica (arachnoidea)
Arteria	Artery	Artère	Arteria	Arterija
Arteria coronaria	Coronary artery	Artère coronaire	Arteria coronaria	Koronarna arterija
Arteria polmonare	Pulmonary artery	Artère pulmonaire	Arteria pulmonar (tronco pulmonar, tronco de las pulmonares)	Plućna arterija
Arteriola	Arteriole	Artériole	Arteriola	Arteriola
Articolazione	Joint	Articulation	Articulación	Zglob
Articolazione del gomito	Elbow joint	Articulation oléacranienne	Articulación del codo	Lakatni zglob
Articolazione dell'anca	Hip joint	Hanche	Articulación de la cadera	Kuk (zglob kuka)
Articolazione della spalla	Shoulder joint	Complexe articulaire de l'épaule	Articulación del hombro	Rameni zglob
Arto inferiore	Leg	Membre inférieur	Miembro inferior	Noga
Ascella	Armpit (axilla, underarm)	Aisselle	Sobaco (axila)	Pazuh (aksila)
Astrocita	Astrocyte	Astrocyte	Astrocito	Astrocit
Atrio	Cardiac atrium	Oreillette	Aurícula cardíaca (atrio)	Srčana pretklijetka (atrij)
Avambraccio	Forearm	Avant-bras	Antebrazo	Podlaktica
Bacino	Innominate bone (pelvis)	Bassin osseux	Pelvis	Zdjelica
Barccio	Upper arm	Partie supérieure du bras	Parte superior del brazo	Nadlaktica
Base del cranio	Skull base	Base du crâne	Base del cráneo	Baza lubanje
Bicipite femorale	Biceps femoris muscle	Muscle biceps fémoral	Músculo bíceps crural	Dvoglavi bedreni mišić
Bile	Gall (bile)	Bile	Bilis	Žuč
Bilirubina	Bilirubin	Bilirubine	Bilirrubina	Bilirubin
Bocca	Mouth	Bouche	Boca	Usta
Borsa sierosa	Synovial bursa	Bourse séreuse	Bursa (bolsa sinovial)	Sluzna vreća (bursa)
Braccio	Arm	Bras	Brazo	Ruka
Bronchiolo	Bronchiole	Bronchiole	Bronquiolo	Bronhiola
Bronco	Bronchus	Bronche	Bronquio	Dušnica (bronh)
Bulbo (midollo allungato, encefalo)	Medulla oblongata	Moelle allongée (medulla oblongata, bulbe rachidien, myélencéphale)	Bulbo raquídeo (médula oblongada, miencéfalo)	Produžena moždina
Bulbo oculare	Eyeball	Globe oculaire	Globo ocular	Očna jabučica
Calcagno	Calcaneus	Calcanéus (calcanéum)	Calcáneo	Petna kost (kalkaneus)
Calcitonina	Calcitonin	Calcitonine	Calcitonina	Kalcitonin
Canale di Schlemm	Canal of Schlemm	Canal de Schlemm	Canal de Schlemm	Schlemmov kanal
Canale naso-lacrimale	Nasolacrimal duct (tear duct)	Canal lacrymonasal (canal lacrimal, canal des larmes)	Conducto nasolagrimal	Suzno-nosni kanal
Canino	Canine tooth	Canine	Canino (diente colmillo)	Očnjak (kanin)
Capelli	Hair	Cheveu	Cabello	Kosa
Capezzolo	Nipple	Mamelon (papille)	Pezón	Bradavica
Capillare	Capillary	Capillaire	Capilar	Kapilara
Capsula articolare	Articular capsule (joint capsule)	Capsule articulaire	Cápsula articular	Zglobna čahura
Carboidrato (glucide)	Carbohydrate	Hidrate de carbone (glucide)	Carbohidrato	Ugljikohidrat
Carpo	Carpus	Carpe	Carpo	Zapešće
Cartilagine	Cartilage	Cartilage	Cartílago	Hrskavica

Italiano	Inglese	Francese	Spagnolo	Croato
Cartilagine articolare	Joint cartilage	Cartilage articulaire	Cartílago articular	Zglobna hrskavica
Cassa del timpano	Tympanic cavity	Cavité tympanique	Cavidad timpánica	Bubnjište
Catecolamina	Catecholamine	Catécholamine	Catecolamina	Katekolamin
Caviglia	Ankle joint	Cheville (cou-de pied)	Tobillo	Skočni zglob (gležanj)
Cavità orale	Mouth cavity (oral cavity)	Cavité buccale	Cavidad bucal (cavidad oral)	Usna šupljina
Cellula	Cell	Cellule	Célula	Stanica
Cemento	Cementum	Cément	Cemento dental	Zubni cement
Cerume	Earwax (cerumen)	Cire de l'oreille (cérumen)	Cerumen (cerilla)	Ušna mast (ušna smola, cerumen)
Cervelletto	Cerebellum	Cervelet	Cerebelo	Mali mozak
Cervello	Brain	Cerveau	Cerebro	Mozak
Cheratina	Keratin	Kératine	Queratina	Keratin
Ciglia	Eyelash	Cil	Pestaña	Trepavica
Cistifellea	Gall bladder	Vésicule biliare (cholécyste)	Vesícula biliar	Žućni mjehur
Clavicola	Collarbone (clavicle)	Clavicule	Clavícula	Ključna kost (klavikula)
Clitoride	Clitoris	Clitoris	Clítoris	Dražica (klitoris)
Coccige	Tailbone (coccyx)	Coccyx	Cóccix (coxis)	Trtica
Coclea	Cochlea	Cochlée	Cóclea (caracol)	Pužnica
Coledoco	Bile duct	Voie biliaire	Vía biliar	Žučovod
Colesterolo	Cholesterol	Cholestérol	Colesterol	Kolesterol
Collagene	Collagen	Collagène	Colágeno	Kolagen
Collo	Neck	Cou	Cuello	Vrat
Colonna vertebrale	Spine (spinal column, backbone)	Colonne vertébrale (rachis)	Columna vertebral	Kralježnica
Corda vocale	Vocal chord	Corde vocale	Cuerda vocal	Glasnica
Cornea	Cornea	Cornée	Córnea	Rožnica
Coroide	Choroid	Choroïde	Coroides	Žilnica
Corona del dente	Crown of a tooth	Couronne de la dent	Corona del diente	Kruna zuba
Corpo luteo	Corpus luteum	Corps jaune	Cuerpo lúteo (cuerpo amarillo)	Žuto tijelo
Corteccia cerebrale	Cerebral cortex	Cortex cérébral (écorce cérébrale)	Corteza cerebral	Moždana kora
Corticosteroide	Corticosteroid	Corticostéroïde	Corticosteroide	Kortikosteroid
Corticosterone	Corticosterone	Corticostérone	Corticosterona	Kortikosteron
Corticotropina (ormone adrenocorticotropo)	Corticotropin (adrenocorticotropic hormone)	Hormone corticotrope (adrenocorticotropic hormone, ACTH)	Hormona adrenocorticotropa (corticotropina, corticotrofina)	Kortikotropin
Cortisolo	Cortisol	Cortisol (hydro-cortisone)	Cortisol (hidrocortisona)	Kortizol
Cortisone	Cortisone	Cortisone	Cortisona	Kortizon
Coscia	Thigh	Cuisse	Muslo (región femoral)	Natkoljenica (bedro)
Costola (costa)	Rib	Côte	Costilla	Rebro
Cotile (acetabolo)	Acetabulum	Acetabulum	Acetábulo	Čašica zdjelične kosti (acetabulum)
Cranio	Skull	Crâne	Calavera (cráneo)	Lubanja
Cristallino	Lens	Cristallin	Cristalino	Leća
Cuoio capelluto	Scalp	Cuir chevelu	Cuero cabelludo (capa capilar)	Vlasište
Cuore	Heart	Coeur	Corazón	Srce
Dendrite	Dendrite	Dendrite	Dendrita	Dendrit
Dente	Tooth	Dent	Diente	Zub
Dente da latte	Milk tooth	Dent temporaire	Diente de leche	Mliječni zub
Dentina	Dentin	Dentine (ivoire)	Dentina	Zubni dentin
Diencefalo	Diencephalon	Diencéphale	Diencéfalo	Međumozak
Digiuno	Jejunum	Jéjunum	Yeyuno	Jejunum
Disco intervertebrale	Intervertebral disc	Disque intervertébral	Disco intervertebral	Međukralježnični disk
Dito del piede	Toe	Orteil	Dedo del pie	Nožni prst
Dito della mano	Finger	Doigt	Dedo de la mano	Ručni prst
Dito indice	Forefinger	Index	Dedo índice	Kažiprst
Dito medio	Middle finger	Majeur	Dedo corazón	Srednji prst
Dotto eiaculatore	Ejaculatory duct	Canal éjaculateur	Conducto eyaculador	Sjemenovod
Duodeno	Duodenum	Duodénum	Duodeno	Dvanaesnik (duodenum)
Dura madre (pachimeninge)	Dura mater	Dure-mère	Duramadre	Tvrda moždana ovojnica
Elastina	Elastin	Élastine	Elastina	Elastin
Elettrolita	Electrolyte	Électrolyte	Electrolito	Elektrolit
Emoglobina	Hemoglobin	Hémoglobine	Hemoglobina	Hemoglobin
Eosinofilo	Eosinophil	Éosinophile	Eosinófilo	Eozinofil
Epididimo	Epididymis	Épididyme	Epidídimo	Pasjemenik
Eritrocita (globulo rosso)	Erythrocyte (red blood cell)	Érythrocyte (hématie, globule rouge)	Eritrocito (glóbulo rojo)	Eritrocit (crveno krvno tjelešce)
Esofago	Gullet (oesophagus)	Oesophage	Esófago	Jednjak
Estradiolo	Estradiol	Estradiol	Estradiol	Folikulin (estradiol)
Estrogeno	Estrogen	Estrogène	Estrógeno	Estrogen
Falange	Phalanx bone	Phalange	Falange	Kost prsta (falanga)
Faringe	Pharynx (gullet, gorge)	Pharynx	Faringe	Ždrijelo

Italiano	Inglese	Francese	Spagnolo	Croato
Fascia muscolare	Muscular fascia	Fascia musculaire (périmysium)	Fascia profunda	Mišićna fascija
Fascio di His	Bundle of His	Faisceau de His	Haz de His	Hisov snopić
Fattore Rh negativo	Rh factor negative	Système Rhésus négatif	Factor Rh negativo	Negativan Rh faktor
Fattore Rh positivo	Rh factor positive	Système Rhésus positif	Factor Rh positivo	Pozitivan Rh faktor
Feci	Stool (feces)	Fèces	Excrementos (heces)	Stolica (feces, izmet)
Fegato	Liver	Foie	Hígado	Jetra
Femore	Thighbone (femur)	Os de la cuisse (fémur)	Fémur	Bedrena kost (femur)
Fibrina	Fibrin	Fibrine	Fibrina	Fibrin
Fibrinogeno	Fibrinogen	Fibrinogène	Fibrinógeno	Fibrinogen
Fibroblasto	Fibroblast	Fibroblaste	Fibroblasto (célula fija)	Fibroblast
Fluido corporale	Body fluid	Fluide corporel	Fluido corporal	Tjelesna tekućina
Fosfolipide	Phospholipid	Phospholipide	Fosfolípido	Fosfolipid
Fronte	Forehead	Front	Frente	Čelo
Gabbia toracica	Rib cage	Cage thoracique	Caja torácica	Grudni koš
Gamba	Lower leg	Jambe	Pierna	Potkoljenica
Gas	Gas	Gaz	Gas	Plin
Gengiva	Gums (gingiva)	Gencive	Encía	Desni
Ghiandola	Gland	Glande	Glándula	Žlijezda
Ghiandola bulbouretrale (ghiandola di Cowper)	Bulbourethral gland (Cowper's gland)	Glande de Cowper (glande bulbo-uretrale)	Glándula bulbouretral (glándula de Cowper)	Bulbouretralna žlijezda (Cowperova žlijezda)
Ghiandola di Bartolini	Bartholin's gland	Glande de Bartholin	Glándula de Bartolino	Bartolinova žlijezda
Ghiandola lacrimale	Lachrymal gland	Glande lacrymale	Glándula lagrimal	Suzna žlijezda
Ghiandola pineale (epifisi)	Pineal body (pineal gland, epiphysis)	Glande pinéale (épiphyse)	Glándula pineal (epífisis)	Pinealna žlijezda (epifiza)
Ghiandola salivare	Salivary gland	Glande salivaire	Glándula salival	Žlijezda slinovnica
Ghiandola sebacea	Sebaceous gland	Glande sébacée	Glándula sebácea	Žlijezda lojnica
Ghiandola sudoripara	Sweat gland	Glande sudoripare (sudorale)	Glándula sudorípara	Žlijezda znojnica
Ginocchio	Knee	Genou	Rodilla	Koljeno
Glande	Glans	Gland	Glande	Glavić
Glicogeno	Glycogen	Glycogène	Glucógeno	Glikogen
Globulina	Globulin	Globuline	Globulina	Globulin
Glomerulo	Glomerulus	Glomérule	Glomérulo	Glomerul
Glucagone	Glucagon	Glucagon	Glucagón	Glukagon
Glucocorticoide	Glucocorticoid	Glucocorticoïde	Glucocorticoide	Glukokortikoid
Glucosio	Glucose	Glucose	Glucosa	Glukoza
Gola	Throat	Gorge	Garganta	Grlo
Gomito	Elbow	Coude	Codo	Lakat
Gonade	Sex gland (gonad)	Gonade	Gónada	Spolna žlijezda
Gonadotropina	Gonadotrophin	Gonadotrophine	Gonadotropina	Gonadotropin
Granulocita	Granulocyte	Granulocyte (polynucléaire)	Granulocito	Granulocit
Granulocita basofilo	Basophil granulocyte	Granulocyte basophile	Basófilo	Bazofilni granulocit
Gruppo sanguigno	Blood group	Groupe sanguin	Grupo sanguíneo	Krvna grupa
Gruppo sanguigno A	Blood group A	Groupe sanguin A	Grupo sanguíneoA	Krvna grupa A
Gruppo sanguigno AB	Blood group AB	Groupe sanguin AB	Grupo sanguíneo AB	Krvna grupa AB
Gruppo sanguigno B	Blood group B	Groupe sanguin B	Grupo sanguíneo B	Krvna grupa B
Gruppo sanguigno 0	Blood group 0	Groupe sanguin 0	Grupo sanguíneo 0	Krvna grupa 0
Guancia	Cheek	Joue	Mejilla (carrillo)	Obraz
Ileo	Ileum	Iléon (ileum)	Íleon	Ileum
Imene	Hymen	Hymen	Himen	Djevičnjak (himen)
Immunoglobulina	Immunoglobulin	Immunoglobuline	Inmunoglobulina	Imunoglobulin
Incisivo	Incisor	Incisive	Incisivo	Sjekutić (inciziv)
Incudine	Anvil (incus)	Enclume	Yunque	Nakovanj
Inguine	Groin	Aine	Ingle	Prepona
Insulina	Insulin	Insuline	Insulina	Inzulin
Intestino	Intestine	Intestin	Intestin	Crijevo
Intestino crasso (colon)	Large intestine (colon)	Gros intestin (côlon)	Intestino grueso (colon)	Debelo crijevo
Intestino tenue (piccolo intestino)	Small intestine	Intestin grêle	Intestino delgado	Tanko crijevo
Ipòfisi (ghiandola pituitaria)	Hypophysis (pituitary gland)	Hypophyse (glande pituitaire)	Hipófisis (glándula pituitaria)	Hipofiza
Ipotalamo	Hypothalamus	Hypothalamus	Hipotálamo	Hipotalamus
Iride	Iris	Iris	Iris	Šarenica
Ischio	Ischium	Ischium	Isquión	Sjedna kost
Labbro	Lip	Lèvre	Labio	Usna
Lacrima	Tear	Larme	Lágrima	Suza
Laringe	Larynx	Larynx	Laringe	Grkljan
Legamento	Ligament	Ligament	Ligamento	Ligament
Leucocita	Leukocyte	Leucocyte	Leucocito	Leukocit
Linfa	Lymph	Lymphe	Linfa	Limfa
Linfocita	Lymphocyte	Lymphocyte	Linfocito	Limfocit
Linfonodo	Lymph gland (lymph node)	Ganglion lymphatique (noeud lymphatique)	Ganglio linfático	Limfna žlijezda
Lingua	Tongue	Langue	Lengua	Jezik
Lipidi	Fat	Matière grasse	Grasa	Mast

Italiano	Inglese	Francese	Spagnolo	Croato
Liquido cefalorachidiano (liquor, liquido cerebrospinale)	Cerebrospinal fluid	Liquide cérébro-spinal	Líquido cefalorraquídeo (líquido cerebrospinal)	Moždana tekućina (likvor)
Liquido extracellulare	Interstitial fluid	Liquide interstitiel	Líquido intersticial (líquido tisular)	Međustanična tekućina
Liquido sinoviale (sinovia)	Synovial fluid (synovia)	Liquide synovial	Líquido sinovial	Zglobna tekućina (sinovijalna tekućina)
Lombo	Loin	Lombes	Espalda baja	Križa
Mammella	Breast	Sein	Mama	Dojka
Mandibola	Lower jaw (mandible)	Mandibule	Mandíbula	Donja čeljust (mandibula)
Mano	Hand	Main	Mano	Šaka
Martello	Hammer (malleus)	Marteau (malléus)	Martillo (malleus)	Čekić (malleus)
Meato acustico esterno	Auditory canal (ear canal)	Conduit auditif externe (canal auriculaire)	Conducto auditivo externo	Slušni kanal
Melanina	Melanin	Mélanine	Melanina	Melanin
Melatonina	Melatonin	Mélatonine (hormone du sommeil)	Melatonina	Melatonin
Membrana mucosa	Mucous membrane	Muqueuse	Mucosa	Sluznica
Membrana sinoviale	Synovial membrane	Membrane synoviale	Membrana sinovial	Sinovijalna opna
Meninge	Meninx	Méninge	Meninge	Moždana ovojnica
Menisco	Meniscus	Ménisque	Menisco	Zglobni menisk
Mento	Chin	Menton	Barbilla (mentón)	Brada
Metacarpo	Metacarpus	Métacarpe	Metacarpo	Pest (metakarpus)
Metatarso	Metatarsus	Métatarse	Metatarso	Donožje (metatarzus)
Midollo cerebrale	Brain marrow	Moelle du cerveau	Médula cerebral	Moždana srž
Midollo osseo	Bone marrow	Moelle osseuse	Médula ósea	Koštana srž
Midollo spinale	Spinal cord	Moelle épinière (moelle spinale)	Médula espinal	Kralježnična moždina
Mignolo	Little finger (pinky)	Auriculaire (petit doigt)	Dedo meñique	Mali prst
Milza	Spleen	Rate	Bazo	Slezena
Mineralcorticoide	Mineralcorticoid	Minéralcorticoïde	Mineralocorticoide	Mineralkortikoid (Na-hormon)
Miocardio	Cardiac muscle (myocardium)	Myocarde	Miocardio	Srčani mišić (miokard)
Molare	Molar	Molaire	Molar	Kutnjak (molar)
Monocita	Monocyte	Monocyte	Monocito	Monocit
Muco	Mucus	Mucus	Moco	Sluz
Mucosa gastrica	Gastric mucous membrane	Muqueuse gastrique	Mucosa estomacal	Želučana sluznica
Muscolo	Muscle	Muscle	Músculo	Mišić
Muscolo adduttore	Adductor muscle	Muscle adducteur	Músculo aductor	Mišić primicač
Muscolo bicipite brachiale	Biceps brachii muscle	Muscle biceps brachial	Músculo bíceps braquial	Dvoglavi mišić nadlaktice
Muscolo brachiale	Brachialis muscle	Muscle brachial	Braquial anterior	Nadlaktični mišić
Muscolo ciliare	Ciliary muscle	Muscle ciliaire	Músculo ciliar	Cilijarni mišić
Muscolo deltoide	Deltoid muscle	Muscle deltoïde	Músculo deltoides	Rameni mišić (deltoideus)
Muscolo diaframma	Diaphragm	Diaphragme	Diafragma	Ošit (dijafragma)
Muscolo gluteo	Gluteal muscle	Muscle glutéal	Músculo glúteo	Sjedni mišić
Muscolo grande pettorale	Pectoralis major muscle	Muscle grand pectoral	Músculo pectoral mayor	Veliki prsni mišić
Muscolo intercostale	Intercostal muscle	Muscle intercostal	Músculo intercostal	Međurebreni mišić
Muscolo massetere	Masseter muscle	Muscle masséter	Músculo masetero	Žvakaći mišić
Musculo obliquo dell'addome	Abdominal oblique muscle	Muscle oblique de l'abdomen	Músculo oblicuo del abdomen	Kosi trbušni mišić
Muscolo piccolo pettorale	Pectoralis minor muscle	Muscle petit pectoral	Músculo pectoral menor	Mali prsni mišić
Muscolo quadricipite femorale	Quadriceps femoris muscle	Muscle quadriceps fémoral	Músculo cuádriceps crural	Četveroglavi bedreni mišić
Muscolo retto dell'addome	Rectus abdominis muscle	Muscle droit de l'abdomen	Músculo recto mayor del abdomen	Ravni trbušni mišić
Muscolo romboide	Rhomboid muscle	Muscle rhomboïde	Músculo romboides	Romboidni mišić
Muscolo sartorio	Tailor's muscle (sartorius muscle)	Muscle couturier (muscle sartorius)	Músculo sartorio	Krojački mišić
Muscolo semimembranoso	Semimembranosus muscle	Muscle semi-membraneux	Músculo semimembranoso	Poluopnasti mišić
Muscolo semitendinoso	Semitendinosus muscle	Muscle semi-tendineux	Músculo semitendinoso	Polutetivni mišić
Muscolo striato	Striated muscle	Muscle strié	Músculo estriado	Poprečno-prugasti mišić
Muscolo trapezio	Trapezius muscle	Muscle trapèze	Músculo trapecio	Trapezni mišić
Muscolo tricipite del braccio	Triceps brachii muscle	Muscle triceps brachial	Músculo tríceps braquial	Troglavi mišić nadlaktice
Muscolo tricipite della sura	Triceps surae muscle	Muscle triceps sural	Músculo tríceps sural	Troglavi mišić potkoljenice
Narice	Nostril	Narine	Narina	Nosnica
Naso	Nose	Nez	Nariz	Nos
Nervo	Nerve	Nerf	Nervio	Živac
Nervo cranico	Cranial nerve	Nerf crânien	Nervio craneal	Moždani živac
Nervo ottico	Optic nerve	Nerf optique	Nervio óptico	Vidni živac
Nervo spinale	Spinal nerve	Nerf spinal	Nervio espinal	Spinalni živac
Nervo vestibolococleare (nervo stato-acustico)	Acoustic nerve (vestibulocochlear nerve)	Nerf vestibulocochléaire (nerf auditif)	Nervio auditivo (ner-vio vestibulococlear, nervio estatoacústico)	Slušni živac
Nodo atrioventricolare	Atrioventricular node	Noeud atrio-ventriculaire	Nódulo auriculoventricular	Atrioventrikularni čvor

Italiano	Inglese	Francese	Spagnolo	Croato
Noradrenalina	Noradrenaline	Noradrénaline	Noradrenalina	Noradrenalin
Nuca	Nape (occiput)	Nuque	Nuca	Zatiljak
Occhio	Eye	Oeil	Ojo	Oko
Ombelico	Navel (belly button)	Ombilic (nombril)	Ombligo (pupo)	Pupak
Omero	Upper arm bone (humerus)	Humérus	Húmero	Nadlaktična kost (humerus)
Orbita oculare	Eye orbit	Orbite de l'oeil	Órbita	Očna šupljina
Orecchio	Ear	Oreille	Óido	Uho
Orecchio medio	Middle ear	Oreille moyenne	Oído medio	Srednje uho
Organo	Organ	Organe	Órgano	Organ
Ormone	Hormone	Hormone	Hormona	Hormon
Ormone antidiuretico (vasopressina)	Antidiuretic hormone (vasopressin)	Hormone antidiuré-tique (vasopressine)	Hormona anidiurética (arginina vasopresina)	Antidiuretski hormon (vazopresin)
Ormone luteinizzante	Luteinising hormone	Hormne lutéinisante	Hormona luteinizante (lutropina)	Luteinizirajući hormon
Ormone melanotropo	Melanotropin	Hormone mélanotrope (mélanocortine, mélanotropine)	Melanotropina	Melanotropin
Ossitocina	Oxytocin	Ocytocine (oxytocine)	Oxitocina	Oksitocin
Osso	Bone	Os	Hueso	Kost
Osso carpale	Wrist bone (carpal bone)	Os du carpe	Hueso del carpo	Kost zapešća (karpalna kost)
Osso dell'anca	Hip bone	Os coxal	Hueso coxal	Kost kuka
Osso etmoide	Ethmoid bone	Os ethmoïde	Hueso etmoides	Sitasta kost (etmoidna kost)
Osso frontale	Frontal bone	Os frontal	Hueso frontal	Čeona kost
Osso iliaco	Ilium	Ilion (ilium)	Ilion	Crijevna kost
Osso ioide	Hyoid bone (lingual bone)	Os hyoïde (os lingual)	Hueso hioides	Podjezična kost
Osso lacrimale	Lachrymal bone	Os lacrymal (unguis)	Unguis (hueso lacrimal)	Suzna kost
Osso mascellare	Upper jaw (maxilla)	Os maxillaire	Hueso maxilar superior (maxila)	Gornja čeljust (maksila)
Osso metacarpale	Metacarpal bone	Os métacarpe	Hueso del metacarpo	Kost pesti (metakarpalna kost)
Osso metatarsale	Metatarsal bone	Os du métatarse	Hueso del metatarso	Kost donožja (metatarzalna kost)
Osso nasale	Nasal bone	Os nasal	Hueso proprio de la nariz (hueso nasal)	Nosna kost
Osso occipitale	Occipital bone	Os occipital	Hueso occipital	Zatiljna kost
Osso palatino	Palatine bone	Os palatin	Hueso palatino	Nepčana kost
Osso parietale	Parietal bone	Os pariétal	Hueso parietal	Tjemena kost
Osso sesamoide	Sesamoid bone	Os sésamoïde	Hueso sesamoide	Sezamska kost
Osso sfenoide	Sphenoid bone	Os sphénoïde	Hueso esfenoides	Klinasta kost (leptirasta kost)
Osso tarsale	Tarsal bone	Os du tarse	Hueso del tarso	Kost zastoplja (kost tarzusa)
Osso temporale	Temporal bone	Os temporal	Hueso temporal	Sljepoočna kost
Osso zigomatico	Zygoma (cheekbone, malar bone)	Os zygomatique (zygoma)	Hueso cigomático (malar)	Sponična kost
Ovaia	Ovary	Ovaire	Ovario	Jajnik
Padiglione auricolare	Pinna (auricle)	Pavillon auriculaire	Pabellón auricular (aurícula)	Ušna školjka
Palato	Palate	Palaise	Paladar	Nepce
Palato duro (volta palatina)	Hard palate	Palais osseux	Paladar óseo	Tvrdo nepce
Palato molle	Soft palate	Voile du palais	Úvula	Meko nepce
Palmo	Palm	Paume	Palma	Dlan
Palpebra	Eyelid	Paupière	Párpado	Kapak
Pancreas	Pancreas	Pancréas	Páncreas	Gušterača
Papilla gustativa	Taste bud	Papille gustative	Papila gustativa	Okusni pupoljak
Paratiroide	Parathyroid gland	Parathyroïde	Glándula paratiroides	Doštitnjača
Paratormone (ormone paratiroideo)	Parathyroid hormone	Parathormone (hormone parathyroïdienne)	Parathormona (hormona paratiroidea, paratirina)	Paratireoidni hormon
Parete addominale	Abdominal wall	Face de la cavité abdominale	Pared abdominal	Trbušna stijenka
Pelle (cute)	Skin	Peau	Piel	Koža
Pelo	Hair	Poil	Pelo	Dlaka
Pene	Penis	Pénis	Pene (falo)	Penis
Pericardio	Pericardium	Péricarde	Pericardio	Osrčje (perikard)
Perineo	Perineum	Périnée	Periné (perineo)	Međica (perineum)
Peritoneo	Peritoneum	Péritoine	Peritoneo	Potrbušnica (peritoneum)
Perone (fibula)	Fibula (calf bone)	Fibula (péroné)	Peroné (fíbula)	Lisna kost (fibula)
Pia madre	Pia mater	Pie-mère	Piamadre	Meka moždana ovojnica
Pianta del piede	Sole	Plante	Planta del pie	Taban
Piede	Foot	Pied	Pie	Stopalo
Plasma	Plasma	Plasma sanguin	Plasma sanguíneo	Plazma
Pleura (pleure)	Pleura	Plèvre	Pleura	Pleura
Pleura parietale	Parietal pleura	Plèvre pariétale	Pleura parietal	Porebrica (parijetalna pleura)
Pleura viscerale	Visceral pleura	Plèvre viscérale	Pleura visceral	Poplućnica (visceralna pleura)

Italiano	Inglese	Francese	Spagnolo	Croato
Pollice	Thumb	Pouce	Dedo pulgar (pólice)	Palac
Polmone	Lung	Poumon	Pulmón	Plućno krilo
Polmoni	Lungs	Poumons	Pulmones	Pluća
Polpa dentaria	Dental pulp	Pulpe dentaire	Pulpa dentaria	Središte zuba (pulpa)
Polpaccio	Calf	Mollet	Pantorrilla	List
Polso	Wrist	Poignet	Muñeca	Ručni zglob
Pomo d'Adamo	Adam's apple	Pomme d'Adam	Nuez de Adán	Adamova jabučica
Poro	Pore	Pore	Poro	Pora
Premolare	Premolar	Prémolaire	Premolar	Pretkutnjak (premolar)
Prepuzio	Foreskin (prepuce)	Prépuce	Prepucio	Prepucij
Progesterone	Progesterone	Progestérone	Progesterona	Progesteron
Prostata	Prostate	Prostate	Próstata	Prostata
Proteina	Protein	Protéine	Proteína	Bjelančevina (protein)
Pube (osso pubico)	Pubis (pubic bone)	Os pubien	Pubis	Stidna kost
Pupilla	Pupil	Pupille	Pupila	Zjenica
Radice del dente	Root of a tooth	Racine dentaire	Raíz del diente	Korijen zuba
Radio	Radius	Radius	Radio	Palčana kost
Rene	Kidney	Rein	Riñón	Bubreg
Rètina	Retina	Rétine	Retina	Mrežnica (retina)
Rotula (patella)	Kneecap (patella)	Rotule (patella)	Rótula (patela)	Iver (patela)
Saliva	Saliva (spit, slobber)	Salive	Saliva	Slina (pljuvačka)
Sangue	Blood	Sang	Sangre	Krv
Scapola (omoplata)	Shoulder blade (scapula)	Omoplate (scapula)	Omóplato (escápula)	Lopatica (skapula)
Scheletro	Skeleton	Squelette	Esqueleto	Kostur
Scheletro della bocca	Jaw	Mâchoire	Quijada	Čeljust
Schiena (dorso)	Back	Dos	Espalda	Leđa
Schiena alto	Upper back	Parti supérieur du dos	Espalda superior	Gornji dio leđa
Sclera	Sclera	Sclère	Eclerótica	Bjeloočnica
Sebo	Sebum	Sébum	Sebo cutáneo	Loj
Seno	Sinus	Sinus	Seno	Sinus
Sfintere	Sphincter	Sphincter	Esfínter	Kružni mišić (sfinkter)
Sigma (colon sigmoideo)	Sigmoid colon	Côlon sigmoïde	Colon sigmoide	Sigmoidni dio debelog crijeva
Sinapsi (bottone sinaptico)	Synapse	Synapse	Sinapsis	Sinapsa
Sistema nervoso parasimpatico	Parasympathetic nervous system	Système nerveux parasympatique (système vagal)	Sistema nervioso parasimpático	Parasimpatikus
Sistema nervoso simpatico	Sympathetic nervous system	Système nerveux orthosympathique (système nerveux sympathique)	Sistema nervioso simpático	Simpatikus
Smalto	Tooth enamel	Émail dentaire	Esmalte dental	Zubna caklina
Somatotropina	Growth hormone (somatotrophin)	Hormone de croissance (somatotropine)	Hormona de crecimi-ento somatotropa	Hormon rasta (somatotropin)
Sopracciglio	Eyebrow	Sourcils	Ceja	Obrva
Spalla	Shoulder	Épaule	Hombro	Rame
Sperma	Semen	Sperme	Semen (esperma)	Sperma
Spermatozoo	Sperm (spermatozoon)	Spermatozoïde	Espermatozoide	Spermij
Staffa (columella)	Stirrup (stapes)	Étrier	Estribo	Stremen
Sterno	Breastbone (sternum)	Sternum	Esternón	Prsna kost (sternum)
Stomaco	Stomach	Estomac	Estómago	Želudac
Succo gastrico	Gastric juice	Suc gastrique	Jugo gástrico	Želučani sok
Succo intestinale	Intestinal juice	Suc intestinal	Jugo intestinal	Crijevni sok
Succo pancreatico	Pancreatic juice	Suc pancréatique	Jugo pancreático	Sok gušterače
Sudore	Sweat	Sueur	Sudor	Znoj
Surrene	Adrenal gland	Glande surrénale	Glándula suprarrenal	Nadbubrežna žlijezda
Talamo	Thalamus	Thalamus	Tálamo	Talamus
Tallone	Heel	Talon	Talón (calcañar)	Peta
Tarso	Tarsus	Tarse	Tarso	Zastoplje
Telencefalo (cervello)	Cerebrum (telencephalon)	Télencéphale (cerveau)	Telencéfalo	Veliki mozak (telencefalon)
Tempia	Temple	Tempe	Sien	Sljepoočnica
Tendine	Tendon (sinew)	Tendon	Tendón	Tetiva
Tessuto	Tissue	Tissu	Tejido	Tkivo
Tessuto adiposo	Fat tissue	Tissu adipeux (masse grasse)	Tejido graso (tejido adiposo)	Masno tkivo
Tessuto muscolare liscio	Smooth muscle	Muscle lisse	Músculo liso	Glatki mišić
Testa	Head	Tête	Cabeza	Glava
Testicolo	Testicle	Testicule	Testículo	Jaje (mudo, testis)
Testosterone	Testosterone	Testostérone	Testosterona	Testosteron
Tibia	Shinbone (tibia)	Tibia	Tibia	Goljenica (tibija)
Timo	Thymus	Thymus	Timo	Grudna žlijezda (timus)
Timpano (membrana timpanica)	Eardrum (tympanic membrane)	Tympan	Tímpano	Bubnjić
Tiroide	Thyroid	Thyroïde	Tiroides	Štitnjača
Tirotropina (ormone tireostimolante)	Thyroid-stimulating hormone (TSH, thyrotropin)	Thyréostimuline (thyréotropine)	Tirotropina (TSH, hormona estimulante de la tiroides)	Tireotropin (TSH)
Tiroxina	Thyroxine	Thyroxine	Tiroxina (tetrayodotironina, T4)	Tiroksin

Italiano	Inglese	Francese	Spagnolo	Croato
Tonsille	Tonsil	Tonsille	Amígdala	Krajnik
Torace	Chest	Torse	Pecho	Grudište (prsa)
Trachea	Windpipe (trachea)	Trachée	Tráquea	Dušnik
Trigliceride	Triglyceride	Triglycéride	Triglicérido	Triglicerid
Triiodotironina	Triiodothyronine	Triiodothyronine	Triiodotironina	Trijodtironin
Trombocita (piastrina)	Thrombocyte	Thrombocyte	Plaqueta (trombocito)	Trombocit
Tronco	Trunk (torso)	Tronc	Tronco	Trup (torzo)
Tronco encefalico	Brain stem	Tronc cérébral	Tronco del encéfalo	Moždano stablo
Tuba di Falloppio	Fallopian tube (oviduct)	Trompe de Fallope	Trompa de Falopio (tuba uterina, oviducto)	Jajovod
Ulna (cubito)	Ulna	Ulna (cubitus)	Cúbito (ulna)	Lakatna kost (ulna)
Unghia	Nail	Ongle	Uña	Nokat
Uovo	Ovum	Ovule	Óvulo	Jajašce
Urea	Urea	Urée (carbamide)	Urea	Mokraćevina (urea, ureja)
Uretere	Ureter	Uretère	Uréter	Mokraćovod (ureter)
Uretra	Urethra	Urètre	Uretra	Vanjska mokraćna cijev (uretra)
Urina	Urine	Urine	Orina	Mokraća (urin)
Utero	Womb (uterus)	Utérus	Matriz (útero, seno materno)	Maternica (uterus)
Vagina	Vagina	Vagin	Vagina (colpos)	Rodnica (vagina)
Valvola	Valve (valvula)	Valve	Válvula	Zalistak
Valvola cardiaca	Heart valve (cardiac valve)	Valve cardiaque	Válvula cardiaca (válvula de corazón)	Srčani zalistak
Valvola mitrale (valvola bicuspide)	Mitral valve (bicuspid valve)	Valve mitrale (valve bicuspide)	Válvula bicúspide (válvula mitral)	Mitralni zalistak (bikuspidalni zalistak)
Valvola semilunare aortica	Aortic valve	Valve aortique	Válvula sigmoidea aórtica	Polumjesečasti aortni zalistak
Valvola tricuspide	Tricuspid valve	Valve tricuspide	Válvula tricúspide	Trolisni zalistak
Vaso linfatico	Lymph vessel	Vaisseau lymphatique	Vaso linfático	Limfna žila
Vaso sanguigno	Blood vessel	Vaisseau sanguin	Vaso sanguíneo	Krvna žila
Vena	Vein	Veine	Vena	Vena
Vena cava inferiore	Inferior vena cava	Veine cave inférieure	Vena cava inferior	Donja šuplja vena
Vena cava superiore	Superior vena cava	Veine cave supérieure	Vena cava superior	Gornja šuplja vena
Vena porta	Portal vein	Veine porte	Vena porta	Portalna vena
Ventricolo	Ventricle	Ventricule	Ventrículo	Klijetka
Ventricolo cardiaco	Cardiac ventricle	Ventricule cardiaque	Ventrículo cardíaco	Srčana klijetka
Ventricolo cerebrale	Brain ventricle	Ventricule cérébral	Ventrículo cerebral	Moždana klijetka
Venula	Venule	Veinule (vénule)	Vénula	Venula
Vertebra	Vertebra	Vertèbre	Vértebra	Kralježak
Vertebra coccigea	Coccygeal vertebra	Vertèbre coccygienne	Vértebra coccígea	Trtični kralježak
Vertebra lombare	Lumbar vertebra	Vertèbre lombale	Vértebra lumbar	Slabinski kralježak (lumbalni kralježak)
Vertebra sacrale	Sacral vertebra	Vertèbre sacrale	Vértebra sacra	Krstačni kralježak (sakralni kralježak)
Vertebra toracica	Thoracic vertebra	Vertèbre thoracique	Vértebra torácica	Leđni kralježak (grudni ili torakalni kralježak)
Vertice della testa	Vertex (crown of head)	Vertex	Vértice craneal	Tjeme
Vescica urinaria	Urinary bladder	Vessie	Vejiga urinaria	Mokraćni mjehur
Vescicola seminale	Seminal vesicle	Vésicule séminale (glande vésiculeuse)	Vesícula seminal	Sjemena vrećica
Vestibolo	Vestibule	Vestibule	Vestíbulo	Predvorje (vestibulum)
Villo intestinale	Intestinal villus	Villosité intestinale	Vellosidad intestinal	Crijevna resica
Viso	Face	Visage	Cara (faz)	Lice
Vomere	Vomer	Vomer	Vómer	Raonik (vomer)
Vulva	Vulva	Vulve	Vulva	Stidnica
I SINTOMI, FERITE E MALATTIE:	**SYMPTOMS, INJURIES AND DISEASES:**	**LES SYMPTÔMES, BLESSURES ET MALADIES:**	**SÍNTOMAS, HERIDAS Y ENFERMEDADES:**	**SIMPTOMI, OZLJEDE I BOLESTI:**
Abbassamento della pressione del sangue	Blood pressure fall	Pression artérielle effondrée	Caída de la presión arterial	Pad krvnog tlaka
Abilità di muoversi	Movement ability	Capacité de mouvement	Capacidad de movimiento	Sposobnost kretanja
Abitudine di mangiare le unghie (onicofagia)	Nail biting (onychophagia)	Se ronger les ongles (onychophagie)	Comerse las uñas (onicofagia)	Griženje noktiju (onikofagija)
Abrasione (escoriazione)	Abrasion	Écorchure	Abrasión (escoriación)	Ojedina (abrazija)
Abulia	Aboulia (disorder of diminished motivation)	Aboulie	Abulia	Abulija (poremećaj umanjene motivacije)
Acariasi	Acariasis	Acariase	Acariasis	Akarijaza
Acidosi	Acidosis	Acidose	Acidosis	Acidoza
Acidosi metabolica	Metabolic acidosis	Acidose métabolique	Acidosis metabólica	Metabolička acidoza
Acidosi renale tubulare	Renal tubular acidosis	Acidose tubulaire rénale	Acidosis tubular renal	Renalna tubularna acidoza
Acloridria	Achlorhydria	Achlorhydrie	Aclorhidria	Aklorhidrija
Acne	Acne	Acné	Acné	Akne
Acne miliare	Milia (milk spots)	Milium (grutum, acné miliaire)	Milium (milia)	Milije (dječje akne)
Acne volgare (acne)	Acne vulgaris	Acné papulo-pustuleuse	Acné común (acne vulgaris)	Vulgarne akne
Acondroplasia	Achondroplasia	Achondroplasie	Acondroplasia	Ahondroplazija

Italiano	Inglese	Francese	Spagnolo	Croato
Acrocianosi	Acrocyanosis	Acrocyanose	Acrocianosis	Akrocijanoza
Acrofobia (paura dei luoghi e levati)	Acrophobia (fear of heights)	Acrophobie (peur des hauteurs)	Acrofobia (miedo a las alturas)	Akrofobija (strah od visine)
Acromegalia	Acromegaly	Acromégalie	Acromegalia	Akromegalija
Actinomicosi	Actinomycosis	Actinomycose	Actinomicosis	Aktinomikoza
Addome acuto	Acute abdomen	Abdomen aigu	Abdomen agudo	Akutni abdomen
Adenocarcinoma	Adenocarcinoma	Adénocarcinome	Adenocarcinoma	Adenokarcinom
Adenoma	Adenoma	Adénome	Adenoma	Adenom
Adenoma epatocellulare	Hepatocellular adenoma	Adénome hépatocellulaire	Adenoma hepático (adenoma hepatocelular)	Hepatocelularni adenom
Adenoma tubulare	Tubular adenoma	Adénome tubulaire	Adenoma tubular	Tubularni adenom
Adenopatia	Adenopathy	Adénopathie	Adenopatía	Adenopatija
Adenosi sclerosante	Sclerosing adenosis	Adénose sclérosante	Adenosis esclerosante	Sklerozirajuća adenoza
Affogamento	Drowning	Noyade	Ahogamiento	Utapanje
Afta (ulcera all'interno della cavità orale)	Aphtha (mouth ulcer)	Aphte (ulcère de la muqueuse buccale)	Afta (úlcera en la mucosa oral)	Afte (ulceracija sluznice usta)
Agenesia (mancanza di un organo)	Agenesis (absence of an organ)	Agénésie	Agenesia (ausencia de un órgano)	Agenezija (nedostatak jednog organa)
Agenesia renale	Renal agenesis	Agénésie rénale	Agenesia renal	Agenezija bubrega
Agranulocitosi	Agranulocytosis	Agranulocytose	Agranulocitosis	Agranulocitoza
Albinismo	Albinism	Albinisme	Albinismo	Albinizam
Albuminuria	Albuminuria	Albuminurie	Albuminuria	Albuminurija
Alcalosi	Alkalosis	Alcalose	Alcalosis	Alkaloza
Alcalosi respiratoria	Respiratory alkalosis	Alcalose respiratoire	Alcalosis respiratoria	Respiratorna alkaloza
Alcolismo	Alcoholism	Alcoolisme	Alcoholismo	Alkoholizam
Algodistrofia	Algodystrophy	Algodystrophie	Algodistrofia	Algodistrofija
Allergia	Allergy	Allergie	Alergia	Alergija
Allergia a farmaci	Drug allergy	Allergie aux médicaments	Alergia al medicamento	Alergija na lijekove
Allergia a pello di animali	Fur allergy	Allergie aux animaux à poils	Alergia al pelo de los animales	Alergija na životinjsku dlaku
Allergia a polvere	Dust allergy	Allergie à la poussière	Alergia al polvo	Alergija na prašinu
Allergia alimentare	Food allergy	Allergie alimentaire	Alergia a alimentos	Alergija na hranu
Allergia alle piume	Feather allergy	Allergie aux plumes	Alergia a las plumas	Alergija na perje
Allergia da poline	Pollen allergy	Allergie au pollen	Alergia al polen	Alergija na pelud
Alluce valgo	Bunion	Hallux valgus	Bunión (hallux valgus)	Čukalj
Allucinazione	Hallucination	Hallucination	Alucinación	Halucinacija
Alopecia	Alopecia	Alopécie	Alopecia	Ćelavost
Alopecia areata	Alopecia areata	Alopécie areata	Alopecia areata	Alopecia areata
Alopecia universale	Alopecia universalis	Alopécie universalis	Alopecia areata universal	Opća alopecija
Alterazione della conoscenza	Changes in consciousness	Changements de conscience	Cambios en la conciencia	Promjene stanja svijesti
Alterazioni dello stato psihico	Psychic changes	Changements psychiques	Cambios psíquicos	Psihičke promjene
Ambliopia	Lazy eye (amblyopia)	Mal-voyance (amblyopie)	Ojo vago (ambliopía)	Slabovidnost
Amebiasi	Amebiasis (amebic dysentery)	Amibiase (dysenterie amibienne)	Disentería amebiana (amebiasis)	Amebijaza
Amiloidosi	Amyloidosis	Amylose (amyloïdose, maladie orpheline)	Amiloidosis	Amiloidoza
Ammaccatura (ecchimosi)	Bruise (ecchymosis)	Ecchymose	Moretón (equimosis)	Modrica (ekhimoza)
Amnesia	Amnesia	Amnésie	Amnesia	Amnezija
Amputazione	Amputation	Amputation	Amputación	Amputacija
Anafilassi	Anaphylactic shock	Choc anaphylactique	Choque anafiláctico	Anafilaktični šok
Analgesia	Analgesia (loss of pain sensation)	Analgésie	Analgesia	Analgezija (neosjetljivost na bol)
Anchilosi	Ankylosis (joint stiffness)	Ankylose	Anquilosis	Ankiloza (ukočenje zgloba)
Anchilostomiasi	Ancylostomiasis	Ankylostomose	Anquilostomiasis	Ankilostomijaza
Androblastoma	Androblastoma (Sertoli-Leydig cell tumor)	Androblastome (tumeur à cellule de Sertoli et Leydig)	Tumor de células de Sertoli-Leydig (arrenoblastoma)	Androblastom (tumor Sertoli-Leydigovih stanica)
Anemia	Anemia	Anémie	Anemia	Slabokrvnost (anemija)
Anemia aplastica	Aplastic anemia	Anémie aplasique	Anemia aplásica	Aplastična anemija
Anemia da carenza di ferro	Iron deficiency anemia (sideropenic anemia)	Anémie ferriprive	Anemia ferropénica	Anemija radi deficita željeza (sideropenična anemija)
Anemia da malattia cronica	Anemia of chronic disease	Anémie des maladies chroniques	Anemia de enfermedades crónicas	Anemija kronične bolesti
Anemia drepanocitica	Sickle-cell disease (sickle-cell anemia)	Drépanocytose (anémie à cellules falciformes)	Anemia falciforme (anemia drepanocítica)	Anemija srpastih stanica
Anemia emolitica	Hemolytic anemia	Anémie hémolytique	Anemia hemolítica	Hemolitična anemija
Anemia ipocromica	Hypochromic anemia	Anémie hypochrome	Anemia hipocrómica	Hipokromna anemija
Anemia megaloblastica	Megaloblastic anemia	Anémie mégaloblastique	Anemia megaloblástica	Megaloblastična anemija (anemija radi deficita vitamina)
Anemia perniciosa	Pernicious anemia	Anémie pernicieuse	Anemia perniciosa	Perniciozna anemija
Anencefalia	Anencephaly	Anencéphalie	Anencefalia	Anencefalija
Aneurisma	Aneurysm (aneurism)	Anévrisme (anévrysme)	Aneurisma	Aneurizma
Aneurisma aortica	Aortic aneurysm	Anévrisme de l'aorte	Aneurisma de aorta	Aneurizma aorte

Italiano	Inglese	Francese	Spagnolo	Croato
Aneurisma arteriosa congenita alla base dell'encefalo	Congenital aneurysm of arteries at the base of the brain	Anévrisme congénital de l'artère à la base du cerveau	Aneurisma congénito arterial de la base del cerebro	Urođena aneurizma arterija baze mozga
Aneurisma cerebrale	Cerebral aneurysm	Anévrisme intra-crânien	Aneurisma cerebral	Cerebralna aneurizma
Aneurisma cerebrale sferica	Ball-shaped aneurysm of the brain artery	Anévrisme intra-crânien en forme de sac	Aneurisma cerebral arterial sacular	Kuglasta aneurizma arterije mozga
Aneurisma dell'aorta addominale	Abdominal aortic aneurysm	Anévrisme de l'aorte abdominale	Aneurisma de aorta abdominal	Aneurizma abdominalne aorte
Aneurisma dell'aorta toracica	Thoracic aortic aneurysm	Anévrisme aortique thoracique	Aneurisma de aorta torácica	Aneurizma torakalne aorte
Angina	Angina	Angine	Angina	Angina
Angina di Prinzmetal	Prinzmetal's angina	Angine de Prinzmetal	Angina de Prinzmetal	Prinzmetalova angina
Angina pectoris	Angina pectoris	Angine de poitrine (angor)	Angina de pecho (angor, angor pectoris)	Angina pektoris
Angioedema (edema di Quincke, edema angioneurotico)	Angioedema (angioneurotic edema)	Oedème de Quincke (angio-oedème)	Angioedema (edema de Quincke)	Angioedem (Quinckeov edem, angioneurotski edem)
Angioma	Angioma	Angiome	Angioma	Angiom
Angioma a ragno	Spider angioma (spider nevus)	Angiome stellaire	Angioma en araña (angioma aracnoideo)	Paukoliki angiom (spider nevus)
Angiosarcoma	Angiosarcoma	Angiosarcome	Angiosarcoma	Angiosarkom
Anisakidosi	Anisakiasis	Anisakiase	Anisakiasis (anisakidosis)	Anisakijaza
Anomalia cerebrovascolare	Cerebrovascular anomaly	Anomalie cérébrovasculaire	Malformación arteriovenosa cerebral	Anomalija moždanih krvnih žila
Anomalia di sviluppo del sistema nervoso	Brain development anomaly	Anomalie du développement cérébral	Malformación del desarrollo cerebral	Anomalija u razvoju mozga
Anomalie di sviluppo	Development anomalies	Anomalies de développement	Anomalías del desarrollo	Razvojne anomalije
Anoressia	Anorexia	Anorexie	Anorexia	Anoreksija
Anormale perdita di sangue durante il ciclo mestruale (menorragia)	Abnormally heavy menstrual period (menorrhagia)	Cycle menstruel anormalement excessice (ménorragie)	Pérdida de sangre mayor durante la menstruación (menorragia)	Abnormalno velik gubitak krvi tijekom mjesečnice (menoragija)
Ansia (ansietà)	Anxiety	Anxiété	Ansiedad	Nemir (anksioznost)
Antrace	Anthrax	Charbon	Carbunco (ántrax)	Antraks (bedrenica, crni prišt)
Antracosi	Anthracosis	Anthracose	Antracosis	Antrakoza
Anuria (produzione di urina < 100 ml nelle 24 ore)	Anuria (passage of urine < 100 ml in 24 hours)	Anurie (volume urinaire < 100 ml par 24 heures)	Anuria (menos de 100ml de orina en 24h)	Anurija (lučenje urina < 100 ml u 24 sata)
Aplasia	Aplasia	Aplasie	Aplasia	Aplazija
Apoplessia	Apoplexy	Apoplexie (attaque d'apoplexie)	Apoplejía (golpe apoplético)	Moždano krvarenje (apopleksija)
Appendicite acuta	Acute appendicitis	Appendicite aiguë	Apendicitis aguda	Akutna upala crvuljka
Appetito	Appetite	Appétit	Apetito	Apetit
Aritmia	Arrhythmia	Arythmie	Arrítmia	Aritmija
Aritmia cardiaca	Cardiac arrhythmia	Arythmie cardiaque	Arrítmia cardíaca	Srčana aritmija
Arresto cardiaco	Cardiac arrest (cardiopulmonary arrest)	Arrêt cardiaque (arrêt ventilatoire, arrêt cardio-respiratoire)	Paro cardiaco (parada cardiorrespiratoria)	Zastoj srca (srčani arest)
Arteriosclerosi	Arteriosclerosis	Artérosclérose	Arteriosclerosis	Arterioskleroza
Arterite temporale (arterite di Horton)	Giant cell arteritis (temporal arteritis)	Artérite giganto-cellulaire (maladie de Horton, artérite temporale)	Arteritis de células gigantes (arteritis de la temporal)	Arteritis divovskih stanica (temporalni arteritis)
Articolazione doloroso (artralgia)	Joint pain (arthralgia)	Douleur articulaire (arthralgie)	Dolor en articulación (artralgia)	Bol u zglobu (artralgija)
Artrite idiopatica giovanile	Juvenile rheumatoid arthritis	Arthrite chronique juvénile	Artritis juvenil	Mladenački reumato-idni artritis (juvenilni reumatoidni artritis)
Artrite psoriasica	Psoriatic arthritis	Arthrite psoriatique	Artritis psoriásica	Psorijatični artritis
Artrite reumatoide	Rheumatoid arthritis	Arthrite rhumatoïde	Artritis reumatoide	Reumatoidni artritis
Artrite settica	Infectious arthritis (septic arthritis)	Arthrite septique	Artritis infecciosa (artritis séptica)	Infekcijski artritis (septički artritis)
Artrite tubercolare	Tuberculous arthritis	Arthrite tuberculeuse	Artritis tuberculosa	Tuberkulozni artritis
Artrogriposi	Arthrogryposis	Arthrogypose	Artrogriposis	Artrogripoza
Artropatia	Arthropathy	Arthropathie	Artropatía	Artropatija
Artropatia emofilica	Hemophiliac arthropathy	Arthropathie hémophile	Artropatía hemofílca	Hemofilična artropatija
Artrosi	Arthrosis (osteoarthritis, degenerative arthritis)	Arthrose (arthropathie chronique dégénérative)	Artrosis	Artroza (osteoartritis, degenerativni artritis)
Artrosi al piede	Foot arthrosis	Arthrose du pied	Artrosis del pie	Artroza stopala
Artrosi della mano	Hand arthrosis	Arthrose de le main	Artrosis de mano	Artroza šake
Artrosi di anca	Hip arthrosis	Arthrose de hanche (coxarthrose)	Artrosis de cadera (coxartrosis)	Artroza kuka (koksartroza)
Artrosi di caviglia	Ankle arthrosis	Arthrose de cheville	Artrosis de tobillo	Artroza skočnog zgloba
Artrosi di ginocchio	Knee arthrosis	Arthrose du genou (gonarthrose)	Artrosis de rodilla (gonartrosis)	Artroza koljena (gonartroza)
Artrosi gleno-omerale	Shoulder arthrosis	Arthrose de l'épaule	Artrosis del hombro	Artroza ramena

Italiano	Inglese	Francese	Spagnolo	Croato
Artrosi di gomito	Elbow arthrosis	Arthrose du coude	Artrosis de codo	Artroza lakta
Artrosi di polso	Wrist arthrosis	Arthrose du poignet	Artrosis de muñeca	Artroza ručnog zgloba
Asbestosi	Asbestosis	Asbestose (amiantose)	Asbestosis	Azbestoza
Ascaridiasi	Ascaridosis	Ascaridiose	Ascaridiasis	Askaridijaza
Ascesso	Abscess	Abcès	Absceso	Apsces
Ascesso anale	Anal abscess	Abcès anale	Absceso anal	Analni apsces
Ascesso cerebrale	Brain abscess	Abcès cérébral	Absceso cerebral	Apsces mozga
Ascesso di Brodie	Brodie abscess	Abcès de Brodie	Absceso de Brodie	Brodijev apsces
Ascesso epatico	Liver abscess	Abcès hépatique	Absceso hepático	Apsces jetre
Ascesso perianale	Perianal abscess	Abcès périanal	Absceso perianal	Perianalni apsces
Ascesso perinefrico	Perinephric abscess	Abcès périnéphrique	Absceso perinéfrico	Paranefritički apsces
Ascesso peritonsillare	Quinsy (peritonsillar abscess)	Abcès périamygdalien	Absceso peritonsilar	Gnojna upala krajnika
Ascesso polmonare	Lung abscess	Abcès pulmonaire	Absceso pulmonar	Apsces pluća
Ascite	Ascites	Ascite	Ascitis	Ascites
Asfissia	Asphyxia	Asphyxie	Asfixia	Asfiksija
Asma	Asthma	Asthme	Asma	Astma
Aspergilloma (micetoma)	Aspergilloma (mycetoma, fungus ball)	Aspergillome	Aspergiloma (micetoma)	Aspergilom
Aspergillosi	Aspergillosis	Aspergillose	Aspergilosis	Aspergiloza
Assenza di mestruazioni (amenorrea)	Absence of menstrual period (amenorrhea)	Absence des règles (aménorrhée)	Ausencia de la menstruación (amenorrea)	Izostanak mjesečnice (amenoreja)
Assenza di respirazione (apnea)	Suspension of external breathing (apnea)	Arrêt respiratoire (apnée)	Falta de respiración (apnea)	Zastoj disanja (apnea)
Astigmatismo	Astigmatism	Astigmatisme	Astigmatismo	Astigmatizam
Astrocitoma	Astrocytoma	Astrocytome	Astrocitoma	Astrocitom
Atassia ereditaria	Hereditary ataxia	Ataxie héréditaire	Ataxia de Friidreich (ataxia hereditaria)	Heredoataksija
Atelectasia polmonare	Pulmonary atelectasis	Atélectasie pulmonaire	Atelectasia pulmonar	Atelektaza pluća
Aterosclerosi	Atherosclerosis	Athérosclérose	Ateroesclerosis	Ateroskleroza
Atetosi	Athetosis	Athétose	Atetosis	Atetoza
Atonia muscolare	Atony (atonia)	Atonie	Atonía	Atonija
Atresia anale	Anal atresia	Atrésie anale	Atresia anal	Atrezija anusa
Atresia biliare	Bile duct atresia	Atrésie biliare	Atresia biliar	Atrezija žučnih vodova
Atresia duodenale	Duodenal atresia	Atrésie duodénale	Atresia duodenal	Atrezija dvanaesnika
Atresia esofagea	Esophageal atresia	Atrésie de l'oesophage	Atresia esofágica	Atrezija jednjaka
Atresia intestinale	Intestinal atresia	Atrésie intestinale	Atresia intestinal	Crijevna atrezija
Atrofia	Atrophy	Atrophie	Atrofia	Atrofija
Atrofia di Sudeck	Sudeck's atrophy	Atrophie de Sudeck	Atrofia de Sudeck	Sudeckova distrofija
Atrofia multi-sistemica	Multiple system atrophy	Atrophie multisystématisée	Atrofia multisistémica	Multipla sistemska atrofija
Attaco di panico	Panic attack	Crise de panique	Ataque de pánico	Napadaj panike
Aumentata emissione di urina (poliuria)	Passage of large volumes of urine (polyuria)	Sécrétion d'urine en quantité abondante (polyurie)	Gasto urinario excesivo (poliuria)	Učestalo mokrenje velikih količina mokraće (poliurija)
Aumento del ritmo respiratorio (tachipnea)	Rapid breathing (tachypnea)	Respiration accélérée (tachypnée)	Respiración rápida (taquipnea)	Ubrzano disanje (tahipnea)
Aumento del senso della sete (polidipsia)	Increased thirst senasation (polydipsia)	Soif excessive (polydipsie)	Aumento anormal de la sed (polidipsia)	Pojačan osjećaj žeđi (polidipsija)
Aumento della distanza fra due parti del corpo (ipertelorismo)	Increased distance between two organs or parts of the body (hypertelorism)	Élargissement de la distance des organes (hypertélorisme)	Aumento de la separación de los organos (hipertelorismo)	Povećan razmak izmedu dva organa ili dijela tijela (hipertelorizam)
Aumento della pelosità (ipertricosi)	Increased hairiness (hypertrichosis)	Pilosité excessive (hypertrichose)	Exceso de cabello (hipertricosis)	Pojačana dlakavost
Aumento della sudorazione (iperidrosi)	Excessive sweating (hyperhidrosis)	Sudation excessive (hyperhidrose)	Excesiva producción de sudor (hiperhidrosis)	Prekomjerno znojenje (hiperhidroza)
Aumento di perdita di capelli	Increased hair loss	Perte de cheveux excessive	Aumento de la cáida del cabello	Pojačano opadanje kose
Aumento di volume del fegato (epatomegalia)	Enlarged liver (hepatomegaly)	Augmentation du foie (hépatomégalie)	Aumento del tamaño del hígado (hepatomegalia)	Povećanje jetre (hepatomegalija)
Aumento incontrollato dell'appetito (polifagia)	Excessive hunger (polyphagia)	Faim excessive (polyphagie)	Aumento anormal de la necesidad de comer (polifagia)	Neumjerena glad
Aumento incontrollato di assunzione di cibo (iperfagia)	Abnormally large intake of food (hyperphagia)	Prise excessive d'aliments (hyperphagie)	Ingestas descontroladas de alimentos (hiperfagia)	Prekomjerno jedenje (hiperfagija)
Autismo	Autism	Autisme	Autismo	Autizam
Autolesionismo	Self-harm	Automutilation	Autolesión (automutilación)	Samoozljeđivanje
Aviofobia (paura di volare)	Aviophobia (fear of flying)	Aerophobie (peur de l'avion)	Aerofobia (miedo a volar)	Aerofobija (strah od letenja)
Avitaminosi	Avitaminosis	Avitaminose	Avitaminosis	Avitamonoza
Avvelenamento (intossicazione)	Poisoning (toxication)	Empoisonnement (toxicité)	Envenenamiento (intoxicación)	Trovanje
Avvelenamento da alcali	Alkali poisoning	Empoisonnement par alcalis	Intoxicación por álcalis	Trovanje alkalima
Avvelenamento da alcool	Alcohol poisoning	Empoisonnement par l'alcool	Intoxicación por alcohol	Trovanje alkoholom
Avvelenamento da amianto	Asbestos poisoning	Empoisonnement par l'amiante	Envenenamiento por asbesto	Trovanje azbestom

Italiano	Inglese	Francese	Spagnolo	Croato
Avvelenamento da armi chimiche	Chemical warfare poisoning	Intoxcation par arme chimique	Intoxicación por armas químicas	Trovanje kemijskim oružjem
Avvelenamento da arsenico	Arsenic poisoning	Empoisonnement à l'arsenic	Envenenamiento por arsénico	Trovanje arsenom
Avvelenamento da cadmio	Cadmium poisoning	Empoisonnement au cadmium	Envenenamiento por cadmio	Trovanje kadmijem
Avvelenamento da cianuro	Cyanide poisoning	Empoisonnement au cyanure	Envenenamiento por cianuro	Trovanje cijanidom
Avvelenamento da cibo	Food poisoning	Empoisonnement alimentaires	Intoxicación alimentaria	Trovanje hranom
Avvelenamento da ferro	Iron poisoning	Empoisonnement au fer	Intoxicación por hierro	Trovanje željezom
Avvelenamento da funghi	Mushroom poisoning	Empoisonnement par des champignons	Envenenamiento por setas	Trovanje gljivama
Avvelenamento da gas	Gas poisoning	Empoisonnement au gaz	Envenenamiento por gas	Trovanje plinom
Avvelenamento da gas tossico	Warfare gases poisoning	Intoxication par gaz de combat	Intoxicación por armas gaseosas	Trovanje bojnim otrovima
Avvelenamento da insetticidi	Insecticide poisoning	Empoisonnement au insecticide	Envenenamiento por insecticidas	Trovanje insekticidima
Avvelenamento da litio	Lithium poisoning	Empoisonnement au lithium	Intoxicación por litio	Trovanje litijem
Avvelenamento da mercurio	Mercury poisoning	Empoisonnement au mercure	Envenenamiento por mercurio	Trovanje živom
Avvelenamento da metanolo	Methanol poisoning	Empoisonnement au méthanol	Intoxicación por metanol	Trovanje metanolom
Avvelenamento da molluschi	Shellfish poisoning	Intoxication par des coquillages	Intoxicación por mariscos	Trovanje školjkašima
Avvelenamento da monossido di carbonio	Carbon monoxide poisoning	Empoisonnement au monoxyde de carbone	Intoxicación por monóxido de carbono	Trovanje ugljičnim monoksidom
Avvelenamento da paracetamolo	Paracetamol poisoning	Intoxication par le paracétamol	Intoxicación por paracetamol	Trovanje paracetamolom
Avvelenamento da pesci	Fish poisoning	Empoisonnement du poisson	Intoxicación por pescado	Trovanje ribom
Avvelenamento da piombo (saturnismo)	Lead poisoning	Empoisonnement au plomb	Envenenamiento por plomo	Trovanje olovom
Avvelenamento da radiazione	Radiation poisoning	Empoisonnement par radiations	Envenenamiento por radiación	Trovanje zračenjem
Avvelenamento da salicilati	Salicylate poisoning	Empoisonnement au salicylate	Intoxicación por salicilatos	Trovanje salicilatima
Avvelenamento da tallio	Thallium poisoning	Empoisonnement au thallium	Envenenamiento por talio	Trovanje talijem
Barcollamento	Shuffling gait	Démarche traînante	Marcha arrastrando los pies	Teturav nesiguran hod
Barotrauma	Barotrauma	Barotraumatisme	Barotraumatismo (barotrauma)	Barotrauma
Bartonellosi	Bartonellosis	Bartonellose	Bartonelosis	Bartoneloza
Basalioma (carcinoma basocellulare)	Basal cell carcinoma	Carcinome basocellulaire	Carcinoma de células basales (basilioma)	Karcinom bazalnih stanica (bazaliom)
Basofilia	Basophilia	Basophilie	Basofilia	Bazofilija
Bassa pressione arteriosa (ipotensione)	Low blood pressure (hypotension)	Baisse de la pression artérielle (hypotension artérielle)	Presión sanguínea baja (hipotensión)	Nizak krvni tlak (hipotenzija)
Bassa temperatura corporea (ipotermia)	Decreased body temperature (hypothermia)	Température corporelle basse (hypothermie)	Temperatura corporal baja (hipotermia)	Snižena temperatura tijela (hipotermija)
Basso metabolismo basale	Slow basal metabolism	Métabolisme basal diminué	Metabolismo basal lento	Usporen bazalni metabolizam
Batteriemia	Bacteremia	Bactériémie	Bacteriemia (bacteremia)	Bakterijemija
Batteriuria	Bacteriuria	Bactériurie	Bacteriuria	Bakteriurija
Bissinosi	Byssinosis (Monday fever)	Byssinose	Bisinosis (fiebre del lunes)	Bisinoza
Blastoma	Blastoma	Blastome	Blastoma	Blastom
Blastomicosi	Blastomycosis	Blastomycose	Blastomicosis	Blastomikoza
Blefarite	Blepharitis	Blépharite	Blefaritis	Blefaritis
Blocco atrioventricolare	Atrioventricular block (AV block)	Bloc auriculo-ventriculaire	Bloqueo auriculoventricular	Atrijskoventrikularni blok
Blocco di branca	Bundle branch block	Bloc de branche	Bloqueo de rama	Blok grane Hisovog snopića
Blocco trifascicolare	Trifascicular block	Bloc trifasciculaire	Bloqueo trifascicular	Trifasikularni blok
Borborigmo	Stomach growling (borborygmus)	Gargouillements (borborygme)	Sonidos de tripas (borborigmo)	Kruljenje u želucu
Borreliosi	Borreliosis	Borréliose	Borreliosis	Borelioza
Botulismo	Botulism	Botulisme	Botulismo	Botulizam
Brachialgia	Brachial syndrome	Brachialgie	Síndrome braquial	Brahijalni sindrom bolne nadlaktice
Brivido	Shivering	Frissonnement	Escalofrío (tiritón)	Zimica (tresavica)
Bronchiectasia	Bronchiectasis	Bronchectasie (dilatation des bronches)	Bronquiectasia	Bronhiektazije
Bronchite cronica	Chronic obstructive pulmonary disease	Broncho-pneumopathie chronique obstructive	Enfermedad pulmonar obstructiva crónica	Kronična opstruktivna plućna bolest
Broncopolmonite	Bronchopneumonia	Bronchopneumonie	Neumonía bronquial	Bronhopneumonija
Broncospasmo	Bronchospasm	Bronchospasme	Broncoespasmo	Bronhospazam

Italiano	Inglese	Francese	Spagnolo	Croato
Brucellosi	Brucellosis	Brucellose (fièvre de Malte, fièvre méditerranéenne)	Brucelosis	Bruceloza (malteška ili sredozemna groznica, Bangova bolest)
Bruciore di stomaco (pirosi)	Heartburn	Brûlure de l'estomac (pyrosis)	Ardor de estómago (acidez, pirosis)	Žgaravica
Bruciore urinario	Urinary burning	Brûlures à la miction	Ardor al orinar	Pećenje za vrijeme mokrenja
Bulimia	Bulimia	Boulimie	Bulimia	Bulimija
Cachessia	Cachexia	Cachexie	Caquexia	Kaheksija
Calazio	Stye (chalazion)	Chalazion	Orzuelo	Ječmenac
Calcificazione	Calcification	Calcification	Calcificación	Ovapnjenje (kalcifikacija)
Calcolo biliare	Gallstone (cholelithiasis)	Calcul biliaire (cholélithiase)	Cálculo biliar (litiasis biliar)	Žučni kamenac (holelitijaza)
Calcolo ureterale	Ureteral stone (ureterolithiasis)	Calcul dans l'uretère	Cálculo en el uréter (ureterolitiasis)	Ureteralni kamenac (ureterolitijaza)
Calcolo urinario (urolitiasi)	Bladder stone (urolithiasis)	Calcul urinaire (urolithiase)	Cálculo en el tracto urinario (urolitiasis)	Kamenac mokraćnog mjehura
Calcolosi renale (nefrolitiasi)	Kidney stone (nephrolithiasis)	Calcul rénal (néphrolithiase, lithiase urinaire)	Piedra en el riñon (cálculo renal, litiasis renal)	Bubrežni kamenac (nefrolitijaza)
Calicosi	Chalicosis	Chalicose	Calicosis	Kalikoza
Callo (vescica, bolla)	Blister (corn)	Cor (cal)	Ampolla (callo)	Žulj (plik, kurje oko)
Callosità (callo)	Callosity (thickening)	Callosité	Callosidad (callo)	Zadebljanje kože
Cambiamenti della mucosa	Changes in mucous membrane	Changement de la muqueuse	Cambios en la membrana mucosa	Promjene na sluznici
Cambiamenti della sensazione tattile	Changes in tactile sensation	Changements des sensations tactiles	Cambios en la sensibilidad táctil	Promjene osjeta dodira
Cambiamenti delle sensazoni olfattive	Changes in olfactory sensation	Changements des sensations olfactives	Cambios en la sensibilidad olfatoria	Promjene osjeta mirisa
Cambiamenti di nevi	Changes in moles	Changements dans les grains de beauté	Cambios en los lunares	Promjene na madežima
Cambiamenti di personalità	Personality changes	Changements de personnalité	Cambios de personalidad	Promjene osobnosti
Cambiamenti nell'appetito	Appetite changes	Changements d'appétit	Cambios en el apetito	Promjene apetita
Cambiamenti nella forma delle ossa	Changes in shape of bones	Changements dans la forme des os	Cambios en la forma de los huesos	Promjene oblika kosti
Cambiamenti nelle sensazioni del gusto	Changes in taste sensation	Changements de sensation de goût	Cambios en la sensación de sabores	Promjene osjeta okusa
Cambiamento d'umore	Mood swing	Saute d'humeur	Oscilaciones del humor	Promjene raspoloženja
Cambiamento di colore della pelle	Skin color changes	Changements de couleur de la peau	Cambios en el color de la piel	Promjene boje kože
Cambiamento di voce	Voice changes	Changements de voix	Cambios en la voz	Promjene glasa
Cancrena	Gangrene	Gangrène	Gangrena	Gangrena
Cancro della cervice uterina	Cervical cancer	Cancer du col utérin	Cáncer del cuello uterino (cáncer cervical)	Rak grlića maternice
Cancro della mammella	Breast cancer	Cancer du sein	Cáncer de mama	Rak dojke
Cancro della prostata	Prostate cancer	Cancer de la prostate	Cáncer de próstata	Rak prostate
Cancro dello stomaco (cancro gastrico)	Stomach cancer (gastric cancer)	Cancer de l'estomac	Cáncer de estómago (cáncer gástrico)	Rak želuca
Candidosi (candidiasi)	Candidiasis (thrush)	Candidiase	Candidiasis	Kandidijaza
Capezzolo invertito	Inverted nipple	Téton ombiliqué	Pezón invertido	Uvućena bradavica
Capogiro (vertigine)	Dizziness (vertigo)	Vertige	Vértigo	Vrtoglavica
Capsulite adesiva	Frozen shoulder (adhesive capsulitis of shoulder)	Épaule bloquée (périarthrite scapulo-humérale)	Capsulitis adhesiva del hombro	Sindrom bolnog ramena (adhezivni kapsulitis ramena, smrznuto rame)
Carbonchio (pustola)	Carbuncle	Anthrax	Ántrax (carbunco)	Karbunkul
Carcinoide	Carcinoid	Carcinoïde	Carcinoide	Karcinoid
Carcinoide bronchiale	Bronchial carcinoid	Carcinoïde bronchiale	Carcinoide bronquial	Karcinoid bronha
Carcinoma	Carcinoma	Carcinome	Carcinoma	Karcinom
Carcinoma a cellule renali	Renal cell carcinoma (hypernephroma)	Carcinome à cellules rénales	Carcinoma de células renales	Hipernefrom
Carcinoma a cellule squamose	Squamous cell carcinoma (planocellular carcinoma)	Carcinome spinocellulaire	Carcinoma de células escamosas	Planocelularni karcinom
Carcinoma anaplastico	Anaplastic carcinoma	Carcinome anaplastique	Carcinoma anaplásico	Anaplastični karcinom
Carcinoma bronchiale	Bronchial carcinoma	Carcinome bronchique	Carcinoma bronquial	Karcinom bronha
Carcinoma della cervice uterina	Cervical carcinoma	Carcinome du col utérin	Carcinoma del cuello uterino	Karcinom grlića maternice
Carcinoma della prostata	Prostate carcinoma	Carcinome de la prostate	Carcinoma de próstata	Karcinom prostate
Carcinoma embrionale	Embryonal carcinoma	Carcinome embryonnaire	Carcinoma embrional	Embrionalni karcinom
Carcinoma endometriale	Endometrial carcinoma	Carcinome de l'endomètre	Carcinoma de endometrio	Karcinom endometrija
Carcinoma epatocellulare	Hepatocellular carcinoma	Carcinome hépatocellulaire	Carcinoma hepatocelular	Hepatocelularni karcinom
Carcinoma epiteliale	Epithelial carcinoma	Carcinome épithélial	Carcinoma epitelial	Karcinom pokrovnog epitela
Carcinoma gastrico	Gastric carcinoma	Carcinome de l'estomac	Carcinoma gástrico	Karcinom želuca
Carcinoma mammario	Breast carcinoma	Carcinome du sein	Carcinoma de mama	Karcinom dojke
Carcinoma midollare	Medullary carcinoma	Carcinome médullaire	Carcinoma medular	Medularni karcinom
Carcinoma papillare	Papillary carcinoma	Carcinome papillaire	Carcinoma papilar	Papilarni karcinom

Carcinoma transizionale	Transitional cell carcinoma	Carcinome à cellules de transition	Carcinoma de células transicionales	Tranzicionalni karc
Carcinosi (carcinomatosi, cancerosi)	Carcinosis	Carcinose	Carcinosis	Karcinoza
Carcinosi pericardiale	Pericardial carcinosis	Carcinose péricardique	Carcinosis pericárdica	Karcinoza perikard
Carcinosi peritoneale	Peritoneal carcinosis	Carcinose péritonéale	Carcinosis peritoneal	Karcinoza peritone
Carcinosi pleurica	Pleural carcinosis	Carcinose pleurale	Carcinosis pleural	Karcinoza pleure
Cardiomiopatia	Cardiomyopathy	Cardiomyopathie	Miocardiopatía	Kardiomiopatija
Cardiomiopatia dilatativa	Dilated cardiomyopathy	Cardiomyopathie dilatée	Miocardiopatía dilatada	Dilatacijska kardio
Cardiomiopatia ipertrofica	Hypertrophic cardiomyopathy	Cardiomyopathie hypertrophique	Miocardiopatía hipertrófica	Hipertrofijska kardiomiopatija
Cardiomiopatia restrittiva	Restrictive cardiomyopathy	Cardiomyopathie restrictive	Cardiomiopatía restrictiva	Restriktivna kardio
Cardiomiopatia tossica	Cardiotoxicity	Cardiotoxicité	Cardiotoxicidad	Toksična kardiomic
Cardiopalmo (palpitazione)	Palpitation	Palpitation	Palpitación	Lupanje srca (palpi
Cardiopatia congenita	Congenital heart disease (congenital cardiopathy)	Cardiopathie congénitale	Cardiopatía congénita	Urođena srčana bo (kongenitalna kardi
Cardiopatia reumatica	Rheumatic heart disease	Cardite rhumatismale	Cardiopatía reumática	Reumatska bolest s
Carenza di estrogeno	Estrogen deficiency	Carence oestrogénique	Deficiencia de estrógenos	Manjak estrogena
Carenza di fattore di coagulazione	Coagulation factor deficiency	Déficit en facteur de la coagulation	Deficiencia de factor de coagulación	Manjak faktora koa
Carenza di vitamine	Vitamin deficiency	Carence en vitamine	Carencia de vitamina	Manjak vitamina
Carenza di vitamina A	Vitamin A deficiency	Carence en vitamine A	Carencia de vitamina A	Manjak vitamina A
Carenza di vitamina B1	Vitamin B1 deficiency	Carence en vitamine B1	Carencia de vitamina B1	Manjak vitamina B
Carenza di vitamina B2	Vitamin B2 deficiency	Carence en vitamine B2	Carencia de vitamina B2	Manjak vitamina B
Carenza di vitamina B3	Vitamin B3 deficiency	Carence en vitamine B3	Carencia de vitamina B3	Manjak vitamina B
Carenza di vitamina B12	Vitamin B12 deficiency	Carence en vitamine B12	Carencia de vitamina B12	Manjak vitamina B
Carenza di vitamina C	Vitamin C deficiency	Carence en vitamine C	Carencia de vitamina C	Manjak vitamina C
Carenza di vitamina D	Vitamin D deficiency	Carence en vitamine D	Carencia de vitamina D	Manjak vitamina D
Carenza di vitamina K	Vitamin K deficiency	Carence en vitamine K	Carencia de vitamina K	Manjak vitamina K
Carie dentaria	Dental caries	Carie dentaire	Caries	Zubni karijes
Catalessia	Catalepsy	Catalepsie	Catalepsia	Katalepsija
Cataplessia	Cataplexy	Cataplexie	Cataplexia (cataplejía)	Katapleksija
Cataratta	Cataract	Cataracte	Catarata	Mrena (katarakta)
Catarro	Catarrh	Catarrhe	Catarro	Katar
Cecità	Blindness	Cécité	Ceguera	Sljepoća
Cecità notturna (nictalopia)	Night blindness (nyctalopia)	Cécité nocturne (héméralopie)	Ceguera nocturna (nictalopia)	Noćno sljepilo
Cefalea a grappolo	Cluster headache	Algie vasculaire de la face	Cefalea en racimos	Cluster glavobolja
Cefalea di tipo tensivo	Tension headache	Céphalée de tension	Cefalea tensional	Tenzijska glavobolj
Cefalea post-traumatica	Post-traumatic headache	Céphalée post-traumatique	Cefalea postraumática	Posttraumatska gla
Cefalocèle	Cephalocele	Céphalocèle	Cefalocele	Cefalokela
Celiachia (malattia caliacha)	Coeliac disease (celiac disease)	Maladie coeliaque	Celiaquía (enfermedad celíaca)	Celijakija
Cellulite	Cellulitis	Cellulite	Celulitis	Celulitis
Cellulite orbitale	Orbital cellulitis	Cellulite orbitale	Celulitis orbital	Celulitis orbite
Cercaria	Cercaria	Cercaire	Cercaria	Cerkarija
Cheloide	Keloid	Chéloïde	Queloide	Keloid
Cheratosi	Keratosis	Kératose (kératodermie)	Keratosis	Keratoza
Cheratosi seborroica	Seborrheic keratosis	Kératose séborrhéïque	Queratosis seborreica	Seboreična keratoz
Cheratosi solare	Actinic keratosis	Kératose actinique	Queratosis actínica	Aktinička keratoza
Chetoacidosi diabetica	Diabetic ketoacidosis	Cétoacidose diabétique	Cetoacidosis diabética	Dijabetična ketoaci
Chikungunya	Chikungunya	Chikungunya	Chikungunya	Chikungunya virus
Chilotorace	Chylothorax	Chylothorax	Quilotórax	Hilotoraks
Cianosi	Cyanosis	Cyanose	Cianosis	Cijanoza
Cicatrice (sfregio)	Scar	Cicatrice	Cicatriz	Ožiljak
Cifoscoliosi	Kyphoscoliosis	Cypho-scoliose	Cifoescoliosis	Kifoskolioza
Cifosi	Kyphosis	Cyphose	Cifosis	Kifoza
Cirrosi	Liver cirrhosis	Cirrhose hépatique	Cirrosis hepática	Ciroza jetre
Cirrosi alcolica	Alcoholic cirrhosis	Cirrhose alcoolique	Cirrosis alcohólica	Alkoholna ciroza
Cirrosi biliare	Biliary cirrhosis	Cirrhose biliaire	Cirrosis biliar	Bilijarna ciroza
Cirrosi criptogenica	Cryptogenic cirrhosis	Cirrhose cryptogénique	Cirrosis criptogénica	Kriptogena ciroza
Cirrosi post-necrotica	Post-necrotic cirrhosis	Cirrhose postnecrotique	Cirrosis postnecrótica	Postnekrotična ciro
Cistadenocarcinoma	Cystadenocarcinoma	Cystadénocarcinome	Cistadenocarcinoma	Cistadenokarcinom
Cistadenofibroma	Cystadenofibroma	Cystadénofibrome	Cistadenofibroma	Cistadenofibrom
Cistadenoma	Cystadenoma	Cystadénome	Cistadenoma	Cistadenom
Cisti (ciste)	Cyst	Kyste	Quiste	Cista
Cisti del dotto tiroglosso	Thyroglossal duct cyst	Kyste du canal thyréoglosse	Quiste tirogloso	Cista na tireoglosn
Cisti dermoide	Dermoid cyst	Kyste dermoïde	Quiste dermoide	Dermoidna cista
Cisti ovarica	Ovarian cyst	Kyste ovarien	Quiste ovárico	Cista na jajniku
Cisti pancreatica	Pancreatic cyst	Kyste du pancréas	Quiste de páncreas	Cista na gušterači
Cisti pilonidale	Pilonidal cyst	Kyste pilonidal	Quiste pilonidal	Pilonidalna cista
Cisti renale	Renal cyst	Kyste rénal	Quiste de riñón	Cista na bubregu
Cisti sebacea	Sebaceous cyst (wen)	Kyste sébacé	Quiste sebáceo	Lojna cista
Cisti tiroidea	Thyroid cyst	Kyste thyroïdien	Quiste de tiroides	Cista na štitnjači

Italiano	Inglese	Francese	Spagnolo	Croato
Cisticercosi	Cysticercosis	Cysticercose	Cisticercosis	Cisticerkoza
Cistoma	Cystoma	Kystome	Cistoma	Cistom
Claudicatio intermittens	Intermittent claudication	Claudication intermittente	Claudicación intermitente	Intermitentna klaudikacija
Claustrofobia (paura di luoghi chiusi)	Claustrophobia (fear of closed space)	Claustrophobie	Claustrofobia (miedo a los espacios cerrados)	Klaustrofobija (strah od zatvorenog prostora)
Cleptomania	Kleptomania	Cleptomanie	Cleptomanía	Kleptomanija
Clonorchiasi	Clonorchiasis	Clonorchiase	Clonorquiasis (clonorquiosis)	Klonorkijaza
Coagulazione intravascolare disseminata	Disseminated intra-vascular coagulation	Coagulation intra-vasculaire disséminée	Coagulación intra-vascular diseminada	Diseminirana intravaskularna koagulacija
Coartazione dell'aorta	Coarctation of the aorta	Coarctation de l'aorte	Coartación de la aorta	Koarktacija aorte
Coccidiomicosi	Coccidioidomycosis (San Joaquin Valley fever)	Coccidioïmycose (fièvre de la vallée de San Joaquín, fièvre du désert)	Coccidioidomicosis	Kokcidioidomikoza (San Joaquin Valley vrućica)
Coccigodinia	Coccygodynia	Coccygodynie (douleur coccygienne)	Coccigodinia (dolor de coxis)	Kokcigodinija
Colangiocarcinoma (carcinoma colangiocellulare)	Cholangiocellular carcinoma	Cholangiocarcinome	Carcinoma de las vías biliares (colangiocarcinoma)	Kolangiocelularni karcinom
Colera	Cholera	Choléra	Cólera	Kolera
Colica	Colic	Colique	Cólico	Kolika
Colica addominale	Abdominal colic	Colique abdominale	Cólico abdominal	Trbušna kolika (abdominalna kolika)
Colica biliare	Biliary colic	Colique biliaire	Cólico biliar	Žučna kolika
Colica renale	Renal colic	Colique néphrétique	Cólico nefrítico (cólico renal)	Bubrežna kolika (renalna kolika)
Coliche del neonato	Baby colic	Coliques de bébé	Cólico del recién nacido	Novorođenačke kolike
Collaso circolatorio (shock)	Shock	Choc	Choque (shock)	Šok
Collasso	Collapse	Collapsus	Colapso	Kolaps
Colon trasverso	Transverse colon	Côlon transverse	Colon transverso	Poprečno debelo crijevo
Colpo apoplettico	Stroke (cerebrovascular accident)	Attaque cérébrale (accident vasculaire cérébral)	Derrame cerebral (accidente cerebrovascular)	Moždani udar
Coma	Coma	Coma	Coma	Koma
Coma diabetico	Diabetic coma	Coma diabétique	Coma diabético	Dijabetična koma
Commozione cerebrale	Brain concussion	Commotion cérébrale	Conmoción cerebral	Potres mozga
Compressione cerebrale	Brain compression	Compression cérébrale	Compresión cerebral	Kompresija mozga
Compressone del nervo	Nerve compression (pinched nerve)	Compression du nerf	Compresión del nérvio	Kompresija živca (uklješten živac)
Condiloma	Genital wart	Verrue génitale	Verruga genital (condiloma acuminata)	Genitalna bradavica (venerična bradavica)
Condroblastoma	Chondroblastoma	Chondroblastome	Condroblastoma	Hondroblastom
Condroma	Chondroma	Chondrome	Condroma	Hondrom
Condrosarcoma	Chondrosarcoma	Chondrosarcome	Condrosarcoma	Hondrosarkom
Confusione (disordine)	Confusion	Confusion	Confusión	Smetenost
Congelamento	Frostbite	Gelure	Congelamiento	Ozeblina
Congestione nasale	Nasal congestion (stuffy nose)	Congestion nasale	Congestión nasal	Začepljeni nos
Congestione polmonare	Pulmonary congestion	Congestion pulmonaire	Congestión pulmonar	Plućna kongestija
Congiuntivite allergica	Allergic conjunctivitis	Conjonctivite allergique	Conjuntivitis alérgica	Alergijski konjuktivitis
Congiuntivite batterica	Bacterial conjunctivitis	Conjonctivite bactérienne	Conjuntivitis bacteriana	Bakterijski konjuktivitis
Congiuntivite irritativa da agenti chimici	Chemical conjunctivitis	Conjonctivite chimique	Conjuntivitis química	Kemijski konjuktivitis
Congiuntivite irritativa da corpi estranei	Conjunctival foreign body	Conjonctivite due à un corps étranger	Conjuntivitis por cuerpo extraño	Konjuktivitis izazvan stranim tijelom
Congiuntivite virale	Viral conjuctivitis	Conjonctivite virale	Conjuntivitis viral	Virusni konjuktivitis
Consistenza acquosa delle feci	Watery stool	Selles aqueuses	Heces acuosas	Vodenasta stolica
Contrattura	Contracture	Contracture	Contractura	Kontraktura
Contrattura articolare	Joint contracture	Contracture articulaire	Contractura articular	Kontraktura zgloba
Contrattura ischemica di Volkmann	Volkmann's ischemic contracture	Syndrome de Volkmann	Contractura isquémica de Volkmann	Volkmannova ishemična kontraktura
Contrattura muscolare	Muscular contracture	Contracture musculaire	Contractura muscular	Kontraktura mišića
Contusione	Contusion	Contusion	Contusión	Nagnječenje (zgnječenje, kontuzija)
Contusione cerebrale	Cerebral contusion	Contusion cérébrale	Contusión cerebral	Nagnječenje mozga
Convulsioni	Convulsions	Convulsions	Convulsiones	Konvulzije
Convulsioni febbrili	Febrile convulsions	Convulsion hyperthermique	Convulsiones febriles	Febrilne konvulzije
Coprolalia	Involuntary swearing (coprolalia)	Tic de langage à dire des mots vulgaires (coprolalie)	Expresión vocal involuntaria de obscenidades (coprolalia)	Nekontrolirano psovanje (koprolalija)
Coreoatetosi	Choreoathetosis	Choréoathétose	Coreoatetosis	Koreoatetoza
Coriocarcinoma	Choriocarcinoma	Choriocarcinome	Coriocarcinoma	Koriokarcinom
Coriomeningite linfocitaria	Lymphocytic choriomeningitis	Chorioméningite lymphocytaire	Coriomeningitis linfocítica	Limfocitni koriomeningitis
Coronaropatia	Coronary disease	Maladie coronarienne	Enfermedad coronaria	Koronarna bolest (koronaropatija)
Corpo estraneo nel naso	Foreign body in nose	Corps étranger dans le nez	Cuerpo extraño en la nariz	Strano tijelo u nosu

Italiano	Inglese	Francese	Spagnolo	Croato
Corpo estraneo nell'orecchio	Foreign body in ear	Corps étranger dans l'oreille	Cuerpo extraño en el oído	Strano tijelo u uhu
Costa cervicale	Cervical rib	Côte cervicale	Costilla cervical	Vratno rebro
Crampo notturno alle gambe	Nocturnal leg cramps	Crampes nocturnes des jambes	Calambres nocturnos en las piernas	Noćni grčevi u nogama
Crepitazione	Crepitation	Crépitation	Crepitación	Krepitacija
Criptococcosi	Cryptococcosis	Cryptococcose	Criptococcosis	Kriptokokoza
Criptorchidismo	Cryptorchidism	Cryptorchidie	Criptorquidismo	Retencija testisa (kriptorhizam)
Crisi d'astinenza	Withdrawal	Sevrage	Síndrome de abstinencia	Apstinencijska kriza
Crisi tonico-clonica	Tonic-clonic seizure	Crise tonico-clonique	Crisis tónico-clónica	Toničko-klonički napadaj
Cromomicosi (cromoblastomicosi)	Chromoblastomycosis (chromomycosis, Pedroso's disease)	Chromomycose	Cromomicosis (cromoblastomicosis)	Kromomikoza
Crosta (escara)	Crust (scab)	Croûte	Costra	Krasta
Croup (laringite acuta ostruttiva)	Croup (acute obstructive laryngitis)	Croup (laryngotrachéo-bronchite)	Crup (laringotraqueo-bronquitis)	Krup (akutni opstruktivni laringitis)
Cuore dell'atleta (ipertrofia cardiaca da sport)	Athlete's heart (cardiac hypertrophy)	Hypertrophie cardiaque du sportif (coeur d'athlète)	Corazón de atleta (hipertrofia del corazón del deportista)	Sportsko srce
Cuore polmonare	Pulmonary heart disease	Coeur pulmonaire	Enfermedad cardíaca pulmonar (cor pulmonale)	Plućno srce
Cuore polmonare acuto	Acute pulmonary heart	Coeur pulmonaire aigu	Cor pulmonale agudo	Akutno plućno srce
Cupololitiasi (canalolitiasi)	Benign positional vertigo	Vertige paroxystique positionnel bénin	Vértigo posicional paroxístico benigno	Benigna pozicijska vrtoglavica
Daltonismo	Daltonism	Daltonisme	Daltonismo	Daltonizam
Debolezza	Weakness	Faiblesse	Debilidad	Slabost
Decompensazione cardiaca	Cardiac decompensation	Décompensation cardiaque	Descompensación cardíaca	Srčana dekompenzacija
Deformità di Madelung	Madelung's deformity	Déformation de Madelung	Deformidad de Madelung	Madelungov deformitet
Deformità di Sprengel	Sprengel's deformity	Anomalie de Sprengel	Deformidad de Sprengel	Sprengelova bolest (scapula alta)
Degenerazione della retina	Retinal degeneration	Dégénérescence de la rétine	Degeneración retinal	Degeneracija mrežnice
Degenerazione maculare	Macular degeneration	Dégénérescence maculaire	Degeneración macular	Degeneracija makule
Degenerazione spinale	Spinal deformity	Difformité spinale	Deformidad vertebral	Deformacija kralježnice
Deglutizione dolorosa (odinofagia)	Painful swallowing (odynophagia)	Déglutition douloureuse (odynophagie)	Dolor al tragar (odinofagia)	Bolno gutanje (odinofagija)
Delirio	Delirium	Délirium	Delirio	Delirij
Demenza	Dementia	Démence	Demencia	Demencija
Demineralizzazione	Demineralization	Déminéralisation	Desmineralización	Demineralizacija
Dengue	Dengue fever	Dengue (grippe tropicale, dengue hémorragique)	Dengue	Dengue groznica
Dente guasto	Rotten tooth	Dent pourri	Diente podrido	Pokvareni zub
Depressione	Depression	Dépression	Depresión	Depresija
Dermatite allergica	Allergic contact dermatitis	Dermite de contact allergique	Dermatitis alérgica de contacto	Alergijski kontaktni dermatitis
Dermatite da contatto	Contact dermatitis	Dermite de contact	Dermatitis de contacto	Kontaktni dermatitis
Dermatite erpetiforme di Duhring	Dermatitis herpetiformis (Duhring's disease)	Dermatite herpétiforme	Dermatitis herpetiforme (enfermedad de Duhring)	Duhringova bolest (dermatitis herpetiformis)
Dermatite irritativo da contatto	Irritant contact dermatitis	Dermite de contact irritative	Dermatitis irritante de contacto	Iritantni kontaktni dermatitis
Dermatite nummulare	Nummular dermatitis	Dermatite nummulaire	Dermatitis numular	Numularni dermatitis
Dermatite seborroica infantile	Cradle cap (infantile seborrhoeic dermatitis)	Dermite séborrhéique infantile	Dermatitis seborreica infantil	Tjemenica (dojenačka seboreja)
Dermatomicosi	Dermatomycosis	Dermatomycose	Dermatomicosis	Dermatomikoza
Dermatomiosite	Dermatomyositis	Dermatomyosite	Dermatomiositis	Dermatomiozitis
Deviazione del setto nasale	Nasal septum deviation	Déviation du septum nasal	Desviación del tabique nasal	Devijacija nosnog septuma
Diabete	Diabetes	Diabète	Diabetes	Dijabetes
Diabete insipido	Diabetes insipidus	Diabète insipide	Diabetes insípida	Dijabetes insipidus
Diabete mellito	Diabetes mellitus	Diabète sucré	Diabetes mellitus (diabetes sacarina)	Dijabetes melitus
Diabete mellito di tipo 1	Diabetes mellitus type 1	Diabète sucré de type 1 (diabète insulino-dépendant)	Diabetes mellitus tipo 1	Dijabetes melitus tip 1
Diabete mellito di tipo 2	Diabetes mellitus type 2	Diabète sucré de type 2 (diabète insulinorésistant)	Diabetes mellitus tipo 2	Dijabetes melitus tip 2
Diarrea	Diarrhea	Diarrhée	Diarrea	Proljev (dijarea)
Difetto cardiaco congenito	Congenital heart defect	Malformation congénitale du coeur	Malformación cardiaca congénita	Urođena srčana greška
Difetto del piede	Foot deformity	Difformité du pied	Deformidad del pie	Deformacija stopala
Difetto del setto interatriale	Atrial septal defect	Communication inter-auriculaire	Comunicación interauricular	Atrijski septalni defekt
Difetto del setto ventricolare	Ventricular septal defect	Communication inter-ventriculaire	Comunicación interventricular	Ventrikularni septalni defekt
Difficoltà a defecare (tenesmo)	Difficult defecation (tenesmus)	Difficulté à déféquer (ténesme)	Dificultad para la defecación (tenesmo rectal)	Otežano pražnjenje crijeva (otežana defekacija)
Difficoltà a deglutire (disfagia)	Difficult swallowing (dysphagia)	Difficulté de deglutition (dysphagie)	Dificultad para tragar (disfagia)	Otežano gutanje (disfagija)

Italiano	Inglese	Francese	Spagnolo	Croato
Difterite	Diphtheria	Diphtérie	Difteria	Difterija
Dilatazione gastrica acuta	Acute gastric dilatation	Dilatation aiguë de l'estomac	Dilatación aguda del estómago	Akutna dilatacija želuca
Dimagramento	Weight loss (weight reduction)	Amaigrissement	Pérdida de peso	Mršavljenje
Diminuita escrezione urinaria (oliguria)	Decreased production of urine (oliguria)	Raréfaction du volume des urines (oligurie)	Disminución de producción de orina (oliguria)	Smanjeno izlučivanje urina (oligurija)
Dipendenza	Addiction	Dépendance (addiction)	Adicción (dependencia)	Ovisnost
Dipendenza sessuale	Sexual addiction	Sexualité compulsive	Adicción sexual	Ovisnost o seksu
Discartrosi (discopatia degenerativa)	Discarthrosis (degenerative disc disease)	Arthrose du disque intervertébral	Discartrosis	Diskartroza
Discondroplasia	Dyschondroplasia	Dyschondroplasie	Discondroplasia	Dishondroplazija
Diseguaglianza del diametro delle pupille (anisocoria)	Unequal size of pupils (anisocoria)	Différence de taille entres les pupilles (anisocorie)	Asimetría del tamaño de las pupilas (anisocoria)	Nejednaka veličina zjenica (anizokorija)
Disgenesia gonadica	Testicular dysgenesis	Dysgénésie testiculaire	Disgénesis testicular	Testikularna disgeneza
Disgerminoma	Dysgerminoma	Dysgerminome	Disgerminoma	Disgerminom
Disidratazione	Dehydration	Déshydratation	Deshidratación	Dehidracija
Disidrosi	Dyshidrosis	Dyshidrose	Eczema dishidrótico	Dishidroza
Dislessia	Dyslexia	Dyslexie	Dislexia	Disleksija
Dislocazione dei frammenti	Dislocated fragments	Fragments deboîtées	Dislocación de los fragmentos	Dislokacija ulomaka
Disordine della differenziazione sessuale	Sexual differentiation disorder	Trouble de la différenciation sexuelle	Trastorno de la diferenciación sexual	Poremećaj spolne diferencijacije
Disordine del movimento	Movement disorder	Trouble du mouvement	Trastorno de movimiento	Poremećaj kretanja
Disorientamento	Disorientation	Désorientation	Desorientación	Dezorijentiranost
Dispepsia	Dyspepsia (upset stomach)	Dyspepsie	Dispepsia (indigestión)	Dispepsija (nervozni želudac)
Displasia cervicale	Cervical dysplasia	Dysplasie du col de l'utérus	Displasia del cuello uterino	Cervikalna displazija
Displasia fibrosa	Fibrous dysplasia	Dysplasie fibreuse	Displasia fibrosa	Fibrozna displazija
Displasia ventricolare destra aritmogena	Arrhytmogenic right ventricular dysplasia	Dysplasie ventriculair droite arythmogène	Displasia arritmogénica ventricular derecha	Aritmogena displazija desne klijetke
Dispnea parossistica notturna	Cardiac asthma (paroxysmal nocturnal dyspnea)	Dyspnée chez un cardiaque	Disnea paroxística nocturna	Srčana astma (paroksizmalna dispneja)
Dissecazione aortica	Aortic dissection	Dissection aortique	Disección aórtica	Disekcija aorte
Dissenteria	Dysentery (flux)	Dysenterie	Disentería	Dizenterija
Distacco di retina	Retinal ablation (retinal detachment)	Décollement de la rétine	Desprendimiento de retina	Odvajanje mrežnice (ablacija retine)
Distonia	Dystonia	Dystonie	Distonía	Distonija
Distorsione	Joint distortion	Distorsion articulaire	Distorsión articular	Uganuće zgloba (distorzija zgloba)
Distorsione alla caviglia	Ankle distortion	Distorsion de la cheville	Distorsión del tobillo	Uganuće skočnog zgloba
Distrofia	Dystrophy	Dystrophie	Distrofia	Distrofija
Distrofia di Duchenne	Duchenne muscular dystrophy	Myopathie de Duchenne	Distrofia muscular de Duchenne	Duchenneova mišićna distrofija
Distrofia muscolare	Muscular dystrophy	Dystrophie musculaire	Distrofia muscular	Mišićna distrofija
Distrofia muscolare progressiva	Progressive muscular dystrophy	Dystrophie musculaire progressive	Distrofia muscular	Progresivna mišićna distrofija
Disturbi mestruali	Menstrual disorder	Troubles du cycle menstruel	Trastorno menstrual	Menstrualne smetnje
Disturbo borderline di personalità	Borderline personality disorder	Personnalité borderline	Trastorno límite de la personalidad	Granični poremećaj osobnosti
Disturbo del comportamento alimentare	Eating disorder	Trouble de conduite alimentaire	Trastorno alimentario	Poremećaj ishrane
Disturbo del linguaggio verbale (afasia)	Speech difficulty (dysphasia)	Trouble de l'apprentissage du langage (dysphasie)	Trastorno del lenguaje (disfasia)	Otežan govor (disfazija)
Disturbo del sonno	Sleeping disorder	Trouble du sommeil	Trastorno del sueño	Poremećaj spavanja
Disturbo dell'equilibrio	Balance disorder	Trouble de l'équilibre	Trastorno del equilibrio	Poremećaj ravnoteže
Disturbo dell'udito	Hearing disorder	Trouble de l'audition	Trastorno de la audición	Poremećaj sluha
Disturbo dell'umore	Behavioral disorder	Trouble du comportement	Trastorno del comportamiento	Poremećaj ponašanja
Disturbo della concentrazione	Attention deficit disorder	Trouble déficit de l'attention	Trastorno por déficit de atención	Poremećaj koncentracije
Disturbo della coordinazione muscolare (atassia)	Lack of coordination of muscle movements (ataxia)	Trouble de coordination des mouvements musculaires (ataxie)	Descoordinación en el movimientos musculares (ataxia)	Poremećaj koordinacije mišićnih pokreta (ataksija)
Disturbo della minzione	Urination disorder	Trouble de la miction	Trastorno de la micción	Poremećaj mokrenja
Disturbo della vista	Sight disorder	Trouble de la vue	Trastorno de la visión	Poremećaj vida
Disturbo di apprendimento	Learning disability	Trouble de l'apprentissage	Dificultad del aprendizaje	Poremećaj učenja
Disturbo di personalità	Personality disorder	Trouble de la personnalité	Trastorno de personalidad	Poremećaj osobnosti
Disturbo post traumatico da stress	Posttraumatic stress disorder	Trouble de stress post-traumatique	Trastorno por estrés postraumático	Posttraumatski stresni poremećaj (PTSP)
Dita ippocratiche (dita a bacchetta di tamburo)	Finger clubbing (digital clubbing)	Hippocratisme digital (doigts en baguettes de tambour)	Acropaquia (hipocratismo digital)	Batićasti prsti
Diverticolite	Diverticulitis	Diverticulite	Diverticulitis	Divertikulitis

Italiano	Inglese	Francese	Spagnolo	Croato
Diverticolo	Diverticulum	Diverticule	Divertículo	Divertikul
Diverticolo del colon	Colon diverticulum	Diverticule du côlon	Divertículo del colon	Divertikul na debelom crijevu
Diverticolo di Meckel	Small intestine diverticulum	Diverticule de Meckel	Divertículo de Meckel	Divertikul tankog crijeva
Diverticolo duodenale	Duodenal diverticulum	Diverticule duodenal	Divertículo duodenal	Divertikul na dvanaesniku
Diverticolosi	Diverticulosis	Diverticulose	Enfermedad diverticular	Divertikuloza
Dolore	Pain	Douleur	Dolor	Bol
Dolore acuto	Acute pain	Douleur aiguë	Dolor agudo	Akutna bol
Dolore addominale	Abdominal pain	Douleur abdominale	Dolor abdominal	Bol u trbuhu
Dolore al seno (mastalgia)	Breast pain (mastalgia)	Douleur au sein (mastodynie)	Dolor en la mama (mastalgia)	Bol u dojci (mastalgija)
Dolore auricolare (otalgia)	Ear pain (otalgia)	Mal à l'oreille (otalgie)	Dolor en oído (otalgia)	Bol u uhu (otalgija)
Dolore cronico	Chronic pain	Douleur chronique	Dolor crónico	Kronična bol
Dolore durante rapporto sessuale (dispareunia)	Painful sexual intercourse (dyspareunia)	Douleur lors du rapport sexuel (dyspareunie)	Relación sexual dolorosa (coitalgia, dispareunia)	Bol pri snošaju
Dolore fantomatico	Phantom pain	Douleur du membre fantôme	Dolor del miembro fantasma	Fantomska bol
Dolore muscolare (mialgia)	Muscle pain (myalgia)	Douleur musculaire (myalgie)	Dolor muscular (mialgia)	Bol u mišiću (mijalgija)
Dolore ottuso	Dull pain	Douleur sourde	Dolor sordo	Tupa bol
Dolore ovulatorio (mittelschmerz)	Ovulation pain (mittelschmerz)	Douleurs ovulatoires (mittelschmerz)	Ovulación dolorosa	Bolna ovulacija (mittelschmerz)
Dolore pulsante	Pulsing pain	Douleur pulsatile	Dolor pulsante	Pulsirajuća bol
Dolore pungente	Twinging pain	Élancement	Dolor tipo punzada	Probadajuća bol
Dolore tagliente	Sharp pain	Douleur tranchante	Dolor afilado	Oštra bol
Dolore toracico	Chest pain	Douleur thoracique	Dolor torácico	Bol u prsištu
Dotto arterioso di Botallo	Ductus arteriosus (ductus Botalli shunt)	Canal artériel	Ductus arteriosus (conducto arterioso de Botal)	Ductus Botalli
Dotto arterioso persistente (ductus arteriosus persistente)	Patent ductus arteriosus (persistent ductus arteriosus)	Persistance du canal artériel	Ductus arterioso persistente (conducto arterioso persistente)	Otvoreni ductus arteriosus (Ductus arteriosus persistens)
Dracunculiasi	Dracunculiasis	Dracunculose	Dracunculiasis	Drakunkulijaza
Ebola	Ebola hemorrhagic fever	Fièvre Ébola	Fiebre hemorrágica viral de Ébola	Groznica Ebola
Eccessiva crescita della lingua (macroglossia)	Enlarged tongue (macroglossia)	Augmentation de la langue (macroglossie)	Lengua más grande de lo normal (macroglosia)	Uvećani jezik (makroglosija)
Eccesso di colesterolo nel sangue (ipercolesterolemia)	High blood cholesterol (hypercholesterolemia)	Choléstérol sanguin élévée (hypercholestérolémie)	Colesterol elevado de la sangre (hipercolesterolemia)	Povišeni kolesterol u krvi (hiperkolesterolemija)
Eccesso di glucosio nel sangue (iperglicemia)	High blood sugar (hyperglicemia)	Taux de sucre dans le sang élevé (hyperglycémie)	Cantidad excesiva de glucosa en la sangre (hiperglucemia, hiperglicemia)	Povišeni šećer u krvi (hiperglikemija)
Echinococcosi (idatidosi)	Echinococcosis (hydatid disease)	Échinococcose	Hidatidosis (equinococosis)	Ehinokokoza
Echinococcosi epatica	Hepatic echinococcosis	Échinococcose hépatique	Hidatidosis hepática	Ehinokokoza jetre
Echinococcosi polmonare	Pulmonary echinococcosis	Échinococcose pulmonaire	Hidatidosis pulmonar	Ehinokokoza pluća
Ecolalia	Echolalia	Écholalie	Ecolalia	Eholalija
Ecoprassia (imitazione spontanea di movimenti osservati)	Echopraxia (involuntary repetition of the observed movements of another)	Échopraxie (tendance spontanée à répéter les mouvements d'une autre personne)	Ecopraxia (repetición de los movimientos de otra persona)	Ehopraksija (nevoljno ponavljanje tuđih pokreta)
Eczema	Eczema	Eczéma	Eccema (eczema)	Ekcem
Edema	Edema	Oedème	Edema (hidropesía)	Edem
Edema cerebrale	Cerebral edema	Oedème cérébral	Edema cerebral	Edem mozga
Edema diffuso (anasarca)	Generalized edema (anasarca)	Oedème généralisé (anasarque)	Anasarca	Generalizirani edem (anasarka)
Edema polmonare	Pulmonary edema	Oedème pulmonaire	Edema pulmonar	Plućni edem
Edema posturale	Postural edema	Oedème postural	Edema postural	Posturalni edem (statički edem)
Eiaculazione precoce	Premature ejaculation	Éjaculation précoce	Eyaculación precoz	Prijevremena ejakulacija
Elefantiasi	Elephantiasis (lymphedema)	Éléphantiasis (filariose lymphatique)	Elefantiasis	Elefantijaza (limfedem)
Elettrosensibilità	Electromagnetic hypersensitivity	Sensibilité électromagnétique	Hipersensibilidad electromagnética	Elektromagnetska hipersenzibilnost
Elevata pressione intracranica	Intracranial hypertension	Hypertension intra-crânienne	Hipertensión intracraneal	Intrakranijalna hipertenzija
Emangioendotelioma	Hemangioendo-thelioma	Hémangio-endothéliome	Hemangioendotelioma	Hemangioendoteliom
Emangioma	Hemangioma	Hémangiome	Hemangioma	Hemangiom
Emangioma capillare	Capillary hemangioma (infantile hemangioma, strawberry hemangioma)	Hémangiome capillaire	Hemangioma capilar (marca de fresa)	Kapilarni hemangiom
Emangioma cavernoso	Cavernous hemangioma	Cavernome (angiome caverneux)	Hemangioma cavernoso	Kavernozni hemangiom
Emartro	Bleeding into joint space (hemarthrosis)	Épanchement de sang à l'intérieur d'une articu-lation (hémarthrose)	Sangrado interno de las articulaciones (hemartrosis)	Krvarenje u zglob (hemartroza)
Ematoma	Hematoma	Hématome	Hematoma	Hematom

Italiano	Inglese	Francese	Spagnolo	Croato
Ematoma cerebrale	Intracerebral hematoma	Hématome intracérébral	Hematoma intracerebral	Intracerebralni hematom
Ematoma epidurale	Epidural hematoma	Hématome épidural	Hematoma epidural	Epiduralni hematom
Ematoma subdurale	Subdural hematoma	Hématome subdural	Hematoma subdural	Subduralni hematom
Ematuria	Blood in urine (hematuria)	Sang dans les urines (hématurie)	Sangre en la orina (hematuria)	Krv u urinu (hematurija)
Embolia adiposa	Fat embolism	Embolie de cholestérol	Embolismo graso	Masna embolija
Embolia dell'arteria	Arterial embolism	Embolie artérielle	Embolia arterial	Arterijska embolija
Embolia gassosa	Air embolism (gas embolism)	Embolie gazeuse	Embolia gaseosa	Zračna embolija
Embolia polmonare	Pulmonary embolism	Embolie pulmonaire	Embolia pulmonar	Plućna embolija
Embolismo (embolia)	Embolism	Embolie	Embolia	Embolija
Emeralopia	Day blindness (hemeralopia)	Héméralopie	Falta de visión en luz brillante (hemeralopia)	Kokošje sljepilo (hemeralopija)
Emesi emorragica (ematemesi)	Vomiting of blood (hematemesis)	Vomissement de sang (hématémèse)	Vómito de sangre (hematemesis)	Povraćanje krvi (hematemeza)
Emicrania	Migraine	Migraine	Migraña (jaqueca)	Migrena
Emicrania cronica parossistica	Chronic paroxysmal hemicrania (Sjaastad syndrome)	Hémicrânie paroxystique chronique	Hemicránea crónica paroxismal	Kronična paroksizmalna hemikranija (Sjaastadov sindrom)
Emissione di urine con difficoltà (disuria)	Difficult urination (dysuria)	Difficulté à uriner (dysurie)	Dificultad al orinar (disuria)	Otežano usporeno mokrenje (dizurija)
Emivertebra	Hemivertebrae	Hémivertèbre	Hemivértebra	Hemivertebra
Emocromatosi	Hemochromatosis	Hémochromatose	Hemocromatosis	Hemokromatoza
Emofilia	Hemophilia	Hémophilie	Hemofilia	Hemofilija
Emopneumotorace	Hemopneumothorax	Hémopneumothorax	Hemoneumotórax	Hemopneumotoraks
Emorragia	Bleeding (haemorrhage)	Saignement (hémorragie)	Desangramiento (hemorragia)	Krvarenje (hemoragija)
Emorragia arteriosa	Arterial bleeding	Hémorragie artérielle	Hemorragia arterial	Arterijsko krvarenje
Emorragia cerebrale	Intracerebral hemorrhage	Hémorragie intracérébrale	Hemorragia intracerebral	Intracerebralno krvarenje
Emorragia epidurale	Epidural bleeding	Hémorragie épidurale	Hemorragia epidural	Epiduralno krvarenje
Emorragia esterna	External bleeding	Saignement externe (hémorragie externe)	Sangrado externo (hemorragia externa)	Vanjsko krvarenje
Emorragia interna	Internal bleeding	Saignement interne (hémorragie interne)	Sangrado interno (hemorragia interna)	Unutarnje krvarenje
Emorragia subaracnoidea	Subarachnoid hemorrhage	Hémorragie sous arachnoïdienne	Hemorragia subaracnoidea	Subarahnoidalno krvarenje
Emorragia subdurale	Subdural hemorrhage	Subdural hemorrhage	Hemorragia subdural	Subduralno krvarenje
Emorragia venosa	Venous bleeding	Saignement veineux	Sangrado venoso (hemorragia venosa)	Vensko krvarenje
Emorroidi	Hemorrhoids	Hémorroïdes	Hemorroides	Hemoroidi
Emosiderosi	Hemosiderosis	Hémosidérosis	Hemosiderosis	Hemosideroza
Emotorace	Hemothorax	Hémothorax	Hemotórax	Hemotoraks
Empiema	Empyema	Empyème	Empiema	Empijem
Encefalite trasmessa da zecche	Tick-borne meningoencephalitis	Méningoencéphalite à tique	Meningoencefalitis de garrapata	Krpeljni meningoencefalitis
Encefalocele	Encephalocele	Encéphalocèle	Encefalocele	Encefalokela
Encefalopatia	Encephalopathy	Encéphalopathie	Encefalopatía	Encefalopatija
Encondroma	Enchondroma	Enchondrome	Encondroma	Enhondrom
Enconpresi	Encopresis	Encoprésie	Encopresis	Enkopreza
Endocardite batterica	Bacterial endocarditis	Endocardite bactérienne	Endocarditis bacteriana	Bakterijski endokarditis
Endometriosi	Endometriosis	Endométriose	Endometriosis	Endometrioza
Enfisema	Emphysema	Emphysème	Enfisema	Emfizem
Enfisema sottocutaneo	Subcutaneous emphysema	Emphisème sous-cutané	Enfisema subcutáneo	Potkožni emfizem
Entesopatia	Enthesopathy	Enthésiopathie	Entesopatía	Entezopatija
Eosinofilia	Eosinophilia	Éosinophilie	Eosinofilia	Eozinofilija
Epatite virale	Viral hepatitis	Hépatite virale	Hepatitis viral	Virusni hepatitis
Epatite virale A	Hepatitis A	Hépatite A	Hepatitis A	Hepatitis A
Epatite virale B	Hepatitis B	Hépatite B	Hepatitis B	Hepatitis B
Epatite virale C	Hepatitis C	Hépatite C	Hepatitis C	Hepatitis C
Epatite virale D	Hepatitis D	Hépatite D	Hepatitis D	Hepatitis D
Epatite virale E	Hepatitis E	Hépatite E	Hepatitis E	Hepatitis E
Ependimoma	Ependymoma	Épendymome	Ependimoma	Ependimom
Epifisiolisi della testa femorale	Epiphyseolysis capitis femoris	Épiphysiolyse de l'extrémité supérieure du fémur	Epifisario de la cabeza femoral (epifisiolisis capitis femoris)	Epifizeoliza glave bedrene kosti
Epilessia	Epilepsy	Épilepsie	Epilepsia	Epilepsija
Epispadia	Epispadias	Épispadias	Epispadia	Epispadija
Epistassi (rinorragia)	Nose bleeding (epistaxis)	Saignement de nez (épistaxis)	Pérdida de sangre por la nariz (epistaxis)	Krvarenje iz nosa (epistaksa)
Erezione persistente dolorosa (priapismo)	Long-lasting painful erection (priapism)	Érection persistente douloureuse (priapisme)	Erección sostenida y dolorosa (priapismo)	Dugotrajna bolna erekcija (prijapizam)
Erisipela	Erysipelas (Ignis sacer, St. Anthony's fire)	Érysipèle (érésipèle)	Erisipela	Crveni vjetar (vrbanac, erizipel)
Erisipeloide	Erysipeloid	Érysipéloïde	Erisipeloide	Erizipeloid
Eritema	Redness of the skin (erythema)	Érythème (rougeur de la peau)	Enrojecimiento de la piel (eritema)	Crvenilo kože (eritem)

Italiano	Inglese	Francese	Spagnolo	Croato
Eritema infettivo (quinta malattia)	Infectious erythema (fifth disease)	Érythème infectieux (cinquième maladie)	Eritema infeccioso (quinta enfermedad)	Infektivni eritem (peta bolest)
Eritroblastosi fetale (malattia emolitica del neonato)	Rh incompatibility (hemolytic disease of the newborn)	Maladie hémolytique du nouveau-né	Enfermedad hemolítica del recién nacido (incompatibilidad Rh)	Rh-inkompatibilnost (hemolitička bolest novorođenčeta)
Eritromelalgia	Erythromelalgia (acromelalgia)	Érythromelalgie	Eritromelalgia	Eritromelalgija
Eritroplachia (eritroplasia)	Erythroplakia (erythroplasia)	Érythroplasie	Eritroplasia	Eritroplazija
Eritroplasia di Queyrat	Erythroplasia of Queyrat	Érythroplasie de Queyrat	Eritroplasia de Queyrat	Eritroplazija Queyrat
Ermafroditismo	Hermaphroditism	Hermaphrodisme	Hermafroditismo	Dvospolnost
Ernia	Hernia	Hernie	Hernia	Kila (bruh, hernija)
Ernia del disco	Spinal disc herniation	Hernie discale	Hernia discal	Hernija intervertrebralnog diska
Ernia diaframmatica	Diaphragmatic hernia	Hernie diaphragmatique	Hernia diafragmática	Dijafragmalna kila
Ernia esterna addominale	External abdominal wall hernia	Hernie de la paroi abdominale (hernie abdominale externe)	Hernia de la pared abdominal	Kila vanjske trbušne stijenke
Ernia iatale	Hiatus hernia	Hernie hiatale	Hernia de hiato	Hijatusna kila
Ernia inguinale	Inguinal hernia	Hernie inguinale	Hernia inguinal	Preponska kila
Ernia ombelicale	Umbilical hernia	Hernie ombilicale	Hernia umbilical	Pupčana kila (umbilikalna hernija)
Erosione cervicale	Cervical erosion	Érosion du col de l'utérus	Erosión cervical	Cervikalna erozija
Erpangina (faringite vescicolare)	Herpangina (mouth blisters)	Herpangine	Herpangina	Herpangina
Eruttazione	Burping (belching)	Rot (renvoi, éructation)	Eructo	Podrigivanje
Esantema	Exanthem	Exanthème	Exantema	Egzantem
Esasperazione (irritazione)	Exasperation	Exaspération (irritation)	Exasperación	Razdražljivost
Esoftalmo	Bulging eyes (exophthalmos)	Exophtalmie (proptose)	Exoftalmos	Izbuljene oči (egzoftalmus)
Esostosi	Exostosis	Exostose	Exostosis	Egzostoza
Esostosi multipla ereditaria	Hereditary multiple exostoses	Maladie des exostoses multiples	Exostosis múltiple hereditaria	Multiple egzostoze
Espettorazione di sangue (emottisi)	Expectoration of blood (hemoptysis)	Rejet de sang issu des voies aériennes (hémoptysie)	Expectoración de sangre (hemoptisis)	Iskašljavanje krvi (hemoptiza, hemoptoja)
Esposizione alle radiazioni ionizzanti	Ionising irradiation	Irradiation ionisante	Exposición a las radiaciones ionizantes	Ionizirajuća ozračenost
Fame	Hunger	Faim	Hambre	Glad
Fame d'aria (dispnea, respirazione difficoltosa)	Shortness of breath (dyspnea)	Difficulté respiratoire (dyspnée)	Falta de aire (disnea)	Zaduha (nedostatak daha, dispneja)
Faringite streptococcica	Streptococcal pharyngitis	Pharyngite streptococcique	Faringitis por estreptococo	Streptokokna angina
Fasciosi plantare	Plantar fasciitis	Fasciite plantaire	Fascitis plantar	Plantarni fasciitis
Fascite necrotizzante	Necrotizing fasciitis	Fasciite nécrosante	Fascitis necrotizante	Nekrotizirajući fasciitis
Febbre	Fever	Fièvre	Fiebre	Groznica (vrućica)
Febbre da fieno	Farmer's lung	Maladie du poumon de fermier	Pulmón de granjero	Farmerska pluća
Febbre da inalazione di fumi metallici	Metal fume fever	Fièvre des métaux	Fiebre de los vapores metálicos	Metalna groznica
Febbre da morso di ratto	Rat-bite fever	Fièvre de la morsure de rat	Fiebre por mordedura de rata	Groznica štakorskog ugriza
Febbre da pappataci (febbre da Flebotomi)	Pappataci fever (phlebotomus fever, sandfly fever)	Fièvre pappataci (fièvre à phlébotomes)	Fiebre pappataci	Papatači-groznica
Febbre da zecca del Colorado	Colorado tick fever (mountain tick fever)	Fièvre à tiques du Colorado (fièvre à tiques des montagnes)	Fiebre del Colorado por garrapatas (fiebre de montaña americana por garrapatas)	Groznica planinskog krpelja
Febbre del Nilo occidentale	West Nile fever	Fièvre du Nil occidental	Fiebre del Nilo Occidental	Groznica zapadnog Nila
Febbre della Rift Valley	Rift Valley fever	Fièvre de la vallée du Rift	Fiebre de Rift Valley	Rift Valley groznica
Febbre di Lassa	Lassa fever	Fièvre de Lassa	Fiebre de Lassa	Groznica Lassa
Febbre di Oroya	Oroya fever (Carrion's disease)	Fièvre d'Oroya (maladie de Carrion)	Fiebre de la Oroya (enfermedad de Carrión, verruga peruana)	Oroya groznica (Carrionova bolest)
Febbre emorragica	Viral hemorrhagic fever	Fièvre hémorragique virale	Fiebre hemorrágica viral	Virusna hemoragijska groznica
Febbre emorragica con sindrome renale (febbre emorragica coreana)	Hemorrhagic fever with renal syndrome (Korean hemorrhagic fever)	Fièvre hémorragique avec syndrome rénal (fièvre hémorragique de Corée)	Fiebre hemorrágica con síndrome renal (fiebre hemorrágica coreana)	Hemoragijska groznica s renalnim sindromom (korejska hemoragijska groznica)
Febbre emorragica Crimean-Congo	Crimean-Congo hemorrhagic fever	Fièvre hémorragique de Congo-Crimée	Fiebre hemorrágica de Crimea-Congo	Krimska hemoragijska groznica
Febbre emorragica di Marburg	Marburg hemorrhagic fever	Fièvre hémorragique de Marbourg	Fiebre hemorrágica de Marburgo	Marburška hemoragijska groznica
Febbre gialla	Yellow fever	Fièvre jaune	Fiebre amarilla	Žuta groznica
Febbre mediterranea familiare	Familial Mediterranean fever	Fièvre méditerranéenne familiale	Fiebre mediterránea familiar	Obiteljska mediteranska groznica

Italiano	Inglese	Francese	Spagnolo	Croato
Febbre paratifoide	Paratyphoid fever	Fièvre paratyphoïde	Fiebre paratifoidea	Trbušni paratifus
Febbre Q	Q fever	Fièvre Q	Fiebre Q	Q-groznica
Febbre reumatica	Rheumatic fever	Rhumatisme articulaire aigu (maladie de Bouillaud)	Fiebre reumática	Reumatska groznica
Febbre ricorrente	Relapsing fever	Fièvre récurrente	Fiebre reincidente	Povratna groznica
Febbre tifoide (tifo)	Typhoid fever (typhoid)	Fièvre typhoïde (typhus abdominal)	Fiebre tifoidea (fiebre entérica)	Tifusna groznica (tifus)
Febbre Zika	Zika fever	Fièvre Zika	Fiebre del Zika	Zika groznica
Feci di colore rosso	Red colored stool	Selles rouges	Heces de color rojo	Crvena stolica
Feci di colore verde	Green stool	Selles vertes	Heces verdes	Zelenkasta stolica
Feci gialle	Yellow stool	Selles jaunes	Heces amarillas	Žuta stolica
Feci picee (melena)	Black stool (melena)	Selles noir (melanea, méléna)	Heces negras (melena)	Crna stolica (melena)
Fenilchetonuria	Phenylketonuria	Phénylcétonurie	Fenilcetonuria	Fenilketonurija
Fenomeno di Bell	Bell's phenomenon	Phénomène de Bell	Fenómeno de Bell	Bellov fenomen
Feocromocitoma	Pheochromocytoma	Phéochromocytome	Feocromocitoma	Feokromocitom (tumor srži nadbubrežne žlijezde)
Ferita	Wound (injury, lesion)	Plaie	Herida	Rana
Ferita chimica	Chemical injuries	Altération d'origine chimique	Lesiones químicas	Kemijske ozljede
Ferita da arma da fuoco	Gunshot wound	Blessure par balle	Herida de bala	Prostrijelna rana
Ferita da morso	Bite wound	Blessure par morsure	Herida por mordedura	Ugrizna rana
Ferita da punta	Stab wound	Coup de couteau	Estocada	Ubodna rana
Ferita da taglio	Cut wound	Plaie par objet tranchant	Herida por corte	Rezna rana (posjekotina)
Ferita esplosiva	Explosive wound	Blessure par explosion	Lesión por explosión	Eksplozivna rana
Ferita termica	Thermal wound	Blessure thermique	Herida térmica	Termička rana
Ferite provocate da esplosioni termonucleari	Thermonuclear injuries	Lésions provoquées par une explosion thermonucléaire	Lesiones por una explosión termonuclear	Termonuklearne ozljede
Fibrillazione atriale	Atrial fibrillation	Fibrillation auriculaire	Fibrilación auricular	Atrijska fibrilacija
Fibrillazione ventricolare	Ventricular fibrillation	Fibrillation ventriculaire	Fibrilación ventricular	Ventrikularna fibrilacija
Fibroadenoma	Fibroadenoma	Fibroadénome	Fibroadenoma	Fibroadenom
Fibroelastosi endocardica	Endocardial fibroelastosis	Fibroélastose endocardique	Fibroelastosis endocardial	Fibroelastoza endokarda
Fibroistiocitoma benigno	Fibrous histiocytoma	Histiocytome fibreux	Histiocitoma fibroso	Fibrozni histiocitom
Fibroma	Fibroma	Fibrome	Fibroma	Fibrom
Fibroma condromixoide	Chondromyxoid fibroma	Fibrome chondromyxoïde	Fibroma condromixoide	Hondromiksoidni fibrom
Fibromialgia	Fibromyalgia	Fibromyalgie	Fibromialgia	Fibromialgija
Fibrosarcoma	Fibrosarcoma (fibroblastic sarcoma)	Fibrosarcome	Fibrosarcoma	Fibrosarkom
Fibrosi	Fibrosis	Fibrose	Fibrosis	Fibroza
Fibrosi cistica	Cystic fibrosis	Mucoviscidose (fibrose kystique)	Fibrosis quística (mucoviscidosis)	Cistična fibroza
Fibrosi polmonare idiopatica	Idiopathic pulmonary fibrosis	Fibrose pulmonaire idiopathique	Fibrosis pulmonar idiopática	Plućna idiopatska fibroza
Fibrosi retroperitoneale	Retroperitoneal fibrosis (Ormond's disease)	Fibrose rétropéritonéale (maladie d'Ormond)	Fibrosis retroperitoneal	Retroperitonealna fibroza (Ormondova bolest)
Fibrosi tendinea	Tendinous fibrositis	Fibrosite du tendon	Fibrositis de tendón	Fibrozitis tetive
Fibrosite di mano	Hand fibrositis	Fasciite de la main (fasciite palmaire)	Fibrositis de la mano	Fibrozitis šake
Fibrosite muscolare	Muscular fibrositis	Fibrosite musculaire	Fibrositis (reumatismo muscular)	Fibrozitis mišića
Filariasi	Filariasis	Filariose	Filariasis	Filarijaza
Fimosi	Phimosis	Phimosis	Fimosis	Fimoza
Fissura anale	Anal fissure	Fissure anale	Fisura anal	Analna fisura
Fistola	Fistula	Fistule	Fístula	Fistula
Fistola anale	Anal fistula	Fistule anale	Fístula anal	Analna fistula
Fistola broncopleurica	Bronchopleural fistula	Fistule bronchopleurale	Fístula bronco-pleural	Bronhopleuralna fistula
Flebotrombosi	Phlebothrombosis	Phlébothrombose	Flebotrombosis	Flebotromboza
Flemmone	Phlegmon	Phlegmon	Flegmón	Flegmona
Flusso di sangue nella tuba di Falloppio	Bleeding into the fallopian tube (hematosalpinx)	Collection de sang dans la trompe de Fallope (hématosalpinx)	Colección de sangre en la trompa de Falopio (hematosalpinx)	Krvarenje u jajovod (hematosalpinks)
Fobia	Phobia	Phobie	Fobia	Fobija
Folgorazione (elettrocuzione)	Electrical injuries (electric shock)	Électrisation	Lesiones por corriente eléctrica	Ozljede električnom strujom (strujni udar)
Follicolite	Folliculitis	Folliculite	Foliculitis	Folikulitis
Follicoloma	Granulosa cell tumor	Tumeur de la granulosa	Tumor de células de la granulosa (tumor de teca-granulosa)	Granuloza tumor
Forfora	Dandruff	Pellicule	Caspa	Perut
Foruncolo	Furuncle (boil)	Furoncle	Forúnculo (furúnculo)	Furunkul (čir na koži)
Fotofobia	Photophobia (fear of light)	Photophobie (crainte de la lumière)	Fotofobia (intolerancia a la luz)	Fotofobija (strah od svjetla)
Framboesia	Yaws (pian)	Pian	Pian (frambesia)	Frambezija
Frattura	Broken bone (bone fracture)	Fracture des os	Fractura de hueso	Prijelom kosti (fraktura kosti)
Frattura a legno verde	Greenstick fracture	Fracture en bois vert	Fractura en rama verde	Prijelom mlade kosti
Frattura a spirale	Spiral fracture	Fracture en spirale	Fractura espiral	Spiralni prijelom kosti

Italiano	Inglese	Francese	Spagnolo	Croato
Frattura aperta (frattura esposta)	Open fracture (compound fracture)	Fracture ouverte	Fractura abierta	Otvoreni prijelom kosti
Frattura comminuta	Comminuted fracture	Fracture comminutive	Fractura cominuta	Kominutivni prijelom kosti
Frattura con dislocazione	Fracture with displacement	Fracture à déplacement	Fractura-dislocación	Prijelom kosti s pomakom
Frattura da stress	Stress fracture	Fracture de fatigue	Fractura por estrés	Prijelom zamora
Frattura da stress della tibia	Tibia stress fracture	Fracture de fatigue du tibia	Fractura por estrés de la tibia	Prijelom zamora goljenične kosti
Frattura del bacino	Broken pelvis (pelvis fracture)	Fracture du bassin	Fractura de pelvis	Prijelom zdjelice
Frattura del calcagno	Broken heel bone (calcaneus fracture)	Fracture du calcanéus	Fractura del calcáneo	Prijelom petne kosti
Frattura del capitello radiale	Radial head fracture (radial capitulum fracture)	Fracture de la tête radiale	Fractura de la cabeza del radio	Prijelom glavice palčane kosti
Frattura del collo del femore	Femoral neck fracture	Fracture du col du fémur	Fractura de cuello del fémur	Prijelom vrata bedrene kosti
Frattura del collo dell'omero	Humeral neck fracture	Fracture du col de l'humérus	Fractura de cuello del húmero	Prijelom vrata nadlaktične kosti
Frattura del corpo vertebrale	Broken vertebral body (vertebral corpus fracture)	Fracture du plateau vertébral	Fractura de cuerpo vertebral	Prijelom trupa kralješka
Frattura del femore	Broken thighbone (femur fracture)	Fracture du fémur	Fractura de fémur	Prijelom bedrene kosti
Frattura del metatarso	Broken foot (metatarsal fracture)	Fracture métatarsienne	Fractura de metatarso	Prijelom kosti stopala
Frattura del radio	Radius fracture	Fracture du radius	Fractura del radio	Prijelom palčane kosti
Frattura del terzo distale di tibia e perone	Supramaleolar fracture of tibia and fibula	Fracture tibia péroné sus-malléolaire	Fractura supramaleolar de tibia y peroné	Supramaleolarni prijelom potkoljenice
Frattura dell'alluce	Broken big toe (fractured hallux)	Fracture du gros orteil	Fractura de los huesos del dedo gordo del pie	Prijelom falange nožnog palca
Frattura dell'epicondilo omerale	Epicondylar elbow fracture	Fracture du condyle huméral	Fractura de epicóndilo humeral	Prijelom kondila nadlaktične kosti
Frattura dell'olecrano	Broken elbow (olecranon fracture)	Fracture de l'olécrâne	Fractura de olécranon	Prijelom lakatnog vrha (prijelom olekranona)
Frattura dell'omero	Broken upper arm (humerus fracture)	Fracture de l'humérus	Fractura del húmero	Prijelom nadlaktice
Frattura dell'osso navicolare	Broken navicular bone (navicular fracture)	Fracture du scaphoïde	Fractura de escafoides (fractura navicular)	Prijelom navikularne kosti
Frattura dell'ulna	Broken ulna (ulna fracture)	Fracture de l'ulna	Fractura-cúbito	Prijelom lakatne kosti
Frattura della base del cranio	Base of skull fracture (basal skull fracture)	Fracture de la base du crâne	Fractura de la base del cráneo	Prijelom baze lubanje
Frattura della caviglia	Broken ankle (ankle fracture)	Fracture de la cheville	Fractura de tobillo	Prijelom gležnja
Frattura della clavicola	Broken collarbone (clavicle fracture)	Fracture de la clavicule	Fractura de clavícula	Prijelom ključne kosti
Frattura della costola	Broken rib (rib fracture)	Fracture de côte	Fractura de costilla	Prijelom rebra
Frattura della diafisi femorale	Diaphyseal tightbone fracture	Fracture de la diaphyse fémorale	Fractura de la diáfisis del fémur	Prijelom dijafize bedrene kosti
Frattura della falange del dito	Broken finger (finger fracture)	Fracture du doigt	Fractura de falange del dedo	Prijelom članka prsta
Frattura della fibula	Broken fibula (fibula fracture)	Fracture de la fibula	Fractura del peroné	Prijelom lisne kosti
Frattura della mascella e/o della mandibola	Upper and/or lower jaw fracture (broken upper/lower jaw)	Fracture du maxillaire et/ou de la mandibule	Fractura de maxilar y/o mandíbula	Prijelom gornje i/ili donje čeljusti
Frattura della rotula	Broken knee cap (patellar fracture)	Fracture de rotule	Fractura de la rótula	Prijelom ivera (prijelom patele)
Frattura della scapola	Broken shoulder blade (scapula fracture)	Fracture de la scapula	Fractura de escápula	Prijelom lopatice
Frattura della tibia	Broken shinbone (tibia fracture)	Fracture du tibia	Fractura de tibia	Prijelom goljenične kosti
Frattura di Pouteau-Colles (frattura delle metafisi radiali distali)	Distal radial fracture	Fracture de l'extrémité inferieure du radius (fracture de Pouteau-Colles)	Fractura distal del radio	Prijelom palčane kosti loco typico
Frattura di radio e ulna	Broken forearm (fractured ulna and radius)	Fracture du radius et du cubitus	Fractura de radio y cúbito	Prijelom obje podlaktične kosti
Frattura di tibia e perone	Broken lower leg bones (fractured tibia and fibula)	Fracture du tibia et de la fibula	Fractura de tibia y peroné	Prijelom obje kosti potkoljenice
Frattura diafisaria dell'omero	Diaphyseal humeral fracture	Fracture diaphysaire de l'humérus	Fractura diafisaria del húmero	Prijelom nadlaktice u području dijafize
Frattura incompleta (infrazione)	Incomplete fracture	Fracture incomplète	Fractura incompleta	Nepotpuni prijelom kosti (napuknuće kosti)
Frattura obliqua	Oblique fracture	Fracture oblique	Fractura obliqua	Kosi prijelom kosti
Frattura ripetuta	Refracturing (repeated fracture)	Fracture répétée	Fractura repetida	Opetovani prijelom kosti
Frattura semplice	Simple bone fracture	Fracture simple	Fractura simple	Jednostavni prijelom kosti
Frattura sovracondiloidea del femore	Supracondylar femoral fracture	Fracture supracondylienne du fémur	Fractura supracondilar del fémur	Suprakondilarni prijelom bedrene kosti

Italiano	Inglese	Francese	Spagnolo	Croato
Frattura sovracondiloidea di omero	Supracondylar humerus fracture	Fracture supracondylienne de l'humérus	Fractura supracondilar del húmero	Suprakondilarni prijelom nadlaktice
Frattura trasversale	Transverse fracture	Fracture transversale	Fractura transversal	Poprečni prijelom kosti
Fratture spontanee	Spontaneous fractures	Fractures spontanées	Fracturas espontáneas	Spontane frakture
Frigidità	Frigidity	Frigidité	Frigidez	Frigidnost
Fuoriuscita (scolo)	Discharge	Sécrétion (suintement, écoulement)	Flujo (descarga, secreción)	Iscjedak
Fuoriuscita di sangue dall'orecchio (otorragia)	Ear bleeding	Saignement de l'oreille	Hemorragia de oído (otorragia)	Krvarenje iz uha
Fuoriuscita vaginale	Vaginal discharge	Pertes vaginales	Flujo vaginal	Vaginalni iscjedak
Fusione di vertebre cervicali (Sindrome di Klippel Feil)	Congenital fusion of cervical vertebrae (Klippel-Feil syndrome)	Fusion congénitale de vertèbres cervicales (Syndrome de Klippel-Feil)	Fusión congenita de vértebras cervicales (síndrome de Klippel-Feil)	Srašteni vrat (sindrom Klippel-Feil)
Galattorrea	Galactorrhea	Galactorrhée	Galactorrea	Galaktoreja
Gangrena di Fournier	Fournier gangrene	Gangrène de Fournier	Gangrena de Fournier	Fournierova gangrena
Gangrena secca	Dry gangrene	Gangrène sèche	Gangrena seca	Suha gangrena
Gangrena umida	Wet gangrene	Gangrène humide	Gangrena húmeda	Vlažna gangrena
Gangrene gassosa	Gas gangrene	Gangrène gazeuse	Gangrena gaseosa	Plinska gangrena
Gastralgia	Epigastric pain	Douleur épigastrique	Dolor epigástrico	Bol u epigastriju
Gastroenterite	Gastroenteritis	Gastroentérite	Gastroenteritis	Gastroenteritis
Giardiasi (lambliasi)	Lambliasis (giardiasis)	Lambliase (giardiase)	Giardiasis (lambliasis)	Lamblijaza (giardijaza)
Gibbo (gobba, gibbosità)	Hunchback	Bossu	Joroba	Grba
Gigantismo	Gigantism	Gigantisme	Gigantismo	Divovski stas
Ginecomastia	Gynecomastia	Gynécomastie	Ginecomastia	Ginekomastija
Ginocchio del nuotatore a rana (stiramento cronico del legamento mediale)	Swimmer's knee	Syndrome du brasseur aux genoux	Rodilla de nadador de pecho (bursitis de la pata de ganso)	Plivačko koljeno
Ginocchio valgo	Knock knees (genu valgum)	Genou cagneux (genu valgum, genou en X)	Genu valgo	Genu valgum
Ginocchio varo (genu varum)	Bow legs (genu varum)	Genu varum	Genu varum	Genu varum
Giocco d'azzardo patologico	Gambling addiction (ludomania)	Jeu pathologique (jeu compulsif)	Adicción a jugar (ludopatía, ludomanía)	Ovisnost o kockanju (ludopatija)
Glaucoma	Glaucoma	Glaucome	Glaucoma	Glaukom
Glicosuria (mellituria)	Glucose in urine (glycosuria)	Sucre dans les urines (glycosurie)	Azúcar en orina (glucosuria)	Šećer u urinu (glikozurija)
Glioblastoma	Glioblastoma	Glioblastome	Glioblastoma	Glioblastom
Glioma	Glioma	Gliome	Glioma	Gliom
Gliosi	Gliosis	Gliose	Gliosis	Glioza
Glomangioma (paraganglioma)	Glomus tumor (glomangioma)	Tumeur glomique (glomangiome)	Tumor glómico (glomangioma)	Glomus-tumor
Glomerulonefrite	Glomerulonephritis	Gloméluronéphrite	Glomerulonefritis	Glomerulonefritis
Gomito del tennista (epicondilite)	Tennis elbow	Épicondylite latérale	Codo del tenista (epicondilitis lateral)	Teniski lakat
Gonadoblastoma	Gonadoblastoma	Gonadoblastome	Gonadoblastoma	Gonadoblastom
Gonfiezza e venti (flatulenza)	Bloating and gases (flatulence)	Ballonnements et vesse (flatulence)	Hinchazón y gases (flatulencia, ventosidad)	Nadutost i vjetrovi
Gonfiore	Swelling	Gonflement (enflure)	Hinchazón	Oteklina
Gonorrea (blenorragia)	Gonorrhea	Gonorrhée (blennorragie, chaude-pisse)	Gonorrea (blenorragia, blenorrea)	Gonoreja (kapavac, triper)
Gotta	Gout (gouty arthritis)	Goutte	Gota (enfermedad gotosa)	Ulozi (giht)
Gozzo	Goiter	Goitre	Bocio (coto)	Guša (struma)
Gozzo multinodulare	Nodular goiter	Goitre multinodulaire	Bocio nodular	Čvorasta guša (nodularna struma)
Graffio (graffiatura)	Scratch	Égratignure	Rasguño	Ogrebotina
Granulocitosi	Granulocytosis	Polynucléose	Granulocitosis	Granulocitoza
Gravidanza ectopica	Ectopic pregnancy (extrauterine pregnancy)	Grossesse extra-utérine	Embarazo ectópico	Izvanmaternična trudnoća (ektopična trudnoća)
Herpes genitalis	Genital herpes	Herpès génital	Herpes genital	Genitalni herpes
Herpes simplex	Herpes simplex	Herpès (infection herpétique)	Herpes simple	Herpes simpleks
Herpes zoster	Herpes zoster	Zona	Herpes zóster (herpes zona)	Herpes zoster
Ictus emorragico	Hemorrhagic brain infarction	Infarctus cérébral hémorragique	Infarto cerebral hemorrágico	Hemoragijski infarkt mozga
Idremia	Hydremia	Hydrémie	Hidremia	Hidremija
Idrocefalo	Hydrocephalus	Hydrocéphalie	Hidrocefalia	Hidrocefalus
Idrocele	Hydrocele	Hydrocèle	Hidrocele	Hidrokela
Idrofobia	Aquaphobia	Aquaphobie	Acuafobia	Hidrofobija
Idronefrosi	Hydronephrosis	Hydronéphrose	Hidronefrosis	Hidronefroza
Idrope	Hydrops	Hydrops	Hidrops	Hidrops
Idrope della colecisti	Gallbladder hydrops	Hydrops de la vésicule biliaire	Hidrops vesicular	Hidrops žučnog mjehura
Idropericardio	Pericardial effusion (hydropericard)	Épanchement péricardique	Derrame pericárdico	Hidroperikard
Idrotorace	Hydrothorax	Hydrothorax	Hidrotórax	Hidrotoraks
Ifema	Hyphema	Hyphème	Hipema	Hifema
Igroma	Hygroma	Hygroma	Higroma	Higrom

Italiano	Inglese	Francese	Spagnolo	Croato
Ileo	Ileus	Iléus	Íleo	Ileus
Imbecillità	Imbecility	Imbécillité	Imbecilidad	Slaboumnost
Immunodeficienza	Immunodeficiency	Immunodéficience	Inmunodeficiencia	Sniženi imunitet
Impetigine	Impetigo	Impétigo	Impétigo	Impetigo
Impotenza	Impotency	Impotence	Impotencia	Impotencija
Impulso a vomitare	Urge to vomit	Envie de vomir	Ganas de vomitar	Podražaj na povraćanje
Incapacità di percipire gli odori (disosmia)	Loss of olfaction (anosmia)	Perte de la sensibilité aux odeurs (anosmie)	Pérdida del sentido del olfato (anosmia)	Gubitak osjeta mirisa
Incapacità di percipire i sapori (ageusia)	Loss of the sense of taste (ageusia)	Perte du sens du goût (agueusie)	Pérdida del sentido del gusto (ageusia)	Gubitak osjeta okusa
Incontinenza	Incontinence	Incontinence	Incontinencia	Inkontinencija
Incontinenza urinaria	Urinary incontinence	Incontinence urinaire	Incontinencia urinaria	Urinarna inkotinencija
Incontinenza urinaria da sforzo	Stress urinary incontinence	Incontinence urinarie d'effort	Incontinencia urinaria por estrés	Stres-inkontinencija urina
Incoscienza (stato di incoscienza)	Unconsciousness	Absence de la conscience	Inconsciencia	Nesvjestica
Indigestione	Indigestion	Indigestion	Indigestión	Probavne smetnje
Induratio penis plastica (malattia di Peyronie)	Peyronie's disease (induratio penis plastica)	Maladie de La Peyronie	Enfermedad de La Peyronie (induración plástica del pene)	Plastična induracija penisa
Inedia	Starvation	Famine	Inanición	Izgladnjelost
Infarto	Infarct	Infarctus	Infarto	Infarkt
Infarto miocardico acuto	Heart attack (myocardial infarction)	Infarctus du myocarde	Infarto de miocardio	Infarkt miokarda
Infarto polmonare	Pulmonary infarction	Infarctus pulmonaire	Infarto pulmonar	Infarkt pluća
Infestazione da pidocchi (pediculosi)	Infestation with head lice (pediculosis)	Infestation par des poux (pédiculose)	Infestación por piojos (pediculosis)	Infestacija ušima (ušljivost, pedikuloza)
Infestazione da pidocchi del pube (ftiriasi)	Infestation with pubic lice (phthiriasis)	Infestation par des poux du pubic (phtiriase)	Infestación por ladilla (ftiriasis)	Infestacija stidnim ušima (iftirijaza)
Infestazione da vermi (elmintiasi)	Infestation with intestinal parasitic warms (helminthiasis)	Infestation par des vers parasites intestinaux (helminthiase)	Infestación de gusanos (helmintiasis)	Infestacija crijevnim parazitima (helmintijaza)
Infezione (malattia infettiva)	Infection	Infection	Infección	Infekcija
Infezione batterica	Bacterial infection	Infection bactérienne	Infección bacteriana	Bakterijska infekcija
Infezione da clamidia	Chlamydia infection	Infection à Chlamydia	Infección por clamidia	Klamidijska infekcija
Infezione da Papilloma Virus Umano (HPV)	Human papilloma virus (HPV) infection	Infection par le virus du papillome humain (VPH)	Infeccion por el virus del papilom humano (VPH)	Infekcija humanim papiloma virusom (HPV)
Infezione del tratto respiratorio superiore	Upper respiratory tract infection	Infection respiratoire haute	Infección respiratoria alta	Infekcija gornjih dišnih puteva
Infezione dell'apparato osteo-articolare (osteomielite)	Infection of the bone or bone marrow (osteomyelitis)	Infection osseuse ou de la moelle osseuse (ostéomyélite)	Infección del hueso o médula ósea (osteomielitis)	Infekcija kosti ili koštane srži (osteomijelitis)
Infezione della vagina batterica (vaginosi)	Bacterial vaginosis	Vaginose bactérienne	Vaginosis bacteriana	Bakterijska infekcija rodnice (bakterijska vaginoza)
Infezione fungina	Fungal infection	Infection fongique	Infección por hongos	Gljivična infekcija
Infezione virale	Viral infection	Infection virale	Infección viral	Virusna infekcija
Infiammazione (flogosi)	Inflammation	Inflammation	Inflamación	Upala
Infiammazione articolare (artrite)	Inflammation of the joint (arthritis)	Inflammation des articulations (arthrite)	Inflamación de una articulación (artritis)	Upala zgloba (artritis)
Infiammazione dei bronchi (bronchite)	Inflammation of the bronchi (bronchitis)	Inflammation des bronches des poumons (bronchite)	Inflamación de los bronquios (bronquitis)	Upala bronhija (bronhitis)
Infiammazione dei bronchioli (bronchiolite)	Inflammation of the bronchioles (bronchiolitis)	Inflammation des petites bronches (bronchiolite)	Inflamación de los bronquiolos (bronquiolitis)	Upala bronhiola (bronhiolitis)
Infiammazione dei polmoni (polmonite)	Inflammation of the lung (pneumonia)	Inflammation des poumons (pneumonie)	Inflamación de los pulmones (neumonía, pulmonía, neumonitis)	Upala pluća (pneumonija)
Infiammazione dei reni (nefrite)	Inflammation of the kidney (nephritis)	Inflammation du rein (néphrite)	Inflamación del riñón (nefritis)	Upala bubrega (nefritis)
Infiammazione dei seni paranasali (sinusite)	Inflammation of the paranasal sinuses (sinusitis)	Inflammation du sinus (sinusite)	Inflamación de los senos paranasales (sinusitis)	Upala sinusa (sinusitis)
Infiammazione dei tessuti gengivali (gengivite)	Inflammation of the gums (gingivitis)	Inflammation de la gencive (gingivite)	Inflamación de las encías (gingivitis)	Upala desni (gingivitis)
Infiammazione dei testicoli (orchite)	Inflammation of the testes (orchitis)	Inflammation des testicules (orchite)	Inflamación del testículo (orquitis)	Upala testisa (orhitis)
Infiammazione del cervello (encefalite)	Inflammation of the brain (encephalitis)	Inflammation du cerveau (encéphalite)	Inflamación del encéfalo (encefalitis)	Upala mozga (encefalitis)
Infiammazione del fegato (epatite)	Inflammation of the liver (hepatitis)	Inflammation du foie (hépatite)	Inflamación del hígado (hepatitis)	Upala jetre (hepatitis)
Infiammazione del miocardio (miocardite)	Inflammation of the heart muscle (myocarditis)	Inflammation du myocarde (myocardite)	Inflamación del miocardio (miocarditis)	Upala srčanog mišića (miokarditis)
Infiammazione del nervo (neurite, nevrite)	Inflammation of the nerve (neuritis)	Inflammation du nerf (névrite)	Inflamación del nervio (neuritis)	Upala živca (neuritis)
Infiammazione del pancreas (pancreatite)	Inflammation of the pancreas (pancreatitis)	Inflammation du pancréas (pancréatite)	Inflamación del páncreas (pancreatitis)	Upala gušterače (pankreatitis)
Infiammazione del parametrio (parametrite)	Inflammation of the parametrium (parametritis)	Inflammation du paramètre (paramétrite)	Inflamación del parametrio (parametritis)	Upala parametrija (parametritis)

Italiano	Inglese	Francese	Spagnolo	Croato
Infiammazione del pericardio (pericardite)	Inflammation of the pericardium (pericarditis)	Inflammation du péricarde (péricardite)	Inflamación del pericardio (pericarditis)	Upala osrčja (perikarditis)
Infiammazione del tendine (tendinite)	Inflammation of the tendon (tendinitis, tendonitis)	Inflammation d'un tendon (tendinite)	Inflamación de un tendón (tendinitis)	Upala tetive (tendinitis)
Infiammazione del tessuto muscolare (miosite)	Inflammation of the muscles (myositis)	Inflammation du tissu musculaire (myosite)	Inflamación del músculo esquelético (miositis)	Upala mišića (miozitis)
Infiammazione del timo	Inflammation of the thymus (thymitis)	Inflammation du thymus	Inflamación del timo (timitis)	Upala prsne žlijezde (timitis)
Infiammazione del'epiglottide (epiglottite)	Inflammation of the epiglottis (epiglottitis)	Inflammation de l'épiglotte (épiglottite)	Inflamación de la epiglotis (epiglotitis)	Upala epiglotisa (epiglotitis)
Infiammazione dell'appendice vermiforme (appendicite)	Inflammation of the appendix (appendicitis)	Inflammation de l'appendice iléo-caecal (appendicite)	Inflamación del apéndice (apendicitis)	Upala slijepog crijeva (apendicitis)
Infiammazione dell'endocardio (endocardite)	Inflammation of the endocardium (endocarditis)	Inflammation de l'endocarde (endocardite)	Inflamación del endocardio (endocarditis)	Upala srčane ovojnice (endokarditis)
Infiammazione dell'endometrio (endometrite)	Inflammation of the endometrium (endometritis)	Inflammation de l'endomètre (endométrite)	Inflamación del endometrio (endometritis)	Upala endometrija maternice (endometritis)
Infiammazione dell'epididimo (epididimite)	Inflammation of the epididymis (epididymitis)	Inflammation de l'épididyme (épididymite)	Inflamación del epidídimo (epididimitis)	Upala pasjemenika (epididimitis)
Infiammazione dell'inserzione di muscolo (entesite)	Inflammation of the entheses (enthesitis)	Inflammation de l'enthèse (enthésite)	Inflamación de la zona de inserción de un músculo (entesitis)	Upala hvatišta mišića (entezitis)
Infiammazione dell'uretra (uretrite)	Inflammation of the urethra (urethritis)	Inflammation de l'urètre (urétrite)	Inflamación de la uretra (uretritis)	Upala sluznice mokraćne cijevi (uretritis)
Infiammazione della borsa sierosa di un'articolazione (borsite)	Inflammation of the synovial fluid sac (bursitis)	Inflammation de la bourse séreuse articulaire (hygroma, bursite)	Inflamación de la bursa (bursitis)	Upala sluzne vreće (burzitis)
Infiammazione della colecisti (colecistite)	Inflammation of the gall bladder (cholecystitis)	Inflammation de la vésicule biliaire (cholécystite)	Inflamación de la vesícula biliar (colecistitis)	Upala žučnog mjehura (holecistitis)
Infiammazione della congiuntiva (congiuntivite)	Inflammation of the conjunctiva (conjunctivitis)	Inflammation de la conjonctive (conjonctivite)	Inflamación de la conjuntiva (conjuntivitis)	Upala sluznice oka (konjuktivitis)
Infiammazione della cornea (cheratite)	Inflammation of the cornea (keratitis)	Inflammation de la cornée (kératite)	Inflamación de la córnea (queratitis)	Upala rožnice (keratitis)
Infiammazione della cornea e della congiutiva (cheratocongiuntivite)	Inflammation of the cornea and conjunctiva (keratoconjunctivitis)	Inflammation de la conjonctive et de la cornée (kératoconjonctivite)	Inflamación de la córnea y de la conjuntiva (queratoconjuntivitis)	Upala rožnice i sluznice oka (keratokonjuktivitis)
Infiammazione della fascia (fascite)	Inflammation of the fascia (fasciitis)	Inflammation du fascia (fasciite)	Inflamación de la fascia (fascitis)	Upala fascije (fasciitis)
Infiammazione della ghiandola prostatica (prostatite)	Inflammation of the prostate gland (prostatitis)	Inflammation de la prostate (prostatite)	Inflamación de la próstata (prostatitis)	Upala prostate (prostatitis)
Infiammazione della laringe (laringite)	Inflammation of the larynx (laryngitis)	Inflammation du larynx (laryngite)	Inflamación de la laringe (laringitis)	Upala glasnica (laringitis)
Infiammazione della mammella (mastite)	Inflammation of the breast (mastitis)	Inflammation de la mamelle (mastite)	Inflamación del seno (mastitis)	Upala dojke (mastitis)
Infiammazione della membrana sinoviale (sinovite)	Inflammation of the synovial membrane (synovitis)	Inflammation de la gaine synoviale (synovite)	Inflamación de la membrana sinovial (sinovitis)	Upala tetivne ovojnice (sinovitis)
Infiammazione della mucosa gastrica (gastrite)	Inflammation of the stomach lining (gastritis)	Inflammation de la paroi de l'estomac (gastrite)	Inflamación de la mucosa gástrica (gastritis)	Upala želučane sluznice (gastritis)
Infiammazione della pelle (dermatite)	Inflammation of the skin (dermatitis)	Inflammaton de la peau (dermatite)	Inflamación de la piel (dermatitis)	Upala kože (dermatitis)
Infiammazione della pleura (pleurite)	Inflammation of the pleura (pleuritis)	Inflammation de la plèvre (pleurésie)	Inflamación de la pleura (pleuritis, pleuresía)	Upala plućne ovojnice (pleuritis)
Infiammazione della retina (retinite)	Inflammation of the retina (retinitis)	Inflammation de la rétine (rétinite)	Inflamación de la retina (retinitis)	Upala mrežnice (retinitis)
Infiammazione della sierosa peritoneale (peritonite)	Inflammation of the peritoneum (peritonitis)	Inflammation du péritoine (péritonite)	Inflamación del peritoneo (peritonitis)	Upala potrbušnice (peritonitis)
Infiammazione della testa del glande (balanite)	Inflammation of the glans penis (balanitis)	Inflammation du gland du pénis (balanite)	Inflamación del glande del pene (balanitis)	Upala glavića penisa (balanitis)
Infiammazione della tiroide (tiroidite)	Inflammation of the thyroid gland (thyroiditis)	Inflammation de la glande thyroïde (thyroïdite)	Inflamación de la glándula tiroides (tiroiditis)	Upala štitnjače (tireoiditis)
Infiammazione della trachea (tracheite)	Inflammation of the windpipe (tracheitis)	Inflammation de la trachée (trachéite)	Inflamación de la tráquea (traqueitis)	Upala dušnika (traheitis)
Infiammazione della tunica media dell'occhio (uveite)	Inflammation of the middle layer of the eye (uveitis)	Inflammation de l'uvée (uvéite)	Inflamación de la lámina intermedia del ojo (uveitis)	Upala srednje ovojnice oka (uveitis)
Infiammazione della vagina (vaginite)	Inflammation of the vagina (vaginitis)	Inflammation du vagin (vaginite)	Inflamación de la vagina (vaginitis)	Upala rodnice (vaginitis)
Infiammazione della vescica urinaria (cistite)	Inflammation of the urinary bladder (cystitis)	Inflammation de la vessie (cystite)	Inflamación de la vejiga urinaria (cistitis)	Upala mokraćnog mjehura (cistitis)
Infiammazione della vulva (vulvite)	Inflammation of the vulva (vulvitis)	Inflammation de la vulve (vulvite)	Inflamación de la vulva (vulvitis)	Upala stidnice (vulvitis)

Italiano	Inglese	Francese	Spagnolo	Croato
Infiammazione delle arterie (arterite)	Inflammation of the arterial walls (arteritis)	Inflammation des parois des artères (artérite)	Inflamación de las arterias (arteritis)	Upala stijenke arterije (arteritis)
Infiammazione delle ghiandole linfatiche (linfoadenite)	Inflammation of the lymph node (lymphadenitis)	Inflammation des ganglions (adénite, lymphadénite)	Inflamación de los ganglios linfáticos (linfadenitis)	Upala limfnog čvora (limfadenitis)
Infiammazione delle ghiandole salivari (sialoadenite)	Inflammation of the salivary gland (sialadenitis)	Inflammation des glandes salivaires (sialoadénite)	Inflamación de las glándulas salivales (sialadenitis)	Upala žlijezda slinovnica (sialadenitis)
Infiammazione delle meningi (meningite)	Inflammation of the meninges (meningitis)	Inflammation des méninges (méningite)	Inflamación de las meninges (meningitis)	Upala moždanih ovojnica (meningitis)
Infiammazione delle mucose della bocca (stomatite)	Inflammation of the mouth mucous lining (stomatitis)	Inflammation de la muqueuse buccale (stomatite)	Inflamación de la mucosa bucal (estomatitis)	Upala sluznice usta (stomatitis)
Infiammazione delle tonsille (tonsillite)	Inflammation of the tonsils (tonsillitis)	Inflammation des tonsilles (tonsillite)	Inflamación de las amígdalas palatinas (amigdalitis)	Upala krajnika (tonzilitis)
Infiammazione delle vene (flebite)	Inflammation of the vein (phlebitis)	Inflammation des veines (phlébite)	Inflamación de las venas (flebitis)	Upala vena (flebitis)
Infiammazione di labirinto nell'orecchio interno (labirintite)	Inflammation of the inner ear (labyrinthitis)	Inflammation de l'oreille interne (labyrinthite, otite interne)	Inflamación del laberinto del oído interno (laberintitis)	Upala labirinta u unutarnjem uhu (labirintitis)
Infiammazione di tendine e di guaina tendinea (tenosinovite)	Inflammation of the synovium and tendon (tenosynovitis)	Inflammation d'un tendon et de sa gaine synoviale (ténosynovite)	Inflamación de un tendón y de su vaina (tenosinovitis)	Upala tetive s ovojnicom (tenosinovitis)
Infiammazione granulomatosa	Granulomatous inflammation	Inflammation granulomateuse	Inflamación granulomatosa	Granulomatozna upala (granulom)
Influenza	Flu (influenza)	Grippe (influenza)	Gripe (gripa, influenza)	Gripa (influenca)
Influenza aviaria H5N1	Bird flu (influenzavirus A subtype H5N1)	Grippe aviaire (influenzavirus A sous-type H5N1)	Gripe aviar H5N1	Ptičja gripa podtip H5N1
Influenza spagnola	Spanish flu	Grippe espagnole	Gripe española	Španjolska gripa
Influenza suina	Pig flu (swine influenza, influenzavirus A subtype H1N1)	Grippe porcine	Gripe porcina (influenza porcina, gripe del cerdo)	Svinjska gripa
Infreddatura (raffreddore)	Common cold	Rhume	Resfriado común (resfrío)	Prehlada (hunjavica)
Ingrossamento (divenire grosso)	Gaining weight	Grossissement	Engorde (ganar peso)	Debljanje
Ingrossamento dei linfonodi (linfoadenopatia)	Enlarged lymph nodes (lymphadenopathy)	Augmentation d'un ganglion lymphatique (lymphadénopathie)	Aumento de volumen de los ganglios linfáticos (linfadenopatía)	Povećanje limfnih čvorova (limfadenopatija)
Insolazione (colpo di sole)	Sunstroke (heat stroke)	Coup de soleil (insolation)	Insolación	Sunčanica
Insonnia	Insomnia	Insomnie	Insomnio	Nesanica
Insufficienza epatica	Liver insufficiency	Insuffisance hépatique	Fallo hepático (insuficiencia hepática)	Zatajenje jetre
Insufficienza renale	Kidney failure (renal insufficiency)	Insuffisance rénale	Fallo renal (insuficiencia renal)	Zatajenje bubrega (insuficijencija bubrega)
Insufficienza renale acuta	Acute kidney failure	Insuffisance rénale aiguë	Insuficiencia renal aguda	Akutno zatajenje bubrega
Insufficienza renale cronica	Chronic renal failure	Insuffisance rénale chronique	Insuficiencia renal crónica	Kronično zatajenje bubrega
Insufficienza venosa cronica cerebrospinale	Chronic cerebrospinal venous insufficiency	Insuffisance veineuse cérébro-spinale chronique	Insuficiencia venosa cerebro-espinal crónica	Kronična cerebrospinalna venozna insuficijencija
Intolleranza al glutine	Gluten intolerance	Intolérance au gluten	Intolerancia al gluten	Nepodnošenje glutena
Intolleranza al lattosio	Lactose intolerance	Intolérance au lactose	Intolerancia a la lactosa	Nepodnošenje laktoze (netolerancija laktoze)
Intormentire	Tingling	Fourmillement	Hormigueo	Trnjenje
Intossicazione alimentare da stafilococco	Staphylococcal food poisoning	Intoxication alimentaire staphylococcique	Intoxicación alimentaria por estafilococo dorado	Stafilokokno trovanje hranom
Intossicazione da metalli pesanti	Heavy metal poisoning	Empoisonnement aux métaux lourds	Envenenamiento por metales pesados	Trovanje teškim metalima
Iperaldosteronismo	Aldosteronism (hyperaldosteronism)	Hyperaldostéronisme	Aldosteronismo (hiperaldosteronismo)	Aldosteronizam
Iperattività	Hyperactivity	Hyperactivité	Hiperactividad	Hiperaktivnost
Ipercalcemia	Hypercalcemia	Hypercalcémie	Hipercalcemia	Hiperkalcijemija
Iperestenzione della regione posteriore del tronco (opistotono)	Spastic arching position (opisthotonus)	Contracture sur les muscles extenseurs de sorte que le corps est incurvé en arrière (opisthotonos)	Contracción del cuerpo entero de tal manera que se mantiene encorvado hacia atrás (opistótonos)	Izvijanje mišića vrata i leđa u luk (opistotonus)
Iperinsulinismo	Hyperinsulinism	Hyperinsulinisme	Hiperinsulinismo	Povišen inzulin u krvi (hiperinzulinizam)
Iperkaliemia	Hyperkalemia	Hyperkaliémie	Hiperpotasemia (hipercalemia)	Hiperkalijemija
Ipermetropia	Farsightedness (hyperopia)	Hypermétropie	Hipermetropía	Dalekovidnost
Iperparatiroidismo	Hyperparathyroidism	Hyperparathyroïdie	Hiperparatiroidismo	Hiperparatireoidizam
Iperpituitarismo	Hyperpituitarism	Hyperpituitarisme	Hiperpituitarismo	Hiperpituitarizam
Iperplasia endometriale	Endometrial hyperplasia	Hyperplasie endométriale	Hiperplasia endometrial	Hiperplazija endometrija
Iperplasia pseudoepiteliomatosa	Pseudoepitheliomatous hyperplasia	Hyperplasie pseudo-épithéliomateuse	Hiperplasia pseudoepeliomatosa	Pseudoepiteliematozna hiperplazija

Italiano	Inglese	Francese	Spagnolo	Croato
Ipertensione arteriosa essenziale	Essential hypertension	Hypertension artérielle essentielle	Hipertensión esencial	Esencijalna hipertenzija
Ipertensione arteriosa polmonare	Pulmonary hypertension	Hypertension artérielle pulmonaire	Hipertensión arterial pulmonar	Plućna hipertenzija
Ipertensione arteriosa secondaria	Secondary hypertension (inessential hypertension)	Hypertension secondaire	Hipertensión secundaria	Sekundarna hipertenzija
Ipertensione arteriosa sistemica	High blood pressure (hypertension)	Pression artérielle élevée (hypertension artérielle)	Incremento de la presión sanguínea (hipertensión)	Visoki krvni tlak (hipertenzija)
Ipertensione maligna	Malignant hypertension	Hypertension artérielle maligne	Hipertensión maligna	Maligna hipertenzija
Ipertensione portale	Portal hypertension	Hypertension portale	Hipertensión portal	Portalna hipertenzija
Ipertensione renale	Renovacsular hypertension	Hypertension rénovasculaire	Hipertensión renovascular	Renovaskularna hipertenzija
Ipertermia	Hyperthermia	Hyperthermie	Hipertermia	Hipertermija
Ipertiroidismo	Hyperthyroidism	Hyperthyroïdie	Hipertiroidismo	Hipertireoza
Ipertrofia	Hypertrophy	Hypertrophie	Hipertrofia	Hipertrofija
Ipertrofia prostatica benigna	Benign prostatic hyperthroph	Hypertrophie bénigne de la prostate	Hiperplasia benigna de próstata	Benigna hipertrofija prostate
Ipertrofia ventricolare	Ventricular hypertrophy	Hypertrophie ventriculaire	Hipertrofia ventricular	Ventrikularna hipertrofija
Iperuricemia	Hyperuricemia	Hyperuricémie	Hiperuricemia	Hiperurikemija
Iperventilazione	Hyperventilation	Hyperventilation	Hiperventilación	Hiperventilacija
Ipervitaminosi	Hypervitaminosis	Hypervitaminose	Hipervitaminosis	Hipervitaminoza
Ipervolemia (aumento del volume ematico circolante)	Hypervolemia (increased level of fluid in the blood)	Hypervolémie (augmentation du volume de sang dans les vaisseaux)	Hipervolemia (aumento del volumen de sangre en la circulación)	Hipervolemija (porast volumena krvi u optoku)
Ipoalbuminemia	Hypoalbuminemia	Hypoalbuminémie	Hipoalbuminemia	Hipoalbuminemija
Ipocalcemia	Hypocalcemia	Hypocalcémie	Hipocalcemia	Hipokalcijemija
Ipocondria	Hypochondria	Hypocondrie	Hipocondría	Hipohondrija
Ipoglicemia	Hypoglycemia	Hypoglycémie	Hipoglicemia	Hipoglikemija
Ipoinsulinemia	Hypoinsulinism	Hypoinsulinisme	Hipoinsulinismo	Hipoinzulinizam
Ipokaliemia	Hypokalemia	Hypokaliémie	Hipocaliemia	Hipokalijemija
Ipoparatiroidismo	Hypoparathyroidism	Hypoparathyroïdie	Hipoparatiroidismo	Hipoparatireodizam
Ipopituitarismo	Hypopituitarism	Hypopituitarisme	Hipopituitarismo	Hipopituitarizam
Ipoplasia del tronco polmonare	Pulmonary hypoplasia	Hypoplasie pulmonaire	Hipoplasia pulmonar	Hipoplazija plućnog režnja
Ipospadia	Hypospadias	Hypospadias	Hipospadias	Hipospadija
Ipossia	Hypoxia	Hypoxie	Hipoxia	Hipoksija
Ipotensione e sincope	Hypotension and syncope	Hypotension et syncope	Hipotensión y síncope	Hipotenzija i sinkope
Ipotermia	Hypothermia	Hypothermie	Hipotermia	Pothlađenost (hipotermija)
Ipotiroidismo	Hypothyroidism	Hypothyroïdie	Hipotiroidismo	Hipotireoza
Ipotonia muscolare	Muscular hypotonia	Hypotonie musculaire	Hipotonia muscular	Mišićna hipotonija
Ippersensibilità ai normali stimoli esterni (iperestesia)	Increased sensitivity to stimuli of the senses (hyperesthesia)	Hypersensibilité aux stimuli extérieurs (hyperesthésie)	Sensación exagerada de los estímulos táctiles (hiperestesia)	Preosjetljivost na podražaj (hiperestezija)
Iridodialisi	Iridodialysis (coredialysis)	Iridodialyse	Iridodiálisis	Iridodijaliza
Irite	Iritis	Iritis	Iritis	Iritis
Irradiazione non ionizzante	Non-ionising irradiation	Irradiation non-ionisante	Irradiación no-ionizante	Neionizirajuća ozračenost
Irradiazione radioattiva	Radioactive irradiation	Irradiation par rayons radioactifs (contami-nation radioactive)	Irradiación radioactiva	Radioaktivna ozračenost
Irsutismo	Hirsutism	Hirsutisme	Hirsutismo	Hirzutizam
Ischemia	Ischemia	Ischémie	Isquemia	Ishemija
Ischemia degli arti	Ischemic limbs	Ischémie des membres	Isquemia de miembros	Ishemični udovi
Ischemia miocardica	Ischemic heart disease	Ischémie myocardique	Isquemia miocárdica (angina de pecho)	Ishemijska bolest srca
Isosporiasi	Isosporiasis	Isosporose	Isosporiasis	Izosporijaza
Isteria (isterismo)	Hysteria	Hystérie	Histeria	Histerija
Istoplasmosi	Histoplasmosis (Darling's disease)	Histoplasmose	Histoplasmosis	Histoplazmoza
Ittero (itterizia)	Jaundice (icterus)	Ictère (jaunisse)	Ictericia	Žutica (ikterus)
Ittero neonatale	Neonatal jaundice	Ictère néonatal	Ictericia del recién nacido	Novorođenačka žutica
Ittero ostruttivo	Mechanic icterus (bile duct obstruction)	Ictère par obstruction des voies biliaires	Ictericia obstructiva	Mehanički ikterus
Kala-azar (febbre d'Assam, splenomegalia infantile)	Kala-azar (black fever)	Kala azar (fièvre noire)	Kala azar (fiebre negra)	Kala-azar
Kernittero (encefalopatia bilirubinica)	Kernicterus	Kernictère	Kernicterus (encefalopatía neonatal bilirrubínica)	Žutica moždanih jezgri
Kuru	Kuru	Kuru	Kuru (muerte de la risa)	Kuru (smrtni smijeh)
Labbro leporino	Cleft lip and palate	Fente labiale et fente palatine	Labio leporino (fisura labial)	Rascjep usne i nepca
Lacerazione (strappo)	Laceration (tear)	Lacération	Laceración	Razderotina
Lacerazione cerebrale	Brain laceration	Lacération cérébrale	Laceración cerebral	Laceracija mozga
Laringospasmo	Laryngospasm	Laryngospasme	Laringoespasmo	Laringospazam
Lebbra	Leprosy	Lèpre	Lepra	Lepra (guba)

Italiano	Inglese	Francese	Spagnolo	Croato
Leiomioma	Leiomyoma	Léiomyome	Leiomioma	Lejomiom
Leiomiosarcoma	Leiomyosarcoma	Leiomyosarcome	Leiomiosarcoma	Lejomiosarkom
Leishmaniosi	Leishmaniasis	Leishmaniose	Leishmaniasis	Lišmenijaza
Leishmaniosi cutanea	Cutaneous leishmaniasis (Oriental sore)	Leishmaniose cutanée (bouton d'Orient)	Leishmaniasis cutánea (uta)	Orijentalni ulkus (kožna lišmenijaza)
Lentezza psicofisica	Slow psychophysiological responses	Réponses psychophysiologiques lentes	Respuestas psicofisiológicas lentas	Psihofizička usporenost
Leptospirosi	Leptospirosis	Leptospirose	Leptospirosis	Leptospiroza
Lesione del nervo	Nerve lesion	Lésion du nerf	Lesión de nervio	Oštećenje živca (lezija živca)
Lesione del nervo periferico	Peripheral nerve lesion	Lésion du nerf périphérique	Lesión de nervio periférico	Oštećenje perifernog živca
Lesione ostruttiva dell'intestino tenue	Obstructive lesion of the small intestine	Lésion obstructive de l'intestin grêle	Lesión obstructiva del intestino delgado	Opstruktivna lezija tankog crijeva
Lesioni da scoppio (blast-syndrome)	Blast-syndrome	Syndrome de blast	Síndrome por explosion	Blast-sindrom
Lesioni della testa e del cervello	Head and brain injuries	Blessures à la tête et blessures du cerveau	Lesiones de la cabeza y del cerebro	Ozljede glave i mozga
Lesioni meccaniche	Mechanical injuries	Lésions mécaniques	Lesiones mecánicas	Mehaničke ozljede
Lesioni termiche	Thermal injuries	Lésions thermiques	Lesiones térmicas	Termičke ozljede
Leucemia	Leukemia	Leucémie	Leucemia	Leukemija
Leucemia acuta linfoblastica	Acute lymphoblastic leukemia	Leucémie lymphoblastique aiguë	Leucemia linfoblástica aguda	Akutna limfatična leukemija
Leucemia linfatica	Lymphatic leukemia	Leucémie lymphoïde	Leucemia linfática	Limfatična leukemija
Leucemia linfatica cronica	Chronic lymphocytic leukemia	Leucémie lymphoïde chronique	Leucemia linfocítica crónica	Kronična limfocitna leukemija
Leucemia mieloide	Myeloid leukemia	Leucémie myéloïde	Leucemia mieloide	Mijeloična leukemija
Leucemia mieloide acuta	Acute myeloid leukemia (AML)	Leucémie aiguë myéloblastique	Leucemia mieloide aguda	Akutna mijeloična leukemija
Leucemia mieloide cronica	Chronic myeloid leukemia	Leucémie myéloïde chronique	Leucemia mieloide crónica	Kronična mijeloična leukemija
Leucemia monocitica	Monocytic leukemia	Leucémie monocytique	Leucemia monocítica	Monocitična leukemija
Leucocitosi	Leukocytosis	Leucocytose	Leucocitosis	Leukocitoza
Leucodistrofia	Leukodystrophy	Leucodystrophie	Leucodistrofia	Leukodistrofija
Leucoplachia	Leukoplakia	Leucoplasie	Leucoplaquia	Leukoplakija
Leucorea	Leukorrhea	Leucorrhée	Leucorrea	Bijelo pranje
Lichen planus	Lichen planus	Lichen plan	Liquen plano	Lišaj (lichen planus)
Linfadenite tubercolare	Tuberculous lymphadenitis	Lymphadénite tuberculeuse	Tuberculosis ganglionar (linfadenitis tubercular)	Tuberkuloza limfnih čvorova
Linfangioma	Lymphangioma	Lymphangiome	Linfangioma	Limfangiom
Linfangiosarcoma	Lymphangiosarcoma	Lymphangiosarcome	Linfangiosarcoma	Limfangiosarkom
Linfedema	Lymphedema	Lymphoedème	Linfedema	Limfedem (zastoj limfe)
Linfoma	Lymphoma	Lymphome	Linfoma	Limfom
Linfoma di Hodgkin	Hodgkin's disease	Maladie de Hodgkin	Enfermedad de Hodgkin	Hodgkinova bolest
Linfoma non Hodgkin	Non-Hodgkin's lymphoma	Lymphome non-Hodgkinien	Linfoma no-Hodgkin	Non-Hodgkinov limfom
Lipodistrofia	Lipodystrophy	Lipodystrophie	Lipodistrofia	Lipodistrofija
Lipoma	Lipoma	Lipome	Lipoma	Lipom
Lipomatosi pancreatica	Pancreatic lipomatosis	Lipomatose du pancréas	Lipomatosis pancreática (reemplazo graso del páncreas)	Lipomatoza gušterače (masna infiltracija gusterače)
Liposarcoma	Liposarcoma	Liposarcome	Liposarcoma	Liposarkom
Listeriosi	Listeriosis	Listériose	Listeriosis	Listerioza
Lobster-claw deformità di piede	Split foot (lobster claw foot, ectrodactyly)	Pince de homard (aplasie digitale, ectrodactylie)	Ectrodactilia en pie	Lobster Claw stopalo
Lombaggine	Low back pain (lumbago, lumbosacral syndrome)	Lombalgie	Dolor de espalda baja (lumbalgia)	Križobolja (lumbosakralni sindrom)
Lombalgia dell'atleta	Gymnastics lower back pain	Lombalgie du gymnaste	Espalda del gimnasta	Gimnastičarska bolna križa
Lordosi	Lordosis	Lordose	Lordosis	Lordoza
Lupus eritematoso sistemico	Lupus erythematosus	Lupus érythémateux	Lupus eritematoso sistémico	Sistemski lupus eritematozus
Lussazione	Dislocation (luxation)	Déboîtement (luxation)	Luxación (lujación, dislocación)	Iščašenje (dislokacija, luksacija)
Lussazione acromio-clavicolare	Separated shoulder (acromioclavicular dislocation)	Luxation acromio-claviculaire	Luxación de la articulación acromioclavicular	Iščašenje akromio-klavikularnog zgloba
Lussazione congenita dell'anca (displasia dell'anca)	Congenital dysplasia of the hip (congenital hip dislocation)	Luxation congénitale de la hanche	Displasia congénita de la cadera (luxación congénita de cadera)	Urođeno iščašenje kuka (kongenitalna displazija kuka)
Lussazione del ginocchio	Knee dislocation (luxation of the knee)	Luxation du genou	Luxación de la rodilla	Iščašenje koljena
Lussazione del gomito	Elbow dislocation (luxation of the elbow)	Luxation du coude	Luxación del codo	Iščašenje lakta
Lussazione dell'anca	Dislocation of a hip	Luxation de la hanche	Luxación de la cadera	Iščašenje kuka
Lussazione della caviglia	Dislocated ankle joint	Luxation de la cheville	Luxación del tobillo	Iščašenje skočnog zgloba
Lussazione della mandibola	Mandibular dislocation	Luxation temporo-mandibulaire	Dislocación de la mandibula	Iščašenje vilice
Lussazione della rotula	Luxating patella (trick knee, floating patella)	Luxation de la rotule	Luxación de la rótula	Iščašenje čašice

Italiano	Inglese	Francese	Spagnolo	Croato
Lussazione della spalla	Dislocated shoulder	Luxation de l'épaule	Luxación del hombro	Iščašenje ramena
Lussazione incompleta (sublussazione)	Partial dislocation (subluxation)	Luxation incomplète (subluxation)	Desplazamiento de una articulación (subluxación)	Djelomična dislokacija (subluksacija)
Lussazioni delle atricolazioni della mano e delle dita	Hand and finger joints dislocation	Luxation des doigts et du poignet	Luxaciones de la mano y los dedos	Iščašenje zglobova šake i prstiju
Macchie di Koplik	Koplik's spots	Signe de Koplik	Manchas de Koplik	Koplikove pjege
Mal di denti	Toothache	Mal de dents	Dolor de muelas	Zubobolja
Mal di gola (infiammazione della faringe, faringite)	Sore throat (inflammation of the throat, pharyngitis)	Mal à la gorge (inflammattion du pharinx, pharingite)	Mal de garganta (inflamación de la faringe, faringitis)	Upala grla (grlobolja, faringitis)
Mal di mare	Seasickness	Mal de mer	Mal de mar	Morska bolest
Mal di montagna	Altitude sickness (acute mountain sickness)	Mal aigu des montagnes	Mal de montaña (mal de altura)	Visinska bolest
Mal di schiena (dorsopatia)	Back pain (dorsalgia)	Mal de dos (dorsalgie)	Dolor de espalda (dorsalgia)	Bol u leđima (dorzopatija)
Mal di schiena su base posturale	Postural back pain	Lombalgie posturale	Dolor de espalda postural	Posturalna križobolja
Mal di testa	Headache	Mal de tête (céphalée)	Dolor de cabeza	Glavobolja
Malaria	Malaria	Malaria	Malaria (paludismo)	Malarija
Malassorbimento	Malabsorption	Malabsorption	Malabsorción	Malapsorpcija
Malattia autoimmunitaria	Autoimmune disease	Maladie auto-immune	Enfermedad autoinmune	Autoimunološka bolest
Malattia da vibrazioni	Vibration disease	Maladie des vibrations	Enfermedad de las vibraciones	Vibracijska bolest
Malattia dei riempitori dei silos	Silo-filler's disease	Maladie des ouvriers des silos	Enfermedad de los ensiladores	Silosna pluća
Malattia del cuore (cardiopatia)	Heart disease (cardiopathy)	Maladie cardiaque (cardiopathie)	Enfermedad del corazón (cardiopatía)	Srčana bolest (kardiopatija)
Malattia del motoneurone	Motor neurone disease	Maladie du motoneurone	Enfermedad de la motoneurona	Bolest motornog neurona
Malattia di Bornholm (mialgia epidemica)	Bornholm disease (epidemic myalgia)	Maladie de Bornholm (myalgie épidémique)	Enfermedad de Bornholm (mialgia epidémica)	Bornholmska bolest (epidemijska mialgija)
Malattia di Brill-Zinsser	Brill's disease	Maladie de Brill-Zinserr (typhus résurgent)	Enfermedad de Brill	Brillova bolest (Brill-Zinsserova bolest)
Malattia di Chagas	Chagas disease (American trypanosomiasis)	Maladie de Chagas (trypanosomiase américaine)	Enfermedad de Chagas (tripanosomiasis americana)	Chagasova bolest (americka tripanosomijaza)
Malattia di Charcot-Marie-Tooth	Charcot-Marie-Tooth disease	Maladie de Charcot-Marie-Tooth	Enfermedad de Charcot-Marie Tooth	Bolest Charcot-Marie-Tooth
Malattia di Creutzfeldt-Jakob (cosiddetta "malattia della mucca pazza")	Creutzfeldt-Jakob disease (so called "mad cow disease")	Maladie de Creutzfeldt-Jakob	Enfermedad de Creutzfeldt-Jakob	Creutzfeldt-Jakobova bolest (tzv. "kravlje ludilo")
Malattia di Crohn	Crohn's disease	Maladie de Crohn	Enfermedad de Crohn	Crohnova bolest
Malattia di decompressione (sindrome di Caisson)	Decompression sickness (diver's disease, caisson disease)	Maladie de décompression (maladie des plongeurs, maladie des caissons)	Síndrome de decompresión (enfermedad de los buzos, mal de presión)	Dekompresijska bolest (kesonska bolest)
Malattia di Dupuytren	Dupuytren's contracture	Contracture de Dupuytren	Contractura de Dupuytren	Dupuytrenova kontraktura
Malattia di Freiberg	Freiberg's disease	Maladie de Freiberg	Enfermedad de Freiberg	Freibergova bolest
Malattia di Haglund (deformità di Haglund)	Haglund's disease	Maladie de Haglund	Enfermedad de Haglund (deformidad de Haglund)	Haglundova bolest
Malattia di Hirschsprung (malattia di Mya)	Hirschsprung's disease (congenital aganglionic megacolon)	Maladie de Hirschsprung (mégacolôn)	Enfermedad de Hirschsprung (megacolon agangliónico)	Hirschsprungova bolest (kongenitalni aganglionarni megakolon)
Malattia di Huntington	Huntington's chorea (Huntington's disease)	Chorée de Huntington (maladie de Huntington)	Enfermedad de Huntington (corea de Huntington)	Huntingtonova koreja
Malattia di Köhler	Köhler disease	Maladie de Köhler	Enfermedad de Köhler	Köhlerova bolest
Malattia di Legg-Perthes-Calvé	Legg-Calvé-Perthes disease	Maladie de Legg-Calvé-Perthes (ostéochondrite primitive de hanche)	Síndrome de Legg-Calvé-Perthes	Legg-Calvé-Perthesova bolest
Malattia di Lyme (borreliosi di Lyme)	Lyme disease (lyme borreliosis)	Maladie de Lyme	Enfermedad de Lyme (borreliosis de Lyme)	Lajmska bolest (Lajmska borelioza)
Malattia di Morquio (mucopolisaccaridosi IV)	Morquio's syndrome (mucopolysaccharidosis IV)	Maladie de Morquio (mucopolysaccharidose type IV)	Enfermedad de Morquio (mucopolisacaridosis tipo IV)	Sindrom Morquio (mukopolisaharidoza tip IV)
Malattia di Panner	Panner's disease	Maladie de Panner	Enfermedad de Panner	Pannerova bolest
Malattia di Pellegrini-Stieda	Pellegrini-Stieda disease	Maladie de Pellegrini-Stieda	Enfermedad de Pellegrini-Stieda	Bolest Pellegrini-Stieda
Malattia di Sever	Sever's disease	Maladie de Sever	Enfermedad de Sever	Severova bolest
Malattia di Van Neck	Van Neck disease	Maladie de Van Neck-Odelberg	Enfermedad de Van Neck	Morbus Van Neck
Malattia infiammatoria pelvica	Pelvic inflammatory disease	Maladie pelvienne inflammatoire	Enfermedad pélvica inflamatoria	Upalna bolest zdjelice
Malattia parassitaria (parassitosi)	Parasitic disease (parasitosis)	Maladie parasitique (parasitose)	Enfermedad parasitaria (parasitosis)	Parazitarna bolest (parazitoza)
Malattia professionale	Occupational disease	Maladie professionnelle	Enfermedad profesional	Profesionalno oboljenje

Italiano	Inglese	Francese	Spagnolo	Croato
Malattia sessualmente trasmissibile	Sexually transmitted disease	Maladie vénérienne	Enfermedad de transmisión sexual	Spolno prenosiva bolest
Malattie dei vasi sanguigni	Blood vessel diseases	Maladies des vaisseaux sanguins	Enfermedades de los vasos sanguíneos	Bolesti krvnih žila
Malattie dell'aorta	Diseases of the aorta	Maladies de l'aorte	Enfermedades de la aorta	Bolesti aorte
Malattie delle valvole cardiache	Heart valve diseases	Maladies des valves cardiaques	Enfermedades de las válvulas del corazón	Bolesti srčanih zalistaka
Malattie infettive dei bambini	Childhood infectious diseases	Maladies infectieuses des enfants	Enfermedades infantiles contagiosas	Dječje zarazne bolesti
Mancanza dell'appetito	Loss of appetite	Perte d'appétit	Pérdida del apetito	Gubitak apetita
Mancanza di movimento	Movement inability	Incapacité de se mouvoir	Incapacidad de movimiento	Nemogućnost kretanja
Mancata discesa del testicolo	Undescended testicle	Absence de descente des testicules	Descenso incompleto de testículo	Nespušteni testis
Mancata secrezione di urina	Inability to urinate	Incapacité d'uriner	Incapacidad para orinar	Nemogućnost mokrenja
Mancato sviluppo di un organo (aplasia di un organo)	Absence in development of an organ (aplasia of an organ)	Arrêt du développement d'un organe (aplasie d'un organe)	Desarrollo detenido de un órgano (aplasia de un órgano)	Nerazvijenost organa (aplazija organa)
Mania	Mania	Manie	Manía	Manija
Mastopatia	Mastopathy	Mastopathie	Mastopatía	Mastopatija
Mastopatia fibrocistica	Fibrocystic breast disease	Mastopathie fibrocystique	Mastitis quística crónica (enfermedad fibroquística)	Fibrocistična bolest dojke
Medulloblastoma	Medulloblastoma	Médulloblastome	Meduloblastoma	Meduloblastom
Megacolon	Megacolon	Mégacolôn	Megacolon	Megakolon
Melanoma	Melanoma	Mélanome	Melanoma	Melanom
Melasma	Melasma (chloasma faciei)	Chleuasme (chloasma)	Melasma (cloasma)	Kloazma (melazma)
Melioidosi	Melioidosis (Whitmore disease)	Mélioïdose	Melioidosis	Melioidoza
Meningioma	Meningioma	Méningiome	Meningioma	Meningeom
Meningocele	Meningocele	Méningocèle	Meningocele	Meningokela
Meningoencefalite amebica primaria	Primary amoebic meningoencephalitis	Méningo-encéphalite amibienne primaire	Meningoencefalitis amebiana primaria	Primarni amebni meningoencefalitis
Meningoencefalocele	Meningoencephàlocele	Méningoencphalocèle	Meningoencefalocele	Meningoencefalokela
Meniscopatia	Meniscal disease	Meniscopathie	Meniscopatia	Meniskopatija
Menopausa	Menopause	Ménopause	Menopausia	Menopauza (klimakterij)
Mesotelioma	Mesothelioma	Mésothéliome	Mesotélioma	Mezoteliom
Mesotelioma sarcomatoide	Sarcomatoid mesothelioma	Mésothéliome sarcomatoïde	Mesotélioma sarcomatoide	Mezoteliosarkom
Mestruazione dolorosa (dismenorrea)	Painful menstruation (dysmenorrhea)	Règle douloureuse (dysménorrhée)	Menstruación dolorosa (dismenorrea)	Bolna menstruacija (dismenoreja)
Metabolismo basale accelerato	Accelerated basal metabolism	Metabolisme de base accéléré	Metabolismo basal acelerado	Ubrzan bazalni metabolizam
Metamorfosi grassa del fegato	Fatty liver metamorphosis	Stéatose hépatique	Metamorfosis grasa del hígado	Masna metarmofoza jetre
Metastasi	Metastasis	Métastase	Metástasis	Metastaza
Metatarsalgia	Metatarsalgia (Morton's neuroma)	Métatarsalgie	Metatarsalgia	Metatarzalgija (Mortonova metatarzalgija)
Meteoropatia	Meteoropathy	Météoropathie	Meteoropatía	Meteoropatija
Mialgia cervicale	Neck myalgia	Myalgie cervicale	Mialgia cervical	Mijalgični sindrom vrata
Miastenia gravis	Myasthenia gravis	Myasthénie grave	Miastenia gravis	Miastenija gravis
Micetoma	Mycetoma	Mycétome	Micetoma	Micetoma
Micosi	Mycosis	Mycose	Micosis	Mikoza
Mieloma multiplo	Plasmacytoma (multiple myeloma)	Plasmocytome (myélome multiple)	Plasmacitoma (mieloma múltiple)	Plazmocitom (multipli mijelom)
Mielomeningocele	Meningomyelocele	Myéloméningocèle	Mielomeningocele	Meningomijelokela
Miliaria rubra	Miliaria rubra (sweat rash)	Miliarie rouge	Miliaria rubra (sarpullido por el calor)	Milijarija rubra
Minzione dolorosa (stranguria)	Painful urination (strangury)	Urination douloureuse (strangurie)	Micción dolorosa (angurria)	Bol pri mokrenju (strangurija)
Mioblastoma	Myoblastoma	Rhabdomyome granocellulaire	Mioblastoma	Mioblastom
Miocardiopatia alcolica	Alcoholic cardiomyopathy	Cardiomyopathie alcoolique	Miocardiopatía alcohólica	Alkoholna kardiomiopatja
Mioclono	Myoclonic twitches (myoclonus)	Myoclonie	Mioclono	Miokloničko trzanje (mioklonus)
Miogelosi	Myogelosis	Myogélose	Miogelosis	Miogeloza
Mioma	Myoma	Myome	Mioma	Miom
Miopia	Shortsightedness (myopia)	Myopie	Miopía	Kratkovidnost
Miosarcoma	Myosarcoma	Myosarcome	Miosarcoma	Miosarkom
Miosite ossificante	Myositis ossificans	Myosite ossifiante	Miositis osificante	Osificirajući miozitis
Miosite ossificante progressiva	Myositis ossificans progressiva	Myosite ossifiante progressive	Miositis osificante progresiva	Progresivno okoštavanje mišića
Miscela di gas (flatulenza)	Passing gas (flatulence, farting)	Pet (flatulence, vesse)	Tener gases (flatulencia)	Puštanje vjetra (flatulencija, plinovi)
Mixedema	Myxedema	Myxoedème	Mixedema	Miksedem
Mixoma	Myxoma	Myxome	Mixoma	Miksom
Mixosarcoma	Myxosarcoma	Myxosarcome	Mixosarcoma	Miksosarkom
Mollusco contagioso	Molluscum contagiosum	Molluscum contagiosum	Molusco contagioso	Molusk

Italiano	Inglese	Francese	Spagnolo	Croato
Mollusco pendule (fibroma molle)	Soft fibroma (fibroma molle, acrochordon)	Molluscum pendulum (acrochordon)	Fibroma blando (fibroma molle)	Kožni privjesak (mekani fibrom)
Mononucleosi infettiva (malattia del bacio)	Infectious mononucleosis (Pfeiffer's disease, kissing disease, glandular fever)	Mononucléose infectieuse (maladie du baiser, maladie des amoureux)	Mononucleosis infecciosa (fiebre glandular, enfermedad de Pfeiffer)	Mononukleoza (bolest poljupca)
Morbillo	Measles	Rougeole (1re maladie)	Sarampión	Ospice (morbili)
Morbo di Addison	Addison's disease	Maladie d'Addison	Enfermedad de Addison	Addisonova bolest
Morbo di Alzheimer	Alzheimer's diesase	Maladie d'Alzheimer	Enfermedad de Alzheimer	Alzheimerova bolest
Morbo di Basedow-Graves	Basedow Graves disease	Maladie de Basedow	Enfermedad de Graves Basedow	Basedowljeva bolest
Morbo di Bowen	Bowen's disease (squamous cell carcinoma in situ)	Maladie de Bowen	Enfermedad de Bowen	Bowenova bolest
Morbo di Buerger	Buerger's disease (thromboangiitis obliterans)	Maladie de Buerger (thromboangéite oblitérante)	Enfermedad de Buerger (tromboangeítis obliterante)	Buergerova bolest
Morbo di Kienböck	Kienböck's disease	Maladie de Kienböck	Enfermedad de Kienböck	Kienböckova bolest
Morbo di Paget	Paget's disease	Maladie de Paget	Enfermedad de Paget	Pagetova bolest
Morbo di Parkinson	Parkinson's disease	Maladie de Parkinson	Enfermedad de Parkinson	Parkinsonova bolest
Morbo di Whipple	Whipple's disease	Maladie de Whipple	Enfermedad de Whipple	Whippleova bolest
Morsicatura	Bite	Morsure	Mordedura	Ugriz
Morsicatura di animale rabbioso	Bite by rabies infected animal	Morsure d'un animal infecté par le virus de la rage	Mordedura de un animal enfermo de rabia	Ugriz bijesne životinje
Morsicatura di cane	Dog bite	Morsure de chien	Mordedura de perro	Ugriz psa
Morsicatura di gatto	Cat bite	Morsure de chat	Mordedura de gato	Ugriz mačke
Morsicatura di ragno	Spider bite	Piqûre d'araignée	Picadura de araña	Ugriz pauka
Morsicatura di ratto	Rat bite	Morsure de rat	Mordedura de rata	Ugriz štakora
Morsicatura di serpenti	Snake bite	Morsure de vipère	Mordedura de víbora	Ugriz zmije
Morsicatura di uomo	Human bite	Morsure humaine	Mordedura humana	Ugriz čovjeka (ljudski ugriz)
Morsicatura di zecca infetta	Infected tick bite	Piqûre de tique infectée	Picadura de garrapata infectada	Ugriz zaraženog krpelja
Morso della vedova nera	Black widow bite	Morsure de veuve noire	Mordedura de viuda negra	Ugriz crne udovice
Morte	Death	Mort	Muerte	Smrt
Morte naturale	Natural death	Mort naturelle	Muerte natural	Prirodna smrt
Morte violenta	Violent death	Mort violente	Muerte violenta	Nasilna smrt
Morva umana	Glanders	Morve	Muermo	Sakagija
Movimenti incontrollati degli occhi (opsoclono)	Uncontrolled eye movement (opsoclonus)	Mouvements involontaires anarchiques des globes oculaires (opsoclonus)	Movimientos involuntarios y rápidos de los ojos (opsoclonus)	Nekontrolirani pokreti očiju (opsoklonus)
Movimento anormale	Abnormal flexibility	Flexibilité anormale	Flexibilidad anormal	Abnormalna gibljivost
MSSA (MRSA)	MRSA	SARM	SARM	MRSA
Muco nasale	Nasal secretion (mucus)	Mucus nasal	Moco (mucus) nasal	Sekrecija iz nosa
Muco nelle feci	Mucus in stool	Mucus dans les selles	Moco en las heces	Sluzava stolica
Mucocele	Mucocele	Mucocèle	Mucocele	Mukocela
Mucopolisaccaridosi	Mucopolysacchari-dosis	Mucopolysaccharidose	Mucopolisacaridosis	Mukopolisaharidoza
Mughetto (moniliasi orale)	Thrush (oral candidiasis)	Candidose orale	Candidiasis oral (muguet oral)	Sor (oralna kandidijaza)
Muscolo flaccido	Flaccid muscle (untoned muscle)	Muscle flasque (hypotonie musculaire)	Músculo flácido	Mlohavi mišić
Nanismo	Dwarfism (nanism)	Nanisme	Enanismo	Patuljasti rast (nanizam)
Narcolessia	Narcolepsy	Narcolepsie (maladie de Gélineau)	Narcolepsia (síndrome de Gelineau, epilepsia del sueño)	Narkolepsija
Naso che cola (rinorrea)	Runny nose (rinorrhea)	Écoulement par le nez (rhinorrhée)	Goteo nasal (rinorrea)	Curenje iz nosa (rinoreja)
Nausea	Nausea	Nausée	Náusea	Mučnina
Necrosi	Necrosis	Nécrose	Necrosis	Nekroza
Necrosi fibrinoide	Fibrinoid necrosis	Nécrose fibrinoïde	Necrosis fibrinoide	Fibrinoidna nekroza
Nefrite interstiziale	Interstitial nephritis	Néphrite interstitielle	Nefritis intersticial	Intersticijska upala bubrega
Nefropatia diabetica	Diabetic nephropathy	Néphropathie diabétique	Nefropatía diabética	Dijabetična nefropatija
Nefrosi	Nephrosis	Néphrose	Nefrosis	Nefroza
Neoplasie del tratto urogenitale	Urogenital neoplasm	Tumeur du système uro-génital	Tumor urogenital	Urogenitalni tumor
Neurinoma (Schwannoma)	Neurinoma	Neurinome	Neurinoma	Neurinom
Neuroblastoma	Neuroblastoma	Neuroblastome	Neuroblastoma	Neuroblastom
Neuroborreliosi	Neuroborreliosis	Neuroborréliose	Neuroborreliosis	Neuroborelioza
Neurodermite (dermatite atopica)	Atopic dermatitis	Dermatite atopique	Dermatitis atópica	Atopijski dermatitis
Neurofibromatosi di tipo 1 (malattia di von Recklinghausen)	Neurofibromatosis type1 (Von Recklinghausen's disease)	Neurofibromatose de type 1 (maladie de Von Recklinghausen)	Neurofibromatosis de tipo 1 (enfermedad de Von Recklinghausen)	Von Recklinghausenova bolest
Neuroma	Neuroma	Neurome	Neuroma	Neurom
Neuroma dell'acustico	Acoustic neuroma	Neurome acoustique	Neuroma acústico	Neurom slušnog živca
Neuropatia	Neuropathy	Neuropathie	Neuropatía	Neuropatija
Neuropatia diabetica	Diabetic neuropathy	Neuropathie diabétique	Neuropatía diabética	Dijabetična neuropatija
Nevralgia	Neuralgia	Névralgie	Neuralgia	Neuralgija
Nevralgia del nervo cranico	Cranial neuralgia	Névralgie des nerfs crâniens	Neuralgia craneal	Neuralgija moždanih živaca

Italiano	Inglese	Francese	Spagnolo	Croato
Nevralgia del trigemino	Trigeminal neuralgia	Névralgie du trijumeau (névralgie trigéminale)	Neuralgia del trigémino	Neuralgija trigeminusa
Nevralgia occipitale (nevralgia di Arnold)	Occipital neuralgia (Arnold's neuralgia)	Nèvralgie occipitale	Síndrome occipital (neuralgia occipital)	Okcipitalna neuralgija
Nevrastenia	Neurasthenia	Neurasthénie	Neurastenia	Neurastenija
Nevrosi	Neurosis	Névrose (neurose)	Neurosis	Neuroza
Nistagmo	Nystagmus	Nystagmus	Nistagmo	Nistagmus
Nodo (nodulo)	Knot (lump)	Nodule	Nudo	Kvržica
Noduli di Bouchard	Bouchard's nodes	Nodules de Bouchard	Nudosidades de Bouchard	Bouchardovi čvorići
Noduli di Heberden	Heberden's nodes	Nodules d'Heberden	Nódulos de Heberden	Heberdenovi čvorići
Nodulo di Suor Maria Giuseppa	Sister Mary Joseph nodule	Nodule de Soeur Marie Joseph (métastase cutanée ombilicale)	Nódulo de la hermana María José	Čvor sestre Mary Joseph (umbilikalna metastaza)
Obesità	Obesity	Obésité	Obesidad	Debljina (gojaznost)
Occhi lacrimosi	Watery eyes	Yeux larmoyants	Ojos llorosos	Suzenje očiju
Occhi secchi (xeroftalmia)	Dry eyes (keratoconjuctivitis sicca)	Oeil sec (kérato-conjonctivite sèche)	Sequedad de los ojos (xeroftalmia)	Suhe oči (kseroftalmija)
Occlusione arteria retinica	Retinal artery occlusion	Occlusion de l'artère de la rétine	Oclusión de la arteria de la retina	Blokada mrežnične arterije
Odore sgradevole dell'alito (alitosi, bromopnea)	Bad breath (halitosis)	Mauvaise heleine (halitose)	Mal aliento (halitosis)	Zadah iz usta (halitoza)
Oligodendroglioma	Oligodendroglioma	Oligodendrocytome	Oligodendroglioma	Oligodendrogliom
Oligomenorrea	Oligomenorrhea	Oligoménorrhée	Oligomenorrea	Oligomenoreja
Oncocercosi (cecità fluviale)	Onchocerciasis (river blindness)	Onchocercose (cécité des rivières)	Oncocercosis	Onkocerkijaza (riječno sljepilo)
Orticaria	Hives (urticaria)	Urticaire	Urticaria	Koprivnjača (urtikarija)
Osteitis fibrosa cistica	Osteitis fibrosa cystica	Ostéite fibrokystique	Ostéitis fibrosa quística	Fibrozna cistična upala kosti
Osteoartropatia ipertrofizzante (sindrome di Pierre Marie-Bamberger)	Hypertrophic osteoarthropaty (Pierre Marie-Bamberger syndrome)	Ostéo-arthropathie hypertrophiante de Pierre Marie (syndrome de Marie-Bamberger)	Osteoartropatía hipertrófica (enfermedad de Bamberger-Marie)	Osteoartropatija hipertrofika Pierre Marie
Osteoclastoma (tumore a cellule giganti)	Gigantocellular tumor (osteoclastoma)	Tumeur à cellules géantes	Tumor de células gigantes (osteoclastoma)	Gigantocelularni tumor (osteoklastom)
Osteocondrite dissecante	Juvenile osteochondrosis	Ostéochondrose juvénile	Osteocondrosis juvenil	Juvenilna osteohondroza
Osteocondroma	Osteochondroma	Ostéochondrome	Osteocondroma	Osteohondrom
Osteogenesi imperfetta	Osteogenesis imperfecta (brittle bone disease)	Ostéogenèse imparfaite	Osteogénesis imperfecta (huesos de cristal)	Osteogeneza imperfekta (staklaste kosti)
Osteoma	Osteoma	Ostéome	Osteoma	Osteom
Osteomalacia	Osteomalacia	Ostéomalacie	Osteomalacia	Osteomalacija
Osteomielite fungale	Fungal osteomyelitis	Ostéomyélite fongique	Osteomielitis micótica	Gljivični osteomijelitis
Osteomielite luetica	Luetic osteomyelitis	Ostéomyélite syphilitique	Osteomielitis luética	Luetični osteomijelitis
Osteopetrosi (malattia delle ossa di marmo)	Osteopetrosis (marble bone disease)	Ostéopétrose (os de marbre)	Osteopetrosis (enfermedad de los huesos de marmol)	Osteopetroza (zadebljane kosti, bolest mramornih kostiju)
Osteoporosi	Osteoporosis	Ostéoporose	Osteoporosis	Osteoporoza
Osteosarcoma	Osteosarcoma	Ostéosarcome	Osteosarcoma	Osteosarkom
Osteosclerosi	Osteosclerosis	Ostéosclérose	Osteosclerosis	Osteoskleroza
Ottusità alle estremità	Dullness in limbs	Membres sourds	Torpeza en las extremidades	Tupost u udovima
Overdose di droga	Drug overdose	Surdose de drogue	Sobredosis por droga	Predoziranje drogom
Overdose di farmaci	Medication overdose	Surdose du médicament	Sobredosis de medicamentos	Predoziranje lijekom
Pallore	Paleness (pallor)	Pâleur	Palidez	Bljedilo
Palmi delle mani caldi e sudati	Warm sweaty palms	Paumes des mains chaudes et humides	Palmas de las manos calientes y mojadas	Topli i vlažni dlanovi
Pancraes aberrante	Aberrant pancreas	Pancréas aberrant	Pancreas aberrante	Aberantni pankreas
Papilledema (edema del nervo ottico)	Optic nerve edema	Oedème du nerf optique	Edema del nervio óptico	Otok očnog živca (zastojna papila)
Papilloma	Papilloma	Papillome	Papiloma	Papilom
Paracoccidioidimicosi (blastomicosi sudamericana)	Paracoccidioidomycosis (Brazilian blastomycosis)	Paracoccidioidose brésilienne	Paracoccidioidomicosis	Parakokcidioidomikoza (brazilska blastomikoza)
Parafimosi	Paraphimosis	Paraphimosis	Parafimosis	Parafimoza
Paragonimiasi	Paragonimiasis	Paragonimiase humaine	Paragonimosis (paragonimiasis)	Paragonimijaza
Paralisi	Paralysis	Paralysie	Parálisis	Paraliza (oduzetost, kljenut)
Paralisi cerebrale infantile	Cerebral palsy	Infirmité motorice cérébrale	Parálisis cerebral	Cerebralna paraliza
Paralisi dei arti superiori e inferiori (quadriplegia)	Paralysis of all limbs and torso (quadriplegia, tetraplegia)	Paralysie de quatre membres (tétraplégie)	Parálisis en brazos y piernas (tetraplejía, cuadriplejia)	Oduzetost gornjih i donjih ekstremiteta i torza (kvadriplegija, tetraplegija)
Paralisi di Bell	Bell's palsy	Paralysie de Bell	Parálisis de Bell	Bellova paraliza
Paralisi di parte inferiore del corpo (paraplegia)	Paralysis of lower extremities (paraplegia)	Paralysie des membres inférieurs (paraplégie)	Parálisis de la parte inferior del cuerpo (paraplejía)	Oduzetost donjih ekstremiteta (paraplegija)
Paralisi di una metà del corpo (emiplegia)	Paralysis of one half of a body (hemiplegia)	Paralysie de la moitié du corps (hémiplégie)	Parálisis de una mitad lateral de cuerpo (hemiplejía)	Oduzetost jedne polovine tijela (hemiplegija)
Paralisi di una parte di corpo simmetrica (diplegia)	Paralysis of symmetrical parts of the body (diplegia)	Paralysie des régions symétriques du corps (diplégie)	Parálisis de partes simétricas del cuerpo (diplejía)	Oduzetost simetričnih dijelova tijela (diplegija)

Italiano	Inglese	Francese	Spagnolo	Croato
Paranoia	Paranoia	Paranoïa	Paranoia	Paranoja
Paresi	Paresis	Parésie	Paresis	Pareza
Parestesie delle estremità	Numbness in limbs	Engourdissements dans les membres (paresthésie)	Adormecimiento de las extremidades	Utrnulost udova
Parodontite	Periodontitis	Parodontite	Periodontitis (piorrea)	Parodontoza
Paronichia	Paronychia	Paronychie	Paroniquia	Paronihija
Parotite (orecchioni)	Mumps (epidemic parotitis)	Oreillons (parotidite virale)	Paperas (parotiditis)	Zaušnjaci (mumps, parotitis)
Patereccio	Whitlow (felon)	Panaris	Panadizo	Panaricij
Pemfigo	Pemphigus	Pemphigus	Pénfigo	Pemfigus
Perdita dell'udito dovuta all'avanzamento dell'età (presbiacusia)	Age-related hearing loss (presbycusis)	Perte de l'audition liée à l'age (presbyacousie)	Trastorno de la capacidad para oír de las personas envejecen (presbiacusia)	Staračka nagluhost (prezbiakuzija)
Perdita dello strato superiore della pelle (desquamazione)	Shedding of the skin (desquamation)	Desquamation	Desquamación	Ljuštenje kože (deskvamacija)
Perdita di abilità di produzione del linguaggio verbale (afasia)	Loss of language ability (aphasia)	Perte d'habileté d'expression du langage (mutisme, aphasie)	Pérdida de capacidad de producir lenguaje (afasia)	Gubitak sposobnosti govora (afazija)
Perdita di liquido cerebrospinale dal naso (rinoliquorrea)	Leakage of cerebrospinal fluid through the nose	Écoulement de liquide cérébrospinal par le nez (rhinoliquorrhée)	Salida de líquido cerebroespinal por la nariz (rinoliquorrea)	Curenje likvora na nos (cerebrospinalna rinoreja)
Perdita di liquido cerebrospinale dall'orechio (otoliquorrea)	Leakage of cerebrospinal fluid through the ear	Écoulement de liquide cérébrospinal par l'oreille (otoliquorrhée)	Salida de líquido cerebroespinal por el oído (otoliquorrea)	Curenje likvora na uho (cerebrospinalna otoreja)
Perdita di memoria	Memory loss	Perte de mémoire	Pérdida de la memoria	Gubitak pamćenja
Perdita di metà di campo visivo (emianopsia)	Loss of half of a field of vision (hemianopsia)	Perte de la vue dans une moitié du champ visuel (hémianopsie)	Pérdida de la mitad del campo visual (hemianopsia)	Gubitak polovice vidnog polja (hemianopsija)
Perdita di polso	Absence of pulse	Absence de pouls	Pérdida de pulso	Gubitak pulsa
Perdita di sangue al di fuori della mestruazione (metrorragia)	Uterine bleeding (metrorrhagia)	Saignement de l'utérus (métrorragie)	Pérdida de sangre uterina (metrorragia)	Krvarenje iz maternice (metroragija)
Perdita di sangue dall'ano (rettoragia, proctorragia)	Anal bleeding	Saignement anal (rectorragie)	Pérdida de sangre a través del ano (rectorragia)	Krvarenje iz analnog otvora
Perdita di senso di tocco	Loss of the sense of touch	Perte du sens du toucher	Pérdida del sentido del tacto	Gubitak osjeta dodoira
Perdita di udito	Hearing loss	Perte d'ouïe	Pérdida de la capacidad auditiva	Gubitak sluha
Perforazione del timpano	Perforated eardrum (tympanorrhexis)	Perforation du tympan	Perforación del tímpano	Puknuće bubnjića (perforacija bubnjića, timpanoreksija)
Periostite tibiale (sindrome del muscolo tibiale posteriore)	Tibialis posterior syndrome	Syndrome tibial postérieur	Síndrome del tibial posterior	Sindrom stražnjeg tibijalnog mišića
Peritendite rotulea (ginocchio del saltatore)	Irritated knee (jumper's knee, patellar tendinopathy)	Genou du sauteur (tendinite rotulienne)	Rodilla de saltador (tendinopatía rotuliana)	Podraženo koljeno (skakačko koljeno)
Perniosi	Chilblain (perniosis)	Engelure	Sabañón	Smrzotina
Pertosse	Whooping cough (pertussis)	Coqueluche	Tos ferina (coqueluche)	Hripavac (pasji kašalj, pertussis)
Peste (pestilenza)	Plague (pest)	Peste	Peste	Kuga
Petecchia	Petechia	Pétéchie	Petequia	Petehije
Petto carenato	Pigeon chest (pectus carinatum)	Pectus carinatum	Pectus carinatum	Kokošja prsa
Piaga da decubito (decubito)	Bedsore (decubitus ulcer)	Escarre (plaie de lit, ulcère de décubitus)	Úlcera de decúbito	Dekubitus
Piede calcaneo	Pes calcaneus	Pied calcanéus	Pie calcáneo	Petno stopalo
Piede cavo (pes cavus)	High arches (pes cavus)	Pied creux	Pie cavo (pes cavus)	Izdubljeno stopalo (pes excavatus)
Piede d'atleta (tinea pedis)	Athlete's foot (tinea pedis)	Pied d'athlète (tinea pedis)	Tiña del pie (pie de atleta, tinea pedis)	Atletsko stopalo (gljivična infekcija stopala, tinea pedis)
Piede equino	Dancer's foot (pes equinus)	Pied equin	Pie equino	Balerinsko stopalo (pes equinus)
Piede equino (talipes equinovarus)	Club foot (talipes equinovarus)	Pied-bot (pied-bot équin)	Pie equinovaro (talipes equinovarus, pie bot, pie retorcido)	Čopavo stopalo (uvrnuto stopalo, pes equinovarus)
Piede piatto (pes planus)	Flat foot (pes planus)	Pied plat (pes planus)	Pie plano (pes planus, arcos vencidos)	Spušteno stopalo (pes planus)
Piede piatto valgo (pes valgus)	Pes valgus	Pied valgus	Pie valgo	Izvrnuto stopalo (pes valgus)
Pielonefrite	Pyelonephritis (kidney infection)	Pyélonéphrite (infection bactérienne des voies urinaires hautes)	Pielonefritis (infección urinaria alta)	Pijelonefritis (infekcija bubrega)
Pilorospasmo	Pylorospasm	Spasme du pylore	Pilorospasmo	Pilorospazam
Pinta	Pinta	Pinta	Pinta	Pinta
Pionefrosi	Pyonephrosis	Pyonéphrose (pus dans le rein)	Pionefrosis	Pionefroza

Italiano	Inglese	Francese	Spagnolo	Croato
Pipita	Agnail (hangnail)	Envie de l'ongle	Padrastro	Zanoktica
Piromania	Pyromania	Pyromanie	Piromanía	Piromanija
Pitiriasi versicolor (tinea versicolor)	Tinea versicolor (pityriasis versicolor, haole rot)	Pityriasis versicolor	Tiña versicolor (pitiriasis versicolor)	Pitirijaza (svjetlije mrlje na osunčanoj koži, Tinea versicolor)
Placca (tartaro)	Dental plaque (dental tartar)	Plaque dentaire	Placa dental	Zubni kamenac
Pneumoconiosi	Pneumoconiosis	Pneumoconiose	Neumoconiosis	Pneumokonioza
Pneumopatia interstiziale	Interstitial lung disease	Maladie pulmonaire interstitielle	Enfermedad pulmonar interstitial	Intersticijska bolest pluća
Pneumotorace	Pneumothorax	Pneumothorax	Neumotórax	Pneumotoraks
Policitemia	Polycythemia	Polycythémie	Policitemia	Policitemija
Polidattilia	Polydactyly	Polydactylie	Polidactilia	Polidaktilija
Polimialgia reumatica	Polymyalgia rheumatica	Polymyalgia rheumatica	Polimialgia reumática	Reumatska polimialgija
Polimiosite	Polymyositis	Polymyosite	Polimiositis	Polimiozitis
Poliomielite (polio, paralisi infantile)	Poliomyelitis (polio, infantile paralysis)	Poliomyélite (polio, paralysie spinale infantile)	Poliomielitis (parálisis infantil)	Dječja paraliza (polio, poliomijelitis)
Polipo	Polyp	Polype	Pólipo	Polip
Polipo cervicale	Cervical polyp	Polype au col de l'utérus	Pólipo cervical	Polip na grliću maternice
Polipo del colon	Colon polyp	Polype du côlon	Pólipo de colon	Polip na debelom crijevu
Polipo della corda vocale	Vocal chords polyp	Polype des cordes vocales	Pólipo de las cuerdas vocales	Polip na glasnicama
Polipo endometriale	Endometrial polyp (uterine polyp)	Polype utérin	Pólipo endometrial	Polip maternice
Polipo nasale	Nasal polyp	Polype nasal	Pólipo nasal	Polip u nosu (nosni polip)
Polmonite atipica	Atypical pneumonia	Pneumonie atypique	Neumonía atípica	Atipična upala pluća
Polmonite batterica	Bacterial pneumonia	Pneumonie bactérienne	Neumonía bacteriana	Bakterijska upala pluća
Polmonite da Pneumocisti	Pneumocystis pneumonia (pneumocystosis)	Pneumocystose	Neumonía por Pneumocystis	Pneumocistična upala pluća
Polmonite virale	Viral pneumonia	Pneumonie virale	Neumonía viral	Virusna upala pluća
Polso accelerato	Accelerated pulse rate	Fréquence du pouls accélérée	Pulso acelerado	Ubrzani puls
Porfiria	Porphyria	Porphyrie	Porfiria	Porfirija
Porpora	Purpura	Purpura	Púrpura	Purpura
Porpora trombotica trombocitopenica	Thrombotic thrombocytopenic purpura	Purpura thrombotique thrombocytopénique	Púrpura trombocitopénica trombótica	Trombotska trombocitopenična purpura
Prematuro sviluppo sessuale del sesso opposto	Premature sexual development of the opposite sex	Développement sexuel prématuré du sexe opposé	Desarrollo sexual prematuro del sexo opuesto	Prerano spolno fizičko sazrijevanje suprotnog spola
Prematuro sviluppo sessuale dello stesso sesso	Premature sexual development of the same sex	Développement sexuel prématuré du même sexe	Desarrollo sexual prematuro del mismo sexo	Prerano spolno fizičko sazrijevanje istog spola
Presbiopia (presbitismo)	Age-related long-sightedness (presbyopia)	Mauvaise vision de près liée à l'âge (presbytie)	Vista cansada por la edad (presbiopía)	Staračka dalekovidnost (prezbiopija)
Presenza di emoglobina nelle urine (emoglobinuria)	Hemoglobin in urine (hemoglobinuria)	Hémoglobine dans l'urine (hémoglobinurie)	Hemoglobina en orina (hemoglobinuria)	Hemoglobin u urinu (hemoglobinurija)
Presenza di pus nelle urine (piuria)	Pus in urine (pyuria)	Présence de pus dans l'urine (pyurie)	Presencia de pus en la orina (piuria)	Gnoj u urinu (piurija)
Presenza di pus nello sputo	Pus in sputum	Crachat purulent	Esputo que contiene pus	Gnojni ispljuvak
Primo flusso mestruale (menarca)	First menstrual cycle (menarche)	Première période de menstruations (ménarche)	Primera menstruación (menarquia)	Prva mjesečnica (menarha)
Proctite	Proctitis	Proctite	Proctitis	Proktitis
Produzione di pochi spermatozoi (oligospermia)	Low semen volume (oligospermia)	Présence de spermatozoïdes en quantité faible (oligospermie)	Bajo volumen de semen (oligospermia)	Manjak sperme (oligospermija)
Produzione di saliva eccessiva (ipersalivazione)	Excessive secretion of saliva (hypersalivation)	Sécrétion de la salive excessive	Excesiva producción de saliva (hipersalivación)	Pojačano lučenje sline (hipersalivacija)
Prolasso del retto	Rectal prolapse	Prolapsus rectal	Prolapso rectal	Prolaps rektuma
Prolasso uterino	Uterine prolapse (fallen womb)	Prolapsus de l'utérus	Prolapso del útero	Prolaps maternice (spuštena maternica)
Proteinosi alveolare polmonare	Pulmonary alveolar proteinosis	Protéinose alvéolaire pulmonaire	Proteinosis alveolar pulmonar	Alveolarna proteinoza pluća
Proteinuria	Proteinuria (presence of proteins in urine)	Protéinurie (excès de protéines dans l'urine)	Proteinuria	Bjelančevine u urinu (proteinurija)
Prurito (pizzicore)	Itching	Prurit	Prurito (picazón, comezón, rasquiña)	Svrbež
Psiconevrosi (nevrosi)	Psychoneurosis	Psychonévrose	Psiconeurosis	Psihoneuroza
Psicopatia	Psychopathy	Psychopathie	Psicopatía	Psihopatija
Psicosi	Psychosis	Psychose	Psicosis	Psihoza
Psicosi maniaco-depressiva	Bipolar disorder (manic-depressive psychosis)	Trouble bipolaire (psychose maniaco-dépressive)	Trastorno bipolar (psicosis maníaco-depresiva)	Bipolarni poremećaj (manično-depresivna psihoza)
Psittacosi (psittacornitosi)	Psittacosis (parrot fever)	Psittacose	Psitacosis (fiebre del loro)	Psitakoza
Psoriasi	Psoriasis	Psoriasis	Psoriasis	Psorijaza
Pubalgia dello sportivo	Groin pain syndrome	Pubalgie du sportif	Síndrome de dolor inguinal	Sindrom bolnih prepona

Italiano	Inglese	Francese	Spagnolo	Croato
Pubertà precoce (pubertà prematura)	Precocious puberty (premature puberty)	Puberté précoce	Pubertad precoz	Preuranjeni pubertet
Pubertà tardiva	Delayed puberty	Puberté tardive	Retraso de la pubertad	Zakašnjeli pubertet
Puntura di formiche	Ant sting	Piqûre de fourmi	Picadura de hormiga	Ugriz mrava
Puntura di scorpione	Scorpion sting	Piqûre de scorpion	Picadura de escorpión	Ugriz škorpiona
Puntura di zanzara infetta	Infected mosquito bite	Piqûre de moustique infecté	Picadura de mosquito infectado	Ugriz zaraženog komarca
Pupille costrette	Small pupils	Pupilles diminuées	Pupilas pequeñas	Sužene zjenice
Pupille dilatate	Enlarged pupils	Pupilles dilatées	Pupilas dilatadas	Proširene zjenice
Pus	Pus	Pus	Pus	Gnoj
Pustola	Pustule	Pustule	Pústula	Gnojni mjehurić
R.S.I. (Repetitive Strain Injury)	Repetitive strain injury (cumulative trauma disorder)	Lésion due à un surmenage répétitif	Síndrome de sobreuso	Sindrom prenaprezanja
Rabbia	Rabies	Rage	Rabia	Bjesnoća (rabies)
Rabdomioma	Rhabdomyoma	Rhabdomyome	Rabdomioma	Rabdomiom
Rabdomiosarcoma	Rhabdomyosarcoma	Rhabdomyosarcome	Rabdomiosarcoma	Rabdomiosarkom
Rachitismo	Rickets (rachitis)	Rachitisme	Raquitismo	Rahitis
Rachitismo renale	Renal rickets	Rachitisme rénal	Raquitismo renal	Bubrežni rahitis
Raucedine	Hoarseness	Enrouement	Ronquera	Promuklost
Rene a ferro di cavallo (fusione renale)	Horseshoe kidney (renal fusion)	Rein en fer à cheval	Riñón de herradura (fusión en los riñones)	Potkovičasti bubreg
Rene policistico	Polycystic kidney disease	Rein polykystique	Enfermedad poliquística renal	Policistični bubreg
Respirazione difficoltosa	Breathing difficulty	Difficulté de respiration	Dificultad de respiración	Otežano disanje
Respirazione superficiale	Shallow breathing	Respiration superficielle	Respiración superficial	Površinsko plitko disanje
Respiro di Biot	Biot's respiration	Respiration de Biot	Respiración de Biot	Biotovo disanje
Respiro di Cheyne-Stokes	Periodic breathing (Cheyne-Stokes respiration)	Respiration Cheynes-Stokes	Respiración periódica (respiración de Cheynes-Stokes)	Periodično disanje (Cheyne-Stokesovo disanje)
Respiro di Kussmaul	Kussmaul breathing	Respiration de type Kussmaul	Respiración de Kussmaul	Kussmaulovo disanje
Reticoloendotelioma (reticolosarcoma)	Reticuloendothelial sarcoma	Sarcome réticuloendothélial	Reticulosarcoma (sarcoma reticuloendotelial)	Retikuloendotelijalni sarkom
Retinite pigmentosa	Retinitis pigmentosa (retinal pigment epithelium dystrophy)	Rétinite pigmentaire	Retinitis pigmentosa	Pigmentna distrofija mrežnice
Retinopatia del prematuro	Retinopathy of prematurity (retrolental fibroplasia)	Rétinopathie du prématuré	Retinopatía de la prematuridad	Retrolentalna fibroplazija
Retinopatia diabetica	Diabetic retinopathy	Rétinopathie diabétique	Retinopatía diabética	Dijabetična retinopatija
Retroflessione uterina	Retroverted uterus	Utérus rétroversé	Retroversión del útero	Retrovertirani uterus
Rettocolite ulcerosa	Ulcerative colitis	Colite ulcéreuse	Colitis ulcerosa	Ulcerozni kolitis
Reumatismo extra-articolare	Extrajoint rheumatism	Rhumatisme extraarticulaire	Reumatismo extraarticular	Izvanzglobni reumatizam
Rickettsiosi	Rickettsiosis	Rickettsiose	Rickettsiosis	Rikecioza
Ridotta mobilità articolare	Limited joint mobility	Mobilité atriculaire limitée	Rango de movimiento articular limitado	Ograničena pokretljivost zgloba
Riduzione della forza muscolare (astenia)	Loss of strenght (asthenia)	Affaiblissement de l'organisme (asthénie)	Pérdida de fuerza muscular (astenia)	Gubitak mišiĉne snage (astenija)
Riduzione della frequenza cardiaca (bradicardia)	Slow pulse rate (bradycardia)	Rythme cardiaque bas (bradycardie)	Descenso de la frecuencia cardiaca (bradicardia)	Usporen puls (bradikardija)
Riduzione della frequenza respiratoria (bradipnea)	Slow breathing rate (bradypnea)	Respiration ralentie (bradypnée)	Descenso de la frecuencia respiratoria (bradipnea)	Usporeno disanje (bradipneja)
Rigidità	Stiffness	Raideur	Agarrotamiento	Ukočenost
Rigidità dell'articolazione	Joint stiffness	Raideur articulaire	Rigidez de las articulaciones	Zakočenost zgloba
Rigidità nucale	Nuchal rigidity (stiff neck)	Raideur de nuque (raideur méningée)	Rigidez de nuca (cuello rígido)	Kočenje šije (ukočeni vrat)
Rinite	Rhinitis	Rhinite	Rinitis	Rinitis
Rinite allergica	Allergic rhinitis	Rhinite allergique	Rinitis alérgica	Alergijski rinitis
Rinite vasomotoria	Vasomotor rhinitis	Rhinite vasomotrice	Rinitis vasomotora	Vazomotorni rinitis
Ripugnanza al cibo	Food aversion	Aversion pour la nourriture	Aversión por la comida	Gađenje prema hrani
Risalita di alimenti dallo stomaco alla bocca (rigurgito)	Expulsion of undigested food from the mouth (regurgitation)	Retour à la bouche du contenu de l'estomac (régurgitation)	Regreso del contenido alimentario a través del esófago (regurgitación)	Vraćanje hrane iz želuca u usta (regurgitacija)
Ritardo mentale	Mental retardation	Retard mental (handicap mental)	Retraso mental	Mentalna retardacija
Ritenzione urinaria	Urinary retention (ischuria)	Rétention d'urine	Retención de orina	Zastoj urina (urinarna retencija)
Rizartrosi (artrosi dell'articolazione alla base del police)	Thumb joint arthritis	Rhizarthrose	Rizartrosis	Rizartroza
Ronzio auricolare (acufene, tinnito)	Ringing in ears (tinnitus)	Acouphène	Pitidos en el oído (acúfeno, tinnitus)	Zujanje u ušima (tinitus)
Rosacea	Rosacea	Rosacée (couperose)	Rosácea	Rozacea
Rosolia	German measles (rubella)	Rubéole	Rubéola	Rubeola (crljenac)

Italiano	Inglese	Francese	Spagnolo	Croato
Rottura	Rupture	Rupture	Ruptura (rotura)	Prsnuće (puknuće, razdor, ruptura)
Rottura del legamento	Ligament rupture (torn ligament)	Rupture ligamentaire	Ruptura de ligamento	Puknuće ligamenta
Rottura del legamento crociato anteriore del ginocchio	Anterior cruciate ligament rupture (ACL rupture)	Rupture du ligament croisé antéro-externe (rupture du LCA)	Ruptura de ligamento cruzado anterior	Razdor prednje ukrižene sveze koljenskog zgloba
Rottura del menisco	Meniscus rupture (meniscus tear)	Rupture du ménisque	Ruptura de menisco	Razdor meniskusa
Rottura del tendine	Tendon rupture (torn tendon)	Rupture du tendon	Ruptura del tendón	Puknuće tetive
Rottura del tendine di Achille	Achilles tendon rupture	Rupture du tendon d'Achille	Ruptura del tendón de Aquiles	Puknuće Ahilove tetive
Rottura della cuffia dei rotatori	Rotator cuff rupture (rotator cuff tear)	Rupture de la coiffe des rotateurs	Ruptura del manguito rotador	Razdor rotatorne manžete ramenog zgloba
Rottura della milza	Ruptured spleen	Rupture de la rate	Ruptura del bazo	Ruptura slezene
Rottura della vescica urinaria	Rupture of urinary bladder	Rupture de la vessie	Ruptura de la vejiga urinaria	Rascjep mokraćnog mjehura
Rottura di aneurisma	Aneurysm rupture	Rupture d'anévrisme	Ruptura del aneurisma	Prsnuće aneurizme
Rottura muscolare	Muscle rupture	Rupture musculaire	Ruptura muscular	Rastrgnuće mišića (ruptura mišića)
Ruga	Wrinkle	Ride	Arruga	Bora
Rumore durante la respirazione (stridore)	Breathing sound due to blockage in the airway (stridor)	Bruit anormal émis lors de la respiration (stridor)	Estridor	Glasno otežano disanje (stridor)
Sacco dell'ernia	Hernia sack	Sac herniaire	Saco de hernia (saco herniario)	Kilna vreća
Salmonellosi	Salmonellosis	Salmonellose	Salmonelosis	Salmoneloza
Sangue al liquido cerebrospinale	Blood in cerebrospinal fluid	Sang dans le liquide cérébro-spinal	Sangre en el líquido cefalorraquídeo	Krv u likvoru
Sangue nelle feci (ematochezia)	Blood in stool (hematochezia)	Sang dans les selles (hématochézie)	Sangre en las heces (hematochezia)	Krv u stolici (hematohezija)
Sangue nello sputo (emottisi)	Blood in sputum (hemoptysis)	Sang dans l'expectoration (hémoptysie)	Sangre en el esputo (hemoptisis)	Krvavi iskašljaj (hemoptiza)
Sarcoidosi	Sarcoidosis (sarcoid, Besnier-Boeck disease)	Sarcoïdose (maladie de Besnier-Boeck-Schaumann)	Sarcoidosis (enfermedad de Besnier-Boeck)	Sarkoidoza
Sarcoma	Sarcoma	Sarcome	Sarcoma	Sarkom
Sarcoma botrioide	Botryoid sarcoma	Sarcome botryoïde	Sarcoma botrioide	Botrioidni sarkom
Sarcoma di Ewing	Ewing's sarcoma	Sarcome d'Ewing	Sarcoma de Ewing	Ewing sarkom (endoteliosarkom)
Sarcoma di Kaposi	Kaposi's sarcoma	Sarcome de Kaposi	Sarcoma de Kaposi	Kaposijev sarkom (endoteliosarkom)
Sarcoma sinoviale	Synovial sarcoma	Sarcome synovial	Sarcoma sinovial	Sinovijalni sarkom
Sarcopenia	Sarcopenia	Sarcopénie	Sarcopenia	Sarkopenija
SARS (Sindrome Acuta Respiratoria Severa)	Severe acute respiratory syndrome (SARS)	Syndrome respiratoire aigu sévère (SRAS)	Síndrome respiratorio agudo severo (SRAS, SARS)	Sindrom akutne respiratorne insuficijencije (SARS)
Sbadiglio	Yawn	Bâillement	Bostezo	Zijevanje
Sbavando (ptialismo, scialorrea)	Drooling (ptyalism, sialorrhea, slobbering)	Hypersialorrhée (ptyalisme)	Sialorrea (ptialismo)	Slinjenje
Scabbia (rogna)	Scabies (the itch)	Gale (mal de Sainte-Marie)	Arador de la sarna (escabiosis)	Svrab (skabijes)
Scarlattina	Scarlet fever	Scarlatine (fièvre écarlate)	Escarlatina (fiebre escarlata)	Šarlah (skarlatina)
Scarsa secrezione salivare (xerostomia)	Dry mouth (xerostomia)	Sècheresse de la bouche (xèrostomie)	Sequedad de la boca (xerostomía)	Suha sluznica usta
Schistosomiasi	Schistosomiasis (snail fever)	Schistosomiase (bilharziose)	Esquistosomiasis (bilharziasis)	Šistosomijaza
Schizofrenia	Schizophrenia	Schizophrénie	Esquizofrenia	Šizofrenija
Sciatica	Sciatica	Sciatique	Ciática	Išijas
Sclerodermia	Scleroderma	Sclérodermie	Esclerodermia	Sklerodermija
Sclerosi laterale amiotrofica	Amyotrophic lateral sclerosis	Sclérose latérale amyotrophique (maladie de Charcot)	Esclerosis lateral amiotrófica	Amiotrofična lateralna skleroza
Sclerosi multipla	Multiple sclerosis	Sclérose en plaques	Esclerosis múltiple	Multipla skleroza
Scoliosi	Scoliosis	Scoliose	Escoliosis	Skolioza
Scorbuto	Scurvy	Scorbut	Escorbuto	Skorbut
Scossa muscolare (fasciciolazione)	Muscle twitch (fasciculation)	Fasciculation musculaire	Crispar del músculo (fasciculación)	Trzanje mišića
Scotoma	Scotoma	Scotome	Escotoma	Skotom
Seborrea	Seborrhea	Séborrhée	Seborrea	Seboreja
Semi-coma	Semicoma	Semi-coma	Semicoma	Semikoma
Sensazione bruciante	Burning sensation	Sensation cuisante	Sensación de ardor	Pećenje (žarenje)
Sensibilità al dolore (algesia)	Sensitivity to pain (algesia)	Sensibilité à la douleur (algésie)	Sensibilidad al dolor (algesia)	Osjetljivost na bol (algezija)
Senso della paura	Sensation of fear	Sensation de peur	Sensación de miedo	Osjećaj straha
Senso delle scarpe troppo strette	'Tight shoes' sensation	Sensation des chaussures très serré	Sensación de "zapatos apretados"	Osjećaj "tijesnih cipela"
Sepsi	Sepsis	Sepsis	Sepsis	Sepsa

Italiano	Inglese	Francese	Spagnolo	Croato
Sesta malattia (roseola infantum, esantema subitum)	Exanthema subitum (roseola infantum, sixth disease)	Roséole (exanthème subit, sixième maladie)	Roséola (exantema súbito)	Rozeola infantum (egzantema subitum, šesta bolest)
Sete	Thirst	Soif	Sed	Žed
Setticemia	Septicemia	Septicémie	Septicemia	Septikemija
Sfogo (eruzione cutanea)	Rash (eruption, eczema)	Rash (eczéma)	Sarpullido (erupción, eccema)	Osip
Shigellosi	Shigellosis (bacillary dysentery)	Shigellose	Shigelosis	Šigeloza
Shock cardiogeno	Cardiogenic shock	Choc cardiogénique	Choque cardiogénico	Kardiogeni šok
Shock chirurgico	Surgical shock (postoperative shock)	Choc post-opératoire	Choque quirúrgico	Kirurški šok
Shock endotossico	Endotoxic shock	Choc endotoxique	Choque endotoxico	Endotoksični šok
Shock ipovolemico	Hypovolemic shock	Choc hypovolémique	Choque hipovolémico	Hipovolemički šok
Shock neurogeno	Neurogenic shock	Choc neurogénique	Choque neurogénico	Neurogeni šok
Shock ostruttivo	Obstructive shock	Choc obstructive	Choque obstructivo	Opstruktivni šok
Shock settico	Septic shock	Choc septique	Choque séptico	Septički šok
Shock spinale	Spinal shock	Choc spinal	Choque espinal	Spinalni šok
Shock traumatico	Traumatic shock	Choc traumatique	Choque traumático	Traumatski šok
SIDA (sindrome da ImmunoDeficienza Acquisita, AIDS)	AIDS (acquired immune deficiency syndrome)	SIDA (syndrome d'immunodéficience acquise)	SIDA (síndrome de inmunodeficiencia adquirida)	SIDA (sindrom stečene imunodeficijencije, AIDS)
Siderosi	Siderosis	Sidérose	Siderosis	Sideroza
Sifilide (lue)	Syphilis	Syphilis (vérole)	Sífilis	Sifilis (lues)
Sifiloma	Chancre	Chancre	Chancro	Čankir
Silicosi	Silicosis	Silicose	Silicosis	Silikoza
Sincope	Syncope	Syncope	Síncope	Sinkopa
Sindattilia	Syndactyly	Syndactylie	Sindactilia	Sindaktilija
Sindrome alcolica fetale	Fetal alcohol syndrome	Syndrome d'alcoolisation foetale	Síndrome de alcoholismo fetal	Fetusni alkoholni sindrom
Sindrome cervicale	Cervicocephal syndrome	Syndrome cervical	Síndrome cervical	Cervikocefalni sindrom
Sindrome cervicobrachiale (sindrome spalla-mano)	Cervicobrachial syndrome	Syndrome cervico-brachial	Síndrome cérvico-braquial	Sindrom vrat-rame (cervikobrahijalni sindrom)
Sindrome compartimentale	Compartment syndrome	Syndrome des loges	Síndrome compartimental	Sindrom fascijalnog prostora
Sindrome da carcinoide	Carcinoid syndrome	Syndrome carcinoïde	Síndrome carcinoide	Karcinoidni sindrom
Sindrome da conflitto subacromiale (impingement sub-acromiale)	Shoulder impingement syndrome (subacromial impingement syndrome)	Syndrome du conflit sous-acromial	Síndrome del conflicto subacromial	Sindrom sraza ramena (subakromijalni sindrom sraza)
Sindrome da distress respiratorio	Respiratory distress syndrome	Syndrome de détresse respiratoire	Síndrome de distrés respiratorio	Respiratorni distres sindrom
Sindrome da distress respiratorio del neonato (malattia da membrane ialine polmonari)	Hyaline membrane disease (infant respiratory distress syndrome)	Maladie des membranes hyalines (détresse respiratoire néonatale)	Enfermedad de la membrana hialina (síndrome de distrés respiratorio)	Bolest hijaline membrane (respiratorni sindrom novorođenćeta)
Sindrome da fatica cronica	Chronic fatigue syndrome	Syndrome de fatigue chronique	Síndrome de fatiga crónica	Sindrom kroničnog umora
Sindrome da impingement della caviglia	Ankle impingement syndrome	Conflit antérieur de la cheville	Pinzamiento anterolateral del tobillo	Prednji sindrom sraza gornjeg nožnog zgloba
Sindrome da impingement posteriore di caviglia	Posterior ankle impingement syndrome	Conflit postérieur de la cheville	Síndrome de pinzamiento posterior del tobillo	Sindrom sraza stražnjeg nožnog zgloba
Sindrome da schiacciamento	Crush-syndrome	Syndrome d'écrasement	Síndrome de aplastamiento (síndrome de crush)	Crush-sindrom
Sindrome da stress tibiale mediale	Shin splints	Périostite tibiale	Dolor en las espinillas	Trkačka potkoljenica
Sindrome da vibrazioni mano-braccio	Hand-arm vibration syndrome (vibration white finger)	Syndrome des vibrations du système main-bras	Vibraciones mano bra-zo (dedo blanco indu-cido por vibraciones)	Vibracijski sindrom šaka-ruka
Sindrome degli ischio-crurali (sindrome dell'hamstring)	Tight hamstrings syndrome	Hamstring syndrome	Síndrome de isquiosurales cortos	Sindrom stražnje lože natkoljenice (sindrom hamstringsa)
Sindrome del bambino flaccido	Floppy infant syndrome	Syndrome du bébé mou	Síndrome de bebé flácido	Sindrom mlohavog djeteta
Sindrome del colon irritabile (colon spastico)	Irritable bowel syndrome (spastic colon)	Côlon irritable (côlon spastique)	Síndrome de intestino irritable (colon irritable, colon espástico)	Sindrom iritabilnog crijeva (spastični kolon)
Sindrome del dolore patello-femorale (ginocchio del corridore)	Chondromalacia patellae (runner's knee, patello-femoral pain syndrome)	Chondromalacie rotulienne	Chondromalacia rotuliana (síndrome patelo-femoral)	Hondromalacija patele (trkačko koljeno, sindrom patelofemoralne boli)
Sindrome del grido di gatto	Cat cry syndrome (5p minus syndrome, Lejeune's syndrome)	Maladie du cri du chat (syndrome de Lejeune)	Síndrome del maullido del gato (síndrome de Lejeune)	Sindrom mačjeg krika
Sindrome del tunnel carpale	Carpal tunnel syndrome	Syndrome du canal carpien	Síndrome del túnel carpiano	Sindrom karpalnog tunela
Sindrome del tunnel cubitale	Little league elbow syndrome (LLE syndrome)	Syndrome du tunnel cubital	Síndrome del túnel cubital	Sindrom kopljaškog lakta

Italiano	Inglese	Francese	Spagnolo	Croato
Sindrome del tunnel tarsale	Tarsal tunnel syndrome	Syndrome du canal tarsien	Síndrome del túnel tarsiano	Sindrom tarzalnog kanala
Sindrome della benderella ileotibiale	Iliotibial band friction syndrome	Syndrome de la bandelette iliotibiale (syndrome de l'essuie glace)	Síndrome de fricción de la banda iliotibial	Sindrom trenja iliotibijalnog traktusa
Sindrome della classe economica	Traveller's thrombosis (economy class syndrome)	Thrombose du voyageur	Síndrome de la clase turista	Sindrom ekonomske klase
Sindrome della morte improvvisa del lattante	Sudden infant death syndrome (crib death, cot death)	Syndrome de mort subite du nourrisson	Síndrome de muerte súbita del lactante (muerte en cuna)	Sindrom iznenadne smrti dojenčeta
Sindrome delle apnee nel sonno	Sleep apnea	Apnée du sommeil	Apnea del sueño	Noćna desaturacija
Sindrome dello stretto toracico superiore	Thoracic outlet syndrome	Syndrome de traversée thoraco-cervico-brachiale	Síndrome del estrecho torácico	Torakalni sindrom
Sindrome di Behçet	Behçet's disease	Maladie de Behçet	Síndrome de Behçet	Behçetova bolest
Sindrome di Blount	Blount's disease	Maladie de Blount	Enfermedad de Blount (tibia vara)	Blountova bolest
Sindrome di Cushing (ipercortisolismo)	Cushing's syndrome (hypercorticism)	Syndrome de Cushing (hypercorticisme)	Síndrome de Cushing (hipercortisolismo)	Cushingov sindrom (hiperkortikolizam)
Sindrome di De Quervain	DeQuervain syndrome	Syndrome de DeQuervain (ténosynovite de DeQuervain)	Síndrome de DeQuervain	Sindrom bubnjarskog palca (Morbus DeQuervain)
Sindrome di Down	Down syndrome	Syndrome de Down	Síndrome de Down	Downov sindrom (mongoloidizam)
Sindrome di Edwards	Edwards syndrome (trisomy 18)	Syndrome d'Edwards (trisomie 18)	Síndrome de Edwards (trisomía del 18)	Trisomija 18D (Edwardsov sindrom)
Sindrome di Eisenmenger	Eisenmenger's syndrome	Syndrome d'Eisenmenger	Síndrome de Eisenmenger	Eisenmengerov sindrom
Sindrome di Goodpasture	Goodpasture's syndrome	Syndrome de Goodpasture (maladie des anti-corps anti-membrane basale glomérulaire)	Síndrome de Goodpasture	Goodpastureov sindrom
Sindrome di Guillain-Barré	Guillain-Barré syndrome	Syndrome de Guillain-Barré	Síndrome de Guillain-Barré	Guillain-Barréov sindrom
Sindrome di Hoffa	Hoffa's disease	Maladie de Hoffa	Enfermedad de Hoffa	Morbus Hoffa
Sindrome di Kawasaki	Kawasaki disease	Maladie de Kawasaki	Enfermedad de Kawasaki	Kawasakijeva bolest (mukokutani limfo-glandularni sindrom)
Sindrome di Leriche	Aortoiliac occlusive disease (Leriche's syndrome)	Maladie occlusive aorto-iliaque	Síndrome de Leriche	Lericheov sindrom
Sindrome di Marfan	Marfan syndrome	Syndrome de Marfan	Síndrome de Marfan	Marfanov sindrom
Sindrome di McCune-Albright-Sternberg	McCune-Albright syndrome	Syndrome de McCune-Albright	Síndrome de McCune-Albright	Albrightov sindrom
Sindrome di Menière	Meniere's disease	Maladie de Menière	Enfermedad de Menière	Menierova bolest
Sindrome di Osgood-Schlatter	Osgood-Schlatter disease (rugby knee)	Maladie d'Osgood-Schlatter	Enfermedad de Osgood-Schlatter	Osgood-Schlatterova bolest
Sindrome di Patau	Patau syndrome (trisomy 13)	Syndrome de Patau (trisomie 13)	Síndrome de Patau (trisomía en el par 13)	Trisomija 13D (Patauov sindrom)
Sindrome di Preiser	Preiser disease	Maladie de Preiser	Enfermedad de Preiser	Morbus Preiser
Sindrome di Raynaud	Raynaud's disease	Maladie de Raynaud	Enfermedad de Raynaud	Raynaudova bolest
Sindrome di Reiter	Reactive arthritis (Reiter's syndrome)	Arthrite réactive (syndrome de Reiter)	Síndrome de Reiter (artritis reactiva)	Reiterov sindrom
Sindrome di Reye	Reye's syndrome	Syndrome de Reye	Síndrome de Reye	Reyeov sindrom
Sindrome di Sjögren	Sjögren's syndrome	Syndrome de Sjögren	Síndrome de Sjögren	Sjögrenov sindrom
Sindrome di Tourette	Tourette's syndrome	Syndrome de Tourette	Síndrome de Tourette	Touretteov sindrom
Sindrome di Turner	Turner syndrome	Syndrome de Turner	Síndrome de Turner	Turnerov sindrom
Sindrome dolorosa	Pain syndrome	Syndrome de douleur	Síndrome doloroso	Bolni sindrom
Sindrome epato-renale	Hepatorenal syndrome	Syndrome hépato-rénal	Síndrome hepatorrenal	Hepatorenalni sindrom
Sindrome mielodisplasica	Myelodysplastic syndrome	Syndrome myélodysplasique	Síndrome mielodisplásico (preleucemia)	Mijelodisplastični sindrom
Sindrome nefrosica	Nephrotic syndrome	Syndrome néphrotique	Síndrome nefrótico	Nefrotski sindrom
Sindrome post trombotica	Post-thrombotic syndrome	Syndrome post-thrombotique	Síndrome postrombótico	Posttrombotički sindrom
Sindrome premestruale	Premenstrual syndrome (PMS)	Syndrome prémenstruel (SPM)	Síndrome premenstrual	Predmenstruacijski sindrom (PMS)
Sindrome prodromica	Early symptom (prodrome)	Phase prodromique	Síndrome prodrómico	Predsimptom bolesti prije nego se bolest razvije
Singhiozzo	Hiccup	Hoquet	Hipo	Štucavica
Sinostosi radio-ulnare	Radioulnar synostosis	Synostose radio-ulnaire	Sinostosis radiocubital	Radioulnarna sinostoza
Sinovioma	Synovioma	Synoviome	Sinovioma	Sinoviom
Sinusite	Sinus headache	Douleur des sinus (sinusite)	Dolor de cabeza por sinusitis	Sinusna glavobolja
Siringomielia	Syringomyelia	Syringomyélie	Siringomielia	Siringomijelija
Soffio cardiaco	Heart murmur	Souffle cardiaque	Soplo del corazón	Šum na srcu
Soffocamento (soffocazione, asfissia)	Choking (suffocation)	Suffocation	Atragantamiento	Gušenje

Italiano	Inglese	Francese	Spagnolo	Croato
Sonnambulismo	Sleepwalking (somnambulism)	Somnabulisme	Sonambulismo (noctambulismo)	Mjesečarenje (somnambulizam)
Sonnolenza	Somnolence	Somnolence	Somnolencia	Pospanost (somnolencija)
Soppressione della secrezione di urina	Nonpassage of urine	Arrêt de la sécrétion d'urine	Supresión de la secreción de orina	Prestanak lučenja urina
Sordità	Deafness	Surdité	Sordera	Gluhoća
Sordità parziale	Hard of hearing	Surdité partielle	Corto de oído (parcialmente sordo)	Nagluhost
Sottopeso (grave magrezza)	Underfedness (malnutrition)	Malnutrition	Desnutrición	Neuhranjenost
Spasmo (contrazione involontaria)	Spasm (cramp)	Spasme (crampe)	Espasmo (calambre)	Grč (spazam)
Spasmo di vagina (vaginismo)	Vaginal spasm (vaginismus)	Spasme vaginal (vaginisme)	Espasmo vaginal (vaginismo)	Grč rodnice (vaginizam)
Spasmo facciale	Facial spasm	Spasme facial	Espasmo facial	Grč mišića lica
Spasmo muscolare	Muscular cramp (spasm)	Crampe musculaire (spasme)	Espasmo muscular (calambre)	Mišićni grč (spazam)
Spermatocele (cisti spermatica)	Spermatocele	Spermatocèle	Espermatocele	Spermatokela (cista epididimisa)
Spina bifida	Spina bifida	Spina bifida	Espina bífida	Spina bifida
Spina nel calcagno (spina calcaneare)	Heel spur (calcaneal spur)	Éperon de talon (epine calcaneenne)	Espuela de talón (espuela calcánea)	Petni trn
Splenomegalia	Splenomegaly	Splénomégalie	Esplenomegalia	Splenomegalija
Spondilite	Spondylitis	Spondilite	Espondilitis	Spondilitis
Spondilite anchilosante	Ankylosing spondylitis (Bechterew's syndrome)	Spondylarthrite ankylosante (morbus Bechterew)	Espondilitis anquilosante (morbus Bechterew)	Ankilozantni spondilitis (Bechterewov sindrom)
Spondilite tubercolare (morbo di Pott)	Tuberculous spondylitis (Pott disease)	Mal de Pott (tuberculose vertébrale)	Espondilitis tuberculosa	Tuberkulozni spondilitis (Pottova bolest)
Spondilolistesi	Spondylolisthesis	Spondylolisthésis	Espondilolistesis	Spondilolisteza
Spondilosi	Spondylosis	Spondylose	Espondilosis	Spondiloza
Sporotricosi	Sporotrichosis	Sporotrichose	Esporotricosis	Sporotrihoza
Spostamento del rene (ptosi renale, nefroptosi)	Floating kidney (nephroptosis, renal ptosis)	Syndrome du rein flottant (néphroptose)	Riñón flotante (ptosis renal, nefroptosis)	Spušteni bubreg (putujući bubreg, nefroptoza)
Spostamento della palpebra (palpebra calante, blefaroptosi)	Drooping of the upper eyelid (blepharoptosis)	Abaissement de la paupière supérieure (blépharoptose)	Despredimiento del párpado superior (blefaroptosis)	Spušteni kapak (blefaroptoza)
Sputo schiumoso	Foamy sputum	Crachat spumeux	Esputo espumoso	Pjenušavi ispljuvak
Stanchezza (fatica, astenia)	Fatigue (exhaustion, lethargy)	Fatigue (affaiblissement)	Cansancio (fatiga, letargo, astenia)	Iscrpljenost (umor, fatigo)
Starnuto	Sneezing	Éternuement	Estornudo	Kihanje
Stenosi aortica	Aortic valve stenosis	Sténose valvulaire aortique	Estenosis de la válvula aórtica	Stenoza aortnog ušća
Stenosi dell'arteria polmonare	Stenosis of pulmonary artery	Sténose de l'artère pulmonaire	Estenosis de la arteria pulmonar	Stenoza plućne arterije
Stenosi esofagea	Esophageal stenosis	Sténose oesophagienne	Estenosis esofágica	Stenoza jednjaka
Stenosi ipertrofica del piloro	Hypertrophic pyloric stenosis	Sténose hypertrophique du pylore	Estenosis pilórica hipertrófica	Hipertrofijska stenoza pilorusa
Stenosi mitralica	Mitral stenosis	Sténose mitrale	Estenosis mitral	Stenoza mitralnog ušća
Stenosi pilorica	Pyloric stenosis	Sténose du pylore	Estenosis del píloro	Stenoza pilorusa (pilorostenoza)
Stenosi pilorica congenita	Congenital pyloric stenosis	Sténose congénitale du pylore	Estenosis congénita del píloro	Urođena stenoza pilorusa
Stenosi polmonare	Pulmonary valve stenosis	Sténose de la valve pulmonaire	Estenosis de la válvula pulmonar	Stenoza plućnog ušća (pulmonalna stenoza)
Sterilità (infecondità)	Infertility (sterility)	Infertilité (stérilité)	Infertilidad	Neplodnost (sterilitet)
Stiramento	Strain (sprain, pull)	Déchirure	Desgarro	Istegnuće
Stiramento del legamento	Ligament sprain	Déchirure ligamentaire	Desgarro de ligamento	Istegnuće ligamenta
Stiramento del tendine	Tendon strain	Déchirure au tendon	Desgarro de tendón	Istegnuće tetive (distenzija tetive)
Stitichezza (costipazione)	Constipation (obstipation)	Constipation	Estreñimiento	Zatvor (opstipacija)
Strabismo	Strabismus	Strabisme	Estrabismo	Razrokost (strabizam)
Strangolamento (strozzamento)	Strangulation	Strangulation (étranglement)	Estrangulamiento	Davljenje
Strappo muscolare	Muscle strain (muscle pull)	Déchirure musculaire (claquage)	Desgarro muscular	Istegnuće mišića (distenzija mišića)
Stupor	Sopor	Sopor	Sopor	Sopor
Stupore	Stupor	Stupeur	Estupor	Stupor
Sudorazione (traspirazione)	Sweating	Sudation	Transpiración (sudación)	Znojenje
Sudore notturno	Night sweats	Sueurs nocturnes	Sudor nocturno	Noćno znojenje
Tachicardia	Tachycardia	Tachycardie	Taquicardia	Tahikardija
Talassemia	Thalassemia	Thalassémie	Talasemia	Talasemija
Tamponamento cardiaco	Pericardial tamponade (cardiac tamponade)	Tamponnade cardiaque	Tamponamiento cardíaco (tamponamiento pericárdiaco)	Tamponada perikarda
Tappo di cerume	Impacted cerumen	Bouchon de cérumen	Tapón de cerumen	Ceruminozni čep

Italiano	Inglese	Francese	Spagnolo	Croato
Temperatura corporea elevata	Elevated body temperature	Élévation de la température du corps	Aumento en la temperatura corporal	Povišena tjelesna temperatura
Tendinite dei estensori delle dita del piede	Extensor tendinitis (inflammation of the extensor tendons of the toes)	Tendinite des extenseurs des orteils	Tendinitis de los extensores de los dedos	Tendinitis ekstenzora prstiju stopala
Tendinite del flessore lungo dell'alluce	Dancer's tendinitis (flexor hallucis tendinitis)	Tendinite des danseurs (fléchisseur de l'hallux tendinite)	Tendinitis del flexor hallucis longus	Tendinitis plesača (tendinitis dugog pregibača palca)
Tendinite del muscolo tibiale posteriore	Tibialis posterior tendinitis	Tendinopathie du tibial postérieur	Tendinopatía tibial posterior	Tendinitis stražnjeg tibijalnog mišića
Tendinite del popliteo	Popliteus syndrome	Syndrome poplité douloureux	Tendinitis poplítea	Sindrom m. popliteusa
Tendinite dell'avambraccio	Forearm tendinitis	Tendinite de l'avant-bras	Tendinitis en el antebrazo	Veslačka podlaktica (tendinitis podlaktice)
Tendinopatia Achille da overuse	Achilles tendon overuse injury	Tendinite achilléenne chronique	Tendinitis por sobreuso en el tendón de Aquiles	Sindrom prenaprezanja Ahilove tetive
Tendinopatia achillea (achillodinia)	Achillodynia (Achilles tendinitis)	Tendinite du tendon d'Achille	Tendinitis de Aquiles	Ahilodinija (tendinitis Ahilove tetive)
Tendinosi	Tendinosis (chronic tendon injury)	Tendinose	Tendinosis (lesión crónica del tendón)	Tendinoza (kronična ozljeda tetive)
Tensione di parete addominale	Abdominal wall tension	Tension de la paroi stomacale	Tensión de la pared abdominal	Napetost trbušne stijenke
Teratocarcinoma	Teratocarcinoma	Tératocarcinome	Teratocarcinoma	Teratokarcinom
Teratoma	Teratoma	Tératome	Teratoma	Teratom
Tetania	Tetany	Tétanie	Tetania	Tetanija
Tetano	Tetanus	Tétanos	Tétanos (tétano)	Tetanus (zli grč)
Tetralogia di Fallot	Tetralogy of Fallot	Tétralogie de Fallot	Tetralogía de Fallot	Fallotova tetralogija
Tic	Tic	Tic	Tic	Tik
Tifo esantematico (tifo epidemico)	Epidemic typhus (louse-borne typhus)	Typhus épidémique (typhus à poux, typhus européen)	Tifus exantemático epidémico	Trbušni tifus (epidemjski tifus, pjegavac)
Tifo murino (tifo endemico)	Murine typhus (endemic typhus)	Typhus murin	Tifus endémico murino	Štakorski pjegavac
Tigna (tinea capitis)	Tinea capitis (scalp ringworm)	Teigne (tinea capitis)	Tiña de la cabeza (tinea capitis)	Gljivična infekcija vlasišta (tinea capitis)
Tinea corporis	Tinea corporis	Tinea corporis	Tiña corporal (tinea corporis)	Tinea corporis
Tinea cruris	Crotch itch (tinea cruris)	Eczéma marginé de hebra	Tiña crural (tinea cruris)	Gljivična infekcija prepona (tinea cruris)
Tinea favosa	Favus	Favus	Tiña favosa (favus, tinea favosa)	Tinea favosa (favus)
Tirare su col naso	Sniffing (sniffle)	Renifler	Sorberse la nariz (moqueo)	Šmrcanje
Tireotossicosi	Thyrotoxicosis	Thyréotoxicose	Tirotoxicosis	Tireotoksikoza (tireotoksična oluja)
Tiroidite di Hashimoto	Hashimoto's disease	Thyroïdite de Hashimoto	Tiroiditis de Hashimoto	Hashimotov sindrom
Tiroidite di Riedel	Riedel's thyroiditis	Thyroïdite de Riedel	Tiroiditis de Riedel	Riedelov tireoiditis
Torace a imbuto (petto escavato)	Pectus excavatum	Thorax en entonnoir (pectus excavatum)	Pecho hundido (pectus excavatum)	Udubljena prsa (ljevkasta prsa)
Torcicollo	Wry neck (torticollis)	Torticolis	Tortícolis	Krivi vrat (tortikolis)
Torsione del testicolo	Testicular torsion	Torsion testiculaire	Torsión testicular	Torzija testisa
Torsione dell'osso	Bone bending (bone torsion)	Torsion osseuse	Torsión del hueso	Savijanje kosti
Tosse	Cough	Toux	Tos	Kašalj
Tosse produttiva	Productive cough	Toux productive	Tos productiva	Produktivni kašalj
Tosse secca	Dry cough	Toux sèche	Tos seca (tos perruna)	Suhi kašalj
Tossicodipendenza (tossicomania)	Drug addiction	Toxicomanie	Adicción a las drogas (drogodependencia)	Ovisnost o drogama
Tossinfezione da Clostridium perfringens	Clostridium perfringens toxic infection	Toxi-infection à Clostridium perfringens	Tóxico-infección por Clostridium perfringens	Toksična infekcija Clostridium perfringensom
Toxocariasi	Toxocariasis	Toxocarose	Toxocariasis	Toksokarijaza
Toxoplasmosi	Toxoplasmosis	Toxoplasmose	Toxoplasmosis	Toksoplazmoza
Tracoma	Trachoma	Trachome	Tracoma	Trahom
Trapianto renale	Kidney transplatation	Transplantation rénale	Transplante de riñón	Transplantacija bubrega
Trasposizione dei grossi vasi	Transposition of the great vessels	Transposition des gros vaisseaux	Transposición de los grandes vasos	Transpozicija velikih žila
Trasposizione dell'aorta	Transposition of aorta	Transposition de l'aorte	Transposición de la aorta	Transpozicija aorte
Trasposizione dell'arteria polmonare	Transposition of pulmonary artery	Transposition de l'artère pulmonaire	Transposición de la arteria pulmonar	Transpozicija plućne arterije
Trauma sportivo	Sports injury	Blessure de sportif	Lesión deportiva	Sportska ozljeda
Tremito (tremore)	Tremor	Tremblement	Temblor	Drhtanje (tremor)
Tremore delle mani	Hand tremor	Tremblement des mains	Temblor en las manos	Drhtanje ruku
Trichinosi	Trichinosis (trichinellosis)	Trichinose	Triquinelosis (triquinosis)	Trihinoza (trihineloza)
Trichomonas vaginalis	Trichomonas vaginalis	Trichomonas vaginalis	Trichomonas vaginalis	Trihomonazni vaginitis
Trichomoniasi	Trichomoniasis	Trichomoniase	Trichomoniasis	Trihomonijaza
Tripanosomiasi	Trypanosomiasis	Trypanosomiase	Tripanosomiasis	Tripanosomijaza
Tripanosomiasi africana (malattia del sonno)	African trypanosomiasis (sleeping sickness)	Maladie du sommeil (trypanosomiase africaine)	Tripanosomiasis africana (enfermedad del sueño)	Afrička tripanosomijaza (bolest spavanja)
Trombo	Blood clot (thrombus)	Caillot sanguin (thrombus)	Coágulo sanguíneo (trombo)	Krvni ugrušak (tromb)
Trombocitopenia	Thrombocytopenia	Thrombocytopénie	Trombocitopenia	Trombocitopenija

Italiano	Inglese	Francese	Spagnolo	Croato
Tromboembolia	Thromboembolism	Accident thromboembolique	Tromboembolismo	Tromboembolija
Tromboflebite	Thrombophlebitis	Thrombophlébite	Tromboflebitis	Tromboflebitis
Trombosi	Thrombosis	Thrombose	Trombosis	Tromboza
Trombosi venosa	Venous thrombosis	Thrombose veineuse	Trombosis venosa	Venska tromboza
Tsutsugamushi (tifo fluviale giapponese)	Scrub typhus (Japanese river fever, Tsutsugamushi fever)	Fièvre fluviale du Japon (typhus à chiques)	Tsutsugamushi (fiebre fluvial japonesa, tifus de los matorrales)	Japanska riječna groznica (Tsutsugamushi groznica)
Tubercolosi (tisi)	Tuberculosis (TBC)	Tuberculose	Tuberculosis (tisis, TBC)	Tuberkuloza (sušica, TBC)
Tubercolosi dei reni	Renal tuberculosis	Tuberculose rénale	Tuberculosis renal	Tuberkuloza bubrega
Tubercolosi delle ossa	Bone tuberculosis	Tuberculose des os	Tuberculosis ósea	Tuberkuloza kosti
Tubercolosi epatica	Hepatic tuberculosis	Tuberculose hépatique	Tuberculosis hepática	Tuberkuloza jetre
Tubercolosi intestinale	Intestinal tuberculosis	Tuberculose intestinale	Tuberculosis intestinal	Tuberkuloza crijeva
Tubercolosi polmonare	Pulmonary tuberculosis	Tuberculose pulmonaire	Tuberculosis pulmonar	Tuberkuloza pluća
Tubercolosi urogenitale	Urogenital tuberculosis	Tuberculose urogénitale	Tuberculosis urogenital	Urogenitalna tuberkuloza
Tularemia (febbre dei conigli)	Tularemia (rabbit fever)	Tularémie	Tularemia (fiebre de los conejos)	Tularemija (zečja groznica)
Tumore	Tumor (tumour)	Tumeur	Tumor	Tumor
Tumore benigno	Benign tumor	Tumeur bénigne	Tumor benigno	Dobroćudni tumor (benigni tumor)
Tumore del sacco vitellino	Yolk sac tumor (endodermal sinus tumor)	Tumeur du sac vitellin	Tumor de saco vitelino	Tumor žumanjčane vreće (endodermalni sinus tumor)
Tumore di Brenner	Brenner tumour	Tumeur de Brenner	Tumor de Brenner	Brennerov tumor
Tumore di Wilms (nefroblastoma)	Wilm's tumor (nephroblastoma)	Tumeur de Wilms (néphroblastome)	Tumor de Wilms (nefroblastoma)	Wilmsov tumor (nefroblastom)
Tumore maligno	Malignant tumor (cancer)	Tumeur maligne (cancer)	Tumor maligno (cáncer)	Zloćudni tumor (maligni tumor, rak)
Tumore misto	Mixed tumor	Tumeur mixte	Tumor mixto	Mješoviti tumor
Tumore misto maligno	Malignant mixed tumor	Tumeur mixte malin	Tumor mixto maligno	Mješoviti maligni tumor
Tungiasi (tunga penetrans)	Tungiasis (nigua, pique)	Sarcopsyllose	Tungiasis	Tungijaza
Ulcera (ulcerazione)	Ulcer	Ulcère	Úlcera (llaga)	Čir (ulkus)
Ulcera duodenale	Duodenal ulcer	Ulcère du doudénum	Úlcera duodenal	Čir na dvanaesniku
Ulcera gastrica	Gastric ulcer	Ulcère de l'estomac	Úlcera gástrica	Čir na želucu
Ulcera ischemica	Ischemic ulceration	Ulcère ischémique	Úlcera isquémica	Ishemična ulceracija
Ulcera perforata	Perforated ulcer	Perforation d'ulcère	Úlcera perforada	Puknuće čira (perforacija ulkusa)
Ulcera varicosa	Venous ulcer (varicose ulcer)	Ulcère veineux	Úlcera varicosa	Varikozni ulcer (venski ulcer)
Ulcera venerea (cancroide)	Chancroid (soft chancre)	Chancre mou (chancrelle)	Chancroide (chancro blando)	Meki čankir
Unghia incarnita (onicocriptosi)	Ingrown nail (onychocryptosis, unguis incarnatus)	Ongle incarné (onychocryptose)	Uña encarnada (onicocriptosis)	Urasli nokat (ungvis inkarnatus)
Uremia (accumulo nel sangue di sostanze azotate a causa dell'insufficienza renale)	Uremia (autointoxication due to kidney failure)	Urémie (le taux de l'urée dans le sang)	Uremia (acumulación en la sangre de los productos tóxicos por un fallo renal)	Uremija (autointoksikacija radi nelučenja urina)
Urina di colore rosso	Red urine	Urine rouge	Orina de color rojo	Crveni urin
Urina marrone	Brown urine	Urine marron	Orina de color marrón	Smeđi urin
Urinazione frequente (pollachiuria)	Frequent urination	Miction fréquente	Micción frecuente	Učestalo mokrenje
Urinazione notturna (nicturia)	Frequent urination at night (nocturia)	Excrétion urinaire à prédominance nocturne (nycturie)	Emisión excesiva de orina durante la noche (nicturia)	Noćno mokrenje (nokturija)
Urine torbide	Unclear urine (foggy urine)	Urine opaque	Orina turbia	Mutni urin
Ustione	Burn	Brûlure	Quemadura	Opeklina
Ustione da corrente elettrica	Electric shock burn	Brûlure électrique	Quemadura eléctrica	Opeklina od strujnog udara
Ustione da medusa	Jellyfish sting burn	Brûlure de méduse	Quemadura de medusa	Opeklina od meduze
Vampata di calore	Hot flushes	Bouffée de chaleur	Sofocos	Valovi vrućine (valunzi)
Varicella	Chicken-pox	Varicelle	Varicela	Vodene kozice
Varici degli arti inferiori	Leg varicose veins	Varices des membres inférieurs	Venas varicosas de las piernas	Proširene vene na nogama
Varici esofagee	Esophageal varices	Varices oesophagiennes	Varices esofágicas	Proširene vene jednjaka (flebektazije)
Varicocele	Varicocele	Varicocèle	Varicocele	Varikokela
Varicosi (varici, malattia varicosa)	Varicose veins	Varices	Varices	Proširene vene
Variola vera (vaiolo)	Smallpox	Variole (petite vérole)	Viruela	Velike boginje (crne boginje, variola vera)
Vene varicose del collo	Neck varicose veins	Varice dans le cou	Varices del cuello	Proširene vratne vene
Verruca	Wart	Verrue	Verruga	Bradavica (virusna bradavica)
Vescichetta (bolla)	Blister	Phlyctène (ampoule, cloque)	Ampolla	Plik
Visione doppia (diplopia)	Double vision (diplopia)	Vision double (diplopie)	Visión doble (diplopía)	Dvoslike
Vitiligine	Vitiligo	Vitiligo	Vitiligo	Vitiligo

Italiano	Inglese	Francese	Spagnolo	Croato
Voglia (neo, nevo)	Birthmark (nevus)	Grain de beauté (naevus)	Nevus (nevo)	Madež (nevus)
Volvolo	Abnormal twisting of the intestines (volvulus)	Volvulus	Retorcimiento anormal del intestino (vólvulo)	Zapletaj crijeva
Vomito (emetismo)	Vomiting	Vomissement	Vómito (emesis)	Povraćanje
Vomito senza nausea (vomito a getto, vomito cerebrale)	Vomiting without nausea (cerebral vomiting)	Vomissement en fusée sans effort	Vómito sin náusea (vómito cerebral)	Povraćanje bez mučnine (povraćanje u luku, cerebralno povraćanje)
Xantelasma	Xanthelasma	Xanthelasma	Xantelasma	Ksantelazma
Xantoma	Xanthoma	Xanthome	Xantoma	Ksantom
Zoonosi	Zoonosis	Zoonose	Zoonosis	Zoonoza
Zoppicamento	Limping	Boitillement	Cojera	Šepanje
FARMACIA:	PHARMACY:	PHARMACIE:	FARMACIA:	LJEKARNA:
A digiuno	On an empty stomach (before the meal)	À jeun	En ayunas	Na tašte
A mezzogiorno	At noon	À midi	A mediodía	U podne
Acido borico	Boric acid	Acide borique	Ácido bórico	Borova otopina
Adrenalina	Adrenaline	Adrénaline	Adrenalina	Adrenalin
Aerosol	Aerosol	Aérosol	Aerosol	Aerosol
Ago	Needle	Aiguille	Aguja	Igla
Alcool	Alcohol	Alkohol	Alcol	Alkohol
Allergia a medicamento	Drug allergy	Allergie à un médicament	Alergia al medicamento	Alergija na lijek
Aminofillina	Aminophylline	Aminophylline	Aminofilina	Aminofilin
Ampicillina	Ampicillin	Ampicilline	Ampicilina	Ampicilin
Ampolla (fiala)	Ampoule	Ampoule	Ampolla (recipiente)	Ampula
Analgesico	Analgesic (painkiller)	Analgésique	Analgésico	Analgetik
Anestetico	Anesthetic	Anesthésique	Anestésico	Anestetik
Antiacido	Antacid	Antiacide	Antiácido	Antacid
Antibiotico	Antibiotic	Antibiotique	Antibiótico	Antibiotik
Anticoagulante	Anticoagulant	Anticoagulant	Anticoagulante	Antikoagulans
Anticonvulsante	Anticonvulsant	Antiépileptique (anticonvulsivant)	Anticonvulsivo (antiepiléptico)	Antiepileptik (antikonvulziv)
Antidepressivo	Antidepressant	Antidépresseur	Antidepresivo	Antidepresiv
Antidiabetico	Anti-diabetic drug	Médicament antidiabétique	Antidiabético	Antidiabetik
Antidiaforetico	Antiperspirant	Déodorant	Desodorante	Antiperspirant
Antidiarroici	Antidiarrhoeal drug	Médicament antidiarrhéique	Antidiarréico	Antidiaroik
Antidoto	Antidote	Antidote	Antídoto	Antidot
Antielmintici	Antihelminthic	Antihelminthique	Antihelmíntico	Antihelmintik
Antiemetico	Antiemetic and motion sickness drug	Antiémétique	Antiemético	Lijek protiv mučnine i povraćanja
Antimalarico	Antimalarial drug	Antimalarique	Antimalárico	Antimalarik
Antimicotico	Antimycotic	Antimycosique	Antimicótico (antifúngico)	Antimikotik
Antinfiammatorio	Anti-inflammatory	Anti-inflammatoire	Antiinflamatorio (antiflogístico)	Protuupalno
Antiossidante (sostanza antiossidante)	Antioxidant	Antioxydant	Antioxidante	Antioksidans
Antipiretico	Antipyretic	Antipyrétique	Antipirético	Antipiretik
Antipsicotico	Antipsychotic	Antipsychotique	Antipsicótico	Antipsihotik
Antireumatico	Antirheumatic drug	Médicament antirhumatismal	Antireumático	Antireumatik
Antisettico	Antiseptic	Antiseptique	Antiséptico	Antiseptik
Antisettico urinario	Urinary antiseptic	Antiseptique urinaire	Antiséptico de las vías urinarias	Uroantiseptik
Antisiero	Antiserum	Antisérum	Antisuero	Antiserum
Antistaminico	Antihistamine	Antihistaminique	Antihistamínico	Antihistaminik
Antitossina	Antitoxin	Antitoxine	Antitoxina	Protuotrov
Aspirina	Aspirin	Aspirine	Aspirina	Aspirin
Assorbenti igienici	Sanitary pads (sanitary napkins)	Serviette hygiénique (protège-slip)	Toalla sanitaria (compresa, pantiprotector)	Higijenski ulošci
Assorbenti per l'incontinenza	Incontinence pads (adult diapers)	Slip d'incontinence	Pañal para adultos	Pelene za inkontinenciju
Atropina	Atropine	Atropine	Atropina	Atropin
Barbiturico	Barbiturate	Barbiturique	Barbitúrico	Barbiturat
Bendaggio	Bandage	Bandage	Venda	Zavoj
Bilancia	Scales	Balance	Balanza	Vaga
Bottiglietta (boccetta)	Vial	Fiole	Frasquito	Bočica
Bouillotte (bouilloire)	Hot water bottle	Bouillotte	Bolsa de agua caliente (guatero)	Termofor
Broncodilatatore	Bronchodilator	Bronchodilatateur	Broncodilatador	Bronhodilatator
Burrocacao	Lip balm	Tube de soin pour lèvres	Bálsamo de labios	Grožđana mast
Caffeina	Caffeine	Caféine	Cafeína	Kofein
Calcio	Calcium	Calcium	Calcio	Kalcij
Camomilla	Chamomile	Camomille	Manzanilla	Kamilica
Candelette	Vaginal suppository	Ovule (suppositoire vaginal)	Supositorio vaginal	Vaginaleta
Cannabis terapeutica	Medical cannabis	Cannabis médical	Cannabis medicinal	Medicinski kanabis
Capsula	Capsule	Gélule	Cápsula	Kapsula
Carbone attivo	Activated carbon	Charbon actif	Carbón activado	Aktivni ugljen
Cardiotonico	Cardiotonic agent	Médicament cardiotonique	Cardiotónico	Kardiotonik

Italiano	Inglese	Francese	Spagnolo	Croato
Cefalosporina	Cephalosporin	Céphalosporine	Cefalosporina	Cefalosporin
Cerotto	Plaster (adhesive strip)	Pansement	Tira adhesiva sanitaria	Flaster
Cerotto antifumo	Nicotine patch	Timbre à la nicotine	Parche de nicotina	Nikotinski flaster
Chemioterapia	Chemotherapy	Chimiothérapie	Quimioterapia	Kemoterapija
Citostatico	Cytostatic	Cytostatique	Citostático	Citostatik
Clistere	Enema (clyster)	Clystère	Enema (clisma)	Klizma (klistir)
Cloramfenicolo	Chloramphenicol	Chloramphénicol	Cloranfenicol	Kloramfenikol
Cloro	Chlorine	Chlore	Cloro	Klor
Cobalto	Cobalt	Cobalt	Cobalto	Kobalt
Codeina	Codeine	Codéine	Codeína	Kodein
Collirio	Eye drops	Collyre (gouttes ophtalmiques)	Colirio	Kapi za oči
Collutorio	Mouthwash liquid	Eau dentifrice	Enjuague bucal (colutorio)	Tekućina za ispiranje usne šupljine
Compressa	Compress	Compresse	Compresa	Oblog
Compressa (pasticca, tavoletta)	Tablet	Comprimé	Comprimido	Dražeja (tableta)
Compresse solubili	Water-soluble tablets	Comprimé effervescent	Solubilizantes (comprimidos dispersables en agua)	Šumeće tablete
Contraccettivo	Contraceptive	Contraceptif	Anticonceptivo	Kontraceptiv
Corticosteroide	Corticosteroid	Corticostéroïde	Corticosteroide	Kortikosteroid
Crema	Skin cream	Crème	Crema	Krema
Cucchiaio	Spoon	Cuillère	Cuchara	Žlica
Dentifricio	Tooth paste	Dentifrice	Pasta de dientes (dentífrico)	Pasta za zube
Di mattina	In the morning	Le matin	Por la mañana	U jutro
Diaframma	Diaphragm (Dutch cap)	Diaphragme	Diafragma	Dijafragma
Digestivo	Digestive	Médicament digestif	Digestivo	Digestiv
Dimagrante (farmaco antiobesità)	Anti-obesity medication	Médicament anti-obésité	Fármaco antiobesidad	Dijetetsko sredstvo
Diuretico	Diuretic	Diurétique	Diurético	Diuretik
Dolcificante artificiale	Sugar substitute	Édulcorant	Edulcorante artificial	Umjetno sladilo
Dopo il pasto	After meal	Après-repas	Después de una comida	Nakon jela
Dose	Dose	Dose	Dosis	Doza
Effetti indesiderati da farmaco	Drug side-effects	Effets indésirables d'un médicament	Reacción adversa a medicamento	Nuspojave lijeka
Emostatico	Antihemorrhagic (hemostatic)	Hémostatique	Hemostático	Hemostatik
Emulsione	Emulsion	Émulsion	Emulsión	Emulzija
Eparina	Heparin	Héparine	Heparina	Heparin
Eritromicina	Erythromycin	Érythromycine	Eritromicina	Eritromicin
Espettorante	Expectorant	Expectorant	Expectorante	Sredstvo za iskašljavanje
Farmacista	Pharmacist	Pharmacien	Farmacéutico	Ljekarnik
Farmaco anti-alcol	Antialcoholic drug	Médicament contre la dépendance à l'alcool	Fármaco antialcohólico	Antialkoholik
Farmaco anti-infiammatore non steroide FANS	Non-steroidal anti-inflammatory drug	Anti-inflammatoire non stéroïdien	Antiinflamatorio no esteroideo	Nesteroidni antireumatik
Farmaco antiallergico	Antiallergic drug	Antiallergique	Antialérgico	Antialergik
Farmaco antianemico	Antianemic	Médicament antianémique	Antianémico	Antianemik
Farmaco antiaritmico	Antiarrhythmic agent	Agent antiarythmique	Agente antiarrítmico	Antiaritmik
Farmaco antiipertensivo	Antihypertensive drug	Antihypertenseur	Antihipertensivo	Antihipertenziv
Farmaco antiprotozoico	Antiprotozoal agent	Médicament antiprotozoal	Antiprotozoario	Antiprotozoik
Farmaco antitubercolare	Antitubercular agent	Antituberculeux	Fármaco tuberculostático	Antituberkulotik
Farmaco antivirale	Antiviral drug	Médicament antiviral	Fármaco antiviral	Antivirusni lijek
Fentanyl	Fentanyl	Fentanyl	Fentanilo	Fentanil
Ferro	Iron	Fer	Hierro (fierro)	Željezo
Filo interdentale	Dental floss	Fil dentaire	Seda dental (hilo dental)	Zubni konac
Filtro solare (crema solare ad alta protezione)	Sunscreen (sunblock)	Crème solaire	Protector solar	Sredstvo za zaštitu od sunca
Fitoterapia	Phytotherapy	Phytothérapie	Fitoterapia	Fitoterapija
Fosforo	Phosphorus	Phosphore	Fósforo	Fosfor
Garza	Gauze sponge	Gaze	Gasa	Gaza
Gel	Gel	Gel	Gel	Gel
Gentamicina	Gentamicin	Gentamicine	Gentamicina	Gentamicin
Glucosio	Glucose	Glucose	Glucosa	Glukoza
Gocce	Drops	Gouttes	Gotas	Kapi (kapljice)
Gocce nasali	Nasal drops	Gouttes nasales	Gotas nasales	Kapi za nos
Gocce per il mal di orecchi	Ear drops	Gouttes auriculaires	Gotas óticas	Kapi za uši
Gomma da masticare antifumo	Nicotine gum	Gomme à la nicotine	Goma de mascar de nicotina	Nikotinska guma za žvakanje
Grammo	Gram (gramme)	Gramme	Gramo	Gram
Immunoglobulina	Immunoglobulin	Immunoglobuline	Inmunoglobulina	Imunoglobulin
Immunosoppressivo	Immunosuppressive	Immunosuppresseur	Inmunosupresor	Imunosupresiv
Inalazione (farmaco per inalazioni)	Inhalation	Inhalation	Inhalación	Inhalacija

Italiano	Inglese	Francese	Spagnolo	Croato
Iniezione	Injection	Injection	Inyección	Injekcija
Insettifugo	Insect repellent	Répulsif d'insectes	Repelente de insectos	Sredstvo protiv insekata
Insulina	Insulin	Insuline	Insulina	Inzulin
Interferone	Interferon	Interféron	Interferón	Interferon
Iodio (tintura di iodio)	Iodine	Iode	Yodo (iodo)	Jod
Ipnotico	Hypnotic (soporific)	Hypnotique (somnifère)	Hipnótico	Hipnotik
La sera	In the evening	Le soir	Por la noche	Na večer
Lassativo	Laxative	Laxatif	Laxante	Laksativ
Lente a contatto morbida	Soft contact lens	Lentille de contact souple	Lente de contacto blanda	Meka kontaktna leća
Lente a contatto rigida	Hard contact lens	Lentille de contact rigide	Lente de contacto duro	Tvrda kontaktna leća
Lenti a contatto	Contact lenses	Lentilles de contact	Lentes de contacto (lentillas, pupilentes)	Kontaktne leće
Litro	Litre	Litre	Litro	Litra
Lozione	Lotion	Lotion	Loción	Losion
Lubrificante	Lubricant	Lubrifiant	Lubricante	Lubrikant
Magnesio	Magnesium	Magnésium	Magnesio	Magnezij
Manganese	Manganese	Manganèse	Manganeso	Mangan
Medicamento (farmaco, rimedio)	Medication (remedy, drug)	Médicament	Medicamento (fármaco)	Lijek
Metadone	Methadone	Méthadone	Metadona	Metadon
Microgrammo	Microgram	Microgramme	Microgramo	Mikrogram
Milligrammo	Milligram (milligramme)	Milligramme	Miligramo	Miligram
Millilitro	Millilitre	Millilitre	Mililitro	Mililitar
Minerale	Mineral	Minéral	Mineral	Mineral
Miorilassante	Muscle relaxant	Myorelaxant	Relajante muscular (miorrelajante)	Miorelaksator
Misuratore di pressione (sfigmomanometro)	Blood pressure meter (sphygmomanometer)	Tensiomètre (sphygmomanomètre)	Tensiómetro (esfigmomanómetro)	Tlakomjer
Molibdeno	Molybdenum	Molybdène	Molibdeno	Molibden
Morfina	Morphine	Morphine	Morfina	Morfin
Mucolitico	Mucolytic	Mucolytique	Mucolítico	Mukolitik
Nistatina	Nystatin	Nystatine	Nistatina	Nistatin
Occhiali	Glasses	Lunettes de vue	Gafas	Naočale
Olio di jojoba	Jojoba oil	Huile de jojoba	Aceite de jojoba	Jojobino ulje
Olio di mandorla	Almond oil	Huile d'amande	Aceite de almendras dulces	Bademovo ulje
Olio di ricino	Castor oil	Huile de ricin	Aceite de ricino	Ricinusovo ulje
Olio essenziale (olio eterico)	Essential oil	Huile essentielle	Aceite esencial	Eterično ulje
Olio minerale	Mineral oil	Huile minérale	Aceite mineral	Mineralno ulje
Omega-3 acidi grassi	Omega-3 fatty acid	Acides gras oméga-3	Ácido graso omega 3	Omega-3 masne kiseline
Oppioide	Opioid	Opioïde	Opioide	Opijat (opioid)
Oralmente (per via orale, per bocca)	Orally	Par voie orale	Por vía oral	Na usta
Ossicodone	Oxycodone	Oxycodone	Oxicodona	Oksikodon
Ovatta	Cotton-wool	Ouate (coton hydrophile)	Algodón hidrófilo	Vata
Paracetamolo	Paracetamol	Paracétamol	Paracetamol	Paracetamol
Paraffina	Paraffin	Paraffine	Parafina	Parafin
Pezzo (porzione)	Piece	Morceau	Pieza	Komad
Pasta	Paste	Pâte	Pasta	Pasta
Pasticca (pastiglia)	Pastille (lozenge)	Pastille	Pastilla	Tableta za sisanje (pastila)
Penicillina	Penicillin	Pénicilline	Penicilina	Penicilin
Per l'applicazione esterna	For external application	Pour l'application externe	De uso externo	Za vanjsku primjenu
Pillola anticoncezionale	Contraceptive pill (oral contraceptive)	Contraception orale	Píldora anticonceptiva	Kontracepcijska pilula
Pillola del "giorno doppo" (contraccezione postcoitale, contraccezione di emergenza)	'Morning-after' pill (postcoital contraception, emergency contraception)	Pilule du lendemain (contraception postcoïtale, contraception d'urgence)	Anticonceptivo de emergencia (contracepción poscoital)	Pilula za "dan poslije" (postkoitalna kontracepcija, hitna kontracepcija)
Polvere liquido	Liquid powder	Poudre fluide	Polvo liquido	Tekući puder
Polverina (polvere)	Powder	Poudre	Polvo	Prašak (puder)
Pomata (unguento)	Ointment (fat)	Pommade	Ungüento (pomada)	Pomada (mast)
Potassio	Potassium	Potassium	Potasio	Kalij
Pozione	Potion	Potion	Poción	Ljekoviti napitak
Prescrizione (rimedio prescritto)	Prescription	Ordonnance médicale	Receta	Recept
Preservativo (profilattico, condom)	Condom	Préservatif	Preservativo (condón, profiláctico)	Prezervativ (kondom)
Psicostimulanti	Psychostimulant	Psychostimulant	Psicoestimulante	Psihostimulans
Purgante (purga)	Purgative	Purgatif	Purgante (purgativo)	Purgativ
Rame	Copper	Cuivre	Cobre	Bakar
Repellente antizanzare	Mosquito repellent	Répulsif antimoustiques	Repelente de mosquitos	Sredstvo protiv komaraca
Rettale	Rectal	Rectal	Rectal	Rektalno
Salicilato	Salicylate	Salicylate	Salicilato	Salicilat
Sapone	Soap	Savon	Jabón	Sapun
Schiuma (spuma)	Foam	Mousse	Espuma	Pjena
Schiuma anticoncezionale	Contraceptive foam	Mousse contraceptive	Espuma anticonceptiva	Kontracepcijska pjena

Italiano	Inglese	Francese	Spagnolo	Croato
Sciacquatra (risciacquatura)	Rinsing	Rinçage	Lavado	Ispiranje
Sciroppo	Syrup	Sirop	Jarabe	Sirup
Sedativo (calmante)	Sedative	Sédatif	Sedativo	Sedativ
Siero	Serum	Sérum	Suero	Serum
Siringa per iniezioni	Syringe	Seringue	Jeringa	Šprica
Sistema internazionale di unità di misura	International System of Units	Système international d'unités	Sistema Internacional de Unidades	Sustav međunarodnih mjernih jedinica
Sodio	Sodium	Sodium	Sodio	Natrij
Soluzione	Solution	Solution	Soluto	Otopina
Soluzione fisiologica	Saline solution	Solution physiologique	Suero fisiológico	Fiziološka otopina
Soluzione per pulizia dentiera	Denture cleaning solution	Solution nettoyante pour les prothèses	Solución limpiadora de dentadura	Tekućina za čišćenje umjetnog zubala
Soluzione per pulizia lenti a contatto	Contact lenses cleaning solution	Solution nettoyante pour lentilles	Solución limpiadora de lentes de contacto	Tekućina za čišćenje kontaktnih leća
Sostanza nutriente (sostanza nutritiva)	Nutrient	Nutriment (élément nutritif)	Nutrimento (nutriente)	Nutritiv
Sovradosaggio	Overdose	Surdose	Sobredosis	Predoziranje
Spasmolitico	Spasmolytic	Spasmolytique	Espasmolítico	Spazmolitik
Spermicida	Spermicide	Spermicide	Espermicida	Spermicid
Spruzzo (vaporizzato)	Spray	Spray	Rociada	Sprej
Spugna contraccettiva	Contraceptive sponge	Éponge contraceptive	Esponja anticonceptiva	Kontracepcijska spužva
Sublinguale	Sublingual administration	Sublingual	Vía sublingual	Pod jezik
Sulfamidici (sulfonamidici)	Sulphonamide	Sulfamidé	Sulfonamida	Sulfonamid
Supposta	Suppository	Suppositoire	Supositorio	Čepić
Tampone	Tampon	Tampon hygiénique	Tampón	Tampon
Terapia ormonale sostitutiva	Hormone replacement therapy	Hormonothérapie de substitution	Terapia de sustitución hormonal	Hormonalna nadomjesna terapija
Termometro	Thermometer	Thermomètre	Termómetro	Toplomjer
Test di gravidanza ad uso domiciliare	Home pregnancy test	Test de grossesse	Prueba de embarazo	Kućni test za trudnoću
Tetraciclina	Tetracycline	Tétracycline	Tetraciclina	Tetraciklin
Tintura	Tincture	Teinture	Tintura	Tinktura
Tisana (infuso di erbe)	Herbal tea	Tisane	Tisana (infusión de hierbas)	Biljni čaj
Tonico (ricostituente)	Tonic	Tonique	Tónico	Tonik
Tramadolo	Tramadol	Tramadol	Tramadol	Tramal
Vaccino	Vaccine	Vaccin	Vacuna	Cjepivo
Vasodilatatore	Vasodilator	Vasodilatateur	Vasodilatador	Vazodilatator
Veleno	Poison	Poison	Veneno	Otrov
Viagra (citrato di sildenafil)	Viagra (sildenafil citrate)	Viagra (citrate de sildénafil)	Viagra	Viagra
Vitamina	Vitamin	Vitamine	Vitamina	Vitamin
Vitamina A (retinolo)	Vitamin A (retinol)	Vitamine A (rétinol)	Vitamina A (retinol)	Vitamin A (retinol)
Vitamina B1 (tiamina)	Vitamin B1 (thiamin)	Vitamine B1 (thiamine)	Vitamina B1 (tiamina)	Vitamin B1 (tiamin)
Vitamina B2 (riboflavina)	Vitamin B2 (riboflavin)	Vitamine B2 (riboflavine)	Vitamina B2 (riboflavina)	Vitamin B2 (riboflavin)
Vitamina B3 (niacina, vitamina PP)	Vitamin B3 (niacin)	Vitamine B3 (nicotinamide, PP)	Vitamina B3 (niacina, vitamina PP)	Vitamin B3 (niacin)
Vitamina B4 (adenina)	Vitamin B4 (adenine)	Vitamine B4 (adénine)	Vitamina B4 (adenina)	Vitamin B4 (adenin)
Vitamina B5 (acido pantotenico, vitamina W)	Vitamin B5 (pantothenic acid)	Vitamine B5 (acide pantothénique)	Vitamina B5 (ácido pantoténico)	Vitamin B5 (pantotenska kiselina)
Vitamina B6 (piridossina)	Vitamin B6 (pyridoxine)	Vitamine B6 (pyridoxine)	Vitamina B6 (piridoxina)	Vitamin B6 (piridoksin)
Vitamina B7 (inositolo)	Vitamin B7 (inositol)	Vitamine B7 (inositol)	Vitamina B7 (inositol)	Vitamin B7 (inozitol)
Vitamina B8 (biotina)	Vitamin B8 (biotin)	Vitamine B8 (biotine)	Vitamina B8 (biotina)	Vitamin B8 (biotin)
Vitamina B9 (acido folico)	Vitamin B9 (folic acid)	Vitamine B9 (acide folique)	Vitamina B9 (ácido fólico)	Vitamin B9 (folna kiselina)
Vitamina B10 (vitamina R)	Vitamin B10 (factor-R)	Vitamine B10 (vitamine R)	Vitamina B10 (vitamina R)	Vitamin B10 (faktor-R)
Vitamina B11 (vitamina S)	Vitamin B11 (factor-S)	Vitamine B11 (carnitine)	Vitamina B11 (vitamina S)	Vitamin B11 (faktor-S)
Vitamina B12 (cobalamina)	Vitamin B12 (cobalamin)	Vitamine B12 (cobalamine)	Vitamina B12 (ciancobalamina)	Vitamin B12 (kobalamin)
Vitamina C (acido L-ascorbico)	Vitamin C (L-ascorbic acid)	Vitamine C (acide ascorbique)	Vitamine C (enantiómero L de ácido ascórbico)	Vitamin C (L-askorbinska kiselina)
Vitamina D2 (ergocalciferolo)	Vitamin D2 (ergocalciferol)	Vitamine D2 (ergocalciférol)	Vitamina D2 (ergocalciferol)	Vitamin D2 (ergokalciferol)
Vitamina D3 (colecalciferolo)	Vitamin D3 (cholecalciferol)	Vitamine D3 (cholécalciférol)	Vitamina D3 (colecalciferol)	Vitamin D3 (kolekalciferol)
Vitamina D4 (diidroergocalciferolo)	Vitamin D4	Vitamine D4	Vitamina D4	Vitamin D4
Vitamina D5 (sitocalciferolo)	Vitamin D5 (sitocalciferol)	Vitamine D5 (sitocalciférol)	Vitamina D5 (sitocalciferol)	Vitamin D5 (sitokalciferol)
Vitamina E (tocoferolo)	Vitamin E (tocopherol)	Vitamine E (tocophérol)	Vitamina E (alfatocoferol)	Vitamin E (tokoferol)
Vitamina F (acido linoleico)	Vitamin F (linoleic acid)	Vitamine F (acide linoléique)	Ácido linoleico	Vitamin F (linoleična kiselina)
Vitamina J (colina)	Vitamin J (choline)	Vitamine J (choline)	Vitamina J (colina)	Vitamin J (kolin)
Vitamina K (fillochinone)	Vitamin K (phylloquinone)	Vitamine K (phylloquinone)	Vitamina K (filoquinona)	Vitamin K (filokinon)
Vitamina L1 (acido antranilico)	Vitamin L1 (anthranilic acid)	Vitamine L1 (acide anthranilique)	Vitamina L1 (ácido antranílico)	Vitamin L1 (antranilna kiselina)

Italiano	Inglese	Francese	Spagnolo	Croato
Vitamina P (flavonoidi)	Vitamin P (flavonoids)	Vitamine P (flavonoïde)	Vitamina P (flavonoide)	Vitamin P (flavonoidi)
Zinco	Zinc	Zinc	Zinc (cinc)	Cink
Zinco pasta	Zinc ointment	Pommade à l'oxyde de zinc	Pasta de óxido de zinc	Cinkova pasta
Zolfo	Sulphur	Soufre	Azufre	Sumpor

ISTITUZIONI, PROCEDURE E CURE DI MEDICINA:	MEDICAL FACILITIES, PROCEDURES AND CARE:	ÉTABLISSEMENTS MÉDICAUX, PROCÉDURES ET SOINS:	FACILIDADES MÉDICAS, PROCEDIMIENTOS Y ASISTENCIA MÉDICA:	MEDICINSKE USTANOVE, ZAHVATI I NJEGA:
Accettazione	Reception office	Réception	Mostrador de recepción	Prijemni ured
Acqua	Water	Eau	Agua	Voda
Addentare	Bite	Mordre	Morder	Zagristi
Allarme	Alarm	Alarme	Alarma	Uzbuna (alarm)
Ambulanza	Ambulance (clinic)	Infirmerie	Enfermería	Ambulanta
Amputazione	Amputation	Amputation	Amputación	Amputacija
Anestesia	Anesthesia	Anesthésie	Anestesia	Anestezija (narkoza)
Anestesia generale	General anesthesia	Anesthésie générale	Anestesia general	Opća anestezija
Anestesia locale	Local anesthesia	Anesthésie locale	Anestesia local	Lokalna anestezija
Angioplastica coronarica	Percutaneous coronary intervention (coronary angioplasty)	Angioplastie coronaire (dilatation transluminale)	Intervención coronaria percutánea	Perkutana koronarna angioplastika
Apertura chirurgica del cranio (craniotomia)	Surgical opnening of the cranium (craniotomy)	Ouverture chirurgicale du crâne (craniotomie)	Abertura quirúrgica en el cráneo (craneotomía)	Kirurški zahvat otvaranja lubanje (kraniotomija)
Apertura chirurgica di un articolazione (artrotomia)	Surgical procedure on a joint (arthrotomy)	Ouverture chirurgicale d'une articulation (arthrotomie)	Incisión quirúrgica de una articulación (artrotomía)	Kirurški zahvat na zglobu (artrotomija)
Apparecchio acustico	Hearing assist device	Appareil acoustique	Audífono	Slušni aparat
Aprire	Open	Ouvrir	Abrir	Otvoriti
Armadio (credenza)	Wardrobe (cupboard, cabinet)	Armoire	Armario	Ormar
Artrodesi	Arthrodesis	Arthrodèse	Artrodesis	Artrodeza
Ascensore	Elevator	Ascenseur	Elevador	Dizalo
Aspiratore di secreti	Suction unit (aspirator)	Appareil à succion	Aspirador	Aspirator
Asportazione chirurgica del pancreas (pancreatectomia)	Surgical removal of the pancreas (pancreatectomy)	Ablation chirurgicale du pancréas (pancréatectomie)	Extirpación quirúrgica del páncreas (pancreatectomía)	Kirurško odstranjenje gušterače (pankreatektomija)
Asportazione chirurgica del testicolo (orchiectomia)	Surgical removal of a testicle (orchidectomy)	Amputation chirurgicale d'un ou des deux testicules (orchidectomie, orchiectomie)	Extirpación quirúrgica del testículo (orquidectomía)	Kirurško odstranjenje testisa (orhidektomija)
Asportazione chirurgica del timo (timectomia)	Surgical removal of the thymus (thymectomy)	Ablation chirurgicale du thymus (thymectomie)	Extirpación quirúrgica del timo (timectomía)	Kirurško odstranjenje prsne žlijezde (timektomija)
Asportazione chirurgica dell'appendice (appendicectomia)	Surgical removal of the vermiform appendix (appendectomy)	Ablation chirurgicale de l'appendice iléo-caecal (appendicectomie)	Extirpación quirúrgica del apéndice cecal (apendicectomía)	Kirurško odstranjenje slijepog crijeva (apendektomija)
Asportazione chirurgica dell'utero (isterectomia)	Surgical removal of the uterus (hysterectomy)	Enlèvement chirurgical de l'uterus (hystérectomie)	Extracción quirúrgica del útero (histerectomía)	Kirurško odstranjenje maternice (histerektomija)
Asportazione chirurgica della colecisti (colecistectomia)	Surgical removal of the gallbladder (cholecystectomy)	Enlèvement chirurgical de la vésicule biliaire (cholécystectomie)	Extracción quirúrgica de la vesícula biliar (colecistectomía)	Kirurško odstranjenje žučnog mjehura (kolecistektomija)
Asportazione chirurgica della lamina di vertebre (laminectomia)	Surgical procedure on the spine (laminectomy)	Résection chirurgicale des lames vertébrales (laminectomie)	Extirpación quirúrgica de parte de una vértebra (laminectomía)	Kirurški zahvat na kralježnici (laminektomija)
Asportazione chirurgica della laringe (laringectomia)	Surgical removal of the larynx (laryngectomy)	Ablation chirurgicale du larynx (laryngectomie)	Extirpación quirúrgica de la laringe (laringectomía)	Kirurško odstranjenje grkljana (laringektomija)
Asportazione chirurgica della mammella (mastectomia)	Surgical removal of a breast (mastectomy)	Enlèvement chirurgical d'un sein (mastectomie)	Remoción quirúrgica de seno (mastectomía)	Kirurško odstranjenje dojke (mastektomija)
Asportazione chirurgica della milza (splenectomia)	Surgical removal of the spleen (splenectomy)	Ablation chirurgicale de la rate (splénectomie)	Extirpación quirúrgica del bazo (esplenectomía)	Kirurško odstranjenje slezene (splenektomija)
Asportazione chirurgica della prostata (prostatectomia)	Surgical removal of the prostate gland (prostatectomy)	Ablation chirurgicale de la prostate (prostatectomie)	Extirpación quirúrgica de la próstata (prostatectomía)	Kirurško odstranjenje prostate (prostatektomija)
Asportazione chirurgica della sacca aneurismatica (aneurismectomia)	Surgical removal of the aneurysm (aneurysmectomy)	Résection chirurgicale d'une poche anévrismale (anevrismectomie)	Extirpación quirúrgica de un aneurisma (aneurismectomía)	Kirurško odstranjenje aneurizme (aneurizmektomija)
Asportazione chirurgica della tiroide (tiroidectomia)	Surgical removal of the thyroid gland (thyroidectomy)	Ablation chirurgicale de la thyroïde (thyroïdectomie, isthmectomie)	Extirpación quirúrgica de la glándula tiroides (tiroidectomía)	Kirurško odstranjenje štitne žlijezde (tiroidektomija)
Asportazione chirurgica delle adenoidi (adenoidectomia)	Surgical removal of adenoids (adenoidectomy)	Ablation chirurgicale des végétations adénoïdes (adénoïdectomie)	Extirpación quirúrgica de las adenoides (adenoidectomía)	Kirurško odstranjenje trećeg krajnika (adenoidektomija)
Asportazione chirurgica delle emorroidi (emorroidectomia)	Surgical removal of a hemorrhoid (hemorrhoidectomy)	Ablation chirurgicale des hémorroïdes (hémorroïdectomie)	Extirpación quirúrgica de las hemorroides (hemorroidectomía)	Kirurško odstranjenje hemeroida (hemoroidektomija)
Asportazione chirurgica delle tonsille (tonsillectomia)	Surgical removal of tonsils (tonsillectomy)	Ablation chirurgicale des amygdales palatines (amygdalectomie, tonsillectomie)	Extracción quirúrgica de las amígdalas (tonsilectomía)	Kirurško odstranjenje krajnika (tonzilektomija)

Italiano	Inglese	Francese	Spagnolo	Croato
Asportazione chirurgica dello stomaco (gastrectomia)	Surgical removal of the stomach (gastrectomy)	Ablation chirurgicale de l'estomac (gastrectomie)	Extirpación quirúrgica del estómago (gastrectomía)	Kirurško odstranjenje želuca (gastrektomija)
Asportazione chirurgica di calcolo (litotomia)	Surgical removal of stones (lithotomy)	Extraction chirurgicale des pierres de la vessie (lithotomie)	Extracción quirúrgica de los cálculos (litotomía)	Kirurško odstranjenje kamenca (litotomija)
Asportazione chirurgica di fibromi nell'utero (miomectomia)	Surgical removal of uterine myomas (myomectomy, fibroidectomy)	Ablation chirurgicale des fibromes utérins (myomectomie)	Extirpación quirúrgica de los fibromas uterinos (miomectomía)	Kirurško odstranjenje mioma u maternici (miomektomija)
Asportazione chirurgica di struttura lobale di un organo (lobectomia)	Surgical removal of a lobe of some organ (lobectomy)	Ablation chirurgicale d'un lobe d'organe (lobectomie)	Extirpación quirúrgica de un lóbulo de un órgano (lobectomía)	Kirurško odstranjenje režnja nekog organa (lobektomija)
Asportazione chirurgica di uno o etrambi surreni (surrenectomia, adrenalectomia)	Surgical removal of one or both adrenal glands (adrenalectomy)	Ablation chirurgicale d'une ou des deux glandes surrénales (adrenalectomie)	Extirpación quirúrgica de una glándula suprarrenal (adrenalectomía)	Kirurško odstranjenje nadbubrežne žlijezde (adrenalektomija)
Assicurazione sanitaria	Health insurance	Assurance maladie	Seguro de salud	Zdravstveno osiguranje
Assistenza infermieristica	Nursing (care)	Soins de santé	Asistencia (cuidado)	Njega
Assistenza sanitaria primaria	Primary health care	Soins de santé primaire	Atención primaria de salud	Primarna zdravstvena zaštita
Autoambulanza	Ambulance	Ambulance	Ambulancia	Kola hitne pomoći
Autopsia	Autopsy	Autopsie	Autopsia	Obdukcija
Bagno	Bathroom	Salle de bains	Cuarto de baño	Kupaonica
Barella (lettiga)	Stretcher	Civière	Camilla enrollable	Nosila
Bendaggio gessato	Plaster cast (immobilization plaster)	Plâtre pour immobilisation rigide	Escayola de inmovilización	Gipsana udlaga
Bypass	Bypass	Pontage	By-pass	Premosnica
Cadavere (salma)	Corpse	Cadavre	Cadáver	Leš
Calendario vaccinale	Vaccination schedule	Calendrier des vaccinations	Calendario de vacunación	Kalendar cijepljenja
Cambiarsi	Get changed	Se changer	Cambiarse	Presvući se
Camera di malato	Patient's room	Chambre de malade	Cuarto del paciente	Bolesnička soba
Camicia da notte	Nightgown	Chemise de nuit	Camisón	Spavačica
Camicia protettiva	Protection gown	Blouse de protection	Gabacha desechable	Zaštitna navlaka za odjeću
Cannula	Airway (cannula)	Canule	Cánula	Kanila
Cannula nasale	Nasal cannula	Canule nasale	Cánula nasal	Nosna kanila
Cannula oro-faringea	Oropharyngeal airway	Canule de Guedel	Cánula orofaríngea (tubo de Mayo, cánula de Guédel)	Orofaringealna kanila
Cardiologia	Cardiology	Cardiologie	Cardiología	Kardiologija
Cardiostimolatore (stimolatore cardiaco)	Pacemaker	Stimulateur cardiaque (pacemaker, pile)	Marcapasos	Električni stimulator srca
Carrello	Hospital trolley	Chariot	Camilla	Kolica
Carrell servitore	Overbed table	Table de lit	Mesa para cama	Stolić za serviranje hrane
Cassetta di pronto soccorso	First aid kit	Trousse de secours	Botiquín de primeros auxilios	Kutija prve pomoći
Catetere	Catheter	Cathéter	Catéter	Kateter
Catetere vescicale	Urological catheter	Cathéter urologique	Catéter urinario	Urinarni kateter
Causa di morte	Cause of death	Cause de la mort	Causa de muerte	Uzrok smrti
Cauterizzazione	Cauterization	Cautérisation	Cauterización	Kauterizacija
Cena	Dinner (supper)	Dîner (souper)	Cena	Večera
Centro di medicina	Medical center	Centre médical	Centro médico	Medicinski centar
Chemioterapia	Chemotherapy	Chimiothérapie	Quimioterapia	Kemoterapija
Chirurgia	Surgery	Chirurgie	Cirugía	Kirurgija
Chirurgia laparoscopica	Laparoscopic surgery	Laparoscopie (coelioscopie)	Cirugía laparoscópica	Laparoskopska operacija
Chiudere	Close	Fermer	Cerrar	Zatvoriti
Chiusura delle tube	Surgical sterilization of a woman (tubal ligation)	Stérilisation chirurgicale au femme (ligature des trompes)	Esterilizatióm quirúrgica femenina (ligadura de trompas)	Kirurška sterilizacija žene (podvezivanje jajovoda)
Ciabatte	Slippers	Chausson	Pantuflas	Šlape
Circoncisione	Circumcision	Circoncision	Circuncisión	Obrezivanje
Citologia	Cytology	Cytologie	Citología	Citologija
Colazione	Breakfast	Petit déjeuner	Desayuno	Doručak
Collare cervicale	Neck immobilizer	Support de cou	Collar cervical	Imobilizator vrata
Comodino	Night table (bedside table)	Table de chevet (table de nuit)	Mesilla de noche	Noćni ormarić
Contagioso (infettivo)	Contagious	Contagieux /contagieuse	Contagioso	Zarazno
Coperta	Cover	Couverture	Cubrecama (colcha, manta)	Pokrivač
Corona	Dental crown	Couronne	Corona	Zubna krunica
Crioestrazione	Cryoextraction	Cryo-extraction	Crío-extracción	Krioekstrakcija
Cuffietta protettiva	Protection cap	Charlotte à usage unique	Gorra desechable	Zaštitna kapa
Cuscino	Pillow	Oreiller	Almohada	Jastuk
Deambulatore (tutore per disabili)	Walker (walking frame)	Déambulateur (cadre de marche, gadot)	Andador	Hodalica
Defecazione	Defecation	Défécation	Defecación	Pražnjenje stolice (defekacija)
Defibrillatore	Defibrillator	Défibrillateur	Desfibrilador	Defibrilator
Defibrillatore manuale	Manual defibrillator	Défibrillateur manuel	Desfibrilador manual	Ručni defibrilator
Defibrillazione	Defibrillation	Défibrillation	Desfibrilación	Defibrilacija

Italiano	Inglese	Francese	Spagnolo	Croato
Dentista	Dentist	Dentiste	Dentista	Stomatolog (zubar)
Deposito (magazzino)	Storage	Stockage	Almacenaje	Spremište
Dermatologia	Dermatology	Dermatologie	Dermatología	Dermatologija
Diagnosi	Diagnosis	Diagnostic	Diagnóstico	Dijagnoza
Dialisi	Dialysis	Dialyse	Diálisis	Dijaliza
Dialisi epatica	Liver dialysis	Dialyse hépatique	Diálisis de hígado	Dijaliza jetre
Dialisi renale	Renal dialysis	Dialyse rénale	Diálisis renal	Dijaliza bubrega
Dieta (regime dietetico)	Diet	Régime alimentaire	Régimen (dieta)	Dijeta
Digestione	Digestion	Digestion	Digestión	Probava
Dinamometro	Dynamometer	Dynamomètre	Dinamómetro	Dinamometar
Donatore / donatrice	Donor	Donneur	Donante	Davalac (donator)
Donazione del sangue	Blood donation	Don de sang	Donación de sangre	Darovanje krvi (donacija krvi)
Dottore / dottoressa (medico)	Doctor (physician)	Médecin	Médico	Liječnik
Drenaggio	Drainage	Drainage	Drenaje	Drenaža
Drenaggio posturale	Postural drainage	Drainage postural	Drenaje postural	Drenažni položaj
Elettrochirurgia	Electrosurgery	Électrochirurgie	Electrocirurgía	Elektrokirurgija
Elettrodo	Electrode	Électrode	Electrodo	Elektroda
Elettroterapia	Electrotherapy	Électrothérapie	Electroterapia	Elektroterapija
Esercizi di equilibrio	Balance training	Entraînement de l'equilibre	Entrenamiento del equilibrio	Trening ravnoteže
Esercizi di Kegel	Kegel exercise	Exercice de Kegel	Ejercicios de Kegel	Kegelove vježbe
Esercizi di respirazione	Breathing exercises	Exercice de respiration	Ejercicios de respiración	Vježbe disanja
Esercizio	Exercise	Exercice	Ejercicio	Vježbanje
Estrazione del dente	Dental extraction	Extraction dentaire	Exodoncia dental	Vađenje zuba
Fasciatura (bendaggio)	Dressing	Pansement	Apósito	Previjanje
Fermacapo	Head immobilizer	Immobiliseur de tête	Inmovilizador de cabeza	Imobilizator glave
Finestra	Window	Fenêtre	Ventana	Prozor
Fisioterapia	Physical therapy	Physiothérapie	Fisioterapia	Fizikalna terapija
Fisioterapista	Physiotherapist	Physiothérapeute	Fisioterapeuta	Fizioterapeut
Forbici	Scissors	Ciseau	Tijeras	Škare
Formazione chirurgica di stomia (colostomia)	Surgical procedure of formation of stoma (colostomy)	Formation chirurgicale de la stomie (colostomie)	Exteriorización de una parte de intestino a través de la cavidad abdominal (colostomía)	Kirurški zahvat formiranja stome (kolostomija)
Gel elettro-conduttivo	Electrode conductive gel	Gel électroconductif	Gel conductor	Kontaktni gel za elektrode
Germi	Germs	Germes	Gérmenes	Klice
Gerontologia	Gerontology	Gérontologie	Gerontología	Gerontologija
Ginecologia	Gynecology	Gynécologie	Ginecología	Ginekologija
Goniometro	Goniometer	Goniomètre	Goniómetro	Goniometar
Gruccia (stampella)	Crutch	Béquille	Muleta	Štaka
Guanti protettivi	Protect gloves	Gants à usage unique	Guantes desechables	Zaštitne rukavice
Guarigione (ristabilimento)	Recovery	Guérison	Recuperación	Oporavak
Idroterapia	Hydrotherapy	Hydrothérapie	Hidroterapia	Hidroterapija
Immunologia	Immunology	Immunologie	Inmunología	Imunologija
Incisione chirurgica della trachea (tracheotomia)	Surgical opening of a direct airway on the neck (tracheotomy)	Ouverture chirurgicale dans la trachée (trachéotomie)	Incisión quirúrgica en la tráquea (traqueotomía)	Kirurško otvaranje dišnog puta (traheotomija)
Infermiera /infermiere	Nurse	Infirmier	Enfermera	Medicinska sestra
Infusione	Infusion	Perfusion	Infusión	Infuzija
Iniezione	Injection	Injection	Inyección	Injekcija
Intervento chirurgico dell'orecchio medio (stapedectomia)	Surgical procedure on the middle ear (stapedectomy)	Ablation chirurgicale de l'étrier (stapédectomie)	Cirugía del oído medio (stapedectomía)	Kirurški zahvat na srednjem uhu (stapedektomija)
Intervento chirurgico delle connessioni talamiche (talamotomia)	Surgical procedure on the thalamus (thalamotomy)	Ablation chirurgicale d'une partie du thalamus (thalamotomie)	Cirugía del tálamo (talamotomía)	Kirurški zahvat na talamusu (talamotomija)
Intubazione	Intubation	Intubation	Intubación	Intubacija
Laringoscopio	Laryngoscope	Laryngoscope	Laringoscopio	Laringoskop
Lavanda gastrica	Gastric lavage (stomach pumping)	Lavage gastrique	Lavado gástrico	Ispiranje želuca
Lavanderia	Laundry	Blanchisserie	Lavandería	Večeraj
Lavare (fare il bagno)	Bath (wash)	Laver	Darse un baño	Kupati
Lenzuolo	Sheet	Drap	Sábana	Plahta
Letto	Bed	Lit	Cama	Krevet
Lift facciale (ritidectomia)	Facelift (rhytidectomy)	Lifting facial (rhytidectomie, lissage, remodelage)	Estiramiento de la cara (ritidectomía)	Lifting lica (ritidektomija)
Liposuzione	Liposuction	Liposuccion	Liposucción	Liposukcija
Lobotomia	Lobotomy	Lobotomie	Lobotomía	Lobotomija
Luce	Light	Lumière	Luz	Svjetlo
Manicotto di sfigmomanometro	Manometer cuff	Brassard du manomètre	Manguito de presión arterial	Manšeta tlakomjera
Manovra di Heimlich	Heimlich maneuver (abdominal thrusts)	Méthode de Heimlich	Maniobra de Heimlich	Heimlichov zahvat

Italiano	Inglese	Francese	Spagnolo	Croato
Maschera dell'ossigeno	Oxygen mask	Masque à oxygène	Máscara de oxígeno	Maska za kisik
Maschera laringea	Laryngeal mask airway	Masque laryngé	Máscara laríngea	Laringealna maska
Maschera per rianimazione	CPR mask	Masque de réanimation	Máscara de reanimación	Maska za oživljavanje
Mascherina di protezione	Protection face mask	Masque de protection	Mascarilla desechable	Zaštitna maska za lice
Materassino a depressione	Vacuum mattress	Matelas immobilisateur à dépression	Colchón al vácio	Vakumirani madrac
Materasso	Mattress	Matelas	Colchón	Madrac
Medicina interna	Internal medicine	Médicine interne	Medicina interna	Interna medicina
Medico di medicina generale (medico di famiglia)	General practitioner	Médecin généraliste (médecin omnipraticien)	Médico de cabecera	Liječnik opće prakse
Monitor per parametri vitali	Vital signs monitor	Moniteur de signes vitaux	Monitor de signos vitales	Monitor za praćenje vitalnih znakova
Morire	Die	Mourir	Morir	Umrijeti
Neurologia	Neurology	Neurologie	Neurología	Neurologija
Obitorio (mortorio)	Morgue (mortuary)	Morgue	Depósito de cadáveres (morgue)	Mrtvačnica
Oncologia	Oncology	Oncologie (cancérologie)	Oncología	Onkologija
Operazione (intervento chirurgico)	Operation (surgery)	Opération chirurgicale	Operación quirúrgica	Operacija
Ortopedia	Orthopedics	Orthopédie	Ortopedia	Ortopedija
Ospedale (policlinico)	Hospital	Hôpital	Hospital	Bolnica
Ospite (visitatore/visitatrice)	Visitor	Visiteur	Visitante	Posjetitelj
Otorinolaringoiatria	Otorhinolaryngology	Oto-rhino-laryngologie	Otorrinolaringología	Uho-grlo-nos
Otturazione odontoiatrica	Dental filling	Composite dentaire	Empaste (emplomadura)	Zubna plomba
Padiglione (reparto)	Ward	Salle	Sala (pabellón)	Odjel
Pallone autoespandibile	Ambu bag valve mask	Respirateur manuel type Ambu	Bolsa Ambú de ventilación manual	Ambu balon s maskom
Palpazione	Palpation	Palpation	Palpación	Pregled pipanjem (palpacija)
Patologia	Pathology	Pathologie	Patología	Patologija
Pattumiera	Litter bin	Poubelle	Papelera	Kanta za smeće
Paziente (ammalato)	Patient	Patient (malade)	Paciente	Bolesnik
Pediatria	Pediatrics	Pédiatrie	Pediatría	Pedijatrija
Percussione	Percussion	Percussion	Percusión	Pregled kucanjem (perkusija)
Pessario	Pessary	Pessaire (pessus)	Pesario	Pesar
Piantana portaflebo	Infusion stand	Pied à perfusion	Intravenoso poste	Stalak za infuziju
Pigiama	Pyjamas (pajamas)	Pyjama	Pijama (piyama)	Piđama
Pinzette	Tweezers	Brucelles	Pinzas	Pinceta
Porta	Door	Porte	Puerta	Vrata
Posizionatore	Body positioner	Coussin de positionnement	Almohada de posicionamiento	Udlaga za pozicioniranje
Posizione di Trendelenburg	Trendelenburg position	Position de Trendelenburg	Posición de Trendelenburg	Trendelenburgov položaj
Pranzo	Lunch	Déjeuner	Almuerzo	Ručak
Primo soccorso	First aid	Premiers secours	Primeros auxilios	Prva pomoć
Procedura di chirurgia plastica del naso (rinoplastica)	Plastic surgery of the nose (rhinoplasty)	Opération de chirurgie esthétique du nez (rhinoplastie)	Cirugía estética de la nariz (rinoplastia)	Plastična operacija nosa (rinoplastika)
Procedura di chirurgia plastica del seno (mastoplastica)	Plastic surgery of the breasts (mammoplasty)	Opération de chirurgie esthétique des seins (mammoplastie)	Cirugía estética de los senos (mamoplastia)	Plastična operacija dojke (mastoplastika)
Procedura di chirurgia plastica dell'addome (addominoplastica)	Plastic surgery of the abdomen ("tummy tuck", abdominoplasty)	Opération de chirurgie esthétique de la paroi abdominale (abdominoplastie)	Cirugía estética del abdomen (abdominoplastia)	Plastična operacija trbuha (abdominoplastika)
Procedura di chirurgia plastica della palpebra (blefaroplastica)	Plastic surgery of the eyelid (blepharoplasty)	Opération de chirurgie esthétique des paupières (blépharoplastie)	Cirugía estética de los párpados (blefaroplastia)	Plastična operacija očnog kapka (blefaroplastika)
Proclamazione del tempo della morte	Calling of the time of death	Détermination de l'heure de la mort	Determinación del tiempo de muerte	Proglašenje vremena smrti
Proteggi materasso cerato	Incontinence pad	Protège-matelas	Sábana de hule para la incontinencia	Gumirano platno
Protese mammaria	Breast implant	Implant mammaire	Implante de mama	Umetak za dojku
Protesi dentale	Dentures	Dentier	Prótesis dental	Umjetno zubalo
Provetta	Test tube	Tube à essai	Tubo de ensayo	Epruveta
Psichiatria	Psychiatry	Psychiatrie	Psiquiatría	Psihijatrija
Psicologo	Psychologist	Psychologue	Psicólogo	Psiholog
Pulitura dei denti	Teeth polishing	Vernis à dents	Pulidor de los dientes	Poliranje zuba
Purificazione	Cleansing	Purification	Purificación	Pročišćavanje
Quarantena	Quarantine	Quarantaine	Cuarentena	Karantena
Radiazione	Radiation	Radiation	Radiación	Zračenje
Radiologia	Radiology	Radiographie	Radiología	Radiologija

Italiano	Inglese	Francese	Spagnolo	Croato
Remissione	Remission	Rémission	Fase de remisión	Stadij mirovanja bolesti (remisija)
Reparto di malattie infettive	Infectious disease unit	Salle maladies infectieuses	Pabellón de enfermedades infecciosas	Zarazni odjel
Reparto di oftalmologia	Ophtalmology ward	Salle d'ophtalmologie	Sala de oftalmología	Očni odjel
Reparto polmonare	Pulmonary ward	Salle de pneumologie	Sala de neumología	Plućni odjel
Resezione transuretrale della prostata	Transurethral resection of the prostate	Résection transurétrale de la prostate	Resección transuretral de la próstata	Transuretralna resekcija prostate
Respiratore	Respirator	Appareil respiratoire	Aparato respiratorio	Aparat za disanje (respirator)
Respirazione artificiale	Artificial respiration	Ventilation artificielle	Respiración artificial	Umjetno disanje
Riabilitazione	Rehabilitation (rehab)	Réhabilitation	Rehabilitación	Rehabilitacija
Rianimazione	Reanimation	Réanimation	Reanimación	Oživljavanje (reanimacija)
Ricevente di trapianto	Recipient of an organ	Receveur de greffe	Receptor de un órgano	Primatelj organa
Rinologia	Rhinology	Rhinologie	Rinología	Rinologija
Riposo a letto	Bed rest	Repos au lit	Guardar cama	Mirovanje u krevetu
Rottami	Debris	Débris	Materia de desperdicio	Otpad (otpadni proizvod)
Sala d'aspetto	Waiting-room	Salle d'attente	Sala de espera	Čekaonica
Sala da pranzo (cenàcolo)	Dining-room	Salle à manger	Comedor	Blagavaonica
Sala operatoria	Operating room	Bloc opératoire	Quirófano	Operacijska sala
Sanare (guarire, recuperare)	Recover (heal)	Se remettre (se guérir)	Reponerse (recuperarse)	Ozdraviti
Scalpello	Scalpel	Scalpel	Escalpelo	Skalpel
Sciacquare	Rinse	Rincer	Lavar	Isprati
Secchia	Wash basin	Cuvette	Palangana (ajofaina)	Lavor
Schiavina	Blanket	Couverture	Manta (cobija)	Deka
Sedia a rotelle (carrozzella)	Wheelchair	Fauteuil roulant (charriot, charrette)	Silla de ruedas	Invalidska kolica
Sedia portantina	Escape chair	Chaise d'évacuation	Silla de evacuación	Sjedalica za evakuaciju
Serbatoio di ossigeno	Oxygen storage tank	Réservoir d'oxygène	Tanque de oxígeno	Boca s kisikom
Servizio di urgenza ed emergenza medica	Emergency medical services	Aide médicale urgente	Servicios médicos de emergencia	Hitna služba
Shunt	Shunt	Pontage (shunt)	Shunt	Spoj (skretnica)
Somministrazione dei farmaci	Administration of drugs	Administration des médicaments	Administración de fármacos	Davanje lijekova
Sonda	Sonde	Sonde	Sonda	Sonda
Sonda gastrica per nutrizione	Feeding tube	Sonde d'alimentation	Sonda de alimentación	Sonda za hranjenje
Sovrascarpe protettive	Protection shoe cover	Sur-chaussures à usage unique	Cubrezapatos	Zaštitna navlaka za obuću
Spugna	Sponge	Éponge	Esponja	Spužva
Sputare	Spit	Cracher	Escupir	Pljunuti
Stanza da terapia intensiva	Intensive care unit	Unité de soins intensifs	Unidad de cuidados intensivos	Jedinica intenzivne njege
Sterile	Sterile (aseptic)	Stérile	Estéril	Sterilno
Sterilizzazione	Sterilization	Stérilisation	Esterilización	Sterilizacija
Stetofon endoscopio	Stethoscop	Stéthoscope	Estetoscopio	Stetoskop
Suturare la ferita	Wound stitching	Suture de la plaie	Suturar la herida	Šivanje rane
Talloniere e gomitiere antidecubito	Heel and elbow protectors	Talonnières et coudières	Protectores talón/codo antiescaras	Zaštitnici za pete i laktove
Tavolo (scrivania)	Table (desk)	Table	Mesa (escritorio)	Stol
Tè	Tea	Thé	Té	Čaj
Terapia	Therapy	Thérapie (traitement curatif)	Tratamiento (terapia)	Liječenje (terapija)
Terapia intensiva	Intensive care	Soins intensifs	Cuidados intensivos	Intenzivna njega
Terapia semi-intensiva	Semi-intensive care	Soins semi-intensifs	Cuidados semi-intensivos	Poluintenzivna njega
Terapista occupazionale	Occupational therapist	Ergothérapeute	Terapeuta ocupacional	Radni terapeut
Trapano (trivella)	Drill	Perceuse	Taladro	Bušilica
Trapianto	Transplantation	Greffe (transplantation)	Trasplante	Presađivanje (transplantacija)
Trasfusione	Transfusion	Transfusion	Transfusión	Transfuzija
Trauma	Trauma	Trauma	Trauma	Trauma
Trazione	Traction	Traction	Tracción	Trakcija
Tubo d'aspirazione	Suction catheter	Cathéter à succion	Catéter de succión	Usisni kateter
Tubo di drenaggio	Drain tube	Drain	Sonda de drenaje	Dren
Tubo endotracheale	Endotracheal tube	Sonde d'intubation endotrachéale	Sonda endotraqueal	Endotrahealna kanila
Ufficio del medico	Doctor's office	Bureau du médecin	Consultorio de médico	Liječnička ambulanta
Urinazione	Urination (voiding)	Miction	Micción	Mokrenje (uriniranje)
Urologia	Urology	Urologie	Urología	Urologija
Uso del gabinetto	Using a toilet	Aller aux toilettes	Ir al servicio	Obaviti nuždu
Vaccinazione (inoculazione)	Vaccination (inoculation)	Vaccination (inoculation)	Vacunación	Cijepljenje
Vasectomia	Surgical sterilization of a man (vasectomy)	Ligature des canaux déférents des testicules (vasectomie)	Esterilización quirúrgica masculina (vasectomía)	Kirurška sterilizacija muškarca (vazektomija)
Vaso da notte (pitale)	Chamber-pot	Pot de chambre	Orinal	Noćna posuda

Italiano	Inglese	Francese	Spagnolo	Croato
Vaso sanitario	Toilet (lavatory)	Toilette (cabinet)	Servicio	Nužnik
Visita	Visit	Visite	Visita	Posjeta
ESAMI MEDICI:	**MEDICAL EXAMS:**	**EXAMENS MÉDICAUX:**	**EXÁMENES MÉDICOS:**	**MEDICINSKE PRETRAGE:**
Agoaspirato (biopsia mediante ago sottile)	Fine needle aspiration biopsy	Forage-biopsie	Punción aspiración con aguja fina	Punkcijsko-aspiracijska biopsija
Agoaspirato polmonare percutaneo transtoracico	Transthoracic percutaneous fine needle aspiration	Ponction transthoracique percutanée à l'aiguille fine	Punción transtorácica aspirativa con aguja ultrafina	Perkutana transtorakalna punkcija pluća
Amniocentesi	Amniocentesis	Amniocentèse	Amniocentesis	Amniocenteza
Analisi chimiche delle urine	Urine chemical analysis	Analyse chimique de l'urine	Análisis químico de orina	Kemijska analiza urina
Analisi dei gas nel sangue (emogas analisi)	Blood gas test	Prélèvement des gaz du sang	Prueba de gases en la sangre	Analiza plinova u krvi
Analisi del DNA	DNA analysis	Analyse de l'ADN	Análisis de DNA	DNK analiza
Analisi del liquido cerebro-spinale	Cerebrospinal fluid analysis	Analyse du liquide céphalo-rachidien	Análisis del líquido cefalorraquídeo	Pregled likvora
Angiografia	Angiography	Angiographie	Angiografía	Angiografija
Angiografia cerebrale	Cerebral angiography	Angiographie cérébrale	Angiografía cerebral	Cerebralna angiografija
Angiografia con cateterismo	Catheter angiography	Angiographie interventionnelle utilisant un cathéter	Angiografía por catéter	Kateterska angiografija
Angiografia digitale a sottrazione	Digital subtraction angiography	Angiographie numérique	Angiografía de sustracción digital	Digitalna supstrakcijska angiografija
Angiografia polmonare	Pulmonary angiography	Angiographie pulmonaire	Angiografía pulmonar	Pulmonalna angiografija
Angiografia spinale	Spinal angiography	Angiographie spinale	Angiografía espinal	Spinalna angiografija
Anoscopia	Anoscopy	Anuscopie	Anoscopía	Anoskopija
Antibiogramma	Antibiogram	Antibiogramme	Antibiograma	Antibiogram
Antigene carcino-embrionario (CEA)	Carcinoembryonic antigen (CEA)	Antigène carcino-embryonnaire (ACE)	Antígeno carcinoembrionario	Karcinoembrionski antigen (CEA)
Aortografia	Aortography	Aortographie	Aortografía	Aortografija
Arteriografia	Arteriography	Artériographie	Arteriografía	Arteriografija
Artrografia	Joint X-ray (arthrography)	Arthrographie	Artrografía	Rendgensko snimanje zgloba
Artroscopia	Arthroscopy	Arthroscopie	Artroscopia	Artroskopija
Aspartato transaminasi (SGOT)	Aspartate transaminase (SGOT)	Aspartate transaminase (SGOT)	Aspartato aminotransferasa (AST, transaminasa glutámico-oxalacética GOT)	Transaminaze u serumu
Audiometria	Audiometry	Audiométrie	Audiometría	Audiometrija
Audiometria di discorso	Speech audiometry	Audiométrie vocale	Audiometría del habla	Govorna audiometrija
Azoto ureico nel sangue (BUN)	Blood urea nitrogen test (BUN)	Azote d'urée dans le sang	Nitrógeno ureico en sangre (BUN)	Ostatni dušik u krvi (urea nitrogen test)
Biligrafia venosa	Intravenous biligraphy	Biligraphie intraveineuse	Biligrafia intravenosa	Intravenozna biligrafija
Biomarcatore	Biomarker	Biomarqueur	Marcador biológico	Biomarker
Biopsia	Biopsy	Biopsie	Biopsia	Biopsija
Biopsia cerebrale (biopsia dei ventricoli cerebrali)	Brain ventricle biopsy	Biopsie d'un ventricule cérébral	Biopsia cerebral	Biopsija moždanih klijetki (ventrikulopunkcija)
Biopsia cutanea	Skin biopsy	Biopsie de peau	Biopsia de piel	Biopsija kože
Biopsia del linfonodo	Lymph node biopsy	Biopsie du ganglion lymphatoque	Biopsia de ganglio linfático	Biopsija limfnog čvora
Biopsia del midollo osseo	Bone marrow biopsy	Biopsie ostéomédullaire	Biopsia de médula ósea	Biopsija koštane srži
Biopsia della tiroide	Thyroid biopsy	Biopsie thyroïdienne	Biopsia de tiroides	Biopsija štitnjače
Biopsia endometriale	Endometrial biopsy	Biopsie endométriale	Biopsia endometrial	Biopsija endometrija
Biopsia epatica	Liver biopsy	Biopsie du foie	Biopsia hepática	Biopsija jetre
Biopsia pleurica	Pleural biopsy	Biopsie pleurale	Biopsia pleural	Biopsija pleure
Biopsia renale	Kidney biopsy	Biopsie rénale	Biopsia renal	Biopsija bubrega
Biopsia stereotassica	Stereotactic biopsy	Biopsie stéréotaxique	Biopsia estereotáctica	Stereotaktična biopsija
Broncografia	Bronchography	Bronchographie	Broncografía	Bronhografija
Broncoscopia	Bronchoscopy	Bronchoscopie	Broncoscopia	Bronhoskopija
CA 125 (antigene di carcinoma 125)	CA 125 (cancer antigen 125)	Antigène de cancer CA 125	Marcador tumoral CA 125	CA 125 (karcinomski antigen 125)
CA 19-9 (antigene carboidratico)	CA 19-9 (carbohydrate antigen)	Antigène de cancer CA 19-9 (antigène d'hydrate de carbone)	CA 19-9 (antígeno carbohidrato 19-9)	CA 19-9 (karbohidratni antigen)
Cardiotocografia	Cardiotocography	Cardiotocographie	Cardiotocografía	Kardiotokografija
Cariotipo	Karyotype	Caryotype	Cariotipo	Kariotip
Cateterismo cardiaco (angiocardiografia)	Cardiac catheterization (heart cath, angiocardiography)	Cathétérisme cardiaque	Cateterismo cardíaco	Kateterizacija srca (angiokardiografija)
Cefalometria	Cephalometry	Céphalométrie	Cefalometría	Cefalometrija
Cistografia	Cystography	Cystographie	Cistografia	Cistografija
Cistoscopia	Cystoscopy	Cystoscopie	Cistoscopia	Cistoskopija
Colangio-pancreatografia endoscopica retrograda	Endoscopic retrograde cholangiopancreatography (ERCP)	Cholangiopancréatographie rétrograde endoscopique	Colangiopancreatografia retrógrada endoscópica	Endoskopska retrograd-na kolangiopankreatografija (ERCP)
Colangiografia	Cholangiography	Cholangiographie	Colangiografia	Kolangiografija

Italiano	Inglese	Francese	Spagnolo	Croato
Colecistografia orale	Oral cholecystography	Cholécystographie orale	Colecistografía oral	Rendgensko snimanje žučnog mjehura s kontrastom (peroralna kolecistografija)
Colonscopia	Colonoscopy	Colonoscopie	Colonoscopia	Kolonoskopija
Colposcopia	Colposcopy	Colposcopie	Colposcopia	Kolposkopija
Coltura del liquor	Cerebrospinal fluid culture	Culture du liquide cérébro-spinal	Cultivo de líquido cefalorraquídeo	Mikrobiološki pregled likvora
Coltura di gola	Throat swab culture	Culture de gorge avec le coton-tige	Exudado faríngeo	Mikrobiološki pregled brisa grla
Coltura di microrganismi	Microbiological culture	Culture microbiologique	Cultivo	Mikrobiološki pregled (kultura)
Coltura di sputo	Sputum culture	Culture de crachat	Cultivo de esputo	Mikrobiološki pregled ispljuvka
Coltura vaginale	Vaginal swab culture	Culture vaginale	Cultivo vaginal	Mikrobiološki pregled brisa rodnice
Concentrazione del glucosio nel plasma	Blood sugar concetration (glucose level)	Taux de la glycémie	Concentración de glucosa en sangre	Šećer u krvi
Conizzazione	Cervical conization	Conisation	Conización	Konizacija
Coronarografia	Coronary catheterization (coronarography)	Coronarographie	Coronariografía	Koronarografija
Craniografia	Skull X-ray (craniography)	Craniographie	Craneografía	Rendgensko snimanje lubanje
Defecografia	Defecography	Défécographie	Defecografía	Defekografija
Densità minerale ossea	Bone densitometry (dual energy X-ray absorpriometry)	Ostéodensitométrie	Densitometría ósea	Denzitometrija kostiju (apsorpciometrija kostiju)
Dermatoscopia (dermoscopia)	Dermatoscopy (dermoscopy)	Dermatoscopie (dermoscopie)	Dermatoscopia	Dermatoskopija (dermoskopija)
Diagnosi differenziale	Differential diagnosis	Diagnostic différentiel	Diagnóstico diferencial	Diferencijalna dijagnoza
Dilatazione delle pupille provocando con tropicamide	Drug induced pupillary dilatation	Dilatation des pupilles provoquée par les médicaments	Dilatación pupilar inducida por fármacos	Širenje zjenica potaknuto lijekovima
Ecocardiografia	Cardiac ultrasound (echocardiography)	Échocardiographie	Ecocardiografía	Ultrazvuk srca (ehokardiografija)
Ecocardiografia doppler	Doppler echocardiography	Échocardiographie-doppler	Ecocardiografía doppler	Ultrazvuk srca s dopplerom
Ecoencefalografia	Echoencephalography	Échoencéphalographie	Ecoencefalografia	Ehoencefalografija
Ecografia	Ultrasound (medical ultrasonography)	Échographie	Ultrasonografía (ecografía)	Ultrazvuk
Ecografia addominale	Abdominal ultrasound	Échographie abdominale	Ecografía abdominal (ultrasonido abdominal)	Ultrazvuk abdomena
Ecografia colecisti e vie biliari	Ultrasound of the gallbladder and bile ducts	Échographie la vésicule biliaire et les voies biliaires	Ecografía de vesícula y vías biliares	Ultrazvuk žuči i žučnih vodova
Ecografia della tiroide	Thyroid ultrasound	Échographie thyroïdienne	Ecografía de la tiroides (ultrasonido de la tiroides)	Ultrazvuk štitnjače
Ecografia epatica	Liver ultrasound	Échographie du foie (échographie hépatique)	Ecografía hepática (ultrasonido hepático)	Ultrazvuk jetre
Ecografia mammaria	Breast ultrasound	Échographie mammaire	Ecografía de mama (ultrasonido de mama)	Ultrazvuk dojke
Ecografia pancreatica	Pancreas ultrasound	Échographie du pancréas	Ecografía de páncreas (ultrasonido de páncreas)	Ultrazvuk gušterače
Ecografia renale	Renal ultrasound	Échographie rénale	Ecografía renal (ultrasonido renal)	Ultrazvuk bubrega
Elettrocardiografia	Electrocardiography (ECG)	Électrocardiographie (ECG)	Electrocardiografía (ECG, EKG)	Elektrokardiografija (EKG)
Elettroencefalografia	Electroencephalography (EEG)	Électro-encéphalographie (EEG)	Electroencefalografía	Elektroencefalografija (EEG)
Elettroforesi delle sieroproteine	Serum protein electrophoresis	Électrophorèse des protéines	Electroforesis de proteínas séricas	Elektroforeza proteina u serumu
Elettromiografia	Electromyography (EMG)	Électromyographie	Electromiografía	Elektromiografija (EMG)
Elettroneurografia	Electroneurography	Électroneurographie	Electroneurografía	Elektroneurografija
Elettroretinografia	Electroretinography	Électrorétinographie	Electrorretinografía	Elektroretinografija
Ematocrito	Hematocrit	Hématocrite	Hematocrito	Hematokrit
Emocoltura	Blood culture	Hémoculture	Hemocultivo	Mikrobiološki pregled krvi (hemokultura)
Emocromo (analisi del sangue, esame emocromocitometrico)	Complete blood count	Hémogramme (numération formule sanguine)	Hemograma (conteo sanguíneo completo)	Kompletna krvna slika
Endoscopia	Endoscopy	Endoscopie	Endoscopia	Endoskopija
Enteroscopia	Enteroscopy	Entéroscopie	Enteroscopia	Enteroskopija
Ergometria (ECG sotto sforzo)	Ergometry test	Ergométrie	Ergometría	Test opterećenja (ergometrija)
Esame chimico di succo gastrico	Gastric juice chemical examination	Analyse chimique du suc gastrique	Análisis químico del jugo gástrico	Kemijski pregled želučanog soka
Esame del fundus oculi	Dilated fundus examination	Fond d'oeil	Exámen dilatado de fundus	Pregled očnog fundusa
Esame della mammella	Breast examination	Examen du sein	Exploración física de mama	Pregled dojke
Esame delle urine peso specifico	Urine specific gravity	Poids spécifique de l'urine	Gravedad específica de la orina	Specifična težina urina

Italiano	Inglese	Francese	Spagnolo	Croato
Esame ginecologico	Gynecological examination	Examen gynécologique	Examen ginecológico	Ginekološki pregled
Esami di laboratorio	Laboratory tests	Analyse médicale (examens de biologie médicale)	Pruebas de laboratorio	Laboratorijske pretrage
Esami sierologici	Serology blood tests	Analyse sérologique	Pruebas de serología	Serološke pretrage na antitijela
Esofagogastroduodenoscopia	Esophagogastroduodenoscopy	Endoscopie oeso-gastro-duodénale	Esofagogastroduodenoscopia	Ezofagogastrodoudenoskopija
Esplorazione rettale	Rectal examination	Toucher rectal	Tacto rectal	Rektalni pregled
Flebografia	Phlebography	Phlébographie	Flebografía	Venografija (flebografija)
Fluoroscopia	Fluoroscopy	Fluoroscopie	Fluoroscopia	Fluoroskopija
Fosfatasi alcalina totale	Alkaline phosphatase	Phosphatase alcaline	Fosfatasa alcalina	Alkalna fosfataza
Gastroscopia	Gastroscopy	Gastroscopie	Gastroscopia	Gastroskopija
Glucosio nelle urine	Glucose urine test	Test du sucre dans les urines	Examen de glucosa en orina	Šećer u urinu
Gonioscopia	Gonioscopy	Gonioscopie	Gonioscopia	Gonioskopija
HbsAg (antigene di superficie dell'epatite B)	HbsAg (Hepatitis B surface antigen)	Antigène HbsAg (antigène de surface du virus de l'hépatite B)	HbsAg (antígeno de superficie de la hepatitis B)	HbsAg (hepatitis B površinski antigen)
Imaging a risonanza magnetica (risonanza magnetica tomografica)	Magnetic resonance imaging (MRI)	Imagerie par résonance magnétique (IRM)	Imagen por resonancia magnética (IRM)	Magnetska rezonancija (MR)
Indagini radiologiche del colon con clisma opaco a doppio contrasto	Barium enema	Lavement baryté	Enema de bario con doble contraste	Rendgensko snimanje debelog crijeva i rektuma s kontrastom barija
Isterosalpingografia	Hysterosalpingography	Hystérosalpingographie	Histerosalpingografía	Rendgensko snimanje maternice i jajovoda
Isteroscopia	Hysterescopy	Hystéroscopie	Histeroscopia	Histeroskopija
Laboratorio	Laboratory (lab)	Laboratoire	Laboratorio	Laboratorij
Laparoscopia	Laparoscopy	Laparoscopie	Laparoscopia	Laparoskopija
Laringoscopia	Laryngoscopy	Laryngoscopie	Laringoscopia	Laringoskopija
Linfangiografia (linfografia)	Lymphography (lymphangiography)	Lymphographie	Linfografia	Limfografija
Magnetoencefalografia	Magnetoencephalography (MEG)	Magnétoencéphalographie	Magnetoencefalografía	Magnetoencefalografija (MEG)
Mammografia (mastografia)	Mammography	Mammographie	Mamografia	Mamografija
Manometria esofagea	Esophageal manometry	Manométrie oesophagienne	Manometría esofágica	Manometrija jednjaka
Mantoux test	Mantoux test (PPD test)	Test Mantoux (test PPD)	Test de Mantoux (PPD)	Tuberkulinski kožni test
Marker tumorale	Tumor marker	Marqueur tumoral	Marcador tumoral	Tumorski marker
Mediastinoscopia	Mediastinoscopy	Médiastinoscopie	Mediastinoscopia	Medijastinoskopija
Medicina nucleare	Radioisotope scanning (nuclear medicine)	Médicine nucléaire	Medicina nuclear	Radioizotopna dijagnostika
Mezzo di contrasto	Contrast medium	Produit de contraste	Medio de contraste	Kontrast
Mielografia	Myelography	Myélographie	Mielografia	Mijelografija
Mielografia lombare	Lumbar myelography	Myélographie lombaire	Mielografía lumbar	Lumbalna mijelografija
Mielografia sotto-occipitale	Suboccipital myelography	Myélographie sous-occipitale	Mielografia cervical suboccipital	Subokcipitalna mijelografija
Misurazione del polso	Pulse monitoring	Prise de pouls	Comprobación del pulso	Mjerenje pulsa
Misurazione della pressione arteriosa	Blood pressure monitoring	Monitoring de la pression artérielle	Monitorización de la presión arterial	Mjerenje krvnog pritiska
Oftalmoscopìa	Ophtalmoscopy	Ophtalmoscopie	Oftalmoscopía	Oftalmoskopija
Otoscopia	Otoscopy	Otoscopie	Otoscopía	Otoskopija
Patch test	Patch test	Patch test	Prueba de emplasto (prueba del parche)	Kožni alergološki test flasterom
Pelvigrafia	Pelvigraphy	Pelvigraphie	Pelvigrafía	Rendgensko snimanje zdjelice i porođajnog kanala
Pelvimetria	Pelvimetry	Pelvimétrie	Pelvimetria	Pelvimetrija
Perimetria	Perimetry	Périmétrie	Campimetría (perimetría)	Perimetrija
Pielografia retrograda	Retrograde pyelography	Urétéro-pyélographie rétrograde	Pielografía retrógrada	Retrogradna pijelografija
Pletismografia	Plethysmography	Pléthysmographie	Pletismografia	Pletizmografija
Pneumoencefalografia	Pneumoencephalography	Encéphalographie gazeuse	Neumoencefalografia	Pneumoencefalografija
Polisonnografia	Polysomnography (sleep study)	Polysomnographie (polygraphie du sommeil)	Polisomnografia	Polisomnografija (viseparametarski test u pracenju procesa sna)
Pressione venosa centrale	Central venous pressure (CVP)	Pression veineuse centrale	Presión venosa central	Centralni venozni pritisak (CVP)
Proteine nelle urine	Urine protein test	Protéines dans les urines	Proteínas en la orina	Bjelančevine u urinu
Prova della benzidina	Benzidine stool test	Analyse fécale de benzidine	Prueba de la bencidina	Benzidinski test stolice
Prova di Weber	Weber test	Test de Weber	Prueba de Weber	Weberov test
Punteggio del coma di Glasgow	Glasgow coma scale	Échelle de Glasgow	Escala de coma de Glasgow	Glasgowska skala kome
Puntura lombare (rachicentesi)	Lumbar puncture	Ponction lombaire (rachicentèse)	Punción lumbar	Lumbalna punkcija
Puntura suboccipitale	Suboccipital puncture	Ponction sous-occipitale	Punción suboccipital	Subokcipitalna punkcija
Radiografia	X-ray (radiography)	Radiographie	Radiografía	Rendgen
Radiografia del torace	Chest X-ray	Radiographie de thorax	Radiografía de tórax	Rendgensko snimanje srca i pluća

Italiano	Inglese	Francese	Spagnolo	Croato
Radiografia della colonna vertebrale	Spine X-ray (spine radiography)	Radiographie de la colonne vertébrale	Radiografía de la columna vertebral (radiografía vertebral)	Rendgensko snimanje kralježnice
Radiografia dentale	Dental X-ray	Radiographie dentaire	Radiografía dental	Rendgensko snimanje zuba
Radiografia gastroduodenale con pasto baritato	Barium meal (upper gastrointestinal series)	Radiographie de l'abdomen en bouillie de sulfate de baryum	Radiografía de esófago, estómago y duodeno tomada con comida baritada	Rendgensko snimanje želuca i dvanaesnika barijevom kašom
Radiografia ossea	Bone X-ray (bone radiography)	Radiographie des os	Radiografía de hueso (radiografía ósea)	Rendgensko snimanje kostiju
Rettoscopia	Rectoscopy	Rectoscopie	Rectoscopia	Rektoskopija
Riflesso patellare	Patellar reflex	Réflexe rotulien	Reflejo patelar	Patelarni refleks
Rifrattometria	Refractometry	Réfractométrie	Refractomería	Ispitivanje refrakcije
Risonanza magnetica funzionale	Functional magnetic resonance imaging (functional MRI)	Imagerie par résonance magnétique fonctionnelle (IRMf)	Imagen por resonancia magnética funcional (IRMf)	Funkcionalna magnetska rezonancija (FMR)
Rose Waaler test	Rose Waaler test	Réaction de Waaler Rose	Test de Waaler-Rose	Rose Waaler test
Scintigrafia epatobiliare con tecnezio -99m	Hepatobiliary scintigraphy with technetium -99m	Scintigraphie hépatobiliaire au Technétium 99m	Gammagrafía hepatobiliar con tecnecio 99m	Scintigrafija jetre i žučnih vodova radioaktivnim izotopima
Scintigrafia ossea	Bone scintigraphy	Scintigraphie osseuse	Gammagrafía ósea	Scintigrafija kostiju
Scintigrafia polmonare	Lung scintigraphy	Scintigraphie pulmonaire	Gammagrafía pulmonar	Scintigrafija pluća
Scintigrafia renale	Renal scintigraphy	Scintigraphie rénale	Gammagrafía renal	Scintigrafija bubrega
Scintigrafia splenica con tecnezio -99m	Spleen scintigraphy with technetium -99m	Scintigraphie splénique au Technétium 99m	Gammagrafía de bazo con tecnecio 99m	Scintigrafija slezene radioaktivnim izotopima
Scintigrafia tiroidea	Thyroid scintigraphy	Scintigraphie thyroïdienne	Gammagrafía tiroidea	Scintigrafija štitnjače
Semenogelasi (antigene prostatico specifico)	Prostate specific antigen	Antigène prostatique spécifique	Antígeno prostático específico	Prostatični specifični antigen (PSA)
Seroalbumina	Serum albumin	Albumine dans le sang	Albúmina en la sangre	Albumin u serumu
Sialografia (scialografia)	Sialography	Sialographie	Sialografía	Sijalografija
Sigmoidoscopia	Sigmoidoscopy	Sigmoïdoscopie	Sigmoidoscopia	Sigmoidoskopija
Spermiogramma	Semen analysis	Spermogramme	Espermiograma	Spermogram
Spirometria (pneumometria)	Spirometry (vital capacity test)	Spirométrie	Espirometría	Spirometrija (mjerenje vitalnog kapaciteta)
Tempo di protrombina	Prothrombin time	Taux de prothrombine	Tiempo de protrombina	Protrombinski indeks
Tempo di tromboplastina parziale	Partial thromboplastin time (PTT)	Temps de céphaline activée (TCA)	Tiempo de trombopla-stina parcial activado	Parcijalno tromboplastinsko vrijeme (PTT)
Test alfa-fetoproteina	Alpha-fetoprotein test (AFP test)	Test d'alpha-foetoprotéine	Prueba de alfa-fetoproteína	Alfafetoproteinski test (AFP)
Test alla fenolsulfonftaleina	Phenolsulfonphthalein test (PSP test)	Épruve à la phénolsulfonphtaléine	Prueba de la fenolsulfonftaleína	Fenolsulfoftaleinski test (PSP-test)
Test biochimici di sangue	Biochemical blood tests	Analyse de biochimie du sang	Exámenes bioquímicos de sangre	Biokemijske pretrage krvi
Test cutaneo per le allergie ''prick test''	Skin allergy testing (prick test)	Test de la piqûre	Test cutaneos de alergia (prick)	Alergološko testiranje kože (prick test)
Test del respiro (urea breath test)	Urea breath test	Test respiratoire à l'urée	Prueba del aliento con urea	Urea izdisajni test
Test della bilirubina	Serum bilirubin	Diagnostic différentiel pour bilirubine sérique	Análisis de bilirrubina sérica	Bilirubin u serumu
Test della bromosulfaleina di funzionalità epatica	Bromsulphalein liver function test	Test de la bromesulfonephtaléine	Prueba de la función hepática con bromosulfaleína	Brom-sulfalein test funkcije jetre
Test di agglutinazione	Agglutination tests	Test d'agglutination	Análisis de aglutinación	Test aglutinacije
Test di captazione tiroidea dello iodio 131	Iodine-131 thyroid test	Fixation thyroïdienne de l'iode 131	Captación tiroidea de 131yodo	Test štitnjače na provodljivost radioaktivnog joda 131
Test di Coombs indiretto	Indirect Coombs test	Réaction de Coombs indirecte	Prueba de Coombs indirecta	Indirektni Coombsov test
Test di funzionalità epatica	Liver function tests	Explorations fonctio-nnelles hépatiques	Pruebas de función hepática	Funkcionalne pretrage jetre
Test di gravidanza	Pregnancy test	Test de grossesse	Pruebas de embarazo	Test na trudnoću
Test di ormoni tiroidei nel sangue	Thyroid blood tests	Taux d'hormones thyroïdiennes dans le sang	Concetración de hormonas tiroideas en sangre	Test na hormone štitnjače u krvi
Test di Papanicolaou (Pap test)	Papanicolau test (Pap test)	Test PAP	Prueba de Papanicolau	Papa-test (Papanicolaouova klasifikacija)
Test orale di tolleranca al glucosio (OGTT, curva da carico orale di glucosio)	Oral glucose tolerance test (OGTT)	Test de tolérance orale au glucose (TTOG)	Test de tolerancia oral a la glucosa	Oralni test tolerancije na glukozu (OGTT)
Test rapido dello streptococco	Rapid strep test	Test de diagnostic rapide du streptocoque	Prueba rápida para estreptococo	Brzi test na streptokok (strep-test)
Timpanocentesi	Tympanocentesis	Tympanocentese	Tímpanocentesis	Timpanocenteza
Timpanometria	Tympanometry	Tympanométrie	Timpanometría	Timpanometrija
Tomografia	Tomography	Tomographie	Tomografía	Tomografija
Tomografia ad emissione di positroni	Positron emission tomography	Tomographie par émission de positrons	Tomografía por emisión de positrones	Pozitronska emisijska tomografija (PET)
Tomografia computerizzata (TC)	Computed tomography (CT)	Tomodensitométrie (TDM)	Tomografía computada	Kompjuterizirana tomografija (CT)
Tonometria	Tonometry	Tonométrie oculaire	Tonometría	Tonometrija oka

Italiano	Inglese	Francese	Spagnolo	Croato
Toracoscopia	Thoracoscopy	Thoracoscopie	Toracoscopia	Torakoskopija
Ultrasuono ad alta intensità focalizzato	High intensity focused ultrasound	Ultrasons focalisés de haute intensité	Ultrasonido focalizado de alta intensidad (HIFU)	Fokusirani ultrazvuk visokog intenziteta
Urea clearance (clearance dell'urea)	Urea clearance test	Épruve d'élimination de l'urée sanguine	Prueba de aclaramiento de urea sanguínea	Urea klirens
Ureteroscopia	Ureteroscopy	Urétéroscopie	Ureteroscopía	Ureteroskopija
Uretrografia	Urethrography	Urétrographie	Uretrografia	Uretrografija
Urinocoltura	Urine culture	Uroculture	Urocultivo	Mikrobiološki pregled mokraće (urinokultura)
Urobilinogeno nelle urine	Urobilinogen in urine	Urobilinogène dans les urines	Urobilinógeno en orina	Urobilinogen u urinu
Urografia	Pyelography	Urographie	Urografía	Pijelografija (urografija)
Urografia intravenosa (pielografia intravenosa)	Intravenous pyelography	Urographie intra-veineuse	Urografia intravenosa	Intravenozna pijelografija (i.v. Urografija)
Velocità di eritrosedimentazione	Erythrocyte sedimentation rate	Vitesse de sédimentation	Velocidad de sedimentación globular	Sedimentacija eritrocita
Ventricolografia	Ventriculography	Ventriculographie	Ventriculografia	Ventrikulografija
Volume urinario residuo	Post-void residual urine volume	Volume urinaire résiduel	Volumen residual de orina	Ostatni urin (rezidualni urin)
GRAVIDANZA ED OSTETRICIA:	**PREGNANCY AND OBSTETRICS:**	**GROSSESSE ET OBSTÉTRIQUE:**	**EMBARAZO Y OBSTETRICIA:**	**TRUDNOĆA I PORODNIŠTVO:**
Aborto abituale	Habitual abortion (recurrent miscarriage)	Avortement à répétition	Aborto habitual	Habitualni pobačaj
Aborto spontaneo	Spontaneous abortion (miscarriage)	Fausse couche	Aborto espontáneo	Spontani pobačaj
Amniocentesi	Amniocentesis	Amniocentèse	Amniocentesis	Amniocenteza
Amnios	Amniotic sac	Amnios (sac amniotique)	Saco amniótico	Vodenjak
Amnioscopia	Amnioscopy	Amnioscopie	Amnioscopia	Amnioskopija
Anomalie di sviluppo fetale (anomalie fetali)	Fetal anomalies (fetal abnormalities)	Anomalies foetales	Anomalías fetales	Anomalije fetusa
Anomalie uterine	Uterine anomalies	Malformations utérines	Malformaciones uterinas	Anomalije maternice
Aspiratore a vuoto	Vacuum extractor (ventouse)	Vacuum extractor	Aspirador al vacío	Vakuumski ekstraktor
Asportazione chirurgica dell'utero (isterectomia)	Surgical removal of the uterus (hysterectomy)	Enlèvement chirurgical de l'uterus (hystérectomie)	Extracción quirúrgica del útero (histerectomía)	Kirurško odstranjenje maternice (histerektomija)
Assenza di mestruazioni (amenorrea)	Absence of menstrual period (amenorrhea)	Absence des règles (aménorrhée)	Ausencia de la menstruación (amenorrea)	Izostanak mjesečnice (amenoreja)
Banca del seme	Sperm bank	Banque du sperme	Banco de semen	Banka sperme
Blastocisti	Blastocyst	Blastocyste	Blastocisto	Blastocista
Canale del parto	Birth canal	Canal utérin	Canal del parto	Porodni kanal
Capezzolo	Nipple	Mamelon (papille)	Pezón	Bradavica
Cardiotocografia	Cardiotocography	Cardiotocographie	Cardiotocografia	Kardiotokografija
Ciclo mestruale	Menstrual cycle	Cycle menstruel	Ciclo menstrual	Menstruacijski ciklus
Clinica ostetrica	Maternity hospital	Maternité	Hospital de maternidad	Rodilište
Collo	Neck	Cou	Cuello	Vrat
Complesso TORCH	TORCH infections	Infections TORCH	Infecciones TORCH	TORCH infekcije
Concezione	Conception	Conception (fécondation)	Fecundación (fertilización)	Začeće (oplodnja)
Contrazioni del travaglio	Labor contractions	Contractions utérines du travail	Contracciones del trabajo de parto (contracciones uterinas)	Trudovi
Cordocentesi	Cordocentesis	Cordocentèse	Cordocentesis	Kordocenteza
Coriocarcinoma	Choriocarcinoma	Choriocarcinome	Coriocarcinoma	Koriokarcinom
Corion (corio)	Chorion	Chorion	Corion	Korion
Culatta (deretano)	Breech	Siège	Nalga	Zadak
Depressione post-partum	Postnatal depression (postpartum depression)	Dépression post-natale (dépression post-partum)	Depresión postparto (depresión postnatal)	Postporođajna depresija
Diabete gestazionale	Gestational diabetes	Diabète gestationnel	Diabetes gestacional	Gestacijski dijabetes
Dilatazione della cervice uterina	Cervical dilation	Dilatation cervicale	Dilatación del cuello uterino	Otvaranje ušća maternice
Distacco di placenta (abruptio placentae)	Placental abruption	Abruption placentaire (rupture placentaire)	Desprendimiento prematuro de placenta	Abrupcija posteljice
Dotto galattoforo	Lactiferous duct	Canal galactophore	Conducto mamario (conducto galactóforo)	Mliječni vod
Durata della gravidanza	Duration of pregnancy	Durée de la grossesse	Duración del embarazo	Trajanje trudnoće
Durata di contrazioni	Duration of contraction	Durée de la contraction utérine	Duración de las contracciones uterinas	Trajanje truda
Eclampsia	Eclampsia	Éclampsie	Eclampsia	Eklampsija
Ecografia	Ultrasound (medical ultrasonography)	Échographie	Ultrasonografía (ecografía)	Ultrazvuk
Edema	Edema	Oedème	Edema (hidropesía)	Edem
Eiaculazione	Ejaculation	Éjaculation	Eyaculación	Ejakulat
Embrione	Embryo	Embryon	Embrión	Embrij (zametak)
Emorragia	Bleeding (haemorrhage)	Saignement (hémorragie)	Desangramiento (hemorragia)	Krvarenje (hemoragija)
Episiotomia	Episiotomy	Épisiotomie	Episiotomia	Kirurško proširenje porođajnog kanala (epiziotomija)

Italiano	Inglese	Francese	Spagnolo	Croato
Eritroblastosi fetale (malattia emolitica del neonato)	Hemolytic disease of the newborn	Maladie hémolytique du nouveau-né	Enfermedad hemolítica del recién nacido (eritroblastosis fetal)	Hemolitička bolest novorođenčeta
Espulsione del feto	Expulsion of the baby	Expulsion du bébé	Expulsión del producto	Istiskivanje ploda
Espulsione della placenta	Expulsion of placenta	Expulsion du placenta	Expulsión de la placenta	Istiskivanje posteljice i ovoja
Estrogeno placentare	Placental estrogen	Oestrogène placentaire	Estrógeno de la placenta	Estrogen placente
False contrazioni (contrazioni di Braxton Hicks)	Braxton Hicks contractons	Fausse contraction (contraction de Braxton Hicks)	Contracción de Braxton Hicks	Lažni trudovi
Farmaci abortivi	Abortifacients	Médicaments abortifs	Fármacos abortivos	Abortivni lijekovi
Farmaco con lo scopo di arrestare le contrazioni uterine (tocolisi)	Medication that suppresses premature labor (tocolytic)	Médicament pour interrompre le déclenchement du travail (tocolytique)	Fármaco utilizado para suprimir el trabajo de parto prematuro (tocolítico)	Lijek za sprečavanje trudova (tokolitik)
Fase del parto	Stage of birth	Stade du travail	Etapas del parto	Porodno doba
Febbre puerperale	Puerperal fever	Fièvre puerpérale	Fiebre puerperal	Puerperalna groznica (babinja groznica)
Fecondazione assistita (fecondazione artificiale)	Artificial insemination	Insémination artificielle	Inseminación artificial	Umjetna oplodnja
Fertilizzazione in vitro	In vitro fertilisation	Fécondation in vitro	Fecundación in vitro	Oplodnja in vitro
Feto	Fetus	Foetus	Feto	Fetus
Fetoscopia	Fetoscopy	Foetoscopie	Fetoscopia	Fetoskopija
Follicolo di Graaf	Graafian follicle	Follicule de Graaf	Folículo de Graaf	Graafov folikul
Forcipe	Forceps	Forceps	Fórceps	Forceps (kliješta)
Frequenza di contrazioni uterine	Labor contraction frequency	Fréquence des contractions utérines	Frecuencia de las contracciones uterinas	Frekvencija trudova
Funicolo ombelicale	Umbilical cord	Cordon ombilical	Cordón umbilical	Pupkovina (pupčana vrpca)
Gemelli	Twins	Jumeaux	Gemelos	Blizanci
Gemelli fraterni (gemelli dizigoti)	Dizygotic twins (biovular twins)	Jumeaux dizygotes	Gemelos dicigóticos (mellizos)	Dvojajčani blizanci
Gemell i identici (gemelli monozigoti)	Monozygotic twins (identical twins)	Jumeaux monozygotes	Gemelos monocigóticos	Jednojajčani blizanci
Genitore	Parent	Géniteur	Padre (primario)	Roditelj
Genitore biologico	Biological parent	Parent biologique	Padre biológico	Biološki roditelj
Ginecologia	Gynecology	Gynécologie	Ginecología	Ginekologija
Gonadotropina corionica	Chorion-gonadotrophin	Gonadotrophine chorionique	Gonadotropina coriónica	Korion-gonadotropin
Gravidanza (gestazione)	Pregnancy	Grossesse	Embarazo	Trudnoća
Gravidanza ectopica	Ectopic pregnancy (extrauterine pregnancy)	Grossesse extra-utérine	Embarazo ectópico	Izvanmaternična trudno-ća (ektopična trudnoća)
Gravidanza gemellare	Multiple pregnancy	Grossesse multiple	Embarazo múltiple	Blizanačka trudnoća
Imene	Hymen	Hymen	Himen	Djevičnjak (himen)
Impianto	Implantation	Implantation	Implatación	Implantacija (usađivanje)
Incubatrice	Incubator	Couveuse (incubateur)	Incubadora	Inkubator
Infezione	Infection	Infection	Infección	Infekcija
Infiammazione del sacco amniotico (corioamniosite)	Inflammation of the fetal membranes (chorioamnionitis)	Chorioamnionite	Infección de las membranas placentarias (corioamnionitis)	Upala plodovih ovoja (korioamnionitis)
Infiammazione della vescica urinaria (cistite)	Inflammation of the urinary bladder (cystitis)	Inflammation de la vessie (cystite)	Inflamación de la vejiga urinaria (cistitis)	Upala mokraćnog mjehura (cistitis)
Iniezione intracitoplasmatica dello spermatozoo	Intracytoplasmatic sperm injection	Injection intra-cytoplasmique de spermatozoïdes	Inyección intracitoplasmática de espermatozoídes	Intracitoplazmatska spermalna injekcija
Intensità di contrazione	Intensity of contractions	Intensité des contractions utérines	Intensidad de contracciones uterinas	Snaga trudova
Interruzione di gravidanza (aborto)	Abortion (pregnancy termination)	Avortement	Aborto inducido	Prekid trudnoće (abortus)
Iperemia dell'ovaio	Ovarian hyperemia	Hyperhémie ovarienne	Hiperemia del ovario	Hiperemija jajnika
Iperplasia endometriale	Endometrial hyperplasia	Hyperplasie endométriale	Hiperplasia endometrial	Hiperplazija maternice
Ipertensione arteriosa sistemica	High blood pressure (hypertension)	Pression artérielle élevée (hypertension artérielle)	Incremento de la presión sanguínea (hipertensión)	Visoki krvni tlak (hipertenzija)
Ipertrofia dell'utero	Hypertrophy of uterus	Hypertrophie de l'utérus	Hipertrofia del útero	Hipertrofija maternice
Ipotrofia fetale	Fetal hypotrophy	Hypotrophie foetale	Hipotrofia fetal	Fetalna hipotrofija
Lattazione	Lactation	Lactation	Lactancia	Dojenje (laktacija)
Liquido amniotico	Amniotic fluid	Liquide amniotique	Líquido amniótico	Plodna voda (amnijska tekućina)
Lithopedion	Lithopedion (stone baby)	Lithopédion (enfant pétrifié)	Litopedion	Litopedion (okamenjeno dijete)
Lochi	Lochia	Lochies	Loquios	Lohija (iscjedak u babinjama)
Lunghezza di neonato	Body length of a newborn	Taille corporelle du nouveau-né	Talla de un neonato	Dužina novorođenčeta
Macrosomia fetale	Macrosomia (big baby syndrome)	Macrosomie foetale	Macrosomía fetal	Fetalna hipertrofija
Madre	Mother	Mère	Madre	Majka

246

Italiano	Inglese	Francese	Spagnolo	Croato
Malattia di Hirschsprung (ostruzione del colon congenita)	Meconium ileus	Iléus méconial	Enfermedad de Hirschsprung (megacolon agangliónico)	Mekonijalni ileus
Mammella	Breast	Sein	Mama	Dojka
Mastite puerperale	Puerperal mastitis	Mammite puerpérale	Mastitis puerperal	Puerperalni mastitis
Meconio	Meconium	Méconium	Meconio	Mekonij
Menopausa	Menopause	Ménopause	Menopausia	Menopauza (klimakterij)
Mestruazione	Menstruation	Règle (menstruation)	Menstruación (período)	Menstruacija
Microcefalia	Microcephaly	Microcéphalie	Microcefalia	Mikrocefalija (sitnoglavost)
Mifepristone	Mifepristone	Mifépristone	Mifepristona	Mifepriston
Morula	Morula	Morula	Mórula	Morula
Mucosa interna dell'utero (endometrio)	Inner membrane of the uterus (endometrium)	Muqueuse utérine (endomètre)	Mucosa interior del útero (endometrio)	Sluznica maternice (endometrij)
Nato morto	Stillborn	Mort-né	Nacido muerto	Mrtvorođenče
Nausea	Nausea	Nausée	Náusea	Mučnina
Neonato	Newborn (infant)	Nouveau-né	Neonato (recién nacido)	Novorođenče
Neonato pretermine	Preterm newborn	Nouveau-né prématuré	Recién nacido pre-término	Nedonošče
Neonatologia	Neonatology	Néonatologie	Neonatología	Neonatologija
Ombelico	Navel (belly button)	Ombilic (nombril)	Ombligo (pupo)	Pupak
Ostetrica (levatrice)	Midwife	Sage-femme	Matrona (matrón)	Babica
Ostetricia	Obstetrics	Obstétrique	Obstetricia	Porodništvo
Ostetrico	Obstetrician	Obstétricien	Tocólogo (obstetra)	Porodničar (opstetičar)
Ovaia (ovario)	Ovary	Ovaire	Ovario	Jajnik
Ovidotto (ovidutto)	Fallopian tube (oviduct)	Trompes de Fallope	Trompa de Falopio (tuba uterina, oviducto)	Jajovod
Ovodonazione	Egg donation	Donneuse d'ovule	Donación de ovocitos	Donacija jajašca
Ovogenesi	Oogenesis	Ovogenèse	Ovogénesis	Ovogeneza (oogeneza)
Ovulazione	Ovulation	Ovulation	Ovulación	Ovulacija
Padre	Father	Père	Padre	Otac
Pannolino	Diaper	Couche-culotte	Pañal	Pelena
Parto	Childbirth	Accouchement (naissance)	Parto	Porod
Parto a termine	Full term birth	Accouchement à terme	Parto a término	Ročni porod
Parto nell'acqua	Water birth	Accouchement dans l'eau	Parto en agua	Porod u vodi
Parto patologico	Pathological birth	Accouchement pathologique	Parto patológico	Patološki porod
Parto post-termine	Postmature birth	Naissance après terme	Parto postérmino	Poslijeročni porod
Parto pretermine	Premature birth	Prématurité	Parto pretérmino	Prijevremeni porod
Parto prolungato	Prolonged birth	Accouchement prolongé	Parto prolongado	Produljeni porod
Pelvi ristretto	Contracted pelvis	Bassin contracté	Pelvis contraída	Sužena zdjelica
Pelvimetria	Pelvimetry	Pelvimétrie	Pelvimetría	Pelvimetrija
Peritonite da meconio	Meconium peritonitis	Péritonite méconiale	Peritonitis meconial	Mekonijalni peritonitis
Peso di neonato	Fetal weight (birth mass)	Poids de naissance	Peso al nacer	Težina ploda (porođajna težina)
pH-metria fetale	Fetal pH-metry	pH-métrie foetale	pH-metría fetal	Fetalna pH-metrija
Pielonefrite	Pyelonephritis	Pyélonéphrite	Pielonefritis	Pijelonefritis
Placenta	Placenta	Placenta	Placenta	Posteljica (placenta)
Placenta accreta	Placenta accreta	Placenta accreta	Placenta accreta	Prirasla posteljica (placenta acrreta)
Placenta previa	Placenta previa	Placenta praevia	Placenta previa	Placenta previja
Plagiocefalia	Plagiocephaly	Plagiocéphalie	Plagiocefalia	Plagiocefalija
Pluripara	Multigravida	Multipare	Multigrávida	Višerotkinja
Pompa tiralatte	Breast pump	Tire-lait	Sacaleches	Pumpica za izdajanje
Posizione del feto trasversale	Transverse fetal position	Position transversale du foetus	Feto posición transversal	Kosi položaj ploda
Posizione podalica del feto	Breech position	Présentation podalique (présentation du siège)	Posición de nalgas	Stav zatkom
Preeclampsia (gestosi)	EPH gestosis (pre-eclampsia)	Pré-éclampsie	Preeclampsia	EPH-gestoze (preeklampsija)
Primipara	Primigravida	Primigeste	Primigesta	Prvorotkinja
Procreazione assistita	Medically assisted procreation	Procréation médicalement assistée	Reproducción asistida	Medicinski potpomognuta oplodnja
Produzione di saliva eccessiva (ipersalivazione)	Excessive secretion of saliva (hypersalivation)	Sécrétion de la salive excessive	Excesiva producción de saliva (hipersalivación)	Pojačano lučenje sline (hipersalivacija)
Profilo biofisico fetale	Biophysical profile of the fetus	Profil biophysique foetal	Perfil biofísico fetal	Biofizikalni profil fetusa
Progesterone	Progesterone	Progestérone	Progesterona	Progesteron
Progesterone placentare	Placental progesterone	Progestérone placentaire	Progesterona de placenta	Progesteron placente
Prolasso del funicolo ombelicale	Umbilical cord prolapse	Prolapsus du cordon ombilical	Prolapso del cordón umbilical	Ispala pupkovina (prolaps pupkovine)
Prolattina	Prolactin	Prolactine	Prolactina	Prolaktin
Psicosi post-partum	Postpartum psychosis	Psychose puerpérale	Psicosis postparto	Puerperalna psihoza
Puerperio	Postnatal (postpartum period, puerperium)	Post-partum	Puerperio	Babinje (puerperij)
Quattro gemelli	Quadruplets	Quadruplés	Cuatrillizos	Četvorci
Raschiamento (curetage)	Curettage	Curetage	Legrado	Kiretaža
Respirazione	Breathing	Respiration	Respiración	Disanje
Rischio teratogenico	Pregnancy risk factors	Facteurs de risque de la grossesse	Agentes teratogénicos	Teratogeni faktori rizika

Italiano	Inglese	Francese	Spagnolo	Croato
Ritenzione urinaria	Urinary retention (ischuria)	Rétention d'urine	Retención de orina	Zastoj urina (urinarna retencija)
Rottura delle membrane	Rupture of membranes	Rupture des membranes	Ruptura de membrana	Prsnuće vodenjaka
Rottura precoce delle membrane	Premature rupture of membranes	Rupture prématurée des membranes	Ruptura prematura de membrana	Prijevremeno prsnuće vodenjaka
Sala parto	Delivery room	Salle d'accouchement	Sala de partos	Rađaona
Segno del Chadwick (tinta bluastra alla vagina)	Chadwick's sign	Signe de Chadwick	Signo de Chadwick	Hiperemična sluznica rodnice (Chadwickov znak)
Seme (sperma)	Semen (sperm)	Sperme	Semen (esperma)	Sjemena tekućina (sperma)
Sepsi puerperale	Puerperal sepsis	Septicémie puerpérale	Sepsis puerperal	Puerperalna sepsa
Sindrome da aspirazione di meconio	Meconium aspiration syndrome	Syndrome d'aspiration méconiale	Síndrome de aspiración de meconio	Mekonijalni aspiracijski sindrom
Sindrome del terzo giorno (baby blues)	Maternity blues (baby blues)	Baby blues	Baby blues (leve depresión post parto)	Labilno psihičko raspoloženje (baby blues)
Sopravvivenza di spermatozoo	Sperm viability	Viabilité du sperme	Viabilidad de espermatozoides	Životna sposobnost spermija
Spermatozoo	Spermatozoon (sperm cell)	Spermatozoïde	Espermatozoide	Spermij
Spingere	Push	Pousser	Empujar	Tiskati
Sterilità	Infertility	Stérilité	Infertilidad	Neplodnost (sterilitet)
Surrogazione di maternità	Surrogate mother (womb mother)	Mère porteuse	Madre de alquiler	Surogat majka (zamjenska majka)
Suzione	Suckling	Succion	Succión	Sisanje
Tagliare (intersecare)	Cut	Couper	Cortar	Presjeći
Taglio cesareo	Cesarean section (C-section)	Césarienne	Cesárea	Carski rez
Testa	Head	Tête	Cabeza	Glavica
Translucenza nucale	Nuchal scan (nuchal translucency)	Clarté nucale	Traslucencia nucal	Nuhalna translucencija
Uovo	Ovum	Ovule	Óvulo	Jajašce
Utero	Womb (uterus)	Utérus	Útero (matriz, seno materno)	Maternica (uterus)
Vagina	Vagina	Vagin	Vagina	Rodnica
Varici degli arti inferiori	Leg varicose veins	Varices des membres inférieurs	Venas varicosas de las piernas	Proširene vene na nogama
Villi coriali	Chorionic villi	Villosités choriales	Vellosidades coriónicas	Korionske resice
Villocentesi	Chorionic villus sampling	Choriocentèse	Muestra de vellosidades coriónicas	Uzorak korionskih resica
Vomito (emetismo)	Vomiting	Vomissement	Vómito (emesis)	Povraćanje

VIŠEJEZIČNI RJEČNIK HITNIH MEDICINSKIH INTERVENCIJA

INTERVENCIJA

Hrvatski-Engleski-Francuski-Španjolski-Talijanski

Hrvatski	Engleski	Francuski	Španjolski	Talijanski
BROJEVI:	**NUMBERS:**	**NUMÉROS:**	**NÚMEROS:**	**NUMERI:**
Nula	Zero	Zéro	Cero	Zero
Jedan	One	Un	Uno	Uno
Dva	Two	Deux	Dos	Due
Tri	Three	Trois	Tres	Tre
Četiri	Four	Quatre	Cuatro	Quattro
Pet	Five	Cinq	Cinco	Cinque
Šest	Six	Six	Seis	Sei
Sedam	Seven	Sept	Siete	Sette
Osam	Eight	Huit	Ocho	Otto
Devet	Nine	Neuf	Nueve	Nove
Deset	Ten	Dix	Diez	Dieci
Jedanaest	Eleven	Onze	Once	Undici
Dvanaest	Twelve	Douze	Doce	Dodici
Trinaest	Thirteen	Treize	Trece	Tredici
Četrnaest	Fourteen	Quatorze	Catorce	Quattordici
Petnaest	Fifteen	Quinze	Quince	Quindici
Šesnaest	Sixteen	Seize	Dieciséis	Sedici
Sedamnaest	Seventeen	Dix-sept	Diecisiete	Diciassette
Osamnaest	Eighteen	Dix-huit	Dieciocho	Diciotto
Devetnaest	Nineteen	Dix-neuf	Diecinueve	Diciannove
Dvadeset	Twenty	Vingt	Veinte	Venti
Dvadest i jedan	Twenty-one	Vingt et un	Veintiuno	Ventuno
Dvadeset i dva	Twenty-two	Vingt-deux	Veintidós	Ventidue
Trideset	Thirty	Trente	Treinta	Trenta
Četrdeset	Forty	Quarante	Cuarenta	Quaranta
Pedeset	Fifty	Cinquante	Cincuenta	Cinquanta
Šezdeset	Sixty	Soixante	Sesenta	Sessanta
Sedamdeset	Seventy	Soixante-dix	Setenta	Settanta
Osamdeset	Eighty	Quatre-vingts	Ochenta	Ottanta
Devedeset	Ninety	Quatre-vingt-dix	Noventa	Novanta
Sto	Hundred	Cent	Cien	Cento
Sto jedan	One hundred and one	Cent un	Ciento uno	Centouno
Sto dvadeset i tri	One hundred and twenty-three	Cent vingt-trois	Ciento veintitrés	Centoventitre
Dvjesto	Two hundred	Deux cents	Doscientos	Duecento
Tristo	Three hundred	Trois cents	Trescientos	Trecento
Četristo	Four hundred	Quatre cents	Cuatrocientos	Quattrocento
Petsto	Five hundred	Cinq cents	Quinientos	Cinquecento
Šesto	Six hundred	Six cents	Seiscientos	Seicento
Sedamsto	Seven hundred	Sept cents	Setecientos	Settecento
Osamsto	Eight hundred	Huit cents	Ochocientos	Ottocento
Devetsto	Nine hundred	Neuf cents	Novecientos	Novecento
Tisuća	Thousand	Mille	Mil	Mille
Dvije tisuće	Two thousand	Deux mille	Dos mil	Duemila
Milijun	Million	Million	Millón	Un milione
Milijarda	Milliard (billion)	Milliard	Mil millones (miliarda)	Un miliardo
ORIJENTACIJA U VREMENU:	**ORIENTATION IN TIME:**	**ORIENTATION DANS LE TEMPS:**	**ORIENTACIÓN EN EL TIEMPO:**	**ORIENTAMENTO NEL TEMPO:**
Jučer	Yesterday	Hier	Ayer	Ieri
Danas	Today	Aujourd'hui	Hoy	Oggi
Sutra	Tomorrow	Demain	Día de mañana	Domani
Godina	Year	Année	Año	Anno
Mjesec	Month	Mois	Mes	Mese
Tjedan	Week	Semaine	Semana	Settimana
Dan	Day	Jour	Día	Giorno
Sat	Hour	Heure	Hora	Ora
Minuta	Minute	Minute	Minuto	Minuto
Sekunda	Second	Seconde	Segundo	Secondo
Jutro (prijepodne)	Morning	Matin	Mañana	Mattina
Poslijepodne	Afternoon	Après-midi	Tarde	Pomeriggio
Večer	Evening	Soir	Anochecer	Sera
Noć	Night	Nuit	Noche	Notte
ORIJENTACIJA U PROSTORU:	**ORIENTATION IN SPACE:**	**ORIENTATION DANS L'ESPACE:**	**ORIENTACIÓN EN EL ESPACIO:**	**ORIENTAMENTO NELLO SPAZIO:**
Gore (iznad)	Up (above)	En haut (au-dessus)	Arriba	Su
Dolje (ispod)	Down (below)	En bas (au-dessous)	Abajo	In basso
Lijevo	Left	Gauche	Izquierda	Sinistra
Desno	Right	Droite	Derecha	Destra
Ispred	In front	Devant	Enfrente	Davanti
Iza	Behind	Derrière	Detrás	Dietro
Unutra	Inside	Dedans	Dentro	Dentro
Vani	Outside	Dehors	Fuera	Fuori

Hrvatski	Engleski	Francuski	Španjolski	Talijanski
NESREĆE, KATASTROFE I POGIBELJNE SITUACIJE:	**ACCIDENTS, CATASTROPHES AND DISTRESS:**	**LES ACCIDENTS, CATASTROPHES ET DÉTRESSE:**	**ACCIDENTES, CATÁSTROFES Y ANGUSTIA:**	**GLI ACCIDENTI, CATASTROFI E ANGOSCIA:**
Atomska bomba	Atomic bomb (A-bomb)	Bombe atomique (bombe A)	Bomba atómica (bomba A)	Bomba atomica (bomba A)
Atomsko oružje	Atomic weapons	Arme atomique	Arma atómica	Arma atomica
Atomsko biološko i kemijsko oružje	ABC weapons	Arme nucléaire, biologique et chimique (NBC)	Armas atómicas, biológicas y químicas (ABQ)	Armi nucleari, biologiche e chimiche (NBC)
Automobilska nesreća	Car accident	Accident automobile (accident de la route)	Accidente automovilístico (siniestro de tráfico)	Incidente stradale
Bakterija	Bacteria	Bacteria	Bacteria	Batterio
Biološko oružje	Biological weapon	Arme biologique	Arma biológica	Arma biologica
Bojni otrov (otrovni plin)	Poison gas	Gaz toxique	Gas tóxico	Gas tossico
Bomba	Bomb	Bombe	Bomba	Bomba
Brod	Ship	Navire	Barco	Nave
Civilna zaštita	Civil defense	Sécurité civile	Protección civil	Difesa civile
Čamac za spašavanje	Lifeboat	Canot de secours	Bote salvavidas	Scialuppa
Ekipa za traganje i spašavanje	Search and rescue team	Équpie de recherche et sauvetage	Equipo de búsqueda y rescate	Squadra di ricerca e salvataggio
Eksplozija	Explosion	Explosion	Explosión	Esplosione
Eksploziv	Explosive	Explosif	Explosivo	Esplosivo
Epidemija	Epidemic	Épidémie	Epidemia	Epidemia
Erupcija vulkana	Volcanic eruption	Éruption volcanique	Erupción volcánica	Eruzione vulcanica
Gusar	Pirate	Pirate	Pirata	Pirata
Gusarski napad	Pirate attack	Attaque de pirates	Ataque de piratas	Attacco dei pirati
Helikopter	Helicopter (chopper)	Hélicoptère	Helicóptero	Elicottero
Hidrogenska bomba	Hidrogen bomb (H-bomb)	Bombe à hydrogène (bombe H)	Bomba de hidrógeno (bomba H)	Bomba all'idrogeno (bomba H)
Hladno oružje	Cold weapon	Arme de contact	Arma blanca	Arma bianca
Invazija	Invasion	Invasion	Invasión	Invasione
Izbjeglica	Refugee	Réfugié	Refugiado	Rifugiato
Izbjeglički logor	Refugee camp	Camp de réfugiés	Campamento para refugiados	Campo per rifugiati
Jezero	Lake	Lac	Lago	Lago
Kemijsko oružje	Chemical weapon	Arme chimique	Arma química	Arma chimica
Kemijsko zagađenje	Chemical pollution	Pollution chimique	Polución química	Inquinamento chimico
Kobaltna bomba	Cobalt bomb	Bombe salée	Bomba de cobalto	Bomba al cobalto (bomba gamma, bomba G)
Konvencionalno oružje	Conventional weapon	Arme conventionnelle	Arma convencional	Arma convenzionale
Kopnena mina	Land mine	Mine terrestre	Mina terrestre	Mina terrestre
Kopno	Land	Terre	Tierra	Terra
Lasersko oružje	Laser weapon	Arme de laser	Arma láser	Armi laser
Lava	Lava	Lave	Lava	Lava
Lavina	Avalanche	Avalanche	Avalancha	Valanga
Led	Ice	Glace	Hielo	Ghiaccio
Ledenjak	Iceberg	Iceberg	Témpano de hielo	Ghiacciaio
Ledolomac	Icebreaker	Brise-glace	Rompehielos	Rompighiaccio
Metak	Bullet	Balle	Bala	Pallottola
Mina	Mine	Mine	Mina	Mina
Minsko polje	Mine field	Champ de mines	Campo minero	Campo minato
More	Sea	Mer	Mar	Mare
Morska mina	Naval mine	Mine marine (mine sous-marine)	Mina marina	Mina navale
Morska pijavica	Waterspout	Trombe marine	Managa de agua (tromba marina)	Tromba marina
Napad	Attack	Attaque	Ataque	Attaco
Napad morskog psa	Shark attack	Attaque de requin	Ataque de tiburón	Attacco di squalo
Nasukavanje broda	Stranding of a ship	Échouage du navire	Encallamiento de barco	Incaglio di nave
Nesreća na radu	Occupational accident	Accident du travail	Accidente laboral	Infortunio sul lavoro
Nesreća u kući	Domestic accident	Accident domestique	Accidente doméstico	Infortunio domestico
Neutronska bomba	Neutron bomb	Bombe à neutrons	Bomba de neutrones (bomba N)	Bomba al neutrone (bomba N)
Nevrijeme (oluja)	Storm	Tempête	Tormenta (tempestad)	Tempesta
Nuklearna nesreća	Nuclear accident	Accident nucléaire	Accidente nuclear	Accidente nucleare
Nuklearni otpad (radioaktivni otpad)	Nuclear waste (radioactive waste)	Déchet radioactif (déchet nucléaire)	Desechos nucleares	Scoria nucleare (scoria radioattiva)
Nuklearni pokus	Nuclear weapons testing	Essai nucléaire	Prueba nuclear (ensayo nuclear)	Test nucleare
Nuklearno oružje	Nuclear weapon	Arme nucléaire	Arma nuclear	Arma nucleare
Obogaćeni uranij	Enriched uranium	Uranium enrichi	Uranio einriquecido	Uranio arricchito
Olupina broda	Ship wreck	Épave de navire	Buque naufragado	Relitto
Oružje	Weapon	Arme	Arma	Arma
Oružje za masovno uništavanje	Weapon of mass destruction	Arme de destruction massive	Armas de destrucción masiva	Arma di distruzione di massa
Otmica	Kidnapping	Enlèvement (rapt)	Secuestro	Rapimento
Pad	Fall	Chute	Caída	Cadutta (cascata)
Pad aviona	Airplane crash	Accident aérien	Accidente de aviación	Incidente aereo

Hrvatski	Engleski	Francuski	Španjolski	Talijanski
Padobran	Parachute	Parachute	Paracáidas	Paracadute
Pandemija	Pandemic	Pandémie	Pandemia	Pandemia
Pas za traganje i spašavanje	Search and rescue dog	Chien de sauvetage	Perro de búsqueda y rescate	Cane da ricerca e salvataggio
Pješćana oluja	Sandstorm	Tempête de sable	Tormenta de arena	Tempesta di sabbia
Planina	Mountain	Montagne	Montaña	Montagna
Plimni val	Tidal wave	Onde de marée	Ola de marea	Onda di marea
Plutonij	Plutonium	Plutonium	Plutonio	Plutonio
Pljačka	Robbery	Vol	Robo	Rapina
Pojas za spašavanje	Lifebelt (lifebuoy)	Bouée couronne	Boya salvavidas	Boa di salvataggio
Poplava	Flood	Inondation	Inundación	Inondazione
Potonuće broda	Sinking of a ship	Naufrage du navire	Hundimiento de un barco	Affondamento della nave
Potraga	Search	Recherche	Búsqueda	Ricerca
Potres	Earthquake	Séisme (tremblement de terre)	Terremoto	Terremoto
Poziv u pomoć	Call for help	Appel à l'aide	Llamada de socorro	Chiamata di aiuto
Požar	Fire (conflagration)	Incendie	Incendio (fuego)	Incendio (fuoco)
Prljava bomba	Dirty bomb	Bombe radiologique (bombe sale)	Bomba sucia	Bomba sporca
Prometna nesreća	Traffic accident	Accident sur la voie publique	Accidente de tráfico	Incidente di traffico
Prsluk za spašavanje	Lifejacket (life vest)	Gilet de sauvetage	Chaleco salvavidas	Giubbotto di salvataggio
Rat	War	Guerre	Guerra	Guerra
Razminiranje	Mine clearance (demining)	Déminage	Desminado (eliminación de minas)	Eliminazione di mine (sminamento)
Rijeka	River	Rivière	Río	Fiume
Ropstvo	Slavery	Esclavage	Esclavitud	Schiavitù (prigionia)
Ruševine	Ruins	Ruine	Ruinas	Macerie (rovine)
Samoubojstvo	Suicide	Suicide	Suicidio	Suicidio
Santa leda	Sea ice	Banquise	Banquisa (hielo marino)	Banchisa (ghiaccio marino; banchiglia)
Silovanje	Rape (violation)	Viol	Violación	Violenza sessuale
Sklonište	Shelter	Abri	Abrigo	Rifugio
Snijeg	Snow	Neige	Nieve (zapada)	Neve
Snježna mećava	Snow storm	Tempête de neige	Nevasca (ventisca de nieve)	Bufera di neve (nevicata)
SOS poziv	SOS call	Appel SOS	Llamada de SOS	SOS richiesta
Spasilac	Rescuer	Sauveur	Salvador (rescatador)	Salvatore
Spašavanje	Salvage	Sauvetage	Salvamento	Salvataggio
Spašavanje broda	Marine salvage	Sauvetage en mer	Salvamento marítimo	Salvataggio navale
Stijena	Rock	Roche	Roca	Roccia
Strateško nuklearno oružje	Strategic nuclear weapon	Arme nucléaire stratégique	Arma nuclear estratégica	Arma nucleare strategica
Strujni udar	Electric shock	Électrisation (électrocution)	Choque eléctrico	Folgorazione (elettrocuzione)
Sudar	Collision	Collision	Colisión	Collisione
Špilja	Cave	Grotte	Cueva	Grotta
Šrapnel	Shrapnel	Shrapnel	Metralla	Shrapnel
Tajfun	Typhoon	Typhon	Tifón	Tifone
Taktičko nuklearno oružje	Tactical nuclear weapon	Arme nucléaire tactique (mini-nuke)	Arma nuclear táctica	Arma nucleare tattica
Taoc (talac)	Hostage	Otage	Rehén	Ostaggio
Terorist	Terrorist	Terroriste	Terrorista	Terrorista
Teroristička ćelija	Terrorist cell	Cellule terroriste (cellule dormante)	Célula terrorista	Cellula terroristica
Teroristički napad	Terrorist attack	Attaque terroriste	Ataque terrorista	Attentato terroristico
Tjelesni napad	Physical assault	Attaque physique	Asalto físico	Attacco fisico
Toplotni udar	Heat stroke	Coup de chaleur	Golpe de calor	Colpo di calore
Trgovina ljudima	Human trafficking	Trafic d'êtres humains	Trata de personas	Traffico di esseri umani
Tsunami	Tsunami	Tsunami (raz-de-marée)	Tsunami (maremoto)	Tsunami
Tučnjava	Fight	Combat	Pelea	Combattimento
Ubojstvo	Homicide (murder)	Homicide (assassinat)	Homicidio (asesinato)	Omicidio (uccisione)
Udar groma	Thunderclap	Foudre	Trueno	Percossa dal fulmine
Udarac	Stroke (hit, blow)	Coup	Golpe	Colpo (botta)
"U pomoć!"	"Help!"	"Aide!"	"¡Socorro!"	"Aiuto!"
Uragan	Hurricane	Ouragan	Huracán	Uragano
Uranij	Uranium	Uranium	Uranio	Uranio
Utapanje	Drowning	Noyade	Ahogamiento	Annegamento
Utopljenik	Drowned person	Noyé	Ahogado	Annegato
Uzbuna	Alarm	Alarme	Alarma	Allarme
Uže	Rope	Corde	Cuerda	Cordone
Vatra	Fire	Feu	Fuego	Fuoco
Vatreno oružje	Firearm	Arme à feu	Arma de fuego	Arma da fuoco
Virus	Virus	Virus	Virus	Virus
Voda	Water	Eau	Agua	Acqua
Znak za uzbunu	Alarm signal	Signal d'alarme	Señal de alarma	Segnale di allarme
Zračenje	Radiation	Rayonnement	Radiación	Radiazione
Zračni napad	Air attack	Attaque aérienne	Ataque aéreo	Incursione area

Hrvatski	Engleski	Francuski	Španjolski	Talijanski
Živčani otrov (neurotoksin)	Neurotoxin	Neurotoxine	Neurotoxina	Neurotossina
Žrtva	Victim	Victime	Víctima	Vittima
DIJELOVI LJUDSKOG TIJELA:	PARTS OF THE HUMAN BODY :	PARTIES DU CORPS HUMAIN:	PARTES DEL CUERPO HUMANO:	PARTI DEL CORPO UMANO:
Abdominalna aorta	Abdominal aorta	Aorte abdominale	Aorta abdominal	Aorta addominale
Acetilkolin	Acetylcholine	Acétylcholine	Acetilcolina	Acetilcolina
Adamova jabučica	Adam's apple	Pomme d'Adam	Nuez de Adán	Pomo d'Adamo
Adenohipofiza	Adenohypophysis	Adénohypophyse	Adenohipófisis	Adenoipofisi
Adrenalin	Adrenalin (adrenaline)	Adrénaline	Adrenalina	Adrenalina
Aglutinin	Agglutinin	Agglutinine	Aglutinina	Agglutinine
Aglutinogen	Agglutinogen	Agglutinogène	Aglutinógeno	Agglutinogeno
Albumin	Albumin	Albumine	Albúmina	Albumina
Aldosteron	Aldosterone	Aldostérone	Aldosterona	Aldosterone
Alveola	Alveolus	Alvéole	Alvéolo	Alveolo
Aminokiselina	Amino acid	Acide aminé	Aminoácido	Amminoacido
Amonijak	Ammonia	Ammoniac	Amoníaco	Ammoniaca
Antidiuretski hormon (vazopresin)	Antidiuretic hormone (vasopressin)	Hormone antidiurétique (vasopressine)	Hormona anidiurética (arginina vasopresina)	Ormone antidiuretico (vasopressina)
Aorta	Aorta	Aorte	Aorta	Aorta
Arterija	Artery	Artère	Arteria	Arteria
Arteriola	Arteriole	Artériole	Arteriola	Arteriola
Astrocit	Astrocyte	Astrocyte	Astrocito	Astrocita
Atrioventrikularni čvor	Atrioventricular node	Noeud atrio-ventriculaire	Nódulo auriculoventricular	Nodo atrioventricolare
Bartolinova žlijezda	Bartholin's gland	Glande de Bartholin	Glándula de Bartolino	Ghiandola di Bartolini
Baza lubanje	Skull base	Base du crâne	Base del cráneo	Base del cranio
Bazofilni granulocit	Basophil granulocyte	Granulocyte basophile	Basófilo	Granulocita basofilo
Bedrena kost (femur)	Thighbone (femur)	Os de la cuisse (fémur)	Fémur	Femore
Bilirubin	Bilirubin	Bilirubine	Bilirrubina	Bilirubina
Bjelančevina (protein)	Protein	Protéine	Proteína	Proteina
Bjeloočnica	Sclera	Sclère	Eclerótica	Sclera
Brada	Chin	Menton	Barbilla (mentón)	Mento
Bradavica	Nipple	Mamelon (papille)	Pezón	Capezzolo
Bronhiola	Bronchiole	Bronchiole	Bronquiolo	Bronchiolo
Bubnjić	Eardrum (tympanic membrane)	Tympan	Tímpano	Timpano (membrana timpanica)
Bubnjište	Tympanic cavity	Cavité tympanique	Cavidad timpánica	Cassa del timpano
Bubreg	Kidney	Rein	Riñón	Rene
Bulbouretralna žlijezda (Cowperova žlijezda)	Bulbourethral gland (Cowper's gland)	Glande de Cowper (glande bulbo-uretrale)	Glándula bulbouretral (glándula de Cowper)	Ghiandola bulbouretrale (ghiandola di Cowper)
Cilijarni mišić	Ciliary muscle	Muscle ciliaire	Músculo ciliar	Muscolo ciliare
Crijevna kost	Ilium	Ilion (ilium)	Ilion	Osso iliaco
Crijevna resica	Intestinal villus	Villosité intestinale	Vellosidad intestinal	Villo intestinale
Crijevni sok	Intestinal juice	Suc intestinal	Jugo intestinal	Succo intestinale
Crijevo	Intestine	Intestin	Intestin	Intestino
Čašica zdjelične kosti (acetabulum)	Acetabulum	Acetabulum	Acetábulo	Cotile (acetabolo)
Čekić (malleus)	Hammer (malleus)	Marteau (malléus)	Martillo (malleus)	Martello
Čelo	Forehead	Front	Frente	Fronte
Čeljust	Jaw	Mâchoire	Quijada	Scheletro della bocca
Čeona kost	Frontal bone	Os frontal	Hueso frontal	Osso frontale
Četveroglavi bedreni mišić	Quadriceps femoris muscle	Muscle quadriceps fémoral	Músculo cuádriceps crural	Muscolo quadricipite femorale
Čmar (anus)	Anus	Anus	Ano	Ano
Debelo crijevo	Large intestine (colon)	Gros intestin (côlon)	Intestino grueso (colon)	Intestino crasso (colon)
Dendrit	Dendrite	Dendrite	Dendrita	Dendrite
Desni	Gums (gingiva)	Gencive	Encía	Gengiva
Dezoksiribonukleinska kiselina (DNK)	Deoxyribonucleic acid (DNA)	Acide désoxyribonucléique	Ácido desoxirribonucleico	Acido desossiribonucleico (DNA)
Djevičnjak (himen)	Hymen	Hymen	Himen	Imene
Dlaka	Hair	Poil	Pelo	Pelo
Dlan	Palm	Paume	Palma	Palmo
Dojka	Breast	Sein	Mama	Mammella
Donožje (metatarzus)	Metatarsus	Métatarse	Metatarso	Metatarso
Donja čeljust (mandibula)	Lower jaw (mandible)	Mandibule	Mandíbula	Mandibola
Donja šuplja vena	Inferior vena cava	Veine cave inférieure	Vena cava inferior	Vena cava inferiore
Doštitnjača	Parathyroid gland	Parathyroïde	Glándula paratiroides	Paratiroide
Dražica (klitoris)	Clitoris	Clitoris	Clítoris	Clitoride
Dušnica (bronh)	Bronchus	Bronche	Bronquio	Bronco
Dušnik	Windpipe (trachea)	Trachée	Tráquea	Trachea
Dvanaesnik (duodenum)	Duodenum	Duodénum	Duodeno	Duodeno
Dvoglavi bedreni mišić	Biceps femoris muscle	Muscle biceps fémoral	Músculo bíceps crural	Bicipite femorale
Dvoglavi mišić nadlaktice	Biceps brachii muscle	Muscle biceps brachial	Músculo bíceps braquial	Muscolo bicipite brachiale
Elastin	Elastin	Élastine	Elastina	Elastina
Elektrolit	Electrolyte	Électrolyte	Electrolito	Elettrolita
Eozinofil	Eosinophil	Éosinophile	Eosinófilo	Eosinofilo

Hrvatski	Engleski	Francuski	Španjolski	Talijanski
Eritrocit (crveno krvno tjelešce)	Erythrocyte (red blood cell)	Érythrocyte (hématie, globule rouge)	Eritrocito (glóbulo rojo)	Eritrocita (globulo rosso)
Estrogen	Estrogen	Estrogène	Estrógeno	Estrogeno
Fibrin	Fibrin	Fibrine	Fibrina	Fibrina
Fibrinogen	Fibrinogen	Fibrinogène	Fibrinógeno	Fibrinogeno
Fibroblast	Fibroblast	Fibroblaste	Fibroblasto (célula fija)	Fibroblasto
Folikulin (estradiol)	Estradiol	Estradiol	Estradiol	Estradiolo
Fosfolipid	Phospholipid	Phospholipide	Fosfolípido	Fosfolipide
Glasnica	Vocal chord	Corde vocale	Cuerda vocal	Corda vocale
Glatki mišić	Smooth muscle	Muscle lisse	Músculo liso	Tessuto muscolare liscio
Glava	Head	Tête	Cabeza	Testa
Glavić	Glans	Gland	Glande	Glande
Glikogen	Glycogen	Glycogène	Glucógeno	Glicogeno
Globulin	Globulin	Globuline	Globulina	Globulina
Glomerul	Glomerulus	Glomérule	Glomérulo	Glomerulo
Glukagon	Glucagon	Glucagon	Glucagón	Glucagone
Glukokortikoid	Glucocorticoid	Glucocorticoïde	Glucocorticoide	Glucocorticoide
Glukoza	Glucose	Glucose	Glucosa	Glucosio
Goljenica (tibija)	Shinbone (tibia)	Tibia	Tibia	Tibia
Gonadotropin	Gonadotrophin	Gonadotrophine	Gonadotropina	Gonadotropina
Gornja čeljust (maksila)	Upper jaw (maxilla)	Os maxillaire	Hueso maxilar superior (maxila)	Osso mascellare
Gornja šuplja vena	Superior vena cava	Veine cave supérieure	Vena cava superior	Vena cava superiore
Gornji dio leđa	Upper back	Parti supérieur du dos	Espalda superior	Schiena alto
Granulocit	Granulocyte	Granulocyte (polynucléaire)	Granulocito	Granulocita
Grkljan	Larynx	Larynx	Laringe	Laringe
Grlo	Throat	Gorge	Garganta	Gola
Grudište (prsa)	Chest	Torse	Pecho	Torace
Grudna žlijezda (timus)	Thymus	Thymus	Timo	Timo
Grudni koš	Rib cage	Cage thoracique	Caja torácica	Gabbia toracica
Gušterača	Pancreas	Pancréas	Páncreas	Pancreas
Hemoglobin	Hemoglobin	Hémoglobine	Hemoglobina	Emoglobina
Hipofiza	Hypophysis (pituitary gland)	Hypophyse (glande pituitaire)	Hipófisis (glándula pituitaria)	Ipòfisi (ghiandola pituitaria)
Hipotalamus	Hypothalamus	Hypothalamus	Hipotálamo	Ipotalamo
Hisov snopić	Bundle of His	Faisceau de His	Haz de His	Fascio di His
Hormon	Hormone	Hormone	Hormona	Ormone
Hormon rasta (somatotropin)	Growth hormone (somatotrophin)	Hormone de croissance (somatotropine)	Hormona de crecimiento somatotropa	Somatotropina
Hrskavica	Cartilage	Cartilage	Cartílago	Cartilagine
Hrskavični prsten	Cartilage ring	Cartilage cricoïde	Cartílago circoides	Anello cartilagineo
Ileum	Ileum	Iléon (ileum)	Íleon	Ileo
Imunoglobulin	Immunoglobulin	Immunoglobuline	Inmunoglobulina	Immunoglobulina
Inzulin	Insulin	Insuline	Insulina	Insulina
Iver (patela)	Kneecap (patella)	Rotule (patella)	Rótula (patela)	Rotula (patella)
Jajašce	Ovum	Ovule	Óvulo	Uovo
Jaje (mudo, testis)	Testicle	Testicule	Testículo	Testicolo
Jajnik	Ovary	Ovaire	Ovario	Ovaia
Jajovod	Fallopian tube (oviduct)	Trompe de Fallope	Trompa de Falopio (tuba uterina, oviducto)	Tuba di Falloppio
Jednjak	Gullet (oesophagus)	Oesophage	Esófago	Esofago
Jejunum	Jejunum	Jéjunum	Yeyuno	Digiuno
Jetra	Liver	Foie	Hígado	Fegato
Jezik	Tongue	Langue	Lengua	Lingua
Kalcitonin	Calcitonin	Calcitonine	Calcitonina	Calcitonina
Kapak	Eyelid	Paupière	Párpado	Palpebra
Kapilara	Capillary	Capillaire	Capilar	Capillare
Katekolamin	Catecholamine	Catécholamine	Catecolamina	Catecolamina
Kažiprst	Forefinger	Index	Dedo índice	Dito indice
Keratin	Keratin	Kératine	Queratina	Cheratina
Klijetka	Ventricle	Ventricule	Ventrículo	Ventricolo
Klinasta kost (leptirasta kost)	Sphenoid bone	Os sphénoïde	Hueso esfenoides	Osso sfenoide
Ključna kost (klavikula)	Collarbone (clavicle)	Clavicule	Clavícula	Clavicola
Kolagen	Collagen	Collagène	Colágeno	Collagene
Kolesterol	Cholesterol	Cholestérol	Colesterol	Colesterolo
Koljeno	Knee	Genou	Rodilla	Ginocchio
Korijen zuba	Root of a tooth	Racine dentaire	Raíz del diente	Radice del dente
Koronarna arterija	Coronary artery	Artère coronaire	Arteria coronaria	Arteria coronaria
Kortikosteroid	Corticosteroid	Corticostéroïde	Corticosteroide	Corticosteroide
Kortikosteron	Corticosterone	Corticostérone	Corticosterona	Corticosterone
Kortikotropin	Corticotropin (adrenocorticotropic hormone)	Hormone corticotrope (adrenocorticotropic hormone, ACTH)	Hormona adrenocorticotropa (corticotropina, corticotrofina)	Corticotropina (ormone adrenocorticotropo)
Kortizol	Cortisol	Cortisol (hydro-cortisone)	Cortisol (hidrocortisona)	Cortisolo
Kortizon	Cortisone	Cortisone	Cortisona	Cortisone

Hrvatski	Engleski	Francuski	Španjolski	Talijanski
Kosa	Hair	Cheveu	Cabello	Capelli
Kosi trbušni mišić	Abdominal oblique muscle	Muscle oblique de l'abdomen	Músculo oblicuo del abdomen	Musculo obliquo dell'addome
Kost	Bone	Os	Hueso	Osso
Kost donožja (metatarzalna kost)	Metatarsal bone	Os du métatarse	Hueso del metatarso	Osso metatarsale
Kost kuka	Hip bone	Os coxal	Hueso coxal	Osso dell'anca
Kost pesti (metakarpalna kost)	Metacarpal bone	Os métacarpe	Hueso del metacarpo	Osso metacarpale
Kost prsta (falanga)	Phalanx bone	Phalange	Falange	Falange
Kost zapešća (karpalna kost)	Wrist bone (carpal bone)	Os du carpe	Hueso del carpo	Osso carpale
Kost zastoplja (kost tarzusa)	Tarsal bone	Os du tarse	Hueso del tarso	Osso tarsale
Kostur	Skeleton	Squelette	Esqueleto	Scheletro
Koštana srž	Bone marrow	Moelle osseuse	Médula ósea	Midollo osseo
Koža	Skin	Peau	Piel	Pelle (cute)
Krajnik	Tonsil	Tonsille	Amígdala	Tonsille
Kralježak	Vertebra	Vertèbre	Vértebra	Vertebra
Kralježnica	Spine (spinal column, backbone)	Colonne vertébrale (rachis)	Columna vertebral	Colonna vertebrale
Kralježnična moždina	Spinal cord	Moelle épinière (moelle spinale)	Médula espinal	Midollo spinale
Križa	Loin	Lombes	Espalda baja	Lombo
Krojački mišić	Tailor's muscle (sartorius muscle)	Muscle couturier (muscle sartorius)	Músculo sartorio	Muscolo sartorio
Krstačni kralježak (sakralni kralježak)	Sacral vertebra	Vertèbre sacrale	Vértebra sacra	Vertebra sacrale
Kruna zuba	Crown of a tooth	Couronne de la dent	Corona del diente	Corona del dente
Kružni mišić (sfinkter)	Sphincter	Sphincter	Esfínter	Sfintere
Krv	Blood	Sang	Sangre	Sangue
Krvna grupa	Blood group	Groupe sanguin	Grupo sanguíneo	Gruppo sanguigno
Krvna grupa A	Blood group A	Groupe sanguin A	Grupo sanguíneoA	Gruppo sanguigno A
Krvna grupa AB	Blood group AB	Groupe sanguin AB	Grupo sanguíneo AB	Gruppo sanguigno AB
Krvna grupa B	Blood group B	Groupe sanguin B	Grupo sanguíneo B	Gruppo sanguigno B
Krvna grupa 0	Blood group 0	Groupe sanguin 0	Grupo sanguíneo 0	Gruppo sanguigno 0
Krvna žila	Blood vessel	Vaisseau sanguin	Vaso sanguíneo	Vaso sanguigno
Kuk (zglob kuka)	Hip joint	Hanche	Articulación de la cadera	Articolazione dell'anca
Kutnjak (molar)	Molar	Molaire	Molar	Molare
Lakat	Elbow	Coude	Codo	Gomito
Lakatna kost (ulna)	Ulna	Ulna (cubitus)	Cúbito (ulna)	Ulna (cubito)
Lakatni zglob	Elbow joint	Articulation oléocranienne	Articulación del codo	Articolazione del gomito
Leća	Lens	Cristallin	Cristalino	Cristallino
Leđa	Back	Dos	Espalda	Schiena (dorso)
Ledni kralježak (grudni ili torakalni kralježak)	Thoracic vertebra	Vertèbre thoracique	Vértebra torácica	Vertebra toracica
Leukocit	Leukocyte	Leucocyte	Leucocito	Leucocita
Lice	Face	Visage	Cara (faz)	Viso
Ligament	Ligament	Ligament	Ligamento	Legamento
Limfa	Lymph	Lymphe	Linfa	Linfa
Limfna žila	Lymph vessel	Vaisseau lymphatique	Vaso linfático	Vaso linfatico
Limfna žlijezda	Lymph gland (lymph node)	Ganglion lymphatique (noeud lymphatique)	Ganglio linfático	Linfonodo
Limfocit	Lymphocyte	Lymphocyte	Linfocito	Linfocita
Lisna kost (fibula)	Fibula (calf bone)	Fibula (péroné)	Peroné (fíbula)	Perone (fibula)
List	Calf	Mollet	Pantorrilla	Polpaccio
Loj	Sebum	Sébum	Sebo cutáneo	Sebo
Lopatica (skapula)	Shoulder blade (scapula)	Omoplate (scapula)	Omóplato (escápula)	Scapola (omoplata)
Lubanja	Skull	Crâne	Calavera (cráneo)	Cranio
Luteinizirajući hormon	Luteinising hormone	Hormne lutéinisante	Hormona luteinizante (lutropina)	Ormone luteinizzante
Mali mozak	Cerebellum	Cervelet	Cerebelo	Cervelletto
Mali prsni mišić	Pectoralis minor muscle	Muscle petit pectoral	Músculo pectoral menor	Muscolo piccolo pettorale
Mali prst	Little finger (pinky)	Auriculaire (petit doigt)	Dedo meñique	Mignolo
Masno tkivo	Fat tissue	Tissu adipeux (masse grasse)	Tejido graso (tejido adiposo)	Tessuto adiposo
Mast	Fat	Matière grasse	Grasa	Lipidi
Maternica (uterus)	Womb (uterus)	Utérus	Matriz (útero, seno materno)	Utero
Međica (perineum)	Perineum	Périnée	Periné (perineo)	Perineo
Međukralježnični disk	Intervertebral disc	Disque intervertébral	Disco intervertebral	Disco intervertebrale
Međumozak	Diencephalon	Diencéphale	Diencéfalo	Diencefalo
Međurebreni mišić	Intercostal muscle	Muscle intercostal	Músculo intercostal	Muscolo intercostale
Međustanična tekućina	Interstitial fluid	Liquide interstitiel	Líquido intersticial (líquido tisular)	Liquido extracellulare
Meka moždana ovojnica	Pia mater	Pie-mère	Piamadre	Pia madre
Meko nepce	Soft palate	Voile du palais	Úvula	Palato molle
Melanin	Melanin	Mélanine	Melanina	Melanina

Hrvatski	Engleski	Francuski	Španjolski	Talijanski
Melanotropin	Melanotropin	Hormone mélanotrope (mélanocortine, mélanotropine)	Melanotropina	Ormone melanotropo
Melatonin	Melatonin	Mélatonine (hormone du sommeil)	Melatonina	Melatonina
Mineralkortikoid (Na-hormon)	Mineralcorticoid	Minéralcorticoïde	Mineralocorticoide	Mineralcorticoide
Mišić	Muscle	Muscle	Músculo	Muscolo
Mišić primicač	Adductor muscle	Muscle adducteur	Músculo aductor	Muscolo adduttore
Mišićna fascija	Muscular fascia	Fascia musculaire (périmysium)	Fascia profunda	Fascia muscolare
Mitralni zalistak (bikuspidalni zalistak)	Mitral valve (bicuspid valve)	Valve mitrale (valve bicuspide)	Válvula bicúspide (válvula mitral)	Valvola mitrale (valvola bicuspide)
Mliječni zub	Milk tooth	Dent temporaire	Diente de leche	Dente da latte
Mokraća (urin)	Urine	Urine	Orina	Urina
Mokraćevina (urea, ureja)	Urea	Urée (carbamide)	Urea	Urea
Mokraćni mjehur	Urinary bladder	Vessie	Vejiga urinaria	Vescica urinaria
Mokraćovod (ureter)	Ureter	Uretère	Uréter	Uretere
Monocit	Monocyte	Monocyte	Monocito	Monocita
Mozak	Brain	Cerveau	Cerebro	Cervello
Moždana klijetka	Brain ventricle	Ventricule cérébral	Ventrículo cerebral	Ventricolo cerebrale
Moždana kora	Cerebral cortex	Cortex cérébral (écorce cérébrale)	Corteza cerebral	Corteccia cerebrale
Moždana ovojnica	Meninx	Méninge	Meninge	Meninge
Moždana srž	Brain marrow	Moelle du cerveau	Médula cerebral	Midollo cerebrale
Moždano stablo	Brain stem	Tronc cérébral	Tronco del encéfalo	Tronco encefalico
Moždana tekućina (likvor)	Cerebrospinal fluid	Liquide cérébro-spinal	Líquido cefalorraquídeo (líquido cerebrospinal)	Liquido cefalorachidiano (liquor, liquido cerebrospinale)
Moždani živac	Cranial nerve	Nerf crânien	Nervio craneal	Nervo cranico
Mrežnica (retina)	Retina	Rétine	Retina	Rètina
Nadbubrežna žlijezda	Adrenal gland	Glande surrénale	Glándula suprarrenal	Surrene
Nadlaktica	Upper arm	Partie supérieure du bras	Parte superior del brazo	Barccio
Nadlaktična kost (humerus)	Upper arm bone (humerus)	Humérus	Húmero	Omero
Nadlaktični mišić	Brachialis muscle	Muscle brachial	Braquial anterior	Muscolo brachiale
Nakovanj	Anvil (incus)	Enclume	Yunque	Incudine
Natkoljenica (bedro)	Thigh	Cuisse	Muslo (región femoral)	Coscia
Negativan Rh faktor	Rh factor negative	Système Rhésus négatif	Factor Rh negativo	Fattore Rh negativo
Nepce	Palate	Palais	Paladar	Palato
Nepčana kost	Palatine bone	Os palatin	Hueso palatino	Osso palatino
Noga	Leg	Membre inférieur	Miembro inferior	Arto inferiore
Nokat	Nail	Ongle	Uña	Unghia
Noradrenalin	Noradrenaline	Noradrénaline	Noradrenalina	Noradrenalina
Nos	Nose	Nez	Nariz	Naso
Nosna kost	Nasal bone	Os nasal	Hueso proprio de la nariz (hueso nasal)	Osso nasale
Nosnica	Nostril	Narine	Narina	Narice
Nožni prst	Toe	Orteil	Dedo del pie	Dito del piede
Obraz	Cheek	Joue	Mejilla (carrillo)	Guancia
Obrva	Eyebrow	Sourcils	Ceja	Sopracciglio
Očna jabučica	Eyeball	Globe oculaire	Globo ocular	Bulbo oculare
Očna šupljina	Eye orbit	Orbite de l'oeil	Órbita	Orbita oculare
Očnjak (kanin)	Canine tooth	Canine	Canino (diente colmillo)	Canino
Oko	Eye	Oeil	Ojo	Occhio
Oksitocin	Oxytocin	Ocytocine (oxytocine)	Oxitocina	Ossitocina
Okusni pupoljak	Taste bud	Papille gustative	Papila gustativa	Papilla gustativa
Organ	Organ	Organe	Órgano	Organo
Osrčje (perikard)	Pericardium	Péricarde	Pericardio	Pericardio
Ošit (dijafragma)	Diaphragm	Diaphragme	Diafragma	Muscolo diaframma
Palac	Thumb	Pouce	Dedo pulgar (pólice)	Pollice
Palčana kost	Radius	Radius	Radio	Radio
Parasimpatikus	Parasympathetic nervous system	Système nerveux parasympatique (système vagal)	Sistema nervioso parasimpático	Sistema nervoso parasimpatico
Paratireoidni hormon	Parathyroid hormone	Parathormone (hormone parathyroïdienne)	Parathormona (hormona paratiroidea, paratirina)	Paratormone (ormone paratiroideo)
Pasjemenik	Epididymis	Épididyme	Epidídimo	Epididimo
Paučinasta ovojnica (arachnoidea)	Arachnoid mater	Arachnoïde	Aracnoides	Aracnoide
Pazuh (aksila)	Armpit (axilla, underarm)	Aisselle	Sobaco (axila)	Ascella
Penis	Penis	Pénis	Pene (falo)	Pene
Pest (metakarpus)	Metacarpus	Métacarpe	Metacarpo	Metacarpo
Peta	Heel	Talon	Talón (calcañar)	Tallone
Petna kost (kalkaneus)	Calcaneus	Calcanéus (calcanéum)	Calcáneo	Calcagno
Pinealna žlijezda (epifiza)	Pineal body (pineal gland, epiphysis)	Glande pinéale (épiphyse)	Glándula pineal (epífisis)	Ghiandola pineale (epifisi)

Hrvatski	Engleski	Francuski	Španjolski	Talijanski
Plazma	Plasma	Plasma sanguin	Plasma sanguíneo	Plasma
Pleura	Pleura	Plèvre	Pleura	Pleura (pleure)
Plin	Gas	Gaz	Gas	Gas
Pluća	Lungs	Poumons	Pulmones	Polmoni
Plućna arterija	Pulmonary artery	Artère pulmonaire	Arteria pulmonar (tronco pulmonar, tronco de las pulmonares)	Arteria polmonare
Plućno krilo	Lung	Poumon	Pulmón	Polmone
Podjezična kost	Hyoid bone (lingual bone)	Os hyoïde (os lingual)	Hueso hioides	Osso ioide
Podlaktica	Forearm	Avant-bras	Antebrazo	Avambraccio
Poluopnasti mišić	Semimembranosus muscle	Muscle semi-membraneux	Músculo semimembranoso	Muscolo semimembranoso
Polumjesečasti aortni zalistak	Aortic valve	Valve aortique	Válvula sigmoidea aórtica	Valvola semilunare aortica
Polutetivni mišić	Semitendinosus muscle	Muscle semi-tendineux	Músculo semitendinoso	Muscolo semitendinoso
Poplućnica (visceralna pleura)	Visceral pleura	Plèvre viscérale	Pleura visceral	Pleura viscerale
Poprečno-prugasti mišić	Striated muscle	Muscle strié	Músculo estriado	Muscolo striato
Pora	Pore	Pore	Poro	Poro
Porebrica (parijetalna pleura)	Parietal pleura	Plèvre pariétale	Pleura parietal	Pleura parietale
Portalna vena	Portal vein	Veine porte	Vena porta	Vena porta
Potkoljenica	Lower leg	Jambe	Pierna	Gamba
Potrbušnica (peritoneum)	Peritoneum	Péritoine	Peritoneo	Peritoneo
Pozitivan Rh faktor	Rh factor positive	Système Rhésus positif	Factor Rh positivo	Fattore Rh positivo
Predvorje (vestibulum)	Vestibule	Vestibule	Vestíbulo	Vestibolo
Prepona	Groin	Aine	Ingle	Inguine
Prepucij	Foreskin (prepuce)	Prépuce	Prepucio	Prepuzio
Pretkutnjak (premolar)	Premolar	Prémolaire	Premolar	Premolare
Produžena moždina	Medulla oblongata	Moelle allongée (medulla oblongata, bulbe rachidien, myélencéphale)	Bulbo raquídeo (médula oblongada, miencéfalo)	Bulbo (midollo allungato, encefalo)
Progesteron	Progesterone	Progestérone	Progesterona	Progesterone
Prostata	Prostate	Prostate	Próstata	Prostata
Prsna kost (sternum)	Breastbone (sternum)	Sternum	Esternón	Sterno
Prstenjak	Ring finger	Annulaire	Dedo anular	Anulare
Pupak	Navel (belly button)	Ombilic (nombril)	Ombligo (pupo)	Ombelico
Pužnica	Cochlea	Cochlée	Cóclea (caracol)	Coclea
Rame	Shoulder	Épaule	Hombro	Spalla
Rameni mišić (deltoideus)	Deltoid muscle	Muscle deltoïde	Músculo deltoides	Muscolo deltoide
Rameni zglob	Shoulder joint	Complexe articulaire de l'épaule	Articulación del hombro	Articolazione della spalla
Raonik (vomer)	Vomer	Vomer	Vómer	Vomere
Ravni trbušni mišić	Rectus abdominis muscle	Muscle droit de l'abdomen	Músculo recto mayor del abdomen	Muscolo retto dell'addome
Rebro	Rib	Côte	Costilla	Costola (costa)
Ribonukleinska kiselina	Ribonucleic acid	Acide ribonucléique (ARN)	Ácido ribonucleico (ARN)	Acido ribonucleico (ARN)
Rodnica (vagina)	Vagina	Vagin	Vagina (colpos)	Vagina
Romboidni mišić	Rhomboid muscle	Muscle rhomboïde	Músculo romboides	Muscolo romboide
Rožnica	Cornea	Cornée	Córnea	Cornea
Ručni prst	Finger	Doigt	Dedo de la mano	Dito della mano
Ručni zglob	Wrist	Poignet	Muñeca	Polso
Ruka	Arm	Bras	Brazo	Braccio
Schlemmov kanal	Canal of Schlemm	Canal de Schlemm	Canal de Schlemm	Canale di Schlemm
Sezamska kost	Sesamoid bone	Os sésamoïde	Hueso sesamoide	Osso sesamoide
Sigmoidni dio debelog crijeva	Sigmoid colon	Côlon sigmoïde	Colon sigmoide	Sigma (colon sigmoideo)
Simpatikus	Sympathetic nervous system	Système nerveux orthosympathique (système nerveux sympathique)	Sistema nervioso simpático	Sistema nervoso simpatico
Sinapsa	Synapse	Synapse	Sinapsis	Sinapsi (bottone sinaptico)
Sinovijalna opna	Synovial membrane	Membrane synoviale	Membrana sinovial	Membrana sinoviale
Sinus	Sinus	Sinus	Seno	Seno
Sitasta kost (etmoidna kost)	Ethmoid bone	Os ethmoïde	Hueso etmoides	Osso etmoide
Sjedna kost	Ischium	Ischium	Isquión	Ischio
Sjedni mišić	Gluteal muscle	Muscle glutéal	Músculo glúteo	Muscolo gluteo
Sjekutić (inciziv)	Incisor	Incisive	Incisivo	Incisivo
Sjemena vrećica	Seminal vesicle	Vésicule séminale (glande vésiculeuse)	Vesícula seminal	Vescicola seminale
Sjemenovod	Ejaculatory duct	Canal éjaculateur	Conducto eyaculador	Dotto eiaculatore
Skočni zglob (gležanj)	Ankle joint	Cheville (cou-de pied)	Tobillo	Caviglia
Slabinski kralježak (lumbalni kralježak)	Lumbar vertebra	Vertèbre lombale	Vértebra lumbar	Vertebra lombare
Slezena	Spleen	Rate	Bazo	Milza
Slijepo crijevo (crvuljak)	Vermiform appendix (cecal appaendix)	Appendice iléo-caecal (appendice, appendice vermiforme)	Apéndice vermiforme (apéndice cecal, apéndice)	Appendice vermiforme

Hrvatski	Engleski	Francuski	Španjolski	Talijanski
Slina (pljuvačka)	Saliva (spit, slobber)	Salive	Saliva	Saliva
Slušni kanal	Auditory canal (ear canal)	Conduit auditif externe (canal auriculaire)	Conducto auditivo externo	Meato acustico esterno
Slušni živac	Acoustic nerve (vestibulocochlear nerve)	Nerf vestibulocochléaire (nerf auditif)	Nervio auditivo (nervio vestibulococlear, nervio estatoacústico)	Nervo vestibolococleare (nervo stato-acustico)
Sluz	Mucus	Mucus	Moco	Muco
Sluzna vreća (bursa)	Synovial bursa	Bourse séreuse	Bursa (bolsa sinovial)	Borsa sierosa
Sluznica	Mucous membrane	Muqueuse	Mucosa	Membrana mucosa
Sljepoočna kost	Temporal bone	Os temporal	Hueso temporal	Osso temporale
Sljepoočnica	Temple	Tempe	Sien	Tempia
Sok gušterače	Pancreatic juice	Suc pancréatique	Jugo pancreático	Succo pancreatico
Sperma	Semen	Sperme	Semen (esperma)	Sperma
Spermij	Sperm (spermatozoon)	Spermatozoïde	Espermatozoide	Spermatozoo
Spinalni živac	Spinal nerve	Nerf spinal	Nervio espinal	Nervo spinale
Spolna žlijezda	Sex gland (gonad)	Gonade	Gónada	Gonade
Sponična kost	Zygoma (cheekbone, malar bone)	Os zygomatique (zygoma)	Hueso cigomático (malar)	Osso zigomatico
Srce	Heart	Coeur	Corazón	Cuore
Srčana klijetka	Cardiac ventricle	Ventricule cardiaque	Ventrículo cardíaco	Ventricolo cardiaco
Srčana pretklijetka (atrij)	Cardiac atrium	Oreillette	Aurícula cardíaca (atrio)	Atrio
Srčani mišić (miokard)	Cardiac muscle (myocardium)	Myocarde	Miocardio	Miocardio
Srčani zalistak	Heart valve (cardiac valve)	Valve cardiaque	Válvula cardiaca (válvula de corazón)	Valvola cardiaca
Središte zuba (pulpa)	Dental pulp	Pulpe dentaire	Pulpa dentaria	Polpa dentaria
Srednje uho	Middle ear	Oreille moyenne	Oído medio	Orecchio medio
Srednji prst	Middle finger	Majeur	Dedo corazón	Dito medio
Stanica	Cell	Cellule	Célula	Cellula
Stidna kost	Pubis (pubic bone)	Os pubien	Pubis	Pube (osso pubico)
Stidnica	Vulva	Vulve	Vulva	Vulva
Stolica (feces, izmet)	Stool (feces)	Fèces	Excrementos (heces)	Feci
Stopalo	Foot	Pied	Pie	Piede
Stremen	Stirrup (stapes)	Étrier	Estribo	Staffa (columella)
Suza	Tear	Larme	Lágrima	Lacrima
Suzna kost	Lachrymal bone	Os lacrymal (unguis)	Unguis (hueso lacrimal)	Osso lacrimale
Suzna žlijezda	Lachrymal gland	Glande lacrymale	Glándula lagrimal	Ghiandola lacrimale
Suzno-nosni kanal	Nasolacrimal duct (tear duct)	Canal lacrymonasal (canal lacrimal, canal des larmes)	Conducto nasolagrimal	Canale naso-lacrimale
Šaka	Hand	Main	Mano	Mano
Šarenica	Iris	Iris	Iris	Iride
Široka plosnata tetiva (aponeuroza)	Aponeurosis	Aponévrose	Aponeurosis	Aponeurosi
Štitnjača	Thyroid	Thyroïde	Tiroides	Tiroide
Taban	Sole	Plante	Planta del pie	Pianta del piede
Talamus	Thalamus	Thalamus	Tálamo	Talamo
Tanko crijevo	Small intestine	Intestin grêle	Intestino delgado	Intestino tenue (piccolo intestino)
Testosteron	Testosterone	Testostérone	Testosterona	Testosterone
Tetiva	Tendon (sinew)	Tendon	Tendón	Tendine
Tireotropin (TSH)	Thyroid-stimulating hormone (TSH, thyrotropin)	Thyréostimuline (thyréotropine)	Tirotropina (TSH, hormona estimulante de la tiroides)	Tirotropina (ormone tireostimolante)
Tiroksin	Thyroxine	Thyroxine	Tiroxina (tetrayodotironina, T4)	Tiroxina
Tjelesna tekućina	Body fluid	Fluide corporel	Fluido corporal	Fluido corporale
Tjeme	Vertex (crown of head)	Vertex	Vértice craneal	Vertice della testa
Tjemena kost	Parietal bone	Os pariétal	Hueso parietal	Osso parietale
Tkivo	Tissue	Tissu	Tejido	Tessuto
Torakalna aorta	Thoracic aorta	Aorte thoracique	Aorta torácica	Aorta toracica
Trapezni mišić	Trapezius muscle	Muscle trapèze	Músculo trapecio	Muscolo trapezio
Trbuh (abdomen)	Belly (abdomen)	Abdomen	Abdomen (panza)	Addome (ventre, pancia)
Trbušna stijenka	Abdominal wall	Face de la cavité abdominale	Pared abdominal	Parete addominale
Trepavica	Eyelash	Cil	Pestaña	Ciglia
Triglicerid	Triglyceride	Triglycéride	Triglicérido	Trigliceride
Trijodtironin	Triiodothyronine	Triiodothyronine	Triiodotironina	Triiodotironina
Troglavi mišić nadlaktice	Triceps brachii muscle	Muscle triceps brachial	Músculo tríceps braquial	Muscolo tricipite del braccio
Troglavi mišić potkoljenice	Triceps surae muscle	Muscle triceps sural	Músculo tríceps sural	Muscolo tricipite della sura
Trolisni zalistak	Tricuspid valve	Valve tricuspide	Válvula tricúspide	Valvola tricuspide
Trombocit	Thrombocyte	Thrombocyte	Plaqueta (trombocito)	Trombocita (piastrina)
Trtica	Tailbone (coccyx)	Coccyx	Cóccix (coxis)	Coccige
Trtični kralježak	Coccygeal vertebra	Vertèbre coccygienne	Vértebra coccígea	Vertebra coccigea
Trup (torzo)	Trunk (torso)	Tronc	Tronco	Tronco
Tvrda moždana ovojnica	Dura mater	Dure-mère	Duramadre	Dura madre (pachimeninge)
Tvrdo nepce	Hard palate	Palais osseux	Paladar óseo	Palato duro (volta palatina)

Hrvatski	Engleski	Francuski	Španjolski	Talijanski
Ugljikohidrat	Carbohydrate	Hidrate de carbone (glucide)	Carbohidrato	Carboidrato (glucide)
Uho	Ear	Oreille	Óido	Orecchio
Usna	Lip	Lèvre	Labio	Labbro
Usna šupljina	Mouth cavity (oral cavity)	Cavité buccale	Cavidad bucal (cavidad oral)	Cavità orale
Usta	Mouth	Bouche	Boca	Bocca
Ušna mast (ušna smola, cerumen)	Earwax (cerumen)	Cire de l'oreille (cérumen)	Cerumen (cerilla)	Cerume
Ušna školjka	Pinna (auricle)	Pavillon auriculaire	Pabellón auricular (aurícula)	Padiglione auricolare
Vanjska mokraćna cijev (uretra)	Urethra	Urètre	Uretra	Uretra
Veliki mozak (telencefalon)	Cerebrum (telencephalon)	Télencéphale (cerveau)	Telencéfalo	Telencefalo (cervello)
Veliki prsni mišić	Pectoralis major muscle	Muscle grand pectoral	Músculo pectoral mayor	Muscolo grande pettorale
Vena	Vein	Veine	Vena	Vena
Venula	Venule	Veinule (vénule)	Vénula	Venula
Vidni živac	Optic nerve	Nerf optique	Nervio óptico	Nervo ottico
Vlasište	Scalp	Cuir chevelu	Cuero cabelludo (capa capilar)	Cuoio capelluto
Vrat	Neck	Cou	Cuello	Collo
Zalistak	Valve (valvula)	Valve	Válvula	Valvola
Zapešće	Carpus	Carpe	Carpo	Carpo
Zastoplje	Tarsus	Tarse	Tarso	Tarso
Zatiljak	Nape (occiput)	Nuque	Nuca	Nuca
Zatiljna kost	Occipital bone	Os occipital	Hueso occipital	Osso occipitale
Zdjelica	Innominate bone (pelvis)	Bassin osseux	Pelvis	Bacino
Zglob	Joint	Articulation	Articulación	Articolazione
Zglobna čahura	Articular capsule (joint capsule)	Capsule articulaire	Cápsula articular	Capsula articolare
Zglobna hrskavica	Joint cartilage	Cartilage articulaire	Cartílago articular	Cartilagine articolare
Zglobna tekućina (sinovijalna tekućina)	Synovial fluid (synovia)	Liquide synovial	Líquido sinovial	Liquido sinoviale (sinovia)
Zglobni menisk	Meniscus	Ménisque	Menisco	Menisco
Zjenica	Pupil	Pupille	Pupila	Pupilla
Znoj	Sweat	Sueur	Sudor	Sudore
Zub	Tooth	Dent	Diente	Dente
Zubna caklina	Tooth enamel	Émail dentaire	Esmalte dental	Smalto
Zubni cement	Cementum	Cément	Cemento dental	Cemento
Zubni dentin	Dentin	Dentine (ivoire)	Dentina	Dentina
Ždrijelo	Pharynx (gullet, gorge)	Pharynx	Faringe	Faringe
Želučana kiselina	Gastric acid	Acide gastrique	Ácido gástrico	Acido gastrico
Želučana sluznica	Gastric mucous membrane	Muqueuse gastrique	Mucosa estomacal	Mucosa gastrica
Želučani sok	Gastric juice	Suc gastrique	Jugo gástrico	Succo gastrico
Želudac	Stomach	Estomac	Estómago	Stomaco
Žilnica	Choroid	Choroïde	Coroides	Coroide
Živac	Nerve	Nerf	Nervio	Nervo
Žlijezda	Gland	Glande	Glándula	Ghiandola
Žlijezda lojnica	Sebaceous gland	Glande sébacée	Glándula sebácea	Ghiandola sebacea
Žlijezda slinovnica	Salivary gland	Glande salivaire	Glándula salival	Ghiandola salivare
Žlijezda znojnica	Sweat gland	Glande sudoripare (sudorale)	Glándula sudorípara	Ghiandola sudoripara
Žuč	Gall (bile)	Bile	Bilis	Bile
Žućni mjehur	Gall bladder	Vésicule biliare (cholécyste)	Vesícula biliar	Cistifellea
Žučovod	Bile duct	Voie biliaire	Vía biliar	Coledoco
Žuto tijelo	Corpus luteum	Corps jaune	Cuerpo lúteo (cuerpo amarillo)	Corpo luteo
Žvakaći mišić	Masseter muscle	Muscle masséter	Músculo masetero	Muscolo massetere

SIMPTOMI, OZLJEDE I BOLESTI:	SYMPTOMS, INJURIES AND DISEASES:	LES SYMPTÔMES, BLESSURES ET MALADIES:	SÍNTOMAS, HERIDAS Y ENFERMEDADES:	I SINTOMI, FERITE E MALATTIE:
Aberantni pankreas	Aberrant pancreas	Pancréas aberrant	Pancreas aberrante	Pancraes aberrante
Abnormalna gibljivost	Abnormal flexibility	Flexibilité anormale	Flexibilidad anormal	Movimento anormale
Abnormalno velik gubitak krvi tijekom mjesečnice (menoragija)	Abnormally heavy menstrual period (menorrhagia)	Cycle menstruel anormalement excessice (ménorragie)	Pérdida de sangre mayor durante la menstruación (menorragia)	Anormale perdita di sangue durante il ciclo mestruale(menorragia)
Abulija (poremećaj umanjene motivacije)	Aboulia (disorder of diminished motivation)	Aboulie	Abulia	Abulia
Acidoza	Acidosis	Acidose	Acidosis	Acidosi
Addisonova bolest	Addison's disease	Maladie d'Addison	Enfermedad de Addison	Morbo di Addison
Adenokarcinom	Adenocarcinoma	Adénocarcinome	Adenocarcinoma	Adenocarcinoma
Adenom	Adenoma	Adénome	Adenoma	Adenoma
Adenopatija	Adenopathy	Adénopathie	Adenopatía	Adenopatia
Aerofobija (strah od letenja)	Aviophobia (fear of flying)	Aerophobie (peur de l'avion)	Aerofobia (miedo a volar)	Aviofobia (paura di volare)
Afrička tripanosomijaza (bolest spavanja)	African trypanosomiasis (sleeping sickness)	Maladie du sommeil (trypanosomiase africaine)	Tripanosomiasis africana (enfermedad del sueño)	Tripanosomiasi africana (malattia del sonno)

Hrvatski	Engleski	Francuski	Španjolski	Talijanski
Afte (ulceracija sluznice usta)	Aphtha (mouth ulcer)	Aphte (ulcère de la muqueuse buccale)	Afta (úlcera en la mucosa oral)	Afta (ulcera all'interno della cavità orale)
Agenezija (nedostatak jednog organa)	Agenesis (absence of an organ)	Agénésie	Agenesia (ausencia de un órgano)	Agenesia (mancanza di un organo)
Agenezija bubrega	Renal agenesis	Agénésie rénale	Agenesia renal	Agenesia renale
Agranulocitoza	Agranulocytosis	Agranulocytose	Agranulocitosis	Agranulocitosi
Ahilodinija (tendinitis Ahilove tetive)	Achillodynia (Achilles tendinitis)	Tendinite du tendon d'Achille	Tendinitis de Aquiles	Tendinopatia achillea (achillodinia)
Ahondroplazija	Achondroplasia	Achondroplasie	Acondroplasia	Acondroplasia
Akarijaza	Acariasis	Acariase	Acariasis	Acariasi
Aklorhidrija	Achlorhydria	Achlorhydrie	Aclorhidria	Acloridria
Akne	Acne	Acné	Acné	Acne
Akrocijanoza	Acrocyanosis	Acrocyanose	Acrocianosis	Acrocianosi
Akrofobija (strah od visine)	Acrophobia (fear of heights)	Acrophobie (peur des hauteurs)	Acrofobia (miedo a las alturas)	Acrofobia (paura dei luoghi elevati)
Akromegalija	Acromegaly	Acromégalie	Acromegalia	Acromegalia
Aktinička keratoza	Actinic keratosis	Kératose actinique	Queratosis actínica	Cheratosi solare
Aktinomikoza	Actinomycosis	Actinomycose	Actinomicosis	Actinomicosi
Akutna bol	Acute pain	Douleur aiguë	Dolor agudo	Dolore acuto
Akutna dilatacija želuca	Acute gastric dilatation	Dilatation aiguë de l'estomac	Dilatación aguda del estómago	Dilatazione gastrica acuta
Akutna limfatična leukemija	Acute lymphoblastic leukemia	Leucémie lymphoblastique aiguë	Leucemia linfoblástica aguda	Leucemia acuta linfoblastica
Akutna mijeloična leukemija	Acute myeloid leukemia (AML)	Leucémie aiguë myéloblastique	Leucemia mieloide aguda	Leucemia mieloide acuta
Akutna upala crvuljka	Acute appendicitis	Appendicite aiguë	Apendicitis aguda	Appendicite acuta
Akutni abdomen	Acute abdomen	Abdomen aigu	Abdomen agudo	Addome acuto
Akutno plućno srce	Acute pulmonary heart	Coeur pulmonaire aigu	Cor pulmonale agudo	Cuore polmonare acuto
Akutno zatajenje bubrega	Acute kidney failure	Insuffisance rénale aiguë	Insuficiencia renal aguda	Insufficienza renale acuta
Albinizam	Albinism	Albinisme	Albinismo	Albinismo
Albrightov sindrom	McCune-Albright syndrome	Syndrome de McCune-Albright	Síndrome de McCune-Albright	Sindrome di McCune-Albright-Sternberg
Albuminurija	Albuminuria	Albuminurie	Albuminuria	Albuminuria
Aldosteronizam	Aldosteronism (hyperaldosteronism)	Hyperaldostéronisme	Aldosteronismo (hiperaldosteronismo)	Iperaldosteronismo
Alergija	Allergy	Allergie	Alergia	Allergia
Alergija na hranu	Food allergy	Allergie alimentaire	Alergia a alimentos	Allergia alimentare
Alergija na lijekove	Drug allergy	Allergie aux médicaments	Alergia al medicamento	Allergia a farmaci
Alergija na pelud	Pollen allergy	Allergie au pollen	Alergia al polen	Allergia da poline
Alergija na perje	Feather allergy	Allergie aux plumes	Alergia a las plumas	Allergia alle piume
Alergija na prašinu	Dust allergy	Allergie à la poussière	Alergia al polvo	Allergia a polvere
Alergija na životinjsku dlaku	Fur allergy	Allergie aux animaux à poils	Alergia al pelo de los animales	Allergia a pello di animali
Alergijski kontaktni dermatitis	Allergic contact dermatitis	Dermite de contact allergique	Dermatitis alérgica de contacto	Dermatite allergica
Alergijski konjuktivitis	Allergic conjunctivitis	Conjonctivite allergique	Conjuntivitis alérgica	Congiuntivite allergica
Alergijski rinitis	Allergic rhinitis	Rhinite allergique	Rinitis alérgica	Rinite allergica
Algodistrofija	Algodystrophy	Algodystrophie	Algodistrofia	Algodistrofia
Alkaloza	Alkalosis	Alcalose	Alcalosis	Alcalosi
Alkoholizam	Alcoholism	Alcoolisme	Alcoholismo	Alcolismo
Alkoholna ciroza	Alcoholic cirrhosis	Cirrhose alcoolique	Cirrosis alcohólica	Cirrosi alcolica
Alkoholna kardiomiopatja	Alcoholic cardiomyopathy	Cardiomyopathie alcoolique	Miocardiopatía alcohólica	Miocardiopatia alcolica
Alopecia areata	Alopecia areata	Alopécie areata	Alopecia areata	Alopecia areata
Alveolarna proteinoza pluća	Pulmonary alveolar proteinosis	Protéinose alvéolaire pulmonaire	Proteinosis alveolar pulmonar	Proteinosi alveolare polmonare
Alzheimerova bolest	Alzheimer's diesase	Maladie d'Alzheimer	Enfermedad de Alzheimer	Morbo di Alzheimer
Amebijaza	Amebiasis (amebic dysentery)	Amibiase (dysenterie amibienne)	Disentería amebiana (amebiasis)	Amebiasi
Amiloidoza	Amyloidosis	Amylose (amyloïdose, maladie orpheline)	Amiloidosis	Amiloidosi
Amiotrofična lateralna skleroza	Amyotrophic lateral sclerosis	Sclérose latérale amyotrophique (maladie de Charcot)	Esclerosis lateral amiotrófica	Sclerosi laterale amiotrofica
Amnezija	Amnesia	Amnésie	Amnesia	Amnesia
Amputacija	Amputation	Amputation	Amputación	Amputazione
Anafilaktični šok	Anaphylactic shock	Choc anaphylactique	Choque anafiláctico	Anafilassi
Analgezija (neosjetljivost na bol)	Analgesia (loss of pain sensation)	Analgésie	Analgesia	Analgesia
Analna fistula	Anal fistula	Fistule anale	Fístula anal	Fistola anale
Analna fisura	Anal fissure	Fissure anale	Fisura anal	Fissura anale
Analni apsces	Anal abscess	Abcès anal	Absceso anal	Ascesso anale
Anaplastični karcinom	Anaplastic carcinoma	Carcinome anaplastique	Carcinoma anaplásico	Carcinoma anaplastico
Androblastom (tumor Sertoli-Leydigovih stanica)	Androblastoma (Sertoli-Leydig cell tumor)	Androblastome (tumeur à cellule de Sertoli et Leydig)	Tumor de células de Sertoli-Leydig (arrenoblastoma)	Androblastoma
Anemija kronične bolesti	Anemia of chronic disease	Anémie des maladies chroniques	Anemia de enfermedades crónicas	Anemia da malattia cronica
Anemija radi deficita želje-za (sideropenična anemija)	Iron deficiency anemia (sideropenic anemia)	Anémie ferriprive	Anemia ferropénica	Anemia da carenza di ferro

Hrvatski	Engleski	Francuski	Španjolski	Talijanski
Anemija srpastih stanica	Sickle-cell disease (sickle-cell anemia)	Drépanocytose (anémie à cellules falciformes)	Anemia falciforme (anemia drepanocítica)	Anemia drepanocitica
Anencefalija	Anencephaly	Anencéphalie	Anencefalia	Anencefalia
Aneurizma	Aneurysm (aneurism)	Anévrisme (anévrysme)	Aneurisma	Aneurisma
Aneurizma abdominalne aorte	Abdominal aortic aneurysm	Anévrisme de l'aorte abdominale	Aneurisma de aorta abdominal	Aneurisma dell'aorta addominale
Aneurizma aorte	Aortic aneurysm	Anévrisme de l'aorte	Aneurisma de aorta	Aneurisma aortico
Aneurizma torakalne aorte	Thoracic aortic aneurysm	Anévrisme aortique thoracique	Aneurisma de aorta torácica	Aneurisma dell'aorta toracica
Angina	Angina	Angine	Angina	Angina
Angina pektoris	Angina pectoris	Angine de poitrine (angor)	Angina de pecho (angor, angor pectoris)	Angina pectoris
Angioedem (Quinckeov edem, angio-neurotski edem)	Angioedema (angioneurotic edema)	Oedème de Quincke (angio-oedème)	Angioedema (edema de Quincke)	Angioedema (edema di Quincke, edema angioneurotico)
Angiom	Angioma	Angiome	Angioma	Angioma
Angiosarkom	Angiosarcoma	Angiosarcome	Angiosarcoma	Angiosarcoma
Anisakijaza	Anisakiasis	Anisakiase	Anisakiasis (anisakidosis)	Anisakidosi
Ankilostomijaza	Ancylostomiasis	Ankylostomose	Anquilostomiasis	Anchilostomiasi
Ankiloza (ukočenje zgloba)	Ankylosis (joint stiffness)	Ankylose	Anquilosis	Anchilosi
Ankilozantni spondilitis (Bechterewov sindrom)	Ankylosing spondylitis (Bechterew's syndrome)	Spondylarthrite ankylosante (morbus Bechterew)	Espondilitis anquilosante (morbus Bechterew)	Spondilite anchilosante
Anomalija moždanih krvnih žila	Cerebrovascular anomaly	Anomalie cérébrovasculaire	Malformación arteriovenosa cerebral	Anomalia cerebrovascolare
Anomalija u razvoju mozga	Brain development anomaly	Anomalie du développement cérébral	Malformación del desarrollo cerebral	Anomalia di sviluppo del sistema nervoso
Anoreksija	Anorexia	Anorexie	Anorexia	Anoressia
Antrakoza	Anthracosis	Anthracose	Antracosis	Antracosi
Antraks (bedrenica, crni prišt)	Anthrax	Charbon	Carbunco (ántrax)	Antrace
Anurija (lučenje urina < 100 ml u 24 sata)	Anuria (passage of urine < 100 ml in 24 hours)	Anurie (volume urinaire < 100 ml par 24 heures)	Anuria (menos de 100ml de orina en 24h)	Anuria (produzione di urina < 100 ml nelle 24 ore)
Apetit	Appetite	Appétit	Apetito	Appetito
Aplastična anemija	Aplastic anemia	Anémie aplasique	Anemia aplásica	Anemia aplastica
Aplazija	Aplasia	Aplasie	Aplasia	Aplasia
Apsces	Abscess	Abcès	Absceso	Ascesso
Apsces jetre	Liver abscess	Abcès hépatique	Absceso hepático	Ascesso epatico
Apsces mozga	Brain abscess	Abcès cérébral	Absceso cerebral	Ascesso cerebrale
Apsces pluća	Lung abscess	Abcès pulmonaire	Absceso pulmonar	Ascesso polmonare
Apstinencijska kriza	Withdrawal	Sevrage	Síndrome de abstinencia	Crisi d'astinenza
Aritmija	Arrhythmia	Arythmie	Arrítmia	Aritmia
Aritmogena displazija desne klijetke	Arrhytmogenic right ventricular dysplasia	Dysplasie ventriculaire droite arythmogène	Displasia arritmogénica ventricular derecha	Displasia ventricolare destra aritmogena
Arterijska embolija	Arterial embolism	Embolie artérielle	Embolia arterial	Embolia dell'arteria
Arterijsko krvarenje	Arterial bleeding	Hémorragie artérielle	Hemorragia arterial	Emorragia arteriosa
Arterioskleroza	Arteriosclerosis	Artérosclérose	Arteriosclerosis	Arteriosclerosi
Arteritis divovskih stanica (temporalni arteritis)	Giant cell arteritis (temporal arteritis)	Artérite giganto-cellulaire (maladie de Horton, artérite temporale)	Arteritis de células gigantes (arteritis de la temporal)	Arterite temporale (arterite di Horton)
Artrogripoza	Arthrogryposis	Arthrogrypose	Artrogriposis	Artrogriposi
Artropatija	Arthropathy	Arthropathie	Artropatía	Artropatia
Artroza (osteoartritis, degenerativni artritis)	Arthrosis (osteoarthritis, degenerative arthritis)	Arthrose (arthropathie chronique dégénérative)	Artrosis	Artrosi
Artroza koljena (gonartroza)	Knee arthrosis	Arthrose du genou (gonarthrose)	Artrosis de rodilla (gonartrosis)	Artrosi di ginocchio
Artroza kuka (koksartroza)	Hip arthrosis	Arthrose de hanche (coxarthrose)	Artrosis de cadera (coxartrosis)	Artrosi di anca
Artroza lakta	Elbow arthrosis	Arthrose du coude	Artrosis de codo	Artrosi di gomito
Artroza ramena	Shoulder arthrosis	Arthrose de l'épaule	Artrosis del hombro	Artrosi gleno-omerale
Artroza ručnog zgloba	Wrist arthrosis	Arthrose du poignet	Artrosis de muñeca	Artrosi di polso
Artroza skočnog zgloba	Ankle arthrosis	Arthrose de cheville	Artrosis de tobillo	Artrosi di caviglia
Artroza stopala	Foot arthrosis	Arthrose du pied	Artrosis del pie	Artrosi al piede
Artroza šake	Hand arthrosis	Arthrose de le main	Artrosis de mano	Artrosi della mano
Ascites	Ascites	Ascite	Ascitis	Ascite
Asfiksija	Asphyxia	Asphyxie	Asfixia	Asfissia
Askaridijaza	Ascaridosis	Ascaridiose	Ascaridiasis	Ascaridiasi
Aspergilom	Aspergilloma (mycetoma, fungus ball)	Aspergillome	Aspergiloma (micetoma)	Aspergilloma (micetoma)
Aspergiloza	Aspergillosis	Aspergillose	Aspergilosis	Aspergillosi
Astigmatizam	Astigmatism	Astigmatisme	Astigmatismo	Astigmatismo
Astma	Asthma	Asthme	Asma	Asma
Astrocitom	Astrocytoma	Astrocytome	Astrocitoma	Astrocitoma
Atelektaza pluća	Pulmonary atelectasis	Atélectasie pulmonaire	Atelectasia pulmonar	Atelectasia polmonare
Ateroskleroza	Atherosclerosis	Athérosclérose	Ateroesclerosis	Aterosclerosi
Atetoza	Athetosis	Athétose	Atetosis	Atetosi
Atipična upala pluća	Atypical pneumonia	Pneumonie atypique	Neumonía atípica	Polmonite atipica

Hrvatski	Engleski	Francuski	Španjolski	Talijanski
Atletsko stopalo (gljivična infekcija stopala, tinea pedis)	Athlete's foot (tinea pedis)	Pied d'athlète (tinea pedis)	Tiña del pie (pie de atleta, tinea pedis)	Piede d'atleta (tinea pedis)
Atonija	Atony (atonia)	Atonie	Atonía	Atonia muscolare
Atopijski dermatitis	Atopic dermatitis	Dermatite atopique	Dermatitis atópica	Neurodermite (dermatite atopica)
Atrezija anusa	Anal atresia	Atrésie anale	Atresia anal	Atresia anale
Atrezija dvanaesnika	Duodenal atresia	Atrésie duodénale	Atresia duodenal	Atresia duodenale
Atrezija jednjaka	Esophageal atresia	Atrésie de l'oesophage	Atresia esofágica	Atresia esofagea
Atrezija žučnih vodova	Bile duct atresia	Atrésie biliaire	Atresia biliar	Atresia biliare
Atrijska fibrilacija	Atrial fibrillation	Fibrillation auriculaire	Fibrilación auricular	Fibrillazione atriale
Atrijski septalni defekt	Atrial septal defect	Communication inter-auriculaire	Comunicación interauricular	Difetto del setto interatriale
Atrijskoventrikularni blok	Atrioventricular block (AV block)	Bloc auriculo-ventriculaire	Bloqueo auriculoventricular	Blocco atrioventricolare
Atrofija	Atrophy	Atrophie	Atrofia	Atrofia
Autizam	Autism	Autisme	Autismo	Autismo
Autoimunološka bolest	Autoimmune disease	Maladie auto-immune	Enfermedad autoinmune	Malattia autoimmunitaria
Avitamonoza	Avitaminosis	Avitaminose	Avitaminosis	Avitaminosi
Azbestoza	Asbestosis	Asbestose (amiantose)	Asbestosis	Asbestosi
Bakterijemija	Bacteremia	Bactériémie	Bacteriemia (bacteremia)	Batteriemia
Bakterijska infekcija	Bacterial infection	Infection bactérienne	Infección bacteriana	Infezione batterica
Bakterijska infekcija rodnice (bakterijska vaginoza)	Bacterial vaginosis	Vaginose bactérienne	Vaginosis bacteriana	Infezione della vagina batterica (vaginosi)
Bakterijska upala pluća	Bacterial pneumonia	Pneumonie bactérienne	Neumonía bacteriana	Polmonite batterica
Bakterijski endokarditis	Bacterial endocarditis	Endocardite bactérienne	Endocarditis bacteriana	Endocardite batterica
Bakterijski konjuktivitis	Bacterial conjunctivitis	Conjonctivite bactérienne	Conjuntivitis bacteriana	Congiuntivite batterica
Bakteriurija	Bacteriuria	Bactériurie	Bacteriuria	Batteriuria
Balerinsko stopalo (pes equinus)	Dancer's foot (pes equinus)	Pied equin	Pie equino	Piede equino
Barotrauma	Barotrauma	Barotraumatisme	Barotraumatismo (barotrauma)	Barotrauma
Bartoneloza	Bartonellosis	Bartonellose	Bartonelosis	Bartonellosi
Basedowljeva bolest	Basedow Graves disease	Maladie de Basedow	Enfermedad de Graves Basedow	Morbo di Basedow-Graves
Batićasti prsti	Finger clubbing (digital clubbing)	Hippocratisme digital (doigts en baguettes de tambour)	Acropaquia (hipocratismo digital)	Dita ippocratiche (dita a bacchetta di tamburo)
Bazofilija	Basophilia	Basophilie	Basofilia	Basofilia
Behçetova bolest	Behçet's disease	Maladie de Behçet	Síndrome de Behçet	Sindrome di Behçet
Bellov fenomen	Bell's phenomenon	Phénomène de Bell	Fenómeno de Bell	Fenomeno di Bell
Bellova paraliza	Bell's palsy	Paralysie de Bell	Parálisis de Bell	Paralisi di Bell
Benigna hipertrofija prostate	Benign prostatic hyperthroph	Hypertrophie bénigne de la prostate	Hiperplasia benigna de próstata	Ipertrofia prostatica benigna
Benigna pozicijska vrtoglavica	Benign positional vertigo	Vertige paroxystique positionnel bénin	Vértigo posicional paroxístico benigno	Cupololitiasi (canalolitiasi)
Bijelo pranje	Leukorrhea	Leucorrhée	Leucorrea	Leucorea
Bilijarna ciroza	Biliary cirrhosis	Cirrhosis biliaire	Cirrosis biliar	Cirrosi biliare
Biotovo disanje	Biot's respiration	Respiration de Biot	Respiración de Biot	Respiro di Biot
Bipolarni poremećaj (manično-depresivna psihoza)	Bipolar disorder (manic-depressive psychosis)	Trouble bipolaire (psychose maniaco-dépressive)	Trastorno bipolar (psicosis maníaco-depresiva)	Psicosi maniaco-depressiva
Bisinoza	Byssinosis (Monday fever)	Byssinose	Bisinosis (fiebre del lunes)	Bissinosi
Bjelančevine u urinu (proteinurija)	Proteinuria (presence of proteins in urine)	Protéinurie (excès de protéines dans l'urine)	Proteinuria	Proteinuria
Bjesnoća (rabies)	Rabies	Rage	Rabia	Rabbia
Blast-sindrom	Blast-syndrome	Syndrome de blast	Síndrome por explosion	Lesioni da scoppio (blast-syndrome)
Blastom	Blastoma	Blastome	Blastoma	Blastoma
Blastomikoza	Blastomycosis	Blastomycose	Blastomicosis	Blastomicosi
Blefaritis	Blepharitis	Blépharite	Blefaritis	Blefarite
Blok grane Hisovog snopića	Bundle branch block	Bloc de branche	Bloqueo de rama	Blocco di branca
Blokada mrežnične arterije	Retinal artery occlusion	Occlusion de l'artère de la rétine	Oclusión de la arteria de la retina	Occlusione arteria retinica
Blountova bolest	Blount's disease	Maladie de Blount	Enfermedad de Blount (tibia vara)	Sindrome di Blount
Bljedilo	Paleness (pallor)	Pâleur	Palidez	Pallore
Bol	Pain	Douleur	Dolor	Dolore
Bol pri mokrenju (strangurija)	Painful urination (strangury)	Urination douloureuse (strangurie)	Micción dolorosa (angurria)	Minzione dolorosa (stranguria)
Bol u dojci (mastalgija)	Breast pain (mastalgia)	Douleur au sein (mastodynie)	Dolor en la mama (mastalgia)	Dolore al seno (mastalgia)
Bol u epigastriju	Epigastric pain	Douleur épigastrique	Dolor epigástrico	Gastralgia
Bol u leđima (dorzopatija)	Back pain (dorsalgia)	Mal de dos (dorsalgie)	Dolor de espalda (dorsalgia)	Mal di schiena (dorsopatia)
Bol u mišiću (mijalgija)	Muscle pain (myalgia)	Douleur musculaire (myalgie)	Dolor muscular (mialgia)	Dolore muscolare (mialgia)

Hrvatski	Engleski	Francuski	Španjolski	Talijanski
Bol u prsištu	Chest pain	Douleur thoracique	Dolor torácico	Dolore toracico
Bol u uhu (otalgija)	Ear pain (otalgia)	Mal à l'oreille (otalgie)	Dolor en oído (otalgia)	Dolore auricolare (otalgia)
Bol pri snošaju	Painful sexual intercourse (dyspareunia)	Douleur lors du rapport sexuel (dyspareunie)	Relación sexual dolorosa (coitalgia, dispareunia)	Dolore durante rapporto sessuale (dispareunia)
Bol u trbuhu	Abdominal pain	Douleur abdominale	Dolor abdominal	Dolore addominale
Bol u zglobu (artralgija)	Joint pain (arthralgia)	Douleur articulaire (arthralgie)	Dolor en articulación (artralgia)	Articolazione doloroso (artralgia)
Bolest Charcot-Marie-Tooth	Charcot-Marie-Tooth disease	Maladie de Charcot-Marie-Tooth	Enfermedad de Charcot-Marie Tooth	Malattia di Charcot-Marie-Tooth
Bolest hijaline membrane (respiratorni sindrom novorođenćeta)	Hyaline membrane disease (infant respiratory distress syndrome)	Maladie des membranes hyalines (détresse respiratoire néonatale)	Enfermedad de la membrana hialina (síndrome de distrés respiratorio)	Sindrome da distress respiratorio del neonato (malattia da membrane ialine polmonari)
Bolest motornog neurona	Motor neurone disease	Maladie du motoneurone	Enfermedad de la motoneurona	Malattia del motoneurone
Bolest Pellegrini-Stieda	Pellegrini-Stieda disease	Maladie de Pellegrini-Stieda	Enfermedad de Pellegrini-Stieda	Malattia di Pellegrini-Stieda
Bolesti aorte	Diseases of the aorta	Maladies de l'aorte	Enfermedades de la aorta	Malattie dell'aorta
Bolesti krvnih žila	Blood vessel diseases	Maladies des vaisseaux sanguins	Enfermedades de los vasos sanguíneos	Malattie dei vasi sanguigni
Bolesti srčanih zalistaka	Heart valve diseases	Maladies des valves cardiaques	Enfermedades de las válvulas del corazón	Malattie delle valvole cardiache
Bolna menstruacija (dismenoreja)	Painful menstruation (dysmenorrhea)	Règle douloureuse (dysménorrhée)	Menstruación dolorosa (dismenorrea)	Mestruazione dolorosa (dismenorrea)
Bolna ovulacija (mittelschmerz)	Ovulation pain (mittelschmerz)	Douleurs ovulatoires (mittelschmerz)	Ovulación dolorosa	Dolore ovulatorio (mittelschmerz)
Bolni sindrom	Pain syndrome	Syndrome de douleur	Síndrome doloroso	Sindrome dolorosa
Bolno gutanje (odinofagija)	Painful swallowing (odynophagia)	Déglutition doulou-reuse (odynophagie)	Dolor al tragar (odinofagia)	Deglutizione dolorosa (odinofagia)
Bora	Wrinkle	Ride	Arruga	Ruga
Borelioza	Borreliosis	Borréliose	Borreliosis	Borreliosi
Bornholmska bolest (epidemijska mialgija)	Bornholm disease (epidemic myalgia)	Maladie de Bornholm (myalgie épidémique)	Enfermedad de Bornholm (mialgia epidémica)	Malattia di Bornholm (mialgia epidemica)
Botrioidni sarkom	Botryoid sarcoma	Sarcome botryoïde	Sarcoma botrioide	Sarcoma botrioide
Botulizam	Botulism	Botulisme	Botulismo	Botulismo
Bouchardovi čvorići	Bouchard's nodes	Nodules de Bouchard	Nudosidades de Bouchard	Noduli di Bouchard
Bowenova bolest	Bowen's disease (squamous cell carcinoma in situ)	Maladie de Bowen	Enfermedad de Bowen	Morbo di Bowen
Bradavica (virusna bradavica)	Wart	Verrue	Verruga	Verruca
Brahijalni sindrom bolne nadlaktice	Brachial syndrome	Brachialgie	Síndrome braquial	Brachialgia
Brennerov tumor	Brenner tumour	Tumeur de Brenner	Tumor de Brenner	Tumore di Brenner
Brillova bolest (Brill-Zinsserova bolest)	Brill's disease	Maladie de Brill-Zinserr (typhus résurgent)	Enfermedad de Brill	Malattia di Brill-Zinsser
Brodijev apsces	Brodie abscess	Abcès de Brodie	Absceso de Brodie	Ascesso di Brodie
Bronhiektazije	Bronchiectasis	Bronchectasie (dilatation des bronches)	Bronquiectasia	Bronchiectasia
Bronhopleuralna fistula	Bronchopleural fistula	Fistule bronchopleurale	Fístula bronco-pleural	Fistola broncopleurica
Bronhopneumonija	Bronchopneumonia	Bronchopneumonie	Neumonía bronquial	Broncopolmonite
Bronhospazam	Bronchospasm	Bronchospasme	Broncoespasmo	Broncospasmo
Bruceloza (malteška ili sredozemna groznica, Bangova bolest)	Brucellosis	Brucellose (fièvre de Malte, fièvre méditerranéenne)	Brucelosis	Brucellosi
Bubrežna kolika (renalna kolika)	Renal colic	Colique néphrétique	Cólico nefrítico (cólico renal)	Colica renale
Bubrežni kamenac (nefrolitijaza)	Kidney stone (nephrolithiasis)	Calcul rénal (néphrolithiase, lithiase urinaire)	Piedra en el riñon (cálculo renal, litiasis renal)	Calcolosi renale (nefrolitiasi)
Bubrežni rahitis	Renal rickets	Rachitisme rénal	Raquitismo renal	Rachitismo renale
Buergerova bolest	Buerger's disease (thromboangiitis obliterans)	Maladie de Buerger (thromboangéite oblitérante)	Enfermedad de Buerger (tromboangeítis obliterante)	Morbo di Buerger
Bulimija	Bulimia	Boulimie	Bulimia	Bulimia
Cefalokela	Cephalocele	Céphalocèle	Cefalocele	Cefalocèle
Celijakija	Coeliac disease (celiac disease)	Maladie coeliaque	Celiaquía (enfermedad celíaca)	Celiachia (malattia caliacha)
Celulitis	Cellulitis	Cellulite	Celulitis	Cellulite
Celulitis orbite	Orbital cellulitis	Cellulite orbitale	Celulitis orbital	Cellulite orbitale
Cerebralna aneurizma	Cerebral aneurysm	Anévrisme intra-crânien	Aneurisma cerebral	Aneurisma cerebrale
Cerebralna paraliza	Cerebral palsy	Infirmité motorice cérébrale	Parálisis cerebral	Paralisi cerebrale infantile
Cerkarija	Cercaria	Cercaire	Cercaria	Cercaria
Ceruminozni čep	Impacted cerumen	Bouchon de cérumen	Tapón de cerumen	Tappo di cerume
Cervikalna displazija	Cervical dysplasia	Dysplasie du col de l'utérus	Displasia del cuello uterino	Displasia cervicale
Cervikalna erozija	Cervical erosion	Érosion du col de l'utérus	Erosión cervical	Erosione cervicale
Cervikocefalni sindrom	Cervicocephal syndrome	Syndrome cervical	Síndrome cervical	Sindrome cervicale
Chagasova bolest (američka tripanosomijaza)	Chagas disease (American trypanosomiasis)	Maladie de Chagas (trypanosomiase américaine)	Enfermedad de Chagas (tripanosomiasis americana)	Malattia di Chagas

Hrvatski	Engleski	Francuski	Španjolski	Talijanski
Chikungunya virusna bolest	Chikungunya	Chikungunya	Chikungunya	Chikungunya
Cijanoza	Cyanosis	Cyanose	Cianosis	Cianosi
Ciroza jetre	Liver cirrhosis	Cirrhose hépatique	Cirrosis hepática	Cirrosi
Cista	Cyst	Kyste	Quiste	Cisti (ciste)
Cistadenofibrom	Cystadenofibroma	Cystadénofibrome	Cistadenofibroma	Cistadenofibroma
Cistadenokarcinom	Cystadenocarcinoma	Cystadénocarcinome	Cistadenocarcinoma	Cistadenocarcinoma
Cistadenom	Cystadenoma	Cystadénome	Cistadenoma	Cistadenoma
Cista na bubregu	Renal cyst	Kyste rénal	Quiste de riñón	Cisti renale
Cista na gušterači	Pancreatic cyst	Kyste du pancréas	Quiste de páncreas	Cisti pancreatica
Cista na jajniku	Ovarian cyst	Kyste ovarien	Quiste ovárico	Cisti ovarica
Cista na štitnjači	Thyroid cyst	Kyste thyroïdien	Quiste de tiroides	Cisti tiroidea
Cista na tireoglosnom vodu	Thyroglossal duct cyst	Kyste du canal thyréoglosse	Quiste tirogloso	Cisti del dotto tiroglosso
Cisticerkoza	Cysticercosis	Cysticercose	Cisticercosis	Cisticercosi
Cistična fibroza	Cystic fibrosis	Mucoviscidose (fibrose kystique)	Fibrosis quística (mucoviscidosis)	Fibrosi cistica
Cistom	Cystoma	Kystome	Cistoma	Cistoma
Cluster glavobolja	Cluster headache	Algie vasculaire de la face	Cefalea en racimos	Cefalea a grappolo
Creutzfeldt-Jakobova bolest (tzv. "kravlje ludilo")	Creutzfeldt-Jakob disease (so called "mad cow disease")	Maladie de Creutzfeldt-Jakob	Enfermedad de Creutzfeldt-Jakob	Malattia di Creutzfeldt-Jakob (cosiddetta "malattia della mucca pazza")
Crijevna atrezija	Intestinal atresia	Atrésie intestinale	Atresia intestinal	Atresia intestinale
Crna stolica (melena)	Black stool (melena)	Selles noir (melanea, méléna)	Heces negras (melena)	Feci picee (melena)
Crohnova bolest	Crohn's disease	Maladie de Crohn	Enfermedad de Crohn	Malattia di Crohn
Crush-sindrom	Crush-syndrome	Syndrome d'écrasement	Síndrome de aplastamiento (síndrome de crush)	Sindrome da schiacciamento
Crvena stolica	Red colored stool	Selles rouges	Heces de color rojo	Feci di colore rosso
Crveni urin	Red urine	Urine rouge	Orina de color rojo	Urina di colore rosso
Crveni vjetar (vrbanac, erizipel)	Erysipelas (Ignis sacer, St. Anthony's fire)	Érysipèle (érésipèle)	Erisipela	Erisipela
Crvenilo kože (eritem)	Redness of the skin (erythema)	Érythème (rougeur de la peau)	Enrojecimiento de la piel (eritema)	Eritema
Curenje likvora na nos (cerebrospinalna rinoreja)	Leakage of cerebrospinal fluid through the nose	Écoulement de liquide cérébrospinal par le nez (rhinoliquorrhée)	Salida de líquido cerebroespinal por la nariz (rinoliquorrea)	Perdita di liquido cerebrospinale dal naso (rinoliquorrea)
Curenje likvora na uho (cerebrospinalna otoreja)	Leakage of cerebrospinal fluid through the ear	Écoulement de liquide cérébrospinal par l'oreille (otoliquorrhée)	Salida de líquido cerebroespinal por el oído (otoliquorrea)	Perdita di liquido cerebrospinale dall'orechio (otoliquorrea)
Curenje iz nosa (rinoreja)	Runny nose (rinorrhea)	Écoulement par le nez (rhinorrhée)	Goteo nasal (rinorrea)	Naso che cola (rinorrea)
Cushingov sindrom (hiperkortikolizam)	Cushing's syndrome (hypercorticism)	Syndrome de Cushing (hypercorticisme)	Síndrome de Cushing (hipercortisolismo)	Sindrome di Cushing (ipercortisolismo)
Čankir	Chancre	Chancre	Chancro	Sifiloma
Čir (ulkus)	Ulcer	Ulcère	Úlcera (llaga)	Ulcera (ulcerazione)
Čir na dvanaesniku	Duodenal ulcer	Ulcère du doudénum	Úlcera duodenal	Ulcera duodenale
Čir na želucu	Gastric ulcer	Ulcère de l'estomac	Úlcera gástrica	Ulcera gastrica
Čopavo stopalo (uvrnuto stopalo, pes equinovarus)	Club foot (talipes equinovarus)	Pied-bot (pied-bot équin)	Pie equinovaro (talipes equinovarus, pie bot, pie retorcido)	Piede equino (talipes equinovarus)
Čukalj	Bunion	Hallux valgus	Bunión (hallux valgus)	Alluce valgo
Čvor sestre Mary Joseph (umbilikalna metastaza)	Sister Mary Joseph nodule	Nodule de Soeur Marie Joseph (métastase cutanée ombilicale)	Nódulo de la hermana María José	Nodulo di Suor Maria Giuseppa
Čvorasta guša (nodularna struma)	Nodular goiter	Goitre multinodulaire	Bocio nodular	Gozzo multinodulare
Ćelavost	Alopecia	Alopécie	Alopecia	Alopecia
Dalekovidnost	Farsightedness (hyperopia)	Hypermétropie	Hipermetropía	Ipermetropia
Daltonizam	Daltonism	Daltonisme	Daltonismo	Daltonismo
Davljenje	Strangulation	Strangulation (étranglement)	Estrangulamiento	Strangolamento (strozzamento)
Debljanje	Gaining weight	Grossissement	Engorde (ganar peso)	Ingrossamento (divenire grosso)
Debljina (gojaznost)	Obesity	Obésité	Obesidad	Obesità
Deformacija kralježnice	Spinal deformity	Difformité spinale	Deformidad vertebral	Degenerazione spinale
Deformacija stopala	Foot deformity	Difformité du pied	Deformidad del pie	Difetto del piede
Degeneracija makule	Macular degeneration	Dégénérescence maculaire	Degeneración macular	Degenerazione maculare
Degeneracija mrežnice	Retinal degeneration	Dégénérescence de la rétine	Degeneración retinal	Degenerazione della retina
Dehidracija	Dehydration	Déshydratation	Deshidratación	Disidratazione
Dekompresijska bolest (kesonska bolest)	Decompression sickness (diver's disease, caisson disease)	Maladie de décompression (maladie des plongeurs, maladie des caissons)	Síndrome de decompresión (enfermedad de los buzos, mal de presión)	Malattia di decompressione (sindrome di Caisson)
Dekubitus	Bedsore (decubitus ulcer)	Escarre (plaie de lit, ulcère de décubitus)	Úlcera de decúbito	Piaga da decubito (decubito)
Delirij	Delirium	Delirium	Delirio	Delirio
Demencija	Dementia	Démence	Demencia	Demenza

Hrvatski	Engleski	Francuski	Španjolski	Talijanski
Demineralizacija	Demineralization	Déminéralisation	Desmineralización	Demineralizzazione
Dengue groznica	Dengue fever	Dengue (grippe tropicale, dengue hémorragique)	Dengue	Dengue
Depresija	Depression	Dépression	Depresión	Depressione
Dermatomikoza	Dermatomycosis	Dermatomycose	Dermatomicosis	Dermatomicosi
Dermatomiozitis	Dermatomyositis	Dermatomyosite	Dermatomiositis	Dermatomiosite
Dermoidna cista	Dermoid cyst	Kyste dermoïde	Quiste dermoide	Cisti dermoide
Devijacija nosnog septuma	Nasal septum deviation	Déviation du septum nasal	Desviación del tabique nasal	Deviazione del setto nasale
Dezorijentiranost	Disorientation	Désorientation	Desorientación	Disorientamento
Difterija	Diphtheria	Diphtérie	Difteria	Difterite
Dijabetes	Diabetes	Diabète	Diabetes	Diabete
Dijabetes insipidus	Diabetes insipidus	Diabète insipide	Diabetes insípida	Diabete insipido
Dijabetes melitus	Diabetes mellitus	Diabète sucré	Diabetes mellitus (diabetes sacarina)	Diabete mellito
Dijabetes melitus tip 1	Diabetes mellitus type 1	Diabète sucré de type 1 (diabète insulino-dépendant)	Diabetes mellitus tipo 1	Diabete mellito di tipo 1
Dijabetes melitus tip 2	Diabetes mellitus type 2	Diabète sucré de type 2 (diabète insulinorésistant)	Diabetes mellitus tipo 2	Diabete mellito di tipo 2
Dijabetična ketoacidoza	Diabetic ketoacidosis	Cétoacidose diabétique	Cetoacidosis diabética	Chetoacidosi diabetica
Dijabetična koma	Diabetic coma	Coma diabétique	Coma diabético	Coma diabetico
Dijabetična nefropatija	Diabetic nephropathy	Néphropathie diabétique	Nefropatía diabética	Nefropatia diabetica
Dijabetična neuropatija	Diabetic neuropathy	Neuropathie diabétique	Neuropatía diabética	Neuropatia diabetica
Dijabetična retinopatija	Diabetic retinopathy	Rétinopathie diabétique	Retinopatía diabética	Retinopatia diabetica
Dijafragmalna kila	Diaphragmatic hernia	Hernie diaphragmatique	Hernia diafragmática	Ernia diaframmatica
Dilatacijska kardiomiopatija	Dilated cardiomyopathy	Cardiomyopathie dilatée	Miocardiopatía dilatada	Cardiomiopatia dilatativa
Disekcija aorte	Aortic dissection	Dissection aortique	Disección aórtica	Dissecazione aortica
Diseminirana intravaskularna koagulacija	Disseminated intravascular coagulation	Coagulation intravasculaire disséminée	Coagulación intravascular diseminada	Coagulazione intravascolare disseminata
Disgerminom	Dysgerminoma	Dysgerminome	Disgerminoma	Disgerminoma
Dishidroza	Dyshidrosis	Dyshidrose	Eczema dishidrótico	Disidrosi
Dishondroplazija	Dyschondroplasia	Dyschondroplasie	Discondroplasia	Discondroplasia
Diskartroza	Discarthrosis (degenerative disc disease)	Arthrose du disque intervertébral	Discartrosis	Discartrosi (discopatia degenerativa)
Disleksija	Dyslexia	Dyslexie	Dislexia	Dislessia
Dislokacija ulomaka	Dislocated fragments	Fragments deboîtées	Dislocación de los fragmentos	Dislocazione dei frammenti
Dispepsija (nervozni želudac)	Dyspepsia (upset stomach)	Dyspepsie	Dispepsia (indigestión)	Dispepsia
Distonija	Dystonia	Dystonie	Distonía	Distonia
Distrofija	Dystrophy	Dystrophie	Distrofia	Distrofia
Divertikul	Diverticulum	Diverticule	Divertículo	Diverticolo
Divertikul na debelom crijevu	Colon diverticulum	Diverticule du côlon	Divertículo del colon	Diverticolo del colon
Divertikul na dvanaesniku	Duodenal diverticulum	Diverticule duodenal	Divertículo duodenal	Diverticolo duodenale
Divertikul tankog crijeva	Small intestine diverticulum	Diverticule de Meckel	Divertículo de Meckel	Diverticolo di Meckel
Divertikulitis	Diverticulitis	Diverticulite	Diverticulitis	Diverticolite
Divertikuloza	Diverticulosis	Diverticulose	Enfermedad diverticular	Diverticolosi
Divovski stas	Gigantism	Gigantisme	Gigantismo	Gigantismo
Dizenterija	Dysentery (flux)	Dysenterie	Disentería	Dissenteria
Dječja paraliza (polio, poliomijelitis)	Poliomyelitis (polio, infantile paralysis)	Poliomyélite (polio, paralysie spinale infantile)	Poliomielitis (parálisis infantil)	Poliomielite (polio, paralisi infantile)
Dječje zarazne bolesti	Childhood infectious diseases	Maladies infectieuses des enfants	Enfermedades infantiles contagiosas	Malattie infettive dei bambini
Djelomična dislokacija (subluksacija)	Partial dislocation (subluxation)	Luxation incomplète (subluxation)	Desplazamiento de una articulación (subluxación)	Lussazione incompleta (sublussazione)
Dobroćudni tumor (benigni tumor)	Benign tumor	Tumeur bénigne	Tumor benigno	Tumore benigno
Downov sindrom (mongoloidizam)	Down syndrome	Syndrome de Down	Síndrome de Down	Sindrome di Down
Drakunkulijaza	Dracunculiasis	Dracunculose	Dracunculiasis	Dracunculiasi
Drhtanje (tremor)	Tremor	Tremblement	Temblor	Tremito (tremore)
Drhtanje ruku	Hand tremor	Tremblement des mains	Temblor en las manos	Tremore delle mani
Duchenneova mišićna distrofija	Duchenne muscular dystrophy	Myopathie de Duchenne	Distrofia muscular de Duchenne	Distrofia di Duchenne
Ductus Botalli	Ductus arteriosus (ductus Botalli shunt)	Canal artériel	Ductus arteriosus (conducto arterioso de Botal)	Dotto arterioso di Botallo
Dugotrajna bolna erekcija (prijapizam)	Long-lasting painful erection (priapism)	Érection persistente douloureuse (priapisme)	Erección sostenida y dolorosa (priapismo)	Erezione persistente dolorosa (priapismo)
Duhringova bolest (dermatitis herpetiformis)	Dermatitis herpetiformis (Duhring's disease)	Dermatite herpétiforme	Dermatitis herpetiforme (enfermedad de Duhring)	Dermatite erpetiforme di Duhring
Dupuytrenova kontraktura	Dupuytren's contracture	Contracture de Dupuytren	Contractura de Dupuytren	Malattia di Dupuytren
Dvoslike	Double vision (diplopia)	Vision double (diplopie)	Visión doble (diplopía)	Visione doppia (diplopia)
Dvospolnost	Hermaphroditism	Hermaphrodisme	Hermafroditismo	Ermafroditismo
Edem	Edema	Oedème	Edema (hidropesía)	Edema
Edem mozga	Cerebral edema	Oedème cérébral	Edema cerebral	Edema cerebrale

Hrvatski	Engleski	Francuski	Španjolski	Talijanski
Egzostoza	Exostosis	Exostose	Exostosis	Esostosi
Egzantem	Exanthem	Exanthème	Exantema	Esantema
Ehinokokoza	Echinococcosis (hydatid disease)	Échinococcose	Hidatidosis (equinococosis)	Echinococcosi (idatidosi)
Ehinokokoza jetre	Hepatic echinococcosis	Échinococcose hépatique	Hidatidosis hepática	Echinococcosi epatica
Ehinokokoza pluća	Pulmonary echinococcosis	Échinococcose pulmonaire	Hidatidosis pulmonar	Echinococcosi polmonare
Eholalija	Echolalia	Écholalie	Ecolalia	Ecolalia
Ehopraksija (nevoljno ponavljanje tuđih pokreta)	Echopraxia (involuntary repetition of the observed movements of another)	Échopraxie (tendance spontanée à répéter les mouvements d'une autre personne)	Ecopraxia (repetición de los movimientos de otra persona)	Ecoprassia (imitazione spontanea di movimenti osservati)
Eisenmengerov sindrom	Eisenmenger's syndrome	Syndrome d'Eisenmenger	Síndrome de Eisenmenger	Sindrome di Eisenmenger
Ekcem	Eczema	Eczéma	Eccema (eczema)	Eczema
Eksplozivna rana	Explosive wound	Blessure par explosion	Lesión por explosión	Ferita esplosiva
Elefantijaza (limfedem)	Elephantiasis (lymphedema)	Éléphantiasis (filariose lymphatique)	Elefantiasis	Elefantiasi
Elektromagnetska hipersenzibilnost	Electromagnetic hypersensitivity	Sensibilité éléctromagnétique	Hipersensibilidad electromagnética	Elettrosensibilità
Embolija	Embolism	Embolie	Embolia	Embolismo (embolia)
Embrionalni karcinom	Embryonal carcinoma	Carcinome embryonnaire	Carcinoma embrional	Carcinoma embrionale
Emfizem	Emphysema	Emphysème	Enfisema	Enfisema
Empijem	Empyema	Empyème	Empiema	Empiema
Encefalokela	Encephalocele	Encéphalocèle	Encefalocele	Encefalocele
Encefalopatija	Encephalopathy	Encéphalopathie	Encefalopatía	Encefalopatia
Endometrioza	Endometriosis	Endométriose	Endometriosis	Endometriosi
Endotoksični šok	Endotoxic shock	Choc endotoxique	Choque endotoxico	Shock endotossico
Enhondrom	Enchondroma	Enchondrome	Encondroma	Encondroma
Enkopreza	Encopresis	Encoprésie	Encopresis	Enconpresi
Entezopatija	Enthesopathy	Enthésiopathie	Entesopatía	Entesopatia
Eozinofilija	Eosinophilia	Éosinophilie	Eosinofilia	Eosinofilia
Ependimom	Ependymoma	Épendymome	Ependimoma	Ependimoma
Epiduralni hematom	Epidural hematoma	Hématome épidural	Hematoma epidural	Ematoma epidurale
Epiduralno krvarenje	Epidural bleeding	Hémorragie épidurale	Hemorragia epidural	Emorragia epidurale
Epifizeoliza glave bedrene kosti	Epiphyseolysis capitis femoris	Épiphysiolyse de l'extrémité supérieure du fémur	Epifisario de la cabeza femoral (epifisiolisis capitis femoris)	Epifisiolisi della testa femorale
Epilepsija	Epilepsy	Épilepsie	Epilepsia	Epilessia
Epispadija	Epispadias	Épispadias	Epispadia	Epispadia
Eritromelalgija	Erythromelalgia (acromelalgia)	Érythromelalgie	Eritromelalgia	Eritromelalgia
Eritroplazija	Erythroplakia (erythroplasia)	Érythroplasie	Eritroplasia	Eritroplachia (eritroplasia)
Eritroplazija Queyrat	Erythroplasia of Queyrat	Érythroplasie de Queyrat	Eritroplasia de Queyrat	Eritroplasia di Queyrat
Erizipeloid	Erysipeloid	Erysipéloïde	Erisipeloide	Erisipeloide
Esencijalna hipertenzija	Essential hypertension	Hypertension artérielle essentielle	Hipertensión esencial	Ipertensione arteriosa essenziale
Ewing sarkom (endoteliosarkom)	Ewing's sarcoma	Sarcome d'Ewing	Sarcoma de Ewing	Sarcoma di Ewing
Fallotova tetralogija	Tetralogy of Fallot	Tétralogie de Fallot	Tetralogía de Fallot	Tetralogia di Fallot
Fantomska bol	Phantom pain	Douleur du membre fantôme	Dolor del miembro fantasma	Dolore fantomatico
Farmerska pluća	Farmer's lung	Maladie du poumon de fermier	Pulmón de granjero	Febbre da fieno
Febrilne konvulzije	Febrile convulsions	Convulsion hyperthermique	Convulsiones febriles	Convulsioni febbrili
Fenilketonurija	Phenylketonuria	Phénylcétonurie	Fenilcetonuria	Fenilchetonuria
Feokromocitom (tumor srži nadbubrežne žlijezde)	Pheochromocytoma	Phéochromocytome	Feocromocitoma	Feocromocitoma
Fetusni alkoholni sindrom	Fetal alcohol syndrome	Syndrome d'alcoolisation foetale	Síndrome de alcoholismo fetal	Sindrome alcolica fetale
Fibrinoidna nekroza	Fibrinoid necrosis	Nécrose fibrinoïde	Necrosis fibrinoide	Necrosi fibrinoide
Fibroadenom	Fibroadenoma	Fibroadénome	Fibroadenoma	Fibroadenoma
Fibrocistična bolest dojke	Fibrocystic breast disease	Mastopathie fibrocystique	Mastitis quística crónica (enfermedad fibroquística)	Mastopatia fibrocistica
Fibroelastoza endokarda	Endocardial fibroelastosis	Fibroélastose endocardique	Fibroelastosis endocardial	Fibroelastosi endocardica
Fibrom	Fibroma	Fibrome	Fibroma	Fibroma
Fibromialgija	Fibromyalgia	Fibromyalgie	Fibromialgia	Fibromialgia
Fibrosarkom	Fibrosarcoma (fibroblastic sarcoma)	Fibrosarcome	Fibrosarcoma	Fibrosarcoma
Fibroza	Fibrosis	Fibrose	Fibrosis	Fibrosi
Fibrozitis mišića	Muscular fibrositis	Fibrosite musculaire	Fibrositis (reumatismo muscular)	Fibrosite muscolare
Fibrozitis šake	Hand fibrositis	Fasciite de la main (fasciite palmaire)	Fibrositis de la mano	Fibrosite di mano
Fibrozitis tetive	Tendinous fibrositis	Fibrosite du tendon	Fibrositis de tendón	Fibrosi tendinea
Fibrozna cistična upala kosti	Osteitis fibrosa cystica	Ostéite fibrokystique	Ostéitis fibrosa quística	Osteitis fibrosa cistica

Hrvatski	Engleski	Francuski	Španjolski	Talijanski
Fibrozna displazija	Fibrous dysplasia	Dysplasie fibreuse	Displasia fibrosa	Displasia fibrosa
Fibrozni histiocitom	Fibrous histiocytoma	Histiocytome fibreux	Histiocitoma fibroso	Fibroistiocitoma benigno
Filarijaza	Filariasis	Filariose	Filariasis	Filariasi
Fimoza	Phimosis	Phimosis	Fimosis	Fimosi
Fistula	Fistula	Fistule	Fístula	Fistola
Flebotromboza	Phlebothrombosis	Phlébothrombose	Flebotrombosis	Flebotrombosi
Flegmona	Phlegmon	Phlegmon	Flegmón	Flemmone
Fobija	Phobia	Phobie	Fobia	Fobia
Folikulitis	Folliculitis	Folliculite	Foliculitis	Follicolite
Fotofobija (strah od svjetla)	Photophobia (fear of light)	Photophobie (crainte de la lumière)	Fotofobia (intolerancia a la luz)	Fotofobia
Fournierova gangrena	Fournier gangrene	Gangrène de Fournier	Gangrena de Fournier	Gangrena di Fournier
Frambezija	Yaws (pian)	Pian	Pian (frambesia)	Framboesia
Freibergova bolest	Freiberg's disease	Maladie de Freiberg	Enfermedad de Freiberg	Malattia di Freiberg
Frigidnost	Frigidity	Frigidité	Frigidez	Frigidità
Furunkul (čir na koži)	Furuncle (boil)	Furoncle	Forúnculo (furúnculo)	Foruncolo
Gađenje prema hrani	Food aversion	Aversion pour la nourriture	Aversión por la comida	Ripugnanza al cibo
Galaktoreja	Galactorrhea	Galactorrhée	Galactorrea	Galattorrea
Gangrena	Gangrene	Gangrène	Gangrena	Cancrena
Gastroenteritis	Gastroenteritis	Gastroentérite	Gastroenteritis	Gastroenterite
Generalizirani edem (anasarka)	Generalized edema (anasarca)	Oedème généralisé (anasarque)	Anasarca	Edema diffuso (anasarca)
Genitalna bradavica (venerična bradavica)	Genital wart	Verrue génitale	Verruga genital (condiloma acuminata)	Condiloma
Genitalni herpes	Genital herpes	Herpès génital	Herpes genital	Herpes genitalis
Genu valgum	Knock knees (genu valgum)	Genou cagneux (genu valgum, genou en X)	Genu valgo	Ginocchio valgo
Genu varum	Bow legs (genu varum)	Genu varum	Genu varum	Ginocchio varo (genu varum)
Gigantocelularni tumor (osteoklastom)	Gigantocellular tumor (osteoclastoma)	Tumeur à cellules géantes	Tumor de células gigantes (osteoclastoma)	Osteoclastoma (tumore a cellule giganti)
Gimnastičarska bolna križa	Gymnastics lower back pain	Lombalgie du gymnaste	Espalda del gimnasta	Lombalgia dell'atleta
Ginekomastija	Gynecomastia	Gynécomastie	Ginecomastia	Ginecomastia
Glad	Hunger	Faim	Hambre	Fame
Glasno otežano disanje (stridor)	Breathing sound due to blockage in the airway (stridor)	Bruit anormal émis lors de la respiration (stridor)	Estridor	Rumore durante la respirazione (stridore)
Glaukom	Glaucoma	Glaucome	Glaucoma	Glaucoma
Glavobolja	Headache	Mal de tête (céphalée)	Dolor de cabeza	Mal di testa
Glioblastom	Glioblastoma	Glioblastome	Glioblastoma	Glioblastoma
Gliom	Glioma	Gliome	Glioma	Glioma
Glioza	Gliosis	Gliose	Gliosis	Gliosi
Glomerulonefritis	Glomerulonephritis	Glomérulonéphrite	Glomerulonefritis	Glomerulonefrite
Glomus-tumor	Glomus tumor	Tumeur glomique (glomangiome)	Tumor glómico (glomangioma)	Glomangioma (paraganglioma)
Gluhoća	Deafness	Surdité	Sordera	Sordità
Gljivična infekcija	Fungal infection	Infection fongique	Infección por hongos	Infezione fungina
Gljivična infekcija prepona (tinea cruris)	Crotch itch (tinea cruris)	Eczéma marginé de hebra	Tiña crural (tinea cruris)	Tinea cruris
Gljivična infekcija vlasišta (tinea capitis)	Tinea capitis (scalp ringworm)	Teigne (tinea capitis)	Tiña de la cabeza (tinea capitis)	Tigna (tinea capitis)
Gljivični osteomijelitis	Fungal osteomyelitis	Ostéomyélite fongique	Osteomielitis micótica	Osteomielite fungale
Gnoj	Pus	Pus	Pus	Pus
Gnoj u urinu (piurija)	Pus in urine (pyuria)	Présence de pus dans l'urine (pyurie)	Presencia de pus en la orina (piuria)	Presenza di pus nelle urine (piuria)
Gnojna upala krajnika	Quinsy (peritonsillar abscess)	Abcès périamygdalien	Absceso peritonsilar	Ascesso peritonsillare
Gnojni ispljuvak	Pus in sputum	Crachat purulent	Esputo que contiene pus	Presenza di pus nello sputo
Gnojni mjehurić	Pustule	Pustule	Pústula	Pustola
Gonadoblastom	Gonadoblastoma	Gonadoblastome	Gonadoblastoma	Gonadoblastoma
Gonoreja (kapavac, triper)	Gonorrhea	Gonorrhée (blennorragie, chaudepisse)	Gonorrea (blenorragia, blenorrea)	Gonorrea (blenorragia)
Goodpastureov sindrom	Goodpasture's syndrome	Syndrome de Goodpasture (maladie des anticorps antimembrane basale glomérulaire)	Síndrome de Goodpasture	Sindrome di Goodpasture
Granični poremećaj osobnosti	Borderline personality disorder	Personnalité borderline	Trastorno límite de la personalidad	Disturbo borderline di personalità
Granulocitoza	Granulocytosis	Polynucléose	Granulocitosis	Granulocitosi
Granulomatozna upala (granulom)	Granulomatous inflammation	Inflammation granulomateuse	Inflamación granulomatosa	Infiammazione granulomatosa
Granuloza tumor	Granulosa cell tumor	Tumeur de la granulosa	Tumor de células de la granulosa (tumor de teca-granulosa)	Follicoloma
Grba	Hunchback	Bossu	Joroba	Gibbo (gobba, gibbosità)
Grč (spazam)	Spasm (cramp)	Spasme (crampe)	Espasmo (calambre)	Spasmo (contrazione involontaria)

Hrvatski	Engleski	Francuski	Španjolski	Talijanski
Grč mišića lica	Facial spasm	Spasme facial	Espasmo facial	Spasmo facciale
Grč rodnice (vaginizam)	Vaginal spasm (vaginismus)	Spasme vaginal (vaginisme)	Espasmo vaginal (vaginismo)	Spasmo di vagina (vaginismo)
Gripa (influenca)	Flu (influenza)	Grippe (influenza)	Gripe (gripa, influenza)	Influenza
Griženje noktiju (onikofagija)	Nail biting (onychophagia)	Se ronger les ongles (onychophagie)	Comerse las uñas (onicofagia)	Abitudine di mangiare le unghie (onicofagia)
Groznica (vrućica)	Fever	Fièvre	Fiebre	Febbre
Groznica Ebola	Ebola hemorrhagic fever	Fièvre Ébola	Fiebre hemorrágica viral de Ébola	Ebola
Groznica Lassa	Lassa fever	Fièvre de Lassa	Fiebre de Lassa	Febbre di Lassa
Groznica planinskog krpelja	Colorado tick fever (mountain tick fever)	Fièvre à tiques du Colorado (fièvre à tiques des montagnes)	Fiebre del Colorado por garrapatas (fiebre de montaña americana por garrapatas)	Febbre da zecca del Colorado
Groznica štakorskog ugriza	Rat-bite fever	Fièvre de la morsure de rat	Fiebre por mordedura de rata	Febbre da morso di ratto
Groznica zapadnog Nila	West Nile fever	Fièvre du Nil occidental	Fiebre del Nilo Occidental	Febbre del Nilo occidentale
Gubitak apetita	Loss of appetite	Perte d'appétit	Pérdida del apetito	Mancanza dell'appetito
Gubitak mišićne snage (astenija)	Loss of strenght (asthenia)	Affaiblissement de l'organisme (asthénie)	Pérdida de fuerza muscular (astenia)	Riduzione della forza muscolare (astenia)
Gubitak osjeta dodoira	Loss of the sense of touch	Perte du sens du toucher	Pérdida del sentido del tacto	Perdita di senso di tocco
Gubitak osjeta mirisa	Loss of olfaction (anosmia)	Perte de la sensibilité aux odeurs (anosmie)	Pérdida del sentido del olfato (anosmia)	Incapacità di percipire gli odori (disosmia)
Gubitak osjeta okusa	Loss of the sense of taste (ageusia)	Perte du sens du goût (ageusie)	Pérdida del sentido del gusto (ageusia)	Incapacità di percipire i sapori (ageusia)
Gubitak pamćenja	Memory loss	Perte de mémoire	Pérdida de la memoria	Perdita di memoria
Gubitak polovice vidnog polja (hemianopsija)	Loss of half of a field of vision (hemianopsia)	Perte de la vue dans une moitié du champ visuel (hémianopsie)	Pérdida de la mitad del campo visual (hemianopsia)	Perdita di metà di campo visivo (emianopsia)
Gubitak pulsa	Absence of pulse	Absence de pouls	Pérdida de pulso	Perdita di polso
Gubitak sluha	Hearing loss	Perte d'ouïe	Pérdida de la capacidad auditiva	Perdita di udito
Gubitak sposobnosti govora (afazija)	Loss of language ability (aphasia)	Perte d'habileté d'expression du langage (mutisme, aphasie)	Pérdida de capacidad de producir lenguaje (afasia)	Perdita di abilità di produzione del linguaggio verbale (afasia)
Guillain-Barréov sindrom	Guillain-Barré syndrome	Syndrome de Guillain-Barré	Síndrome de Guillain-Barré	Sindrome di Guillain-Barré
Guša (struma)	Goiter	Goitre	Bocio (coto)	Gozzo
Gušenje	Choking (suffocation)	Suffocation	Atragantamiento	Soffocamento (soffocazione, asfissia)
Haglundova bolest	Haglund's disease	Maladie de Haglund	Enfermedad de Haglund (deformidad de Haglund)	Malattia di Haglund (deformità di Haglund)
Halucinacija	Hallucination	Hallucination	Alucinación	Allucinazione
Hashimotov sindrom	Hashimoto's disease	Thyroïdite de Hashimoto	Tiroiditis de Hashimoto	Tiroidite di Hashimoto
Heberdenovi čvorići	Heberden's nodes	Nodules d'Heberden	Nódulos de Heberden	Noduli di Heberden
Hemangioendoteliom	Hemangioendothe-lioma	Hémangio-endothéliome	Hemangioendotelioma	Emangioendotelioma
Hemangiom	Hemangioma	Hémangiome	Hemangioma	Emangioma
Hematom	Hematoma	Hématome	Hematoma	Ematoma
Hemivertebra	Hemivertebrae	Hémivertèbre	Hemivértebra	Emivertebra
Hemofilična artropatija	Hemophiliac arthropathy	Arthropathie hémophile	Artropatía hemofílica	Artropatia emofilica
Hemofilija	Hemophilia	Hémophilie	Hemofilia	Emofilia
Hemoglobin u urinu (hemoglobinurija)	Hemoglobin in urine (hemoglobinuria)	Hémoglobine dans l'urine (hémoglobinurie)	Hemoglobina en orina (hemoglobinuria)	Presenza di emoglobina nelle urine (emoglobinuria)
Hemokromatoza	Hemochromatosis	Hémochromatose	Hemocromatosis	Emocromatosi
Hemolitična anemija	Hemolytic anemia	Anémie hémolytique	Anemia hemolítica	Anemia emolitica
Hemopneumotoraks	Hemopneumothorax	Hémopneumothorax	Hemoneumotórax	Emopneumotorace
Hemoragijska groznica s renalnim sindromom (korejska hemoragijska groznica)	Hemorrhagic fever with renal syndrome (Korean hemorrhagic fever)	Fièvre hémorragique avec syndrome rénal (fièvre hémorragique de Corée)	Fiebre hemorrágica con síndrome renal (fiebre hemorrágica coreana)	Febbre emorragica con sindrome renale (febbre emorragica coreana)
Hemoragijski infarkt mozga	Hemorrhagic brain infarction	Infarctus cérébral hémorragique	Infarto cerebral hemorrágico	Ictus emorragico
Hemoroidi	Hemorrhoids	Hémorroïdes	Hemorroides	Emorroidi
Hemosideroza	Hemosiderosis	Hémosidérose	Hemosiderosis	Emosiderosi
Hemotoraks	Hemothorax	Hémothorax	Hemotórax	Emotorace
Hepatitis A	Hepatitis A	Hépatite A	Hepatitis A	Epatite virale A
Hepatitis B	Hepatitis B	Hépatite B	Hepatitis B	Epatite virale B
Hepatitis C	Hepatitis C	Hépatite C	Hepatitis C	Epatite virale C
Hepatitis D	Hepatitis D	Hépatite D	Hepatitis D	Epatite virale D
Hepatitis E	Hepatitis E	Hépatite E	Hepatitis E	Epatite virale E
Hepatocelularni adenom	Hepatocellular adenoma	Adénome hépatocellulaire	Adenoma hepático (a-denoma hepatocelular)	Adenoma epatocellulare
Hepatocelularni karcinom	Hepatocellular carcinoma	Carcinome hépatocellulaire	Carcinoma hepatocelular	Carcinoma epatocellulare
Hepatorenalni sindrom	Hepatorenal syndrome	Syndrome hépato-rénal	Síndrome hepatorrenal	Sindrome epato-renale
Heredoataksija	Hereditary ataxia	Ataxie héréditaire	Ataxia de Friidreich (ataxia hereditaria)	Atassia ereditaria
Hernija intervertrebralnog diska	Spinal disc herniation	Hernie discale	Hernia discal	Ernia del disco

Hrvatski	Engleski	Francuski	Španjolski	Talijanski
Herpangina	Herpangina (mouth blisters)	Herpangine	Herpangina	Erpangina (faringite vescicolare)
Herpes simpleks	Herpes simplex	Herpès (infection herpétique)	Herpes simple	Herpes simplex
Herpes zoster	Herpes zoster	Zona	Herpes zóster (herpes zona)	Herpes zoster
Hidremija	Hydremia	Hydrémie	Hidremia	Idremia
Hidrocefalus	Hydrocephalus	Hydrocéphalie	Hidrocefalia	Idrocefalo
Hidrofobija	Aquaphobia	Aquaphobie	Acuafobia	Idrofobia
Hidrokela	Hydrocele	Hydrocèle	Hidrocele	Idrocele
Hidronefroza	Hydronephrosis	Hydronéphrose	Hidronefrosis	Idronefrosi
Hidroperikard	Pericardial effusion (hydropericard)	Épanchement péricardique	Derrame pericárdico	Idropericardio
Hidrops	Hydrops	Hydrops	Hidrops	Idrope
Hidrops žučnog mjehura	Gallbladder hydrops	Hydrops de la vésicule biliaire	Hidrops vesicular	Idrope della colecisti
Hidrotoraks	Hydrothorax	Hydrothorax	Hidrotórax	Idrotorace
Hifema	Hyphema	Hyphème	Hipema	Ifema
Higrom	Hygroma	Hygroma	Higroma	Igroma
Hijatusna kila	Hiatus hernia	Hernie hiatale	Hernia de hiato	Ernia iatale
Hilotoraks	Chylothorax	Chylothorax	Quilotórax	Chilotorace
Hiperaktivnost	Hyperactivity	Hyperactivité	Hiperactividad	Iperattività
Hiperkalcijemija	Hypercalcemia	Hypercalcémie	Hipercalcemia	Ipercalcemia
Hiperkalijemija	Hyperkalemia	Hyperkaliémie	Hiperpotasemia (hipercalemia)	Iperkaliemia
Hipernefrom	Renal cell carcinoma (hypernephroma)	Carcinome à cellules rénales	Carcinoma de células renales	Carcinoma a cellule renali
Hiperparatireoidizam	Hyperparathyroidism	Hyperparathyroïdie	Hiperparatiroidismo	Iperparatiroidismo
Hiperpituitarizam	Hyperpituitarism	Hyperpituitarisme	Hiperpituitarismo	Iperpituitarismo
Hiperplazija endometrija	Endometrial hyperplasia	Hyperplasie endométriale	Hiperplasia endometrial	Iperplasia endometriale
Hipertermija	Hyperthermia	Hyperthermie	Hipertermia	Ipertermia
Hipertireoza	Hyperthyroidism	Hyperthyroïdie	Hipertiroidismo	Ipertiroidismo
Hipertrofija	Hypertrophy	Hypertrophie	Hipertrofia	Ipertrofia
Hipertrofijska kardiomiopatija	Hypertrophic cardiomyopathy	Cardiomyopathie hypertrophique	Miocardiopatía hipertrófica	Cardiomiopatia ipertrofica
Hipertrofijska stenoza pilorusa	Hypertrophic pyloric stenosis	Sténose hypertrophique du pylore	Estenosis pilórica hipertrófica	Stenosi ipertrofica del piloro
Hiperurikemija	Hyperuricemia	Hyperuricémie	Hiperuricemia	Iperuricemia
Hiperventilacija	Hyperventilation	Hyperventilation	Hiperventilación	Iperventilazione
Hipervitaminoza	Hypervitaminosis	Hypervitaminose	Hipervitaminosis	Ipervitaminosi
Hipervolemija (porast volumena krvi u optoku)	Hypervolemia (increased level of fluid in the blood)	Hypervolémie (augmentation du volume de sang dans les vaisseaux)	Hipervolemia (aumento del volumen de sangre en la circulación)	Ipervolemia (aumento del volume ematico circolante)
Hipoalbuminemija	Hypoalbuminemia	Hypoalbuminémie	Hipoalbuminemia	Ipoalbuminemia
Hipoglikemija	Hypoglycemia	Hypoglycémie	Hipoglicemia	Ipoglicemia
Hipohondrija	Hypochondria	Hypocondrie	Hipocondría	Ipocondria
Hipoinzulinizam	Hypoinsulinism	Hypoinsulinisme	Hipoinsulinismo	Ipoinsulinemia
Hipokalcijemija	Hypocalcemia	Hypocalcémie	Hipocalcemia	Ipocalcemia
Hipokalijemija	Hypokalemia	Hypokaliémie	Hipocaliemia	Ipokaliemia
Hipokromna anemija	Hypochromic anemia	Anémie hypochrome	Anemia hipocrómica	Anemia ipocromica
Hipoksija	Hypoxia	Hypoxie	Hipoxia	Ipossia
Hipoparatireodizam	Hypoparathyroidism	Hypoparathyroïdie	Hipoparatiroidismo	Ipoparatiroidismo
Hipopituitarizam	Hypopituitarism	Hypopituitarisme	Hipopituitarismo	Ipopituitarismo
Hipoplazija plućnog režnja	Pulmonary hypoplasia	Hypoplasie pulmonaire	Hipoplasia pulmonar	Ipoplasia del tronco polmonare
Hipospadija	Hypospadias	Hypospadias	Hipospadias	Ipospadia
Hipotenzija i sinkope	Hypotension and syncope	Hypotension et syncope	Hipotensión y síncope	Ipotensione e sincope
Hipotireoza	Hypothyroidism	Hypothyroïdie	Hipotiroidismo	Ipotiroidismo
Hipotonija	Hypotonia	Hypotonie	Hipotonía	Ipotonia
Hipovolemički šok	Hypovolemic shock	Choc hypovolémique	Choque hipovolémico	Shock ipovolemico
Hirschsprungova bolest (kongenitalni aganglionarni megakolon)	Hirschsprung's disease (congenital aganglionic megacolon)	Maladie de Hirschsprung (mégacolôn)	Enfermedad de Hirschsprung (megacolon agangliónico)	Malattia di Hirschsprung (malattia di Mya)
Hirzutizam	Hirsutism	Hirsutisme	Hirsutismo	Irsutismo
Histerija	Hysteria	Hystérie	Histeria	Isteria (isterismo)
Histoplazmoza	Histoplasmosis (Darling's disease)	Histoplasmose	Histoplasmosis	Istoplasmosi
Hodgkinova bolest	Hodgkin's disease	Maladie de Hodgkin	Enfermedad de Hodgkin	Linfoma di Hodgkin
Hondroblastom	Chondroblastoma	Chondroblastome	Condroblastoma	Condroblastoma
Hondrom	Chondroma	Chondrome	Condroma	Condroma
Hondromalacija patele (trkačko koljeno, sindrom patelofemoralne boli)	Chondromalacia patellae (runner's knee, patello-femoral pain syndrome)	Chondromalacie rotulienne	Chondromalacia rotuliana (síndrome patelo-femoral)	Sindrome del dolore patello-femorale (ginocchio del corridore)
Hondromiksoidni fibrom	Chondromyxoid fibroma	Fibrome chondromyxoïde	Fibroma condromixoide	Fibroma condromixoide
Hondrosarkom	Chondrosarcoma	Chondrosarcome	Condrosarcoma	Condrosarcoma
Hripavac (pasji kašalj, pertussis)	Whooping cough (pertussis)	Coqueluche	Tos ferina (coqueluche)	Pertosse

Hrvatski	Engleski	Francuski	Španjolski	Talijanski
Huntingtonova koreja	Huntington's chorea (Huntington's disease)	Chorée de Huntington (maladie de Huntington)	Enfermedad de Huntington (corea de Huntington)	Malattia di Huntington
Ileus	Ileus	Iléus	Íleo	Ileo
Impetigo	Impetigo	Impétigo	Impétigo	Impetigine
Impotencija	Impotency	Impotence	Impotencia	Impotenza
Infarkt	Infarct	Infarctus	Infarto	Infarto
Infarkt miokarda	Heart attack (myocardial infarction)	Infarctus du myocarde	Infarto de miocardio	Infarto miocardico acuto
Infarkt pluća	Pulmonary infarction	Infarctus pulmonaire	Infarto pulmonar	Infarto polmonare
Infekcija	Infection	Infection	Infección	Infezione (malattia infettiva)
Infekcija gornjih dišnih puteva	Upper respiratory tract infection	Infection respiratoire haute	Infección respiratoria alta	Infezione del tratto respiratorio superiore
Infekcija humanim papiloma virusom (HPV)	Human papilloma virus (HPV) infection	Infection par le virus du papillome humain (VPH)	Infeccion por el virus del papilom humano (VPH)	Infezione da Papilloma Virus Umano (HPV)
Infekcija kosti ili koštane srži (osteomijelitis)	Infection of the bone or bone marrow (osteomyelitis)	Infection osseuse ou de la moelle osseuse (ostéomyélite)	Infección del hueso o médula ósea (osteomielitis)	Infezione dell'apparato osteo-articolare (osteomielite)
Infekcijski artritis (septički artritis)	Infectious arthritis (septic arthritis)	Arthrite septique	Artritis infecciosa (artritis séptica)	Artrite settica
Infektivni eritem (peta bolest)	Infectious erythema (fifth disease)	Érythème infectieux (cinquième maladie)	Eritema infeccioso (quinta enfermedad)	Eritema infettivo (quinta malattia)
Infestacija crijevnim parazitima (helmintijaza)	Infestation with intestinal parasitic warms (helminthiasis)	Infestation par des vers parasites intestinaux (helminthiase)	Infestación de gusanos (helmintiasis)	Infestazione da vermi (elmintiasi)
Infestacija stidnim ušima (iftirijaza)	Infestation with pubic lice (phthiriasis)	Infestation par des poux du pubic (phtiriase)	Infestación por ladilla (ftiriasis)	Infestazione da pidocchi del pube (ftiriasi)
Infestacija ušima (ušljivost, pedikuloza)	Infestation with head lice (pediculosis)	Infestation par des poux (pédiculose)	Infestación por piojos (pediculosis)	Infestazione da pidocchi (pediculosi)
Inkontinencija	Incontinence	Incontinence	Incontinencia	Incontinenza
Intermitentna klaudikacija	Intermittent claudication	Claudication intermittente	Claudicación intermitente	Claudicatio intermittens
Intersticijska bolest pluća	Interstitial lung disease	Maladie pulmonaire interstitielle	Enfermedad pulmonar intersticial	Pneumopatia interstiziale
Intersticijska upala bubrega	Interstitial nephritis	Néphrite interstitielle	Nefritis intersticial	Nefrite interstiziale
Intracerebralni hematom	Intracerebral hematoma	Hématome intracérébral	Hematoma intracerebral	Ematoma cerebrale
Intracerebralno krvarenje	Intracerebral hemorrhage	Hémorragie intracérébrale	Hemorragia intracerebral	Emorragia cerebrale
Intrakranijalna hipertenzija	Intracranial hypertension	Hypertension intra-crânienne	Hipertensión intracraneal	Elevata pressione intracranica
Ionizirajuća ozračenost	Ionising irradiation	Irradiation ionisante	Exposición a las radiaciones ionizantes	Esposizione alle radiazioni ionizzanti
Iridodijaliza	Iridodialysis (coredialysis)	Iridodialyse	Iridodiálisis	Iridodialisi
Iritantni kontaktni dermatitis	Irritant contact dermatitis	Dermite de contact irritative	Dermatitis irritante de contacto	Dermatite irritativo da contatto
Iritis	Iritis	Iritis	Iritis	Irite
Iscjedak	Discharge	Sécrétion (suintement, écoulement)	Flujo (descarga, secreción)	Fuoriuscita (scolo)
Iscrpljenost (umor, fatigo)	Fatigue (exhaustion, lethargy)	Fatigue (affaiblissement)	Cansancio (fatiga, letargo, astenia)	Stanchezza (fatica, astenia)
Ishemična ulceracija	Ischemic ulceration	Ulcère ischémique	Úlcera isquémica	Ulcera ischemica
Ishemični udovi	Ischemic limbs	Ischémie des membres	Isquemia de miembros	Ischemia degli arti
Ishemija	Ischemia	Ischémie	Isquemia	Ischemia
Ishemijska bolest srca	Ischemic heart disease	Ischémie myocardique	Isquemia miocárdica (angina de pecho)	Ischemia miocardica
Iskašljavanje krvi (hemoptiza, hemoptoja)	Expectoration of blood (hemoptysis)	Rejet de sang issu des voies aériennes (hémoptysie)	Expectoración de sangre (hemoptisis)	Espettorazione di sangue (emottisi)
Istegnuće	Strain (sprain, pull)	Déchirure	Desgarro	Stiramento
Istegnuće ligamenta	Ligament strain	Déchirure ligamentaire	Desgarro de ligamento	Stiramento del legamento
Istegnuće mišića (distenzija mišića)	Muscle strain (muscle pull)	Déchirure musculaire (claquage)	Desgarro muscular	Strappo muscolare
Istegnuće tetive (distenzija tetive)	Tendon strain	Déchirure au tendon	Desgarro de tendón	Stiramento del tendine
Iščašenje (dislokacija, luksacija)	Dislocation (luxation)	Déboîtement (luxation)	Luxación (lujación, dislocación)	Lussazione
Iščašenje akromioklavikularnog zgloba	Separated shoulder (acromioclavicular dislocation)	Luxation acromio-claviculaire	Luxación de la articulación acromioclavicular	Lussazione acromio-clavicolare
Iščašenje čašice	Luxating patella (trick knee, floating patella)	Luxation de la rotule	Luxación de la rótula	Lussazione della rotula
Iščašenje koljena	Knee dislocation (luxation of the knee)	Luxation du genou	Luxación de la rodilla	Lussazione del ginocchio
Iščašenje kuka	Dislocation of a hip	Luxation de la hanche	Luxación de la cadera	Lussazione dell'anca
Iščašenje lakta	Elbow dislocation (luxation of the elbow)	Luxation du coude	Luxación del codo	Lussazione del gomito
Iščašenje ramena	Dislocated shoulder	Luxation de l'épaule	Luxación del hombro	Lussazione della spalla
Iščašenje skočnog zgloba	Dislocated ankle joint	Luxation de la cheville	Luxación del tobillo	Lussazione della caviglia
Iščašenje vilice	Mandibular dislocation	Luxation temporo-mandibulaire	Dislocación de la mandibula	Lussazione della mandibola

Hrvatski	Engleski	Francuski	Španjolski	Talijanski
Iščašenje zglobova šake i prstiju	Hand and finger joints dislocation	Luxation des doigts et du poignet	Luxaciones de la mano y los dedos	Lussazioni delle atricolazioni della mano e delle dita
Išijas	Sciatica	Sciatique	Ciática	Sciatica
Izbuljene oči (egzoftalmus)	Bulging eyes (exophthalmos)	Exophtalmie (proptose)	Exoftalmos	Esoftalmo
Izdubljeno stopalo (pes excavatus)	High arches (pes cavus)	Pied creux	Pie cavo (pes cavus)	Piede cavo (pes cavus)
Izgladnjelost	Starvation	Famine	Inanición	Inedia
Izosporijaza	Isosporiasis	Isosporose	Isosporiasis	Isosporiasi
Izostanak mjesečnice (amenoreja)	Absence of menstrual period (amenorrhea)	Absence des règles (aménorrhée)	Ausencia de la menstruación (amenorrea)	Assenza di mestruazioni (amenorrea)
Izvanmaternična trudnoća (ektopična trudnoća)	Ectopic pregnancy (extrauterine pregnancy)	Grossesse extra-utérine	Embarazo ectópico	Gravidanza ectopica
Izvanzglobni reumatizam	Extrajoint rheumatism	Rhumatisme extraarticulaire	Reumatismo extraarticular	Reumatismo extra-articolare
Izvijanje mišića vrata i leđa u luk (opistotonus)	Spastic arching position (opisthotonus)	Contracture sur les muscles extenseurs de sorte que le corps est incurvé en arrière (opisthotonos)	Contracción del cuerpo entero de tal manera que se mantiene encorvado hacia atrás (opistótonos)	Iperestenzione della regione posteriore del tronco (opistotono)
Izvrnuto stopalo (pes valgus)	Pes valgus	Pied valgus	Pie valgo	Piede piatto valgo (pes valgus)
Japanska riječna groznica (Tsutsugamushi groznica)	Scrub typhus (Japanese river fever, Tsutsugamushi fever)	Fièvre fluviale du Japon (typhus à chiques)	Tsutsugamushi (fiebre fluvial japonesa, tifus de los matorrales)	Tsutsugamushi (tifo fluviale giapponese)
Ječmenac	Stye (chalazion)	Chalazion	Orzuelo	Calazio
Jednostavni prijelom kosti	Simple bone fracture	Fracture simple	Fractura simple	Frattura semplice
Juvenilna osteohondroza	Juvenile osteochondrosis	Ostéochondrose juvénile	Osteocondrosis juvenil	Osteocondrite dissecante
Kaheksija	Cachexia	Cachexie	Caquexia	Cachessia
Kala-azar	Kala-azar (black fever)	Kala azar (fièvre noire)	Kala azar (fiebre negra)	Kala-azar (febbre d'Assam, splenomegalia infantile)
Kalikoza	Chalicosis	Chalicose	Calicosis	Calicosi
Kamenac mokraćnog mjehura	Bladder stone (urolithiasis)	Calcul urinaire (urolithiase)	Cálculo en el tracto urinario (urolitiasis)	Calcolo urinario (urolitiasi)
Kandidijaza	Candidiasis (thrush)	Candidiase	Candidiasis	Candidosi (candidiasi)
Kapilarni hemangiom	Capillary hemangioma (infantile hemangioma, strawberry hemangioma)	Hémangiome capillaire	Hemangioma capilar (marca de fresa)	Emangioma capillare
Kaposijev sarkom (endoteliosarkom)	Kaposi's sarcoma	Sarcome de Kaposi	Sarcoma de Kaposi	Sarcoma di Kaposi
Karbunkul	Carbuncle	Anthrax	Ántrax (carbunco)	Carbonchio (pustola)
Karcinoid	Carcinoid	Carcinoïde	Carcinoide	Carcinoide
Karcinoid bronha	Bronchial carcinoid	Carcinoïde bronchiale	Carcinoide bronquial	Carcinoide bronchiale
Karcinoidni sindrom	Carcinoid syndrome	Syndrome carcinoïde	Síndrome carcinoide	Sindrome da carcinoide
Karcinom	Carcinoma	Carcinome	Carcinoma	Carcinoma
Karcinom bazalnih stanica (bazaliom)	Basal cell carcinoma	Carcinome basocellulaire	Carcinoma de células basales (basilioma)	Basalioma (carcinoma basocellulare)
Karcinom bronha	Bronchial carcinoma	Carcinome bronchique	Carcinoma bronquial	Carcinoma bronchiale
Karcinom dojke	Breast carcinoma	Carcinome du sein	Carcinoma de mama	Carcinoma mammario
Karcinom endometrija	Endometrial carcinoma	Carcinome de l'endomètre	Carcinoma de endometrio	Carcinoma endometriale
Karcinom grlića maternice	Cervical carcinoma	Carcinome du col utérin	Carcinoma del cuello uterino	Carcinoma della cervice uterina
Karcinom pokrovnog epitela	Epithelial carcinoma	Carcinome épithélial	Carcinoma epitelial	Carcinoma epiteliale
Karcinom prostate	Prostate carcinoma	Carcinome de la prostate	Carcinoma de próstata	Carcinoma della prostata
Karcinom želuca	Gastric carcinoma	Carcinome de l'estomac	Carcinoma gástrico	Carcinoma gastrico
Karcinoza	Carcinosis	Carcinose	Carcinosis	Carcinosi (carcinomatosi, cancerosi)
Karcinoza peritoneuma	Peritoneal carcinosis	Carcinose péritonéale	Carcinosis peritoneal	Carcinosi peritoneale
Karcinoza perikarda	Pericardial carcinosis	Carcinose péricardique	Carcinosis pericárdica	Carcinosi pericardiale
Karcinoza pleure	Pleural carcinosis	Carcinose pleurale	Carcinosis pleural	Carcinosi pleurica
Kardiogeni šok	Cardiogenic shock	Choc cardiogénique	Choque cardiogénico	Shock cardiogeno
Kardiomiopatija	Cardiomyopathy	Cardiomyopathie	Miocardiopatía	Cardiomiopatia
Kašalj	Cough	Toux	Tos	Tosse
Katalepsija	Catalepsy	Catalepsie	Catalepsia	Catalessia
Katapleksija	Cataplexy	Cataplexie	Cataplexia (cataplejía)	Cataplessia
Katar	Catarrh	Catarrhe	Catarro	Catarro
Kavernozni hemangiom	Cavernous hemangioma	Cavernome (angiome caverneux)	Hemangioma cavernoso	Emangioma cavernoso
Kawasakijeva bolest (mukokutani limfoglandularni sindrom)	Kawasaki disease	Maladie de Kawasaki	Enfermedad de Kawasaki	Sindrome di Kawasaki
Keloid	Keloid	Chéloïde	Queloide	Cheloide
Kemijske ozljede	Chemical injuries	Altération d'origine chimique	Lesiones químicas	Ferita chimica
Kemijski konjuktivitis	Chemical conjunctivitis	Conjonctivite chimique	Conjuntivitis química	Congiuntivite irritativa da agenti chimici
Keratoza	Keratosis	Kératose (kératodermie)	Keratosis	Cheratosi

Hrvatski	Engleski	Francuski	Španjolski	Talijanski
Kienböckova bolest	Kienböck's disease	Maladie de Kienböck	Enfermedad de Kienböck	Morbo di Kienböck
Kifoskolioza	Kyphoscoliosis	Cypho-scoliose	Cifoescoliosis	Cifoscoliosi
Kifoza	Kyphosis	Cyphose	Cifosis	Cifosi
Kihanje	Sneezing	Éternuement	Estornudo	Starnuto
Kila (bruh, hernija)	Hernia	Hernie	Hernia	Ernia
Kila vanjske trbušne stijenke	External abdominal wall hernia	Hernie de la paroi abdominale (hernie abdominale externe)	Hernia de la pared abdominal	Ernia esterna addominale
Kilna vreća	Hernia sack	Sac herniaire	Saco de hernia (saco herniario)	Sacco dell'ernia
Kirurški šok	Surgical shock (postoperative shock)	Choc post-opératoire	Choque quirúrgico	Shock chirurgico
Klamidijska infekcija	Chlamydia infection	Infection à Chlamydia	Infección por clamidia	Infezione da clamidia
Klaustrofobija (strah od zatvorenog prostora)	Claustrophobia (fear of closed space)	Claustrophobie	Claustrofobia (miedo a los espacios cerrados)	Claustrofobia (paura di luoghi chiusi)
Kleptomanija	Kleptomania	Cleptomanie	Cleptomanía	Cleptomania
Kloazma (melazma)	Melasma (chloasma faciei)	Chleuasme (chloasma)	Melasma (cloasma)	Melasma
Klonorkijaza	Clonorchiasis	Clonorchiase	Clonorquiasis (clonorquiosis)	Clonorchiasi
Koarktacija aorte	Coarctation of the aorta	Coarctation de l'aorte	Coartación de la aorta	Coartazione dell'aorta
Kočenje šije (ukočeni vrat)	Nuchal rigidity (stiff neck)	Raideur de nuque (raideur méningée)	Rigidez de nuca (cuello rígido)	Rigidità nucale
Köhlerova bolest	Köhler disease	Maladie de Köhler	Enfermedad de Köhler	Malattia di Köhler
Kokcidioidomikoza (San Joaquin Valley vrućica)	Coccidioidomycosis (San Joaquin Valley fever)	Coccidioïmycose (fièvre de la vallée de San Joaquin, fièvre du désert)	Coccidioidomicosis	Coccidiomicosi
Kokcigodinija	Coccygodynia	Coccygodynie (douleur coccygienne)	Coccigodinia (dolor de coxis)	Coccigodinia
Kokošja prsa	Pigeon chest (pectus carinatum)	Pectus carinatum	Pectus carinatum	Petto carenato
Kokošje sljepilo (hemeralopija)	Day blindness (hemeralopia)	Héméralopie	Falta de visión en luz brillante (hemeralopia)	Emeralopia
Kolangiocelularni karcinom	Cholangiocellular carcinoma	Cholangiocarcinome	Carcinoma de las vías biliares (colangiocarcinoma)	Colangiocarcinoma (carcinoma colangiocellulare)
Kolaps	Collapse	Collapsus	Colapso	Collasso
Kolera	Cholera	Choléra	Cólera	Colera
Kolika	Colic	Colique	Cólico	Colica
Koma	Coma	Coma	Coma	Coma
Kominutivni prijelom kosti	Comminuted fracture	Fracture comminutive	Fractura cominuta	Frattura comminuta
Kompresija mozga	Brain compression	Compression cérébrale	Compresión cerebral	Compressione cerebrale
Kompresija živca (ukliješten živac)	Nerve compression (pinched nerve)	Compression du nerf	Compresión del nérvio	Compressone del nervo
Kontaktni dermatitis	Contact dermatitis	Dermite de contact	Dermatitis de contacto	Dermatite da contatto
Kontraktura	Contracture	Contracture	Contractura	Contrattura
Kontraktura mišića	Muscular contracture	Contracture musculaire	Contractura muscular	Contrattura muscolare
Kontraktura zgloba	Joint contracture	Contracture articulaire	Contractura articular	Contrattura articolare
Konvulzije	Convulsions	Convulsions	Convulsiones	Convulsioni
Konjuktivitis izazvan stranim tijelom	Conjunctival foreign body	Conjonctivite due à un corps étranger	Conjuntivitis por cuerpo extraño	Congiuntivite irritativa da corpi estranei
Koplikove pjege	Koplik's spots	Signe de Koplik	Manchas de Koplik	Macchie di Koplik
Koprivnjača (urtikarija)	Hives (urticaria)	Urticaire	Urticaria	Orticaria
Koreoatetoza	Choreoathetosis	Choréoathétose	Coreoatetosis	Coreoatetosi
Koriokarcinom	Choriocarcinoma	Choriocarcinome	Coriocarcinoma	Coriocarcinoma
Koronarna bolest (koronaropatija)	Coronary disease	Maladie coronarienne	Enfermedad coronaria	Coronaropatia
Kosi prijelom kosti	Oblique fracture	Fracture oblique	Fractura obliqua	Frattura obliqua
Kožni privjesak (mekani fibrom)	Soft fibroma (fibroma molle, acrochordon)	Molluscum pendulum (acrochordon)	Fibroma blando (fibroma molle)	Mollusco pendule (fibroma molle)
Krasta	Crust (scab)	Croûte	Costra	Crosta (escara)
Kratkovidnost	Shortsightedness (myopia)	Myopie	Miopía	Miopia
Krepitacija	Crepitation	Crépitation	Crepitación	Crepitazione
Krimska hemoragijska groznica	Crimean-Congo hemorrhagic fever	Fièvre hémorragique de Congo-Crimée	Fiebre hemorrágica de Crimea-Congo	Febbre emorragica Crimean-Congo
Kriptogena ciroza	Cryptogenic cirrhosis	Cirrhose cryptogénique	Cirrosis criptogénica	Cirrosi criptogenica
Kriptokokoza	Cryptococcosis	Cryptococcose	Criptococcosis	Criptococcosi
Krivi vrat (tortikolis)	Wry neck (torticollis)	Torticolis	Tortícolis	Torcicollo
Križobolja (lumbosakralni sindrom)	Low back pain (lumbago, lumbosacral syndrome)	Lombalgie	Dolor de espalda baja (lumbalgia)	Lombaggine
Kromomikoza	Chromoblastomycosis (chromomycosis, Pedroso's disease)	Chromomycose	Cromomicosis (cromoblastomicosis)	Cromomicosi (cromoblastomicosi)
Kronična bol	Chronic pain	Douleur chronique	Dolor crónico	Dolore cronico
Kronična cerebrospinalna venozna insuficijencija	Chronic cerebrospinal venous insufficiency	Insuffisance veineuse cérébro-spinale chronique	Insuficiencia venosa cerebro-espinal crónica	Insufficienza venosa cronica cerebrospinale
Kronična limfocitna leukemija	Chronic lymphocytic leukemia	Leucémie lymphoïde chronique	Leucemia linfocítica crónica	Leucemia linfatica cronica

Hrvatski	Engleski	Francuski	Španjolski	Talijanski
Kronična mijeloična leukemija	Chronic myeloid leukemia	Leucémie myéloïde chronique	Leucemia mieloide crónica	Leucemia mieloide cronica
Kronična opstruktivna plućna bolest	Chronic obstructive pulmonary disease	Broncho-pneumopathie chronique obstructive	Enfermedad pulmonar obstructiva crónica	Bronchite cronica
Kronična paroksizmalna hemikranija (Sjaastadov sindrom)	Chronic paroxysmal hemicrania (Sjaastad syndrome)	Hémicrânie paroxystique chronique	Hemicránea crónica paroxismal	Emicrania cronica parossistica
Kronično zatajenje bubrega	Chronic renal failure	Insuffisance rénale chronique	Insuficiencia renal crónica	Insufficienza renale cronica
Krpeljni meningoencefalitis	Tick-borne meningoencephalitis	Méningoencéphalite à tique	Meningoencefalitis de garrapata	Encefalite trasmessa da zecche
Kruljenje u želucu	Stomach growling (borborygmus)	Gargouillements (borborygme)	Sonidos de tripas (borborigmo)	Borborigmo
Krup (akutni opstruktivni laringitis)	Croup (acute obstructive laryngitis)	Croup (laryngotrachéo-bronchite)	Crup (laringotraqueo-bronquitis)	Croup (laringite acuta ostruttiva)
Krv u likvoru	Blood in cerebrospinal fluid	Sang dans le liquide cérébro-spinal	Sangre en el líquido cefalorraquídeo	Sangue al liquido cerebrospinale
Krv u stolici (hematohezija)	Blood in stool (hematochezia)	Sang dans les selles (hématochézie)	Sangre en las heces (hematochezia)	Sangue nelle feci (ematochezia)
Krv u urinu (hematurija)	Blood in urine (hematuria)	Sang dans les urines (hématurie)	Sangre en la orina (hematuria)	Ematuria
Krvarenje (hemoragija)	Bleeding (haemorrhage)	Saignement (hémorragie)	Desangramiento (hemorragia)	Emorragia
Krvarenje iz analnog otvora	Anal bleeding	Saignement anal (rectorragie)	Pérdida de sangre a través del ano (rectorragia)	Perdita di sangue dall'ano (rettoragia, proctorragia)
Krvarenje iz maternice (metroragija)	Uterine bleeding (metrorrhagia)	Saignement de l'utérus (métrorragie)	Pérdida de sangre uterina (metrorragia)	Perdita di sangue al di fuori della mestruazione (metrorragia)
Krvarenje iz nosa (epistaksa)	Nose bleeding (epistaxis)	Saignement de nez (épistaxis)	Pérdida de sangre por la nariz (epistaxis)	Epistassi (rinorragia)
Krvarenje iz uha	Ear bleeding	Saignement de l'oreille	Hemorragia de oído (otorragia)	Fuoriuscita di sangue dall'orecchio (otorragia)
Krvarenje u jajovod (hematosalpinks)	Bleeding into the fallopian tube (hematosalpinx)	Collection de sang dans la trompe de Fallope (hématosalpinx)	Colección de sangre en la trompa de Falopio (hematosalpinx)	Flusso di sangue nella tuba di Falloppio
Krvarenje u zglob (hemartroza)	Bleeding into joint space (hemarthrosis)	Épanchement de sang à l'intérieur d'une articulation (hémarthrose)	Sangrado interno de las articulaciones (hemartrosis)	Emartro
Krvavi iskašljaj (hemoptiza)	Blood in sputum (hemoptysis)	Sang dans l'expectoration (hémoptysie)	Sangre en el esputo (hemoptysis)	Sangue nello sputo (emottisi)
Krvni ugrušak (tromb)	Blood clot (thrombus)	Caillot sanguin (thrombus)	Coágulo sanguíneo (trombo)	Trombo
Ksantelazma	Xanthelasma	Xanthelasma	Xantelasma	Xantelasma
Ksantom	Xanthoma	Xanthome	Xantoma	Xantoma
Kuga	Plague (pest)	Peste	Peste	Peste (pestilenza)
Kuglasta aneurizma arterije mozga	Ball-shaped aneurysm of the brain artery	Anévrisme intra-crânien en forme de sac	Aneurisma cerebral arterial sacular	Aneurisma cerebrale sferica
Kuru (smrtni smijeh)	Kuru	Kuru	Kuru (muerte de la risa)	Kuru
Kussmaulovo disanje	Kussmaul breathing	Respiration de type Kussmaul	Respiración de Kussmaul	Respiro di Kussmaul
Kvržica	Knot (lump)	Nodule	Nudo	Nodo (nodulo)
Laceracija mozga	Brain laceration	Lacération cérébrale	Laceración cerebral	Lacerazione cerebrale
Lajmska bolest (Lajmska borelioza)	Lyme disease (lyme borreliosis)	Maladie de Lyme	Enfermedad de Lyme (borreliosis de Lyme)	Malattia di Lyme (borreliosi di Lyme)
Lamblijaza (giardijaza)	Lambliasis (giardiasis)	Lambliase (giardiase)	Giardiasis (lambliasis)	Giardiasi (lambliasi)
Laringospazam	Laryngospasm	Laryngospasme	Laringoespasmo	Laringospasmo
Legg-Calvé-Perthesova bolest	Legg-Calvé-Perthes disease	Maladie de Legg-Calvé-Perthes (ostéochondrite primitive de hanche)	Síndrome de Legg-Calvé-Perthes	Malattia di Legg-Perthes-Calvé
Lejomiom	Leiomyoma	Léiomyome	Leiomioma	Leiomioma
Lejomiosarkom	Leiomyosarcoma	Leiomyosarcome	Leiomiosarcoma	Leiomiosarcoma
Lepra (guba)	Leprosy	Lèpre	Lepra	Lebbra
Leptospiroza	Leptospirosis	Leptospirose	Leptospirosis	Leptospirosi
Lericheov sindrom	Aortoiliac occlusive disease (Leriche's syndrome)	Maladie occlusive aorto-iliaque	Síndrome de Leriche	Sindrome di Leriche
Leukemija	Leukemia	Leucémie	Leucemia	Leucemia
Leukocitoza	Leukocytosis	Leucocytose	Leucocitosis	Leucocitosi
Leukodistrofija	Leukodystrophy	Leucodystrophie	Leucodistrofia	Leucodistrofia
Leukoplakija	Leukoplakia	Leucoplasie	Leucoplaquia	Leucoplachia
Limfangiom	Lymphangioma	Lymphangiome	Linfangioma	Linfangioma
Limfangiosarkom	Lymphangiosarcoma	Lymphangiosarcome	Linfangiosarcoma	Linfangiosarcoma
Limfatična leukemija	Lymphatic leukemia	Leucémie lymphoïde	Leucemia linfática	Leucemia linfatica
Limfedem (zastoj limfe)	Lymphedema	Lymphoedème	Linfedema	Linfedema
Limfocitni koriomeningitis	Lymphocytic choriomeningitis	Chorioméningite lymphocytaire	Coriomeningitis linfocítica	Coriomeningite linfocitaria
Limfom	Lymphoma	Lymphome	Linfoma	Linfoma
Lipodistrofija	Lipodystrophy	Lipodystrophie	Lipodistrofia	Lipodistrofia
Lipom	Lipoma	Lipome	Lipoma	Lipoma

Hrvatski	Engleski	Francuski	Španjolski	Talijanski
Lipomatoza gušterače (masna infiltracija gušterače)	Pancreatic lipomatosis	Lipomatose du pancréas	Lipomatosis pancreática (reemplazo graso del páncreas)	Lipomatosi pancreatica
Liposarkom	Liposarcoma	Liposarcome	Liposarcoma	Liposarcoma
Listerioza	Listeriosis	Listériose	Listeriosis	Listeriosi
Lišaj (lichen planus)	Lichen planus	Lichen plan	Liquen plano	Lichen planus
Lišmenijaza	Leishmaniasis	Leishmaniose	Leishmaniasis	Leishmaniosi
Lobster Claw stopalo	Split foot (lobster claw foot, ectrodactyly)	Pince de homard (aplasie digitale, ectrodactylie)	Ectrodactilia en pie	Lobster-claw deformità di piede
Lojna cista	Sebaceous cyst (wen)	Kyste sébacé	Quiste sebáceo	Cisti sebacea
Lordoza	Lordosis	Lordose	Lordosis	Lordosi
Luetični osteomijelitis	Luetic osteomyelitis	Ostéomyélite syphilitique	Osteomielitis luética	Osteomielite luetica
Lupanje srca (palpitacije)	Palpitation	Palpitation	Palpitación	Cardiopalmo (palpitazione)
Ljuštenje kože (deskvamacija)	Shedding of the skin (desquamation)	Desquamation	Desquamación	Perdita dello strato superiore della pelle (desquamazione)
Madelungov deformitet	Madelung's deformity	Déformation de Madelung	Deformidad de Madelung	Deformità di Madelung
Madež (nevus)	Birthmark (nevus)	Grain de beauté (naevus)	Nevus (nevo)	Voglia (neo, nevo)
Malapsorpcija	Malabsorption	Malabsorption	Malabsorción	Malassorbimento
Malarija	Malaria	Malaria	Malaria (paludismo)	Malaria
Maligna hipertenzija	Malignant hypertension	Hypertension artérielle maligne	Hipertensión maligna	Ipertensione maligna
Manija	Mania	Manie	Manía	Mania
Manjak estrogena	Estrogen deficiency	Carence oestrogénique	Deficiencia de estrógenos	Carenza di estrogeno
Manjak faktora koagulacije	Coagulation factor deficiency	Déficit en facteur de la coagulation	Deficiencia de factor de coagulación	Carenza di fattore di coagulazione
Manjak sperme (oligospermija)	Low semen volume (oligospermia)	Présence de spermatozoïdes en quantité faible (oligospermie)	Bajo volumen de semen (oligospermia)	Produzione di pochi spermatozoi (oligospermia)
Manjak vitamina	Vitamin deficiency	Carence en vitamine	Carencia de vitamina	Carenza di vitamine
Manjak vitamina A	Vitamin A deficiency	Carence en vitamine A	Carencia de vitamina A	Carenza di vitamina A
Manjak vitamina B1	Vitamin B1 deficiency	Carence en vitamine B1	Carencia de vitamina B1	Carenza di vitamina B1
Manjak vitamina B2	Vitamin B2 deficiency	Carence en vitamine B2	Carencia de vitamina B2	Carenza di vitamina B2
Manjak vitamina B3	Vitamin B3 deficiency	Carence en vitamine B3	Carencia de vitamina B3	Carenza di vitamina B3
Manjak vitamina B12	Vitamin B12 deficiency	Carence en vitamine B12	Carencia de vitamina B12	Carenza di vitamina B12
Manjak vitamina C	Vitamin C deficiency	Carence en vitamine C	Carencia de vitamina C	Carenza de vitamina C
Manjak vitamina D	Vitamin D deficiency	Carence en vitamine D	Carencia de vitamina D	Carenza de vitamina D
Manjak vitamina K	Vitamin K deficiency	Carence en vitamine K	Carencia de vitamina K	Carenza de vitamina K
Marburška hemoragijska groznica	Marburg hemorrhagic fever	Fièvre hémorragique de Marbourg	Fiebre hemorrágica de Marburgo	Febbre emorragica di Marburg
Marfanov sindrom	Marfan syndrome	Syndrome de Marfan	Síndrome de Marfan	Sindrome di Marfan
Masna embolija	Fat embolism	Embolie de cholestérol	Embolismo graso	Embolia adiposa
Masna metarmofoza jetre	Fatty liver metamorphosis	Stéatose hépatique	Metamorfosis grasa del hígado	Metamorfosi grassa del fegato
Mastopatija	Mastopathy	Mastopathie	Mastopatía	Mastopatia
Medularni karcinom	Medullary carcinoma	Carcinome médullaire	Carcinoma medular	Carcinoma midollare
Meduloblastom	Medulloblastoma	Médulloblastome	Meduloblastoma	Medulloblastoma
Megakolon	Megacolon	Mégacolôn	Megacolon	Megacolon
Megaloblastična anemija (anemija radi deficita vitamina)	Megaloblastic anemia	Anémie mégaloblastique	Anemia megaloblástica	Anemia megaloblastica
Mehaničke ozljede	Mechanical injuries	Lésions mécaniques	Lesiones mecánicas	Lesioni meccaniche
Mehanički ikterus	Mechanic icterus (bile duct obstruction)	Ictère par obstruction des voies biliaires	Ictericia obstructiva	Ittero ostruttivo
Meki čankir	Chancroid (soft chancre)	Chancre mou (chancrelle)	Chancroide (chancro blando)	Ulcera venerea (cancroide)
Melanom	Melanoma	Mélanome	Melanoma	Melanoma
Melioidoza	Melioidosis (Whitmore disease)	Mélioïdose	Melioidosis	Melioidosi
Menierova bolest	Meniere's disease	Maladie de Ménière	Enfermedad de Menière	Sindrome di Menière
Meningeom	Meningioma	Méningiome	Meningioma	Meningioma
Meningoencefalokela	Meningoencephalocele	Méningoencephalocèle	Meningoencefalocele	Meningoencefalocele
Meningokela	Meningocele	Méningocèle	Meningocele	Meningocele
Meningomijelokela	Meningomyelocele	Myéloméningocèle	Mielomeningocele	Mielomeningocele
Meniskopatija	Meniscal disease	Meniscopathie	Meniscopatia	Meniscopatia
Menopauza (klimakterij)	Menopause	Ménopause	Menopausia	Menopausa
Menstrualne smetnje	Menstrual disorder	Troubles du cycle menstruel	Trastorno menstrual	Disturbi mestruali
Mentalna retardacija	Mental retardation	Retard mental (handicap mental)	Retraso mental	Ritardo mentale
Metabolička acidoza	Metabolic acidosis	Acidose métabolique	Acidosis metabólica	Acidosi metabolica
Metalna groznica	Metal fume fever	Fièvre des métaux	Fiebre de los vapores metálicos	Febbre da inalazione di fumi metallici
Metastaza	Metastasis	Métastase	Metástasis	Metastasi
Metatarzalgija (Mortonova metatarzalgija)	Metatarsalgia (Morton's neuroma)	Métatarsalgie	Metatarsalgia	Metatarsalgia
Meteoropatija	Meteoropathy	Météoropathie	Meteoropatía	Meteoropatia

Hrvatski	Engleski	Francuski	Španjolski	Talijanski
Mezoteliom	Mesothelioma	Mésothéliome	Mesotélioma	Mesotelioma
Mezoteliosarkom	Sarcomatoid mesothelioma	Mésothéliome sarcomatoïde	Mesotélioma sarcomatoide	Mesotelioma sarcomatoide
Miastenija gravis	Myasthenia gravis	Myasthénie grave	Miastenia gravis	Miastenia gravis
Micetoma	Mycetoma	Mycétome	Micetoma	Micetoma
Migrena	Migraine	Migraine	Migraña (jaqueca)	Emicrania
Mijalgični sindrom vrata	Neck myalgia	Myalgie cervicale	Mialgia cervical	Mialgia cervicale
Mijelodisplastični sindrom	Myelodysplastic syndrome	Syndrome myélodysplasique	Síndrome mielodisplásico (preleucemia)	Sindrome mielodisplasica
Mijeloična leukemija	Myeloid leukemia	Leucémie myéloïde	Leucemia mieloide	Leucemia mieloide
Mikoza	Mycosis	Mycose	Micosis	Micosi
Miksedem	Myxedema	Myxoedème	Mixedema	Mixedema
Miksom	Myxoma	Myxome	Mixoma	Mixoma
Miksosarkom	Myxosarcoma	Myxosarcome	Mixosarcoma	Mixosarcoma
Milijarija rubra	Miliaria rubra (sweat rash)	Miliarie rouge	Miliaria rubra (sarpullido por el calor)	Miliaria rubra
Milije (dječje akne)	Milia (milk spots)	Milium (grutum, acné miliaire)	Milium (milia)	Acne miliare
Mioblastom	Myoblastoma	Rhabdomyome granocellulaire	Mioblastoma	Mioblastoma
Miogeloza	Myogelosis	Myogélose	Miogelosis	Miogelosi
Miokloničko trzanje (mioklonus)	Myoclonic twitches (myoclonus)	Myoclonie	Mioclono	Mioclono
Miom	Myoma	Myome	Mioma	Mioma
Miosarkom	Myosarcoma	Myosarcome	Miosarcoma	Miosarcoma
Mišićna distrofija	Muscular dystrophy	Dystrophie musculaire	Distrofia muscular	Distrofia muscolare
Mišićna hipotonija	Muscular hypotonia	Hypotonie musculaire	Hipotonía muscular	Ipotonia muscolare
Mišićni grč (spazam)	Muscular cramp (spasm)	Crampe musculaire (spasme)	Espasmo muscular (calambre)	Spasmo muscolare
Mjesečarenje (somnambulizam)	Sleepwalking (somnambulism)	Somnabulisme	Sonambulismo (noctambulismo)	Sonnambulismo
Mješoviti maligni tumor	Malignant mixed tumor	Tumeur mixte malin	Tumor mixto maligno	Tumore misto maligno
Mješoviti tumor	Mixed tumor	Tumeur mixte	Tumor mixto	Tumore misto
Mladenački reumatoidni artritis (juvenilni reumatoidni artritis)	Juvenile rheumatoid arthritis	Arthrite chronique juvénile	Artritis juvenil	Artrite idiopatica giovanile
Mlohavi mišić	Flaccid muscle (untoned muscle)	Muscle flasque (hypotonie musculaire)	Músculo flácido	Muscolo flaccido
Modrica (ekhimoza)	Bruise (ecchymosis)	Ecchymose	Moretón (equimosis)	Ammaccatura (ecchimosi)
Molusk	Molluscum contagiosum	Molluscum contagiosum	Molusco contagioso	Mollusco contagioso
Monocitična leukemija	Monocytic leukemia	Leucémie monocytique	Leucemia monocítica	Leucemia monocitica
Mononukleoza (bolest poljupca)	Infectious mononucleosis (Pfeiffer's disease, kissing disease, glandular fever)	Mononucléose infectieuse (maladie du baiser, maladie des amoureux)	Mononucleosis infecciosa (fiebre glandular, enfermedad de Pfeiffer)	Mononucleosi infettiva (malattia del bacio)
Morbus Hoffa	Hoffa's disease	Maladie de Hoffa	Enfermedad de Hoffa	Sindrome di Hoffa
Morbus Preiser	Preiser disease	Maladie de Preiser	Enfermedad de Preiser	Sindrome di Preiser
Morbus Van Neck	Van Neck disease	Maladie de Van Neck-Odelberg	Enfermedad de Van Neck	Malattia di Van Neck
Morska bolest	Seasickness	Mal de mer	Mal de mar	Mal di mare
Moždani udar	Stroke (cerebrovascular accident)	Attaque cérébrale (accident vasculaire cérébral)	Derrame cerebral (accidente cerebrovascular)	Colpo apoplettico
Moždano krvarenje (apopleksija)	Apoplexy	Apoplexie (attaque d'apoplexie)	Apoplejía (golpe apoplético)	Apoplessia
Mrena (katarakta)	Cataract	Cataracte	Catarata	Cataratta
MRSA	MRSA	SARM	SARM	MSSA (MRSA)
Mršavljenje	Weight loss (weight reduction)	Amaigrissement	Pérdida de peso	Dimagramento
Mučnina	Nausea	Nausée	Náusea	Nausea
Mukocela	Mucocele	Mucocèle	Mucocele	Mucocele
Mukopolisaharidoza	Mucopolysaccharido-sis	Mucopolysaccharidose	Mucopolisacaridosis	Mucopolisaccaridosi
Multipla sistemska atrofija	Multiple system atrophy	Atrophie multisystématisée	Atrofia multisistémica	Atrofia multi-sistemica
Multipla skleroza	Multiple sclerosis	Sclérose en plaques	Esclerosis múltiple	Sclerosi multipla
Multiple egzostoze	Hereditary multiple exostoses	Maladie des exostoses multiples	Exostosis múltiple hereditaria	Esostosi multipla ereditaria
Mutni urin	Unclear urine (foggy urine)	Urine opaque	Orina turbia	Urine torbide
Nadutost i vjetrovi	Bloating and gases (flatulence)	Ballonnements et vesse (flatulence)	Hinchazón y gases (flatulencia, ventosidad)	Gonfiezza e venti (flatulenza)
Nagluhost	Hard of hearing	Surdité partielle	Corto de oído (parcialmente sordo)	Sordità parziale
Nagnječenje (zgnječenje, kontuzija)	Contusion	Contusion	Contusión	Contusione
Nagnječenje mozga	Cerebral contusion	Contusion cérébrale	Contusión cerebral	Contusione cerebrale
Napadaj panike	Panic attack	Crise de panique	Ataque de pánico	Attaco di panico
Napetost trbušne stijenke	Abdominal wall tension	Tension de la paroi stomacale	Tensión de la pared abdominal	Tensione di parete addominale

Hrvatski	Engleski	Francuski	Španjolski	Talijanski
Narkolepsija	Narcolepsy	Narcolepsie (maladie de Gélineau)	Narcolepsia (síndrome de Gelineau, epilepsia del sueño)	Narcolessia
Nasilna smrt	Violent death	Mort violente	Muerte violenta	Morte violenta
Nefrotski sindrom	Nephrotic syndrome	Syndrome néphrotique	Síndrome nefrótico	Sindrome nefrosica
Nefroza	Nephrosis	Néphrose	Nefrosis	Nefrosi
Neionizirajuća ozračenost	Non-ionising irradiation	Irradiation non-ionisante	Irradiación no-ionizante	Irradiazione non ionizzante
Nejednaka veličina zjenica (anizokorija)	Unequal size of pupils (anisocoria)	Différence de taille entres les pupilles (anisocorie)	Asimetría del tamaño de las pupilas (anisocoria)	Diseguaglianza del diametro delle pupille (anisocoria)
Nekontrolirani pokreti očiju (opsoklonus)	Uncontrolled eye movement (opsoclonus)	Mouvements involontaires anarchiques des globes oculaires (opsoclonus)	Movimientos involuntarios y rápidos de los ojos (opsoclonus)	Movimenti incontrollati degli occhi (opsoclono)
Nekontrolirano psovanje (koprolalija)	Involuntary swearing (coprolalia)	Tic de langage à dire des mots vulgaires (coprolalie)	Expresión vocal involuntaria de obscenidades (coprolalia)	Coprolalia
Nekrotizirajući fasciitis	Necrotizing fasciitis	Fasciite nécrosante	Fascitis necrotizante	Fascite necrotizzante
Nekroza	Necrosis	Nécrose	Necrosis	Necrosi
Nemir (anksioznost)	Anxiety	Anxiété	Ansiedad	Ansia (ansietà)
Nemogućnost kretanja	Movement inability	Incapacité de se mouvoir	Incapacidad de movimiento	Mancanza di movimento
Nemogućnost mokrenja	Inability to urinate	Incapacité d'uriner	Incapacidad para orinar	Mancata secrezione di urina
Neplodnost (sterilitet)	Infertility (sterility)	Infertilité (stérilité)	Infertilidad	Sterilità (infecondità)
Nepodnošenje glutena	Gluten intolerance	Intolérance au gluten	Intolerancia al gluten	Intolleranza al glutine
Nepodnošenje laktoze (netolerancija laktoze)	Lactose intolerance	Intolérance au lactose	Intolerancia a la lactosa	Intolleranza al lattosio
Nepotpuni prijelom kosti (napuknuće kosti)	Incomplete fracture	Fracture incomplète	Fractura incompleta	Frattura incompleta (infrazione)
Nerazvijenost organa (aplazija organa)	Absence in development of an organ (aplasia of an organ)	Arrêt du développement d'un organe (aplasie d'un organe)	Desarrollo detenido de un órgano (aplasia de un órgano)	Mancato sviluppo di un organo (aplasia di un organo)
Nesanica	Insomnia	Insomnie	Insomnio	Insonnia
Nespušteni testis	Undescended testicle	Absence de descente des testicules	Descenso incompleto de testículo	Mancata discesa del testicolo
Nesvjestica	Unconsciousness	Absence de la conscience	Inconsciencia	Iienza (ncoscstato di incoscienza)
Neuhranjenost	Underfedness (malnutrition)	Malnutrition	Desnutrición	Sottopeso (grave magrezza)
Neumjerena glad	Excessive hunger (polyphagia)	Faim excessive (polyphagie)	Aumento anormal de la necesidad de comer (polifagia)	Aumento incontrollato dell'appetito (polifagia)
Neuralgija	Neuralgia	Névralgie	Neuralgia	Nevralgia
Neuralgija trigeminusa	Trigeminal neuralgia	Névralgie du trijumeau (névralgie trigéminale)	Neuralgia del trigémino	Nevralgia del trigemino
Neuralgija moždanih živaca	Cranial neuralgia	Névralgie des nerfs crâniens	Neuralgia craneal	Nevralgia del nervo cranico
Neurastenija	Neurasthenia	Neurasthénie	Neurastenia	Nevrastenia
Neurinom	Neurinoma	Neurinome	Neurinoma	Neurinoma (Schwannoma)
Neuroblastom	Neuroblastoma	Neuroblastome	Neuroblastoma	Neuroblastoma
Neuroborelioza	Neuroborreliosis	Neuroborréliose	Neuroborreliosis	Neuroborreliosi
Neurogeni šok	Neurogenic shock	Choc neurogénique	Choque neurogénico	Shock neurogeno
Neurom	Neuroma	Neurome	Neuroma	Neuroma
Neurom slušnog živca	Acoustic neuroma	Neurome acoustique	Neuroma acústico	Neuroma dell'acustico
Neuropatija	Neuropathy	Neuropathie	Neuropatía	Neuropatia
Neuroza	Neurosis	Névrose (neurose)	Neurosis	Nevrosi
Nistagmus	Nystagmus	Nystagmus	Nistagmo	Nistagmo
Nizak krvni tlak (hipotenzija)	Low blood pressure (hypotension)	Baisse de la pression artérielle (hypotension artérielle)	Presión sanguínea baja (hipotensión)	Bassa pressione arteriosa (ipotensione)
Noćna desaturacija	Sleep apnea	Apnée du sommeil	Apnea del sueño	Sindrome delle apnee nel sonno
Noćni grčevi u nogama	Nocturnal leg cramps	Crampes nocturnes des jambes	Calambres nocturnos en las piernas	Crampo notturno alle gambe
Noćno mokrenje (nokturija)	Frequent urination at night (nocturia)	Excrétion urinaire à prédominance nocturne (nycturie)	Emisión excesiva de orina durante la noche (nicturia)	Urinazione notturna (nicturia)
Noćno sljepilo	Night blindness (nyctalopia)	Cécité nocturne (héméralopie)	Ceguera nocturna (nictalopia)	Cecità notturna (nictalopia)
Noćno znojenje	Night sweats	Sueurs nocturnes	Sudor nocturno	Sudore notturno
Non-Hodgkinov limfom	Non-Hodgkin's lymphoma	Lymphome non-Hodgkinien	Linfoma no-Hodgkin	Linfoma non Hodgkin
Novorođenačka žutica	Neonatal jaundice	Ictère néonatal	Ictericia del recién nacido	Ittero neonatale
Novorođenačke kolike	Baby colic	Coliques de bébé	Cólico del recién nacido	Coliche del neonato
Numularni dermatitis	Nummular dermatitis	Dermatite nummulaire	Dermatitis numular	Dermatite nummulare
Obiteljska mediteranska groznica	Familial Mediterranean fever	Fièvre méditerranéenne familiale	Fiebre mediterránea familiar	Febbre mediterranea familiare
Oduzetost donjih ekstremiteta (paraplegija)	Paralysis of lower extremities (paraplegia)	Paralysie des membres inférieurs (paraplégie)	Parálisis de la parte inferior del cuerpo (paraplejía)	Paralisi di parte inferiore del corpo (paraplegia)
Oduzetost gornji i donjih ekstremiteta i torza (kvadriplegija, tetraplegija)	Paralysis of all limbs and torso (quadriplegia, tetraplegia)	Paralysie des quatre membres (tétraplégie)	Parálisis en brazos y piernas (tetraplejía, cuadriplejia)	Paralisi dei arti superiori e inferiori(quadriplegia)

Hrvatski	Engleski	Francuski	Španjolski	Talijanski
Oduzetost jedne polovine tijela (hemiplegija)	Paralysis of one half of a body (hemiplegia)	Paralysie de la moitié du corps (hémiplégie)	Parálisis de una mitad lateral de cuerpo (hemiplejía)	Paralisi di una metà del corpo (emiplegia)
Oduzetost simetričnih dijelova tijela (diplegija)	Paralysis of symmetrical parts of the body (diplegia)	Paralysie des régions symétriques du corps (diplégie)	Parálisis de partes simétricas del cuerpo (diplejía)	Paralisi di una parte di corpo simmetrica (diplegia)
Odvajanje mrežnice (ablacija retine)	Retinal ablation (retinal detachment)	Décollement de la rétine	Desprendimiento de retina	Distacco di retina
Ograničena pokretljivost zgloba	Limited joint mobility	Mobilité atriculaire limitée	Rango de movimiento articular limitado	Ridotta mobilità articolare
Ogrebotina	Scratch	Égratignure	Rasguño	Graffio (graffiatura)
Ojedina (abrazija)	Abrasion	Écorchure	Abrasión (escoriación)	Abrasione (escoriazione)
Okcipitalna neuralgija	Occipital neuralgia (Arnold's neuralgia)	Nèvralgie occipitale	Síndrome occipital (neuralgia occipital)	Nevralgia occipitale (nevralgia di Arnold)
Oligodendrogliom	Oligodendroglioma	Oligodendrocytome	Oligodendroglioma	Oligodendroglioma
Oligomenoreja	Oligomenorrhea	Oligoménorrhée	Oligomenorrea	Oligomenorrea
Onkocerkijaza (riječno sljepilo)	Onchocerciasis (river blindness)	Onchocercose (cécité des rivières)	Oncocercosis	Oncocercosi (cecità fluviale)
Opća alopecija	Alopecia universalis	Alopécie universalis	Alopecia areata universal	Alopecia universale
Opeklina	Burn	Brûlure	Quemadura	Ustione
Opeklina od meduze	Jellyfish sting burn	Brûlure de méduse	Quemadura de medusa	Ustione da medusa
Opeklina od strujnog udara	Electric shock burn	Brûlure électrique	Quemadura eléctrica	Ustione da corrente elettrica
Opetovani prijelom kosti	Refracturing (repeated fracture)	Fracture répétée	Fractura repetida	Frattura ripetuta
Opstruktivna lezija tankog crijeva	Obstructive lesion of the small intestine	Lésion obstructive de l'intestin grêle	Lesión obstructiva del intestino delgado	Lesione ostruttiva dell'intestino tenue
Opstruktivni šok	Obstructive shock	Choc obstructive	Choque obstructivo	Shock ostruttivo
Orijentalni ulkus (kožna lišmenijaza)	Cutaneous leishmaniasis (Oriental sore)	Leishmaniose cutanée (bouton d'Orient)	Leishmaniasis cutánea (uta)	Leishmaniosi cutanea
Oroya groznica (Carrionova bolest)	Oroya fever (Carrion's disease)	Fièvre d'Oroya (maladie de Carrion)	Fiebre de la Oroya (enfermedad de Carrión, verruga peruana)	Febbre di Oroya
Osgood-Schlatterova bolest	Osgood-Schlatter disease (rugby knee)	Maladie d'Osgood-Schlatter	Enfermedad de Osgood-Schlatter	Sindrome di Osgood-Schlatter
Osificirajući miozitis	Myositis ossificans	Myosite ossifiante	Miositis osificante	Miosite ossificante
Osip	Rash (eruption, eczema)	Rash (eczéma)	Sarpullido (erupción, eccema)	Sfogo (eruzione cutanea)
Osjećaj "tijesnih cipela"	'Tight shoes' sensation	Sensation des chaussures très serré	Sensación de "zapatos apretados"	Senso delle scarpe troppo strette
Osjećaj straha	Sensation of fear	Sensation de peur	Sensación de miedo	Senso della paura
Osjetljivost na bol (algezija)	Sensitivity to pain (algesia)	Sensibilité à la douleur (algésie)	Sensibilidad al dolor (algesia)	Sensibilità al dolore (algesia)
Ospice (morbili)	Measles	Rougeole (1re maladie)	Sarampión	Morbillo
Osteoartropatija hipertrofika Pierre Marie	Hyperthropic osteoarthropaty (Pierre Marie-Bamberger syndrome)	Ostéo-arthropathie hypertrophiante de Pierre Marie (syndrome de Marie-Bamberger)	Osteoartropatía hipertrófica (enfermedad de Bamberger-Marie)	Osteoartropatia ipertrofizzante (sindrome di Pierre Marie-Bamberger)
Osteogeneza imperfekta (staklaste kosti)	Osteogenesis imperfecta (brittle bone disease)	Ostéogenèse imparfaite	Osteogénesis imperfecta (huesos de cristal)	Osteogenesi imperfetta
Osteohondrom	Osteochondroma	Ostéochondrome	Osteocondroma	Osteocondroma
Osteom	Osteoma	Ostéome	Osteoma	Osteoma
Osteomalacija	Osteomalacia	Ostéomalacie	Osteomalacia	Osteomalacia
Osteopetroza (zadebljane kosti, bolest mramornih kostiju)	Osteopetrosis (marble bone disease)	Ostéopétrose (os de marbre)	Osteopetrosis (enfermedad de los huesos de marmol)	Osteopetrosi (malattia delle ossa di marmo)
Osteoporoza	Osteoporosis	Ostéoporose	Osteoporosis	Osteoporosi
Osteosarkom	Osteosarcoma	Ostéosarcome	Osteosarcoma	Osteosarcoma
Osteoskleroza	Osteosclerosis	Ostéosclérose	Osteosclerosis	Osteosclerosi
Oštećenje perifernog živca	Peripheral nerve lesion	Lésion du nerf périphérique	Lesión de nervio periférico	Lesione del nervo periferico
Oštećenje živca (lezija živca)	Nerve lesion	Lésion du nerf	Lesión de nervio	Lesione del nervo
Oštra bol	Sharp pain	Douleur tranchante	Dolor afilado	Dolore tagliente
Oteklina	Swelling	Gonflement (enflure)	Hinchazón	Gonfiore
Otežan govor (disfazija)	Speech difficulty (dysphasia)	Trouble de l'apprentissage du langage (dysphasie)	Trastorno del lenguaje (disfasia)	Disturbo del linguaggio verbale (afasia)
Otežano disanje	Breathing difficulty	Difficulté de respiration	Dificultad de respiración	Respirazione difficoltosa
Otežano gutanje (disfagija)	Difficult swallowing (dysphagia)	Difficulté de deglutition (dysphagie)	Dificultad para tragar (disfagia)	Difficoltà a deglutire (disfagia)
Otežano pražnjenje crijeva (otežana defekacija)	Difficult defecation (tenesmus)	Difficulté à déféquer (ténesme)	Dificultad para la defecación (tenesmo rectal)	Difficoltà a defecare (tenesmo)
Otežano usporeno mokrenje (dizurija)	Difficult urination (dysuria)	Difficulté à uriner (dysurie)	Dificultad al orinar (disuria)	Emissione di urine con difficoltà (disuria)
Otok očnog živca (zastojna papila)	Optic nerve edema	Oedème du nerf optique	Edema del nervio óptico	Papilledema (edema del nervo ottico)

Hrvatski	Engleski	Francuski	Španjolski	Talijanski
Otvoreni ductus arteriosus (Ductus arteriosus persistens)	Patent ductus arteriosus (persistent ductus arteriosus)	Persistance du canal artériel	Ductus arterioso persistente (conducto arterioso persistente)	Dotto arterioso persistente (ductus arteriosus persistente)
Otvoreni prijelom kosti	Open fracture (compound fracture)	Fracture ouverte	Fractura abierta	Frattura aperta (frattura esposta)
Ovapnjenje (kalcifikacija)	Calcification	Calcification	Calcificación	Calcificazione
Ovisnost	Addiction	Dépendance (addiction)	Adicción (dependencia)	Dipendenza
Ovisnost o drogama	Drug addiction	Toxicomanie	Adicción a las drogas (drogodependencia)	Tossicodipendenza (tossicomania)
Ovisnost o kockanju (ludopatija)	Gambling addiction (ludomania)	Jeu pathologique (jeu compulsif)	Adicción a jugar (ludopatía, ludomanía)	Giocco d'azzardo patologico
Ovisnost o seksu	Sexual addiction	Sexualité compulsive	Adicción sexual	Dipendenza sessuale
Ozeblina	Frostbite	Gelure	Congelamiento	Congelamento
Ozljede električnom strujom (strujni udar)	Electrical injuries (electric shock)	Électrisation	Lesiones por corriente eléctrica	Folgorazione (elettrocuzione)
Ozljede glave i mozga	Head and brain injuries	Blessures à la tête et blessures du cerveau	Lesiones de la cabeza y del cerebro	Lesioni della testa e del cervello
Ožiljak	Scar	Cicatrice	Cicatriz	Cicatrice (sfregio)
Pad krvnog tlaka	Blood pressure fall	Pression artérielle effondrée	Caída de la presión arterial	Abbassamento della pressione del sangue
Pagetova bolest	Paget's disease	Maladie de Paget	Enfermedad de Paget	Morbo di Paget
Panaricij	Whitlow (felon)	Panaris	Panadizo	Patereccio
Pannerova bolest	Panner's disease	Maladie de Panner	Enfermedad de Panner	Malattia di Panner
Papatači- groznica	Pappataci fever (phlebotomus fever, sandfly fever)	Fièvre pappataci (fièvre à phlébotomes)	Fiebre pappataci	Febbre da pappataci (febbre da Flebotomi)
Papilarni karcinom	Papillary carcinoma	Carcinome papillaire	Carcinoma papilar	Carcinoma papillare
Papilom	Papilloma	Papillome	Papiloma	Papilloma
Parafimoza	Paraphimosis	Paraphimosis	Parafimosis	Parafimosi
Paragonimijaza	Paragonimiasis	Paragonimiase humaine	Paragonimosis (paragonimiasis)	Paragonimiasi
Parakokcidioidomikoza (brazilska blastomikoza)	Paracoccidioidomycosis (Brazilian blastomycosis)	Paracoccidioidose brésilienne	Paracoccidioidomicosis	Paracoccidioidimicosi (blastomicosi sudamericana)
Paraliza (oduzetost, kljenut)	Paralysis	Paralysie	Parálisis	Paralisi
Paranefritički apsces	Perinephric abscess	Abcès périnéphrique	Absceso perinéfrico	Ascesso perinefrico
Paranoja	Paranoia	Paranoïa	Paranoia	Paranoia
Parazitarna bolest (parazitoza)	Parasitic disease (parasitosis)	Maladie parasitique (parasitose)	Enfermedad parasitaria (parasitosis)	Malattia parassitaria (parassitosi)
Pareza	Paresis	Parésie	Paresis	Paresi
Parkinsonova bolest	Parkinson's disease	Maladie de Parkinson	Enfermedad de Parkinson	Morbo di Parkinson
Parodontoza	Periodontitis	Parodontite	Periodontitis (piorrea)	Parodontite
Paronihija	Paronychia	Paronychie	Paroniquia	Paronichia
Patuljasti rast (nanizam)	Dwarfism (nanism)	Nanisme	Enanismo	Nanismo
Paukoliki angiom (spider nevus)	Spider angioma (spider nevus)	Angiome stellaire	Angioma en araña (angioma aracnoideo)	Angioma a ragno
Pećenje (žarenje)	Burning sensation	Sensation cuisante	Sensación de ardor	Sensazione bruciante
Pećenje za vrijeme mokrenja	Urinary burning	Brûlures à la miction	Ardor al orinar	Bruciore urinario
Pemfigus	Pemphigus	Pemphigus	Pénfigo	Pemfigo
Perianalni apsces	Perianal abscess	Abcès périanal	Absceso perianal	Ascesso perianale
Periodično disanje (Cheyne-Stokesovo disanje)	Periodic breathing (Cheyne-Stokes respiration)	Respiration Cheynes-Stokes	Respiración periódica (respiración de Cheynes-Stokes)	Respiro di Cheyne-Stokes
Perniciozna anemija	Pernicious anemia	Anémie pernicieuse	Anemia perniciosa	Anemia perniciosa
Perut	Dandruff	Pellicule	Caspa	Forfora
Petehije	Petechia	Pétéchie	Petequia	Petecchia
Petni trn	Heel spur (calcaneal spur)	Éperon de talon (epine calcaneenne)	Espuela de talón (espuela calcánea)	Spina nel calcagno (spina calcaneare)
Petno stopalo	Pes calcaneus	Pied calcanéus	Pie calcáneo	Piede calcaneo
Pigmentna distrofija mrežnice	Retinitis pigmentosa (retinal pigment epithelium dystrophy)	Rétinite pigmentaire	Retinitis pigmentosa	Retinite pigmentosa
Pijelonefritis (infekcija bubrega)	Pyelonephritis (kidney infection)	Pyélonéphrite (infection bactérienne des voies urinaires hautes)	Pielonefritis (infección urinaria alta)	Pielonefrite
Pilonidalna cista	Pilonidal cyst	Kyste pilonidal	Quiste pilonidal	Cisti pilonidale
Pilorospazam	Pylorospasm	Spasme du pylore	Pilorospasmo	Pilorospasmo
Pinta	Pinta	Pinta	Pinta	Pinta
Pionefroza	Pyonephrosis	Pyonéphrose (pus dans le rein)	Pionefrosis	Pionefrosi
Piromanija	Pyromania	Pyromanie	Piromanía	Piromania
Pitirijaza (svjetlije mrlje na osunčanoj koži, Tinea versicolor)	Tinea versicolor (pityriasis versicolor, haole rot)	Pityriasis versicolor	Tiña versicolor (pitiriasis versicolor)	Pitiriasi versicolor (tinea versicolor)
Pjenušavi ispljuvak	Foamy sputum	Crachat spumeux	Esputo espumoso	Sputo schiumoso
Planocelularni karcinom	Squamous cell carcinoma (planocellular carcinoma)	Carcinome spinocellulaire	Carcinoma de células escamosas	Carcinoma a cellule squamose

Hrvatski	Engleski	Francuski	Španjolski	Talijanski
Plantarni fasciitis	Plantar fasciitis	Fasciite plantaire	Fascitis plantar	Fasciosi plantare
Plastična induracija penisa	Peyronie's disease (induratio penis plastica)	Maladie de La Peyronie	Enfermedad de La Peyronie (induración plástica del pene)	Induratio penis plastica (malattia di Peyronie)
Plazmocitom (multipli mijelom)	Plasmacytoma (multiple myeloma)	Plasmocytome (myélome multiple)	Plasmacitoma (mieloma múltiple)	Mieloma multiplo
Plik	Blister	Phlyctène (ampoule, cloque)	Ampolla	Vescichetta (bolla)
Plinska gangrena	Gas gangrene	Gangrène gazeuse	Gangrena gaseosa	Gangrene gassosa
Plivačko koljeno	Swimmer's knee	Syndrome du brasseur aux genoux	Rodilla de nadador de pecho (bursitis de la pata de ganso)	Ginocchio del nuotatore a rana (stiramento cronico del legamento mediale)
Plućna embolija	Pulmonary embolism	Embolie pulmonaire	Embolia pulmonar	Embolia polmonare
Plućna hipertenzija	Pulmonary hypertension	Hypertension artérielle pulmonaire	Hipertensión arterial pulmonar	Ipertensione arteriosa polmonare
Plućna idiopatska fibroza	Idiopathic pulmonary fibrosis	Fibrose pulmonaire idiopathique	Fibrosis pulmonar idiopática	Fibrosi polmonare idiopatica
Plućna kongestija	Pulmonary congestion	Congestion pulmonaire	Congestión pulmonar	Congestione polmonare
Plućni edem	Pulmonary edema	Oedème pulmonaire	Edema pulmonar	Edema polmonare
Plućno srce	Pulmonary heart disease	Coeur pulmonaire	Enfermedad cardíaca pulmonar (cor pulmonale)	Cuore polmonare
Pneumocistična upala pluća	Pneumocystis pneumonia (pneumocystosis)	Pneumocystose	Neumonía por Pneumocystis	Polmonite da Pneumocisti
Pneumokonioza	Pneumoconiosis	Pneumoconiose	Neumoconiosis	Pneumoconiosi
Pneumotoraks	Pneumothorax	Pneumothorax	Neumotórax	Pneumotorace
Podražaj na povraćanje	Urge to vomit	Envie de vomir	Ganas de vomitar	Impulso a vomitare
Podraženo koljeno (skakačko koljeno)	Irritated knee (jumper's knee, patellar tendinopathy)	Genou du sauteur (tendinite rotulienne)	Rodilla de saltador (tendinopatía rotuliana)	Peritendite rotulea (ginocchio del saltatore)
Podrigivanje	Burping (belching)	Rot (renvoi, éructation)	Eructo	Eruttazione
Pojačan osjećaj žeđi (polidipsija)	Increased thirst senasation (polydipsia)	Soif excessive (polydipsie)	Aumento anormal de la sed (polidipsia)	Aumento del senso della sete (polidipsia)
Pojačana dlakavost	Increased hairiness (hypertrichosis)	Pilosité excessive (hypertrichose)	Exceso de cabello (hipertricosis)	Aumento della pelosità (ipertricosi)
Pojačano lučenje sline (hipersalivacija)	Excessive secretion of saliva (hypersalivation)	Sécrétion de la salive excessive	Excesiva producción de saliva (hipersalivación)	Produzione di saliva eccessiva (ipersalivazione)
Pojačano opadanje kose	Increased hair loss	Perte de cheveux excessive	Aumento de la cáída del cabello	Aumento di perdita di capelli
Pokvareni zub	Rotten tooth	Dent pourri	Diente podrido	Dente guasto
Policistični bubreg	Polycystic kidney disease	Rein polykystique	Enfermedad poliquística renal	Rene policistico
Policitemija	Polycythemia	Polycythémie	Policitemia	Policitemia
Polidaktilija	Polydactyly	Polydactylie	Polidactilia	Polidattilia
Polimiozitis	Polymyositis	Polymyosite	Polimiositis	Polimiosite
Polip	Polyp	Polype	Pólipo	Polipo
Polip na debelom crijevu	Colon polyp	Polype du côlon	Pólipo de colon	Polipo del colon
Polip na glasnicama	Vocal chords polyp	Polype des cordes vocales	Pólipo de las cuerdas vocales	Polipo della corda vocale
Polip na grliću maternice	Cervical polyp	Polype au col de l'utérus	Pólipo cervical	Polipo cervicale
Polip maternice	Endometrial polyp (uterine polyp)	Polype utérin	Pólipo endometrial	Polipo endometriale
Polip u nosu (nosni polip)	Nasal polyp	Polype nasal	Pólipo nasal	Polipo nasale
Poprečni prijelom kosti	Transverse fracture	Fracture transversale	Fractura transversal	Frattura trasversale
Poprečno debelo crijevo	Transverse colon	Côlon transverse	Colon transverso	Colon trasverso
Poremećaj ishrane	Eating disorder	Trouble de conduite alimentaire	Trastorno alimentario	Disturbo del comportamento alimentare
Poremećaj koncentracije	Attention deficit disorder	Trouble déficit de l'attention	Trastorno por déficit de atención	Disturbo della concentrazione
Poremećaj koordinacije mišićnih pokreta (ataksija)	Lack of coordination of muscle movements (ataxia)	Trouble de coordina-tion des mouvements musculaires (ataxie)	Descoordinación en el movimientos musculares (ataxia)	Disturbo della coordinazione muscolare (atassia)
Poremećaj kretanja	Movement disorder	Trouble du mouvement	Trastorno de movimiento	Disordine del movimento
Poremećaj mokrenja	Urination disorder	Trouble de la miction	Trastorno de la micción	Disturbo della minzione
Poremećaj osobnosti	Personality disorder	Trouble de la personnalité	Trastorno de personalidad	Disturbo di personalità
Poremećaj ponašanja	Behavioral disorder	Trouble du comportement	Trastorno del comportamiento	Disturbo dell'umore
Poremećaj ravnoteže	Balance disorder	Trouble de l'équilibre	Trastorno del equilibrio	Disturbo dell'equilibrio
Poremećaj sluha	Hearing disorder	Trouble de l'audition	Trastorno de la audición	Disturbo dell'udito
Poremećaj spavanja	Sleeping disorder	Trouble du sommeil	Trastorno del sueño	Disturbo del sonno
Poremećaj spolne diferencijacije	Sexual differentiation disorder	Trouble de la différenciation sexuelle	Trastorno de la diferenciación sexual	Disordine della differenziazione sessuale
Poremećaj učenja	Learning disability	Trouble de l'apprentissage	Dificultad del aprendizaje	Disturbo di apprendimento
Poremećaj vida	Sight disorder	Trouble de la vue	Trastorno de la visión	Disturbo della vista
Porfirija	Porphyria	Porphyrie	Porfiria	Porfiria
Portalna hipertenzija	Portal hypertension	Hypertension portale	Hipertensión portal	Ipertensione portale
Pospanost (somnolencija)	Somnolence	Somnolence	Somnolencia	Sonnolenza
Postnekrotična ciroza	Post-necrotic cirrhosis	Cirrhose postnecrotique	Cirrosis postnecrótica	Cirrosi post-necrotica
Posttraumatska glavobolja	Post-traumatic headache	Céphalée post-traumatique	Cefalea postraumática	Cefalea post-traumatica

Hrvatski	Engleski	Francuski	Španjolski	Talijanski
Posttraumatski stresni poremećaj (PTSP)	Posttraumatic stress disorder	Trouble de stress post-traumatique	Trastorno por estrés postraumático	Disturbo post traumatico da stress
Posttrombotički sindrom	Post-thrombotic syndrome	Syndrome post-thrombotique	Síndrome postrombótico	Sindrome post trombotica
Posturalna križobolja	Postural back pain	Lombalgie posturale	Dolor de espalda postural	Mal di schiena su base posturale
Posturalni edem (statički edem)	Postural edema	Oedème postural	Edema postural	Edema posturale
Pothlađenost (hipotermija)	Hypothermia	Hypothermie	Hipotermia	Ipotermia
Potkovičasti bubreg	Horseshoe kidney (renal fusion)	Rein en fer à cheval	Riñón de herradura (fusión en los riñones)	Rene a ferro di cavallo (fusione renale)
Potkožni emfizem	Subcutaneous emphysema	Emphisème sous-cutané	Enfisema subcutáneo	Enfisema sottocutaneo
Potres mozga	Brain concussion	Commotion cérébrale	Conmoción cerebral	Commozione cerebrale
Povećan razmak između dva organa ili dijela tijela (hipertelorizam)	Increased distance between two organs or parts of the body (hypertelorism)	Élargissement de la distance des organes (hypertélorisme)	Aumento de la separación de los organos (hipertelorismo)	Aumento della distanza fra due parti del corpo (ipertelorismo)
Povećanje jetre (hepatomegalija)	Enlarged liver (hepatomegaly)	Augmentation du foie (hépatomégalie)	Aumento del tamaño del hígado (hepatomegalia)	Aumento di volume del fegato (epatomegalia)
Povećanje limfnih čvorova (limfadenopatija)	Enlarged lymph nodes (lymphadenopathy)	Augmentation d'un ganglion lymphatique (lymphadénopathie)	Aumento de volumen de los ganglios linfáti-cos (linfadenopatia)	Ingrossamento dei linfonodi (linfoadenopatia)
Povišen inzulin u krvi (hiperinzulinizam)	Hyperinsulinism	Hyperinsulinisme	Hiperinsulinismo	Iperinsulinismo
Povišen kolesterol u krvi (hiperkolesterolemija)	High blood cholesterol (hypercholesterolemia)	Cholésterol sanguin élevée (hypercholestérolémie)	Colesterol elevado de la sangre (hipercolesterolemia)	Eccesso di colesterolo nel sangue (ipercolesterolemia)
Povišen šećer u krvi (hiperglikemija)	High blood sugar (hyperglicemia)	Taux de sucre dans le sang élevé (hyperglycémie)	Cantidad excesiva de gluco-sa en la sangre (hipergluce-mia, hiperglicemia)	Eccesso di glucosio nel sangue (iperglicemia)
Povišena tjelesna temperatura	Elevated body temperature	Élévation de la température du corps	Aumento en la temperatura corporal	Temperatura corporea elevata
Povraćanje	Vomiting	Vomissement	Vómito (emesis)	Vomito (emetismo)
Povraćanje bez mučnine (povraćanje u luku, cerebralno povraćanje)	Vomiting without nausea (cerebral vomiting)	Vomissement en fusée sans effort	Vómito sin náusea (vómito cerebral)	Vomito senza nausea (vomito a getto, vomito cerebrale)
Povraćanje krvi (hematemeza)	Vomiting of blood (hematemesis)	Vomissement de sang (hématémèse)	Vómito de sangre (hematemesis)	Emesi emorragica (ematemesi)
Povratna groznica	Relapsing fever	Fièvre récurrente	Fiebre reincidente	Febbre ricorrente
Površinsko plitko disanje	Shallow breathing	Respiration superficielle	Respiración superficial	Respirazione superficiale
Predmenstruacijski sindrom (PMS)	Premenstrual syndrome (PMS)	Syndrome prémenstruel (SPM)	Síndrome premenstrual	Sindrome premestruale
Prednji sindrom sraza gornjeg nožnog zgloba	Ankle impingement syndrome	Conflit antérieur de la cheville	Pinzamiento anterolateral del tobillo	Sindrome da impingement della caviglia
Predoziranje drogom	Drug overdose	Surdose de drogue	Sobredosis por droga	Overdose di droga
Predoziranje lijekom	Medication overdose	Surdose du médicament	Sobredosis de medicamentos	Overdose di farmaci
Predsimptom bolesti prije nego se bolest razvije	Early symptom (prodrome)	Phase prodromique	Síndrome prodrómico	Sindrome prodromica
Prehlada (hunjavica)	Common cold	Rhume	Resfriado común (resfrío)	Infreddatura (raffreddore)
Prekomjerno jedenje (hiperfagija)	Abnormally large intake of food (hyperphagia)	Prise excessive d'aliments (hyperphagie)	Ingestas descontroladas de alimentos (hiperfagia)	Aumento incontrollato di assunzione di cibo (iperfagia)
Prekomjerno znojenje (hiperhidroza)	Excessive sweating (hyperhidrosis)	Sudation excessive (hyperhidrose)	Excesiva producción de sudor (hiperhidrosis)	Aumento della sudorazione (iperidrosi)
Preosjetljivost na podražaj (hiperestezija)	Increased sensitivity to stimuli of the senses (hyperesthesia)	Hypersensibilité aux stimuli extérieurs (hyperesthésie)	Sensación exagerada de los estímulos táctiles (hiperestesia)	Ipersensibilità ai normali stimoli esterni (iperestesia)
Preponska kila	Inguinal hernia	Hernie inguinale	Hernia inguinal	Ernia inguinale
Prerano splono fizičko sazrijevanje istog spola	Premature sexual development of the same sex	Développement sexuel prématuré du même sexe	Desarrollo sexual prematuro del mismo sexo	Prematuro sviluppo sessuale dello stesso sesso
Prerano spolno fizičko sazrijevanje suprotnog spola	Premature sexual development of the opposite sex	Développement sexuel prématuré du sexe opposé	Desarrollo sexual prematuro del sexo opuesto	Prematuro sviluppo sessuale del sesso opposto
Prestanak lučenja urina	Nonpassage of urine	Arrêt de la sécrétion d'urine	Supresión de la secreción de orina	Soppressione della secrezione di urina
Preuranjeni pubertet	Precocious puberty (premature puberty)	Puberté précoce	Pubertad precoz	Pubertà precoce (pubertà prematura)
Prijelom baze lubanje	Base of skull fracture (basal skull fracture)	Fracture de la base du crâne	Fractura de la base del cráneo	Frattura della base del cranio
Prijelom bedrene kosti	Broken thighbone (femur fracture)	Fracture du fémur	Fractura de fémur	Frattura del femore
Prijelom članka prsta	Broken finger (finger fracture)	Fracture du doigt	Fractura de falange del dedo	Frattura della falange del dito
Prijelom dijafize bedrene kosti	Diaphyseal tightbone fracture	Fracture de la diaphyse fémorale	Fractura de la diáfisis del fémur	Frattura della diafisi femorale
Prijelom falange nožnog palca	Broken big toe (fractured hallux)	Fracture du gros orteil	Fractura de los huesos del dedo gordo del pie	Frattura dell'alluce

Hrvatski	Engleski	Francuski	Španjolski	Talijanski
Prijelom glavice palčane kosti	Radial head fracture (radial capitulum fracture)	Fracture de la tête radiale	Fractura de la cabeza del radio	Frattura del capitello radiale
Prijelom gležnja	Broken ankle (ankle fracture)	Fracture de la cheville	Fractura de tobillo	Frattura della caviglia
Prijelom goljenične kosti	Broken shinbone (tibia fracture)	Fracture du tibia	Fractura de tibia	Frattura della tibia
Prijelom gornje i/ili donje čeljusti	Upper and/or lower jaw fracture (broken upper/lower jaw)	Fracture du maxillaire et/ou de la mandibule	Fractura de maxilar y/o mandíbula	Frattura della mascella e/o della mandibola
Prijelom ivera (prijelom patele)	Broken knee cap (patellar fracture)	Fracture de rotule	Fractura de la rótula	Frattura della rotula
Prijelom ključne kosti	Broken collarbone (clavicle fracture)	Fracture de la clavicule	Fractura de clavícula	Frattura della clavicola
Prijelom kondila nadlaktične kosti	Epicondylar elbow fracture	Fracture du condyle huméral	Fractura de epicóndilo humeral	Frattura dell'epicondilo omerale
Prijelom kosti (fraktura kosti)	Broken bone (bone fracture)	Fracture des os	Fractura de hueso	Frattura
Prijelom kosti s pomakom	Fracture with displacement	Fracture à déplacement	Fractura-dislocación	Frattura con dislocazione
Prijelom lakatne kosti	Broken ulna (ulna fracture)	Fracture de l'ulna	Fractura de cúbito	Frattura dell'ulna
Prijelom lakatnog vrha (prijelom olekranona)	Broken elbow (olecranon fracture)	Fracture de l'olécrâne	Fractura de olécranon	Frattura dell'olecrano
Prijelom lisne kosti	Broken fibula (fibula fracture)	Fracture de la fibula	Fractura del peroné	Frattura della fibula
Prijelom lopatice	Broken shoulder blade (scapula fracture)	Fracture de la scapula	Fractura de escápula	Frattura della scapola
Prijelom kosti stopala	Broken foot (metatarsal fracture)	Fracture métatarsienne	Fractura de metatarso	Frattura del metatarso
Prijelom mlade kosti	Greenstick fracture	Fracture en bois vert	Fractura en rama verde	Frattura a legno verde
Prijelom nadlaktice	Broken upper arm (humerus fracture)	Fracture de l'humérus	Fractura del húmero	Frattura dell'omero
Prijelom nadlaktice u području dijafize	Diaphyseal humeral fracture	Fracture diaphysaire de l'humérus	Fractura diafisaria del húmero	Frattura diafisaria dell'omero
Prijelom navikularne kosti	Broken navicular bone (navicular fracture)	Fracture du scaphoïde	Fractura de escafoides (fractura navicular)	Frattura dell'osso navicolare
Prijelom obje kosti potkoljenice	Broken lower leg bones (fractured tibia and fibula)	Fracture du tibia et de la fibula	Fractura de tibia y peroné	Frattura di tibia e perone
Prijelom obje podlaktične kosti	Broken forearm (frac-tured ulna and radius)	Fracture du radius et du cubitus	Fractura de radio y cúbito	Frattura di radio e ulna
Prijelom palčane kosti	Radius fracture	Fracture du radius	Fractura del radio	Frattura del radio
Prijelom palčane kosti loco typico	Distal radial fracture	Fracture de l'extrémité inferieure du radius (fracture de Pouteau-Colles)	Fractura distal del radio	Frattura di Pouteau-Colles (frattura delle metafisi radiali distali)
Prijelom petne kosti	Broken heel bone (calcaneus fracture)	Fracture du calcanéus	Fractura del calcáneo	Frattura del calcagno
Prijelom rebra	Broken rib (rib fracture)	Fracture de côte	Fractura de costilla	Frattura della costola
Prijelom trupa kralješka	Broken vertebral body (vertebral corpus fracture)	Fracture du plateau vertébral	Fractura de cuerpo vertebral	Frattura del corpo vertebrale
Prijelom vrata bedrene kosti	Femoral neck fracture	Fracture du col du fémur	Fractura de cuello del fémur	Frattura del collo del femore
Prijelom vrata nadlaktične kosti	Humeral neck fracture	Fracture du col de l'humérus	Fractura de cuello del húmero	Frattura del collo dell'omero
Prijelom zamora	Stress fracture	Fracture de fatigue	Fractura por estrés	Frattura da stress
Prijelom zamora goljenične kosti	Tibia stress fracture	Fracture de fatigue du tibia	Fractura por estrés de la tibia	Frattura da stress della tibia
Prijelom zdjelice	Broken pelvis (pelvis fracture)	Fracture du bassin	Fractura de pelvis	Frattura del bacino
Prijevremena ejakulacija	Premature ejaculation	Éjaculation précoce	Eyaculación precoz	Eiaculazione precoce
Primarni amebni meningoencefalitis	Primary amoebic meningoencephalitis	Méningo-encéphalite amibienne primaire	Meningoencefalitis amebiana primaria	Meningoencefalite amebica primaria
Prinzmetalova angina	Prinzmetal's angina	Angine de Prinzmetal	Angina de Prinzmetal	Angina di Prinzmetal
Prirodna smrt	Natural death	Mort naturelle	Muerte natural	Morte naturale
Probadajuća bol	Twinging pain	Élancement	Dolor tipo punzada	Dolore pungente
Probavne smetnje	Indigestion	Indigestion	Indigestión	Indigestione
Produktivni kašalj	Productive cough	Toux productive	Tos productiva	Tosse produttiva
Profesionalno oboljenje	Occupational disease	Maladie professionnelle	Enfermedad profesional	Malattia professionale
Progresivna mišićna distrofija	Progressive muscular dystrophy	Dystrophie musculaire progressive	Distrofia muscular progresiva	Distrofia muscolare progressiva
Progresivno okoštavanje mišića	Myositis ossificans progressiva	Myosite ossifiante progressive	Miositis osificante progresiva	Miosite ossificante progressiva
Proktitis	Proctitis	Proctite	Proctitis	Proctite
Prolaps maternice (spuštena maternica)	Uterine prolapse (fallen womb)	Prolapsus de l'utérus	Prolapso del útero	Prolasso uterino
Prolaps rektuma	Rectal prolapse	Prolapsus rectal	Prolapso rectal	Prolasso del retto
Proljev (dijarea)	Diarrhea	Diarrhée	Diarrea	Diarrea
Promjene apetita	Appetite changes	Changements d'appétit	Cambios en el apetito	Cambiamenti nell'appetito
Promjene boje kože	Skin color changes	Changements de couleur de la peau	Cambios en el color de la piel	Cambiamento di colore della pelle

Hrvatski	Engleski	Francuski	Španjolski	Talijanski
Promjene glasa	Voice changes	Changements de voix	Cambios en la voz	Cambiamento di voce
Promjene na madežima	Changes in moles	Changements dans les grains de beauté	Cambios en los lunares	Cambiamenti di nevi
Promjene na sluznici	Changes in mucous membrane	Changement de la muqueuse	Cambios en la membrana mucosa	Cambiamenti della mucosa
Promjene oblika kosti	Changes in shape of bones	Changements dans la forme des os	Cambios en la forma de los huesos	Cambiamenti nella forma delle ossa
Promjene osjeta dodira	Changes in tactile sensation	Changements des sensations tactiles	Cambios en la sensibilidad táctil	Cambiamenti della sensazione tattile
Promjene osjeta mirisa	Changes in olfactory sensation	Changements des sensations olfactives	Cambios en la sensibilidad olfatoria	Cambiamenti delle sensazoni olfattive
Promjene osjeta okusa	Changes in taste sensation	Changements de sensation de goût	Cambios en la sensación de sabores	Cambiamenti nelle sensazioni del gusto
Promjene osobnosti	Personality changes	Changements de personnalité	Cambios de personalidad	Cambiamenti di personalità
Promjene raspoloženja	Mood swing	Saute d'humeur	Oscilaciones del humor	Cambiamento d'umore
Promjene stanja svijesti	Changes in consciousness	Changements de conscience	Cambios en la conciencia	Alterazione della conoscenza
Promuklost	Hoarseness	Enrouement	Ronquera	Raucedine
Prostrijelna rana	Gunshot wound	Blessure par balle	Herida de bala	Ferita da arma da fuoco
Proširene vene	Varicose veins	Varices	Varices	Varicosi (varici, malattia varicosa)
Proširene vene jednjaka (flebektazije)	Esophageal varices	Varices oesophagiennes	Varices esofágicas	Varici esofagee
Proširene vene na nogama	Leg varicose veins	Varices des membres inférieurs	Venas varicosas de las piernas	Varici degli arti inferiori
Proširene vratne vene	Neck varicose veins	Varice dans le cou	Varices del cuello	Vene varicose del collo
Proširene zjenice	Enlarged pupils	Pupilles dilatées	Pupilas dilatadas	Pupille dilatate
Prsnuće (puknuće, razdor, ruptura)	Rupture	Rupture	Ruptura (rotura)	Rottura
Prsnuće aneurizme	Aneurysm rupture	Rupture d'anévrisme	Ruptura del aneurisma	Rottura di aneurisma
Prva mjesečnica (menarha)	First menstrual cycle (menarche)	Première période de menstruations (ménarche)	Primera menstruación (menarquia)	Primo flusso mestruale (menarca)
Pseudoepiteliematozna hiperplazija	Pseudoepitheliomatous hyperplasia	Hyperplasie pseudo-épithéliomateuse	Hiperplasia pseudoepiteliomatosa	Iperplasia pseudoepiteliomatosa
Psihičke promjene	Psychic changes	Changements psychiques	Cambios psíquicos	Alterazioni dello stato psishico
Psihofizička usporenost	Slow psychophysiological responses	Réponses psychophysiologiques lentes	Respuestas psicofisiológicas lentas	Lentezza psicofisica
Psihoneuroza	Psychoneurosis	Psychonévrose	Psiconeurosis	Psiconevrosi (nevrosi)
Psihopatija	Psychopathy	Psychopathie	Psicopatía	Psicopatia
Psihoza	Psychosis	Psychose	Psicosis	Psicosi
Psitakoza	Psittacosis (parrot fever)	Psittacose	Psitacosis (fiebre del loro)	Psittacosi (psittacornitosi)
Psorijatični artritis	Psoriatic arthritis	Arthrite psoriatique	Artritis psoriásica	Artrite psoriasica
Psorijaza	Psoriasis	Psoriasis	Psoriasis	Psoriasi
Ptičja gripa podtip H5N1	Bird flu (influenzavirus A subtype H5N1)	Grippe aviaire (influenzavirus A sous-type H5N1)	Gripe aviar H5N1	Influenza aviaria H5N1
Puknuće Ahilove tetive	Achilles tendon rupture	Rupture du tendon d'Achille	Ruptura del tendón de Aquiles	Rottura del tendine di Achille
Puknuće bubnjića (perforacija bubnjića, timpanoreksija)	Perforated eardrum (tympanorrhexis)	Perforation du tympan	Perforación del tímpano	Perforazione del timpano
Puknuće čira (perforacija ulkusa)	Perforated ulcer	Perforation d'ulcère	Úlcera perforada	Ulcera perforata
Puknuće ligamenta	Ligament rupture (torn ligament)	Rupture ligamentaire	Ruptura de ligamento	Rottura del legamento
Puknuće tetive	Tendon rupture (torn tendon)	Rupture du tendon	Ruptura del tendón	Rottura del tendine
Pulsirajuća bol	Pulsing pain	Douleur pulsatile	Dolor pulsante	Dolore pulsante
Pupčana kila (umbilikalna hernija)	Umbilical hernia	Hernie ombilicale	Hernia umbilical	Ernia ombelicale
Purpura	Purpura	Purpura	Púrpura	Porpora
Puštanje vjetra (flatulencija, plinovi)	Passing gas (flatulence, farting)	Pet (flatulence, vesse)	Tener gases (flatulencia)	Miscela di gas (flatulenza)
Q-groznica	Q fever	Fièvre Q	Fiebre Q	Febbre Q
Rabdomiom	Rhabdomyoma	Rhabdomyome	Rabdomioma	Rabdomioma
Rabdomiosarkom	Rhabdomyosarcoma	Rhabdomyosarcome	Rabdomiosarcoma	Rabdomiosarcoma
Radioaktivna ozračenost	Radioactive irradiation	Irradiation par rayons radioactifs (contamination radioactive)	Irradiación radioactiva	Irradiazione radioattiva
Radioulnarna sinostoza	Radioulnar synostosis	Synostose radio-ulnaire	Sinostosis radiocubital	Sinostosi radio-ulnare
Rahitis	Rickets (rachitis)	Rachitisme	Raquitismo	Rachitismo
Rak dojke	Breast cancer	Cancer du sein	Cáncer de mama	Cancro della mammella
Rak grlića maternice	Cervical cancer	Cancer du col utérin	Cáncer del cuello uterino (cáncer cervical)	Cancro della cervice uterina
Rak prostate	Prostate cancer	Cancer de la prostate	Cáncer de próstata	Cancro della prostata

Hrvatski	Engleski	Francuski	Španjolski	Talijanski
Rak želuca	Stomach cancer (gastric cancer)	Cancer de l'estomac	Cáncer de estómago (cáncer gástrico)	Cancro dello stomaco (cancro gastrico)
Rana	Wound (injury, lesion)	Plaie	Herida	Ferita
Rascjep mokraćnog mjehura	Rupture of urinary bladder	Rupture de la vessie	Ruptura de la vejiga urinaria	Rottura della vescica urinaria
Rascjep usne i nepca	Cleft lip and palate	Fente labiale et fente palatine	Labio leporino (fisura labial)	Labbro leporino
Rastrgnuće mišića (ruptura mišića)	Muscle rupture	Rupture musculaire	Ruptura muscular	Rottura muscolare
Raynaudova bolest	Raynaud's disease	Maladie de Raynaud	Enfermedad de Raynaud	Sindrome di Raynaud
Razderotina	Laceration (tear)	Lacération	Laceración	Lacerazione (strappo)
Razdor meniskusa	Meniscus rupture (meniscus tear)	Rupture du ménisque	Ruptura de menisco	Rottura del menisco
Razdor prednje ukrižene sveze koljenskog zgloba	Anterior cruciate ligament rupture (ACL rupture)	Rupture du ligament croisé antéro-externe (rupture du LCA)	Ruptura de ligamento cruzado anterior	Rottura del legamento crociato anteriore del ginocchio
Razdor rotatorne manžete ramenog zgloba	Rotator cuff rupture (rotator cuff tear)	Rupture de la coiffe des rotateurs	Ruptura del manguito rotador	Rottura della cuffia dei rotatori
Razdražljivost	Exasperation	Exaspération (irritation)	Exasperación	Esasperazione (irritazione)
Razrokost (strabizam)	Strabismus	Strabisme	Estrabismo	Strabismo
Razvojne anomalije	Development anomalies	Anomalies de développement	Anomalías del desarrollo	Anomalie di sviluppo
Reiterov sindrom	Reactive arthritis (Reiter's syndrome)	Arthrite réactive (syndrome de Reiter)	Síndrome de Reiter (artritis reactiva)	Sindrome di Reiter
Renalna tubularna acidoza	Renal tubular acidosis	Acidose tubulaire rénale	Acidosis tubular renal	Acidosi renale tubulare
Renovaskularna hipertenzija	Renovacsular hypertension	Hypertension rénovasculaire	Hipertensión renovascular	Ipertensione renale
Respiratorna alkaloza	Respiratory alkalosis	Alcalose respiratoire	Alcalosis respiratoria	Alcalosi respiratoria
Respiratorni distres sindrom	Respiratory distress syndrome	Syndrome de détresse respiratoire	Síndrome de distrés respiratorio	Sindrome da distress respiratorio
Restriktivna kardiomiopatija	Restrictive cardiomyopathy	Cardiomyopathie restrictive	Cardiomiopatía restrictiva	Cardiomiopatia restrittiva
Retencija testisa (kriptorhizam)	Cryptorchidism	Cryptorchidie	Criptorquidismo	Criptorchidismo
Retikuloendotelijalni sarkom	Reticuloendothelial sarcoma	Sarcome réticuloendothélial	Reticulosarcoma (sarcoma reticuloendotelial)	Reticoloendotelioma (reticolosarcoma)
Retrolentalna fibroplazija	Retinopathy of prematurity (retrolental fibroplasia)	Rétinopathie du prématuré	Retinopatía de la prematuridad	Retinopatia del prematuro
Retroperitonealna fibroza (Ormondova bolest)	Retroperitoneal fibrosis (Ormond's disease)	Fibrose rétropéritonéale (maladie d'Ormond)	Fibrosis retroperitoneal	Fibrosi retroperitoneale
Retrovertirani uterus	Retroverted uterus	Utérus rétroversé	Retroversión del útero	Retroflessione uterina
Reumatoidni artritis	Rheumatoid arthritis	Arthrite rhumatoïde	Artritis reumatoide	Artrite reumatoide
Reumatska bolest srca	Rheumatic heart disease	Cardite rhumatismale	Cardiopatía reumática	Cardiopatia reumatica
Reumatska groznica	Rheumatic fever	Rhumatisme articulaire aigu (maladie de Bouillaud)	Fiebre reumática	Febbre reumatica
Reumatska polimialgija	Polymyalgia rheumatica	Polymyalgia rheumatica	Polimialgia reumática	Polimialgia reumatica
Reyeov sindrom	Reye's syndrome	Syndrome de Reye	Síndrome de Reye	Sindrome di Reye
Rezna rana (posjekotina)	Cut wound	Plaie par objet tranchant	Herida por corte	Ferita da taglio
Rh-inkompatibilnost (hemolitička bolest novorođenčeta)	Rh incompatibility (hemolytic disease of the newborn)	Maladie hémolytique du nouveau-né	Enfermedad hemolítica del recién nacido (incompatibilidad Rh)	Eritroblastosi fetale (malattia emolitica del neonato)
Riedelov tireoiditis	Riedel's thyroiditis	Thyroïdite de Riedel	Tiroiditis de Riedel	Tiroidite di Riedel
Rift Valley groznica	Rift Valley fever	Fièvre de la vallée du Rift	Fiebre de Rift Valley	Febbre della Rift Valley
Rikecioza	Rickettsiosis	Rickettsiose	Rickettsiosis	Rickettsiosi
Rinitis	Rhinitis	Rhinite	Rinitis	Rinite
Rizartroza	Thumb joint arthritis	Rhizarthrose	Rizartrosis	Rizartrosi (artrosi dell'articolazione alla base del police)
Rozacea	Rosacea	Rosacée (couperose)	Rosácea	Rosacea
Rozeola infantum (egzantema subitum, šesta bolest)	Exanthema subitum (roseola infantum, sixth disease)	Roséole (exanthème subit, sixième maladie)	Roséola (exantema súbito)	Sesta malattia (roseola infantum, esantema subitum)
Rubeola (crljenac)	German measles (rubella)	Rubéole	Rubéola	Rosolia
Ruptura slezene	Ruptured spleen	Rupture de la rate	Ruptura del bazo	Rottura della milza
Sakagija	Glanders	Morve	Muermo	Morva umana
Salmoneloza	Salmonellosis	Salmonellose	Salmonelosis	Salmonellosi
Samoozljeđivanje	Self-harm	Automutilation	Autolesión (automutilación)	Autolesionismo
Sarkoidoza	Sarcoidosis (sarcoid, Besnier-Boeck disease)	Sarcoïdose (maladie de Besnier-Boeck-Schaumann)	Sarcoidosis (enfermedad de Besnier-Boeck)	Sarcoidosi
Sarkom	Sarcoma	Sarcome	Sarcoma	Sarcoma
Sarkopenija	Sarcopenia	Sarcopénie	Sarcopenia	Sarcopenia
Savijanje kosti	Bone bending (bone torsion)	Torsion osseuse	Torsión del hueso	Torsione dell'osso
Seboreična keratoza	Seborrheic keratosis	Kératose séborrhéïque	Queratosis seborreica	Cheratosi seborroica
Seboreja	Seborrhea	Séborrhée	Seborrea	Seborrea
Sekrecija iz nosa	Nasal secretion (mucus)	Mucus nasal	Moco (mucus) nasal	Muco nasale

Hrvatski	Engleski	Francuski	Španjolski	Talijanski
Sekundarna hipertenzija	Secondary hypertension (inessential hypertension)	Hypertension secondaire	Hipertensión secundaria	Ipertensione arteriosa secondaria
Semikoma	Semicoma	Semi-coma	Semicoma	Semi-coma
Sepsa	Sepsis	Sepsis	Sepsis	Sepsi
Septički šok	Septic shock	Choc septique	Choque séptico	Shock settico
Septikemija	Septicemia	Septicémie	Septicemia	Setticemia
Severova bolest	Sever's disease	Maladie de Sever	Enfermedad de Sever	Malattia di Sever
SIDA (sindrom stečene imunodeficijencije, AIDS)	AIDS (acquired immune deficiency syndrome)	SIDA (syndrome d'immunodéficience acquise)	SIDA (síndrome de inmunodeficiencia adquirida)	SIDA (sindrome da ImmunoDeficienza Acquisita, AIDS)
Sideroza	Siderosis	Sidérose	Siderosis	Siderosi
Sifilis (lues)	Syphilis	Syphilis (vérole)	Sífilis	Sifilide (lue)
Silikoza	Silicosis	Silicose	Silicosis	Silicosi
Silosna pluća	Silo-filler's disease	Maladie des ouvriers des silos	Enfermedad de los ensiladores	Malattia dei riempitori dei silos
Sindaktilija	Syndactyly	Syndactylie	Sindactilia	Sindattilia
Sindrom akutne respiratorne insuficijencije (SARS)	Severe acute respiratory syndrome (SARS)	Syndrome respiratoire aigu sévère (SRAS)	Síndrome respiratorio agudo severo (SRAS, SARS)	SARS (Sindrome Acuta Respiratoria Severa)
Sindrom bolnih prepona	Groin pain syndrome	Pubalgie du sportif	Síndrome de dolor inguinal	Pubalgia dello sportivo
Sindrom bolnog ramena (adhezivni kapsulitis ramena, smrznuto rame)	Frozen shoulder (adhesive capsulitis of shoulder)	Épaule bloquée (périarthrite scapulo-humérale)	Capsulitis adhesiva del hombro	Capsulite adesiva
Sindrom bubnjarskog palca (Morbus DeQuervain)	DeQuervain syndrome	Syndrome de DeQuervain (ténosynovite de DeQuervain)	Síndrome de DeQuervain	Sindrome di De Quervain
Sindrom ekonomske klase	Traveller's thrombosis (economy class syndrome)	Thrombose du voyageur	Síndrome de la clase turista	Sindrome della classe economica
Sindrom fascijalnog prostora	Compartment syndrome	Syndrome des loges	Síndrome compartimental	Sindrome compartimentale
Sindrom iritabilnog crijeva (spastični kolon)	Irritable bowel syndrome (spastic colon)	Côlon irritable (côlon spastique)	Síndrome de intestino irritable (colon irritable, colon espástico)	Sindrome del colon irritabile (colon spastico)
Sindrom iznenadne smrti dojenčeta	Sudden infant death syndrome (crib death, cot death)	Syndrome de mort subite du nourrisson	Síndrome de muerte súbita del lactante (muerte en cuna)	Sindrome della morte improvvisa del lattante
Sindrom karpalnog tunela	Carpal tunnel syndrome	Syndrome du canal carpien	Síndrome del túnel carpiano	Sindrome del tunnel carpale
Sindrom kopljaškog lakta	Little league elbow syndrome (LLE syndrome)	Syndrome du tunnel cubital	Síndrome del túnel cubital	Sindrome del tunnel cubitale
Sindrom kroničnog umora	Chronic fatigue syndrome	Syndrome de fatigue chronique	Síndrome de fatiga crónica	Sindrome da fatica cronica
Sindrom m. popliteusa	Popliteus syndrome	Syndrome poplité douloureux	Tendinitis poplítea	Tendinite del popliteo
Sindrom mačjeg krika	Cat cry syndrome (5p minus syndrome, Lejeune's syndrome)	Maladie du cri du chat (syndrome de Lejeune)	Síndrome del maullido del gato (síndrome de Lejeune)	Sindrome del grido di gatto
Sindrom mlohavog djeteta	Floppy infant syndrome	Syndrome du bébé mou	Síndrome de bebé flácido	Sindrome del bambino flaccido
Sindrom Morquio (mukopolisaharidoza tip IV)	Morquio's syndrome (mucopolysaccharidosis IV)	Maladie de Morquio (mucopolysaccharidose type IV)	Enfermedad de Morquio (mucopolisacaridosis tipo IV)	Malattia di Morquio (mucopolisaccaridosi IV)
Sindrom prenaprezanja	Repetitive strain injury (cumulative trauma disorder)	Lésion due à un surmenage répétitif	Síndrome de sobreuso	R.S.I (Repetitive Strain Injury)
Sindrom prenaprezanja Ahilove tetive	Achilles tendon overuse injury	Tendinite achilléenne chronique	Tendinitis por sobreuso en el tendón de Aquiles	Tendinopatia Achille da overuse
Sindrom sraza ramena (subakromijalni sindrom sraza)	Shoulder impingement syndrome (subacromial impingement syndrome)	Syndrome du conflit sous-acromial	Síndrome del conflicto subacromial	Sindrome da conflitto subacromiale (impingement subacromiale)
Sindrom sraza stražnjeg nožnog zgloba	Posterior ankle impingement syndrome	Conflit postérieur de la cheville	Síndrome de pinzamiento posterior del tobillo	Sindrome da impingement posteriore di caviglia
Sindrom stražnje lože natkoljenice (sindrom hamstringsa)	Tight hamstrings syndrome	Hamstring syndrome	Síndrome de isquiosurales cortos	Sindrome degli ischiocrurali (sindrome dell'hamstring)
Sindrom stražnjeg tibijalnog mišića	Tibialis posterior syndrome	Syndrome tibial postérieur	Síndrome del tibial posterior	Periostite tibiale (sindrome del muscolo tibiale posteriore)
Sindrom tarzalnog kanala	Tarsal tunnel syndrome	Syndrome du canal tarsien	Síndrome del túnel tarsiano	Sindrome del tunnel tarsale
Sindrom trenja iliotibijalnog traktusa	Iliotibial band friction syndrome	Syndrome de la bandelette iliotibiale (syndrome de l'essuie glace)	Síndrome de fricción de la banda iliotibial	Sindrome della benderella ileotibiale
Sindrom vrat-rame (cervikobrahijalni sindrom)	Cervicobrachial syndrome	Syndrome cervico-brachial	Síndrome cérvico-braquial	Sindrome cervico-brachiale (sindrome spalla-mano)
Sinkopa	Syncope	Syncope	Síncope	Sincope
Sinovijalni sarkom	Synovial sarcoma	Sarcome synovial	Sarcoma sinovial	Sarcoma sinoviale
Sinoviom	Synovioma	Synoviome	Sinovioma	Synovioma

Hrvatski	Engleski	Francuski	Španjolski	Talijanski
Sinusna glavobolja	Sinus headache	Douleur des sinus (sinusite)	Dolor de cabeza por sinusitis	Sinusite
Siringomijelija	Syringomyelia	Syringomyélie	Siringomielia	Siringomielia
Sistemski lupus eritematozus	Lupus erythematosus	Lupus érythémateux	Lupus eritematoso sistémico	Lupus eritematoso sistemico
Sjögrenov sindrom	Sjögren's syndrome	Syndrome de Sjögren	Síndrome de Sjögren	Sindrome di Sjögren
Sklerodermija	Scleroderma	Sclérodermie	Esclerodermia	Sclerodermia
Sklerozirajuća adenoza	Sclerosing adenosis	Adénose sclérosante	Adenosis esclerosante	Adenosi sclerosante
Skolioza	Scoliosis	Scoliose	Escoliosis	Scoliosi
Skorbut	Scurvy	Scorbut	Escorbuto	Scorbuto
Skotom	Scotoma	Scotome	Escotoma	Scotoma
Slabokrvnost (anemija)	Anemia	Anémie	Anemia	Anemia
Slabost	Weakness	Faiblesse	Debilidad	Debolezza
Slaboumnost	Imbecility	Imbécillité	Imbecilidad	Imbecillità
Slabovidnost	Lazy eye (amblyopia)	Mal-voyance (amblyopie)	Ojo vago (ambliopía)	Ambliopia
Slinjenje	Drooling (ptyalism, sialorrhea, slobbering)	Hypersialorrhée (ptyalisme)	Sialorrea (ptialismo)	Sbavando (ptialismo, scialorrea)
Sluzava stolica	Mucus in stool	Mucus dans les selles	Moco en las heces	Muco nelle feci
Sljepoća	Blindness	Cécité	Ceguera	Cecità
Smanjeno izlučivanje urina (oligurija)	Decreased production of urine (oliguria)	Raréfaction du volume des urines (oligurie)	Disminución de producción de orina (oliguria)	Diminuita escrezione urinaria (oliguria)
Smeđi urin	Brown urine	Urine marron	Orina de color marrón	Urina marrone
Smetenost	Confusion	Confusion	Confusión	Confusione (disordine)
Smrt	Death	Mort	Muerte	Morte
Smrzotina	Chilblain (perniosis)	Engelure	Sabañón	Perniosi
Snižena temperatura tijela (hipotermija)	Decreased body temperature (hypothermia)	Température corporelle basse (hypothermie)	Temperatura corporal baja (hipotermia)	Bassa temperatura corporea (ipotermia)
Sniženi imunitet	Immunodeficiency	Immunodéficience	Inmunodeficiencia	Immunodeficienza
Sopor	Sopor	Sopor	Sopor	Stupor
Sor (oralna kandidijaza)	Thrush (oral candidiasis)	Candidose orale	Candidiasis oral (muguet oral)	Mughetto (moniliasi orale)
Spermatokela (cista epididimisa)	Spermatocele	Spermatocèle	Espermatocele	Spermatocele (cisti spermatica)
Spina bifida	Spina bifida	Spina bifida	Espina bífida	Spina bifida
Spinalni šok	Spinal shock	Choc spinal	Choque espinal	Shock spinale
Spiralni prijelom kosti	Spiral fracture	Fracture en spirale	Fractura espiral	Frattura a spirale
Splenomegalija	Splenomegaly	Splénomégalie	Esplenomegalia	Splenomegalia
Spolno prenosiva bolest	Sexually transmitted disease	Maladie vénérienne	Enfermedad de transmisión sexual	Malattia sessualmente trasmissibile
Spondilitis	Spondylitis	Spondilite	Espondilitis	Spondilite
Spondilolisteza	Spondylolisthesis	Spondylolisthésis	Espondilolistesis	Spondilolistesi
Spondiloza	Spondylosis	Spondylose	Espondilosis	Spondilosi
Spontane frakture	Spontaneous fractures	Fractures spontanées	Fracturas espontáneas	Fratture spontanee
Sporotrihoza	Sporotrichosis	Sporotrichose	Esporotricosis	Sporotricosi
Sportska ozljeda	Sports injury	Blessure de sportif	Lesión deportiva	Trauma sportivo
Sportsko srce	Athlete's heart (cardiac hypertrophy)	Hypertrophie cardiaque du sportif (coeur d'athlète)	Corazón de atleta (hipertrofia del corazón del deportista)	Cuore dell'atleta (ipertrofia cardiaca da sport)
Sposobnost kretanja	Movement ability	Capacité de mouvement	Capacidad de movimiento	Abilità di muoversi
Sprengelova bolest (scapula alta)	Sprengel's deformity	Anomalie de Sprengel	Deformidad de Sprengel	Deformità di Sprengel
Spušteni bubreg (putujući bubreg, nefroptoza)	Floating kidney (nephroptosis, renal ptosis)	Syndrome du rein flottant (néphroptose)	Riñón flotante (ptosis renal, nefroptosis)	Spostamento del rene (ptosi renale, nefroptosi)
Spušteni kapak (blefaroptoza)	Drooping of the upper eyelid (blepharoptosis)	Abaissement de la paupière supérieure (blépharoptose)	Despredimiento del párpado superior (blefaroptosis)	Spostamento della palpebra (palpebra calante, blefaroptosi)
Spušteno stopalo (pes planus)	Flat foot (pes planus)	Pied plat (pes planus)	Pie plano (pes planus, arcos vencidos)	Piede piatto (pes planus)
Srašteni vrat (sindrom Klippel-Feil)	Congenital fusion of cervical vertebrae (Klippel-Feil syndrome)	Fusion congénitale de vertèbres cervicales (Syndrome de Klippel-Feil)	Fusión congenita de vértebras cervicales (síndrome de Klippel-Feil)	Fusione di vertebre cervicali (Sindrome di Klippel Feil)
Srčana aritmija	Cardiac arrhythmia	Arythmie cardiaque	Arrítmia cardíaca	Aritmia cardiaca
Srčana astma (paroksizmalna dispneja)	Cardiac asthma (paroxysmal nocturnal dyspnea)	Dyspnée chez un cardiaque	Disnea paroxística nocturna	Dispnea parossistica notturna
Srčana bolest (kardiopatija)	Heart disease (cardiopathy)	Maladie cardiaque (cardiopathie)	Enfermedad del corazón (cardiopatía)	Malattia del cuore (cardiopatia)
Srčana dekompenzacija	Cardiac decompensation	Décompensation cardiaque	Descompensación cardíaca	Decompensazione cardiaca
Stafilokokno trovanje hranom	Staphylococcal food poisoning	Intoxication alimentaire staphylococcique	Intoxicación alimentaria por estafilococo dorado	Intossicazione alimentare da stafilococco
Staračka dalekovidnost (prezbiopija)	Age-related long-sightedness (presbyopia)	Mauvaise vision de près liée à l'âge (presbytie)	Vista cansada por la edad (presbiopía)	Presbiopia (presbitismo)
Staračka nagluhost (prezbiakuzija)	Age-related hearing loss (presbycusis)	Perte de l'audition liée à l'age (presbyacousie)	Trastorno de la capacidad para oír de las personas envejecen (presbiacusia)	Perdita dell'udito dovuta all'avanzamento dell'età (presbiacusia)
Stenoza aortnog ušća	Aortic valve stenosis	Sténose valvulaire aortique	Estenosis de la válvula aórtica	Stenosi aortica
Stenoza jednjaka	Esophageal stenosis	Sténose oesophagienne	Estenosis esofágica	Stenosi esofagea

Hrvatski	Engleski	Francuski	Španjolski	Talijanski
Stenoza mitralnog ušća	Mitral stenosis	Sténose mitrale	Estenosis mitral	Stenosi mitralica
Stenoza pilorusa (pilorostenoza)	Pyloric stenosis	Sténose du pylore	Estenosis del píloro	Stenosi pilorica
Stenoza plućnog ušća (pulmonalna stenoza)	Pulmonary valve stenosis	Sténose de la valve pulmonaire	Estenosis de la válvula pulmonar	Stenosi polmonare
Stenoza plućne arterije	Stenosis of pulmonary artery	Sténose de l'artère pulmonaire	Estenosis de la arteria pulmonar	Stenosi dell'arteria polmonare
Strano tijelo u nosu	Foreign body in nose	Corps étranger dans le nez	Cuerpo extraño en la nariz	Corpo estraneo nel naso
Strano tijelo u uhu	Foreign body in ear	Corps étranger dans l'oreille	Cuerpo extraño en el oído	Corpo estraneo nell'orecchio
Streptokokna angina	Streptococcal pharyngitis	Pharyngite streptococcique	Faringitis por estreptococo	Faringite streptococcica
Stres-inkontinencija urina	Stress urinary incontinence	Incontinence urinarie d'effort	Incontinencia urinaria por estrés	Incontinenza urinaria da sforzo
Stupor	Stupor	Stupeur	Estupor	Stupore
Subarahnoidalno krvarenje	Subarachnoid hemorrhage	Hémorragie sous arachnoïdienne	Hemorragia subaracnoidea	Emorragia subaracnoidea
Subduralni hematom	Subdural hematoma	Hématome subdural	Hematoma subdural	Ematoma subdurale
Subduralno krvarenje	Subdural hemorrhage	Subdural hemorrhage	Hemorragia subdural	Emorragia subdurale
Sudeckova distrofija	Sudeck's atrophy	Atrophie de Sudeck	Atrofia de Sudeck	Atrofia di Sudeck
Suha gangrena	Dry gangrene	Gangrène sèche	Gangrena seca	Gangrena secca
Suha sluznica usta	Dry mouth (xerostomia)	Sècheresse de la bouche (xèrostomie)	Sequedad de la boca (xerostomía)	Scarsa secrezione salivare (xerostomia)
Suhe oči (kseroftalmija)	Dry eyes (keratoconjuctivitis sicca)	Oeil sec (kérato-conjonctivite sèche)	Sequedad de los ojos (xeroftalmia)	Occhi secchi (xeroftalmia)
Suhi kašalj	Dry cough	Toux sèche	Tos seca (tos perruna)	Tosse secca
Sunčanica	Sunstroke (heat stroke)	Coup de soleil (insolation)	Insolación	Insolazione (colpo di sole)
Suprakondilarni prijelom bedrene kosti	Supracondylar femoral fracture	Fracture supracondylienne du fémur	Fractura supracondilar del fémur	Frattura sovracondiloidea del femore
Suprakondilarni prijelom nadlaktice	Supracondylar humerus fracture	Fracture supracondylienne de l'humérus	Fractura supracondilar del húmero	Frattura sovracondiloidea di omero
Supramaleolarni prijelom potkoljenice	Supramaleolar fracture of tibia and fibula	Fracture tibia péroné sus-malléolaire	Fractura supramaleolar de tibia y peroné	Frattura del terzo distale di tibia e perone
Suzenje očiju	Watery eyes	Yeux larmoyants	Ojos llorosos	Occhi lacrimosi
Sužene zjenice	Small pupils	Pupilles diminuées	Pupilas pequeñas	Pupille costrette
Svinjska gripa	Pig flu (swine influenza, influenzavirus A subtype H1N1)	Gripe porcine	Gripe porcina (influenza porcina, gripe del cerdo)	Influenza suina
Svrab (skabijes)	Scabies (the itch)	Gale (mal de Sainte-Marie)	Arador de la sarna (escabiosis)	Scabbia (rogna)
Svrbež	Itching	Prurit	Prurito (picazón, comezón, rasquiña)	Prurito (pizzicore)
Šarlah (skarlatina)	Scarlet fever	Scarlatine (fièvre écarlate)	Escarlatina (fiebre escarlata)	Scarlattina
Šećer u urinu (glikozurija)	Glucose in urine (glycosuria)	Sucre dans les urines (glycosurie)	Azúcar en orina (glucosuria)	Glicosuria (mellituria)
Šepanje	Limping	Boitillement	Cojera	Zoppicamento
Šigeloza	Shigellosis (bacillary dysentery)	Shigellose	Shigelosis	Shigellosi
Šistosomijaza	Schistosomiasis (snail fever)	Schistosomiase (bilharziose)	Esquistosomiasis (bilharziasis)	Schistosomiasi
Šizofrenija	Schizophrenia	Schizophrénie	Esquizofrenia	Schizofrenia
Šmrcanje	Sniffing (sniffle)	Renifler	Sorberse la nariz (moqueo)	Tirare su col naso
Šok	Shock	Choc	Choque (shock)	Collaso circolatorio (shock)
Španjolska gripa	Spanish flu	Grippe espagnole	Gripe española	Influenza spagnola
Štakorski pjegavac	Murine typhus (endemic typhus)	Typhus murin	Tifus endémico murino	Tifo murino (tifo endemico)
Štucavica	Hiccup	Hoquet	Hipo	Singhiozzo
Šum na srcu	Heart murmur	Souffle cardiaque	Soplo del corazón	Soffio cardiaco
Tahikardija	Tachycardia	Tachycardie	Taquicardia	Tachicardia
Talasemija	Thalassemia	Thalassémie	Talasemia	Talassemia
Tamponada perikarda	Pericardial tamponade (cardiac tamponade)	Tamponnade cardiaque	Tamponamiento cardí-aco (tamponamiento pericárdiaco)	Tamponamento cardiaco
Tendinitis ekstenzora prstiju stopala	Extensor tendinitis (inflammation of the extensor tendons of the toes)	Tendinite des extenseurs des orteils	Tendinitis de los extensores de los dedos	Tendinite dei estensori delle dita del piede
Tendiniti s plesača (tendinitis dugog pregibača palca)	Dancer's tendinitis (flexor hallucis tendinitis)	Tendinite des danseurs (fléchisseur de l'hallux tendinite)	Tendinitis del flexor hallucis longus	Tendinite del flessore lungo dell'alluce
Tendinitis stražnjeg tibijalnog mišića	Tibialis posterior tendinitis	Tendinopathie du tibial postérieur	Tendinopatía tibial posterior	Tendinite del muscolo tibiale posteriore
Tendinoza (kronična ozljeda tetive)	Tendinosis (chronic tendon injury)	Tendinose	Tendinosis (lesión crónica del tendón)	Tendinosi
Teniski lakat	Tennis elbow	Épicondylite latérale	Codo del tenista (epicondílitis lateral)	Gomito del tennista (epicondilite)
Tenzijska glavobolja	Tension headache	Céphalée de tension	Cefalea tensional	Cefalea di tipo tensivo
Teratokarcinom	Teratocarcinoma	Tératocarcinome	Teratocarcinoma	Teratocarcinoma
Teratom	Teratoma	Tératome	Teratoma	Teratoma
Termička rana	Thermal wound	Blessure thermique	Herida térmica	Ferita termica

Hrvatski	Engleski	Francuski	Španjolski	Talijanski
Termičke ozljede	Thermal injuries	Lésions thermiques	Lesiones térmicas	Lesioni termiche
Termonuklearne ozljede	Thermonuclear injuries	Lésions provoquées par une explosion thermonucléaire	Lesiones por una explosión termonuclear	Ferite provocate da esplosioni termonucleari
Testikularna disgeneza	Testicular dysgenesis	Dysgénésie testiculaire	Disgénesis testicular	Disgenesia gonadica
Tetanija	Tetany	Tétanie	Tetania	Tetania
Tetanus (zli grč)	Tetanus	Tétanos	Tétanos (tétano)	Tetano
Teturav nesiguran hod	Shuffling gait	Démarche traînante	Marcha arrastrando los pies	Barcollamento
Tifusna groznica (tifus)	Typhoid fever (typhoid)	Fièvre typhoïde (typhus abdominal)	Fiebre tifoidea (fiebre entérica)	Febbre tifoide (tifo)
Tik	Tic	Tic	Tic	Tic
Tinea corporis	Tinea corporis	Tinea corporis	Tiña corporal (tinea corporis)	Tinea corporis
Tinea favosa (favus)	Favus	Favus	Tiña favosa (favus, tinea favosa)	Tinea favosa
Tireotoksikoza (tireotoksična oluja)	Thyrotoxicosis	Thyréotoxicose	Tirotoxicosis	Tireotossicosi
Tjemenica (dojenačka seboreja)	Cradle cap (infantile seborrhoeic dermatitis)	Dermite séborrhéique infantile	Dermatitis seborreica infantil	Dermatite seborroica infantile
Toksična infekcija Clostridium perfringensom	Clostridium perfringens toxic infection	Toxi-infection à Clostridium perfringens	Tóxico-infección por Clostridium perfringens	Tossinfezione da Clostridium perfringens
Toksična kardiomiopatija	Cardiotoxicity	Cardiotoxicité	Cardiotoxicidad	Cardiomiopatia tossica
Toksokarijaza	Toxocariasis	Toxocarose	Toxocariasis	Toxocariasi
Toksoplazmoza	Toxoplasmosis	Toxoplasmose	Toxoplasmosis	Toxoplasmosi
Toničko-klonički napadaj	Tonic-clonic seizure	Crise tonico-clonique	Crisis tónico-clónica	Crisi tonico-clonica
Topli i vlažni dlanovi	Warm sweaty palms	Paumes des mains chaudes et humides	Palmas de las manos calientes y mojadas	Palmi delle mani caldi e sudati
Torakalni sindrom	Thoracic outlet syndrome	Syndrome de traversée thoraco-cervico-brachiale	Síndrome del estrecho torácico	Sindrome dello stretto toracico superiore
Torzija testisa	Testicular torsion	Torsion testiculaire	Torsión testicular	Torsione del testicolo
Touretteov sindrom	Tourette's syndrome	Syndrome de Tourette	Síndrome de Tourette	Sindrome di Tourette
Trahom	Trachoma	Trachome	Tracoma	Tracoma
Transplantacija bubrega	Kidney transplatation	Transplantation rénale	Transplante de riñón	Trapianto renale
Transpozicija aorte	Transposition of aorta	Transposition de l'aorte	Transposición de la aorta	Trasposizione dell'aorta
Transpozicija plućne arterije	Transposition of pulmonary artery	Transposition de l'artère pulmonaire	Transposición de la arteria pulmonar	Trasposizione dell'arteria polmonare
Transpozicija velikih žila	Transposition of the great vessels	Transposition des gros vaisseaux	Transposición de los grandes vasos	Trasposizione dei grossi vasi
Tranzicionalni karcinom	Transitional cell carcinoma	Carcinome à cellules de transition	Carcinoma de células transicionales	Carcinoma transizionale
Traumatski šok	Traumatic shock	Choc traumatique	Choque traumático	Shock traumatico
Trbušna kolika (abdominalna kolika)	Abdominal colic	Colique abdominale	Cólico abdominal	Colica addominale
Trbušni paratifus	Paratyphoid fever	Fièvre paratyphoïde	Fiebre paratifoidea	Febbre paratifoide
Trbušni tifus (epidemjski tifus, pjegavac)	Epidemic typhus (louse-borne typhus)	Typhus épidémique (typhus à poux, typhus européen)	Tifus exantemático epidémico	Tifo esantematico (tifo epidemico)
Trifascikularni blok	Trifascicular block	Bloc trifasciculaire	Bloqueo trifascicular	Blocco trifascicolare
Trihinoza (trihineloza)	Trichinosis (trichinellosis)	Trichinose	Triquinelosis (triquinosis)	Trichinosi
Trihomonazni vaginitis	Trichomonas vaginalis	Trichomonas vaginalis	Trichomonas vaginalis	Trichomonas vaginalis
Trihomonijaza	Trichomoniasis	Trichomoniase	Trichomoniasis	Trichomoniasi
Tripanosomijaza	Trypanosomiasis	Trypanosomiase	Tripanosomiasis	Tripanosomiasi
Trisomija 13D (Patauov sindrom)	Patau syndrome (trisomy 13)	Syndrome de Patau (trisomie 13)	Síndrome de Patau (trisomía en el par 13)	Sindrome di Patau
Trisomija 18D (Edwardsov sindrom)	Edwards syndrome (trisomy 18)	Syndrome d'Edwards (trisomie 18)	Síndrome de Edwards (trisomía del 18)	Sindrome di Edwards
Trkačka potkoljenica	Shin splints	Périostite tibiale	Dolor en las espinillas	Sindrome da stress tibiale mediale
Trnjenje	Tingling	Fourmillement	Hormigueo	Intormentire
Trombocitopenija	Thrombocytopenia	Thrombocytopénie	Trombocitopenia	Trombocitopenia
Tromboembolija	Thromboembolism	Accident thromboembolique	Tromboembolismo	Tromboembolia
Tromboflebitis	Thrombophlebitis	Thrombophlébite	Troboflebitis	Tromboflebite
Trombotska trombocitopenična purpura	Thrombotic thrombocytopenic purpura	Purpura thrombotique thrombocytopénique	Púrpura trombocitopénica trombótica	Porpora trombotica trombocitopenica
Tromboza	Thrombosis	Thrombose	Trombosis	Trombosi
Trovanje	Poisoning (toxication)	Empoisonnement (toxicité)	Envenenamiento (intoxicación)	Avvelenamento (intossicazione)
Trovanje alkalima	Alkali poisoning	Empoisonnement par alcalis	Intoxicación por álcalis	Avvelenamento da alcali
Trovanje alkoholom	Alcohol poisoning	Empoisonnement par l'alcool	Intoxicación por alcohol	Avvelenamento da alcool
Trovanje arsenom	Arsenic poisoning	Empoisonnement à l'arsenic	Envenenamiento por arsénico	Avvelenamento da arsenico
Trovanje azbestom	Asbestos poisoning	Empoisonnement par l'amiante	Envenenamiento por asbesto	Avvelenamento da amianto
Trovanje bojnim otrovima	Warfare gases poisoning	Intoxication par gaz de combat	Intoxicación por armas gaseosas	Avvelenamento da gas tossico
Trovanje cijanidom	Cyanide poisoning	Empoisonnement au cyanure	Envenenamiento por cianuro	Avvelenamento da cianuro

Hrvatski	Engleski	Francuski	Španjolski	Talijanski
Trovanje gljivama	Mushroom poisoning	Empoisonnement par des champignons	Envenenamiento por setas	Avvelenamento da funghi
Trovanje hranom	Food poisoning	Empoisonnement alimentaires	Intoxicación alimentaria	Avvelenamento da cibo
Trovanje insekticidima	Insecticide poisoning	Empoisonnement au insecticide	Envenenamiento por insecticidas	Avvelenamento da insetticidi
Trovanje kadmijem	Cadmium poisoning	Empoisonnement au cadmium	Envenenamiento por cadmio	Avvelenamento da cadmio
Trovanje kemijskim oružjem	Chemical warfare poisoning	Intoxcation par arme chimique	Intoxicación por armas químicas	Avvelenamento da armi chimiche
Trovanje litijem	Lithium poisoning	Empoisonnement au lithium	Intoxicación por litio	Avvelenamento da litio
Trovanje metanolom	Methanol poisoning	Empoisonnement au méthanol	Intoxicación por metanol	Avvelenamento da metanolo
Trovanje olovom	Lead poisoning	Empoisonnement au plomb	Envenenamiento por plomo	Avvelenamento da piombo (saturnismo)
Trovanje paracetamolom	Paracetamol poisoning	Intoxication par le paracétamol	Intoxicación por paracetamol	Avvelenamento da paracetamolo
Trovanje plinom	Gas poisoning	Empoisonnement au gaz	Envenenamiento por gas	Avvelenamento da gas
Trovanje ribom	Fish poisoning	Empoisonnement du poisson	Intoxicación por pescado	Avvelenamento da pesci
Trovanje salicilatima	Salicylate poisoning	Empoisonnement au salicylate	Intoxicación por salicilatos	Avvelenamento da salicilati
Trovanje školjkašima	Shellfish poisoning	Intoxication par des coquillages	Intoxicación por mariscos	Avvelenamento da molluschi
Trovanje talijem	Thallium poisoning	Empoisonnement au thallium	Envenenamiento por talio	Avvelenamento da tallio
Trovanje teškim metalima	Heavy metal poisoning	Empoisonnement aux métaux lourds	Envenenamiento por metales pesados	Intossicazione da metalli pesanti
Trovanje ugljičnim monoksidom	Carbon monoxide poisoning	Empoisonnement au monoxyde de carbone	Intoxicación por monóxido de carbono	Avvelenamento da monossido di carbonio
Trovanje zračenjem	Radiation poisoning	Empoisonnement par radiations	Envenenamiento por radiación	Avvelenamento da radiazione
Trovanje željezom	Iron poisoning	Empoisonnement au fer	Intoxicación por hierro	Avvelenamento da ferro
Trovanje živom	Mercury poisoning	Empoisonnement au mercure	Envenenamiento por mercurio	Avvelenamento da mercurio
Trzanje mišića	Muscle twitch (fasciculation)	Fasciculation musculaire	Crispar del músculo (fasciculación)	Scossa muscolare (fasciciolazione)
Tuberkuloza (sušica, TBC)	Tuberculosis (TBC)	Tuberculose	Tuberculosis (tisis, TBC)	Tubercolosi (tisi)
Tuberkuloza bubrega	Renal tuberculosis	Tuberculose rénale	Tuberculosis renal	Tubercolosi dei reni
Tuberkuloza crijeva	Intestinal tuberculosis	Tuberculose intestinale	Tuberculosis intestinal	Tubercolosi intestinale
Tuberkuloza jetre	Hepatic tuberculosis	Tuberculose hépatique	Tuberculosis hepática	Tubercolosi epatica
Tuberkuloza kosti	Bone tuberculosis	Tuberculose des os	Tuberculosis ósea	Tubercolosi delle ossa
Tuberkuloza limfnih čvorova	Tuberculous lymphadenitis	Lymphadénite tuberculeuse	Tuberculosis ganglionar (linfadenitis tubercular)	Linfadenite tubercolare
Tuberkuloza pluća	Pulmonary tuberculosis	Tuberculose pulmonaire	Tuberculosis pulmonar	Tubercolosi polmonare
Tuberkulozni artritis	Tuberculous arthritis	Arthrite tuberculeuse	Artritis tuberculosa	Artrite tubercolare
Tuberkulozni spondilitis (Pottova bolest)	Tuberculous spondylitis (Pott disease)	Mal de Pott (tuberculose vertébrale)	Espondilitis tuberculosa	Spondilite tubercolare (morbo di Pott)
Tubularni adenom	Tubular adenoma	Adénome tubulaire	Adenoma tubular	Adenoma tubulare
Tularemija (zečja groznica)	Tularemia (rabbit fever)	Tularémie	Tularemia (fiebre de los conejos)	Tularemia (febbre dei conigli)
Tumor	Tumor (tumour)	Tumeur	Tumor	Tumore
Tumor žumanjčane vreće (endodermalni sinus tumor)	Yolk sac tumor (endodermal sinus tumor)	Tumeur du sac vitellin	Tumor de saco vitelino	Tumore del sacco vitellino
Tungijaza	Tungiasis (nigua, pique)	Sarcopsyllose	Tungiasis	Tungiasi (tunga penetrans)
Tupa bol	Dull pain	Douleur sourde	Dolor sordo	Dolore ottuso
Tupost u udovima	Dullness in limbs	Membres sourds	Torpeza en las extremidades	Ottusità alle estremità
Turnerov sindrom	Turner syndrome	Syndrome de Turner	Síndrome de Turner	Sindrome di Turner
Ubodna rana	Stab wound	Coup de couteau	Estocada	Ferita da punta
Ubrzan bazalni metabolizam	Accelerated basal metabolism	Metabolisme de base accéléré	Metabolismo basal acelerado	Metabolismo basale accelerato
Ubrzani puls	Accelerated pulse rate	Fréquence du pouls accélérée	Pulso acelerado	Polso accelerato
Ubrzano disanje (tahipnea)	Rapid breathing (tachypnea)	Respiration accélérée (tachypnée)	Respiración rápida (taquipnea)	Aumento del ritmo respiratorio (tachipnea)
Učestalo mokrenje	Frequent urination	Miction fréquente	Micción frecuente	Urinazione frequente (pollachiuria)
Učestalo mokrenje velikih količina mokraće (poliurija)	Passage of large volumes of urine (polyuria)	Sécrétion d'urine en quantité abondante (polyurie)	Gasto urinario excesivo (poliuria)	Aumentata emissione di urina (poliuria)
Udubljena prsa (ljevkasta prsa)	Pectus excavatum	Thorax en entonnoir (pectus excavatum)	Pecho hundido (pectus excavatum)	Torace a imbuto (petto escavato)
Uganuće zgloba (distorzija zgloba)	Joint distortion	Distorsion articulaire	Distorsión articular	Distorsione
Uganuće skočnog zgloba	Ankle distortion	Distorsion de la cheville	Distorsión del tobillo	Distorsione alla caviglia

Hrvatski	Engleski	Francuski	Španjolski	Talijanski
Ugriz	Bite	Morsure	Mordedura	Morsicatura
Ugriz bijesne životinje	Bite by rabies infected animal	Morsure d'un animal infecté par le virus de la rage	Mordedura de un animal enfermo de rabia	Morsicatura di animale rabbioso
Ugriz crne udovice	Black widow bite	Morsure de veuve noire	Mordedura de viuda negra	Morso della vedova nera
Ugriz čovjeka (ljudski ugriz)	Human bite	Morsure humaine	Mordedura humana	Morsicatura di uomo
Ugriz mačke	Cat bite	Morsure de chat	Mordedura de gato	Morsicatura di gatto
Ugriz mrava	Ant sting	Piqûre de fourmi	Picadura de hormiga	Puntura di formiche
Ugriz pauka	Spider bite	Piqûre d'araignée	Picadura de araña	Morsicatura di ragno
Ugriz psa	Dog bite	Morsure de chien	Mordedura de perro	Morsicatura di cane
Ugriz škorpiona	Scorpion sting	Piqûre de scorpion	Picadura de escorpión	Puntura di scorpione
Ugriz štakora	Rat bite	Morsure de rat	Mordedura de rata	Morsicatura di ratto
Ugriz zaraženog komarca	Infected mosquito bite	Piqûre de moustique infecté	Picadura de mosquito infectado	Puntura di zanzara infetta
Ugriz zaraženog krpelja	Infected tick bite	Piqûre de tique infectée	Picadura de garrapata infectada	Morsicatura di zecca infetta
Ugriz zmije	Snake bite	Morsure de vipère	Mordedura de víbora	Morsicatura di serpenti
Ugrizna rana	Bite wound	Blessure par morsure	Herida por mordedura	Ferita da morso
Ukočenost	Stiffness	Raideur	Agarrotamiento	Rigidità
Ulcerozni kolitis	Ulcerative colitis	Colite ulcéreuse	Colitis ulcerosa	Rettocolite ulcerosa
Ulozi (giht)	Gout (gouty arthritis)	Goutte	Gota (enfermedad gotosa)	Gotta
Unutarnje krvarenje	Internal bleeding	Saignement interne (hémorragie interne)	Sangrado interno (hemorragia interna)	Emorragia interna
Upala	Inflammation	Inflammation	Inflamación	Infiammazione (flogosi)
Upala bronhija (bronhitis)	Inflammation of the bronchi (bronchitis)	Inflammation des bronches des poumons (bronchite)	Inflamación de los bronquios (bronquitis)	Infiammazione dei bronchi (bronchite)
Upala bronhiola (bronhiolitis)	Inflammation of the bronchioles (bronchiolitis)	Inflammation des petites bronches (bronchiolite)	Inflamación de los bronquiolos (bronquiolitis)	Infiammazione dei bronchioli (bronchiolite)
Upala bubrega (nefritis)	Inflammation of the kidney (nephritis)	Inflammation du rein (néphrite)	Inflamación del riñón (nefritis)	Infiammazione dei reni (nefrite)
Upala desni (gingivitis)	Inflammation of the gums (gingivitis)	Inflammation de la gencive (gingivite)	Inflamación de las encías (gingivitis)	Infiammazione dei tessuti gengivali (gengivite)
Upala dojke (mastitis)	Inflammation of the breast (mastitis)	Inflammation de la mamelle (mastite)	Inflamación del seno (mastitis)	Infiammazione della mammella (mastite)
Upala dušnika (traheitis)	Inflammation of the windpipe (tracheitis)	Inflammation de la trachée (trachéite)	Inflamación de la tráquea (traqueitis)	Infiammazione della trachea (tracheite)
Upala endometrija maternice (endometritis)	Inflammation of the endometrium (endometritis)	Inflammation de l'endomètre (endométrite)	Inflamación del endometrio (endometritis)	Infiammazione dell'endometrio (endometrite)
Upala epiglotisa (epiglotitis)	Inflammation of the epiglottis (epiglottitis)	Inflammation de l'épiglotte (épiglottite)	Inflamación de la epiglotis (epiglotitis)	Infiammazione dell'epi-glottide (epiglottite)
Upala fascije (fasciitis)	Inflammation of the fascia (fasciitis)	Inflammation du fascia (fasciite)	Inflamación de la fascia (fascitis)	Infiammazione della fascia (fascite)
Upala glasnica (laringitis)	Inflammation of the larynx (laryngitis)	Inflammation du larynx (laryngite)	Inflamación de la laringe (laringitis)	Infiammazione della laringe (laringite)
Upala glavića penisa (balanitis)	Inflammation of the glans penis (balanitis)	Inflammation du gland du pénis (balanite)	Inflamación del glande del pene (balanitis)	Infiammazione della testa del glande (balanite)
Upala grla (grlobolja, faringitis)	Sore throat (inflammation of the throat, pharyngitis)	Mal à la gorge (inflamma-ttion du pharinx, pharingite)	Mal de garganta (inflama-ción de la faringe, faringitis)	Mal di gola (infiammazione della faringe, faringite)
Upala gušterače (pankreatitis)	Inflammation of the pancreas (pancreatitis)	Inflammation du pancréas (pancréatite)	Inflamación del páncreas (pancreatitis)	Infiammazione del pancreas (pancreatite)
Upala hvatišta mišića (entezitis)	Inflammation of the entheses (enthesitis)	Inflammation de l'enthèse (enthésite)	Inflamación de la zona de inserción de un músculo (entesitis)	Infiammazione dell'inserzione di muscolo (entesite)
Upala jetre (hepatitis)	Inflammation of the liver (hepatitis)	Inflammation du foie (hépatite)	Inflamación del hígado (hepatitis)	Infiammazione del fegato (epatite)
Upala kože (dermatitis)	Inflammation of the skin (dermatitis)	Inflammaton de la peau (dermatite)	Inflamación de la piel (dermatitis)	Infiammazione della pelle (dermatite)
Upala krajnika (tonzilitis)	Inflammation of the tonsils (tonsillitis)	Inflammation des tonsilles (tonsillite)	Inflamación de las amígdalas palatinas (amigdalitis)	Infiammazione delle tonsille (tonsillite)
Upala labirinta u unutarnjem uhu (labirintitis)	Inflammation of the inner ear (labyrinthitis)	Inflammation de l'oreille interne (labyrinthite, otite interne)	Inflamación del laberinto del oído interno (laberintitis)	Infiammazione di labirinto nell'orecchio interno (labirintite)
Upala limfnog čvora (limfadenitis)	Inflammation of the lymph node (lymphadenitis)	Inflammation des ganglions (adénite, lymphadénite)	Inflamación de los ganglios linfáticos (linfadenitis)	Infiammazione delle ghiandole linfatiche (linfoadenite)
Upala mišića (miozitis)	Inflammation of the muscles (myositis)	Inflammation du tissu musculaire (myosite)	Inflamación del músculo esquelético (miositis)	Infiammazione del tessuto muscolare (miosite)
Upala mokraćnog mjehura (cistitis)	Inflammation of the urinary bladder (cystitis)	Inflammation de la vessie (cystite)	Inflamación de la vejiga urinaria (cistitis)	Infiammazione della vescica urinaria (cistite)
Upala mozga (encefalitis)	Inflammation of the brain (encephalitis)	Inflammation du cerveau (encéphalite)	Inflamación del encéfalo (encefalitis)	Infiammazione del cervello (encefalite)
Upala moždanih ovojnica (meningitis)	Inflammation of the meninges (meningitis)	Inflammation des méninges (méningite)	Inflamación de las meninges (meningitis)	Infiammazione delle meningi (meningite)
Upala mrežnice (retinitis)	Inflammation of the retina (retinitis)	Inflammation de la rétine (rétinite)	Inflamación de la retina (retinitis)	Infiammazione della retina (retinite)

Hrvatski	Engleski	Francuski	Španjolski	Talijanski
Upala osrčja (perikarditis)	Inflammation of the pericardium (pericarditis)	Inflammation du péricarde (péricardite)	Inflamación del pericardio (pericarditis)	Infiammazione del pericardio (pericardite)
Upala parametrija (parametritis)	Inflammation of the parametrium (parametritis)	Inflammation du paramètre (paramétrite)	Inflamación del parametrio (parametritis)	Infiammazione del parametrio (parametrite)
Upala pasjemenika (epididimitis)	Inflammation of the epididymis (epididymitis)	Inflammation de l'épididyme (épididymite)	Inflamación del epidídimo (epididimitis)	Infiammazione dell'epididimo (epididimite)
Upala plućne ovojnice (pleuritis)	Inflammation of the pleura (pleuritis)	Inflammation de la plèvre (pleurésie)	Inflamación de la pleura (pleuritis, pleuresía)	Infiammazione della pleura (pleurite)
Upala pluća (pneumonija)	Inflammation of the lung (pneumonia)	Inflammation des poumons (pneumonie)	Inflamación de los pulmones (neumonía, pulmonía, neumonitis)	Infiammazione dei polmoni (polmonite)
Upala potrbušnice (peritonitis)	Inflammation of the peritoneum (peritonitis)	Inflammation du péritoine (péritonite)	Inflamación del peritoneo (peritonitis)	Infiammazione dela sierosa peritoneale (peritonite)
Upala prostate (prostatitis)	Inflammation of the prostate gland (prostatitis)	Inflammation de la prostate (prostatite)	Inflamación de la próstata (prostatitis)	Infiammazione della ghiandola prostatica (prostatite)
Upala prsne žlijezde (timitis)	Inflammation of the thymus (thymitis)	Inflammation du thymus	Inflamación del timo (timitis)	Infiammazione del timo
Upala rodnice (vaginitis)	Inflammation of the vagina (vaginitis)	Inflammation du vagin (vaginite)	Inflamación de la vagina (vaginitis)	Infiammazione della vagina (vaginite)
Upala rožnice (keratitis)	Inflammation of the cornea (keratitis)	Inflammation de la cornée (kératite)	Inflamación de la córnea (queratitis)	Infiammazione della cornea (cheratite)
Upala rožnice i sluznice oka (keratokonjuktivitis)	Inflammation of the cornea and conjunctiva (keratoconjunctivitis)	Inflammation de la conjonctive et de la cornée (kératoconjonctivite)	Inflamación de la córnea y de la conjuntiva (queratoconjuntivitis)	Infiammazione della cornea e della congiutiva (cheratocongiuntivite)
Upala sinusa (sinusitis)	Inflammation of the paranasal sinuses (sinusitis)	Inflammation du sinus (sinusite)	Inflamación de los senos paranasales (sinusitis)	Infiammazione dei seni paranasali (sinusite)
Upala slijepog crijeva (apendicitis)	Inflammation of the appendix (appendicitis)	Inflammation de l'appendice iléo-caecal (appendicite)	Inflamación del apéndice (apendicitis)	Infiammazione dell'appendice vermiforme (appendicite)
Upala sluzne vreće (burzitis)	Inflammation of the synovial fluid sac (bursitis)	Inflammation de la bourse séreuse articulaire (hygroma, bursite)	Inflamación de la bursa (bursitis)	Infiammazione della borsa sierosa di un'articolazione (borsite)
Upala sluznice mokraćne cijevi (uretritis)	Inflammation of the urethra (urethritis)	Inflammation de l'urètre (urétrite)	Inflamación de la uretra (uretritis)	Infiammazione dell'uretra (uretrite)
Upala sluznice oka (konjuktivitis)	Inflammation of the conjunctiva (conjunctivitis)	Inflammation de la conjonctive (conjonctivite)	Inflamación de la conjuntiva (conjuntivitis)	Infiammazione della congiuntiva (congiuntivite)
Upala sluznice usta (stomatitis)	Inflammation of the mouth mucous lining (stomatitis)	Inflammation de la muqueuse buccale (stomatite)	Inflamación de la mucosa bucal (estomatitis)	Infiammazione delle mucose della bocca (stomatite)
Upala srčane ovojnice (endokarditis)	Inflammation of the endocardium (endocarditis)	Inflammation de l'endocarde (endocardite)	Inflamación del endocardio (endocarditis)	Infiammazione dell'endocardio (endocardite)
Upala srčanog mišića (miokarditis)	Inflammation of the heart muscle (myocarditis)	Inflammation du myocarde (myocardite)	Inflamación del miocardio (miocarditis)	Infiammazione del miocardio (miocardite)
Upala srednje ovojnice oka (uveitis)	Inflammation of the middle layer of the eye (uveitis)	Inflammation de l'uvée (uvéite)	Inflamación de la lámina intermedia del ojo (uveítis)	Infiammazione della tunica media dell'occhio (uveite)
Upala stidnice (vulvitis)	Inflammation of the vulva (vulvitis)	Inflammation de la vulve (vulvite)	Inflamación de la vulva (vulvitis)	Infiammazione della vulva (vulvite)
Upala stijenke arterije (arteritis)	Inflammation of the arterial walls (arteritis)	Inflammation des parois des artères (artérite)	Inflamación de las arterias (arteritis)	Infiammazione delle arterie (arterite)
Upala štitnjače (tireoiditis)	Inflammation of the thyroid gland (thyroiditis)	Inflammation de la glande thyroïde (thyroïdite)	Inflamación de la glándula tiroides (tiroiditis)	Infiammazione della tiroide (tiroidite)
Upala testisa (orhitis)	Inflammation of the testes (orchitis)	Inflammation des testicules (orchite)	Inflamación del testículo (orquitis)	Infiammazione dei testicoli (orchite)
Upala tetive (tendinitis)	Inflammation of the tendon (tendinitis, tendonitis)	Inflammation d'un tendon (tendinite)	Inflamación de un tendón (tendinitis)	Infiammazione del tendine (tendinite)
Upala tetive s ovojnicom (tenosinovitis)	Inflammation of the synovium and tendon (tenosynovitis)	Inflammation d'un tendon et de sa gaine synoviale (ténosynovite)	Inflamación de un tendón y de su vaina (tenosinovitis)	Infiammazione di tendine e di guaina tendinea (tenosinovite)
Upala tetivne ovojnice (sinovitis)	Inflammation of the synovial membrane (synovitis)	Inflammation de la gaine synoviale (synovite)	Inflamación de la membrana sinovial (sinovitis)	Infiammazione della membrana sinoviale (sinovite)
Upala vena (flebitis)	Inflammation of the vein (phlebitis)	Inflammation des veines (phlébite)	Inflamación de las venas (flebitis)	Infiammazione delle vene (flebite)
Upala zgloba (artritis)	Inflammation of the joint (arthritis)	Inflammation des articulations (arthrite)	Inflamación de una articulación (artritis)	Infiammazione articolare (artrite)
Upala želučane sluznice (gastritis)	Inflammation of the stomach lining (gastritis)	Inflammation de la paroi de l'estomac (gastrite)	Inflamación de la mucosa gástrica (gastritis)	Infiammazione della mucosa gastrica (gastrite)
Upala živca (neuritis)	Inflammation of the nerve (neuritis)	Inflammation du nerf (névrite)	Inflamación del nervio (neuritis)	Infiammazione del nervo (neurite, nevrite)
Upala žlijezda slinovnica (sialadenitis)	Inflammation of the salivary gland (sialadenitis)	Inflammation des glandes salivaires (sialoadénite)	Inflamación de las glándulas salivales (sialadenitis)	Infiammazione delle ghiandole salivari (sialoadenite)
Upala žučnog mjehura (holecistitis)	Inflammation of the gall bladder (cholecystitis)	Inflammation de la vésicule biliaire (cholécystite)	Inflamación de la vesícula biliar (colecistitis)	Infiammazione della colecisti (colecistite)
Upalna bolest zdjelice	Pelvic inflammatory disease	Maladie pelvienne inflammatoire	Enfermedad pélvica inflamatoria	Malattia infiammatoria pelvica

Hrvatski	Engleski	Francuski	Španjolski	Talijanski
Urasli nokat (ungvis inkarnatus)	Ingrown nail (onychocryptosis, unguis incarnatus)	Ongle incarné (onychocryptose)	Uña encarnada (onicocriptosis)	Unghia incarnita (onicocriptosi)
Uremija (autointoksikacija radi nelučenja urina)	Uremia (autointoxication due to kidney failure)	Urémie (le taux de l'urée dans le sang)	Uremia (acumulación en la sangre de los productos tóxicos por un fallo renal)	Uremia (accumulo nel sangue di sostanze azotate a causa dell'insufficienza renale)
Ureteralni kamenac (ureterolitijaza)	Ureteral stone (ureterolithiasis)	Calcul dans l'uretère	Cálculo en el uréter (ureterolitiasis)	Calcolo ureterale
Urinarna inkotinencija	Urinary incontinence	Incontinence urinaire	Incontinencia urinaria	Incontinenza urinaria
Urođena aneurizma arterija baze mozga	Congenital aneurysm of arteries at the base of the brain	Anévrisme congénital de l'artère à la base du cerveau	Aneurisma congénito arterial de la base del cerebro	Aneurisma arteriosa congenita alla base dell'encefalo
Urođena srčana bolest (kongenitalna kardiopatija)	Congenital heart disease (congenital cardiopathy)	Cardiopathie congénitale	Cardiopatía congénita	Cardiopatia congenita
Urođena srčana greška	Congenital heart defect	Malformation congénitale du coeur	Malformación cardiaca congénita	Difetto cardiaco congenito
Urođena stenoza pilorusa	Congenital pyloric stenosis	Sténose congénitale du pylore	Estenosis congénita del píloro	Stenosi pilorica congenita
Urođeno iščašenje kuka (kongenitalna displazija kuka)	Congenital dysplasia of the hip (congenital hip dislocation)	Luxation congénitale de la hanche	Displasia congénita de la cadera (luxación congénita de cadera)	Lussazione congenita dell'anca (displasia dell'anca)
Urogenitalna tuberkuloza	Urogenital tuberculosis	Tuberculose urogénitale	Tuberculosis urogenital	Tubercolosi urogenitale
Urogenitalni tumor	Urogenital neoplasm	Tumeur du système uro-génital	Tumor urogenital	Neoplasie del tratto urogenitale
Usporen bazalni metabolizam	Slow basal metabolism	Métabolisme basal diminué	Metabolismo basal lento	Basso metabolismo basale
Usporen puls (bradikardija)	Slow pulse rate (bradycardia)	Rythme cardiaque bas (bradycardie)	Descenso de la frecuencia cardiaca (bradicardia)	Riduzione della frequenza cardiaca (bradicardia)
Usporeno disanje (bradipneja)	Slow breathing rate (bradypnea)	Respiration ralentie (bradypnée)	Descenso de la frecuencia respiratoria (bradipnea)	Riduzione della frequenza respiratoria (bradipnea)
Utapanje	Drowning	Noyade	Ahogamiento	Affogamento
Utrnulost udova	Numbness in limbs	Engourdissements dans les membres (paresthésie)	Adormecimiento de las extremidades	Parestesie delle estremità
Uvećani jezik (makroglosija)	Enlarged tongue (macroglossia)	Augmentation de la langue (macroglossie)	Lengua más grande de lo normal (macroglosia)	Eccessiva crescita della lingua (macroglossia)
Uvučena bradavica	Inverted nipple	Téton ombiliqué	Pezón invertido	Capezzolo invertito
Vaginalni iscjedak	Vaginal discharge	Pertes vaginales	Flujo vaginal	Fuoriuscita vaginale
Valovi vrućine (valunzi)	Hot flushes	Bouffée de chaleur	Sofocos	Vampata di calore
Vanjsko krvarenje	External bleeding	Saignement externe (hémorragie externe)	Sangrado externo (hemorragia externa)	Emorragia esterna
Varikokela	Varicocele	Varicocèle	Varicocele	Varicocele
Varikozni ulcer (venski ulcer)	Venous ulcer (varicose ulcer)	Ulcère veineux	Úlcera varicosa	Ulcera varicosa
Vazomotorni rinitis	Vasomotor rhinitis	Rhinite vasomotrice	Rinitis vasomotora	Rinite vasomotoria
Velike boginje (crne boginje, variola vera)	Smallpox	Variole (petite vérole)	Viruela	Variola vera (vaiolo)
Venska tromboza	Venous thrombosis	Thrombose veineuse	Trombosis venosa	Trombosi venosa
Vensko krvarenje	Venous bleeding	Saignement veineux	Sangrado venoso (hemorragia venosa)	Emorragia venosa
Ventrikularna fibrilacija	Ventricular fibrillation	Fibrillation ventriculaire	Fibrilación ventricular	Fibrillazione ventricolare
Ventrikularna hipertrofija	Ventricular hypertrophy	Hypertrophie ventriculaire	Hipertrofia ventricular	Ipertrofia ventricolare
Ventrikularni septalni defekt	Ventricular septal defect	Communication inter-ventriculaire	Comunicación interventricular	Difetto del setto ventricolare
Veslačka podlaktica (tendinitis podlaktice)	Forearm tendinitis	Tendinite de l'avant-bras	Tendinitis en el antebrazo	Tendinite dell'avambraccio
Vibracijska bolest	Vibration disease	Maladie des vibrations	Enfermedad de las vibraciones	Malattia da vibrazioni
Vibracijski sindrom šaka-ruka	Hand-arm vibration syndrome (vibration white finger)	Syndrome des vibrations du système main-bras	Vibraciones mano bra-zo (dedo blanco indu-cido por vibraciones)	Sindrome da vibrazioni mano-braccio
Virusna hemoragijska groznica	Viral hemorrhagic fever	Fièvre hémorragique virale	Fiebre hemorrágica viral	Febbre emorragica
Virusna infekcija	Viral infection	Infection virale	Infección viral	Infezione virale
Virusna upala pluća	Viral pneumonia	Pneumonie virale	Neumonía viral	Polmonite virale
Virusni hepatitis	Viral hepatitis	Hépatite virale	Hepatitis viral	Epatite virale
Virusni konjuktivitis	Viral conjuctivitis	Conjonctivite virale	Conjuntivitis viral	Congiuntivite virale
Visinska bolest	Altitude sickness (acute mountain sickness)	Mal aigu des montagnes	Mal de montaña (mal de altura)	Mal di montagna
Visoki krvni tlak (hipertenzija)	High blood pressure (hypertension)	Pression artérielle élevée (hypertension artérielle)	Incremento de la presión sanguínea (hipertensión)	Ipertensione arteriosa sistemica
Vitiligo	Vitiligo	Vitiligo	Vitiligo	Vitiligine
Vlažna gangrena	Wet gangrene	Gangrène humide	Gangrena húmeda	Gangrena umida
Vodenasta stolica	Watery stool	Selles aqueuses	Heces acuosas	Consistenza acquosa delle feci
Vodene kozice (variričela)	Chicken-pox	Varicelle	Varicela	Varicella

Hrvatski	Engleski	Francuski	Španjolski	Talijanski
Volkmannova ishemična kontraktura	Volkmann's ischemic contracture	Syndrome de Volkmann	Contractura isquémica de Volkmann	Contrattura ischemica di Volkmann
Von Recklinghausenova bolest	Neurofibromatosis type1 (Von Recklinghausen's disease)	Neurofibromatose de type 1 (maladie de Von Recklinghausen)	Neurofibromatosis de tipo 1 (enfermedad de Von Recklinghausen)	Neurofibromatosi di tipo1 (malattia di von Recklinghausen)
Vraćanje hrane iz želuca u usta (regurgitacija)	Expulsion of undigested food from the mouth (regurgitation)	Retour à la bouche du contenu de l'estomac (régurgitation)	Regreso del contenido alimentario a través del esófago (regurgitación)	Risalita di alimenti dallo stomaco alla bocca (rigurgito)
Vratno rebro	Cervical rib	Côte cervicale	Costilla cervical	Costa cervicale
Vrtoglavica	Dizziness (vertigo)	Vertige	Vértigo	Capogiro (vertigine)
Vulgarne akne	Acne vulgaris	Acné papulo-pustuleuse	Acné común (acne vulgaris)	Acne volgare (acne)
Whippleova bolest	Whipple's disease	Maladie de Whipple	Enfermedad de Whipple	Morbo di Whipple
Wilmsov tumor (nefroblastom)	Wilm's tumor (nephroblastoma)	Tumeur de Wilms (néphroblastome)	Tumor de Wilms (nefroblastoma)	Tumore di Wilms (nefroblastoma)
Začepljeni nos	Nasal congestion (stuffy nose)	Congestion nasale	Congestión nasal	Congestione nasale
Zadah iz usta (halitoza)	Bad breath (halitosis)	Mauvaise heleine (halitose)	Mal aliento (halitosis)	Odore sgradevole dell'alito (alitosi, bromopnea)
Zadebljanje kože	Callosity (thickening)	Callosité	Callosidad (callo)	Callosità (callo)
Zaduha (nedostatak daha, dispneja)	Shortness of breath (dyspnea)	Difficulté respiratoire (dyspnée)	Falta de aire (disnea)	Fame d'aria (dispnea, respirazione difficoltosa)
Zakašnjeli pubertet	Delayed puberty	Puberté tardive	Retraso de la pubertad	Pubertà tardiva
Zakočenost zgloba	Joint stiffness	Raideur articulaire	Rigidez de las articulaciones	Rigidità dell'articolazione
Zanoktica	Agnail (hangnail)	Envie de l'ongle	Padrastro	Pipita
Zapletaj crijeva	Abnormal twisting of the intestines (volvulus)	Volvulus	Retorcimiento anormal del intestino (vólvulo)	Volvolo
Zastoj disanja (apnea)	Suspension of external breathing (apnea)	Arrêt respiratoire (apnée)	Falta de respiración (apnea)	Assenza di respirazione (apnea)
Zastoj urina (urinarna retencija)	Urinary retention (ischuria)	Rétention d'urine	Retención de orina	Ritenzione urinaria
Zastoj srca (srčani arest)	Cardiac arrest (cardiopulmonary arrest)	Arrêt cardiaque (arrêt ventilatoire, arrêt cardio-respiratoire)	Paro cardiaco (parada cardiorrespiratoria)	Arresto cardiaco
Zatajenje bubrega (insuficijencija bubrega)	Kidney failure (renal insufficiency)	Insuffisance rénale	Fallo renal (insuficiencia renal)	Insufficienza renale
Zatajenje jetre	Liver insufficiency	Insuffisance hépatique	Fallo hepático (insuficiencia hepática)	Insufficienza epatica
Zatvor (opstipacija)	Constipation (obstipation)	Constipation	Estreñimiento	Stitichezza (costipazione)
Zaušnjaci (mumps, parotitis)	Mumps (epidemic parotitis)	Oreillons (parotidite virale)	Paperas (parotiditis)	Parotite (orecchioni)
Zelenkasta stolica	Green stool	Selles vertes	Heces verdes	Feci di colore verde
Zijevanje	Yawn	Bâillement	Bostezo	Sbadiglio
Zika groznica	Zika fever	Fièvre Zika	Fiebre del Zika	Febbre Zika
Zimica (tresavica)	Shivering	Frissonnement	Escalofrío (tiritón)	Brivido
Zloćudni tumor (maligni tumor, rak)	Malignant tumor (cancer)	Tumeur maligne (cancer)	Tumor maligno (cáncer)	Tumore maligno
Znojenje	Sweating	Sudation	Transpiración (sudación)	Sudorazione (traspirazione)
Zoonoza	Zoonosis	Zoonose	Zoonosis	Zoonosi
Zračna embolija	Air embolism (gas embolism)	Embolie gazeuse	Embolia gaseosa	Embolia gassosa
Zubni kamenac	Dental plaque (dental tartar)	Plaque dentaire	Placa dental	Placca (tartZub
Zubni karijes	Dental caries	Carie dentaire	Caries	Carie dentaria
Zubobolja	Toothache	Mal de dents	Dolor de muelas	Mal di denti
Zujanje u ušima (tinitus)	Ringing in ears (tinnitus)	Acouphène	Pitidos en el oído (acúfeno, tinnitus)	Ronzio auricolare (acufene, tinnito)
Žed	Thirst	Soif	Sed	Sete
Žgaravica	Heartburn	Brûlure de l'estomac (pyrosis)	Ardor de estómago (acidez, pirosis)	Bruciore di stomaco (pirosi)
Žučna kolika	Biliary colic	Colique biliaire	Cólico biliar	Colica biliare
Žučni kamenac (holelitijaza)	Gallstone (cholelithiasis)	Calcul biliaire (cholélithiase)	Cálculo biliar (litiasis biliar)	Calcolo biliare
Žulj (plik, kurje oko)	Blister (corn)	Cor (cal)	Ampolla (callo)	Callo (vescica, bolla)
Žuta groznica	Yellow fever	Fièvre jaune	Fiebre amarilla	Febbre gialla
Žuta stolica	Yellow stool	Selles jaunes	Heces amarillas	Feci gialle
Žutica (ikterus)	Jaundice (icterus)	Ictère (jaunisse)	Ictericia	Ittero (itterizia)
Žutica moždanih jezgri	Kernicterus	Kernictère	Kernicterus (encefalopatía neonatal bilirrubínica)	Kernittero (encefalopatia bilirubinica)
LJEKARNA:	PHARMACY:	PHARMACIE:	FARMACIA:	FARMACIA:
Adrenalin	Adrenaline	Adrénaline	Adrenalina	Adrenalina
Aerosol	Aerosol	Aérosol	Aerosol	Aerosol
Aktivni ugljen	Activated carbon	Charbon actif	Carbón activado	Carbone attivo
Alergija na lijek	Drug allergy	Allergie à un médicament	Alergia al medicamento	Allergia a medicamento
Alkohol	Alcohol	Alcool	Alcohol	Alcol
Aminofilin	Aminophylline	Aminophylline	Aminofilina	Aminofillina
Ampicilin	Ampicillin	Ampicilline	Ampicilina	Ampicillina
Ampula	Ampoule	Ampoule	Ampolla (recipiente)	Ampolla (fiala)
Analgetik	Analgesic (painkiller)	Analgésique	Analgésico	Analgesico

Hrvatski	Engleski	Francuski	Španjolski	Talijanski
Anestetik	Anesthetic	Anesthésique	Anestésico	Anestetico
Antacid	Antacid	Antiacide	Antiácido	Antiacido
Antialergik	Antiallergic drug	Antiallergique	Antialérgico	Farmaco antiallergico
Antialkoholik	Antialcoholic drug	Médicament contre la dépendance à l'alcool	Fármaco antialcohólico	Farmaco anti-alcol
Antianemik	Antianemic	Médicament antianémique	Antianémico	Farmaco antianemico
Antiaritmik	Antiarrhythmic agent	Agent antiarythmique	Agente antiarrítmico	Farmaco antiaritmico
Antibiotik	Antibiotic	Antibiotique	Antibiótico	Antibiotico
Antidepresiv	Antidepressant	Antidépresseur	Antidepresivo	Antidepressivo
Antidiabetik	Anti-diabetic drug	Médicament antidiabétique	Antidiabético	Antidiabetico
Antidiaroik	Antidiarrhoeal drug	Médicament antidiarrhéique	Antidiarréico	Antidiarroici
Antidot	Antidote	Antidote	Antídoto	Antidoto
Antiepileptik (antikonvulziv)	Anticonvulsant	Antiépileptique (anticonvulsivant)	Anticonvulsivo (antiepiléptico)	Anticonvulsante
Antihelmintik	Antihelminthic	Antihelminthique	Antihelmíntico	Antielmintici
Antihipertenziv	Antihypertensive drug	Antihypertenseur	Antihipertensivo	Farmaco antiipertensivo
Antihistaminik	Antihistamine	Antihistaminique	Antihistamínico	Antistaminico
Antikoagulans	Anticoagulant	Anticoagulant	Anticoagulante	Anticoagulante
Antimalarik	Antimalarial drug	Antimalarique	Antimalárico	Antimalarico
Antimikotik	Antimycotic	Antimycosique	Antimicótico (antifúngico)	Antimicotico
Antioksidans	Antioxidant	Antioxydant	Antioxidante	Antiossidante (sostanza antiossidante)
Antiperspirant	Antiperspirant	Déodorant	Desodorante	Antidiaforetico
Antipiretik	Antipyretic	Antipyrétique	Antipirético	Antipiretico
Antiprotozoik	Antiprotozoal agent	Médicament antiprotozoal	Antiprotozoario	Farmaco antiprotozoico
Antipsihotik	Antipsychotic	Antipsychotique	Antipsicótico	Antipsicotico
Antireumatik	Antirheumatic drug	Médicament antirhumatismal	Antireumático	Antireumatico
Antiseptik	Antiseptic	Antiseptique	Antiséptico	Antisettico
Antiserum	Antiserum	Antisérum	Antisuero	Antisiero
Antituberkulotik	Antitubercular agent	Antituberculeux	Fármaco tuberculostático	Farmaco antitubercolare
Antivirusni lijek	Antiviral drug	Médicament antiviral	Fármaco antiviral	Farmaco antivirale
Aspirin	Aspirin	Aspirine	Aspirina	Aspirina
Atropin	Atropine	Atropine	Atropina	Atropina
Bademovo ulje	Almond oil	Huile d'amande	Aceite de almendras dulces	Olio di mandorla
Bakar	Copper	Cuivre	Cobre	Rame
Barbiturat	Barbiturate	Barbiturique	Barbitúrico	Barbiturico
Biljni čaj	Herbal tea	Tisane	Tisana (infusión de hierbas)	Tisana (infuso di erbe)
Bočica	Vial	Fiole	Frasquito	Bottiglietta (boccetta)
Borova otopina	Boric acid	Acide borique	Ácido bórico	Acido borico
Bronhodilatator	Bronchodilator	Bronchodilatateur	Broncodilatador	Broncodilatatore
Cefalosporin	Cephalosporin	Céphalosporine	Cefalosporina	Cefalosporina
Cink	Zinc	Zinc	Zinc (cinc)	Zinco
Cinkova pasta	Zinc ointment	Pommade à l'oxyde de zinc	Pasta de óxido de zinc	Zinco pasta
Citostatik	Cytostatic	Cytostatique	Citostático	Citostatico
Cjepivo	Vaccine	Vaccin	Vacuna	Vaccino
Čepić	Suppository	Suppositoire	Supositorio	Supposta
Digestiv	Digestive	Médicament digestif	Digestivo	Digestivo
Dijafragma	Diaphragm (Dutch cap)	Diaphragme	Diafragma	Diaframma
Dijetetsko sredstvo	Anti-obesity medication	Médicament anti-obésité	Fármaco antiobesidad	Dimagrante (farmaco antiobesità)
Diuretik	Diuretic	Diurétique	Diurético	Diuretico
Doza	Dose	Dose	Dosis	Dose
Dražeja (tableta)	Tablet	Comprimé	Comprimido	Compressa (pasticca, tavoletta)
Emulzija	Emulsion	Émulsion	Emulsión	Emulsione
Eritromicin	Erythromycin	Érythromycine	Eritromicina	Eritromicina
Eterično ulje	Essential oil	Huile essentielle	Aceite esencial	Olio essenziale (olio eterico)
Fentanil	Fentanyl	Fentanyl	Fentanilo	Fentanyl
Fitoterapija	Phytotherapy	Phytothérapie	Fitoterapia	Fitoterapia
Fiziološka otopina	Saline solution	Solution physiologique	Suero fisiológico	Soluzione fisiologica
Flaster	Plaster (adhesive strip)	Pansement	Tira adhesiva sanitaria	Cerotto
Fosfor	Phosphorus	Phosphore	Fósforo	Fosforo
Gaza	Gauze sponge	Gaze	Gasa	Garza
Gel	Gel	Gel	Gel	Gel
Gentamicin	Gentamicin	Gentamicine	Gentamicina	Gentamicina
Glukoza	Glucose	Glucose	Glucosa	Glucosio
Gram	Gram (gramme)	Gramme	Gramo	Grammo
Grožđana mast	Lip balm	Tube de soin pour lèvres	Bálsamo de labios	Burrocacao
Hemostatik	Antihemorrhagic (hemostatic)	Hémostatique	Hemostático	Emostatico
Heparin	Heparin	Héparine	Heparina	Eparina
Higijenski ulošci	Sanitary pads (sanitary napkins)	Serviette hygiénique (protège-slip)	Toalla sanitaria (compresa, pantiprotector)	Assorbenti igienici
Hipnotik	Hypnotic (soporific)	Hypnotique (somnifère)	Hipnótico	Ipnotico

Hrvatski	Engleski	Francuski	Španjolski	Talijanski
Hormonalna nadomjesna terapija	Hormone replacement therapy	Hormonothérapie de substitution	Terapia de sustitución hormonal	Terapia ormonale sostitutiva
Igla	Needle	Aiguille	Aguja	Ago
Imunoglobulin	Immunoglobulin	Immunoglobuline	Inmunoglobulina	Immunoglobulina
Imunosupresiv	Immunosuppressive	Immunosuppresseur	Inmunosupresor	Immunosoppressivo
Inhalacija	Inhalation	Inhalation	Inhalación	Inalazione (farmaco per inalazioni)
Interferon	Interferon	Interféron	Interferón	Interferone
Inzulin	Insulin	Insuline	Insulina	Insulina
Injekcija	Injection	Injection	Inyección	Iniezione
Ispiranje	Rinsing	Rinçage	Lavado	Sciacquatra (risciacquatura)
Jod	Iodine	Iode	Yodo (iodo)	Iodio (tintura di iodio)
Jojobino ulje	Jojoba oil	Huile de jojoba	Aceite de jojoba	Olio di jojoba
Kalcij	Calcium	Calcium	Calcio	Calcio
Kalij	Potassium	Potassium	Potasio	Potassio
Kamilica	Chamomile	Camomille	Manzanilla	Camomilla
Kapi (kapljice)	Drops	Gouttes	Gotas	Gocce
Kapi za nos	Nasal drops	Gouttes nasales	Gotas nasales	Gocce nasali
Kapi za oči	Eye drops	Collyre (gouttes ophtalmiques)	Colirio	Collirio
Kapi za uši	Ear drops	Gouttes auriculaires	Gotas óticas	Gocce per il mal di orecchi
Kapsula	Capsule	Gélule	Cápsula	Capsula
Kardiotonik	Cardiotonic agent	Médicament cardiotonique	Cardiotónico	Cardiotonico
Kemoterapija	Chemotherapy	Chimiothérapie	Quimioterapia	Chemioterapia
Klizma (klistir)	Enema (clyster)	Clystère	Enema (clisma)	Clistere
Klor	Chlorine	Chlore	Cloro	Cloro
Kloramfenikol	Chloramphenicol	Chloramphénicol	Cloranfenicol	Cloramfenicolo
Kobalt	Cobalt	Cobalt	Cobalto	Cobalto
Kodein	Codeine	Codéine	Codeína	Codeina
Kofein	Caffeine	Caféine	Cafeína	Caffeina
Komad	Piece	Morceau	Pieza	Pezzo (porzione)
Kontaktne leće	Contact lenses	Lentilles de contact	Lentes de contacto (lentillas, pupilentes)	Lenti a contatto
Kontracepcijska pilula	Contraceptive pill (oral contraceptive)	Contraception orale	Píldora anticonceptiva	Pillola anticoncezionale
Kontracepcijska pjena	Contraceptive foam	Mousse contraceptive	Espuma anticonceptiva	Schiuma anticoncezionale
Kontracepcijska spužva	Contraceptive sponge	Éponge contraceptive	Esponja anticonceptiva	Spugna contraccettiva
Kontraceptiv	Contraceptive	Contraceptif	Anticonceptivo	Contraccettivo
Kortikosteroid	Corticosteroid	Corticostéroïde	Corticosteroide	Corticosteroide
Krema	Skin cream	Crème	Crema	Crema
Kućni test za trudnoću	Home pregnancy test	Test de grossesse	Prueba de embarazo	Test di gravidanza ad uso domiciliare
Laksativ	Laxative	Laxatif	Laxante	Lassativo
Lijek	Medication (remedy, drug)	Médicament	Medicamento (fármaco)	Medicamento (farmaco, rimedio)
Lijek protiv mučnine i povraćanja	Antiemetic and motion sickness drug	Antiémétique	Antiemético	Antiemetico
Litra	Litre	Litre	Litro	Litro
Losion	Lotion	Lotion	Loción	Lozione
Lubrikant	Lubricant	Lubrifiant	Lubricante	Lubrificante
Ljekarnik	Pharmacist	Pharmacien	Farmacéutico	Farmacista
Ljekoviti napitak	Potion	Potion	Poción	Pozione
Magnezij	Magnesium	Magnésium	Magnesio	Magnesio
Mangan	Manganese	Manganèse	Manganeso	Manganese
Medicinski kanabis	Medical cannabis	Cannabis médical	Cannabis medicinal	Cannabis terapeutica
Meka kontaktna leća	Soft contact lens	Lentille de contact souple	Lente de contacto blanda	Lente a contatto morbida
Metadon	Methadone	Méthadone	Metadona	Metadone
Mikrogram	Microgram	Microgramme	Microgramo	Microgrammo
Miligram	Milligram (milligramme)	Milligramme	Miligramo	Milligrammo
Mililitar	Millilitre	Millilitre	Mililitro	Millilitro
Mineral	Mineral	Minéral	Mineral	Minerale
Mineralno ulje	Mineral oil	Huile minérale	Aceite mineral	Olio minerale
Miorelaksator	Muscle relaxant	Myorelaxant	Relajante muscular (miorrelajante)	Miorilassante
Molibden	Molybdenum	Molybdène	Molibdeno	Molibdeno
Morfin	Morphine	Morphine	Morfina	Morfina
Mukolitik	Mucolytic	Mucolytique	Mucolítico	Mucolitico
Na tašte	On an empty stomach (before the meal)	À jeun	En ayunas	A digiuno
Na usta	Orally	Par voie orale	Por vía oral	Oralmente (per via orale, per bocca)
Na večer	In the evening	Le soir	Por la noche	La sera
Nakon jela	After meal	Après-repas	Después de una comida	Dopo il pasto
Naočale	Glasses	Lunettes de vue	Gafas	Occhiali
Natrij	Sodium	Sodium	Sodio	Sodio
Nesteroidni antireumatik	Non-steroidal anti-inflammatory drug	Anti-inflammatoire non stéroïdien	Antiinflamatorio no esteroideo	Farmaco anti-infiammatore non steroide-FANS

Hrvatski	Engleski	Francuski	Španjolski	Talijanski
Nikotinska guma za žvakanje	Nicotine gum	Gomme à la nicotine	Goma de mascar de nicotina	Gomma da masticare antifumo
Nikotinski flaster	Nicotine patch	Timbre à la nicotine	Parche de nicotina	Cerotto antifumo
Nistatin	Nystatin	Nystatine	Nistatina	Nistatina
Nuspojave lijeka	Drug side-effects	Effets indésirables d'un médicament	Reacción adversa a medicamento	Effetti indesiderati da farmaco
Nutritiv	Nutrient	Nutriment (élément nutritif)	Nutrimento (nutriente)	Sostanza nutriente (sostanza nutritiva)
Oblog	Compress	Compresse	Compresa	Compressa
Oksikodon	Oxycodone	Oxycodone	Oxicodona	Ossicodone
Omega -3 masne kiseline	Omega-3 fatty acid	Acides gras oméga-3	Ácido graso omega 3	Omega-3 acidi grassi
Opijat (opioid)	Opioid	Opioïde	Opioide	Oppioide
Otopina	Solution	Solution	Soluto	Soluzione
Otrov	Poison	Poison	Veneno	Veleno
Paracetamol	Paracetamol	Paracétamol	Paracetamol	Paracetamolo
Parafin	Paraffin	Paraffine	Parafina	Paraffina
Pasta	Paste	Pâte	Pasta	Pasta
Pasta za zube	Tooth paste	Dentifrice	Pasta de dientes (dentífrico)	Dentifricio
Pelene za inkontinenciju	Incontinence pads (adult diapers)	Slip d'incontinence	Pañal para adultos	Assorbenti per l'incontinenza
Penicilin	Penicillin	Pénicilline	Penicilina	Penicillina
Pilula za "dan poslije" (postkoitalna kontracepcija, hitna kontracepcija)	'Morning-after' pill (postcoital contraception, emergency contraception)	Pilule du lendemain (contraception postcoïtale, contraception d'urgence)	Anticonceptivo de emergencia (contracepción poscoital)	Pillola del "giorno doppo" (contraccezione postcoitale, contraccezione di emergenza)
Pjena	Foam	Mousse	Espuma	Schiuma (spuma)
Pod jezik	Sublingual administration	Sublingual	Vía sublingual	Sublinguale
Pomada (mast)	Ointment (fat)	Pommade	Ungüento (pomada)	Pomata (unguento)
Prašak (puder)	Powder	Poudre	Polvo	Polverina (polvere)
Predoziranje	Overdose	Surdose	Sobredosis	Sovradosaggio
Prezervativ (kondom)	Condom	Préservatif	Preservativo (condón, profiláctico)	Preservativo (profilattico, condom)
Protuotrov	Antitoxin	Antitoxine	Antitoxina	Antitossina
Protuupalno	Anti-inflammatory	Anti-inflammatoire	Antiinflamatorio (antiflogístico)	Antinfiammatorio
Psihostimulans	Psychostimulant	Psychostimulant	Psicoestimulante	Psicostimulanti
Purgativ	Purgative	Purgatif	Purgante (purgativo)	Purgante (purga)
Recept	Prescription	Ordonnance médicale	Receta	Prescrizione (rimedio prescritto)
Rektalno	Rectal	Rectal	Rectal	Rettale
Ricinusovo ulje	Castor oil	Huile de ricin	Aceite de ricino	Olio di ricino
Salicilat	Salicylate	Salicylate	Salicilato	Salicilato
Sapun	Soap	Savon	Jabón	Sapone
Sedativ	Sedative	Sédatif	Sedativo	Sedativo (calmante)
Serum	Serum	Sérum	Suero	Siero
Sirup	Syrup	Sirop	Jarabe	Sciroppo
Spazmolitik	Spasmolytic	Spasmolytique	Espasmolítico	Spasmolitico
Spermicid	Spermicide	Spermicide	Espermicida	Spermicida
Sprej	Spray	Spray	Rociada	Spruzzo (vaporizzato)
Sredstvo protiv insekata	Insect repellent	Répulsif d'insectes	Repelente de insectos	Insettifugo
Sredstvo protiv komaraca	Mosquito repellent	Répulsif antimoustiques	Repelente de mosquitos	Repellente antizanzare
Sredstvo za iskašljavanje	Expectorant	Expectorant	Expectorante	Espettorante
Sredstvo za zaštitu od sunca	Sunscreen (sunblock)	Crème solaire	Protector solar	Filtro solare (crema so-lare ad alta protezione)
Sulfonamid	Sulphonamide	Sulfamidé	Sulfonamida	Sulfamidici (sulfonamidici)
Sumpor	Sulphur	Soufre	Azufre	Zolfo
Sustav međunarodnih mjernih jedinica	International System of Units	Système international d'unités	Sistema Internacional de Unidades	Sistema internazionale di unità di misura
Šprica	Syringe	Seringue	Jeringa	Siringa per iniezioni
Šumeće tablete	Water-soluble tablets	Comprimé effervescent	Solubilizantes (comprimidos dispersables en agua)	Compresse solubili
Tableta za sisanje (pastila)	Pastille (lozenge)	Pastille	Pastilla	Pasticca (pastiglia)
Tampon	Tampon	Tampon hygiénique	Tampón	Tampone
Tekući puder	Liquid powder	Poudre fluide	Polvo liquido	Polvere liquido
Tekućina za čišćenje kontaktnih leća	Contact lenses cleaning solution	Solution nettoyante pour lentilles	Solución limpiadora de lentes de contacto	Soluzione per pulizia lenti a contatto
Tekućina za čišćenje umjetnog zubala	Denture cleaning solution	Solution nettoyante pour les prothèses	Solución limpiadora de dentadura	Soluzione per pulizia dentiera
Tekućina za ispiranje usne šupljine	Mouthwash liquid	Eau dentifrice	Enjuague bucal (colutorio)	Collutorio
Termofor	Hot water bottle	Bouillotte	Bolsa de agua caliente (guatero)	Bouillotte (bouilloire)
Tetraciklin	Tetracycline	Tétracycline	Tetraciclina	Tetraciclina
Tinktura	Tincture	Teinture	Tintura	Tintura
Tlakomjer	Blood pressure meter (sphygmomanometer)	Tensiomètre (sphygmomanomètre)	Tensiómetro (esfigmomanómetro)	Misuratore di pressione (sfigmomanometro)

Hrvatski	Engleski	Francuski	Španjolski	Talijanski
Tonik	Tonic	Tonique	Tónico	Tonico (ricostituente)
Toplomjer	Thermometer	Thermomètre	Termómetro	Termometro
Tramal	Tramadol	Tramadol	Tramadol	Tramadolo
Tvrda kontaktna leća	Hard contact lens	Lentille de contact rigide	Lente de contacto duro	Lente a contatto rigida
U jutro	In the morning	Le matin	Por la mañana	Di mattina
U podne	At noon	À midi	A mediodía	A mezzogiorno
Umjetno sladilo	Sugar substitute	Édulcorant	Edulcorante artificial	Dolcificante artificiale
Uroantiseptik	Urinary antiseptic	Antiseptique urinaire	Antiséptico de las vías urinarias	Antisettico urinario
Vaga	Scales	Balance	Balanza	Bilancia
Vaginaleta	Vaginal suppository	Ovule (suppositoire vaginal)	Supositorio vaginal	Candelette
Vata	Cotton-wool	Ouate (coton hydrophile)	Algodón hidrófilo	Ovatta
Vazodilatator	Vasodilatator	Vasodilatador	Vasodilatador	Vasodilatatore
Viagra	Viagra (sildenafil citrate)	Viagra (citrate de sildénafil)	Viagra	Viagra (citrato di sildenafil)
Vitamin	Vitamin	Vitamine	Vitamina	Vitamina
Vitamin A (retinol)	Vitamin A (retinol)	Vitamine A (rétinol)	Vitamina A (retinol)	Vitamina A (retinolo)
Vitamin B1 (tiamin)	Vitamin B1 (thiamin)	Vitamine B1 (thiamine)	Vitamina B1 (tiamina)	Vitamina B1 (tiamina)
Vitamin B2 (riboflavin)	Vitamin B2 (riboflavin)	Vitamine B2 (riboflavine)	Vitamina B2 (riboflavina)	Vitamina B2 (riboflavina)
Vitamin B3 (niacin)	Vitamin B3 (niacin)	Vitamine B3 (nicotinamide, PP)	Vitamina B3 (niacina, vitamina PP)	Vitamina B3 (niacina, vitamina PP)
Vitamin B4 (adenin)	Vitamin B4 (adenine)	Vitamine B4 (adénine)	Vitamina B4 (adenina)	Vitamina B4 (adenina)
Vitamin B5 (pantotenska kiselina)	Vitamin B5 (pantothenic acid)	Vitamine B5 (acide pantothénique)	Vitamina B5 (ácido pantoténico)	Vitamina B5 (acido pantotenico, vitamina W)
Vitamin B6 (piridoksin)	Vitamin B6 (pyridoxine)	Vitamine B6 (pyridoxine)	Vitamina B6 (piridoxina)	Vitamina B6 (piridossina)
Vitamin B7 (inozitol)	Vitamin B7 (inositol)	Vitamine B7 (inositol)	Vitamina B7 (inositol)	Vitamina B7 (inositolo)
Vitamin B8 (biotin)	Vitamin B8 (biotin)	Vitamine B8 (biotine)	Vitamina B8 (biotina)	Vitamina B8 (biotina)
Vitamin B9 (folna kiselina)	Vitamin B9 (folic acid)	Vitamine B9 (acide folique)	Vitamina B9 (ácido fólico)	Vitamina B9 (acido folico)
Vitamin B10 (faktor-R)	Vitamin B10 (factor-R)	Vitamine B10 (vitamine R)	Vitamina B10 (vitamina R)	Vitamina B10 (vitamina R)
Vitamin B11 (faktor-S)	Vitamin B11 (factor-S)	Vitamine B11 (carnitine)	Vitamina B11 (vitamina S)	Vitamina B11 (vitamina S)
Vitamin B12 (kobalamin)	Vitamin B12 (cobalamin)	Vitamine B12 (cobalamine)	Vitamina B12 (ciancobalamina)	Vitamina B12 (cobalamina)
Vitamin C (L-askorbinska kiselina)	Vitamin C (L-ascorbic acid)	Vitamine C (acide ascorbique)	Vitamine C (enantiómero L de ácido ascórbico)	Vitamina C (acido L-ascorbico)
Vitamin D2 (ergokalciferol)	Vitamin D2 (ergocalciferol)	Vitamine D2 (ergocalciférol)	Vitamina D2 (ergocalciferol)	Vitamina D2 (ergocalciferolo)
Vitamin D3 (kolekalciferol)	Vitamin D3 (cholecalciferol)	Vitamine D3 (cholécalciférol)	Vitamina D3 (colecalciferol)	Vitamina D3 (colecalciferolo)
Vitamin D4	Vitamin D4	Vitamine D4	Vitamina D4	Vitamina D4 (diidroergocalciferolo)
Vitamin D5 (sitokalciferol)	Vitamin D5 (sitocalciferol)	Vitamine D5 (sitocalciférol)	Vitamina D5 (sitocalciferol)	Vitamina D5 (sitocalciferolo)
Vitamin E (tokoferol)	Vitamin E (tocopherol)	Vitamine E (tocophérol)	Vitamina E (alfatocoferol)	Vitamina E (tocoferolo)
Vitamin F (linoleična kiselina)	Vitamin F (linoleic acid)	Vitamine F (acide linoléique)	Ácido linoleico	Vitamina F (acido linoleico)
Vitamin J (kolin)	Vitamin J (choline)	Vitamine J (choline)	Vitamina J (colina)	Vitamina J (colina)
Vitamin K (filokinon)	Vitamin K (phylloquinone)	Vitamine K (phylloquinone)	Vitamina K (filoquinona)	Vitamina K (fillochinone)
Vitamin L1 (antranilna kiselina)	Vitamin L1 (anthranilic acid)	Vitamine L1 (acide anthranilique)	Vitamina L1 (ácido antranílico)	Vitamina L1 (acido antranilico)
Vitamin P (flavonoidi)	Vitamin P (flavonoids)	Vitamine P (flavonoïde)	Vitamina P (flavonoide)	Vitamina P (flavonoidi)
Za vanjsku primjenu	For external application	Pour l'application externe	De uso externo	Per l'applicazione esterna
Zavoj	Bandage	Bandage	Venda	Bendaggio
Zubni konac	Dental floss	Fil dentaite	Seda dental (hilo dental)	Filo interdentale
Željezo	Iron	Fer	Hierro (fierro)	Ferro
Žlica	Spoon	Cuillère	Cuchara	Cucchiaio

MEDICINSKE USTANOVE, ZAHVATI I NJEGA:	**MEDICAL FACILITIES, PROCEDURES AND CARE:**	**ÉTABLISSEMENTS MÉDICAUX, PROCÉDURES ET SOINS:**	**FACILIDADES MÉDICAS, PROCEDIMIENTOS Y ASISTENCIA MÉDICA:**	**ISTITUZIONI, PROCEDURE E CURE DI MEDICINA:**
Ambu balon s maskom	Ambu bag valve mask	Respirateur manuel type Ambu	Bolsa Ambú de ventilación manual	Pallone autoespandibile
Ambulanta	Ambulance (clinic)	Infirmerie	Enfermería	Ambulanza
Amputacija	Amputation	Amputation	Amputación	Amputazione
Anestezija (narkoza)	Anesthesia	Anesthésie	Anestesia	Anestesia
Aparat za disanje (respirator)	Respirator	Appareil respiratoire	Aparato respiratorio	Respiratore
Artrodeza	Arthrodesis	Arthrodèse	Artrodesis	Artrodesi
Aspirator	Suction unit (aspirator)	Appareil à succion	Aspirador	Aspiratore di secreti
Blagavaonica	Dining-room	Salle à manger	Comedor	Sala da pranzo (cenàcolo)
Boca s kisikom	Oxygen storage tank	Réservoir d'oxygène	Tanque de oxígeno	Serbatoio di ossigeno
Bolesnička soba	Patient's room	Chambre de malade	Cuarto del paciente	Camera di malato
Bolesnik	Patient	Patient (malade)	Paciente	Paziente (ammalato)
Bolnica	Hospital	Hôpital	Hospital	Ospedale (policlinico)
Bušilica	Drill	Perceuse	Taladro	Trapano (trivella)
Cijepljenje	Vaccination (inoculation)	Vaccination (inoculation)	Vacunación	Vaccinazione (inoculazione)
Citologija	Cytology	Cytologie	Citología	Citologia
Čaj	Tea	Thé	Té	Tè

Hrvatski	Engleski	Francuski	Španjolski	Talijanski
Čekaonica	Waiting-room	Salle d'attente	Sala de espera	Sala d'aspetto
Darovanje krvi (donacija krvi)	Blood donation	Don de sang	Donación de sangre	Donazione del sangue
Davalac (donator)	Donor	Donneur	Donante	Donatore/donatrice
Davanje lijekova	Administration of drugs	Administration des médicaments	Administración de fármacos	Somministrazione dei farmaci
Defibrilacija	Defibrillation	Défibrillation	Desfibrilación	Defibrillazione
Defibrilator	Defibrillator	Défibrillateur	Desfibrilador	Defibrillatore
Deka	Blanket	Couverture	Manta (cobija)	Schiavina
Dermatologija	Dermatology	Dermatologie	Dermatología	Dermatologia
Dijagnoza	Diagnosis	Diagnostic	Diagnóstico	Diagnosi
Dijaliza	Dialysis	Dialyse	Diálisis	Dialisi
Dijaliza bubrega	Renal dialysis	Dialyse rénale	Diálisis renal	Dialisi renale
Dijaliza jetre	Liver dialysis	Dialyse hépatique	Diálisis de hígado	Dialisi epatica
Dijeta	Diet	Régime alimentaire	Régimen (dieta)	Dieta (regime dietetico)
Dinamometar	Dynamometer	Dynamomètre	Dinamómetro	Dinamometro
Dizalo	Elevator	Ascenseur	Elevador	Ascensore
Doručak	Breakfast	Petit déjeuner	Desayuno	Colazione
Dren	Drain tube	Drain	Sonda de drenaje	Tubo di drenaggio
Drenaža	Drainage	Drainage	Drenaje	Drenaggio
Drenažni položaj	Postural drainage	Drainage postural	Drenaje postural	Drenaggio posturale
Električni stimulator srca	Pacemaker	Stimulateur cardiaque (pacemaker, pile)	Marcapasos	Cardiostimolatore (stimolatore cardiaco)
Elektroda	Electrode	Électrode	Electrodo	Elettrodo
Elektrokirurgija	Electrosurgery	Électrochirurgie	Electrocirurgía	Elettrochirurgia
Elektroterapija	Electrotherapy	Électrothérapie	Electroterapia	Elettroterapia
Endotrahealna kanila	Endotracheal tube	Sonde d'intubation endotrachéale	Sonda endotraqueal	Tubo endotracheale
Epruveta	Test tube	Tube à essai	Tubo de ensayo	Provetta
Fizikalna terapija	Physical therapy	Physiothérapie	Fisioterapia	Fisioterapia
Fizioterapeut	Physiotherapist	Physiothérapeute	Fisioterapeuta	Fisioterapista
Gerontologija	Gerontology	Gérontologie	Gerontología	Gerontologia
Ginekologija	Gynecology	Gynécologie	Ginecología	Ginecologia
Gipsana udlaga	Plaster cast (immobilization plaster)	Plâtre pour immobilisation rigide	Escayola de inmovilización	Bendaggio gessato
Goniometar	Goniometer	Goniomètre	Goniómetro	Goniometro
Gumirano platno	Incontinence pad	Protège-matelas	Sábana de hule para la incontinencia	Proteggi materasso cerato
Heimlichov zahvat	Heimlich maneuver (abdominal thrusts)	Méthode de Heimlich	Maniobra de Heimlich	Manovra di Heimlich
Hidroterapija	Hydrotherapy	Hydrothérapie	Hidroterapia	Idroterapia
Hitna služba	Emergency medical services	Aide médicale urgente	Servicios médicos de emergencia	Servizio di urgenza ed emergenza medica
Hodalica	Walker (walking frame)	Déambulateur (cadre de marche, gadot)	Andador	Deambulatore (tutore per disabili)
Imobilizator glave	Head immobilizer	Immobiliseur de tête	Inmovilizador de cabeza	Fermacapo
Imobilizator vrata	Neck immobilizer	Support de cou	Collar cervical	Collare cervicale
Imunologija	Immunology	Immunologie	Inmunología	Immunologia
Infuzija	Infusion	Perfusion	Infusión	Infusione
Intenzivna njega	Intensive care	Soins intensifs	Cuidados intensivos	Terapia intensiva
Interna medicina	Internal medicine	Médicine interne	Medicina interna	Medicina interna
Intubacija	Intubation	Intubation	Intubación	Intubazione
Invalidska kolica	Wheelchair	Fauteuil roulant (charriot, charrette)	Silla de ruedas	Sedia a rotelle (carrozzella)
Injekcija	Injection	Injection	Inyección	Iniezione
Ispiranje želuca	Gastric lavage (stomach pumping)	Lavage gastrique	Lavado gástrico	Lavanda gastrica
Isprati	Rinse	Rincer	Lavar	Sciacquare
Jastuk	Pillow	Oreiller	Almohada	Cuscino
Jedinica intenzivne njege	Intensive care unit	Unité de soins intensifs	Unidad de cuidados intensivos	Stanza da terapia intensiva
Kalendar cijepljenja	Vaccination schedule	Calendrier des vaccinations	Calendario de vacunación	Calendario vaccinale
Kanila	Airway (cannula)	Canule	Cánula	Cannula
Kanta za smeće	Litter bin	Poubelle	Papelera	Pattumiera
Karantena	Quarantine	Quarantaine	Cuarentena	Quarantena
Kardiologija	Cardiology	Cardiologie	Cardiología	Cardiologia
Kateter	Catheter	Cathéter	Catéter	Catetere
Kauterizacija	Cauterization	Cautérisation	Cauterización	Cauterizzazione
Kegelove vježbe	Kegel exercise	Exercice de Kegel	Ejercicios de Kegel	Esercizi di Kegel
Kemoterapija	Chemotherapy	Chimiothérapie	Quimioterapia	Chemioterapia
Kirurgija	Surgery	Chirurgie	Cirugia	Chirurgia
Kirurška sterilizacija muškarca (vazektomija)	Surgical sterilization of a man (vasectomy)	Ligature des canaux déférents des testicules (vasectomie)	Esterilización quirúrgica masculina (vasectomía)	Vasectomia
Kirurška sterilizacija žene (podvezivanje jajovoda)	Surgical sterilization of a woman (tubal ligation)	Stérilisation chirurgicale au femme (ligature des trompes)	Esterilizatióm quirúrgica femenina (ligadura de trompas)	Chiusura delle tube

Hrvatski	Engleski	Francuski	Španjolski	Talijanski
Kirurški zahvat formiranja stome (kolostomija)	Surgical procedure of formation of stoma (colostomy)	Formation chirurgicale de la stomie (colostomie)	Exteriorización de una parte de intestino a través de la cavidad abdominal (colostomía)	Formazione chirurgica di stomia (colostomia)
Kirurški zahvat na kralježnici (laminektomija)	Surgical procedure on the spine (laminectomy)	Résection chirurgicale des lames vertébrales (laminectomie)	Extirpación quirúrgica de parte de una vértebra (laminectomía)	Asportazione chirurgica della lamina di vertebre (laminectomia)
Kirurški zahvat na srednjem uhu (stapedektomija)	Surgical procedure on the middle ear (stapedectomy)	Ablation chirurgicale de l'étrier (stapédectomie)	Cirugía del oído medio (stapedectomía)	Intervento chirurgico dell'orecchio medio (stapedectomia)
Kirurški zahvat na talamusu (talamotomija)	Surgical procedure on the thalamus (thalamotomy)	Ablation chirurgicale d'une partie du thalamus (thalamotomie)	Cirugía del tálamo (talamotomía)	Intervento chirurgico delle connessioni talamiche (talamotomia)
Kirurški zahvat na zglobu (artrotomija)	Surgical procedure on a joint (arthrotomy)	Ouverture chirurgicale d'une articulation (arthrotomie)	Incisión quirúrgica de una articulación (artrotomía)	Apertura chirurgica di un articolazione (artrotomia)
Kirurški zahvat otvaranja lubanje (kraniotomija)	Surgical opnening of the cranium (craniotomy)	Ouverture chirurgicale du crâne (craniotomie)	Abertura quirúrgica en el cráneo (craneotomía)	Apertura chirurgica del cranio (craniotomia)
Kirurško odstranjenje aneurizme (aneurizmektomija)	Surgical removal of the aneurysm (aneurysmectomy)	Résection chirurgicale d'une poche anévrismale (anevrismectomie)	Extirpación quirúrgica de un aneurisma (aneurismectomía)	Asportazione chirurgica della sacca aneurismatica (aneurismectomia)
Kirurško odstranjenje dojke (mastektomija)	Surgical removal of a breast (mastectomy)	Enlèvement chirurgical d'un sein (mastectomie)	Remoción quirúrgica de seno (mastectomía)	Asportazione chirurgica della mammella (mastectomia)
Kirurško odstranjenje grkljana (laringektomija)	Surgical removal of the larynx (laryngectomy)	Ablation chirurgicale du larynx (laryngectomie)	Extirpación quirúrgica de la laringe (laringectomía)	Asportazione chirurgica della laringe (laringectomia)
Kirurško odstranjenje gušterače (pankreatektomija)	Surgical removal of the pancreas (pancreatectomy)	Ablation chirurgicale du pancréas (pancréatectomie)	Extirpación quirúrgica del páncreas (pancreatectomía)	Asportazione chirurgica del pancreas (pancreatectomia)
Kirurško odstranjenje hemeroida (hemoroidektomija)	Surgical removal of a hemorrhoid (hemorrhoidectomy)	Ablation chirurgicale des hémorroïdes (hémorroïdectomie)	Extirpación quirúrgica de las hemorroides (hemorroidectomía)	Asportazione chirurgica delle emorroidi (emorroidectomia)
Kirurško odstranjenje kamenca (litotomija)	Surgical removal of stones (lithotomy)	Extraction chirurgicale des pierres de la vessie (lithotomie)	Extracción quirúrgica de los cálculos (litotomía)	Asportazione chirurgica di calcolo (litotomia)
Kirurško odstranjenje krajnika (tonzilektomija)	Surgical removal of tonsils (tonsillectomy)	Ablation chirurgicale des amygdales palati-nes (amygdalectomie, tonsillectomie)	Extracción quirúrgica de las amígdalas (tonsilectomía)	Asportazione chirurgica delle tonsille (tonsillectomia)
Kirurško odstranjenje maternice (histerektomija)	Surgical removal of the uterus (hysterectomy)	Enlèvement chirurgical de l'uterus (hystérectomie)	Extracción quirúrgica del útero (histerectomía)	Asportazione chirurgica dell'utero (isterectomia)
Kirurško odstranjenje mioma u maternici (miomektomija)	Surgical removal of uterine myomas (myomectomy, fibroidectomy)	Ablation chirurgicale des fibromes utérins (myomectomie)	Extracción quirúrgica de los fibromas uterinos (miomectomía)	Asportazione chirurgica di fibromi nell'utero (miomectomia)
Kirurško odstranjenje nadbubrežne žlijezde (adrenalektomija)	Surgical removal of one or both adrenal glands (adrenalectomy)	Ablation chirurgicale d'une ou des deux glandes surrénales (adrenalectomie)	Extirpación quirúrgica de una glándula suprarrenal (adrenalectomía)	Asportazione chirurgi-ca di uno o etrambi surreni(surrenectomia, adrenalectomia)
Kirurško odstranjenje prostate (prostatektomija)	Surgical removal of the prostate gland (prostatectomy)	Ablation chirurgicale de la prostate (prostatectomie)	Extirpación quirúrgica de la próstata (prostatectomía)	Asportazione chirurgica della prostata (prostatectomia)
Kirurško odstranjenje prsne žlijezde (timektomija)	Surgical removal of the thymus (thymectomy)	Ablation chirurgicale du thymus (thymectomie)	Extirpación quirúrgica del timo (timectomía)	Asportazione chirurgica del timo (timectomia)
Kirurško odstranjenje režnja nekog organa (lobektomija)	Surgical removal of a lobe of some organ (lobectomy)	Ablation chirurgicale d'un lobe d'organe (lobectomie)	Extirpación quirúrgica de un lóbulo de un órgano (lobectomía)	Asportazione chirurgica di struttura lobale di un organo (lobectomia)
Kirurško odstranjenje slezene (splenektomija)	Surgical removal of the spleen (splenectomy)	Ablation chirurgicale de la rate (splénectomie)	Extirpación quirúrgica del bazo (esplenectomía)	Asportazione chirurgica della milza (splenectomia)
Kirurško odstranjenje slijepog crijeva (apendektomija)	Surgical removal of the vermiform appendix (appendectomy)	Ablation chirurgicale de l'appendice iléocaecal (appendicectomie)	Extirpación quirúrgica del apéndice cecal (apendicectomía)	Asportazione chirurgica dell'appendice (appendicectomia)
Kirurško odstranjenje štitne žlijezde (tiroidektomija)	Surgical removal of the thyroid gland (thyroidectomy)	Ablation chirurgicale de la thyroïde (thyroïdectomie, isthmectomie)	Extirpación quirúrgica de la glándula tiroides (tiroidectomía)	Asportazione chirurgica della tiroide (tiroidectomia)
Kirurško odstranjenje testisa (orhidektomija)	Surgical removal of a testicle (orchidectomy)	Amputation chirurgi-cale d'un ou des deux testicules (orchidectomie, orchiectomie)	Extirpación quirúrgica del testículo (orquidectomía)	Asportazione chirurgica del testicolo (orchiectomia)
Kirurško odstranjenje trećeg krajnika (adenoidektomija)	Surgical removal of adenoids (adenoidectomy)	Ablation chirurgicale des végétations adénoïdes (adénoïdectomie)	Extirpación quirúrgica de las adenoides (adenoidectomía)	Asportazione chirurgica delle adenoidi (adenoidectomia)
Kirurško odstranjenje želuca (gastrektomija)	Surgical removal of the stomach (gastrectomy)	Ablation chirurgicale de l'estomac (gastrectomie)	Extirpación quirúrgica del estómago (gastrectomía)	Asportazione chirurgica dello stomaco (gastrectomia)
Kirurško odstranjenje žučnog mjehura (kolecistektomija)	Surgical removal of the gallbladder (cholecystectomy)	Enlèvement chirurgical de la vésicule biliaire (cholécystectomie)	Extracción quirúrgica de la vesícula biliar (colecistectomía)	Asportazione chirurgica della colecisti (colecistectomia)

Hrvatski	Engleski	Francuski	Španjolski	Talijanski
Kirurško otvaranje dišnog puta (traheotomija)	Surgical opening of a direct airway on the neck (tracheostomy)	Ouverture chirurgicale dans la trachée (trachéotomie)	Incisión quirúrgica en la tráquea (traqueotomía)	Incisione chirurgica della trachea (tracheotomia)
Klice	Germs	Germes	Gérmenes	Germi
Kola hitne pomoći	Ambulance	Ambulance	Ambulancia	Autoambulanza
Kolica	Hospital trolley	Chariot	Camilla	Carrello
Kontaktni gel za elektrode	Electrode conductive gel	Gel électroconductif	Gel conductor	Gel elettro-conduttivo
Krevet	Bed	Lit	Cama	Letto
Krioekstrakcija	Cryoextraction	Cryo-extraction	Crío-extracción	Crioestrazione
Kupaonica	Bathroom	Salle de bains	Cuarto de baño	Bagno
Kupati	Bath (wash)	Laver	Darse un baño	Lavare (fare il bagno)
Kutija prve pomoći	First aid kit	Trousse de secours	Botiquín de primeros auxilios	Cassetta di pronto soccorso
Laparoskopska operacija	Laparoscopic surgery	Laparoscopie (coelioscopie)	Cirugía laparoscópica	Chirurgia laparoscopica
Laringealna maska	Laryngeal mask airway	Masque laryngé	Máscara laríngea	Maschera laringea
Laringoskop	Laryngoscope	Laryngoscope	Laringoscopio	Laringoscopio
Lavor	Wash basin	Cuvette	Palangana (ajofaina)	Secchia
Leš	Corpse	Cadavre	Cadáver	Cadavere (salma)
Lifting lica (ritidektomija)	Facelift (rhytidectomy)	Lifting facial (rhytidectomie, lissage, remodelage)	Estiramiento de la cara (ritidectomía)	Lift facciale (ritidectomia)
Liječenje (terapija)	Therapy	Thérapie (traitement curatif)	Tratamiento (terapia)	Terapia
Liječnička ambulanta	Doctor's office	Bureau du médecin	Consultorio de médico	Ufficio del medico
Liječnik	Doctor (physician)	Médecin	Médico	Dottore/dottoressa (medico)
Liječnik opće prakse	General practitioner	Médecin généraliste (médecin omnipraticien)	Médico de cabecera	Medico di medicina generale (medico di famiglia)
Liposukcija	Liposuction	Liposuccion	Liposucción	Liposuzione
Lobotomija	Lobotomy	Lobotomie	Lobotomía	Lobotomia
Lokalna anestezija	Local anesthesia	Anesthésie locale	Anestesia local	Anestesia locale
Madrac	Mattress	Matelas	Colchón	Materasso
Manšeta tlakomjera	Manometer cuff	Brassard du manomètre	Manguito de presión arterial	Manicotto di sfigmomanometro
Maska za kisik	Oxygen mask	Masque à oxygène	Máscara de oxígeno	Maschera dell'ossigeno
Maska za oživljavanje	CPR mask	Masque de réanimation	Máscara de reanimación	Maschera per rianimazione
Medicinska sestra	Nurse	Infirmier	Enfermera	Infermiera/infermiere
Medicinski centar	Medical center	Centre médical	Centro médico	Centro di medicina
Mirovanje u krevetu	Bed rest	Repos au lit	Guardar cama	Riposo a letto
Mokrenje (uriniranje)	Urination (voiding)	Miction	Micción	Urinazione
Monitor za praćenje vitalnih znakova	Vital signs monitor	Moniteur de signes vitaux	Monitor de signos vitales	Monitor per parametri vitali
Mrtvačnica	Morgue (mortuary)	Morgue	Depósito de cadáveres (morgue)	Obitorio (mortorio)
Neurologija	Neurology	Neurologie	Neurología	Neurologia
Noćna posuda	Chamber-pot	Pot de chambre	Orinal	Vaso da notte (pitale)
Noćni ormarić	Night table (bedside table)	Table de chevet (table de nuit)	Mesilla de noche	Comodino
Nosila	Stretcher	Civière	Camilla enrollable	Barella (lettiga)
Nosna kanila	Nasal cannula	Canule nasale	Cánula nasal	Cannula nasale
Nužnik	Toilet (lavatory)	Toilette (cabinet)	Servicio	Vaso sanitario
Njega	Nursing (care)	Soins de santé	Asistencia (cuidado)	Assistenza infermieristica
Obaviti nuždu	Using a toilet	Aller aux toilettes	Ir al servicio	Uso del gabinetto
Obdukcija	Autopsy	Autopsie	Autopsia	Autopsia
Obrezivanje	Circumcision	Circoncision	Circuncisión	Circoncisione
Očni odjel	Ophtalmology ward	Salle d'ophtalmologie	Sala de oftalmología	Reparto di oftalmologia
Odjel	Ward	Salle	Sala (pabellón)	Padiglione (reparto)
Onkologija	Oncology	Oncologie (cancérologie)	Oncología	Oncologia
Opća anestezija	General anesthesia	Anesthésie générale	Anestesia general	Anestesia generale
Operacija	Operation (surgery)	Opération chirurgicale	Operación quirúrgica	Operazione (intervento chirurgico)
Operacijska sala	Operating room	Bloc opératoire	Quirófano	Sala operatoria
Oporavak	Recovery	Guérison	Recuperación	Guarigione (ristabilimento)
Ormar	Wardrobe (cupboard, cabinet)	Armoire	Armario	Armadio (credenza)
Orofaringealna kanila	Oropharyngeal airway	Canule de Guedel	Cánula orofaríngea (tubo de Mayo, cánula de Guédel)	Cannula oro-faringea
Ortopedija	Orthopedics	Orthopédie	Ortopedia	Ortopedia
Otpad (otpadni proizvod)	Debris	Débris	Materia de desperdicio	Rottami
Otvoriti	Open	Ouvrir	Abrir	Aprire
Ozdraviti	Recover (heal)	Se remettre (se guérir)	Reponerse (recuperarse)	Sanare (guarire, recuperare)
Oživljavanje (reanimacija)	Reanimation	Réanimation	Reanimación	Rianimazione
Patologija	Pathology	Pathologie	Patología	Patologia
Pedijatrija	Pediatrics	Pédiatrie	Pediatría	Pediatria
Perkutana koronarna angioplastika	Percutaneous coronary intervention (coronary angioplasty)	Angioplastie coronaire (dilatation transluminale)	Intervención coronaria percutánea	Angioplastica coronarica
Pesar	Pessary	Pessaire (pessus)	Pesario	Pessario

Hrvatski	Engleski	Francuski	Španjolski	Talijanski
Piđama	Pyjamas (pajamas)	Pyjama	Pijama (piyama)	Pigiama
Pinceta	Tweezers	Brucelles	Pinzas	Pinzette
Plahta	Sheet	Drap	Sábana	Lenzuolo
Plastična operacija dojke (mastoplastika)	Plastic surgery of the breasts (mammoplasty)	Opération de chirurgie esthétique des seins (mammoplastie)	Cirugía estética de los senos (mamoplastia)	Procedura di chirurgia plastica del seno (mastoplastica)
Plastična operacija nosa (rinoplastika)	Plastic surgery of the nose (rhinoplasty)	Opération de chirurgie esthétique du nez (rhinoplastie)	Cirugía estética de la nariz (rinoplastia)	Procedura di chirurgia plastica del naso (rinoplastica)
Plastična operacija očnog kapka (blefaroplastika)	Plastic surgery of the eyelid (blepharoplasty)	Opération de chirurgie esthétique des paupières (blépharoplastie)	Cirugía estética de los párpados (blefaroplastia)	Procedura di chirurgia plastica della palpebra (blefaroplastica)
Plastična operacija trbuha (abdominoplastika)	Plastic surgery of the abdomen ("tummy tuck", abdominoplasty)	Opération de chirurgie esthétique de la paroi abdominale (abdominoplastie)	Cirugía estética del abdomen (abdominoplastia)	Procedura di chirurgia plastica dell'addome (addominoplastica)
Plućni odjel	Pulmonary ward	Salle de pneumologie	Sala de neumología	Reparto polmonare
Pljunuti	Spit	Cracher	Escupir	Sputare
Pokrivač	Cover	Couverture	Cubrecama (colcha, manta)	Coperta
Poliranje zuba	Teeth polishing	Vernis à dents	Pulidor de los dientes	Pulitura dei denti
Poluintenzivna njega	Semi-intensive care	Soins semi-intensifs	Cuidados semi-intensivos	Terapia semi-intensiva
Posjeta	Visit	Visite	Visita	Visita
Posjetitelj	Visitor	Visiteur	Visitante	Ospite (visitatore/visitatrice)
Pražnjenje stolice (defekacija)	Defecation	Défécation	Defecación	Defecazione
Pregled kucanjem (perkusija)	Percussion	Percussion	Percusión	Percussione
Pregled pipanjem (palpacija)	Palpation	Palpation	Palpación	Palpazione
Premosnica	Bypass	Pontage	By-pass	Bypass
Presađivanje (transplantacija)	Transplantation	Greffe (transplantation)	Trasplante	Trapianto
Presvući se	Get changed	Se changer	Cambiarse	Cambiarsi
Previjanje	Dressing	Pansement	Apósito	Fasciatura (bendaggio)
Prijemni ured	Reception office	Réception	Mostrador de recepción	Accettazione
Primarna zdravstvena zaštita	Primary health care	Soins de santé primaire	Atención primaria de salud	Assistenza sanitaria primaria
Primatelj organa	Recipient of an organ	Receveur de greffe	Receptor de un órgano	Ricevente di trapianto
Probava	Digestion	Digestion	Digestión	Digestione
Pročišćavanje	Cleansing	Purification	Purificación	Purificazione
Proglašenje vremena smrti	Calling of the time of death	Détermination de l'heure de la mort	Determinación del tiempo de muerte	Proclamazione del tempo della morte
Prozor	Window	Fenêtre	Ventana	Finestra
Prva pomoć	First aid	Premiers secours	Primeros auxilios	Primo soccorso
Psihijatrija	Psychiatry	Psychiatrie	Psiquiatría	Psichiatria
Psiholog	Psychologist	Psychologue	Psicólogo	Psicologo
Radiologija	Radiology	Radiographie	Radiología	Radiologia
Radni terapeut	Occupational therapist	Ergothérapeute	Terapeuta ocupacional	Terapista occupazionale
Rehabilitacija	Rehabilitation (rehab)	Réhabilitation	Rehabilitación	Riabilitazione
Rinologija	Rhinology	Rhinologie	Rinología	Rinologia
Ručak	Lunch	Déjeuner	Almuerzo	Pranzo
Ručni defibrilator	Manual defibrillator	Défibrillateur manuel	Desfibrilador manual	Defibrillatore manuale
Sjedalica za evakuaciju	Escape chair	Chaise d'évacuation	Silla de evacuación	Sedia portantina
Skalpel	Scalpel	Scalpel	Escalpelo	Scalpello
Slušni aparat	Hearing assist device	Appareil acoustique	Audífono	Apparecchio acustico
Sonda	Sonde	Sonde	Sonda	Sonda
Sonda za hranjenje	Feeding tube	Sonde d'alimentation	Sonda de alimentación	Sonda gastrica per nutrizione
Spavačica	Nightgown	Chemise de nuit	Camisón	Camicia da notte
Spoj (skretnica)	Shunt	Pontage (shunt)	Shunt	Shunt
Spremište	Storage	Stockage	Almacenaje	Deposito (magazzino)
Spužva	Sponge	Éponge	Esponja	Spugna
Stadij mirovanja bolesti (remisija)	Remission	Rémission	Fase de remisión	Remissione
Stalak za infuziju	Infusion stand	Pied à perfusion	Intravenoso poste	Piantana portaflebo
Sterilizacija	Sterilization	Stérilisation	Esterilización	Sterilizzazione
Sterilno	Sterile (aseptic)	Stérile	Estéril	Sterile
Stetoskop	Stethoscop	Stéthoscope	Estetoscopio	Stetofonendoscopio
Stol	Table (desk)	Table	Mesa (escritorio)	Tavolo (scrivania)
Stolić za serviranje hrane	Overbed table	Table de lit	Mesa para cama	Carrello servitore
Stomatolog (zubar)	Dentist	Dentiste	Dentista	Dentista
Svjetlo	Light	Lumière	Luz	Luce
Šivanje rane	Wound stitching	Suture de la plaie	Suturar la herida	Suturare la ferita
Škare	Scissors	Ciseau	Tijeras	Forbici
Šlape	Slippers	Chausson	Pantuflas	Ciabatte
Štaka	Crutch	Béquille	Muleta	Gruccia (stampella)
Trakcija	Traction	Traction	Tracción	Trazione

Hrvatski	Engleski	Francuski	Španjolski	Talijanski
Transfuzija	Transfusion	Transfusion	Transfusión	Trasfusione
Transuretralna resekcija prostate	Transurethral resection of the prostate	Résection transurétrale de la prostate	Resección transuretral de la próstata	Resezione transuretrale della prostata
Trauma	Trauma	Trauma	Trauma	Trauma
Trendelenburgov položaj	Trendelenburg position	Position de Trendelenburg	Posición de Trendelenburg	Posizione di Trendelenburg
Trening ravnoteže	Balance training	Entraînement de l'equilibre	Entrenamiento del equilibrio	Esercizi di equilibrio
Udlaga za pozicioniranje	Body positioner	Coussin de positionnement	Almohada de posicionamiento	Posizionatore
Uho-grlo-nos	Otorhinolaryngology	Oto-rhino-laryngologie	Otorrinolaringología	Otorinolaringoiatria
Umetak za dojku	Breast implant	Implant mammaire	Implante de mama	Protese mammaria
Umjetno disanje	Artificial respiration	Ventilation artificielle	Respiración artificial	Respirazione artificiale
Umjetno zubalo	Dentures	Dentier	Prótesis dental	Protesi dentale
Umrijeti	Die	Mourir	Morir	Morire
Urinarni kateter	Urological catheter	Cathéter urologique	Catéter urinario	Catetere vescicale
Urologija	Urology	Urologie	Urología	Urologia
Usisni kateter	Suction catheter	Cathéter à succion	Catéter de succión	Tubo d'aspirazione
Uzbuna (alarm)	Alarm	Alarme	Alarma	Allarme
Uzrok smrti	Cause of death	Cause de la mort	Causa de muerte	Causa di morte
Vađenje zuba	Dental extraction	Extraction dentaire	Exodoncia dental	Estrazione del dente
Vakumirani madrac	Vacuum mattress	Matelas immobilisateur à dépression	Colchón al vácio	Materassino a depressione
Večera	Dinner (supper)	Dîner (souper)	Cena	Cena
Vešeraj	Laundry	Blanchisserie	Lavandería	Lavanderia
Vježbanje	Exercise	Exercice	Ejercicio	Esercizio
Vježbe disanja	Breathing exercises	Exercice de respiration	Ejercicios de respiración	Esercizi di respirazione
Voda	Water	Eau	Agua	Acqua
Vrata	Door	Porte	Puerta	Porta
Zagristi	Bite	Mordre	Morder	Addentare
Zarazni odjel	Infectious disease unit	Salle maladies infectieuses	Pabellón de enfermedades infecciosas	Reparto di malattie infettive
Zarazno	Contagious	Contagieux/ contagieuse	Contagioso	Contagioso (infettivo)
Zaštitna kapa	Protection cap	Charlotte à usage unique	Gorra desechable	Cuffietta protettiva
Zaštitna maska za lice	Protection face mask	Masque de protection	Mascarilla desechable	Mascherina di protezione
Zaštitna navlaka za obuću	Protection shoe cover	Sur-chaussures à usage unique	Cubrezapatos	Sovrascarpe protettive
Zaštitna navlaka za odjeću	Protection gown	Blouse de protection	Gabacha desechable	Camicia protettiva
Zaštitne rukavice	Protect gloves	Gants à usage unique	Guantes desechables	Guanti protettivi
Zaštitnici za pete i laktove	Heel and elbow protectors	Talonnières et coudières	Protectores talón/codo antiescaras	Talloniere e gomitiere antidecubito
Zatvoriti	Close	Fermer	Cerrar	Chiudere
Zdravstveno osiguranje	Health insurance	Assurance maladie	Seguro de salud	Assicurazione sanitaria
Zračenje	Radiation	Radiation	Radiación	Radiazione
Zubna krunica	Dental crown	Couronne	Corona	Corona
Zubna plomba	Dental filling	Composite dentaire	Empaste (emplomadura)	Otturazione odontoiatrica
MEDICINSKE PRETRAGE:	MEDICAL EXAMS:	EXAMENS MÉDICAUX:	EXÁMENES MÉDICOS:	ESAMI MEDICI:
Albumin u serumu	Serum albumin	Albumine dans le sang	Albúmina en la sangre	Seroalbumina
Alergološko testiranje kože (prick test)	Skin allergy testing (prick test)	Test de la piqûre	Test cutaneos de alergia (prick)	Test cutaneo per le allergie "prick test"
Alfafetoproteinski test (AFP)	Alpha-fetoprotein test (AFP test)	Test d'alpha-foetoprotéine	Prueba de alfa-fetoproteína	Test alfa-fetoproteina
Alkalna fosfataza	Alkaline phosphatase	Phosphatase alcaline	Fosfatasa alcalina	Fosfatasi alcalina totale
Amniocenteza	Amniocentesis	Amniocentèse	Amniocentesis	Amniocentesi
Analiza plinova u krvi	Blood gas test	Prélèvement des gaz du sang	Prueba de gases en la sangre	Analisi dei gas nel san-gue (emogas analisi)
Angiografija	Angiography	Angiographie	Angiografía	Angiografia
Anoskopija	Anoscopy	Anuscopie	Anoscopía	Anoscopia
Antibiogram	Antibiogram	Antibiogramme	Antibiograma	Antibiogramma
Aortografija	Aortography	Aortographie	Aortografía	Aortografia
Arteriografija	Arteriography	Artériographie	Arteriografía	Arteriografia
Artroskopija	Arthroscopy	Arthroscopie	Artroscopia	Artroscopia
Audiometrija	Audiometry	Audiométrie	Audiometría	Audiometria
Benzidinski test stolice	Benzidine stool test	Analyse fécale de benzidine	Prueba de la bencidina	Prova della benzidina
Bilirubin u serumu	Serum bilirubin	Diagnostic différentiel pour bilirubine sérique	Análisis de bilirrubina sérica	Test della bilirubina
Biokemijske pretrage krvi	Biochemical blood tests	Analyse de biochimie du sang	Exámenes bioquímicos de sangre	Test biochimici di sangue
Biomarker	Biomarker	Biomarqueur	Marcador biológico	Biomarcatore
Biopsija	Biopsy	Biopsie	Biopsia	Biopsia
Biopsija bubrega	Kidney biopsy	Biopsie rénale	Biopsia renal	Biopsia renale
Biopsija jetre	Liver biopsy	Biopsie du foie	Biopsia hepática	Biopsia epatica
Biopsija endometrija	Endometrial biopsy	Biopsie endométriale	Biopsia endometrial	Biopsia endometriale
Biopsija koštane srži	Bone marrow biopsy	Biopsie ostéomédullaire	Biopsia de médula ósea	Biopsia del midollo osseo
Biopsija kože	Skin biopsy	Biopsie de peau	Biopsia de piel	Biopsia cutanea
Biopsija limfnog čvora	Lymph node biopsy	Biopsie du ganglion lymphatoque	Biopsia de ganglio linfático	Biopsia del linfonodo

Hrvatski	Engleski	Francuski	Španjolski	Talijanski
Biopsija moždanih klijetki (ventrikulopunkcija)	Brain ventricle biopsy	Biopsie d'un ventricule cérébral	Biopsia cerebral	Biopsia cerebrale (biopsia dei ventricoli cerebrali)
Biopsija pleure	Pleural biopsy	Biopsie pleurale	Biopsia pleural	Biopsia pleurica
Biopsija štitnjače	Thyroid biopsy	Biopsie thyroïdienne	Biopsia de tiroides	Biopsia della tiroide
Bjelančevine u urinu	Urine protein test	Protéines dans les urines	Proteínas en la orina	Proteine nelle urine
Brom-sulfalein test funkcije jetre	Bromsulphalein liver function test	Test de la bromesulfonephtaléine	Prueba de la función hepática con bromosulfaleína	Test dela bromosulfaleina di funzionalità epatica
Bronhografija	Bronchography	Bronchographie	Broncografía	Broncografia
Bronhoskopija	Bronchoscopy	Bronchoscopie	Broncoscopia	Broncoscopia
Brzi test na streptokok (strep-test)	Rapid strep test	Test de diagnostic rapide du streptocoque	Prueba rápida para estreptococo	Test rapido dello streptococco
CA 19-9 (karbohidratni antigen)	CA 19-9 (carbohydrate antigen)	Antigène de cancer CA 19-9 (antigène d'hydrate de carbone)	CA 19-9 (antigeno carbohidrato 19-9)	CA 19-9 (antigene carboidratico)
CA 125 (karcinomski antigen 125)	CA 125 (cancer antigen 125)	Antigène de cancer CA 125	Marcador tumoral CA 125	CA 125 (antigene di carcinoma 125)
Cefalometrija	Cephalometry	Céphalométrie	Cefalometría	Cefalometria
Centralni venozni pritisak (CVP)	Central venous pressure (CVP)	Pression veineuse centrale	Presión venosa central	Pressione venosa centrale
Cerebralna angiografija	Cerebral angiography	Angiographie cérébrale	Angiografía cerebral	Angiografia cerebrale
Cistografija	Cystography	Cystographie	Cistografia	Cistografia
Cistoskopija	Cystoscopy	Cystoscopie	Cistoscopia	Cistoscopia
Defekografija	Defecography	Défécographie	Defecografía	Defecografia
Denzitometrija kostiju (apsorpciometrija kostiju)	Bone densitometry (dual energy X-ray absorpriometry)	Ostéodensitométrie	Densitometría ósea	Densità minerale ossea
Dermatoskopija (dermoskopija)	Dermatoscopy (dermoscopy)	Dermatoscopie (dermoscopie)	Dermatoscopia	Dermatoscopia (dermoscopia)
Diferencijalna dijagnoza	Differential diagnosis	Diagnostic différentiel	Diagnóstico diferencial	Diagnosi differenziale
Digitalna supstrakcijska angiografija	Digital subtraction angiography	Angiographie numérique	Angiografía de sustracción digital	Angiografia digitale a sottrazione
DNK analiza	DNA analysis	Analyse de l'ADN	Análisis de DNA	Analisi del DNA
Ehoencefalografija	Echoencephalography	Échoencéphalographie	Ecoencefalografia	Ecoencefalografia
Elektroencefalografija (EEG)	Electroencephalography (EEG)	Électro-encéphalographie (EEG)	Electroencefalografia	Elettroencefalografia
Elektroforeza proteina u serumu	Serum protein electrophoresis	Électrophorèse des protéines	Electroforesis de proteínas séricas	Elettroforesi delle sieroproteine
Elektrokardiografija (EKG)	Electrocardiography (ECG)	Électrocardiographie (ECG)	Electrocardiografia (ECG, EKG)	Elettrocardiografia
Elektromiografija (EMG)	Electromyography (EMG)	Électromyographie	Electromiografia	Elettromiografia
Elektroneurografija	Electroneurography	Électroneurographie	Electroneurografia	Elettroneurografia
Elektroretinografija	Electroretinography	Électrorétinographie	Electrorretinografia	Elettroretinografia
Endoskopija	Endoscopy	Endoscopie	Endoscopia	Endoscopia
Endoskopska retrogradna kolangiopankreatografija (ERCP)	Endoscopic retrograde cholangiopancreatography (ERCP)	Cholangiopancréatographie rétrograde endoscopique	Colangiopancreatografia retrógrada endoscópica	Colangio-pancreatografia endoscopica retrograda
Enteroskopija	Enteroscopy	Entéroscopie	Enteroscopia	Enteroscopia
Ezofagogastroduode-noskopija	Esophagogastroduode-noscopy	Endoscopie oeso-gastro-duodénale	Esofagogastroduode-noscopia	Esofagogastroduode-noscopia
Fenolsulfoftaleinski test (PSP-test)	Phenolsulfonphthalein test (PSP test)	Épruve à la phénolsulfonphtaléine	Prueba de la fenolsulfonftaleína	Test alla fenolsulfonftaleina
Fluoroskopija	Fluoroscopy	Fluoroscopie	Fluoroscopia	Fluoroscopia
Fokusirani ultrazvuk visokog intenziteta	High intensity focused ultrasound	Ultrasons focalisés de haute intensité	Ultrasonido focalizado de alta intensidad (HIFU)	Ultrasuono ad alta intensità focalizzato
Funkcionalna magnetska rezonancija (FMR)	Functional magnetic resonance imaging (functional MRI)	Imagerie par résonance magnétique fonctionnelle (IRMf)	Imagen por resonancia magnética funcional (IRMf)	Risonanza magnetica funzionale
Funkcionalne pretrage jetre	Liver function tests	Explorations fonctionnelles hépatiques	Pruebas de función hepática	Test di funzionalità epatica
Gastroskopija	Gastroscopy	Gastroscopie	Gastroscopia	Gastroscopia
Ginekoliški pregled	Gynecological examination	Examen gynécologique	Examen ginecológico	Esame ginecologico
Glasgowska skala kome	Glasgow coma scale	Échelle de Glasgow	Escala de coma de Glasgow	Punteggio del coma di Glasgow
Gonioskopija	Gonioscopy	Gonioscopie	Gonioscopia	Gonioscopia
Govorna audiometrija	Speech audiometry	Audiométrie vocale	Audiometría del habla	Audiometria di discorso
HbsAg (hepatitis B površinski antigen)	HbsAg (Hepatitis B surface antigen)	Antigène HbsAg (antigène de surface du virus de l'hépatite B)	HbsAg (antigeno de superficie de la hepatitis B)	HbsAg (antigene di superficie dell'epatite B)
Hematokrit	Hematocrit	Hématocrite	Hematocrito	Ematocrito
Histeroskopija	Hysteroscopy	Hystéroscopie	Histeroscopia	Isteroscopia
Indirektni Coombsov test	Indirect Coombs test	Réaction de Coombs indirecte	Prueba de Coombs indirecta	Test di Coombs indiretto
Intravenozna bilirafija	Intravenous biligraphy	Biligraphie intraveineuse	Biligrafia intravenosa	Biligrafia venosa
Intravenozna pijelografija (i.v. Urografija)	Intravenous pyelography	Urographie intra-veineuse	Urografia intravenosa	Urografia intravenosa (pielografia intravenosa)
Ispitivanje refrakcije	Refractometry	Réfractométrie	Refractomería	Rifrattometria

Hrvatski	Engleski	Francuski	Španjolski	Talijanski
Karcinoembrionski antigen (CEA)	Carcinoembryonic antigen (CEA)	Antigène carcino-embryonnaire (ACE)	Antígeno carcinoembrionario	Antigene carcino-embrionario (CEA)
Kardiotokografija	Cardiotocography	Cardiotocographie	Cardiotocografia	Cardiotocografia
Kariotip	Karyotype	Caryotype	Cariotipo	Cariotipo
Kateterizacija srca (angiokardiografija)	Cardiac catheterization (heart cath, angiocardiography)	Cathétérisme cardiaque	Cateterismo cardíaco	Cateterismo cardiaco (angiocardiografia)
Kateterska angiografija	Catheter angiography	Angiographie interventio-nnelle utilisant un cathéter	Angiografía por catéter	Angiografia con cateterismo
Kemijska analiza urina	Urine chemical analysis	Analyse chimique de l'urine	Análisis químico de orina	Analisi chimiche delle urine
Kemijski pregled želučanog soka	Gastric juice chemical examination	Analyse chimique du suc gastrique	Análisis químico del jugo gástrico	Esame chimico di succo gastrico
Kolangiografija	Cholangiography	Cholangiographie	Colangiografía	Colangiografia
Kolonoskopija	Colonoscopy	Colonoscopie	Colonscopia	Colonscopia
Kolposkopija	Colposcopy	Colposcopie	Colposcopia	Colposcopia
Kompjuterizirana tomografija (CT)	Computed tomography (CT)	Tomodensitométrie (TDM)	Tomografía computada	Tomografia computerizzata (TC)
Kompletna krvna slika	Complete blood count	Hémogramme (numération formule sanguine)	Hemograma (conteo sanguíneo completo)	Emocromo (analisi del sangue, esame emocromocitometrico)
Konizacija	Cervical conization	Conisation	Conización	Conizzazione
Kontrast	Contrast medium	Produit de contraste	Medio de contraste	Mezzo di contrasto
Koronarografija	Coronary catheterization (coronarography)	Coronarographie	Coronariografía	Coronarografia
Kožni alergološki test flasterom	Patch test	Patch test	Prueba de emplasto (prueba del parche)	Patch test
Laboratorij	Laboratory (lab)	Laboratoire	Laboratorio	Laboratorio
Laboratorijske pretrage	Laboratory tests	Analyse médicale (examens de biologie médicale)	Pruebas de laboratorio	Esami di laboratorio
Laparoskopija	Laparoscopy	Laparoscopie	Laparoscopia	Laparoscopia
Laringoskopija	Laryngoscopy	Laryngoscopie	Laringoscopia	Laringoscopia
Limfografija	Lymphography (lymphangiography)	Lymphographie	Linfografía	Linfangiografia (linfografia)
Lumbalna mijelografija	Lumbar myelography	Myélographie lombaire	Mielografía lumbar	Mielografia lombare
Lumbalna punkcija	Lumbar puncture	Ponction lombaire (rachicentèse)	Punción lumbar	Puntura lombare (rachicentesi)
Magnetoencefalografija (MEG)	Magnetoencephalography (MEG)	Magnétoencéphalographie	Magnetoencefalografía	Magnetoencefalografia
Magnetska rezonancija (MR)	Magnetic resonance imaging (MRI)	Imagerie par résonance magnétique (IRM)	Imagen por resonancia magnética (IRM)	Imaging a risonanza magnetica (risonanza magnetica tomografica)
Mamografija	Mammography	Mammographie	Mamografía	Mammografia (mastografia)
Manometrija jednjaka	Esophageal manometry	Manométrie oesophagienne	Manometría esofágica	Manometria esofagea
Medijastinoskopija	Mediastinoscopy	Médiastinoscopie	Mediastinoscopia	Mediastinoscopia
Mijelografija	Myelography	Myélographie	Mielografía	Mielografia
Mikrobiološki pregled (kultura)	Microbiological culture	Culture microbiologique	Cultivo	Coltura di microrganismi
Mikrobiološki pregled brisa grla	Throat swab culture	Culture de gorge avec le coton-tige	Exudado faríngeo	Coltura di gola
Mikrobiološki pregled brisa rodnice	Vaginal swab culture	Culture vaginale	Cultivo vaginal	Coltura vaginale
Mikrobiološki pregled ispljuvka	Sputum culture	Culture de crachat	Cultivo de esputo	Coltura di sputo
Mikrobiološki pregled krvi (hemokultura)	Blood culture	Hémoculture	Hemocultivo	Emocoltura
Mikrobiološki pregled likvora	Cerebrospinal fluid culture	Culture du liquide cérébro-spinal	Cultivo de líquido cefalorraquídeo	Coltura del liquor
Mikrobiološki pregled mokraće (urinokultura)	Urine culture	Uroculture	Urocultivo	Urinocoltura
Mjerenje krvnog pritiska	Blood pressure monitoring	Monitoring de la pression artérielle	Monitorización de la presión arterial	Misurazione della pressione arteriosa
Mjerenje pulsa	Pulse monitoring	Prise de pouls	Comprobación del pulso	Misurazione del polso
Oftalmoskopija	Ophtalmoscopy	Ophtalmoscopie	Oftalmoscopia	Oftalmoscopia
Oralni test tolerancije na glukozu (OGTT)	Oral glucose tolerance test (OGTT)	Test de tolérance orale au glucose (TTOG)	Test de tolerancia oral a la glucosa	Test orale di tolleranca al glucosio (OGTT, curva da carico orale di glucosio)
Ostatni urin (rezidualni urin)	Post-void residual urine volume	Volume urinaire résiduel	Volumen residual de orina	Volume urinario residuo
Ostatni dušik u krvi (urea nitrogen test)	Blood urea nitrogen test (BUN)	Azote d'urée dans le sang	Nitrógeno ureico en sangre (BUN)	Azoto ureico nel sangue (BUN)
Otoskopija	Otoscopy	Otoscopie	Otoscopia	Otoscopia
Papa-test (Papanicolaouova klasifikacija)	Papanicolau test (Pap test)	Test PAP	Prueba de Papanicolau	Test di Papanicolaou (Pap test)
Parcijalno tromboplastinsko vrijeme (PTT)	Partial thromboplastin time (PTT)	Temps de céphaline activée (TCA)	Tiempo de tromboplastina parcial activado	Tempo di tromboplastina parziale

Hrvatski	Engleski	Francuski	Španjolski	Talijanski
Patelarni refleks	Patellar reflex	Réflexe rotulien	Reflejo patelar	Riflesso patellare
Pelvimetrija	Pelvimetry	Pelvimétrie	Pelvimetria	Pelvimetria
Perimetrija	Perimetry	Périmétrie	Campimetría (perimetría)	Perimetria
Perkutana transtorakalna punkcija pluća	Transthoracic percutaneous fine needle aspiration	Ponction transthoracique percutanée à l'aiguille fine	Punción transtorácica aspirativa con aguja ultrafina	Agoaspirato polmonare percutaneo transtoracico
Pijelografija (urografija)	Pyelography	Urographie	Urografía	Urografia
Pletizmografija	Plethysmography	Pléthysmographie	Pletismografía	Pletismografia
Pneumoencefalografija	Pneumoencephalography	Encéphalographie gazeuse	Neumoencefalografia	Pneumoencefalografia
Polisomnografija (višeparametarski test u praćenju procesa sna)	Polysomnography (sleep study)	Polysomnographie (polygraphie du sommeil)	Polisomnografia	Polisonnografia
Pozitronska emisijska tomografija (PET)	Positron emission tomography	Tomographie par émission de positrons	Tomografía por emisión de positrones	Tomografia ad emissione di positroni
Pregled dojke	Breast examination	Examen du sein	Exploración física de mama	Esame della mammella
Pregled likvora	Cerebrospinal fluid analysis	Analyse du liquide céphalo-rachidien	Análisis del líquido cefalorraquídeo	Analisi del liquido cerebro-spinale
Pregled očnog fundusa	Dilated fundus examination	Fond d'oeil	Exámen dilatado de fundus	Esame del fundus oculi
Prostatični specifični antigen (PSA)	Prostate specific antigen	Antigène prostatique spécifique	Antígeno prostático específico	Semenogelasi (antigene prostatico specifico)
Protrombinski indeks	Prothrombin time	Taux de prothrombine	Tiempo de protrombina	Tempo di protrombina
Pulmonalna angiografija	Pulmonary angiography	Angiographie pulmonaire	Angiografía pulmonar	Angiografia polmonare
Punkcijsko-aspiracijska biopsija	Fine needle aspiration biopsy	Forage-biopsie	Punción aspiración con aguja fina	Agoaspirato (biopsia mediante ago sottile)
Radioizotopna dijagnostika	Radioisotope scanning (nuclear medicine)	Médicine nucléaire	Medicina nuclear	Medicina nucleare
Rektalni pregled	Rectal examination	Toucher rectal	Tacto rectal	Esplorazione rettale
Rektoskopija	Rectoscopy	Rectoscopie	Rectoscopia	Rettoscopia
Rendgen	X-ray (radiography)	Radiographie	Radiografía	Radiografia
Rendgensko snimanje debelog crijeva i rektuma s kontrastom barija	Barium enema	Lavement baryté	Enema de bario con doble contraste	Indagini radiologiche del colon con clisma opaco a doppio contrasto
Rendgensko snimanje kostiju	Bone X-ray (bone radiography)	Radiographie des os	Radiografía de hueso (radiografía ósea)	Radiografia ossea
Rendgensko snimanje kralježnice	Spine X-ray (spine radiography)	Radiographie de la colonne vertébrale	Radiografía de la columna vertebral (radiografía vertebral)	Radiografia della colonna vertebrale
Rendgensko snimanje lubanje	Skull X-ray (craniography)	Craniographie	Craneografía	Craniografia
Rendgensko snimanje maternice i jajovoda	Hysterosalpingography	Hystérosalpingogra-phie	Histerosalpingografía	Isterosalpingografia
Rendgensko snimanje srca i pluća	Chest X-ray	Radiographie de thorax	Radiografía de tórax	Radiografia del torace
Rendgensko snimanje zdjelice i porođajnog kanala	Pelvigraphy	Pelvigraphie	Pelvigrafía	Pelvigrafia
Rendgensko snimanje zgloba	Joint X-ray (arthrography)	Arthrographie	Artrografía	Artrografia
Rendgensko snimanje zuba	Dental X-ray	Radiographie dentaire	Radiografía dental	Radiografia dentale
Rendgensko snimanje želuca i dvanaesnika barijevom kašom	Barium meal (upper gastrointestinal series)	Radiographie de l'abdomen en bouillie de sulfate de baryum	Radiografía de esófago, estómago y duodeno tomada con comida baritada	Radiografia gastroduodenale con pasto baritato
Rendgensko snimanje žučnog mjehura s kontrastom (peroralna kolecistografija)	Oral cholecystography	Cholécystographie orale	Colecistografía oral	Colecistografia orale
Retrogradna pijelografija	Retrograde pyelography	Urétéro-pyélographie rétrograde	Pielografía retrógrada	Pielografia retrograda
Rose Waaler test	Rose Waaler test	Réaction de Waaler Rose	Test de Waaler-Rose	Rose Waaler test
Scintigrafija bubrega	Renal scintigraphy	Scintigraphie rénale	Gammagrafía renal	Scintigrafia renale
Scintigrafija jetre i žučnih vodova radioaktivnim izotopima	Hepatobiliary scintigraphy with technetium -99m	Scintigraphie hépato-biliaire au Technétium 99m	Gammagrafía hepatobiliar con tecnecio 99m	Scintigrafia epatobiliare con tecnezio -99m
Scintigrafija kostiju	Bone scintigraphy	Scintigraphie osseuse	Gammagrafía ósea	Scintigrafia ossea
Scintigrafija pluća	Lung scintigraphy	Scintigraphie pulmonaire	Gammagrafía pulmonar	Scintigrafia polmonare
Scintigrafija slezene radioaktivnim izotopima	Spleen scintigraphy with technetium -99m	Scintigraphie splénique au Technétium 99m	Gammagrafía de bazo con tecnecio 99m	Scintigrafia splenica con tecnezio -99m
Scintigrafija štitnjače	Thyroid scintigraphy	Scintigraphie thyroïdienne	Gammagrafía tiroidea	Scintigrafia tiroidea
Sedimentacija eritrocita	Erythrocyte sedimentation rate	Vitesse de sédimentation	Velocidad de sedimentación globular	Velocità di eritrosedimentazione
Serološke pretrage na antitijela	Serology blood tests	Analyse sérologique	Pruebas de serología	Esami sierologici
Sigmoidoskopija	Sigmoidoscopy	Sigmoïdoscopie	Sigmoidoscopia	Sigmoidoscopia
Sijalografija	Sialography	Sialographie	Sialografía	Sialografia (scialografia)
Specifična težina urina	Urine specific gravity	Poids spécifique de l'urine	Gravedad específica de la orina	Esame delle urine peso specifico

Hrvatski	Engleski	Francuski	Španjolski	Talijanski
Spermogram	Semen analysis	Spermogramme	Espermiograma	Spermiogramma
Spinalna angiografija	Spinal angiography	Angiographie spinale	Angiografía espinal	Angiografia spinale
Spirometrija (mjerenje vitalnog kapaciteta)	Spirometry (vital capacity test)	Spirométrie	Espirometría	Spirometria (pneumometria)
Stereotaktična biopsija	Stereotactic biopsy	Biopsie stéréotaxique	Biopsia estereotáctica	Biopsia stereotassica
Subokcipitalna mijelografija	Suboccipital myelography	Myélographie sous-occipitale	Mielografía cervical suboccipital	Mielografia sotto-occipitale
Subokcipitalna punkcija	Suboccipital puncture	Ponction sous-occipitale	Punción suboccipital	Puntura suboccipitale
Šećer u krvi	Blood sugar concetra-tion (glucose level)	Taux de la glycémie	Concentración de glucosa en sangre	Concentrazione del glucosio nel plasma
Šećer u urinu	Glucose urine test	Test du sucre dans les urines	Examen de glucosa en orina	Glucosio nelle urine
Širenje zjenica potaknuto lijekovima	Drug induced pupillary dilatation	Dilatation des pupilles provoquée par les médicaments	Dilatación pupilar inducida por fármacos	Dilatazione delle pupille provocando con tropicamide
Test aglutinacije	Agglutination tests	Test d'agglutination	Análisis de aglutinación	Test di agglutinazione
Test na hormone štitnjače u krvi	Thyroid blood tests	Taux d'hormones thyroïdiennes dans le sang	Concetración de hormonas tiroideas en sangre	Test di ormoni tiroidei nel sangue
Test na trudnoću	Pregnancy test	Test de grossesse	Pruebas de embarazo	Test di gravidanza
Test opterećenja (ergometrija)	Ergometry test	Ergométrie	Ergometría	Ergometria (ECG sotto sforzo)
Test štitnjače na provodljivost radioaktivnog joda 131	Iodine-131 thyroid test	Fixation thyroïdienne de l'iode 131	Captación tiroidea de 131yodo	Test di captazione tiroidea dello iodio 131
Timpanocenteza	Tympanocentesis	Tympanocentese	Timpanocentesis	Timpanocentesi
Timpanometrija	Tympanometry	Tympanométrie	Timpanometría	Timpanometria
Tomografija	Tomography	Tomographie	Tomografía	Tomografia
Tonometrija oka	Tonometry	Tonométrie oculaire	Tonometría	Tonometria
Torakoskopija	Thoracoscopy	Thoracoscopie	Toracoscopia	Toracoscopia
Transaminaze u serumu	Aspartate transaminase (SGOT)	Aspartate transaminase (SGOT)	Aspartato aminotransferasa (AST, transaminasa glutámico-oxalacética GOT)	Aspartato transaminasi (SGOT)
Tuberkulinski kožni test	Mantoux test (PPD test)	Test Mantoux (test PPD)	Test de Mantoux (PPD)	Mantoux test
Tumorski marker	Tumor marker	Marqueur tumoral	Marcador tumoral	Marker tumorale
Ultrazvuk	Ultrasound (medical ultrasonography)	Échographie	Ultrasonografía (ecografía)	Ecografia
Ultrazvuk abdomena	Abdominal ultrasound	Échographie abdominale	Ecografia abdominal (ultrasonido abdominal)	Ecografia addominale
Ultrazvuk bubrega	Renal ultrasound	Échographie rénale	Ecografia renal (ultrasonido renal)	Ecografia renale
Ultrazvuk dojke	Breast ultrasound	Échographie mammaire	Ecografía de mama (ultrasonido de mama)	Ecografia mammaria
Ultrazvuk gušterače	Pancreas ultrasound	Échographie du pancréas	Ecografía de páncreas (ultrasonido de páncreas)	Ecografia pancreatica
Ultrazvuk jetre	Liver ultrasound	Échographie du foie (échographie hépatique)	Ecografía hepática (ultrasonido hepático)	Ecografia epatica
Ultrazvuk srca (ehokardiografija)	Cardiac ultrasound (echocardiography)	Échocardiographie	Ecocardiografia	Ecocardiografia
Ultrazvuk srca s dopplerom	Doppler echocardiography	Échocardiographie-doppler	Ecocardiografia doppler	Ecocardiografia doppler
Ultrazvuk štitnjače	Thyroid ultrasound	Échographie thyroïdienne	Ecografía de la tiroides (ultrasonido de la tiroides)	Ecografia della tiroide
Ultrazvuk žuči i žučnih vodova	Ultrasound of the gallbladder and bile ducts	Échographie la vésicule biliaire et les voies biliaires	Ecografía de vesícula y vías biliares	Ecografia colecisti e vie biliari
Urea klirens	Urea clearance test	Épruve d'élimination de l'urée sanguine	Prueba de aclaramiento de urea sanguínea	Urea clearance (clearance dell'urea)
Urea izdisajni test	Urea breath test	Test respiratoire à l'urée	Prueba del aliento con urea	Test del respiro (urea breath test)
Uretrografija	Urethrography	Urétrographie	Uretrografía	Uretrografia
Ureteroskopija	Ureteroscopy	Urétéroscopie	Ureteroscopía	Ureteroscopia
Urobilinogen u urinu	Urobilinogen in urine	Urobilinogène dans les urines	Urobilinógeno en orina	Urobilinogeno nelle urine
Venografija (flebografija)	Phlebography	Phlébographie	Flebografía	Flebografia
Ventrikulografija	Ventriculography	Ventriculographie	Ventriculografia	Ventricolografia
Weber test	Weber test	Test de Weber	Prueba de Weber	Prova di Weber
TRUDNOĆA I PORODNIŠTVO:	**PREGNANCY AND OBSTETRICS:**	**GROSSESSE ET OBSTÉTRIQUE:**	**EMBARAZO Y OBSTETRICIA:**	**GRAVIDANZA ED OSTETRICIA:**
Abortivni lijekovi	Abortifacients	Médicaments abortifs	Fármacos abortivos	Farmaci abortivi
Abrupcija posteljice	Placental abruption	Abruption placentaire (rupture placentaire)	Desprendimiento prematuro de placenta	Distacco di placenta (abruptio placentae)
Amniocenteza	Amniocentesis	Amniocentèse	Amniocentesis	Amniocentesi
Amnioskopija	Amnioscopy	Amnioscopie	Amnioscopia	Amnioscopia
Anomalije fetusa	Fetal anomalies (fetal abnormalities)	Anomalies foetales	Anomalías fetales	Anomalie di sviluppo fetale (anomalie fetali)
Anomalije maternice	Uterine anomalies	Malformations utérines	Malformaciones uterinas	Anomalie uterine
Babica	Midwife	Sage-femme	Matrona (matrón)	Ostetrica (levatrice)
Babinje (puerperij)	Postnatal (postpartum period, puerperium)	Post-partum	Puerperio	Puerperio

Hrvatski	Engleski	Francuski	Španjolski	Talijanski
Banka sperme	Sperm bank	Banque du sperme	Banco de semen	Banca del seme
Biofizikalni profil fetusa	Biophysical profile of the fetus	Profil biophysique foetal	Perfil biofísico fetal	Profilo biofísico fetale
Biološki roditelj	Biological parent	Parent biologique	Padre biológico	Genitore biologico
Blastocista	Blastocyst	Blastocyste	Blastocisto	Blastocisti
Blizanačka trudnoća	Multiple pregnancy	Grossesse multiple	Embarazo múltiple	Gravidanza gemellare
Blizanci	Twins	Jumeaux	Gemelos	Gemelli
Bradavica	Nipple	Mamelon (papille)	Pezón	Capezzolo
Carski rez	Cesarean section (C-section)	Césarienne	Cesárea	Taglio cesareo
Četvorci	Quadruplets	Quadruplés	Cuatrillizos	Quattro gemelli
Disanje	Breathing	Respiration	Respiración	Respirazione
Djevičnjak (himen)	Hymen	Hymen	Himen	Imene
Dojenje (laktacija)	Lactation	Lactation	Lactancia	Lattazione
Dojka	Breast	Sein	Mama	Mammella
Donacija jajašca	Egg donation	Donneuse d'ovule	Donación de ovocitos	Ovodonazione
Dužina novorođenčeta	Body length of a newborn	Taille corporelle du nouveau-né	Talla de un neonato	Lunghezza di neonato
Dvojajčani blizanci	Dizygotic twins (biovular twins)	Jumeaux dizygotes	Gemelos dicigóticos (mellizos)	Gemelli fraterni (gemelli dizigoti)
Edem	Edema	Oedème	Edema (hidropesía)	Edema
Ejakulat	Ejaculation	Éjaculation	Eyaculación	Eiaculazione
Eklampsija	Eclampsia	Éclampsie	Eclampsia	Eclampsia
Embrij (zametak)	Embryo	Embryon	Embrión	Embrione
EPH-gestoze (preeklampsija)	EPH gestosis (pre-eclampsia)	Pré-éclampsie	Preeclampsia	Preeclampsia (gestosi)
Estrogen placente	Placental estrogen	Oestrogène placentaire	Estrógeno de la placenta	Estrogeno placentare
Fetalna hipertrofija	Macrosomia (big baby syndrome)	Macrosomie foetale	Macrosomía fetal	Macrosomia fetale
Fetalna hipotrofija	Fetal hypotrophy	Hypotrophie foetale	Hipotrofia fetal	Ipotrofia fetale
Fetalna pH-metrija	Fetal pH-metry	pH-métrie foetale	pH-metría fetal	pH-metria fetale
Fetoskopija	Fetoscopy	Foetoscopie	Fetoscopia	Fetoscopia
Fetus	Fetus	Foetus	Feto	Feto
Forceps (kliješta)	Forceps	Forceps	Fórceps	Forcipe
Trudovi	Labor contractions	Contractions utérines du travail	Contracciones del trabajo de parto (contracciones uterinas)	Contrazioni del travaglio
Gestacijski dijabetes	Gestational diabetes	Diabète gestationnel	Diabetes gestacional	Diabete gestazionale
Ginekologija	Gynecology	Gynécologie	Ginecología	Ginecologia
Glavica	Head	Tête	Cabeza	Testa
Graafov folikul	Graafian follicle	Follicule de Graaf	Folículo de Graaf	Follicolo di Graaf
Habitualni pobačaj	Habitual abortion (recurrent miscarriage)	Avortement à répétition	Aborto habitual	Aborto abituale
Hemolitička bolest novorođenčeta	Hemolytic disease of the newborn	Maladie hémolytique du nouveau-né	Enfermedad hemolítica del recién nacido (eritroblastosis fetal)	Eritroblastosi fetale (malattia emolitica del neonato)
Hiperemična sluznica rod-nice (Chadwickov znak)	Chadwick's sign	Signe de Chadwick	Signo de Chadwick	Segno del Chadwick (tinta bluastra alla vagina)
Hiperemija jajnika	Ovarian hyperemia	Hyperhémie ovarienne	Hiperemia del ovario	Iperemia dell'ovaio
Hiperplazija maternice	Endometrial hyperplasia	Hyperplasie endométriale	Hiperplasia endometrial	Iperplasia endometriale
Hipertrofija maternice	Hypertrophy of uterus	Hypertrophie de l'utérus	Hipertrofia del útero	Ipertrofia dell'utero
Implantacija (usađivanje)	Implantation	Implantation	Implatación	Impianto
Infekcija	Infection	Infection	Infección	Infezione
Inkubator	Incubator	Couveuse (incubateur)	Incubadora	Incubatrice
Intracitoplazmatska spermalna injekcija	Intracytoplasmatic sperm injection	Injection intracytoplasmique de spermatozoïdes	Inyección intracitoplasmá-tica de espermatozoides	Iniezione intracitoplasma-tica dello spermatozoo
Ispala pupkovina (prolaps pupkovine)	Umbilical cord prolapse	Prolapsus du cordon ombilical	Prolapso del cordón umbilical	Prolasso del funicolo ombelicale
Istiskivanje ploda	Expulsion of the baby	Expulsion du bébé	Expulsión del producto	Espulsione del feto
Istiskivanje posteljice i ovoja	Expulsion of placenta	Expulsion du placenta	Expulsión de la placenta	Espulsione della placenta
Izostanak mjesečnice (amenoreja)	Absence of menstrual period (amenorrhea)	Absence des règles (aménorrhée)	Ausencia de la menstruación (amenorrea)	Assenza di mestruazioni (amenorrea)
Izvanmaternična trudnoća (ektopična trudnoća)	Ectopic pregnancy (extrauterine pregnancy)	Grossesse extra-utérine	Embarazo ectópico	Gravidanza ectopica
Jajašce	Ovum	Ovule	Óvulo	Uovo
Jajnik	Ovary	Ovaire	Ovario	Ovaia (ovario)
Jajovod	Fallopian tube (oviduct)	Trompes de Fallope	Trompa de Falopio (tuba uterina, oviducto)	Ovidotto (ovidutto)
Jednojajčani blizanci	Monozygotic twins (identical twins)	Jumeaux monozygotes	Gemelos monocigóticos	Gemelli identici (gemelli monozigoti)
Kardiotokografija	Cardiotocography	Cardiotocographie	Cardiotocografía	Cardiotocografia
Kiretaža	Curettage	Curetage	Legrado	Raschiamento (curetage)
Kirurško odstranjenje maternice (histerektomija)	Surgical removal of the uterus (hysterectomy)	Enlèvement chirurgical de l'uterus (hystérectomie)	Extracción quirúrgica del útero (histerectomía)	Asportazione chirurgica dell'utero (isterectomia)
Kirurško proširenje porođajnog kanala (epiziotomija)	Episiotomy	Épisiotomie	Episiotomía	Episiotomia

Hrvatski	Engleski	Francuski	Španjolski	Talijanski
Kordocenteza	Cordocentesis	Cordocentèse	Cordocentesis	Cordocentesi
Koriokarcinom	Choriocarcinoma	Choriocarcinome	Coriocarcinoma	Coriocarcinoma
Korion	Chorion	Chorion	Corion	Corion (corio)
Korion-gonadotropin	Chorion-gonadotrophin	Gonadotrophine chorionique	Gonadotropina coriónica	Gonadotropina corionica
Korionske resice	Chorionic villi	Villosités choriales	Vellosidades coriónicas	Villi coriali
Kosi položaj ploda	Transverse fetal position	Position transversale du foetus	Feto posición transversal	Posizione del feto trasversale
Krvarenje (hemoragija)	Bleeding (haemorrhage)	Saignement (hémorragie)	Desangramiento (hemorragia)	Emorragia
Labilno psihičko raspoloženje (baby blues)	Maternity blues (baby blues)	Baby blues	Baby blues (leve depresión post parto)	Sindrome del terzo giorno (baby blues)
Lažni trudovi	Braxton Hicks contractons	Fausse contraction (contraction de Braxton Hicks)	Contracción de Braxton Hicks	False contrazioni (contrazioni di Braxton Hicks)
Lijek za sprečavanje trudova (tokolitik)	Medication that suppresses premature labor (tocolytic)	Médicament pour interrompre le déclenchement du travail (tocolytique)	Fármaco utilizado para suprimir el trabajo de parto prematuro (tocolítico)	Farmaco con lo scopo di arrestare le contrazioni uterine (tocolisi)
Litopedion (okamenjeno dijete)	Lithopedion (stone baby)	Lithopédion (enfant pétrifié)	Litopedion	Lithopedion
Lohija (iscjedak u babinjama)	Lochia	Lochies	Loquios	Lochi
Majka	Mother	Mère	Madre	Madre
Maternica (uterus)	Womb (uterus)	Utérus	Útero (matriz, seno materno)	Utero
Medicinski potpomognuta oplodnja	Medically assisted procreation	Procréation médicalement assistée	Reproducción asistida	Procreazione assistita
Mekonij	Meconium	Méconium	Meconio	Meconio
Mekonijalni aspiracijski sindrom	Meconium aspiration syndrome	Syndrome d'aspiration méconiale	Síndrome de aspiración de meconio	Sindrome da aspirazione di meconio
Mekonijalni ileus	Meconium ileus	Iléus méconial	Enfermedad de Hirschsprung (megacolon agangliónico)	Malattia di Hirschsprung (ostruzione del colon congenita)
Mekonijalni peritonitis	Meconium peritonitis	Péritonite méconiale	Peritonitis meconial	Peritonite da meconio
Menopauza (klimakterij)	Menopause	Ménopause	Menopausia	Menopausa
Menstruacija	Menstruation	Règle (menstruation)	Menstruación (período)	Mestruazione
Menstruacijski ciklus	Menstrual cycle	Cycle menstruel	Ciclo menstrual	Ciclo mestruale
Mikrocefalija (sitnoglavost)	Microcephaly	Microcéphalie	Microcefalia	Microcefalia
Mifepriston	Mifepristone	Mifépristone	Mifepristona	Mifepristone
Mliječni vod	Lactiferous duct	Canal galactophore	Conducto mamario (conducto galactóforo)	Dotto galattoforo
Morula	Morula	Morula	Mórula	Morula
Mrtvorođenče	Stillborn	Mort-né	Nacido muerto	Nato morto
Mučnina	Nausea	Nausée	Náusea	Nausea
Nedonošće	Preterm newborn	Nouveau-né prématuré	Recién nacido pre-término	Neonato pretermine
Neonatologija	Neonatology	Néonatologie	Neonatología	Neonatologia
Neplodnost (sterilitet)	Infertility	Stérilité	Infertilidad	Sterilità
Novorođenče	Newborn (infant)	Nouveau-né	Neonato (recién nacido)	Neonato
Nuhalna translucencija	Nuchal scan (nuchal translucency)	Clarté nucale	Traslucencia nucal	Translucenza nucale
Oplodnja in vitro	In vitro fertilisation	Fécondation in vitro	Fecundación in vitro	Fertilizzazione in vitro
Otac	Father	Père	Padre	Padre
Otvaranje ušća maternice	Cervical dilation	Dilatation cervicale	Dilatación del cuello uterino	Dilatazione della cervice uterina
Ovogeneza (oogeneza)	Oogenesis	Ovogenèse	Ovogénesis	Ovogenesi
Ovulacija	Ovulation	Ovulation	Ovulación	Ovulazione
Patološki porod	Pathological birth	Accouchement pathologique	Parto patológico	Parto patologico
Pelena	Diaper	Couche-culotte	Pañal	Pannolino
Pelvimetrija	Pelvimetry	Pelvimétrie	Pelvimetría	Pelvimetria
Pijelonefritis	Pyelonephritis	Pyélonéphrite	Pielonefritis	Pielonefrite
Placenta previja	Placenta previa	Placenta praevia	Placenta previa	Placenta previa
Plagiocefalija	Plagiocephaly	Plagiocéphalie	Plagiocefalia	Plagiocefalia
Plodna voda (amnijska tekućina)	Amniotic fluid	Liquide amniotique	Líquido amniótico	Liquido amniotico
Pojačano lučenje sline (hipersalivacija)	Excessive secretion of saliva (hypersalivation)	Sécrétion de la salive excessive	Excesiva producción de saliva (hipersalivación)	Produzione di saliva eccessiva (ipersalivazione)
Porod	Childbirth	Accouchement (naissance)	Parto	Parto
Porod u vodi	Water birth	Accouchement dans l'eau	Parto en agua	Parto nell'acqua
Porodni kanal	Birth canal	Canal utérin	Canal del parto	Canale del parto
Porodničar (opstetičar)	Obstetrician	Obstétricien	Tocólogo (obstetra)	Ostetrico
Porodništvo	Obstetrics	Obstétrique	Obstetricia	Ostetricia
Porodno doba	Stage of birth	Stade du travail	Etapas del parto	Fase del parto
Poslijeročni porod	Postmature birth	Naissance après terme	Parto postérmino	Parto post-termine
Posteljica (placenta)	Placenta	Placenta	Placenta	Placenta
Postporođajna depresija	Postnatal depression (postpartum depression)	Dépression post-natale (dépression post-partum)	Depresión postparto (depresión postnatal)	Depressione post-partum

Hrvatski	Engleski	Francuski	Španjolski	Talijanski
Povraćanje	Vomiting	Vomissement	Vómito (emesis)	Vomito (emetismo)
Prekid trudnoće (abortus)	Abortion (pregnancy termination)	Avortement	Aborto inducido	Interruzione di gravidanza (aborto)
Presjeći	Cut	Couper	Cortar	Tagliare (intersecare)
Prijevremeni porod	Premature birth	Prématurité	Parto pretérmino	Parto pretermine
Prijevremeno prsnuće vodenjaka	Premature rupture of membranes	Rupture prématurée des membranes	Ruptura prematura de membrana	Rottura precoce delle membrane
Prirasla posteljica (placenta acrreta)	Placenta accreta	Placenta accreta	Placenta accreta	Placenta accreta
Produljeni porod	Prolonged birth	Accouchement prolongé	Parto prolongado	Parto prolungato
Progesteron	Progesterone	Progestérone	Progesterona	Progesterone
Progesteron placente	Placental progesterone	Progestérone placentaire	Progesterona de placenta	Progesterone placentare
Prolaktin	Prolactin	Prolactine	Prolactina	Prolattina
Proširene vene na nogama	Leg varicose veins	Varices des membres inférieurs	Venas varicosas de las piernas	Varici degli arti inferiori
Prsnuće vodenjaka	Rupture of membranes	Rupture des membranes	Ruptura de membrana	Rottura delle membrane
Prvorotkinja	Primigravida	Primigeste	Primigesta	Primipara
Puerperalna groznica (babinja groznica)	Puerperal fever	Fièvre puerpérale	Fiebre puerperal	Febbre puerperale
Puerperalna psihoza	Postpartum psychosis	Psychose puerpérale	Psicosis postparto	Psicosi post-partum
Puerperalna sepsa	Puerperal sepsis	Septicémie puerpérale	Sepsis puerperal	Sepsi puerperale
Puerperalni mastitis	Puerperal mastitis	Mammite puerpérale	Mastitis puerperal	Mastite puerperale
Pumpica za izdajanje	Breast pump	Tire-lait	Sacaleches	Pompa tiralatte
Pupak	Navel (belly button)	Ombilic (nombril)	Ombligo (pupo)	Ombelico
Pupkovina (pupčana vrpca)	Umbilical cord	Cordon ombilical	Cordón umbilical	Funicolo ombelicale
Rađaona	Delivery room	Salle d'accouchement	Sala de partos	Sala parto
Ročni porod	Full term birth	Accouchement à terme	Parto a término	Parto a termine
Rodilište	Maternity hospital	Maternité	Hospital de maternidad	Clinica ostetrica
Roditelj	Parent	Géniteur	Padre (primario)	Genitore
Rodnica	Vagina	Vagin	Vagina	Vagina
Sisanje	Suckling	Succion	Succión	Suzione
Sjemena tekućina (sperma)	Semen (sperm)	Sperme	Semen (esperma)	Seme (sperma)
Sluznica maternice (endometrij)	Inner membrane of the uterus (endometrium)	Muqueuse utérine (endomètre)	Mucosa interior del útero (endometrio)	Mucosa interna dell'utero (endometrio)
Snaga trudova	Intensity of contractions	Intensité des contractions utérines	Intensidad de contracciones uterinas	Intensità di contrazione
Spermij	Spermatozoon (sperm cell)	Spermatozoïde	Espermatozoide	Spermatozoo
Spontani pobačaj	Spontaneous abortion (miscarriage)	Fausse couche	Aborto espontáneo	Aborto spontaneo
Stav zatkom	Breech position	Présentation podalique (présentation du siège)	Posición de nalgas	Posizione podalica del feto
Surogat majka (zamjenska majka)	Surrogate mother (womb mother)	Mère porteuse	Madre de alquiler	Surrogazione di maternità
Sužena zdjelica	Contracted pelvis	Bassin contracté	Pelvis contraída	Pelvi ristretto
Teratogeni faktori rizika	Pregnancy risk factors	Facteurs de risque de la grossesse	Agentes teratogénicos	Rischio teratogenico
Težina ploda (porođajna težina)	Fetal weight (birth mass)	Poids de naissance	Peso al nacer	Peso di neonato
Tiskati	Push	Pousser	Empujar	Spingere
TORCH infekcije	TORCH infections	Infections TORCH	Infecciones TORCH	Complesso TORCH
Trajanje trudnoće	Duration of pregnancy	Durée de la grossesse	Duración del embarazo	Durata della gravidanza
Trajanje truda	Duration of contraction	Durée de la contraction utérine	Duración de las contracciones uterinas	Durata di contrazioni
Trudnoća	Pregnancy	Grossesse	Embarazo	Gravidanza (gestazione)
Frekvencija trudova	Labor contraction frequency	Fréquence des contractions utérines	Frecuencia de las contracciones uterinas	Frequenza di contrazioni uterine
Ultrazvuk	Ultrasound (medical ultrasonography)	Échographie	Ultrasonografía (ecografía)	Ecografia
Umjetna oplodnja	Artificial insemination	Insémination artificielle	Inseminación artificial	Fecondazione assistita (fecondazione artificiale)
Upala mokraćnog mjehura (cistitis)	Inflammation of the urinary bladder (cystitis)	Inflammation de la vessie (cystite)	Inflamación de la vejiga urinaria (cistitis)	Infiammazione della vescica urinaria (cistite)
Upala plodovih ovoja (korioamnionitis)	Inflammation of the fetal membranes (chorioamnionitis)	Chorioamnionite	Infección de las membranas placentarias (corioamnionitis)	Infiammazione del sacco amniotico (corioamniosite)
Urinarna inkotinencija	Urinary incontinence	Incontinence urinaire	Incontinencia urinaria	Incontinenza urinaria
Uzorak korionskih resica	Chorionic villus sampling	Choriocentèse	Muestra de vellosidades coriónicas	Villocentesi
Vakuumski ekstraktor	Vacuum extractor (ventouse)	Vacuum extractor	Aspirador al vacío	Aspiratore a vuoto
Visoki krvni tlak (hipertenzija)	High blood pressure (hypertension)	Pression artérielle élevée (hypertension artérielle)	Incremento de la presión sanguínea (hipertensión)	Ipertensione arteriosa sistemica
Višerotkinja	Multigravida	Multipare	Multigrávida	Pluripara
Vodenjak	Amniotic sac	Amnios (sac amniotique)	Saco amniótico	Amnios
Vrat	Neck	Cou	Cuello	Collo

Hrvatski	Engleski	Francuski	Španjolski	Talijanski
Začeće (oplodnja)	Conception	Conception (fécondation)	Fecundación (fertilización)	Concezione
Zadak	Breech	Siège	Nalga	Culatta (deretano)
Zastoj urina (urinarna retencija)	Urinary retention (ischuria)	Rétention d'urine	Retención de orina	Ritenzione urinaria
Životna sposobnost spermija	Sperm viability	Viabilité du sperme	Viabilidad de espermatozoides	Sopravvivenza di spermatozoo

ABOUT THE AUTHOR

Edita Ciglenečki is medical translator with Academic degrees in Biomedical Sciences and Public Health Sciences. Besides Croatian, being her mother tongue, she is a holder of international diplomas in English, French and Italian language. For many years she worked as a medical professional inside the travel industry. This dictionary is the product of her own working experience built on her passion for traveling, medicine and language skills.

www.ingramcontent.com/pod-product-compliance
Lightning Source LLC
Chambersburg PA
CBHW080759180526
45168CB00006B/2263